Principles of
MEDICAL
PHARMACOLOGY

Fifth Edition

Principles of
MEDICAL
PHARMACOLOGY

Fifth Edition

HAROLD KALANT, M.D., PH.D.

Department of Pharmacology
University of Toronto Faculty of Medicine
Toronto, Ontario

WALTER H.E. ROSCHLAU, M.D.

Department of Pharmacology
University of Toronto Faculty of Medicine
Toronto, Ontario

1989
B.C. Decker Inc • Toronto • Philadelphia

Publisher

B.C. Decker Inc
3228 South Service Road
Burlington, Ontario L7N 3H8

B.C. Decker Inc
320 Walnut Street
Suite 400
Philadelphia, Pennsylvania 19106

Sales and Distribution

United States and Puerto Rico
The C.V. Mosby Company
11830 Westline Industrial Drive
Saint Louis, Missouri 63146

Canada
University of Toronto
The Secretary, Department of Pharmacology
Medical Sciences Building
Toronto, Ontario M5S 1A8

Australia
McGraw-Hill Book Company Australia Pty. Ltd.
4 Barcoo Street
Roseville East 2069
New South Wales, Australia

Brazil
Editora McGraw-Hill do Brasil, Ltda.
rua Tabapua, 1.105, Itaim-Bibi
Sao Paulo, S.P. Brasil

Colombia
Interamericana/McGraw-Hill de Colombia, S.A.
Apartado Aereo 81078
Bogota, D.E. Colombia

Europe
McGraw-Hill Book Company GmbH
Lademannbogen 136
D-2000 Hamburg 63
West Germany

France
MEDSI/McGraw-Hill
6, avenue Daniel Lesueur
75007 Paris, France

Hong Kong and China
McGraw-Hill Book Company
Suite 618, Ocean Centre
5 Canton Road
Tsimshatsui, Kowloon
Hong Kong

India
Tata McGraw-Hill Publishing Company, Ltd.
12/4 Asaf Ali Road, 3rd Floor
New Delhi 110002, India

Indonesia
P.O. Box 122/JAT
Jakarta, 1300 Indonesia

Italy
McGraw-Hill Libri Italia, s.r.l.
Piazza Emilia, 5
I-20129 Milano MI
Italy

Japan
Igaku-Shoin Ltd.
Tokyo International P.O. Box 5063
1-28-36 Hongo, Bunkyo-ku,
Tokyo 113, Japan

Korea
C.P.O. Box 10583
Seoul, Korea

Malaysia
No. 8 Jalan SS 7/6B
Kelana Jaya
47301 Petaling Jaya
Selangor, Malaysia

Mexico
Interamericana/McGraw-Hill de Mexico, S.A. de C.V.
Cedro 512, Colonia Atlampa
(Apartado Postal 26370)
06450 Mexico, D.F., Mexico

New Zealand
McGraw-Hill Book Co. New Zealand Ltd.
5 Joval Place, Wiri
Manukau City, New Zealand

Panama
Editorial McGraw-Hill Latinoamericana, S.A.
Apartado Postal 2036
Zona Libre de Colon
Colon, Republica de Panama

Portugal
Editora McGraw-Hill de Portugal, Ltda.
Rua Rosa Damasceno 11A–B
1900 Lisboa, Portugal

South Africa
Libriger Book Distributors
Warehouse Number 8
"Die Ou Looiery"
Tannery Road
Hamilton, Bloemfontein 9300

Southeast Asia
McGraw-Hill Book Co.
348 Jalan Boon Lay
Jurong, Singapore 2261

Spain
McGraw-Hill/Interamericana de Espana, S.A.
Manuel Ferrero, 13
28020 Madrid, Spain

Taiwan
P.O. Box 87–601
Taipei, Taiwan

Thailand
632/5 Phaholyothin Road
Sapan Kwai
Bangkok 10400
Thailand

United Kingdom, Middle East and Africa
McGraw-Hill Book Company (U.K.) Ltd.
Shoppenhangers Road
Maidenhead, Berkshire
SL6 2QL England

Venezuela
McGraw-Hill/Interamericana, C.A.
2da. calle Bello Monte
(entre avenida Casanova y Sabana Grande)
Apartado Aereo 50785
Caracas 1050, Venezuela

NOTICE

The authors and publisher have made every effort to ensure that the patient care recommended herein, including choice of drugs and drug dosages, is in accord with the accepted standards and practice at the time of publication. However, since research and regulation constantly change clinical standards, the reader is urged to check the product information sheet included in the package of each drug, which includes recommended doses, warnings, and contraindications. This is particularly important with new or infrequently used drugs.

Principles of Medical Pharmacology
Fifth Edition

ISBN 1–55664–125–7

Library of Congress catalog card number: 88–51748

10 9 8 7 6 5 4 3 2 1

The Department of Pharmacology
dedicates
the fifth edition of this book to
the memory of

EDWARD ALEXANDER SELLERS
(1916–1986)

An outstanding scientist, teacher, humane and
generous colleague, and gracious gentleman—
he was the principal agent of the department's
growth and modernization.

Contributors

From the Department of Pharmacology, Faculty of Medicine, University of Toronto (including Cross-Appointments):

W.M. Burnham, Ph.D.
Department of Psychiatry

F.J. Carmichael, M.D., Ph.D.
Department of Anaesthesia

L. Endrenyi, Ph.D.
Department of Preventive Medicine and Biostatistics

C. Erlichman, M.D.
Department of Medicine

K.V. Flattery, M.D.

C. Forster, Ph.D.
Department of Medicine

S.R. George, M.D.
Department of Medicine

L.A. Grupp, D.Sc.
Addiction Research Foundation of Ontario

D. Kadar, Ph.D.

H. Kalant, M.D., Ph.D.
Addiction Research Foundation of Ontario

W. Kalow, M.D.

I.G. Kerr, M.D.
Department of Medicine

J.S. Keystone, M.D.
Department of Medicine

J.M. Khanna, Ph.D.
Addiction Research Foundation of Ontario

S.M. MacLeod, M.D., Ph.D.
Departments of Medicine and Pediatrics,
McMaster University, Hamilton, Ontario

W.A. Mahon, M.D.
Department of Medicine

A. Marquez-Julio, M.D.
Department of Medicine

M.A. McGuigan, M.D.
Department of Pediatrics

M.G. Myers, M.D.
Department of Medicine

C.A. Naranjo, M.D.
Department of Medicine, Addiction Research
Foundation of Ontario

R.I. Ogilvie, M.D.
Department of Medicine

A.B. Okey, Ph.D.
Department of Pediatrics

H. Orrego, M.D.
Department of Medicine, Addiction Research
Foundation of Ontario

C.R. Pace-Asciak, Ph.D.
Department of Pediatrics

W.H.E. Roschlau, M.D.

B.P. Schimmer, Ph.D.
Banting and Best Department of Medical Research

P. Seeman, M.D., Ph.D.
Department of Psychiatry

E.M. Sellers, M.D., Ph.D.
Department of Medicine, Addiction Research
Foundation of Ontario

L. Spero, Ph.D.

S.P. Spielberg, M.D., Ph.D.
Department of Pediatrics

W.C. Sturtridge, M.D., Ph.D., D.D.S.
Department of Medicine; Faculty of Dentistry,
University of Toronto

F.A. Sunahara, Ph.D.
Faculty of Dentistry, University of Toronto

J. Uetrecht, M.D., Ph.D.
Faculty of Pharmacy, University of Toronto

P.G. Wells, Ph.D.
Faculty of Pharmacy, University of Toronto

From Other Departments and Institutions:

M.J. Baigent, Ph.D.
Department of Nutritional Sciences, Faculty of Medicine, University of Toronto

U. Busto, Pharm.D.
Faculty of Pharmacy, University of Toronto, Addiction Research Foundation of Ontario

P. Dorian, M.D., M.Sc.
Department of Medicine, Faculty of Medicine, University of Toronto

E.L. Ford-Jones, M.D.
Department of Pediatrics, Faculty of Medicine, University of Toronto

E. Janecek, B.Sc.Pharm.
Faculty of Pharmacy, University of Toronto

C. Prober, M.D.
Department of Pediatrics, Stanford University School of Medicine, Stanford, California

P. Rajchgot, M.D.C.M., M.Sc.
Department of Pediatrics, Faculty of Medicine, University of Toronto

J. Tetiuk, B.Sc.Pharm.
Women's College Hospital, Toronto, Ontario

S.L. Walmsley, M.D.
Department of Microbiology, Mount Sinai Hospital, Toronto, Ontario

C. Whiteside, M.D., Ph.D.
Department of Medicine, Faculty of Medicine, University of Toronto

Preface

This book had its origin over 25 years ago in the form of detailed lecture notes that were distributed by members of the Department of Pharmacology to students in Medicine, Dentistry, and Pharmacy, and later to undergraduate Arts and Science students enrolled in specialist programs in pharmacology and toxicology. The lecture assignments to individual staff members changed from year to year, so that the notes gradually came to reflect the combined approaches of the whole Department.

In 1975 the notes were edited to provide greater uniformity of organization and were combined into the first edition of this book. It was intended as a working text for students, not as an exhaustive reference work or an advanced treatise for senior clinicians and researchers, whose needs are better met by a variety of specialized publications. The illustrations were simple line drawings, and the list of suggested readings following each chapter was not intended to document each point in the chapter, but only to provide sources of additional information for those readers who were interested in learning more about the subject.

The book has matured and expanded through four successive editions under the overall supervision of the departmental Book Committee, and a progression of editors:

   1st edition, 1975: P. Seeman and E.M. Sellers

   2nd edition, 1976: P. Seeman and E.M. Sellers

   3rd edition, 1979: P. Seeman, E.M. Sellers, and W.H.E. Roschlau

   4th edition, 1985: H. Kalant, W.H.E. Roschlau, and E.M. Sellers.

However, its primary purpose and general character remained unchanged. The emphasis has continued to be on solid basics. Very recent research developments, controversial issues, and unproven hypotheses are mentioned only briefly, if at all, to alert the reader to possible future developments that might become clinically important at a later time. It is a textbook of basic pharmacology rather than of therapeutics, and the clinical aspects covered in most chapters are meant only to amplify or illustrate basic pharmacologic concepts.

The present edition, the 5th, retains this general didactic approach, but has undergone a major change in content and style. It is the first edition of this work to be published by B.C. Decker Inc., and it reflects the imagination and drive of Mr. Brian Decker and his staff, who have strongly supported the educational philosophy of the book while giving it a totally new face. The unique illustrations in the 4th edition (1985) had been conceived and masterfully executed by Mr. Seward Hung, who was at that time a student in this department. For the present edition, Ms. Jean Calder has adapted many of Mr. Hung's line drawings, converting them into full-color illustrations. Most of the line graphs have also been highlighted by the use of color. This has undoubtedly given the book a much more pleasing appearance. The editors hope that it will also add to the clarity and didactic value of the illustrations; the readers will be the ultimate judges.

Three new chapters—*Hyperlipoproteinemias and Antihyperlipidemic Drugs, The Eicosanoids,* and *Sources of Variation in Drug Response*—have been added. The first two were previously included as short sections of other chapters, but have now been expanded into new chapters with new authors. The chapter *Neuron-Inhibitory Amino Acids* in the 4th edition has now been incorporated into the chapter *Antiseizure Drugs*. Several other chapters have undergone major revision by new authors.

Consistent with their adoption by the health care systems in many countries, SI (système international) units have been used as much as possible in the book, but are accompanied in most instances by the traditional units with which many teachers and clinicians continue to be more comfortable. As in previous editions, drugs are discussed under their non-proprietary (i.e., official or "generic") names, but examples of proprietary names are usually given for convenience. In the few instances in which differences exist between Canadian and U.S. official nomenclature or usage, both forms are now given in the text (e.g., Canadian and British "adrenaline" and U.S. "epinephrine"). The text has been reviewed by Dr. D. Craig Brater, Director of Clinical Pharmacology, Wishard Memorial Hospital, Indianapolis, Indiana, to ensure that American terminology and usage are appropriately represented. Dr. Brater's numerous additional comments and valuable suggestions are gratefully acknowledged by the editors.

Previous editions of this book have been well received not only throughout Canada but also in a growing number of medical schools in the United States and other countries. The editors and publisher believe that the changes described above will enable the present edition to serve better the needs of students and practitioners in many more countries.

The editors express their gratitude to the chapter authors for the care, cooperation, and patience they have shown in updating the text; to Mr. Orest Podolsky for his capable preparation and processing of the manuscript; to Mr. Brian Decker for his enthusiastic and confident support of this project; to Ms. Helga Kelly and the publisher's editorial staff, who worked tirelessly to see this new edition through its period of gestation; and to Mr. Dennis Boyes and Ms. Jean Calder for their cooperation in the countless revisions made to both text and illustrations during production of the book.

Spring 1989   The Editors

Contents

AUTONOMIC NERVOUS SYSTEM AND NEUROMUSCULAR JUNCTION

CENTRAL NERVOUS SYSTEM

AUTACOIDS AND MEDIATORS / MODIFIERS OF TISSUE RESPONSES

CARDIOVASCULAR SYSTEM

RESPIRATORY, RENAL, AND BLOOD SYSTEMS

ENDOCRINE SYSTEMS

GASTROINTESTINAL SYSTEM

CHEMOTHERAPY

SPECIAL TOPICS

GENERAL PRINCIPLES

—

Chapter 1

Introduction to General Pharmacology

H. Kalant

What Is Pharmacology?

The word **pharmacology** is derived from the Greek words *pharmakon* (a drug or poison) and *logos* (word or discourse), and means the science (discourse) that deals with the fate of drugs in the body and their actions on the body. It overlaps extensively with **pharmacy** (the science of preparation of drugs) and with **therapeutics** (the treatment of disease, by drugs and other means). Some of the areas of overlap will be mentioned below.

Pharmacology is both a basic science and a clinically applied one. As a basic science, it deals with the fate and actions of drugs at various levels (molecular, cellular, organ, and whole-body, in any animal species) in the same way as biochemistry, physiology, biophysics, and other divisions of biologic science. As an applied science, it deals with the same questions, but in the specific context of the human species and the use of drugs in the treatment of disease. This book includes both aspects of the subject.

What Is a Drug?

No definition of "drug" yet offered is entirely satisfactory. Perhaps the nearest we can come to one is the following: A drug is any substance, other than a normal constituent of the body or one that is required for normal bodily function (e.g., food, water, oxygen), that, when applied to or introduced into a living organism, has the effect of altering body function(s). This alteration may prove useful in the treatment of disease (therapeutic application) or it may cause disease (toxicity), but these outcomes are quite a separate matter from the definition of "drug."

Cold and hay-fever remedies bought off a supermarket shelf, penicillin given on prescription, and LSD bought illicitly on the street are all drugs. Vitamin C in orange juice is a food, but pure ascorbic acid injected in large doses to alter fibroblast activity is a drug. Hydrocortisone secreted by the adrenal cortex is a hormone, but when administered in large doses to suppress inflammatory or immune responses it is a drug. These actions may be useful in treating such diseases as rheumatoid arthritis or asthma, or they may cause Cushing's disease.

Pharmacology is not concerned *primarily* with what the drug may be used for, but with what actions it has.

SCOPE AND SUBDIVISIONS OF PHARMACOLOGY

The best way to convey an idea of the various subdivisions of pharmacology, and of how and where it overlaps with pharmacy and therapeutics, is to show schematically what happens when a drug enters the body (Fig. 1–1).

1. Whether the drug was given as a tablet or capsule by mouth, a vapor or aerosol by inhalation, a crystalline suspension by subcutaneous injection, or in any other form, it must first go into free solution at the site of administration. Preparation of the drug form, and adjustment of its physical properties so that the drug will dissolve at the desired rate, are problems of **pharmacy.**

2. The dissolved drug must be absorbed, into the portal blood if it is given by mouth, directly into the systemic circulation if it is given by injection or by inhalation. Absorption of the drug can involve a variety of different mechanisms that enable it to cross cell membranes, not only in the gastrointestinal tract but in all tissues. The absorption of a drug is strongly influenced

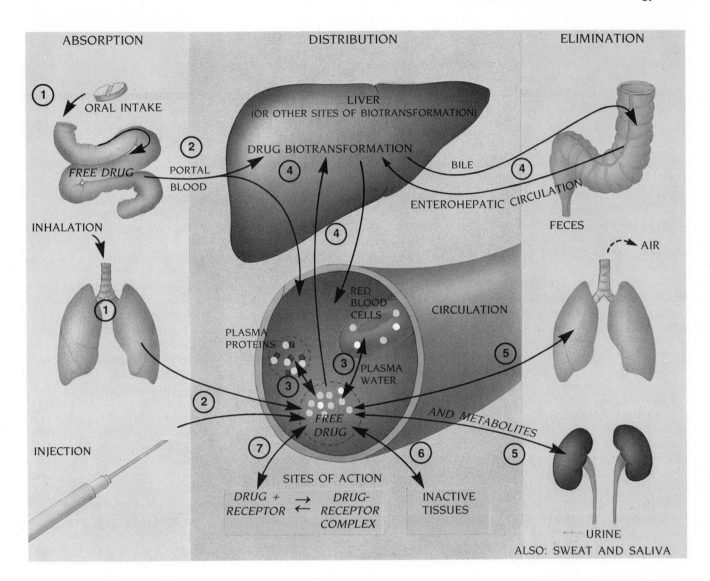

Figure 1–1   Schematic outline of the fate of a drug in the body. Numbers refer to the successive steps described in this section.

by its molecular size, lipid solubility, ionization, and other physicochemical properties. These questions are discussed in detail in Chapter 2. From the portal blood, some of the drug is taken up by the liver, but some goes on into the systemic circulation. This is considered in detail in Chapter 7, *Drug Clearance by Specific Organs*. The study of drug absorption and uptake by the liver is part of **pharmacology.**

Bioavailability of a drug, *i.e.*, the proportion of an administered dose that eventually reaches the systemic circulation in unchanged form, depends on both (1) and (2), and therefore is of concern to **both pharmacy and pharmacology**. It is considered in Chapter 5.

3. Once in the systemic blood, the free drug dissolved in the plasma water may be reversibly taken up into red cells, or reversibly bound to plasma proteins.

4. It may be taken up into the liver or other tissues where it can be converted into metabolites of the original drug. These may be eliminated in the bile, and thus reach the intestine, where they can either be excreted in the feces or be reabsorbed and carried in the portal blood back to the liver (enterohepatic circulation). Alternatively, the metabolites (and the original drug itself) may pass back from the liver into the general circulation and be carried to all other organs and tissues.

5. Among these other organs is the kidney, where both the drug and its metabolites may be filtered by the glomerulus or secreted by the tubule into the urine. However, depending on the concentration, the degree of ionization of the drug at the pH of the urine, and other factors, some of the drug may be reabsorbed from the urine by the tubule and pass back into the blood. This is discussed in greater detail in Chapter 7. Another organ to which the drug is carried is the lung. If the drug or its metabolite is volatile, it can pass from the blood into the alveolar air and be eliminated in the breath. This is particularly important for terminating the action of volatile anaesthetics (*see* Chapter 23), and is also the basis of the Breathalyzer test for blood alcohol level (*see* Chapter 25).

6. Among the tissues and organs to which the drug passes, some are not affected by it, and therefore simply act as reservoirs forming part of the drug's volume of distribution. This influences the equilibrium concentration of drug in the plasma after administration of a specified dose.

All of the processes mentioned in (2) to (6) above determine the rate at which the concentrations of the drug and its metabolites in the plasma and tissues rise and fall, as well as the maximum concentrations reached after a given dose. Together, these factors control the speed of onset and duration of drug effects. The study of the time course of drug concentration, and of the factors affecting it, is called **pharmacokinetics**, which is discussed in detail in Chapter 5. The pharmacokinetic features of a drug determine the dosage schedule that is used clinically (*see* Chapter 6), and therefore influence the **therapeutic** program.

7. Most (but not all) drugs bind to relatively specific receptors on the surface or in the interior of the tissue cells on which the drugs act. The binding of a drug to its receptor may initiate biochemical or biophysical changes that lead to its characteristic effects on body functions, and the drug is called an **agonist** at that receptor. In other cases, a drug may bind to a receptor without initiating any change, but prevent another substance from gaining access to the receptor where it normally acts; many drugs function in this way as **receptor blockers** or **antagonists**.

The study of these mechanisms of drug action is called **pharmacodynamics**, and the quantitative study of the relation among drug dose, concentration, and the magnitude of its effects is called **pharmacometrics**. These topics are discussed in Chapters 8 and 9. The ability of a drug to combine with its receptor depends on specific features of the drug's molecular structure. Therefore the study of pharmacodynamics overlaps with the field of **pharmaceutical chemistry**, which deals with the chemical synthesis of drugs and the study of their **structure-activity relationships**.

In addition to these basic divisions of the subject matter of pharmacology, there are other sets of divisions based on different criteria. For example, pharmacology may be divided according to:

1. The organ system of primary interest, *e.g.*, neuropharmacology, cardiovascular pharmacology, renal pharmacology, *etc.*
2. The techniques used, *e.g.*, biochemical pharmacology, molecular pharmacology, behavioral pharmacology, immunopharmacology, *etc.*
3. The purpose or application to which the knowledge is put, *e.g.*,
   - clinical pharmacology, the study of pharmacokinetics and pharmacodynamics in patients receiving drugs for the treatment of disease; therefore it includes the effect of disease on the action and disposition of the drug;
   - pharmacogenetics, the study of genetic factors causing variation in the response to drugs;
   - toxicology, the study of drugs that are acting as poisons rather than as agents for the treatment of disease; it includes specialized subdivisions such as forensic toxicology, clinical toxicology, industrial and environmental toxicology, behavioral toxicology, *etc.*;
   - agricultural pharmacology, the use of drugs for pest control.

DRUG CLASSIFICATIONS

Classification Based on Origin

Throughout human history there have been keen observers who, by chance observation or by systematic trial and error, were able to recognize that certain substances had interesting or useful drug effects. But such individuals were exceptions; most "drugs" used through the centuries were based on symbolic or magical thinking. For example, a plant with liver-shaped leaves was used to "treat" illnesses thought to arise in the liver.

With the growth of modern science in the last two centuries, systematic observation of the effects of exogenous substances on the body gave rise to techniques for screening possible new drugs. At first, the substances screened were natural materials gathered by botanists, anthropologists, explorers, *etc.* Later, chemists extracted and purified the active ingredients of these natural materials, and later still they synthesized wholly new compounds that did not exist in nature, but that, by analogy with natural compounds, might be expected to have drug effects.

On the basis of their origin, drugs may be classed in the following four broad categories.

Natural Preparations or Galenicals

These are relatively crude preparations obtained by drying or extracting plant or animal materials (*e.g.*, digitalis leaf, tincture of belladonna, and desiccated thyroid). This type of medicine, originally prepared by medicine men or priest-physicians, and later by apothecaries or physicians, dates back to prehistoric times. One of the first careful and systematic descriptions of all such drugs that were then known was written by the Greek physician Galen (130–200 A.D.), who practiced in Rome and in whose honor such drugs became known later as "Galenicals." Even now, new drugs are found from such materials, but they are no longer likely to be used as Galenicals; pharmaceutical chemistry is more likely to carry them immediately to the next stage shown below.

Pure Compounds

These are isolated, by physical and chemical extraction and purification procedures, from natural sources. A number of classical examples are shown in Table 1–1. The first to be isolated was morphine, which Sertürner

purified from opium in 1806. Many important drugs have come from natural sources, even in the last few years. Modern examples include penicillin and numerous other antibiotics from a variety of molds or fungi, and various anticancer and antileukemic chemotherapeutic drugs such as vinblastine and vincristine from certain varieties of periwinkle plant.

Semisynthetic Substances

These are obtained by chemical modification of the pure compounds obtained from natural sources. For example, acetylating two hydroxyl groups in morphine yields diacetylmorphine (heroin). Changing a side-group in penicillin yields oxacillin. Inserting a fluorine atom in the adrenal steroid hydrocortisone yields fludrocortisone. Many such semisynthetic modifications are dramatic improvements over the parent compounds with respect to potency, specificity, and duration of action.

Purely Synthetic Compounds

This is the most recent class. The first barbiturate was synthesized in 1902. Most drugs are now synthetic. Some of these were synthesized for other purposes, and medical uses were discovered accidentally; *e.g.*, disulfiram was invented as an agent for vulcanizing rubber, and its use as an antialcoholism drug came about through the observation that workers in the rubber factories got very bad reactions when they drank alcohol. In contrast, other drugs (*e.g.*, B.A.L., an antidote for arsenic or mercury poisoning) have been synthesized deliberately on the basis of predicted chemical properties. Still others have been synthesized on the basis of knowledge gained from the study of semisynthetic modifications of existing compounds. By learning which molecular features were necessary for which drug actions, pharmaceutical chemists have sometimes been able to "custom-design" a molecule to produce a desired pharmacologic effect.

Classification Based on Use

Most textbooks of pharmacology, particularly those intended for students and practitioners of medicine, dentistry, pharmacy, nursing, and other health sciences, classify drugs according to the organ systems upon which they exert their most prominent actions, or the therapeutic uses to which they are put. For example, drugs are classed as antibiotics, antiarrhythmic agents, diuretics, anticonvulsants, and so forth. There are some valid arguments against this method of classification, including the fact that almost every drug has more than one effect, and acts in more than one tissue, and the fact that different drugs may produce a similar therapeutic effect by quite different means. Nevertheless, this is still the commonest system of classification, and in deference to tradition and clinical usefulness it is also employed in this book.

TABLE 1–1   Some Examples of Drugs Derived from Plant Materials in Various Parts of the World

Plant Material or Galenical Preparation	Pure Compound	Original Source
Tincture of belladonna	Atropine	Orient (ancient)
Coca leaves	Cocaine	Peru, Bolivia
Curare	d-Tubocurarine	Amazon basin
Digitalis leaf, tincture	Digoxin, *etc.*	England
Ephedra	Ephedrine	China
Calabar bean	Eserine	West Africa
Opium	Morphine	Greece (ancient)
Tobacco	Nicotine	North and Central America
Cinchona bark	Quinine	Peru
Rauwolfia	Reserpine	India

Operational Classification

Drugs can also be classified on a totally different basis from the preceding ones. This refers to the circumstances under which they will be used or prescribed.

Drugs for Emergencies, To Be Known Perfectly by the Physician

Some tools one has to know very well. These are the tools that the physician uses in emergencies when immediate and exact action is required. Every physician must know the effects, the dangers, the dosages, and the modes of administration of drugs such as morphine and adrenaline,* because, whatever the physician's specialty, one may suddenly be faced with a patient whose life can be saved only by the immediate and correct use of one of these drugs.

Drugs of Frequent Use, To Be Known in Main Outline

There is a much longer list of drugs with whose characteristics you will become very familiar, but that are used in circumstances that will give you the opportunity of refreshing your memory if you need to; this list will vary with your area of practice.

Drugs Used Occasionally, After Checking Details

There is a third list of drugs that you will never administer without checking the details of actions, interactions, effects, and dosages. This list includes all drugs that you do not use frequently, and all new drugs.

Drugs To Be Used Only by Experts

There is a fourth list that you will use only after special training and experience. For example, there are a number of anaesthetics that should be administered only by an anaesthetist. You need to know about such drugs, but you cannot possibly carry all their details in your mind or acquire skill in their use without special training and repeated practice.

DRUGS AND SOCIETY

Our society comes into contact with drugs in many different ways, which are related to different uses and different problems:

1. **Medical prescription** or therapeutic use. This is the way that receives most attention in medical teaching, but it is by no means the commonest.

2. **Over-the-counter sale**, without prescription. This is also intended primarily for "therapeutic" purposes, even though it is most commonly not under medical supervision. There is a huge range of cough remedies, analgesics, topical antiseptics, local anaesthetics, antihistamines, hypnotics and so forth, that can be bought in this way. Many of them are quite potent and can give rise to serious toxicity if used improperly.

3. **Social use.** This includes alcohol, cannabis, and a wide range of other psychoactive substances (*i.e.,* that affect mood, perception, psychomotor performance, and emotional responses). Some are legally available, some are diverted from legal production to the illicit market, and some are manufactured illegally. All such use carries the risk of abuse, with the attendant problems of toxicity and dependence (*see* Chapter 67).

4. **Industrial use.** Many preservatives, artificial flavorings, colorings, fillers, *etc.*, are added to processed foods. Though each is kept to a level considered to be safe in any individual product, there is very little known about cumulative totals, or interactions between substances and what they may contribute to low-grade toxicity.

5. **Agricultural use.** Widespread use of pesticides has contributed greatly to increased agricultural productivity in many parts of the world. However, pesticides, weed-killers, and herbicides, together with industrial wastes, automobile exhaust fumes, and other products of human industry, all contribute to the total of environmental toxicity.

6. **Accident.** Apart from the obvious cases of accidental poisoning, which come to hospital emergency rooms, or deliberate suicidal or homicidal poisonings, which are dealt with by forensic toxicologists as well as hospitals, there are natural accidents. For example, a certain fungus growth on peanuts can generate a very potent carcinogen (aflatoxin); another fungus growth on rye generates ergot alkaloids, which on occasion cause serious poisoning.

All of these manners of exposure to drugs have become vastly more common as a result of population growth, chemical inventiveness, improved means of communication, and industrialization. Apart from the accident category, the other forms of exposure all carry certain benefits and certain hazards, but the optimum balance of benefits versus risks is often hard to define. It depends to a large extent on the scale of social values. This is particularly true of the third, fourth, and fifth categories above, but is also true of the first and second.

Therefore most societies have imposed governmental controls on the availability, quality, and permitted uses of drugs. Such controls are generally pragmatic, rather than theoretical. To a large extent they are handled by administrative regulation, but certain broad principles and policies are laid down in legislation. This subject is covered in Chapter 73.

---

* epinephrine

DRUG STANDARDS AND REFERENCES

The rapid progress in the chemical industry in the past half-century has altered the nature of pharmacy, pharmacology, and therapeutics. Because most drugs used nowadays are potent pure chemicals, they must be prepared and used under strict controls. Therefore, their definition and standardization are regulated by law in terms of name, purity, potency, and preparation, and so is their distribution to the public.

Not only the active drugs themselves, but also the forms in which they are dispensed, must be carefully controlled if the effectiveness of drug treatment is to be assured. For application in drug therapy, most chemicals have to be put into tablets, capsules, ampuls, aerosols, ointments, solutions, or suppositories. The drug must have the highest purity compatible with chemical stability and economic feasibility. It must have appropriate crystal size. It must be compatible with ingredients usually necessary to give bulk to a tablet, to regulate its hardness, cohesiveness, and its rate of disintegration in gastric or intestinal juice. The tablet may have to be protected from light and withstand storage in tropical climates. It may require a corrective for taste. It should not explode in the patient's stomach (as have some tablets used in the treatment of tuberculosis). Above all, it must release the drug in such a manner that the drug will be absorbed at a suitable rate. There are equivalent problems in compounding drug vehicles other than tablets. All this is the domain of **pharmacy**, and all of it is subject to controls and standards.

The standards are published in **pharmacopoeias** such as the British Pharmacopoeia (B.P.), the U.S. Pharmacopeia (U.S.P.), the Codex Français, and the International Pharmacopoeia. These books are revised periodically and supplements to them may be issued between editions. A drug listed in a pharmacopoeia is termed an "official" drug because it enjoys official recognition by a government. Canada has no pharmacopoeia of its own, but other pharmacopoeias that have official status as defined in the Food and Drugs Act (*see* Chapter 73, *Drug Development and Regulations*) may be used. However, any drug offered under the B.P. name must conform to the B.P. standard unless the label states that it conforms to another acceptable standard, *e.g.*, U.S.P. From time to time, names are published in the form of regulations under the Federal Food and Drugs Act, and these names take precedence over those given in foreign pharmacopoeias.

There are also a number of reference books that do not have official status in every province of Canada:

Pediatric Dosage Handbook. American Pharmaceutical Association.

European Pharmacopoeia.

U.S. National Formulary (N.F.). American Pharmaceutical Society.

American Medical Association Drug Evaluations.

Accepted Dental Therapeutics (A.D.T.). Published annually by the American Dental Association. Convenient and useful for dentists, it includes information on (1) drugs of recognized value in dentistry, (2) drugs of uncertain status more recently proposed for use by dentists, and (3) some drugs now generally regarded as obsolete.

Compendium of Pharmaceuticals and Specialties (C.P.S.). Published annually by the Canadian Pharmaceutical Association. For Canadian readers, this publication is very useful; it describes many of the prescription drugs available in Canada, their uses, contraindications, adverse reactions, and doses.

Drug Benefit Formulary (PARCOST). Published by the Ontario Department of Health, comparing the prices of all principal brands of prescription drugs commonly used and available in Ontario, and meeting government standards of quality and uniformity.

DRUG NOMENCLATURE

There are many names given to drugs that are often confusing to those who are not familiar with the nomenclature system. When a drug is first synthesized and subjected to initial screening, it is usually referred to, in the scientific literature, by its chemical name or by a code number indicating the manufacturer and test document file number (*e.g.*, RO15–4513, EN–2234A). When it reaches the stage of clinical testing, it usually receives a more convenient but unofficial short name. After it comes into general use, it may receive other names indicative of different levels of medical or official approval. When a pharmaceutical company finally receives permission to bring the new drug on to the market, usually a proprietary (trade or brand) name is given to it. The use of this name is protected by law and is restricted to the firm that introduces the preparation; it carries the symbol ®. Thus, the same drug may be known (unfortunately) under several different names at the same time:

1. Chemical name.
2. Nonproprietary drug name (sometimes called "generic name"):
   - Official names (in pharmacopoeias);
   - Approved names (not yet in pharmacopoeias):
     - Canadian Proper Names;
     - Approved names, British Pharmacopoeial Commission;
     - U.S. Adopted Name (USAN; Joint Committee of AMA, U.S. Pharmacopeial Commission, and American Pharmaceutical Association).
3. Proprietary name: manufacturer's trade name, registered by owner, somewhat like a copyright.
4. Common name.

Examples:

1. *Chemical names*: 1-methyl-4-phenyl-4-carbethoxy piperidine; 1-methyl-4-phenyl-isonipecotic acid ethyl ester.

Official names: pethidine (B.P.), meperidine (U.S.P.), isonipecaine (I.P.).
Proprietary names: Demerol, Dolantin, Dolantol, Eudolal.

2. *Chemical name*: ortho-acetoxybenzoic acid.
Official names: acetylsalicylic acid (B.P.), aspirin (U.S.P.).
Proprietary names: Aspirin (in Canada only), Acetophen, Empirin, and many more.

It is in the financial interest of the manufacturer to popularize and use the trade name only, because the patent will last only 17 years in the United States, but the trade name registration for at least 50. The time from patenting to marketing is usually 8–10 years and the cost of development is typically $100 million or more per drug. In addition, the patent may not be valid because someone else may have published an article or own a patent with close to the same idea. If the drug is really very good, it will also be produced in a country that does not have reciprocal patent laws, *e.g.*, Italy, Argentina, or Hungary. It is easy to appreciate why a company that has spent millions of dollars for drug development will encourage the use of its own brand, or proprietary, name. As a rule, the trade name was chosen to be simple and euphonious, while the nonproprietary name tended to be difficult and did not suggest its use or chemical nature. A combined **Committee on Nomenclature of the American Medical Association, American Pharmaceutical Association, and U.S. Pharmacopeial Commission** has made good progress in correcting this situation, so that the United States Adopted Name (USAN) is easier to remember and suggests the nature of the drug. The names, chemical structures, and uses of newly introduced drugs are published in the *Journal of the American Medical Association (JAMA)*.

We recommend the use of official, proper (Canada), approved (U.K.), or USAN (U.S.A.) names, which are used in most reputable journals, and which are almost always the same because of international cooperation in naming. If a drug becomes official, the proper, approved, or USAN name will almost certainly become the official name.

We advise against using trade names because they lead to an artificially complex vocabulary, which hinders medical communication; the same product is often produced by several reliable manufacturers, all using different brand names; and the use of trade names encourages high pricing.

In fairness to pharmaceutical firms it must be pointed out that there have been occasional instances where nonbrand preparations failed to be reliable. Certain trade name preparations have standards that are often higher than those called for by pharmacopoeial specification. Unreliability of certain types of drugs can be extremely serious. It may be desirable, therefore, to depend on the reputation of the company producing them. This can be done by specifying the brand or the company in your prescription.

OTHER SOURCES OF INFORMATION

The material in this book is only a **starting point** in learning about drug actions and drug use. All medical students should consider, and have access to, the following reference text:

- Goodman and Gilman's *The Pharmacological Basis of Therapeutics*. Editors: A.G. Gilman, L.S. Goodman, T.W. Rall, and F. Murad. Seventh Edition. Macmillan Publishing Co., New York/Collier Macmillan Canada Ltd., Toronto (1985).

Other books that can be consulted include:

- *Principles of Drug Action—The Basis of Pharmacology*. A. Goldstein *et al*. Second Edition. Wiley Medical Publishers (1974). [Deals with more basic aspects of drug action.]
- *Drugs, Society and Personal Choice*. H. Kalant and O.J. Kalant. Addiction Research Foundation of Ontario (1971). [A short book, mainly about nonmedical use of drugs and social control policy.]

For anyone with special interest in drugs or drug research, there are numerous scientific journals, such as:

- *Drugs;*
- *Pharmacological Reviews;*
- *Journal of Pharmacology and Experimental Therapeutics;*
- *British Journal of Pharmacology and Chemotherapy;*
- *European Journal of Clinical Pharmacology;*
- *Canadian Journal of Physiology and Pharmacology;*
- *Clinical Pharmacokinetics.*

Most of the major medical journals continue to present drug information in the form of editorials or reviews.
The Medical Letter on Drugs and Therapeutics represents a specialized effort to provide practising physicians and medical students with unbiased data and critical information on newly introduced drugs. It compares new drugs with older agents and critically analyses claims put forth by manufacturers. The information presented is concise and usually very up to date.

For those who wish to know more about the origins and history of drugs, two very interesting books are:

- *Readings in Pharmacology*. Editors: B. Holmstedt and G. Liljestrand. Macmillan, New York, 1963.
- *Ethnopharmacologic Search for Psychoactive Drugs*. Editors: D.H. Efron, B. Holmstedt, and N.S. Kline. U.S. Dept. of Health, Education and Welfare, Washington, D.C., 1967.

Chapter 2

DRUG SOLUBILITY, ABSORPTION, AND MOVEMENT ACROSS BODY MEMBRANES

P. Seeman and H. Kalant

In Chapter 1, a general outline of the fate of drugs in the body was given, beginning with absorption from the site of administration, and going on to distribution throughout the body, including the sites of action, biotransformation, and elimination (see Fig. 1–1). It was pointed out that all these processes together determine the speed of onset of drug action, its intensity, and its duration. In general, the intensity of action is most directly related to the concentration of drug at the site of action (''receptor'' in the broadest sense; see Chapter 9), while the duration of action is related to the speed of biotransformation and elimination of the drug, and hence of its removal from the site of action.

When a drug is used therapeutically, the main concern is to get an adequate concentration to the site of action as quickly as possible, and to maintain that concentration as continuously as possible. However, it is not possible to hold a constant concentration unless the drug is given by continuous intravenous infusion at exactly the same rate at which it is being eliminated. Any other mode of administration that involves repeated but separate doses results in some fluctuation of drug concentration. This is discussed in detail in Chapter 5, *Pharmacokinetics*. At this stage we shall merely provide a framework for understanding how the route and rate of administration are chosen, and what factors affect the speed with which the drug reaches its sites of action and elimination.

ROUTES OF DRUG ADMINISTRATION

Topical

The simplest mode of administration is direct local application of the drug to the place where it must act. Such local application is called topical (from the Greek *topos* = a place). In practice this most often means direct application to an accessible body surface. Examples include the use of ointments, creams, lotions, powders, or sprays applied to the **skin**; **eye** drops and ophthalmic ointments; **nose** drops and sprays; **ear** drops; and solutions or sprays for use in the **mouth, throat, rectum, vagina,** and **urethra.**

However, drugs applied to mucous membranes can often be absorbed rapidly enough to produce actions in the rest of the body. When cocaine was first used as a local anaesthetic, it was widely adopted in rectal and urologic surgery and used in large volumes that gave rise to many poisonings, including fatal ones. Topical use refers to the application of sufficiently small volumes and low concentrations to ensure that the drug acts **only** at that site.

Occasionally, drugs are injected directly into **body cavities** for local action at those sites. For example, corticosteroids may be injected into a joint or a bursa for treatment of a sharply localized arthritis or bursitis not caused by infection. Antibiotics may be injected into the pleural space or into an abscess cavity for treatment of a local pocket of infection surrounded by fibrous tissue that prevents the antibiotic from getting there *via* the blood stream. The doses injected in such cases are enough to produce fairly high local concentrations, but not so large as to produce significant levels in the circulating blood when the drug diffuses away from the site of injection.

Percutaneous

Drug absorption through the intact skin is proportional to the lipid solubility of the drug (the epidermis behaves as a lipoid barrier, the dermis is freely permeable). Absorption can be enhanced by suspending the drug in an oily vehicle (''inunction''). Other than for local effects, this is probably the least effective and least economical route of administration (huge quantities of drug are required to get some of it absorbed). However, a few drugs are now marketed, or under consideration, for percutaneous administration, such as nitroglycerin ointment to treat angina pectoris, scopolamine plasters to prevent motion sickness, and a proposed hormone cream for male contraception.

Even though the skin is an effective barrier that hinders the transport of almost all substances, letting no molecule through readily, there are very few substances to which it is totally impermeable. Even a heavy metal like mercury can be absorbed to some degree through the skin. Indeed, absorption through the skin represents one of the most common routes by which poisoning in humans and animals occurs following accidental exposure to foreign chemicals. For example, many insecticides, particularly those containing parathion, malathion, or nicotine, may cause serious poisoning as a result of percutaneous absorption following inadvertent contamination of the skin or clothing.

Gastrointestinal Tract

Oral Mucosa (Sublingual)

The mouth is capable of serving as a site for the absorption of drugs. A familiar example is nitroglycerin, made into small tablets that are placed under the tongue (sublingual). The drug is rapidly absorbed through the thin mucosa there, giving rapid relief of anginal attacks. Drugs absorbed sublingually or buccally are not exposed to gastric and intestinal digestive juices. In addition, drugs absorbed from the mouth are not subject to immediate passage through the liver (*i.e.*, no prior transformation) before they circulate throughout the body. Many drugs, however, are not capable of penetrating the oral mucosa in significant amounts and others are too irritating to be held in the mouth.

Stomach and Intestine (Oral, per os, p.o., PO)

Absorption, and the resulting attainment of drug effects, depends on many factors, such as pH, gastric emptying, intestinal motility, solubility of solid drugs, concentration of drug solutions, stability of drugs in gastrointestinal fluids, and binding to gastrointestinal contents.

The considerable blood supply of the stomach, combined with the potential for prolonged contact of an agent with the relatively large epithelial surface, are conducive to the absorption of various drugs. The length of time a substance remains in the stomach, however, is the greatest variable affecting the extent of gastric absorption. The rate at which the stomach empties its contents into the small intestine is influenced by the volume, viscosity, and constituents of those contents; by physical activity and the position of the body; by the ingested drugs themselves; and by many other factors. Only when a drug is taken with water on a relatively empty stomach is it possible to say that it will reach the small intestine fairly rapidly (Fig. 2–1).

Rectal Mucosa (Suppositories, Enemas)

Even though the function of the colon is not fundamentally that of absorption, drugs which escape absorption in the small intestine may continue to be absorbed during their passage out of the body. Moreover, the terminal segment of the large intestine, the rectum, can serve as a useful site for drug adminis-

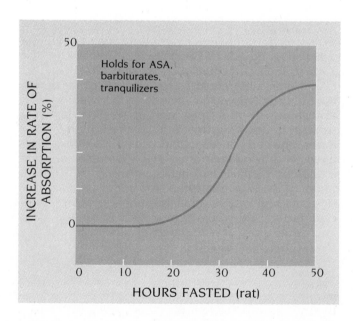

Figure 2–1 Relationship of drug absorption rate to presence of gastrointestinal contents in rats.

tration, particularly when the oral route is unsuitable. Rectal administration is advantageous in the unconscious patient, in patients unable to retain material given by mouth, and for drugs with objectionable taste or odor or those destroyed by digestive enzymes. This route protects susceptible drugs not only from alteration but also from the biotransformation reactions occurring in the liver (*see* Chapter 4), because the blood draining the lower part of the rectum passes into the inferior vena cava *via* the internal pudendal veins rather than through the portal vein and liver. However, absorption by this route is often irregular and incomplete. Many drugs cause irritation of the rectal mucosa.

Pulmonary Epithelium

Gases, vapors, or aerosols can be inhaled and absorbed through the alveolar surface or the bronchial mucosa, giving rapid access to the circulation. The drugs may be intended for local action (*e.g.*, antiasthmatic agents) or for action elsewhere in the body (*e.g.*, general anaesthetics, amyl nitrite for angina pectoris).

Injection

This is also called parenteral administration (from the Greek *para* = beside, *i.e.*, not in, and *enteron* = gut). Usual advantages are more rapid and more predictable absorption and more accurate dose selection. General disadvantages are the need for strict asepsis, the possibility of pain, and some difficulty in self-administration of drugs by injection. Moreover, injectable drugs are usually more expensive.

Subcutaneous Injection (s.c., SC, subcut.)

Only nonirritating drugs can be administered in this way. Large volumes may be painful because of tissue distention. This route provides for even and slow absorption to obtain sustained drug effects. Vasoconstrictors, such as adrenaline (epinephrine), greatly decrease the rate of absorption from a subcutaneous injection site. The enzyme hyaluronidase, by virtue of its ability to break down mucopolysaccharides in connective tissue, increases the spread of drug solutions injected subcutaneously and leads to a much faster absorption.

Intramuscular Injection (i.m., IM)

Aqueous solutions are rapidly absorbed from deep intramuscular injection sites. Slow and even absorption becomes possible if the drugs are suspended or dissolved in oil, which forms a depot in the muscle. Irritating substances or large volumes may cause pain, and drugs that dissolve only at very low or very high pH can cause sterile abscesses if injected intramuscularly.

Intravenous Administration (i.v., IV)

Rapid injection. The desired blood concentration of a drug is obtained accurately and immediately, without variation due to prior absorption or passage through the liver.

The dangers lie in the fact that once the drug is injected, its rapid removal is impossible. There is also the risk of transmission of infections, occurrence of vascular injury, or extravasation of drug into surrounding tissues.

Slow infusion. In addition to the general advantages of intravenous administration, with slow infusion (over 20 minutes or more) the level of the drug in the blood can be "titrated" by proper adjustments of flow rate and drug concentration. Infusions are particularly useful to maintain constant blood levels of drugs over extended periods of time. This lessens the risk of irrevocable administration of an overdose. However, expertise is required to minimize the risk of vascular injury, infection, and accidents (severing of infusion lines, bleeding, air embolism, *etc.*)

Intra-arterial Injection (i.a.)

This method is occasionally employed to direct small volumes of drug solutions at high concentrations to specific target tissues or organs, increasing the drug uptake at those sites but minimizing the effects elsewhere by subsequent drug dilution in the general circulation (*see* Chapter 10, *Specificity of Drug Action*).

Intrathecal Injection (i.th.)

This method is employed to administer drugs directly into the cerebrospinal fluid (CSF) bathing the central nervous system, bypassing the blood–brain barrier and the blood–CSF barrier.

Injection into Body Cavities

The peritoneum provides a large absorbing surface that permits rapid entry of drugs into the circulation. **Intraperitoneal (i.p., IP)** injection is a common laboratory procedure, but it is seldom used clinically because of dangers of infection, intestinal or vascular injury, and adhesions.

CHOICE OF ROUTE

Regardless of the route of administration, a drug must be absorbed, reach its site of action, and interact in some way with the target tissue. These processes occur at very different speeds, depending on the route of administration. This question will be dealt with in detail later (*see* Chapter 5), but Figure 2–2 illustrates

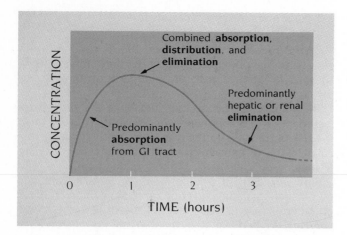

Figure 2–2 Components of the concentration-time curve after oral drug administration.

the order of magnitude of the times that may be required.

The choice of route may depend on therapeutic objectives. For example, intravenous injection or inhalation may be selected to produce a rapid, intense, but rather short-lived effect, while oral dosage may be better and more convenient for long-lasting effects of relatively moderate and even intensity.

The choice of routes is sometimes limited by the properties of the drug in question. Barbiturates (anaesthetic or hypnotic agents) and phenytoin (anticonvulsant), for example, will dissolve only in rather strongly alkaline solution. If they have to be given by injection for rapid effect, they can be injected intravenously (the blood buffers the pH of the drug solution). In contrast, if they are injected intramuscularly or subcutaneously there is not sufficient local buffering by tissue fluids, and the alkaline solution causes pain and local tissue damage. EDTA (a chelating agent for treating heavy-metal poisoning) is poorly absorbed from the gastrointestinal tract and is therefore generally given by intravenous injection or infusion. Ordinary penicillin G is rapidly inactivated by gastric HCl. Therefore, if given by mouth, it must be given in huge doses to allow for the high percentage destroyed. In serious infections, this may introduce too much uncertainty, and the penicillin is more likely to be given by intramuscular or intravenous injection to ensure that high enough blood levels are reached.

MOLECULAR SIZE, SOLUBILITY, AND DRUG DISTRIBUTION

Once a drug has been administered, the processes of uptake and distribution depend largely upon the physical properties of the drug. It must usually pass from the site of administration across capillary walls into the circulation, and from the circulation it must again cross capillary walls to reach the site(s) of action (Fig. 2–3). The only exceptions are those instances in which the drug is applied directly to the site of action (topical application). Even here, however, the drug will often have to cross cell membranes to reach specific intracellular sites of action, such as an enzyme or a nuclear receptor.

The ability of the drug to cross capillary walls, cell membranes, and other barriers to free movement depends to a large extent upon its molecular size and shape and its solubility in aqueous and lipid phases.

Molecular Size

Most drugs, excluding peptides, have molecular weights of the order of 300. Among the lightest are the anaesthetic gas nitrous oxide, and ethanol, which have molecular weights of 44 and 46 respectively. The muscle relaxant tubocurarine (curare) is exceptionally heavy and has a molecular weight of about 700. Small peptides like ADH (antidiuretic hormone) are in the 1000 to 2000 MW range. Insulin, a small protein, has a MW of 6000; that of albumin is 65,000, while the MW of the heavier proteins may range into the hundreds of thousands or the millions (such as botulinum toxin). Thus, compared to the protein molecules, which are the main building blocks of the body, most drug molecules are small (5–10 Å long). The significance of this fact, with respect to drug distribution, is discussed below in the section on passive diffusion of water-soluble drugs.

Drug Solubility

To be pharmacologically active, a drug must have some solubility within the body fluids. Although the water molecule as a whole is electrically neutral, the distribution of electrons between oxygen and hydrogen is such that the O region of the molecule has a slight preponderance of negative charge while the two H regions are preponderant in positive charge. Drugs that are positively or negatively charged, therefore, readily associate with water molecules, and we refer to such drugs as being water-soluble or hydrophilic. In general, any chemical substituent group, when attached to a drug molecule, will affect the electron distribution within the drug and make that molecule either more water-soluble (and less lipid-soluble) or less water-soluble (and more lipid-soluble or lipophilic).

In the pharmacologic literature, the absolute solubility of a drug is not often mentioned, but its relative solubility in lipid and water may be stressed. This is very important, because when a drug molecule arrives at the cell membrane, this relative solubility determines whether it is more likely to stay in the water phase

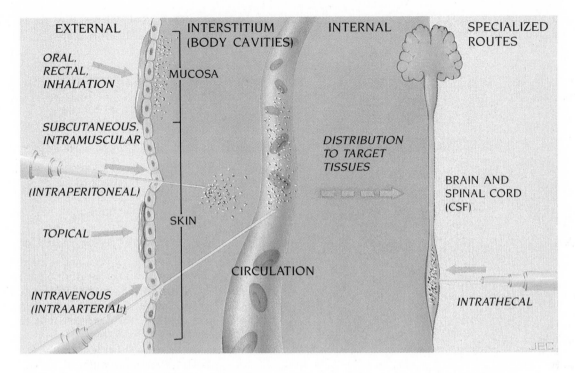

Figure 2–3 Routes of drug administration, in relation to biologic barriers to drug diffusion.

or to permeate into the fatty material of the cell membrane. Relative solubility of a drug is measured by its partition coefficient. Oil and water, when shaken together, form an unstable mixture that afterwards separates into a two-phase system containing oil on the top and water on the bottom. If a drug is added to this system before shaking, the drug will be finally found in both phases. The oil/water partition coefficient is the ratio of the drug concentration in the oil phase over that in the water phase:

$$P_{oil/water} = \frac{C_{oil}}{C_{water}}.$$

Using radioisotopes, it is now also possible to measure and speak of the membrane/buffer partition coefficient of a drug:

$$P_{mem/buffer} = \frac{C_{membrane}}{C_{buffer\ or\ water}}.$$

The membrane/buffer partition coefficients of various drugs can be arithmetically derived, starting with the $P_{m/b}$ values of the "parent drug" structures shown in Table 2–1.

TABLE 2–1 Membrane-Buffer Partition Coefficients of Some Basic Structures

Parent Structure	$P_{m/b}$
CH_4 (Methane)	0.6
Benzene ring	25
Cyclohexane	16

Table 2–2 (Partition Factors) lists a series of chemical substituent groups and the factor by which each substituent increases the membrane/buffer partition coefficient. For example, if the partition (P) factor for a substituent is greater than 1, this means that the substituent increases the solubility of the drug in the membrane (or in fat, or in oil, or in octanol) by the factor listed in the Table. However, if the P factor of the substituent is less than 1, this means that the substituent reduces the solubility of the drug in the membrane (or oil) phase.

TABLE 2–2 Partition Factors of Substituent Groups in Drug Molecules

Substituent Group	Partition Factor	
	If on Aromatic Parent	If on Aliphatic Parent
$-I$	$\times 13$	$\times 10$
$-Br$	$\times 7.3$	$\times 6$
$-Cl$	$\times 5$	$\times 2.5$
$-CH_2$ or $-CH_3$	$\times 3$	$\times 3$
$-F$	$\times 1.4$	$\times 0.7$
$-SH$	$\times 1.3$	$\times 0.9$
$-OCH_3$	$\times 0.95$	$\times 0.34$
$-NO_2$	$\times 0.53$	$\times 0.14$
$=S=O$	$\times 0.3$	$\times 0.3$
$-COOH$	$\times 0.52$	$\times 0.2$
$-OH$	$\times 0.2$	$\times 0.07$
$-C\equiv N$	$\times 0.27$	$\times 0.15$
$-NH_2$ or $-NH-$ or $-NH_3^+$	$\times 0.06$	$\times 0.064$
$-C=O$	$\times 0.09$	$\times 0.062$

= (double bond)	$\times 0.5$
Branching in C chain	$\times 0.63$
Ring closure	$\times 0.9$

The following examples illustrate how it is possible to derive the approximate value for the membrane/buffer partition coefficient (or $P_{m/b}$) for any particular drug, using the data given in Tables 2–1 and 2–2.

Example #1. ETHANOL:

$$CH_3CH_2OH$$

The $P_{m/b}$ for ethanol is derived from the parent methane, which has a $P_{m/b}$ of 0.6. Hence, the $P_{m/b}$ for ethanol will be the product of 0.6 and the partition factors for $-CH_2$ and $-OH$, as follows:

$$P_{m/b}(EtOH) = P_{m/b} \text{ (methane)} \times P_{CH_2} \times P_{OH}$$
$$= 0.6 \times 3 \times 0.07 = 0.13.$$

(Note: The real experimental value has not yet been obtained for ethanol, but the triolein/water partition coefficient is 0.035.)

Example #2. ISO-BUTANOL:

$$CH_3 - CH - CH_2OH$$
$$\mid$$
$$CH_3$$

The $P_{m/b}$ for iso-butanol will be

$$= P_{m/b} \text{ (methane)} \times (P_{CH_2})^3 \times P_{branch} \times P_{OH}$$
$$= 0.6 \times 3^3 \times 0.63 \times 0.07 = 0.71.$$

Example #3. PENTOBARBITAL:

Barbital

$$
\begin{array}{c}
C_2H_5 \quad CO-NH \\
\diagdown \diagup \qquad \diagdown \\
\qquad C \qquad\qquad C=O \\
\diagup \diagdown \qquad \diagup \\
C_2H_5 \quad CO-NH
\end{array}
$$

Pentobarbital

$$
\begin{array}{c}
C_2H_5 \quad CO-NH \\
\diagdown \diagup \qquad \diagdown \\
\qquad C \qquad\qquad C=O \\
\diagup \diagdown \qquad \diagup \\
CH_3CH_2CH_2-CH \quad CO-NH \\
\mid \\
CH_3
\end{array}
$$

The membrane/buffer partition coefficient of pentobarbital can be arithmetically derived from the $P_{m/b}$ of barbital (which happens to be approximately 1.0). It will be the product of $P_{m/b}$ for barbital, the partition factors of three extra $-CH_2$ groups, and the partition factor of a C branch, as follows:

$$= P_{m/b} \text{ (barbital)} \times (P_{CH_2})^3 \times P_{branch}$$
$$= 1.0 \times 3^3 \times 0.63 = 17.$$

(Note: The real value is approximately 15.)

MOLECULAR MECHANISMS OF DRUG ABSORPTION

Of the following eight molecular mechanisms of drug passage across membranes, only the first four are of major significance:

- Passive diffusion of water-soluble drugs.
- Passive diffusion of lipid-soluble drugs.
- Active transport.
- Pinocytosis/phagocytosis.
- Facilitated diffusion.
- Passive filtration.
- Adsorption of drugs to cell contents.
- Drug passage *via* gap junctions.

Each of these mechanisms will now be explained in turn.

Passive Diffusion of Water-Soluble Drugs

The passive diffusion of water-soluble drugs into cells largely depends on the molecular size of the drug. This is because the aqueous channels of the cell membrane are only about 8 Å wide and will restrict passage of any molecules larger than those with MW 150–200. These channels in the cell membrane consist of pathways through the membrane proteins and between the oscillating lipid molecules (Fig. 2–4). Since most drugs are either lipid-soluble or have molecular weights greater than 150–200, passive diffusion through aqueous channels is not the major permeation mechanism.

Drugs that are highly water-soluble have low membrane/water partition coefficients, with values less than 3. Examples of such highly water-soluble drugs that enter cells by this mechanism of simple passive diffusion *via* aqueous channels are shown in Table 2–3.

As shown in Figure 2–5, the permeation rate of water-soluble drugs falls as the MW of the drug becomes larger. The mechanism of tetracycline permeation is puzzling, since it is quite water-soluble but has a high molecular weight.

TABLE 2–3 Examples of Water-Soluble Drugs That Enter Cells Through Aqueous Channels in the Membrane

Drug	MW	$P_{m/b}$
Acetylsalicylic acid	180	3
Nicotine	162	3
Salts (*e.g.*, Li_2CO_3)	~70	0.0002
Caffeine	194	0.17
Ephedrine	165	1.6
Low MW diuretics (*e.g.*, furosemide)	~100	
Ascorbic acid (vitamin C)	176	0.02
Sulfanilamide	172	0.03
Hydrogen peroxide	34	0.02
Nicotinamide (vitamin B_3)	122	0.02
Saccharin	183	1.7
Amino acids	100–150	0.02

Passive Diffusion of Lipid-Soluble Drugs

The majority of lipid-soluble drugs permeate across cell membranes by passive diffusion between the lipid molecules of the cell membrane (*see* Fig. 2–4). The permeation rate of a lipid-soluble drug depends on the following factors:

- Concentration (or dose) of drug.
- Oil/water partition coefficient of drug.
- The concentration of protons (cH^+).
- The area for drug diffusion.

Unlike the situation with highly water-soluble drugs (previous section), the permeation rate of lipid-soluble drugs does not vary systematically with the size of the molecule. However, extremely large drug molecules of around MW 1000 or more can be absorbed only by pinocytosis.

Dependence on the Concentration (or Dose) of the Drug

The overall rate of drug permeation increases if the amount of drug administered is increased; this simply means that "the more you give, the more becomes absorbed." However, the relation between dosage and

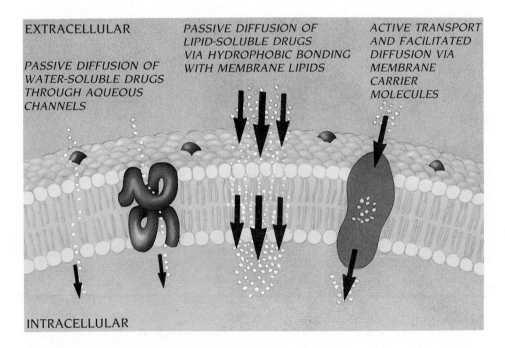

Figure 2–4 Pathways of drug permeation across cell membranes. Aqueous channels occur between lipids and in the interstices of proteins.

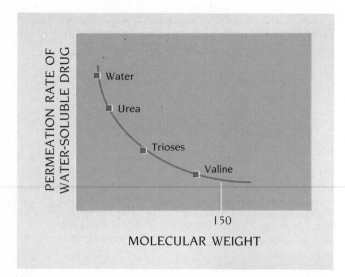

Figure 2–5   Indicating that larger water-soluble drugs permeate more slowly. Those above MW 150 permeate extremely slowly and need other mechanisms to traverse the membrane barriers.

absorption is not simple. Some drugs are absorbed in direct proportion to the amount given, while other drugs have a nonlinear relation (Fig. 2–6). This creates serious difficulties in trying to regulate the drug dosage for a particular patient.

Role of the Oil/Water (or Membrane/Buffer) Partition Coefficient

The oil/water partition coefficient of a drug is the principal factor determining the absorption of drugs in the

body. In general, if a drug has a high oil/water partition coefficient (or a high membrane/buffer partition coefficient), then it will be absorbed more rapidly across cell membranes and tissue barriers. Examples of this general rule may be found in the case of barbiturates permeating the colon, or sedative-hypnotics (e.g., carbamates) permeating the stomach epithelium (Fig. 2–7).

The situation is apparently not so simple, however, since in the case of the small intestine, where the bulk of drug absorption occurs (because of the large surface area involved), there is an optimum value for the oil/water partition coefficient. An example of such an optimum is shown in Figure 2–8.

The explanation of this optimum has to do with the fact that there is a hydrophilic barrier to drugs before

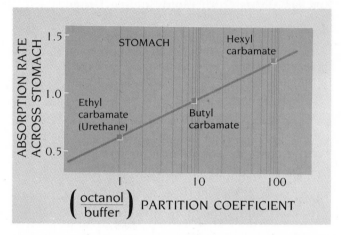

Figure 2–7   The more lipid-soluble anaesthetics permeate more easily across the stomach wall.

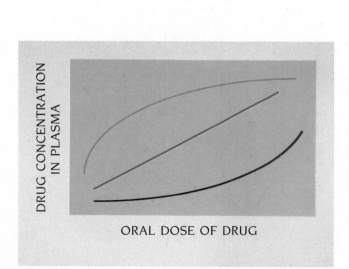

Figure 2–6   Three types of relations between the oral drug dosage and plasma drug concentration.

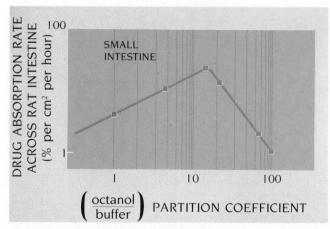

Figure 2–8   Indicating that, although increasing the lipid solubility of a drug generally increases the absorption rate of the drug, there is a limit to this (see Fig. 2–9 for explanation).

the drug molecules actually have a chance to permeate across the cell membrane itself. This hydrophilic barrier is composed of the unstirred water between the microvilli and immediately next to the surface sugar coat of the cell membrane, as shown in Figure 2–9. This means that, in order to permeate a tissue barrier such as the intestinal mucosal epithelium, a drug must have some water solubility as well as some lipid solubility. If the drug has a very high lipid solubility and very low water solubility, then it will be blocked by the water barrier or hydrophilic barrier, even though its extremely high lipid/water partition coefficient would otherwise enable it to cross the membrane itself very readily. Sometimes, this is referred to as the "cut-off" phenomenon of drug absorption. The point at which the "cut-off" occurs will vary with the cytologic features of the membrane involved. For the colon and gastric mucosa, in which the glycocalix is not nearly as thick as in the small intestine, it does not occur until the partition coefficient is at least 1000. For human skin, it lies somewhere between 100 and 1000 (Fig. 2–10).

Do lipid-soluble drugs permeate quickly because they are attracted by the membrane? The chemical force that causes lipid-soluble drugs to move readily across membranes is termed the hydrophobic force (or bond). It is not that the membrane or the drug have any particular attraction to one another, but the force is based on the fact that water "repels" the lipid-soluble drug, thus driving it into the membrane. Since the cell membrane is extremely thin (75 Å), it becomes fully loaded in a few milliseconds. Some of the drug molecules in the membrane then spill over and go into the water on the other side of the membrane, that is, they go

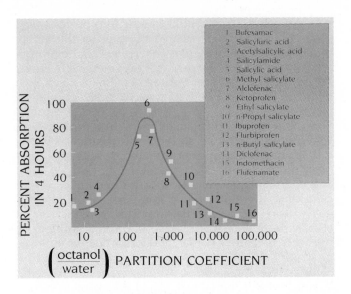

Figure 2–10 Rate of diffusion of various nonsteroidal anti-inflammatory agents across unbroken skin in humans, as a function of the octanol/water partition coefficient. Absorption "cut-off" corresponds to a coefficient of about 240.

into the cytoplasm, and the permeation process is thus completed.

Dependence of Drug Absorption on the pH and Drug Protonation

The net electrical charge on a drug molecule is very important in determining the rate of its absorption across cell membranes and tissue barriers. With respect to the net electrical charge on a drug molecule, almost all drugs fall into one of the following three categories:

- uncharged drugs,
- organic acids, or
- organic amines (tertiary and quaternary).

Consider, first of all, the case of a tertiary amine type of drug. This type of compound can exist in two forms, with or without a proton attached:

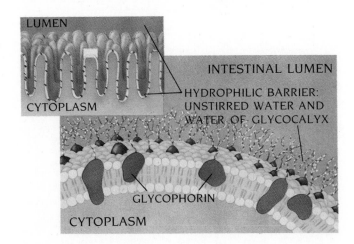

Figure 2–9 Indicating that the cell membrane surface of the small intestine is extensively covered with a rich glycocalyx (*i.e.*, surface sugar coat). The membrane glycophorins (*i.e.*, protein-sugar molecules) are heavily hydrated with water molecules "frozen" to the sugar hydroxyls. The ice-like water forms a hydrophilic barrier accounting for the limiting permeation effect described in Figure 2–8.

INTESTINE (High pH = Low cH^+)	STOMACH (Low pH = High cH^+)
$R-N{\scriptstyle\diagup R \atop \diagdown R}$ ⇌	$\underset{H}{\overset{R}{\diagup}}\overset{+}{N}{\overset{R}{\diagdown}}R$
Non-protonated	Protonated
Uncharged	Charged
High $P_{oil/water}$	Low $P_{oil/water}$
High permeability	Low permeability

In a medium containing very few free protons (*i.e.*, high pH or low cH+), such as the fluid in the lumen of the duodenum, the tertiary amine will not be protonated, and will be uncharged, as shown on the left above. This uncharged form of the tertiary amine has a high oil/water partition coefficient and readily permeates membranes.

But in a medium containing many free protons (*i.e.*, low pH or high cH+), such as the gastric juice, the tertiary amine becomes protonated, resulting in a net positive charge for the molecule. This charged form of the tertiary amine has a low oil/water partition coefficient and, therefore, has a low permeation rate.

A striking example of the importance of the role of cH+ in determining drug absorption is illustrated by the work of Travell (1940). He noted that large doses of strychnine (a tertiary amine) produced no toxic effects on the cat if the strychnine was placed in the stomach and if the stomach fluid was kept at a high cH+ of about 10^{-2} moles of protons per litre (=pH 2). However, when the contents of the stomach were made alkaline by reducing the cH+ to 10^{-8} M (=pH 8), the strychnine molecules lost their protons, became uncharged, permeated the stomach, and killed the cat.

In the case of an organic acid, the same general principles apply. The organic acid molecules can exist in two forms, as shown below:

INTESTINE (High pH = Low cH+)	STOMACH (Low pH = High cH+)
$R-COO^-$	$R-COOH$
Non-protonated	Protonated
Charged	Uncharged
Low $P_{oil/water}$	High $P_{oil/water}$
Low permeability	High permeability

The protonated organic acid, however, is a neutral molecule and thus permeates the tissues readily. Hence, organic acids such as barbiturates, acetylsalicylic acid, phenytoin, dicumarol, phenylbutazone, sulfonamides, and thyroxine have a higher absorption rate in the stomach where the cH+ is high.

It is important to point out that the form of the drug (*i.e.*, charged or uncharged) in the tablet or the vial or the ampul does not matter. Rather, we are interested in the degree of ionization of the drug in the gastrointestinal contents or other body fluid, and this depends upon the relation between the pH (*i.e.*, $-\log[H^+]$) of the fluid in question and the pK$_a$ of the drug. K$_a$ is the acidic dissociation constant, *i.e.*, the equilibrium constant for the dissociation that yields free hydrogen ions:

$$R-\overset{\overset{O}{\|}}{C}-OH \xrightleftharpoons{K_a} R-\overset{\overset{O}{\|}}{C}-O^- + H^+$$
Acidic Drugs

$$R-\overset{+}{N}H_3 \xrightleftharpoons{K_a} R-NH_2 + H^+$$
Basic Drugs

Obviously this dissociation will be affected by the cH+ in the medium in which it is occurring, as illustrated in Figure 2–11. High cH+ (low pH) will drive the equilibrium to the left, in accordance with the law of mass action. The higher the pH of the fluid, the higher is the ionization of acidic drugs and the lower that of basic drugs; the lower the pH, the lower is the ionization of acidic drugs and the higher that of basic drugs. Put in other terms, basic drugs tend to accept protons, and to give them up only when the cH+ of the surrounding fluid is very low. Therefore the K$_a$ of basic drugs is low, and the pK$_a$ (*i.e.*, $-\log K_a$) is high. Conversely, acidic drugs (by definition) give up protons readily, so that their K$_a$ values are high, or their pK$_a$ values low. The pK$_a$ of a drug can be calculated from the Henderson-Hasselbalch equation. When the pK$_a$ of a drug equals the pH of the surrounding fluid, equal numbers of ionized and unionized molecules of the drug will be present, *i.e.*, **the pK$_a$ = pH at which 50% ionization occurs**. Table 2–4 illustrates some examples of drugs of which the absorption depends on the pH of the stomach contents.

Role of Surface Area in Absorption

It should be obvious that more drug is absorbed if there is more area available for absorption. On the other hand, in certain diseases, such as Crohn's disease (regional ileitis), the surgeon may have to remove much of the inflamed intestine, thus drastically reducing the surface area available for absorption of nutrients, vitamins, and drugs.

For any substance that can penetrate the gastrointestinal epithelium in measurable amounts, the small intestine represents the greatest area for absorption. This is true whether the molecule is charged or un-

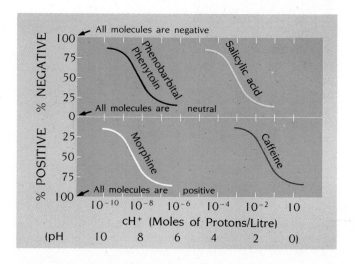

Figure 2–11 Showing that organic amines are positively charged (*i.e.*, protonated) at high concentrations of protons (*i.e.*, high cH+ or low pH). Organic acids are also protonated at high cH+, which makes them become uncharged.

TABLE 2–4 Effect of Local pH on Drug Absorption from Stomach

Drug	% Absorbed in Presence of 0.1 M HCl $cH^+ = 10^{-1}$ M	% Absorbed in Presence of NaHCO$_3$ $cH^+ = 10^{-8}$ M
Salicylic acid	60	13
Thiopental	46	34
Caffeine	24	>24
Morphine	0	16

charged. Table 2–5 illustrates that ethanol, although considerably absorbed by the stomach, is absorbed about eight times faster from the small intestine. Phenobarbital is absorbed 17 times more rapidly from the intestine than from the stomach.

The great epithelial area of the intestine provided by the many villi and microvilli is much larger than the surface of the gastric mucosa. This great intestinal area more than compensates for the decreased tendency to absorb the organic acids. It follows from this that the rate at which the stomach empties its contents into the intestine markedly affects the overall rate at which drugs reach the general circulation after oral administration. The absorption of tertiary amines, which constitute the majority of commonly used drugs, would be particularly dependent on the speed with which they arrive in the intestine. But for all drugs, it is essentially valid to say that slowing the rate at which the stomach empties will decrease the overall rate of gastrointestinal absorption, and *vice versa*. That is why so many agents are administered on an empty stomach with sufficient water to ensure their rapid passage into the intestine.

Active Transport of Drugs

Although the principal mechanism for drug permeation is passive diffusion, more and more examples of active transport of drugs across cell membranes are being discovered. Active transport is defined as a process that moves the drug against the concentration gradient, that can be blocked by inhibiting metabolism or by reducing ATP levels, and that can be saturated.

TABLE 2–5 Dominant Role of Surface Area in Drug Absorption

Drug	% Absorbed from Stomach in 1 Hour	% Absorbed from Small Intestine in 10 Minutes
Ethanol	38	64
Phenobarbital	17	52

Using these criteria, the following drugs are among those actively transported:

- penicillin by the kidney;
- 5-fluorouracil by the intestine;
- nitrogen mustard by lymphocytes;
- melphalan by lymphocytes;
- digitalis glycosides by the liver;
- pentazocine, narcotic antagonists by leukocytes (as in Fig. 2–12).

Pinocytosis and Phagocytosis of Drugs

Drugs with large molecular weights, generally over MW 900, enter cells or cross tissue barriers by means of pinocytosis or phagocytosis. Substances normally absorbed in this manner include proteins, tetanus toxin, diphtheria toxin, botulinum toxin, milk antigens, and other antigens. Drugs tightly bound to plasma proteins can also enter in the same way. These substances enter the lysosomal system (Fig. 2–13) and may be digested within the lysosome. If adequate amounts of the foreign substance enter, however, the lysosomal protective mechanism is overwhelmed, and the agent may enter the organism by exocytosis.

Facilitated Diffusion of Drugs

Diffusion along a transmembrane concentration gradient is, for some substances, facilitated by the presence of relatively selective carrier molecules in the membrane. These carrier molecules combine with the sub-

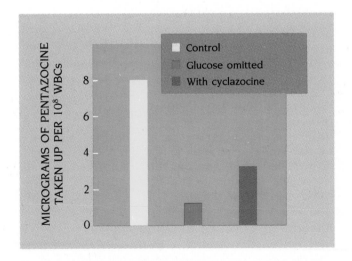

Figure 2–12 Active uptake of pentazocine by white blood cells is dependent upon an energy supply (glucose), and can be inhibited by cyclazocine, which competes for the same transport mechanism.

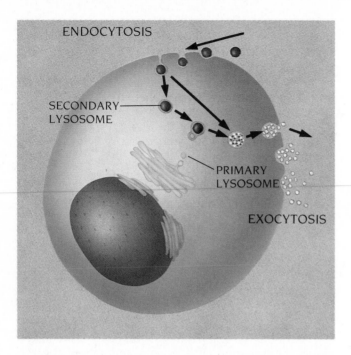

Figure 2–13 Pinocytosis or endocytosis of proteins results in a secondary lysosome, which in turn fuses with a primary lysosome. After hydrolysis within the fused vesicle, the products may be released by exocytosis.

stances in question, forming complexes that can diffuse more rapidly across the membrane than the free substances themselves, but that dissociate on the other side of the membrane to release the free substances into the cell. This is known as facilitated diffusion. Drugs that permeate by facilitated diffusion include:

- amino acids into brain (*e.g.*, L-dopa);
- adenosine-like compounds;
- antimetabolic nucleotides (used in cancer or antiviral chemotherapy).

Passive Filtration of Drugs

This is an important mechanism for drug elimination by the kidney glomerulus. Note that only the free, or unbound, drug and metabolites are available for glomerular filtration.

Adsorption of Drugs to Cytoplasm

In the same way as many drugs bind to plasma proteins, most drugs, once having entered the cell, adsorb reversibly to cell proteins and lipids. Since the concentration of cell proteins is very high, the cytoplasmic concentration of the drug can achieve a level many times higher than that in the plasma. Drug adsorption, however, is not a drug transport mechanism, but rather

a drug reservoir mechanism. As with plasma proteins, this drug reservoir serves to smooth out the time course of drug action, so that the drug is not quickly biotransformed and excreted.

Drug Passage *via* Gap Junctions

There are gap junctions between epithelial cells of the same tissue, and of endothelial cells of the same tissue, as well as mesothelial cells of the same tissue (such as smooth muscle cells). It is known that small molecules (MW < 500) can move from cell to cell through these gap junctions. It is thought that the actual channels exist within the centres of the membrane particles, as represented schematically in Figure 2–14.

TYPES OF TISSUE BARRIERS TO DRUGS

Table 2–6, at the end of this chapter, summarizes the types of tissue barriers to drug permeation.

Gastrointestinal Mucosa

The epithelial cells lining the lumen of the gastrointestinal tract are all joined to one another by occluding zonulae. These zonulae are continuous tight junctions made up of rows of membrane particles of one cell that are fused to rows of membrane particles of the adjacent cell. Thus, these zonulae completely block off the intercellular spaces, as shown in Figure 2–15.

Because these membrane particles form a continuous closed junction around the cell (somewhat similar

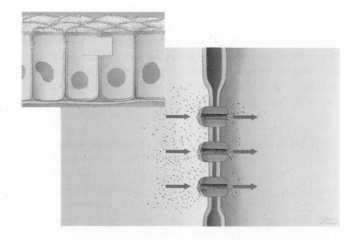

Figure 2–14 Cell-to-cell passage of drugs through gap junctions, as has been demonstrated by Loewenstein using fruit-fly salivary glands.

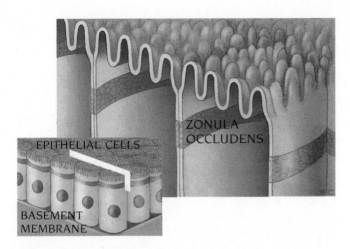

Figure 2-15 The continuous tight junctions between adjacent cells, separating the outside world from the body spaces, are composed of a "necklace" of membrane proteins.

Capillaries with Maculae

These include all capillaries in the body except those with fenestrae and those with occluding zonulae. This means, for example, that such macular capillaries are found in muscles, skin, gastrointestinal tract (and peritoneum), bone, liver, heart, *etc*. These capillaries are characterized by having macular junctions, or "spot-junctions," between the cells. This is shown in Figure 2-16. Such maculae do not form a continuous belt but only exist as a patch of membrane particles on one cell membrane fused to another set of particles on the second cell membrane. Hence, there are intercellular spaces around these maculae.

In addition to the intercellular spaces, these capillaries are rich in pinocytotic vesicles. Some of these vesicles transiently extend through the entire cytoplasm, forming a transient window (fenestra) or open channel

to a necklace of pearls), drug molecules are forced to permeate the cell membrane and go through the cell rather than go between the cells. This is why drugs must be membrane-soluble or lipid-soluble in order to permeate the gastrointestinal barrier. Large molecules, as explained previously, must be pinocytosed in order to traverse the barrier. The basement membrane, adjacent to all epithelial cells, is composed of a loose carbohydrate-protein matrix and offers no resistance to drug permeation.

Epithelial Barriers of Skin, Cornea, and Urinary Bladder

All these epithelial barriers seal the external world off by having occluding zonulae between the cells. Hence, only lipid-soluble drugs permeate readily; there is no between-the-cells permeation.

Capillary Barriers to Drugs

There are three types of capillary structures in the body:

- Capillaries with maculae.
- Fenestrated capillaries: kidney, pituitary, and exocrine glands.
- Capillaries with occluding zonulae: all capillaries in the brain except those in the choroid plexus, the median eminence, the area postrema, the pineal gland, and the pituitary gland.

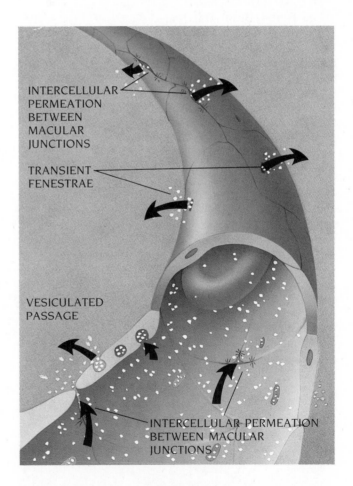

Figure 2-16 Solute and drug permeation across capillary walls occurs *via* intercellular spaces and transient windows or fenestrae.

from the capillary lumen all the way to the basement membrane. All drugs, regardless of solubility, readily pass through these transient fenestrae and the intercellular spaces. Drug molecules with MW greater than 100,000 must be pinocytosed and then transported by the vesicles moving within the cells.

Tissues with Fenestrated Capillaries

The excretory and secretory organs generally have fenestrated capillaries. Such tissues include the kidney glomeruli (Fig. 2–17), thyroid, pituitary, salivary glands, and pancreas. The fenestrae or "windows" through the cytoplasm of the cell may be covered by a few Å of non-membrane material, which essentially offers no barrier to any drug or solute existing free and unbound in the plasma. The basement membrane only holds back molecules greater than about MW 45,000.

Tissues with Occluded Capillaries:
The Blood–Brain Barrier

The only capillaries in the body that have their intercellular spaces completely occluded by occluding zonulae are the brain capillaries. As mentioned briefly earlier, all brain capillary endothelial cells are connected to one another by these occluding zonulae, which thus constitute the "blood–brain barrier" (Fig. 2–18). There are five regions of the brain, however, where

no occluding zonulae exist, and consequently these regions are relatively permeable. These regions are:

- the pituitary gland;
- the pineal body;
- the area postrema;
- the median eminence;
- the choroid plexus capillaries.

The area postrema contains the vomiting control centre, and since the capillaries there are fenestrated, the vomiting centre thus readily monitors the circulating level of foreign substances such as toxins and drugs. Hence, there is clearly a "purpose" for the area postrema to be readily exposed to substances in plasma; in addition, the rest of the brain capillaries with occluding zonulae serve the function of protecting the brain from circulating toxins, drugs, and harmful solutes.

A second important feature contributing to the blood–brain barrier is that these brain capillaries have very few vesicles; consequently, there are no transient fenestrae.

Cerebrospinal Fluid Barriers to Drugs

The cerebrospinal fluid (CSF) is a secretion formed from the epithelial cells of the choroid plexus, which are in contact with the brain ventricular spaces. These

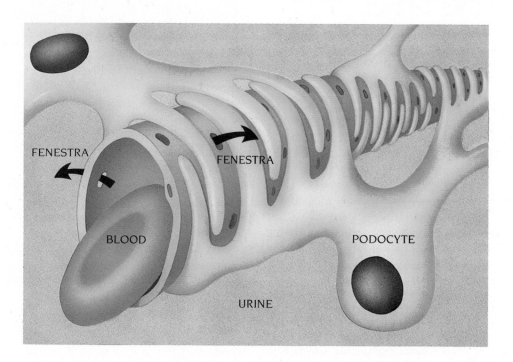

Figure 2–17 Capillaries in the kidney glomerulus are of the fenestrated type.

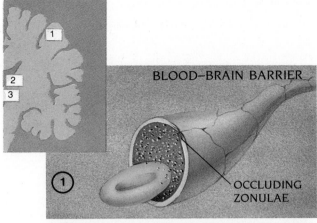

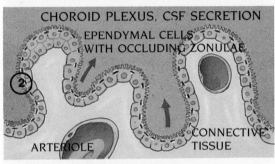

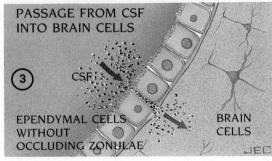

Figure 2-18   Blood-brain and CSF-brain barriers.

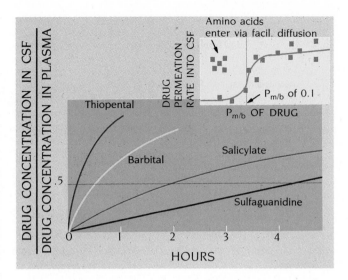

Figure 2-19 Indicating that the more lipid-soluble drugs (thiopental, *etc.*) equilibrate more readily between CSF and plasma. The inset illustrates the general relation between drug permeation rate and the membrane/buffer partition coefficient. Thus, some amino acids (*e.g.*, L-dopa) have partition coefficients below 0.1 and would not enter the brain, were it not for the fact that the brain capillaries have special facilitated diffusion mechanisms for these drugs.

epithelial cells of the choroid plexus are connected by occluding zonulae (*see* Fig. 2-18). This means that for any drug to get into the CSF from the blood, the drug should be lipid-soluble, as shown in Figure 2-19.

The CSF-brain barrier is composed of epithelial cells lining the ventricles, and these cells are not connected by occluding zonulae (*see* Fig. 2-18, bottom). Hence, the CSF-brain barrier is extremely permeable, offering unrestricted passage of drug molecules from the CSF to the brain cells. Clinically, advantage may be taken of this fact. For example, penicillin is not very lipid-soluble and, therefore, penetrates poorly from the blood into the brain. Hence, to obtain a high penicillin concentration in the brain when treating a brain infection or abscess, intrathecal injections directly into the CSF are the most effective means.

Permeation of Drugs Across the Placenta

Because there is a limited amount of maternal blood flowing into the placenta, the fastest time for drug equilibration between mother and fetus is in the order of 10-15 minutes (*see* Chapter 68). This is a useful fact, since it indicates that it is possible to anaesthetize the mother, during the final stages of labor, with a margin of safety (about 10 minutes), avoiding a serious depression of the baby's breathing. (It is also worth noting that newborn babies have a higher requirement for general anaesthesia, so that it takes more than the usual amount of general anaesthetic to depress their breathing.)

The following are half-times for equilibration of various drugs between maternal blood and fetal cord blood:

Anaesthetics	8 minutes
Secobarbital	8 minutes
Sulfadiazine	1 hour
Curare	4 hours
Penicillin	10 hours
Streptomycin	18 hours

Until proven otherwise, it is safe to assume that all drugs cross the placenta, and that all drugs enter the breast milk. Children of morphine-addicted mothers may be born with depressed respiration and pinpoint pupils. Antipsychotic drugs are transferred across the placenta, and if the mother is on rather high dosage,

TABLE 2–6 Summary of Types of Tissue Barriers to Drug Permeation

Tissue	Barrier	Permeability
Outside World: Gastrointestinal Mucosa, Skin, Cornea, Lung, Urinary Bladder	Occluding zonulae (continuous tight junctions)	Complete blockage of intercellular spaces; drugs must permeate cell membranes
Capillaries	Maculae	Open intercellular spaces
Except: Glomeruli, Excretory and Secretory Organs	Fenestrae	Free passage of MW < 45,000
Blood–Brain Barrier	Occluding zonulae	Drugs permeate membranes
CSF Barriers: Choroid Plexus Cells→CSF CSF→Brain	Occluding zonulae No barrier	Difficult passage Very easy passage
Placenta	Limited by blood flow	Slow equilibration
Peritoneum	Maculae	Free passage

the offspring may be born with extrapyramidal signs (*see* Chapter 27). Erythromycin and tetracyclines cross the placenta in appreciable amounts and also appear in the milk.

Drug Permeation Across the Peritoneum

The cells of the peritoneum and of the capillaries in the peritoneum are connected by macular ("spot") junctions. Hence, drugs and other solutes injected intraperitoneally have rapid and unrestricted access to the bloodstream (Fig. 2–20). All drugs, whether lipid-soluble or not, whether charged or uncharged, readily permeate between the cells. Large molecules, however, are pinocytosed across the peritoneum.

Drug Permeation Across the Lung

As with all epithelial barriers against the outside world, the alveolar cells are also held together by continuous occluding zonular junctions. The cells are exceedingly rich in vesicles and the cytoplasm is very thin. It may be, therefore, that there are many moments when a transient fenestra exists by the momentary fusion of a vesicle on both sides of the cell. This would account for the ready alveolar permeation of a highly water-soluble compound like nicotine (Fig. 2–21).

General anaesthetics have no difficulty crossing the lung barrier since these drugs are rather lipid-soluble.

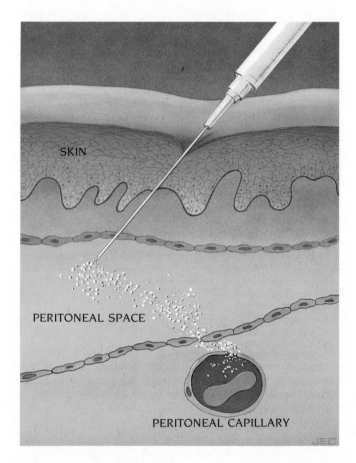

Figure 2–20 Drug movement across the peritoneum.

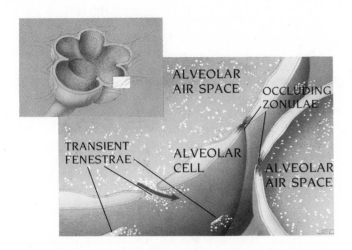

ALVEOLAR AIR SPACE

OCCLUDING ZONULAE

TRANSIENT FENESTRAE

ALVEOLAR CELL

ALVEOLAR AIR SPACE

Figure 2–21 The lung barrier.

is about 40×10^{-9} moles of protons per litre of blood).

However, not all of the morphine molecules will be protonated; some of them will be uncharged. These neutral molecules will readily permeate into all the body spaces including the stomach lumen. The cH^+ of the stomach contents, however, is about 10^{-2} M and thus, any morphine molecules which happen to diffuse across from the bloodstream into the lumen of the stomach will be instantly protonated. Once the molecules are protonated, however, they are trapped and cannot be reabsorbed.

Hence, washing out the stomach, following a morphine overdose from intravenous injection, can remove some of the morphine and prevent it from being reabsorbed by the intestine later. (Since the development of specific opiate antagonists such as naloxone [see Chapter 22], gastric lavage is seldom used in cases of morphine overdose.)

Question

A semi-conscious patient is brought to the emergency room, and a diagnosis of morphine overdosage is made. Although it is known that the morphine was self-administered by intravenous injection, the intern decides to wash out the patient's stomach. Is the intern merely confused, or "taking no chances," or does the intern have some reason for doing this procedure?

Answer

The injected morphine enters the blood and most of the morphine molecules will be protonated and charged at the pH of blood which, in terms of cH^+, is 40 nmol/L (i.e., the proton concentration in blood

SUGGESTED READING

Houston JB, Upshall DG, Bridges JW. A re-evaluation of the importance of partition coefficients in the gastrointestinal absorption of nutrients. J Pharmacol Exp Ther 1974; 189:244–254.

Leo A, Hansch C, Elkins D. Partition coefficients. Chem Rev 1971; 71:525–616.

Mattocks AM, El-Bassiouni EA. Peritoneal dialysis: a review. J Pharm Sci 1971; 60:1767–1782.

Schanker LS. Physiological transport of drugs. In: Harper NJ, Simmonds AB, eds. Advances in drug research. London: Academic Press, 1964:71–106.

Yano T, Nakagawa A, Tsuji M, Noda K. Skin permeability of various non-steroidal anti-inflammatory drugs in man. Life Sci 1986; 39:1043–1050.

Chapter 3

DRUG DISTRIBUTION

L. Endrenyi

The administration of a drug to a patient is analogous to sprinkling salt all over one's plate with the hope that enough of the salt will land on the potatoes. In fact, most of it will land on other parts of the meal. In understanding drug distribution one has to consider the pattern of "scatter" of the amount of drug in the body, as indicated schematically in Figure 3–1.

The body fluids act as solvents and carriers for the great majority of drugs, so that they reach their sites of action dissolved in the water that bathes the cells. The crudest division of the total body water is into intracellular and extracellular water, with subdivision of the extracellular water into plasma and interstitial fluid. But some parts of the extracellular water, such as the inaccessible water in bone and the slowly accessible water in tendon and cartilage, are not reached by drugs; so the distribution volumes to be discussed are not necessarily identical with the volumes truly occupied by water in the body. In short, the distribution compartments discussed here are usually physiologic rather than anatomical entities (Fig. 3–2).

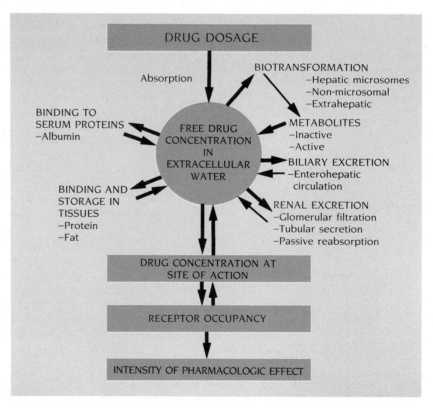

Figure 3–1 Pathways of drug disposition.

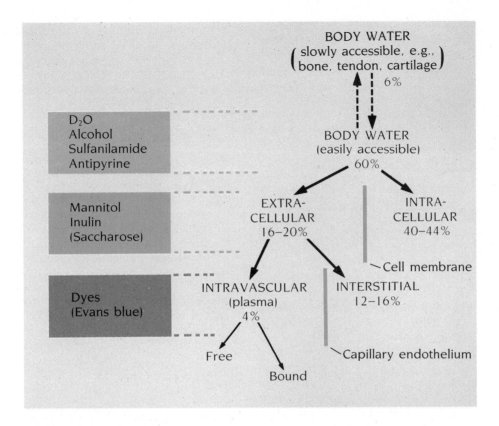

Figure 3–2 Various spaces (compartments) and volumes of distribution (approximate, as percent of total body mass, assuming average body fat). The boxes on the left show agents that typically distribute into the respective compartments. Consequently, these substances are used as indicators for the apparent volumes of these spaces.

TERMINOLOGY

Actual Volume of Distribution

This is the anatomical volume accessible to the drug. For example, a charged compound, which cannot enter cells, will have as its volume of distribution the extracellular space of about 12 litres. A nonpolar compound will spread through the total body water of about 40 litres (about 60% of the weight of a 70 kg man). Very few therapeutic drugs are confined to such a simply identified space as plasma.

Apparent Volume of Distribution

The apparent volume of distribution is a calculated value. First, recall the simple relationship between mass (amount of drug), volume, and concentration. Let them

be designated by M, V, and C respectively. Concentration is mass per unit volume, or, as a formula:

$$C = M/V.$$

Knowing any two, one can always calculate the third. For example, to calculate a volume when the mass of a drug and a concentration are given:

$$V = M/C.$$

The apparent volume of a drug's distribution can be determined by injecting the drug intravenously. If a plot of the logarithmic concentration versus time yields a straight line, extrapolation to zero time gives the theoretical initial serum concentration of the drug (C_0), assuming instantaneous distribution (Fig. 3–3).

Once an apparent volume of distribution is known for a particular drug, the amount of drug that must be given to achieve a desired concentration can be determined. It is important to realize that this approach

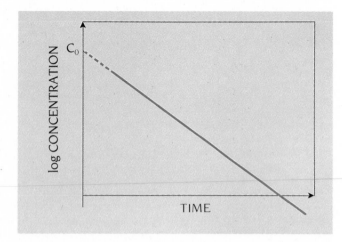

Figure 3–3   Determination of a drug's apparent volume of distribution. $V = Dose/C_0$ (*see* text).

is a mathematical convenience that works quite well in practice, but that says virtually nothing about where the drug really is in the body.

SITES OF DRUG DISTRIBUTION

Total Body Water

Ethyl alcohol is the most commonly consumed drug that equilibrates with the total body water (TBW), although the pharmacologic effects experienced are due to some molecules attaching to susceptible structures. If, for the sake of simple arithmetic, a lean young man weighing 70 kg has a total body water of 50 litres (70% of body weight), then a 15 g drink of alcohol (*i.e.*, 0.21 g/kg) would give a concentration of 15 g per 50 litres of total body water. This is the same as 30 g per 100 litres, or 0.3 g per litre. Since alcohol does not bind significantly to plasma proteins and plasma is about 93% water, one can therefore expect a concentration in plasma of 0.28 g per litre.

However, the body water in an obese elderly female is usually only about one-half of her body weight. If she also weighs 70 kg, she will have only 35 litres of body water. Therefore the same dose of 15 g of alcohol (*i.e.*, 0.21 g/kg) would produce, in her, an alcohol concentration more than 40% higher than it did in the 70 kg lean man.

Antipyrine is another drug that spreads throughout the total body water without concentrating in any one area. It is an old synthetic analgesic, and this drug as well as some of its derivatives are now often used to

determine the volume of total body water. If a known amount of the drug is injected intravenously into the subject and the plasma concentration is measured after equilibrium is reached, the total water in which the drug is now diluted can be calculated.

Extracellular Water

The cell membrane acts as a barrier, but capillary walls are permeable to all but very large molecules (*see* Chapter 2). For such substances, therefore, the plasma and interstitial fluid can be regarded as a unit called the extracellular fluid (ECF). Since many drugs act upon the cell surface, but are inert once inside the cell, drug distribution in extracellular fluid is pharmacologically very important.

Mannitol is a saccharide that is often used to measure extracellular fluid volume because it does not enter cells, is not transformed in the body, but is readily excreted through the kidney by glomerular filtration.

In a study of mannitol distribution, 50 g of the substance was administered to a 70 kg man. From repeated observations, referenced to plasma water, an extrapolated initial concentration of 4.46 g per litre of water was measured. Consequently, the apparent volume of distribution is 50/4.46 = 11.2 litres. This is 16% of the body weight, or 160 mL/kg. In a series of investigations of healthy adult males, the mannitol distribution volume averaged 160 mL/kg but ranged from 141 to 187 mL/kg. Hence the concentration of a drug which distributes in extracellular space may vary considerably from person to person, even if all other factors are equal.

Many drugs spread through extracellular fluid in less time than it takes them to penetrate cell membranes. There is, therefore, an initial transient period when their extracellular concentration is high compared to their intracellular concentration. If they are drugs that act on the cell surface, their onset of action will, therefore, be more rapid than if they are drugs whose site of action is within the cell.

Blood

Even within the blood, the distribution of a drug could be uneven. Thus, while a proportion of the drug molecules could be dissolved in water, others could be attached to various constituents of blood. These intravascular distribution processes will be considered briefly.

Intravascular Distribution

Drug concentrations are typically measured in plasma and/or serum. Unless the drug is equally partitioned between red cells (and other cells) and plasma, drug concentrations will be dependent on the protein concentration and/or the hematocrit value (the proportion, by volume, of red blood cells in the whole blood).

Since the distribution of ethanol between plasma and cells is a passive one, it follows that the ethanol content of a tissue is determined by its water content. This has important consequences for blood analysis, as cells contain less water than plasma. The average values are about 68% and 94%, respectively. Since cells occupy about half of the blood volume (hematocrit $\simeq$ 0.5), the whole blood contains about 81% water. The commonly accepted conversion factor for calculating plasma ethanol from blood ethanol is 1.16 (= 94/81), though this will obviously vary with the hematocrit value. Hence a whole blood alcohol value of 50 mg/100 mL implies a plasma ethanol concentration of about 58 mg/100 mL.

The situation becomes even more complex if variations in plasma composition are taken into account. A volume of 100 mL of human blood plasma contains 4–9 g protein, about 0.1 g sugars, and 0.4–0.6 g lipids, which, after a fatty meal, may rise to over 1 g/100 mL. Hence the normal variation in plasma water is from about 89% to about 96%.

Serum and Plasma Protein Binding

Most drugs are carried from their sites of absorption to their sites of action and elimination by the circulating blood. Some drugs are simply dissolved in serum water, but many others are partly associated with blood constituents such as albumin, globulins, lipoproteins, and erythrocytes. For the great majority of drugs binding to serum constituents, **albumin** is quantitatively the most important macromolecule and often accounts for almost the entire drug binding. For example, Evans Blue binds so strongly to plasma albumin that almost the whole dose is retained in the plasma, and so its plasma concentration provides a measure of plasma volume. Recently it has been found that some basic drugs bind extensively to α_1-acid glycoproteins.

Plasma protein binding influences the fate of drugs in the body. Only the unbound or free drug diffuses through capillary walls, reaches the site of drug action, and is subject to elimination from the body. Since drug binding to albumin is readily reversible, the albumin-drug complex serves as a circulating drug reservoir that releases more drug as free drug is biotransformed or excreted. Thus, albumin binding decreases the maximum intensity, but increases the duration, of action of many drugs.

Misleadingly small distribution volumes can be obtained for highly bound drugs when their total concentration (bound + unbound) is measured in the plasma. However, it is the free drug in the plasma water that equilibrates with the rest of the body. Consequently, the volume of distribution should be evaluated, for meaningful interpretation, from the concentration of the unbound drug.

Protein binding of drugs is dealt with specifically in the section of this chapter entitled Plasma and Serum Protein Binding of Drugs.

Body Fat

Adipose tissue is capable of storing large amounts of lipid-soluble drugs. Since blood flow to fat is relatively low per gram of tissue, a long period of time will be required for equilibrium to be achieved between the concentrations of unbound drug in plasma and in fat. In the reverse direction, drug stored in fat may require a long time to be removed completely from the body. Thus, body fat generally becomes an important site of storage after prolonged exposure to a drug or chemical. For example, the insecticide DDT is now stored in the body fat of nearly every living creature on earth. Some wild animals have died suddenly from the DDT released when their fat depots were depleted by starvation, although no physiologic damage to humans from DDT has yet been demonstrated.

Tissue Binding

If the tissue concentration of a drug is greater than its concentration in the plasma free water, tissue localization has occurred. If the binding site has a large capacity for the drug, the presence of the binding site is equivalent to an increase in the effective volume of distribution of the drug. The end result can be a marked prolongation of the life of the material in the body. One example is radioactive strontium (^{90}Sr). It is so strongly bound to sites in the bone (which is poorly perfused anyway) that it has a tissue half-life of years.

Enterohepatic Circulation as a "Reservoir"

The enterohepatic circulation is another potential site of drug distribution. Phenolphthalein, for example, which is used as a popular laxative as well as a pH indicator, is rapidly extracted from the body by the liver, excreted *via* the biliary system into the gut, and then reabsorbed across the intestinal mucosa back into the blood. This circulating quantity of phenolphthalein thus acts as a reservoir, and the drug stays in the body for days instead of the few hours it would persist without this recirculation. Unfortunately, little is known of the relative rates of biliary excretion and the intestinal reabsorption of drugs, so that the general significance of the enterohepatic cycle as a drug reservoir is difficult to assess. Enterohepatic circulation is discussed in greater detail in Chapter 7.

PLASMA AND SERUM PROTEIN BINDING OF DRUGS

Affinity and Extent of Binding

The interaction of a drug with a binding site on a protein may be considered a reversible reaction obeying the law of mass action. The total measured drug concentration in serum is the sum of the unbound and bound drug concentrations (Fig. 3–4).

In the reaction shown in Figure 3–4, k_1 and k_2 are the rate constants of the forward and reverse reactions. The processes of association and dissociation of drug and protein have half-times of a few milliseconds.

The affinity between a drug and its binding sites is accurately expressed as the concentration ratio of the drug in the bound form to the product of unbound drug and albumin,

$$\frac{[\text{drug-protein complex}]}{[\text{unbound drug}] \times [\text{protein}]} = \frac{k_1}{k_2}.$$

The ratio of the rate constants k_1/k_2 is the association constant (K_a), and its units are litres per mole. The greater the affinity between drug and protein, the larger is the K_a. Affinity is more frequently expressed in terms of the dissociation constant (K_d). This is equal to k_2/k_1, its units are moles per litre, and it is inversely proportional to the affinity. The dissociation constant equals the free drug concentration at which 50% of the corresponding binding site on the protein is saturated. The relation between association and dissociation constants is exemplified by warfarin (an anti-

coagulant) binding to albumin with a K_a of 1.6×10^5 litres per mole and a K_d of 6.2×10^{-6} moles per litre.

At high drug concentrations, almost all binding sites on the protein molecule become saturated. When a drug binds with different affinities at several sites in the protein molecule, several different equilibria are involved. Each of these is characterized by a dissociation constant. The maximum possible binding capacity of a protein for a given drug equals the molar albumin concentration multiplied by the number of binding sites for that drug.

Figure 3–5 illustrates the effect of three variables on the free concentration of a hypothetical drug, with a molecular weight of 300, binding to a single site on albumin. At any given drug and albumin concentrations, the unbound fraction of the total drug rises with decreasing affinity (increasing dissociation constant, K_d). With any given affinity, the fraction of free drug

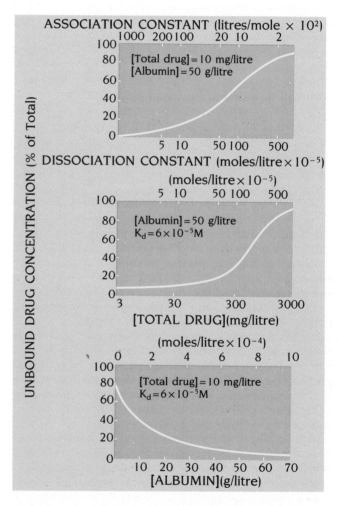

Figure 3–5 Effect on drug-albumin interaction of changes in dissociation constant (*top*), total drug concentration (*middle*), and albumin concentration (*bottom*). Albumin has a molecular weight of 69,000; the assumed molecular weight of the drug is 300 (*see* text).

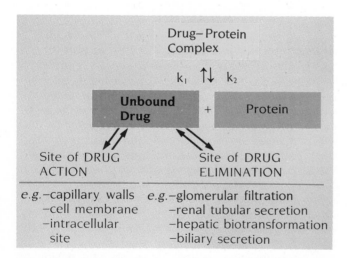

Figure 3–4 Effect of protein binding on drug disposition. Only the unbound drug is available for eliciting an effect and for elimination (*see* text).

rises when total drug concentration increases or when albumin concentration falls. If the albumin concentration is in the normal range, the binding affinity very high (K_d very low), and total drug concentration low, practically all the drug in the serum will be present in the bound complex. Even with very high binding affinity and normal albumin concentration, the binding capacity becomes saturated at high drug concentrations, and the free drug concentration rises rapidly.

A glance at the two lower panels of Figure 3–5 makes it obvious that statements about ''the percentage of drug bound to serum albumin'' are of limited value unless the concentrations of drug and albumin are stated. When they are specified, the statement applies only to that situation. However, at low drug concentrations, the fractions of the drug being either bound or unbound approach their limiting values. These are important characterizations of the extent of binding of the drug to plasma proteins under the given conditions.

The considerable differences among normal persons in the affinity of some drugs to serum proteins are not yet fully understood. Age appears to be one factor, with binding relatively low in neonates and perhaps in old age. Appreciable sex differences in affinity have not been found. Temperature, pH, and ionic strength can affect the number of binding sites and their dissociation constants *in vitro*, and even clinically encountered variations in these factors may be of importance. Competition for plasma protein binding sites by endogenous substances, such as free fatty acids or other organic acids, may play a role.

Protein Binding and Drug Distribution

Whatever the route of administration, almost all therapeutic agents reach their sites of action *via* the systemic circulation. Only the fraction of the drug in the bloodstream that is not bound to plasma proteins can leave the circulation, distribute throughout the body, and reach the sites of action. Because the equilibrium between bound and free drug is constantly maintained, some of the drug-albumin complex continuously dissociates as free drug diffuses out of the blood through capillary membranes.

Once drug distribution is complete, the drug concentration throughout the extracellular water will equal that in serum water (the free drug concentration in serum). It is not the total, but rather the free, drug concentration in the serum that correlates with the concentration at the sites of action. It does not usually matter in this regard whether the active site is at the cell surface or lies intracellularly.

For highly albumin-bound drugs the free drug concentration in serum is only a small percentage of the total concentration. For example, during phenylbutazone therapy the total serum concentration of the drug is nearly 100 times greater than its concentration in serum water and extracellular fluid. With such exten-

sive binding most of the drug in the body may at all times be sequestered in the drug-albumin complex. The exact fraction that is free depends on the specific drug, on drug and albumin concentrations, and on any interference with binding by endogenous substances or other drugs.

An important example of the difference between total drug concentrations in the serum and in extravascular fluids is furnished by cerebrospinal fluid (CSF). Indeed, it was the much lower concentration of some sulfonamides in CSF than in serum that called attention to the reversible binding of drugs by serum proteins. The concentration in CSF of a sulfonamide that is 75% bound to serum albumin is only one-fourth of the total drug concentration in serum. Similarly, the CSF concentration of phenytoin in subjects with normal serum albumin averages only 9–10% of the total serum level when the latter is in the therapeutic range. What is true for CSF also applies to other less easily obtained extravascular fluids. However, to the extent that they contain albumin, their total drug concentration will be higher than that of CSF.

Protein Binding and Drug Elimination

The kidneys remove drugs and their metabolites from the blood by glomerular filtration and/or by tubular secretion. The first process is dependent on diffusion; the second often involves an active transport mechanism. Drug binding to albumin has entirely different effects on glomerular and tubular excretion of drugs.

Since albumin does not appreciably pass through the glomerular membrane, neither does drug bound to albumin. In contrast, the free fraction of almost all drugs is readily filtered. The concentration of drugs in the glomerular filtrate generally equals the free drug concentration in the serum. Thus, as blood passes through the glomeruli, no change occurs in the free drug concentration except for the minute effect of the increased albumin concentration. It follows that there is little stimulus for dissociation of the drug-albumin complex, and that **albumin-bound drug is completely protected from glomerular filtration**. In addition, binding to serum albumin can further decrease the rate of elimination of drugs that are lipid-soluble at the pH of tubular fluid by increasing their back-diffusion from the glomerular filtrate into blood.

The rate of glomerular filtration of a drug is therefore inversely proportional to the extent of drug-albumin binding. Glomerular elimination of highly albumin-bound drugs can be extremely slow. This is most important for drugs that are also slowly biotransformed and poorly excreted by the renal tubules. For example, diazoxide is primarily eliminated by glomerular filtration, but its 90% binding to serum albumin renders this route relatively ineffective and results in a half-life of approximately 30 hours. The slow elimination from the body of some benzothiadiazide diuretics and anti-infective sulfonamides partly reflects their extensive binding to albumin and their consequent slow filtration by the glomeruli.

Unlike their crucial effect on glomerular filtration, drug-albumin interactions have variable effects on, and do not generally limit, the **tubular elimination** of drugs. Only free drug can be secreted by the tubules but, in contrast to glomerular filtration, active tubular secretion decreases the serum concentration of free drug. Because equilibrium between free and bound drug is always maintained, a decrease in the concentration of free drug immediately causes dissociation of some of the drug-albumin complex and thus makes further drug available for tubular elimination. The interaction between drug and albumin is so rapidly reversible that any free drug withdrawn from serum by active transport mechanisms is instantly replaced. As a consequence, even drugs such as certain penicillins, which are more than 90% bound to serum albumin at therapeutic concentrations, can be removed almost completely from the blood by tubular secretory mechanisms during a single passage through the kidneys. (*See also* Chapter 7, *Drug Clearance by Specific Organs*.)

The importance of binding to albumin is generally analogous in the case of **hepatic biotransformation** of drugs. Drugs that enter the hepatocyte by simple diffusion are protected from biotransformation to the extent of their binding to serum albumin. The greater the extent of albumin binding, the less drug will be available at any one time at the site of hepatic biotransformation. Coumarin anticoagulants, phenylbutazone, and certain sulfonamides are among the drugs whose rate of hepatic transformation has been shown to be inversely proportional to the extent of their albumin binding.

On the other hand, hepatic biotransformation or biliary secretion of drugs that are concentrated in the hepatic cell by active transport mechanisms may not be limited by albumin binding. Free drug molecules withdrawn from the serum are immediately replaced by more free drug resulting from the dissociation of the drug-albumin complex. This explains the rapid hepatic clearance of some highly albumin-bound substances such as sulfobromophthalein and propranolol. The quantitative aspects of hepatic metabolism are considered in greater detail in Chapter 7.

Protein Binding and Pharmacologic Actions

Only free drug can reach the sites of action and exert a pharmacologic effect. (*See* Table 3–1 for a partial list of drugs that are extensively bound in human serum.) Binding to serum albumin decreases the maximum intensity of action of a single dose of most drugs because it lowers the peak drug concentration achieved at the sites of action. The magnitude of this decrease is directly proportional to the fraction of the administered dose bound to serum albumin. If 50% of the dose becomes albumin-bound, the achievement of

TABLE 3–1 Approximate Drug Binding in Human Serum (Examples of Highly Bound Drugs)

Drug	% Free
Anticoagulants	
Warfarin	0.5
Bishydroxycoumarin	1
Anti-infectives	
Cloxacillin	5
Oxacillin	8
Doxycycline	10
Sulfadimethoxine	10
Sulfisoxazole	10
Anti-inflammatory	
Fenoprofen	1
Phenylbutazone	3
Oxyphenbutazone	3
Indomethacin	10
Salicylic acid	18
Cardiovascular	
Digitoxin	5
Propranolol	7
Diazoxide	9
Quinidine	15
Central Nervous System	
Diazepam	1
Amitriptyline	4
Imipramine	4
Chlorpromazine	4
Chlordiazepoxide	5
Nortriptyline	6
Desipramine	8
Phenytoin	10
Thiopental	15
Diuretics and Uricosurics	
Probenecid	1
Furosemide	3
Chlorothiazide	5
Sulfinpyrazone	5
Ethacrynic acid	10
Oral Hypoglycemics	
Tolbutamide	5
Tolazamide	6
Chlorpropamide	13
Miscellaneous	
Clofibrate	5

any given peak intensity of pharmacologic action will require approximately twice the dose that would be necessary in the absence of any albumin binding.

Because albumin binding slows the elimination of drugs that are removed from the serum by glomerular filtration or by diffusion to the hepatic biotransformation site, it increases the duration of action of a single dose of such drugs. The duration of action of some diuretics, sulfonamides, and tetracyclines tends to correlate with the degree of their albumin binding. However, this may be due only in part to a direct effect of albumin binding. The amount of such drugs bound to tissue proteins may correlate with the extent of their binding to albumin, and a high degree of such **binding at inactive tissue sites** would also lead to a long half-life and duration of action. In contrast to its effect on ''passively'' eliminated drugs, binding to plasma proteins can facilitate the transport of drugs within the blood stream. Therefore, it may shorten the duration of action of drugs that are actively transported into renal tubular or hepatic cells, just as it can decrease their half-lives.

Clinically Important Aspects of Serum Protein Binding

- Free drug concentration is lower, pharmacologic activity is decreased, drug clearance by glomerular filtration and passive processes is decreased in the presence of protein binding.
- One highly protein-bound drug may be competitively displaced by another highly bound drug. The pharmacologic effect of the displaced drug will increase, as will its renal clearance.
- Endogenous substances with high affinity for protein binding sites (*e.g.*, bilirubin, fatty acids) may displace a highly bound drug.
- In disease states characterized by hypoalbuminemia (*e.g.*, hepatic failure or nephrotic syndrome) the concentration of free, active drug will be higher at any given total concentration.

DRUG DISTRIBUTION FOLLOWING RAPID INTRAVENOUS INJECTION

We have considered so far the general conditions for the distribution of a drug some time after its administration (say, at steady state). We shall discuss now a few aspects of the time course for approaching these conditions.

The concentration in blood following a rapid intravenous injection is at its highest value initially and then falls ultimately to zero (Fig. 3–6). The time course of drug concentrations can be divided into three stages: initial dilution; distribution; elimination (renal and metabolic). (*See also* Chapter 5.)

Initial Dilution

A drug rapidly injected in a small volume will, for approximately 2 or 3 circulation times, be distributed in a ''bolus'' within the circulation (Fig. 3–7). If the drug has a very narrow margin of safety and acts on receptors within sensitive, vital systems, serious toxicity

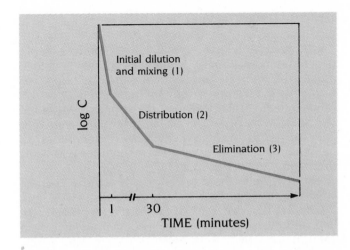

Figure 3–6 Time course of drug concentration following intravenous drug injection.

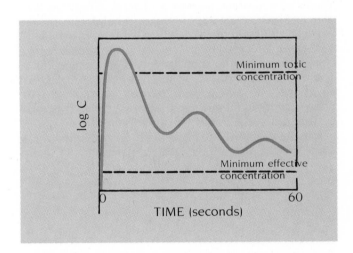

Figure 3–7 Mixing of drug after rapid intravenous injection (*i.e.*, dissipation of bolus effect over 2 to 3 circulation times).

may occur if injection is too rapid (*e.g.*, isoproterenol and cardiac arrhythmias; thiopental and medullary respiratory depression). Generally, drugs should be injected slowly (*e.g.*, diazepam at less than 2.5 mg/minute). Conversely, for a few drugs with a high threshold, rapid bolus injection may be required to initiate a response. A special situation applies if the rapidly injected drug is highly protein-bound. During the ''bolus'' phase, drug binding sites on albumin will be saturated, and free drug concentration will be much greater relative to total drug concentration than after complete redistribution has occurred. Highly protein-bound drugs for which such kinetics may be important include quinidine, phenytoin, and diazoxide.

Redistribution

If the drug is injected rapidly, the total dose is distributed in only a small volume of blood. As this blood moves through the lungs and out into the body, the drug mixes in a larger volume of blood, and when this blood reaches the capillaries the drug is distributed by diffusion to the extracellular space (and into cells if it can cross the cell membrane). After about 15 minutes or so, the drug will be distributed fairly evenly throughout the extracellular fluid space. (There are exceptions to this—the drug will not reach the average concentration in poorly perfused tissues.)

Different tissues in the body have different blood perfusion rates. Hence, drugs reach equilibrium quickly in some tissues and more slowly in others. The effects on different groups of tissues can be demonstrated by inhaling a constant concentration of halothane (a general anaesthetic) and measuring the time course for the amount taken up by the whole body. As shown in Figure 3–8, the uptake of halothane by the whole body generally can be subdivided into 3 phases: a rapid-uptake phase, which reflects the uptake of halothane by the **vessel-rich group of tissues** (VRG) (brain, heart, liver); a phase of intermediate rates, which shows the uptake of halothane by the **muscle group of tissues** (MG); and a very slow phase, which reflects the uptake of halothane into **vessel-poor tissues** (VPG) (fat, skin, bone, ligaments, teeth, hair). After stopping exposure to the drug, the rates for the declining amount of halothane demonstrate again the presence of the three tissue groups. (Note the qualitative similarity of the pic-

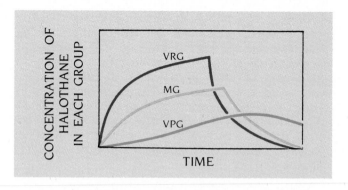

Figure 3–9 Concentration of halothane in various tissue groups while undergoing redistribution (*cf.* Fig. 3–8).

ture shown in Fig. 3–8 to that illustrated in Fig. 3–6.)

It is the organs and tissues of the vessel-rich group that are the targets in most drug therapy, and the rate of onset of drug action in them can be very fast. But it is important to remember that blood flow can be different in various parts of the same organ. For example, the blood flow to the gray matter of the brain is almost four times as great as to the white matter, so that drugs that are able to cross the blood–brain barrier reach the cortex and brain nuclei much faster than the rest of the brain.

The muscle group fills up with drug more slowly than the vessel-rich group, and because of relative concentrations, drugs that have initially gone to vessel-rich organs can be carried out of them again by the circulation and moved on to relocate in the muscle and fat groups of tissues. This **redistribution** is shown in Figure 3–9 in a general way, and various specific examples are given in succeeding chapters.

SUGGESTED READING

Goldstein A, Aronow L, Kalman SM. Principles of drug action, 2nd ed. New York: Wiley Medical Publishers, 1974.

Jusko WJ, Gretch M. Plasma and tissue protein binding of drugs in pharmacokinetics. Drug Metab Rev 1976; 5:43.

Koch-Weser J, Sellers EM. Importance of drug-protein binding. N Engl J Med 1976; 294:311–316 (part 1), 526–531 (part 2).

Levy R, Shand D, eds. Clinical implications of drug-protein binding. Clin Pharmacokinet 1984; 9(Suppl 1):1–104.

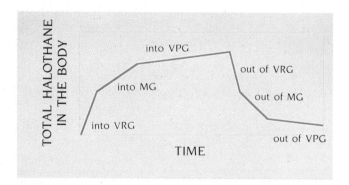

Figure 3–8 Uptake and distribution of a drug (halothane) in various tissue groups depending on blood perfusion rates (*see* text). VRG = vessel-rich group; MG = muscle group; VPG = vessel-poor group.

Chapter 4

DRUG BIOTRANSFORMATION

H. Kalant

Metabolism is a term that refers to the total fate of a drug in the body, including its absorption, distribution, biotransformation, and excretion. For example, one talks of ''electrolyte metabolism'' even though electrolytes can not undergo any biotransformation.

Biotransformation means chemical transformation of the drug within the living organism, usually by enzyme-catalysed reactions. Many authors use the terms ''drug metabolism'' and ''drug biotransformation'' interchangeably, but this is incorrect.

BIOLOGIC SIGNIFICANCE

All foods that animals eat contain traces of potentially toxic materials. This is particularly true of plants, which lack excretory mechanisms and therefore accumulate metabolic excretory products in vacuoles inside their cells. Many plants produce alkaloids that are potent pharmacologic agents. Those toxic or pharmacologically active materials in the food that have high lipid solubility are the most likely to be absorbed from the gastrointestinal tract and the least likely to be excreted. They may be filtered in the glomerulus and reabsorbed in the renal tubule, or excreted in the bile and reabsorbed in the intestine, remaining in the body for long periods of time.

In fish and most other aquatic animals (except whales and other marine mammals), this is not a serious problem because there is a large gill surface or other dialysing surface across which toxic materials, even quite lipid-soluble ones, can diffuse into the infinitely large volume of water surrounding them. When terrestrial animals evolved, however, conservation of water was essential for survival, and the kidney developed mechanisms for producing a highly concentrated urine.

This would favor reabsorption of lipid-soluble materials in the tubule by increasing the concentration gradient from lumen to blood. As a protective measure, therefore, amphibians and higher animals developed an enzymatic mechanism in the liver that intercepts foreign compounds (''xenobiotics'') that have entered the portal venous blood from the gut and transforms them into more polar, and hence more water-soluble, substances. This permits more efficient excretion in a limited volume of water in the urine or bile.

Although the liver is the major site of biotransformation of drugs and toxins, for the reasons given above, it is by no means the only site. Many other organs and tissues have enzymes that normally biotransform endogenous substrates, but that are also capable of acting on exogenous substances if these have enough molecular resemblance to the natural substrates.

In general, highly water-soluble materials, such as the obligatory ion tetramethylammonium, do not require biotransformation and there are no enzymes that transform them. In contrast, very nonpolar drugs may undergo a great many different reactions, all yielding products more polar than the precursors.

These biotransformation reactions may have three different **consequences with respect to pharmacologic activity:**

Activation. An inactive precursor is converted into a pharmacologically active drug, *e.g.*, the insecticide parathion (inactive) is converted by the liver into paraoxon (active, toxic); L-dopa (inactive) is converted to dopamine (active) in the basal ganglia.

Maintenance of activity. An active substance is converted into another active substance, which may be more strongly or less strongly active, *e.g.*,
- strongly active metabolites: diazepam is converted to oxazepam; trimethadione is converted to dimethadione;
- weakly active metabolites: acetophenetidin is converted to *p*-hydroxyacetanilid.

Inactivation. An active drug is converted to inactive products, *e.g.*, pentobarbital is converted to hydroxypentobarbital and glucosylpentobarbital.

The only feature common to all these reactions is that the products of biotransformation are more water-soluble than the original drugs.

METHODS OF STUDY

In vivo, drug **metabolism** is often studied by measuring the rate of disappearance of the drug from the plasma. However, this does not necessarily differentiate distribution from biotransformation or excretion of the drug. This is somewhat easier if a semilogarithmic plot yields a biphasic disappearance curve, with a rapid phase of distribution from plasma into tissues, and a slow phase of elimination (Fig. 4–1). However, even this slow phase can not differentiate biotransformation from excretion, unless the biotransformation products can be isolated, identified, and measured in the plasma, urine, and/or bile. If the rate of disappearance of the original drug equals the rate of appearance of the transformation product(s), this is good evidence that the slow phase of disappearance corresponds to the rate of biotransformation. Even then, however, this approach gives no information about the organ(s) or process(es) involved, the mechanism, or the rate-controlling factors.

In vitro, many different preparations can be used to explore these latter questions. Perfused organs, tissue slices, isolated cell suspensions, homogenates, sub-cellular fractions (cytosol, nuclei, mitochondria, and microsomes) and purified enzyme systems all permit direct study of the reaction mechanism(s) and identification of the products. However, the *in vitro* reaction is usually studied under optimal conditions of substrate and cofactor concentrations, *etc.*, and the rate of reaction may be quite different from that seen under the influence of rate-limiting factors *in vivo*.

Drug biotransformation may occur in almost any tissue in the body, and at almost any subcellular site within those tissues. However, the most important organ of biotransformation is the liver, and the most important site within the liver cell is the endoplasmic reticulum, which is broken up into "microsomes" when the liver is homogenized.

It has been shown that drug biotransforming activity predominates in the smooth endoplasmic reticulum (SER) rather than the rough (RER). For example, the demethylation of ethylmorphine occurs at a rate of 2.8 nmol per mg of protein per minute in SER as compared to 0.65 nmol per mg per minute in RER. Ribosomes are not essential to drug oxidation. Treatment of hepatic microsomes with ribonuclease, which stops protein synthesis, does not alter microsomal enzyme activity. Treatment with deoxycholic acid, which destroys lipoid membranes, usually destroys enzyme activity. Rupture of the ER vesicles osmotically or ultrasonically does not solubilize the enzymes. It thus appears that the enzymes are membrane-bound, and probably arranged in a specific sequence, as are the constituents of the mitochondrial electron transport chain.

DRUG BIOTRANSFORMATION REACTIONS

Drug biotransformation reactions, especially those in the liver, are commonly grouped into two phases. Phase 1, involving microsomal enzymes, includes oxidation, reduction, or hydrolysis reactions that may activate the drugs, inactivate them, or leave activity unchanged. However, the products of phase 1 reactions may contain hydroxyl, amine, carboxyl, or other groups capable of undergoing further reactions, referred to as phase 2 reactions. These may be catalysed by microsomal, mitochondrial, or cytoplasmic enzymes, or combinations of these, and usually consist of conjugation or other synthetic reactions. Phase 2 reactions almost always result in inactivation of the drug, if it has not already been inactivated by phase 1 reactions. Some drugs originally contain reactive groups capable of being conjugated, and may therefore undergo phase 2 reactions immediately, without having to go through phase 1. These relationships are summarized in Figure 4–2.

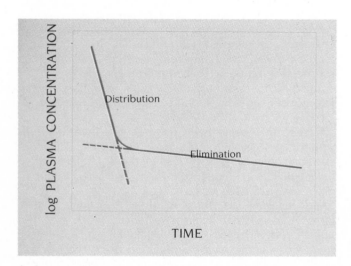

Figure 4–1 Biphasic drug disappearance curve.

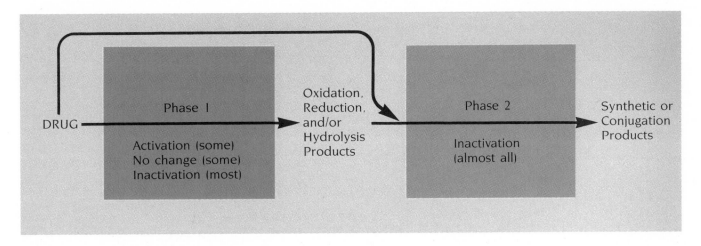

Figure 4–2 Sequence and biologic effects of phase 1 and phase 2 drug biotransformation reactions.

Phase 1 Reactions

Nature of the Reaction

The basic process in phase 1 reactions in liver microsomes is hydroxylation, catalysed by the cytochrome P-450 system, and requiring NADPH, NADH and molecular oxygen. This is not a "new" system developed exclusively in the liver of terrestrial animals, but a specialization of a system that already existed in liver and other tissues, serving other functions. In adrenal mitochondria it carries out hydroxylation as a step in the biosynthesis of corticosteroids. In the liver it hydroxylates fatty acids before they are desaturated, and even in the liver of the rainbow trout this system has some ability to hydroxylate the insecticide permethrin, to yield a hydroxy metabolite that undergoes subsequent conjugation. The hydroxylating system is also found in the kidney, where its original function is not wholly clear.

In essence, this is an oxidative pathway analogous to the mitochondrial electron transport chain, with the central role played by a heme protein (cytochrome P-450) catalysing the redox change. The H and electrons come from NADPH and NADH, and the H acceptor is O_2 (forming water), but because one atom of the O_2 also goes to a drug substrate (RH_2) the enzyme is called a "mixed-function oxidase". The term "monooxygenase" has also been used. The term "polysubstrate monooxygenase (trivial name, P-450)" was adopted recently as the official nomenclature for this biotransformation system to emphasize the great variety of substrates on which it acts. The overall balance of the reaction is as follows:

$$NADH + NADPH + RH_2 + O_2 \rightarrow$$
$$NADP^+ + NAD^+ + RHOH + H_2O.$$

The final oxidase in this system is called cytochrome P-450 because it can bind to CO, yielding a product with an absorption spectrum showing an intense maximum at, or close to, 450 nm. When bound to CO it can not catalyse the oxidative reaction; the CO-binding is used only as an analytical method for measuring the cytochrome. Cyto-P-450 is a constituent part of the liver SER, making up 20% of the total protein of the SER.

Actual Reaction Pathway

This is much more complex than is shown in the overall balance equation given above. The pathway is outlined in Figure 4–3, in which the circled numbers correspond to the major steps described below:

1. The drug (RH_2) combines with cytochrome P-450 in the oxidized state (*i.e.*, with Fe^{3+} in the cytochrome) to form a drug-cyto-P-450$_{ox}$ complex.
2. NADPH is formed from NADP by the action of glucose-6-phosphate dehydrogenase and other NADP-linked oxidative enzymes.
3. The drug-cyto-P-450$_{ox}$ complex is converted to drug-cyto-P-450$_{red}$ (*i.e.*, its iron is reduced to the Fe^{2+} state) by the flavoprotein NADPH-cyto-P-450 reductase, which transfers a proton and two electrons from the NADPH. This transfer requires the presence of a heat-stable phospholipid fraction of the SER membrane, together with Mg^{2+} and O_2, but the exact role of this phospholipid is not known.
4. The drug-cyto-P-450$_{red}$ complex is oxidized by a molecule of O_2 and undergoes an internal rearrangement.
5. NADH-cytochrome b_5 reductase (also a flavoprotein) transfers a second proton and two electrons from NADH to cytochrome b_5.
6. In the absence of NADH and NADH-cyto-b_5 reduc-

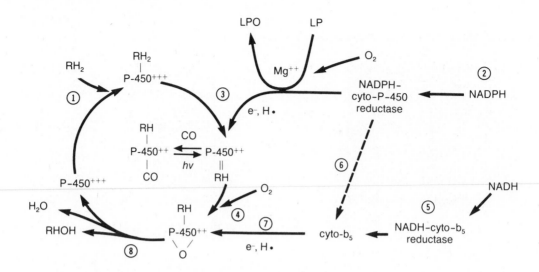

Figure 4–3 Scheme of mixed-function oxidase reaction pathway catalysed by cytochrome P-450 system in hepatic smooth endoplasmic reticulum. *See* text for the meaning of numbers in circles.

tase, the cytochrome b_5 can be reduced by NADPH-cyto-P-450 reductase, which transfers the additional proton and electrons from NADPH. However, this is less efficient than the NADH pathway, and probably occurs only *in vitro*, because there is never likely to be a deficiency of NADH in the living organism.

7. Cytochrome b_5 has a redox potential such that it readily passes the reducing equivalents on to the oxygenated drug-cyto-P-450 complex, which undergoes further internal rearrangement.

8. The complex finally splits into a molecule of hydroxylated drug (RHOH), a molecule of water, and the free oxidized cytochrome P-450, which is then ready to recommence the cycle with a new molecule of drug.

Cytochrome P-450 Multiplicity; Drug Binding Spectra

The term cyto-P-450 is really applied to a **group** of heme proteins that differ slightly from each other, with respect to their molecular weights, CO-binding spectra, electrophoretic and immunologic properties, and catalytic activities toward different drugs. The best-known variant is P-448 (CO-absorption spectrum has a maximum at 448 nm instead of 450 nm), but at least two dozen distinct "P-450" species have been purified and characterized from mammalian tissues (*see also* Chapter 12).

These were originally separated by polyacrylamide gel electrophoresis and other physical techniques. However, rapid progress has occurred as a result of the development of **monoclonal antibodies** (MAbs) that are specific for single epitopes (*i.e.*, antigenic sequences in the molecule). An individual cytochrome in the P-450

family may have several different epitopes and thus react with several different MAbs. Conversely, the same epitope may occur in several different cytochromes, all of which will react with the same MAb. However, each cytochrome has a unique "fingerprint" combination of epitopes, so that typing with a variety of MAbs provides a distinctive spectrum for each variety of cytochrome P-450. In addition, the MAbs can be used in affinity chromatography to isolate the pure cytochrome varieties. Combination with an MAb usually abolishes the enzymatic activity of the cyto-P-450; therefore, by studying the biotransformation of a variety of different drugs by a cyto-P-450 mixture treated with different MAb combinations, it is possible to identify which isozyme is mainly responsible for the biotransformation of a particular drug. This has been done in human liver tissue specimens. The various cytochromes have preferential affinities for different drugs, but as a group they also show a major difference in binding properties with two broad groups of substrates that are designated as Type I and Type II binders.

As shown in Figure 4–3, the drug or other substrate binds to oxidized cytochrome P-450, forming a drug-cyto-P-450$_{ox}$ complex. This is then reduced by electrons transferred from the NADPH-cytochrome P-450 reductase, yielding a drug-cyto-P-450$_{red}$. Binding of the drug to the oxidized cytochrome P-450 has a marked effect on its ability to undergo this initial reduction.

Substrates may be divided into two groups according to the type of spectral change produced when they are added to liver microsomes, *i.e.*, when they are bound to cytochrome P-450. This is illustrated by the "difference spectra" shown in Figure 4–4.

These are not absorption spectra; rather, they are the **difference** between the absorption spectrum of the cytochrome alone, and that of the cytochrome-drug complex, and the two difference curves are the basis

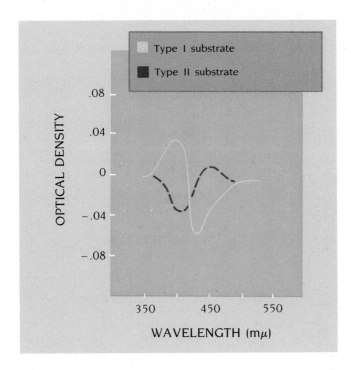

Figure 4–4 Difference spectra resulting from binding of substrates to cytochrome P-450.

for classifying drugs as either Type I or Type II. Type I substrates range from simple alkanes to complex heterocyclic chemicals including tertiary amines. Most of the common drugs are Type I substrates; examples include pentobarbital, aminopyrine, meprobamate, tolbutamide, and warfarin. Type II compounds are generally pyridine derivatives and primary aromatic amines (aniline is the best example), including some drugs and many polycyclic hydrocarbons, some of which are procarcinogens. Type I substrates facilitate the reduction of cytochrome P-450 by the NADPH-cyto-P-450 reductase. Type II substrates have the opposite effect, *i.e.*, they retard the reduction of cytochrome P-450, and are thus poor substrates for hepatic microsomal drug biotransforming enzymes. Moreover, they may even be potent inhibitors (*e.g.*, DPEA or dichlorophenylphenoxyethylamine) of the hydroxylation of Type I substrates, by tying up the cytochrome P-450 in a slowly reducible complex.

Rate-Limiting Factors

Since there are a number of essential factors and critical steps in the whole reaction sequence, different steps may limit the overall reaction rate *in vivo* and *in vitro*:

1. Hepatic circulation may be limiting under some circumstances, if it is reduced enough to impair delivery of drug and of O_2 to the liver. Similarly, severe lung disease and consequent reduction of arterial

PO_2 might impair drug hydroxylation in the liver.
2. There appear to be between 5 and 20 molecules of cytochrome P-450 to each molecule of NADPH-cyto-P-450 reductase, depending on the methods used to measure them. Therefore the reductase is more likely to be rate-limiting than the cytochrome P-450 itself.
3. The rate of NADPH and NADH production is normally ample to supply this reaction sequence. However, it is possible that prolonged fasting, with depletion of hepatic glycogen and other substrates, might reduce the availability of the reduced nucleotides.
4. As noted in the preceding section, the drug-cyto-P-450$_{ox}$ complex is more rapidly reducible when the drug is a Type I binder than when it is a Type II binder. This step may therefore become rate-limiting in the hydroxylation of a Type I drug if a Type II substrate is present at the same time.

Reaction Products

The phase 1 reaction catalysed by the cytochrome P-450 system is referred to as a drug hydroxylation reaction. Yet there is a wide range of products formed from the many drug substrates of this system, and only some of them are hydroxy derivatives. How does this come about? The answer appears to be that the initial product in every case is a hydroxy derivative, but some of these are unstable and promptly break down into the recognized end products. This process is illustrated in Figure 4–5.

Aromatic hydroxylation (*see* Fig. 4–5) proceeds by first attaching an oxygen atom to two neighboring carbons of the aromatic ring. The resulting "arene oxide," an epoxide, is an unstable radical that sometimes during its brief life can combine covalently with cell constituents such as nucleic acids or proteins, causing such problems as hepatic necrosis (*see* Chapter 62) or cancer. This may account for the carcinogenic properties of benzpyrene and other chemically inert hydrocarbons (*see* Chapter 63, *Carcinogenesis and Mutagenesis*).

Another example of an oxidative reaction is oxidative deamination (*see* Fig. 4–5). Many weak bases that have an amino group are biotransformed in this way. The amino group is removed and the compound simultaneously converted into an aldehyde, which may then be further oxidized to an acid. Oxidative deaminations occur not only in microsomes, but also in mitochondria and in plasma; these are discussed under phase 2 reactions.

Removal of methyl, ethyl, or alkyl groups of longer chain length is carried out by dealkylation reactions (*see* Fig. 4–5). An alkyl group may be removed from nitrogen, oxygen, or sulfur. This is a route of metabolic degradation of many analgesic and hypnotic drugs. Methyl groups are most readily removed, whereas the removal of ethyl groups is always slow, and longer alkyl chains can rarely be detached. The degree to which dealkylation enhances water-solubility depends on the nature of the compound undergoing dealkylation.

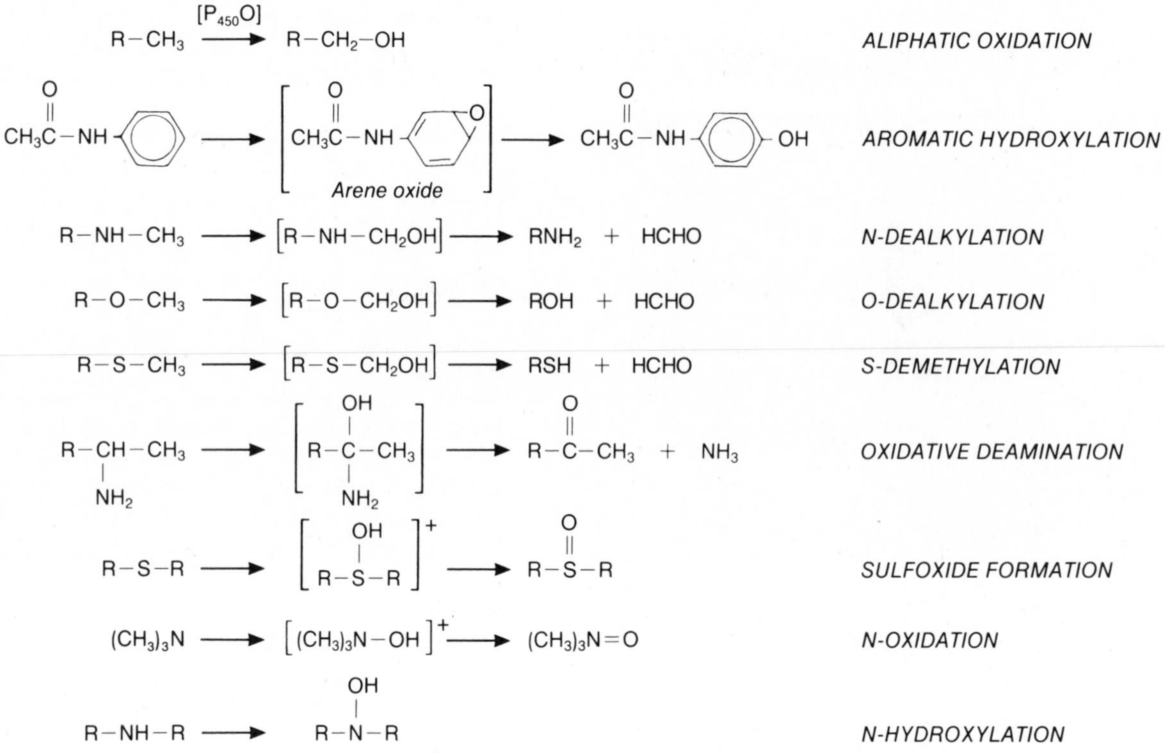

R−CH₃ $\xrightarrow{[P_{450}O]}$ R−CH₂−OH   *ALIPHATIC OXIDATION*

$CH_3\overset{O}{\overset{\|}{C}}-NH-\bigcirc \longrightarrow \left[CH_3\overset{O}{\overset{\|}{C}}-NH-\bigcirc O \right] \longrightarrow CH_3\overset{O}{\overset{\|}{C}}-NH-\bigcirc-OH$ *AROMATIC HYDROXYLATION*

Arene oxide

R−NH−CH₃ ⟶ [R−NH−CH₂OH] ⟶ RNH₂ + HCHO   *N-DEALKYLATION*

R−O−CH₃ ⟶ [R−O−CH₂OH] ⟶ ROH + HCHO   *O-DEALKYLATION*

R−S−CH₃ ⟶ [R−S−CH₂OH] ⟶ RSH + HCHO   *S-DEMETHYLATION*

$\underset{NH_2}{R-\overset{}{C}H-CH_3} \longrightarrow \left[\underset{NH_2}{R-\overset{OH}{\underset{|}{C}}-CH_3} \right] \longrightarrow R-\overset{O}{\overset{\|}{C}}-CH_3 + NH_3$ *OXIDATIVE DEAMINATION*

$R-S-R \longrightarrow \left[R-\overset{OH}{\underset{|}{S}}-R \right]^+ \longrightarrow R-\overset{O}{\overset{\|}{S}}-R$ *SULFOXIDE FORMATION*

$(CH_3)_3N \longrightarrow \left[(CH_3)_3N-OH \right]^+ \longrightarrow (CH_3)_3N=O$ *N-OXIDATION*

$R-NH-R \longrightarrow R-\overset{OH}{\underset{|}{N}}-R$ *N-HYDROXYLATION*

Figure 4–5   Drug biotransformation reactions catalysed by cytochrome P-450 system, and their relation to hydroxylation.

Cytochrome P-450-Catalysed Reduction Reactions

Under anaerobic conditions, the same P-450 system can function as a reductase, particularly with substrates that already contain a reducible oxygen. This is illustrated by the reduction of the nitro group in chloramphenicol (Fig. 4–6). The steps in the process are illustrated in the reaction scheme in Figure 4–7. There are three major differences to be noted between this type of cytochrome P-450 reaction and the aerobic hydroxylation reaction: (1) the drug binds **after** reduction of the cyto-P-450, rather than before, (2) two additional H₂ equivalents are required, and (3) the overall reaction yields **two** reduced drug metabolites rather than one. This reductase activity is, in an evolutionary sense, probably as old as the cyto-P-450 system itself: the housefly shows an NADPH-dependent nitroreductase activity that can reduce the insecticide parathion to aminoparathion:

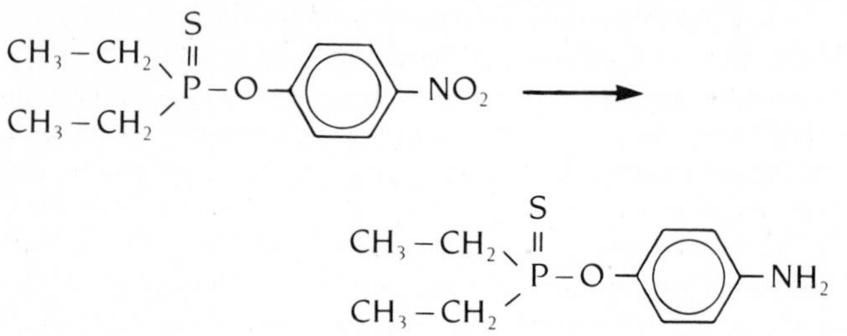

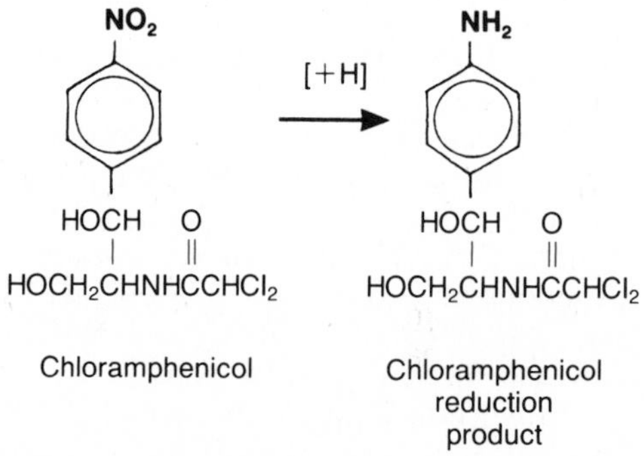

Figure 4–6   Microsomal reduction of chloramphenicol.

Induction

Many enzymes, sometimes called "adaptive enzymes," are able to increase in amount and activity in response to certain substances known as inducers. An inducer may actively stimulate synthesis of an enzyme, or it may bind to, and inactivate, a repressor molecule that inhibits the synthesis. In many cases, an inducer is also a substrate for the enzyme it induces, but some substrates are not good inducers and some inducers are not substrates.

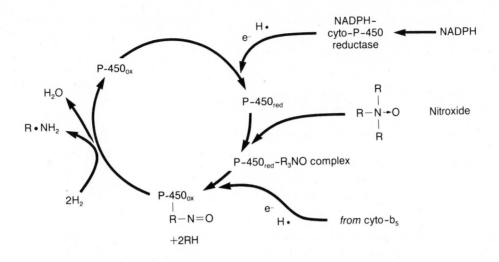

Figure 4–7 Anaerobic reduction of a nitroxide by cytochrome P-450 system.

The liver microsomal cytochrome P-450 system is readily induced by many drugs and other exogenous compounds. When this happens, there is a large increase in the amount of smooth endoplasmic reticulum visible by electron microscopy, and large increases occur in the amounts of all chemical components of the system, including the cytochromes, the cytochrome reductases, and the lipoproteins of the membranes.

A number of **drugs** are known to be efficient enzyme-inducing agents. Pentobarbital stimulates formation of the enzyme that causes its own hydroxylation, so that tolerance develops (*see* Chapter 26). However, as noted above, ability to induce enzyme formation is not confined to compounds that are substrates of these enzymes. For example, phenobarbital is only slightly biotransformed in man, yet it increases the metabolism of aminopyrine, griseofulvin, dicumarol, phenytoin, hydrocortisone, and many other drugs. The drug must have a long enough half-life, *i.e.*, it must remain in the body long enough, to act as an effective inducer. Therefore a substrate that is biotransformed and eliminated rapidly is not likely to be a good inducer unless it is given by continuous infusion or in very frequent doses. Other drugs, including phenylbutazone, glutethimide and phenytoin, have been shown to induce microsomal enzyme formation in man. Animal experiments have shown that some of the strongest inducers are polycyclic hydrocarbon insecticides such as DDT and chlordane.

Induction of the liver microsomal system results in relatively selective increase of one or another cyto-P-450 isozyme, depending on which inducer is acting. This relative specificity has been confirmed by the use of monoclonal antibodies. In general, Type I binding drugs tend to induce different patterns of cyto-P-450

increase than Type II binders do. The pattern of induced activity can also vary with the dose of inducer used. For example, low doses of clotrimazole (an antifungal agent; *see* Chapter 54) induce a 48 kd protein and increase the *p*-nitroanisole demethylase and aniline hydroxylase activities, whereas high doses of clotrimazole induce a 51 kd protein with erythromycin demethylase and ethylmorphine demethylase activities. Such findings illustrate the complexity of the cytochrome P-450 system.

Hydrocarbons in **tobacco smoke** are very strong inducers of the microsomal drug-metabolizing system. Several studies have shown that smokers have more rapid biotransformation of many drugs (shorter plasma half-life) than nonsmokers do. Inducibility decreases with age: this effect of smoking is seen in the young and middle-aged, but not in the elderly. Among the many drugs affected are antipyrine, d-propoxyphene, diazepam, chlordiazepoxide, phenobarbital, and chlorpromazine. The shortening of half-lives is proportional to the amount of smoking, and results in reduced efficacy of standard clinical doses of these drugs. If the patients stop smoking, the drug half-lives return toward normal over a period of weeks or months.

Alcohol appears to act as a nonspecific inducer of SER production in the liver, increasing the protein, cyto-P-450, and all other constituents of the cyto-P-450 system. It also alters the lipid composition of the SER membrane. Chronic ingestion of alcohol leads to moderately increased hydroxylation of both Type I and Type II ligands, and increased oxidation of alcohols and various organic solvents. It is not a strong inducer like phenobarbital, producing only a one- to two-fold increase in enzyme activity versus a twenty- to forty-fold increase by phenobarbital. The mechanism is not entirely clear. One hypothesis is that the alcohol effect is due as much to activation of existing enzyme (by altering the lipid matrix of the SER membrane) as to true induction. The other view, based on recent evidence obtained by the use of monoclonal antibodies, is that there really is induction of a distinct cyto-P-450$_{alc}$ with a rather low substrate specificity (*see* Chapter 25).

Numerous **environmental contaminants**, such as polycyclic aromatic hydrocarbons and chlorinated hydrocarbons, are good inducers. For example, polychlorinated biphenyls (PCBs) have been found as inducers in the livers of deep-sea fish, as a result of oceanic contamination from land-based sources. Several years ago it was reported that laboratory rats suddenly showed a large increase in drug biotransforming ability of the liver when the type of wood shavings used as bedding in their cages was changed. The new shavings contained a volatile aromatic constituent that the rats inhaled, and that acted as an inducer.

Diet is a factor, both in experimental animals and in humans. A high-protein diet usually increases drug biotransformation capacity, and a low-protein diet reduces it. This has been shown to have a substantial influence on the rate of biotransformation of such varied drugs as theophylline, antipyrine, testosterone, and estradiol. Charcoal broiling of beef has been reported to produce a potent inducer, which may be important in converting inactive substances into carcinogens. Certain indole compounds found in Brussels sprouts are also active inducers.

Phase 2 Reactions

As noted earlier, the hydroxylation products produced by phase 1 biotransformation reactions are often capable of undergoing further reactions (phase 2) that usually inactivate the drugs if they are not already inactive, and that make them even more water-soluble. Some of these further reactions are catalysed by cytoplasmic enzymes, and some by microsomal enzymes, acting separately or in combination.

Combination Reactions (Cytoplasmic + Microsomal)

One of the most important of these is **glucuronic acid conjugation**. Free glucuronic acid will not couple with drugs, but uridine diphosphoglucuronic acid (UDPGA) is able to combine with drugs in the presence of a transferring enzyme. Like cyto-P-450, glucuronyl transferase is actually a family of isozymes with differing substrate specificities, *i.e.*, that can transfer glucuronic acid from UDPGA to different acceptor molecules. The reaction involves two essential components: (1) synthesis of UDPGA, which is carried out by cytoplasmic enzymes, and (2) the glucuronyl transferase activity in the microsomes. These steps are illustrated schematically in Figure 4–8.

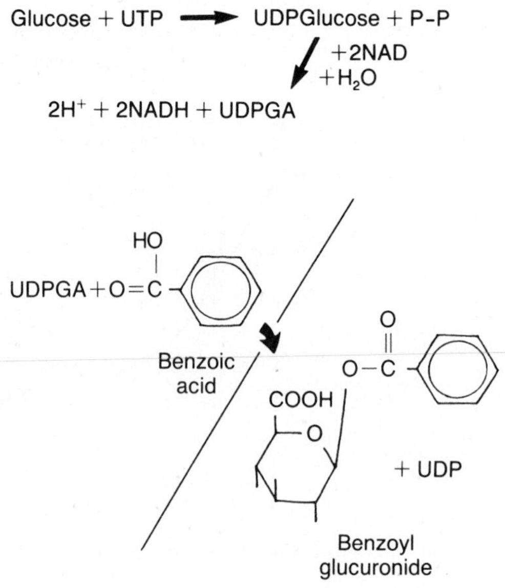

Figure 4–8 Reaction sequence for glucuronic acid conjugation of benzoic acid.

The acceptor (drug) molecule may be among other things a weak acid or base, a phenol, or an alcohol. Since the donor is derived from glucose, it is usually readily available. However, certain genetic defects may cause a transferase to be absent. Also, premature infants have a decreased capacity for glucuronide conjugation of drugs. In some premature infants this has been a contributing factor to poisoning by the antibiotic chloramphenicol. In contrast, inducers of the cyto-P-450 system also tend to induce the glucuronyl transferase activity of the hepatic SER.

Glutathione conjugation, which may lead to various products including mercapturic acids, is another combination reaction that can involve up to five different steps (Fig. 4–9). Glutathione is a tripeptide (gamma-glutamyl-cysteinyl-glycine) that plays an extremely important role in protecting hepatocytes, erythrocytes, and other cells against toxic injury (*see* Chapters 62 and 63). The glutathione is activated by a kinase in the cytoplasm. Enzyme activity in both the cytoplasm and microsomes then conjugates the drug substrate (e.g., an arene oxide, *see* Fig. 4–5) with the cysteine portion of the glutathione (*see* Fig. 4–9). The glutamate and glycine portions are then split off by gamma-glutamyl transpeptidase and cysteinyl glycinase respectively, and the free cysteine-drug conjugate is finally acetylated by a cytoplasmic acetyltransferase to form a mercapturic acid, which is excreted.

Cytoplasmic Reactions

A soluble **sulfotransferase** catalyses a sulfate conjugation, which yields "ethereal sulfates" of various aro-

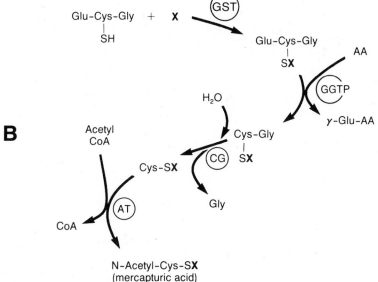

Figure 4–9 Role of glutathione in detoxification reactions. (*A*) Structural formula of glutathione (γ Glu-Cys-Gly). (*B*) Pathway of mercapturic acid formation. X is an electrophilic drug metabolite or epoxide reacting with glutathione. Enzymes catalysing the successive steps are: glutathione-S-transferase (GST); gamma-glutamyl transpeptidase (GGTP); cysteinyl glycinase (CG); acetyltransferase (AT).

matic and aliphatic hydroxyl compounds, such as phenol, chloramphenicol, and androgens and estrogens. Sulfatation is also a multistage reaction (Fig. 4–10) that actually involves several enzymes, but all are located in the cytoplasmic compartment.

Acylation reactions (*e.g.*, acetylation) are carried out by acyl transferases, with acyl-CoA as the donor, as shown in Figure 4–11A. In contrast to conjugation with glucuronide and sulfate, acetylation does not convert drugs into acids. The most prominent drugs to be acetylated are some sulfonamides, isoniazid, dapsone, hydralazine, salicylazopyrine, and phenelzine.

Glycine or glutamine conjugation is essentially the same reaction, also involving CoA and an acyl or aryl transferase, but the carboxylic acid is regarded as the substrate, and the amine (glycine) is considered to be the conjugator, as shown in Figure 4–11B.

Other Phase 2 Reactions

Additional phase 2 reactions can be carried out by mitochondrial, lysosomal, or microsomal enzymes, and by enzymes of uncertain localization. It is more convenient to consider these by type than by compartmental location.

Hydrolysis can be effected by many different physiologically important enzymes which may act in phase 1 or phase 2 reactions (*e.g.*, proteases). The best known hydrolytic enzymes are cholinesterases including acetylcholinesterase, which catalyses the breakdown of acetylcholine. There are, however, in addition microsomal esterases and others that have been less well characterized. Drugs such as procaine and meperidine are examples of esters whose activity is destroyed by

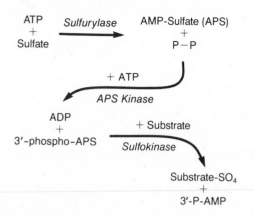

Figure 4–10   Reaction sequence in the phase 2 sulfate conjugation reaction.

hydrolysis to an alcohol and an acid. Amides such as procainamide are hydrolysed at a much lower rate.

There are three important groups of drugs that are esters that can be readily hydrolysed: (1) some local anaesthetics, (2) various analgesics, and (3) esters of choline. The choline esters are of special interest. Since choline and all of its esters are quaternary ammonium compounds, they are strongly ionized and highly water-soluble. Hence the enzymes that hydrolyse them, the cholinesterases, must have extracellular locations. One of these, the acetylcholinesterase, is located on membrane surfaces wherever acetylcholine is exerting its transmitter action. Hydrolysis of acetylcholine and termination of its action are, therefore, closely related processes. The choline ester that has the widest clinical use is the muscle relaxant succinylcholine. In humans this is destroyed by cholinesterase in plasma, so that its metabolic degradation is also an extracellular

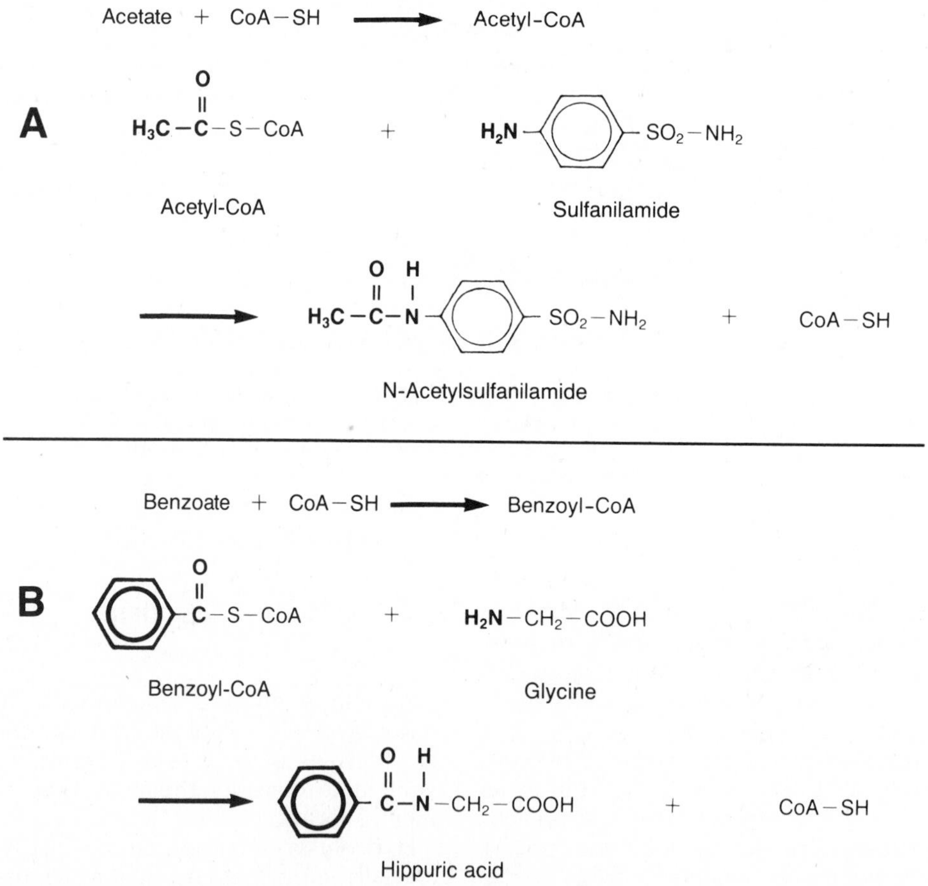

Acetate + CoA—SH ⟶ Acetyl-CoA

A

$$H_3C-\overset{\overset{\displaystyle O}{\|}}{C}-S-CoA \quad + \quad H_2N-\bigcirc-SO_2-NH_2$$

Acetyl-CoA   Sulfanilamide

$$\longrightarrow \quad H_3C-\overset{\overset{\displaystyle O}{\|}}{C}-\overset{\overset{\displaystyle H}{|}}{N}-\bigcirc-SO_2-NH_2 \quad + \quad CoA-SH$$

N-Acetylsulfanilamide

Benzoate + CoA—SH ⟶ Benzoyl-CoA

B

$$\bigcirc-\overset{\overset{\displaystyle O}{\|}}{C}-S-CoA \quad + \quad H_2N-CH_2-COOH$$

Benzoyl-CoA   Glycine

$$\longrightarrow \quad \bigcirc-\overset{\overset{\displaystyle O}{\|}}{C}-\overset{\overset{\displaystyle H}{|}}{N}-CH_2-COOH \quad + \quad CoA-SH$$

Hippuric acid

Figure 4–11   CoA-dependent peptide bond synthesis in phase 2 drug biotransformations. (A) Acetylation of an exogenous amide by endogenous acetate. (B) Conjugation of an endogenous amino acid with exogenous benzoic acid.

4. Drug Biotransformation

process. There are rare genetic variants of plasma cholinesterase which fail to hydrolyse the drug in the human body (*see* Chapter 12). The plasma cholinesterase also hydrolyses procaine and similar local anaesthetics (Fig. 4–12).

Oxidases of various types are found in the cytoplasm (*e.g.*, alcohol dehydrogenase) and in the mitochondria (*e.g.*, aldehyde dehydrogenase, monoamine oxidase). The monoamine oxidase in mitochondria is especially capable of deaminating adrenaline* and other sympathomimetic amines. Inhibitors of monoamine oxidase were the first antidepressant drugs. The aminooxidase of plasma is known as diaminooxidase and catalyses in particular the biotransformation of histamine. These are not ordinarily regarded as phase 2 reactions, but they can function as such in special cases. For example, the oral hypoglycemic agent tolbutamide, and the minor tranquilizer meprobamate, are converted to monohydroxy derivatives by the cytochrome P-450 system (phase 1). The hydroxy derivatives are then oxidized to aldehydes by alcohol dehydrogenase + NAD, functioning as a phase 2 system.

Biologic Importance of Phase 2 Reactions

Conjugation reactions are, for numerous drugs, the most important detoxication steps. This is illustrated by the much higher toxicity of phenol, paracetamol, and benzoic acid in the cat, which has a genetic deficiency of the glucuronyl transferase system, than in the rat or rabbit, which have a very active glucuronidation system. In humans, the glutathione conjugation system is the rate-limiting factor in the detoxication of the ac-

* epinephrine

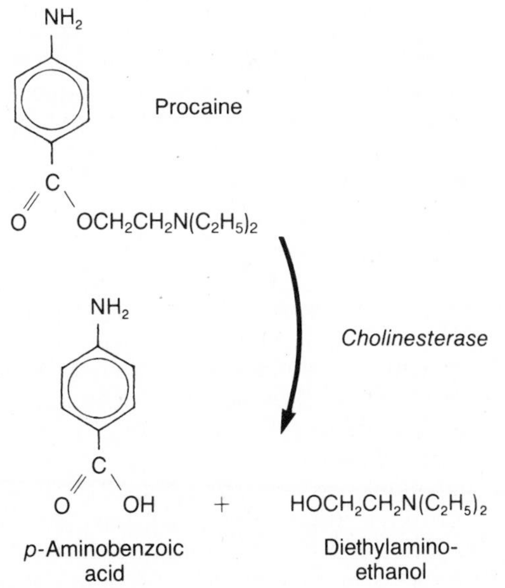

Figure 4–12 Nonmicrosomal hydrolysis (restricted to esters and amides).

tive metabolites of paracetamol, bromobenzene, and various other agents capable of covalent binding to cell constituents. A deficiency of the glutathione conjugation system renders the person susceptible to liver cell necrosis caused by these drugs (*see* Chapter 62, *Drugs and the Liver*).

The biologic importance of phase 2 reactions is very well illustrated by two serious drug-induced conditions seen in newborn infants. The cyto-P-450 activity in the fetal liver has a V_{max} less than 5% of that in the adult, and it is still low at birth, but increases rapidly in the postnatal period. However, the glucuronyl transferase activity remains low for several weeks after birth, so that drug conjugation reactions are inadequate. This results in susceptibility to a condition known as **kernicterus**. At birth, there is a massive breakdown of fetal-type hemoglobin (physiologic jaundice of the newborn), but the resulting bile pigment can not be excreted because it can not be converted to glucuronic acid conjugates. Therefore it is carried in circulation, bound to plasma albumin. If the infant receives a drug that competes for the binding sites, the bile pigment is displaced and precipitates in certain brain nuclei ("Kern" = nucleus; "icterus" = jaundice) where it causes serious or fatal damage. Drugs capable of causing kernicterus are of many different pharmacologic types. Examples include sulfonamides and various antibiotics, analgesic-antipyretic agents, nonsteroidal anti-inflammatory drugs, diuretics, anticonvulsants, barbiturates, benzodiazepines, and X-ray contrast media.

The second problem is that the low capacity and high K_m of both the cyto-P-450 and glucuronic acid conjugation systems in the newborn result in a marked increase in the toxicity of the antibiotic chloramphenicol. This drug can be life-saving in infants with serious *Haemophilus influenzae* infections (*see* Chapter 55), but the margin of safety is small because of the inadequacy of both major biotransformation reactions responsible for detoxication of chloramphenicol. Excessive plasma levels of the unconjugated drug cause a shock-like state with failure of peripheral circulation. The combination of pallor and cyanosis of the skin in this state gave rise to the name **gray baby syndrome**.

In adults, a genetically determined inadequacy of the acetylation system is responsible for many of the toxic reactions to isoniazid (antituberculosis agent), sulfonamides, and phenelzine (antidepressant).

Despite what has been said above, there are a few instances in which even phase 2 reaction products remain pharmacologically active, or are even more active than their precursors. Morphine-6-glucuronide has a longer-lasting analgesic effect than morphine itself. The N-acetyl derivative of the β-adrenoceptor blocker acebutolol still has β-blocking activity. It is not clear, in these and other instances, whether the conjugated derivatives are active directly or act as storage and transport forms that are split by glucuronidases or esterases to re-form the original drug. Some evidence for this latter possibility is provided by examples of renal toxicity caused by deconjugation reactions in the tubular epithelium. The compound trifluoro-chloroethene is detoxified by the glutathione conjugation reaction to yield a cysteine conjugate as the final product. This is excreted in the urine, but a β-lyase in the renal tubule splits the conjugate to yield a free radical, which acts as an alkylating agent to produce local damage:

$$F_2C=CFCl \xrightarrow{\text{Glutathione conjugation}} Cys-S-CF_2-CFClH$$

$$\xrightarrow{\beta\text{-lyase}} \text{Pyruvate} + NH_3 + \cdot S-CF_2-CFClH$$

(Alkylating agent)

The most important role of conjugation reactions, however, is to make the derivatives more water-soluble, and often more acidic, than the original drugs. This favors their excretion in urine and bile, and has a marked effect on the plasma half-life of the drug. Many drugs undergo two or more phase 2 reactions simultaneously; since many of these reactions are saturable at rather low substrate concentrations, the spectrum of excretion products of a particular drug, and its elimination half-life at any given plasma concentration, will depend on which reaction is the rate-limiting one at that concentration. Acetylsalicylic acid (ASA, Aspirin®) illustrates this well. It has a longer half-life at high plasma levels than at low levels, because the more rapid conjugation reaction is saturated at high levels, and a slower reaction becomes the rate-determining one.

DRUG BIOTRANSFORMATION IN OTHER TISSUES

Many of the enzymes that carry out drug biotransformation reactions are found not only in the liver but in other organs as well. Among these are the gastrointestinal epithelium and the kidney. This activity in the intestinal epithelium may be responsible for a substantial part of the "first-pass effect" (see Chapter 2) with certain drugs, such as diazepam. However, drug biotransformation in two other sites has received special attention, viz., the lung and the plasma.

Lung

The unique position of the lungs between the venous and arterial systems, as well as the large surface area of the pulmonary vascular-alveolar tree, may alter the disposition and activity of many drugs and endogenous substances. Pulmonary macrophages or histiocytes contain substantial concentrations of microsomal cytochrome P-450, and can play a significant role in the biotransformation of some drugs and toxins, especially those that are inhaled. For example, it has been suggested that tetrahydrocannabinol in cannabis smoke can be activated to 11-hydroxy-tetrahydrocannabinol in the lung itself. Although the concentration of cyto-P-450 per gram of microsomal tissue is eight times as high in the liver as in the lung, the lung:liver ratio of microsomal hydroxylation activity can be quite high for some drugs, e.g., 1.23:1 for benzphetamine and 1.19:1 for biphenyl.

In addition, pulmonary vascular endothelium and Type II alveolar cells contain substantial amounts of enzymes involved in the biotransformation of endogenous substances. These enzymes can also act on exogenous drugs that resemble the natural substrates.

As a result, the lung can carry out a wide range of drug biotransformation reactions with different pharmacological consequences. **Activation** reactions are seen in the case of various peptides, such as the conversion of angiotensin I to angiotensin II, or of prostaglandins (see Chapter 30) which are synthesized from arachidonic acid in the lung and other tissues. **Inactivation** is illustrated by further proteolytic reactions (e.g., aminopeptidase) that degrade angiotensin II, and by the dehydrogenases that inactivate prostaglandins.

The presence of both activation and inactivation reactions in the same tissue suggests that the enzymes are primarily involved in the rapid turnover of locally acting endogenous substances. Not surprisingly, therefore, the lung has a high capacity for uptake and degradation of various neurotransmitters, including catecholamines, serotonin, and acetylcholine, and of steroids.

Drug-biotransforming enzymes in the lung are also inducible, and one question of current interest is whether hydrocarbons in tobacco smoke can induce the cytochrome P-450 reactions that convert procarcinogens into active carcinogens that cause lung cancer.

Blood

Some drugs are extensively metabolized in the plasma or blood cells, e.g., succinylcholine and procaine are hydrolysed by pseudocholinesterase; chloral hydrate is oxidized by erythrocytes; acetylsalicylic acid and heroin are deacetylated rapidly. Drugs that are biotransformed intravascularly will have very short half-lives. Their pharmacologic effect may be influenced by the rate of intravenous injection if enzyme-saturating concentrations of drug are achieved during injection (cf. saturation of serum protein binding sites).

DRUG INTERACTIONS IN BIOTRANSFORMATION PROCESSES

In view of the large numbers of drugs that share the same enzymatic mechanisms of biotransformation, it is not surprising that interactions among them are very common. In general, acute interactions tend to be inhibitory, *i.e.*, one drug competes with another for the available enzyme binding sites, and each thus inhibits the biotransformation of the other.

A number of drugs have now been identified as inhibitors of drug biotransformation enzymes both in the hepatic microsomes and at other sites. These include the following: (1) MAO inhibitors; (2) dopa decarboxylase inhibitors; (3) isoniazid; (4) para-aminosalicylic acid; (5) procarbazine; (6) neuroleptics; (7) tricyclic antidepressants; (8) allopurinol; (9) chloramphenicol; (10) bishydroxycoumarin; (11) tolbutamide; (12) SKF 525A; (13) alcohol; (14) cannabinoids; and others.

Oral administration of tetrahydrocannabinol (THC), 60–180 mg/day for 2 weeks to healthy volunteers, lengthened the half-life of antipyrine and of pentobarbital by 20–25% and retarded the oxidation of alcohol by 12%.

In contrast, chronic administration of many drugs can lead to induction of drug biotransformation enzymes, as discussed above, and thus reduce the half-life and the duration of action of many other drugs.

Alcohol affects drug biotransformation reactions in various ways. As a substrate of alcohol dehydrogenase (ADH), it competitively inhibits the biotransformation of other drugs that are also acted upon by ADH, such as chloral hydrate, or the hydroxy derivatives of tolbutamide or meprobamate. As a precursor of acetyl-CoA (formed from ethanol *via* acetaldehyde), it increases the rate of acetylation of isoniazid. By a nonspecific physicochemical effect on the lipids of the SER, it inhibits the binding of many drugs to cytochrome P-450, but when ingested chronically it induces the formation of SER.

Drug interactions can also be due to remote effects. For example, catecholamines and vasopressin, by altering splanchnic circulation, can alter delivery of drugs to the liver, and thus affect the rate of biotransformation. Hypnotics and other potential respiratory depressants may impair pulmonary gas exchange, and thus reduce O_2 delivery to the liver, where it is required for drug hydroxylation.

SOURCES OF VARIATION IN DRUG BIOTRANSFORMATION

If drug metabolism were a biologic constant, so that one could count on it being the same all the time, the clinician could afford not to worry about it. However, there are striking differences between people and also in the same person from time to time. Among the factors responsible for inter-individual and intra-individual variations in drug biotransformation are: (1) genetics, (2) age, (3) fever, (4) endocrine status, (5) liver disease, and (6) drug distribution.

Genetic factors are dealt with in Chapter 12. Important examples in this area are those of pseudocholinesterase deficiency as a determinant of succinylcholine toxicity, and acetylator phenotype as a determinant of isoniazid activity and toxicity.

The **influence of age** is most important in very young and very old patients. Examples of important differences in newborns have been given above, and further detail is provided in Chapter 68. Recent work has shown that most elderly patients also have reduced drug biotransformation activity, as indicated by long half-lives of antipyrine, digitoxin, and phenylbutazone.

Fever has been known to increase the half-life of antipyrine in most, but not all, patients. It is not clear whether the change is a direct effect of temperature elevation, or a toxic effect of the pyrogens which are responsible for the fever.

Thyroid hormones in particular may be major endocrine determinants of drug biotransformation activity. Antipyrine half-life has been shown to be prolonged in patients who are hypothyroid.

Liver disease is another potentially important factor in determining drug biotransformation activity. For example, the half-life of diazepam is prolonged three-fold in patients with cirrhosis. These changes in clearance have not always been demonstrably associated with diminished drug biotransformation capacity in the hepatocytes; in part, at least, changes are due to alterations in the architecture and blood flow of the liver.

Changes in drug distribution may also influence drug biotransformation. For example, patients in renal failure, who have quantitative and qualitative changes in plasma protein, may show altered distribution of phenytoin, so that more of the anticonvulsant is free in the circulation and is available for biotransformation. This has been shown to be associated with a shortened half-life of phenytoin in uremic patients.

SUGGESTED READING

Benowitz NL, Jones RT. Effects of delta-9-tetrahydrocannabinol on drug distribution and metabolism: antipyrine, pentobarbital and ethanol. Clin Pharmacol Ther 1977; 22:259–268.

Caldwell J. The significance of phase II (conjugation) reactions in drug disposition and toxicity. Life Sci 1979; 24: 571–578.

Conney AH. Induction of microsomal cytochrome P-450 enzymes. Life Sci 1986; 39:2493–2518.

Cooper DY, Rosenthal O, Snyder R. Wittmer C, eds. Cytochromes P-450 and b_5: structure, function and interaction. New York: Plenum Press, 1975.

Friedman FK, Park SS, Gelboin HY. The application of monoclonal antibodies for studies on cytochrome P-450. Rev Drug Metabol Drug Interact 1985; 5:159–192.

Hietanen E, Laitinen M, Hänninen O, eds. Cytochrome P-450, biochemistry, biophysics and environmental implications. Amsterdam: Elsevier Biomedical, 1982.

Jakoby WB, ed. Enzymatic basis of detoxication. Vol I and II. New York: Academic Press, 1980.

Jenner P, Testa B, eds. Concepts in drug metabolism. Parts A and B. New York: Marcel Dekker, 1980.

Vestal RE, Wood AJJ. Influence of age and smoking on drug kinetics in man. Clin Pharmacokinet 1980; 5:309–319.

Chapter 5

PHARMACOKINETICS

L. Endrenyi

RATIONALE AND BACKGROUND

Aims of Pharmacokinetics

Pharmacokinetics describes quantitatively the rates of the various steps of drug disposition. These steps include, as seen in the preceding chapters, (1) the absorption of drugs which enables them to reach the systemic circulation, (2) their distribution to various organs and tissues in the body, and (3) their elimination by biotransformation and excretion.

The rates of these processes are used for two main purposes. First, they are of great interest by themselves for pharmacologists since they characterize in some detail the fate of a drug in the body. Second, physicians use pharmacokinetic data for calculating and predicting methods, doses, and frequencies of drug administration.

Such pharmacokinetic assessments are particularly essential in the view of clinicians when, for a given drug, the doses eliciting toxic side effects are not much higher than those required for therapeutic action. Similar care must be exercised when the responses of different patients to a given dose of a drug show large variation. The variability can appear in various forms: In addition to a generally large variation between the responses of various people, with some drugs a few subjects may respond very differently from the majority, or the responses may be separated into two or more groups indicating genetically affected differences. In all these cases, a pharmacokinetic study of an individual patient is desirable for the optimal adjustment of the doses of the drug.

Relation of Dose, Serum Drug Concentration, and Effect

A particular amount (dose) of an administered drug will produce an effect according to the following sequence:

Dosage
↓
Concentration in serum water
↓
Concentration at site of action
↓
Intensity of effect

The intensity of drug action is most frequently related to the concentration of the drug at the site of action ("receptor"). Similarly, the duration of the drug effect is related to the greater or lesser persistence of its presence at this site. The concentration at the receptors changes, in turn, as the drug enters, is distributed in, and leaves various parts of the body, and as it undergoes biotransformation (metabolic degradation) reactions.

Pharmacodynamic investigations examine the intensity and the time courses of responses to drugs. Unfortunately, it is often very difficult to characterize these responses quantitatively. Therefore, we frequently assume that the intensity of pharmacologic action correlates better with the concentration of free drug in serum than with the dose, and evaluate in pharmacokinetic studies the time course of drug concentrations in the serum (and in other body fluids) following various routes of drug administration. As an important application, the efficacy of drug therapy can be improved, and toxicity decreased, by using serum drug concentrations as an aid in adjusting drug dosage.

In some situations, however, the relation between serum concentration and effect is difficult to interpret, *e.g.,* irreversibly acting drugs (phenoxybenzamine); acute, chronic, or cross tolerance (barbiturates); combinations of drugs with synergistic or antagonistic actions (barbiturate + amphetamine); active metabolites present (*e.g.,* diazepam and desmethyldiazepam).

Methodology of Pharmacokinetics

Whenever the fate of a drug in the body is described qualitatively or quantitatively, a **model** of the body is assumed. Figure 5–1 illustrates a fairly general model characterizing the fate of drugs in the body. (Note the similarity with Figures 1–1 and 3–1, which state the same concepts with slightly different emphasis.)

Hypothesizing a model should be a deliberate, conscious process, which is in fact implicitly performed even when the physician or the experimenter is not aware of this. Such a hypothesis, however, is entirely useless unless it is verified by experimental observations. To achieve this goal, the mathematical consequences of the model are derived first by considering material and rate balances. Solution of the resulting system of differential equations is difficult or occasionally impossible for even moderately complicated models and requires the use of computers. The mathematical predictions of the model must then be compared with the experimental observations: agreement suggests, but does not prove, that the assumptions involving the model have been correct.

KINETICS OF DRUG DISPOSITION PROCESSES

Elimination Following Intravenous Injection: One-Compartment Model

We shall assume first-order drug disposition. This means that the rate at any given time is proportional to the concentration at that time. Consequently, after the intravenous introduction of a drug, its concentration (C) in the plasma decreases at a rate that is proportional at all times (t) to the concentration itself. This statement is described mathematically by:

$$-dC/dt = kC$$

(**k** is the proportionality or rate constant). The solution of this differential equation is (on the assumption of an initial concentration, C_0):

$$C = C_0\, e^{-kt}$$

(here **e** is the base of the natural logarithms). The exponentially moderated decrease of the plasma concentration is shown in Figure 5–2A.

In practice a more convenient form of this equation is obtained by using logarithms to the base 10, rather than natural logarithms:

$$\log_{10}C = \log_{10}C_0 - \frac{k}{2.303} \cdot t$$

($2.303 = \log_e 10$, often written as ln 10). Thus, if we

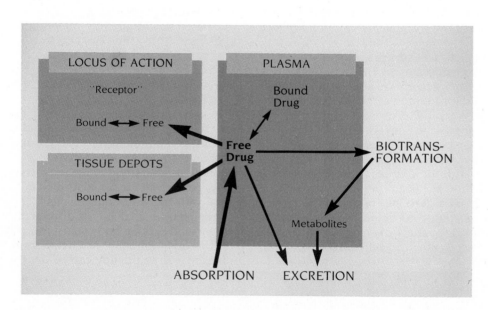

Figure 5–1   Scheme depicting the fate of drugs in the body.

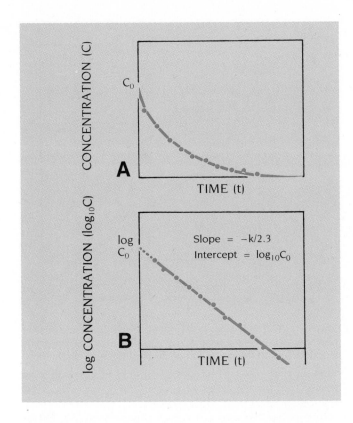

Figure 5–2 Time dependence of a drug concentration in blood after an intravenous injection. The drug concentration is plotted on a linear (*A*) and on a logarithmic (*B*) scale.

plot the logarithm of the concentrations (log C) against the times of their observation (t), we should obtain a straight line (Fig. 5–2B). The plot provides the values of k and C_0 at once, since the slope of the line equals $-k/2.303$ and the intercept is log C_0.

From the latter and from the injected dose (D_0) the **volume of distribution (V)** can be calculated:

$V = D_0/C_0$.

Also another important quantity, the **half-life of elimination (t½)** can be evaluated from the rate constant of elimination:

t½ = 0.693/k

(since 0.693 = ln 2). This is the time period during which the concentration decreases to one-half of its earlier value.
(Note: This treatment is mostly analogous with the usual analysis of first-order chemical reactions.)

Example: A 100 mg dose of a drug was injected intravenously and its concentration (in mg per litre) in the plasma was observed repeatedly. The logarithms

of the concentrations have been plotted against the times (in hours) of their observation. A straight line could be drawn through the points, which had a slope of -0.0751 and an extrapolated intercept of 1.30. Consequently,

$$k = -2.303 \times (-0.0751) = 0.173 \text{ hr}^{-1}$$

and

$$C_0 = \text{antilog } 1.30 = 10^{1.30} = 20 \text{ mg/L}.$$

From these, the half-life of elimination is

$$t½ = 0.693/0.173 = 4.0 \text{ hours},$$

and the volume of distribution

$$V = 100/20 = 5 \text{ L}.$$

The half-life of 4.0 hours means that, 4 hours after the injection of the initial 100 mg, only 50 mg is left in the plasma (and in those parts of the body in which the concentration of this drug is in constant proportion to that in the plasma). After 8 hours 25 mg is left, 12.5 mg remains after 12 hours, and so on. With a distribution volume of 5 L this is equivalent to concentrations of 20, 10, 5, and 2.5 mg/L at 0, 4, 8, and 12 hours after injection, respectively.

The Model: Such simple results are based naturally on the assumption of a very simple model. A single compartment is hypothesized which may possibly refer to the plasma and to all the tissues and receptors in which the drug is in equilibrium with the (free) drug molecules in the plasma. Thus in Figure 5–1, illustrating a model for the fate of drugs in the body, the plasma, tissue, and receptor compartments are now pooled. Absorption is omitted since the drug is introduced directly into the blood stream, and elimination from the plasma includes excretion and possible metabolic degradations. Consequently, we are left with Model 1.

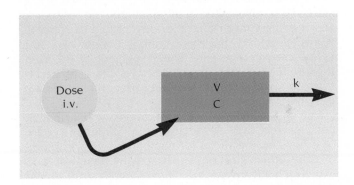

Model 1: One-compartment open model with rapid intravenous injection.

Two Compartments

Distribution and Elimination

After intravenous injection, curvature can often be detected in the early part of the semilogarithmic elimination plot. This is reasonable since, as already indicated, it takes some time for the drug to be redistributed to the extracellular space. During this period the logarithmic concentration decreases more rapidly than in the later, linear, steady-state section of the curve (Fig. 5–3). Therefore, we assume now two compartments (Model 2): a central compartment that may perhaps refer to the plasma, and a peripheral compartment including the extracellular space and, possibly, the equilibrated tissues and receptors.

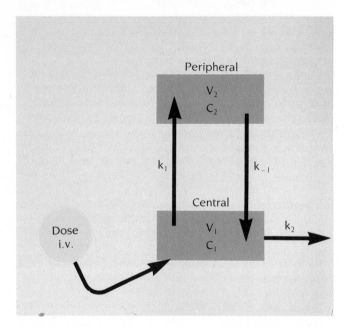

Model 2: Two-compartment open model with rapid intravenous injection.

(A two-compartment system can be described mathematically by two differential equations, the solution of which is the sum or the difference of two exponential terms, provided that the system is "open", *i.e.*, that it has an exit. The final, linear segment of the semilogarithmic elimination plot is always characterized by the term containing the smallest exponent, *i.e.*, the longest half-life.)

One of the most useful applications of pharmacokinetic models involves the prediction of the time course of drug concentrations for compartments and modes of drug administration which actually have not been experimentally investigated. For example, drug concentrations are frequently measured only in the central compartment (including usually the plasma). Still, if a drug displays two-compartmental characteristics, then it is possible to predict the time dependence of its concentration in the peripheral compartment (Fig. 5–3).

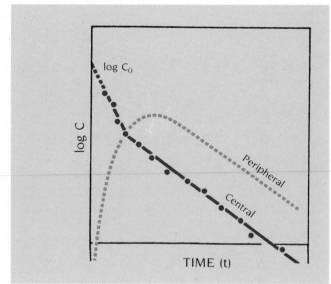

Figure 5–3 Time course of plasma (central) and tissue (peripheral) concentrations of a drug following its intravenous injection, and in the presence of distribution and elimination.

Absorption and Elimination

If the drug is administered not intravenously but, for example, orally, intramuscularly, or subcutaneously, then generally its concentration in the plasma will rise during the initial absorption phase and decrease again when (1) the absorption is complete, (2) the drug is in steady state between the plasma and the peripheral compartments, and (3) the rate of concentration decrease is dominated by the elimination processes (Fig. 5–4). In a semilogarithmic scale the final, descending part of the curve is linear (Fig. 5–4B).

The model is identical with Model 1 with the addition of an absorption compartment (Model 3). This is justified, because it has been found repeatedly that the rate of absorption is proportional to the unabsorbed amount of drug, and so a (first-order) compartment for absorption may be assumed.

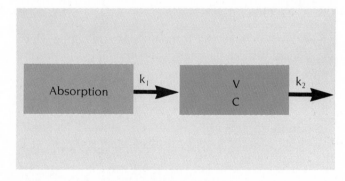

Model 3: Absorption and elimination.

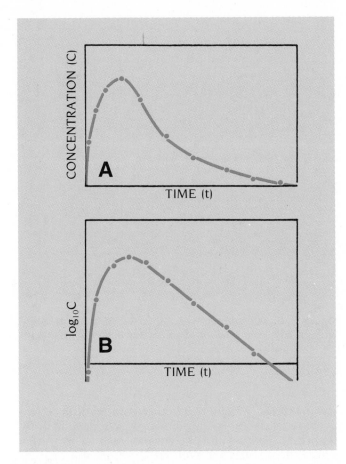

Figure 5–4 Time course of plasma concentration after the oral administration of a drug. The drug concentration is plotted on a linear (A) and on a logarithmic (B) scale.

Concentration Dependence of Rates

We have assumed that the rates of various processes are proportional to the drug concentration in the compartment from which the molecules exit. This is very frequently a reasonable assumption. For example, it is valid for diffusion-controlled processes, since the rate of diffusion is proportional to the concentration gradient (the difference of concentrations on the two sides of a membrane or other barrier), and the concentration of the "receiving" side is usually negligibly small in comparison with the concentration in the "donating" compartment. Similarly, the rate of urinary excretion is usually proportional to the concentration of the (free) drug in plasma water. Certainly, this is true for excretion by glomerular filtration, but in practice it is often valid even for active transfer processes such as tubular secretion or reabsorption, when the drug concentration is low enough that the carrier system is not close to being saturated.

However, the carrier system can become saturated at high concentrations. The rate of urinary excretion

is then constant, independently of the plasma concentration, and thereby conforms to the features of a zero-order process. A linear plot for the time course of concentrations (Fig. 5–5A) shows a constant rate of decline. In contrast, the slope in the semilogarithmic plot of concentrations (Fig. 5–5B) is not constant in this region but gets gradually steeper. Eventually the concentration decreases sufficiently so that the carrier system is not saturated any more. After passing through an intermediate region, the concentration reaches, at its low levels, the range of first-order removal.

Some drugs act therapeutically in the transitional range between the regions of purely zero-order and first-order kinetics (e.g., phenytoin, dicumarol, salicylic acid). Other substances are physiologically effective within the range of zero-order kinetics (e.g., ethanol). Similar considerations apply to biotransformation reactions or to binding to plasma proteins. At high drug concentrations the catalysing enzyme or the binding protein (albumin) becomes saturated with substrate

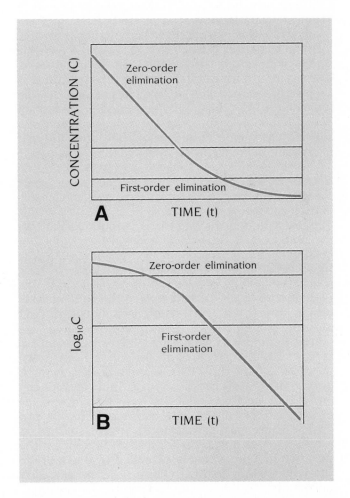

Figure 5–5 Time course of plasma concentration of a drug exhibiting zero-order kinetics at high levels. Linear plot (A) and semilogarithmic plot (B).

(drug) molecules and, therefore, the rate of the appropriate process is independent of the drug concentration. However, at much below saturating concentrations these rates also become proportional to the concentrations.

As mentioned earlier, the rate of absorption is also proportional to the amount of the unabsorbed drug. This is, of course, not so when drug tablets are specially coated to yield slow, sustained-release preparations that are absorbed at a rate independent of the amount of drug remaining in the intestinal lumen.

DURATION OF DRUG ACTION

It is usually assumed that a drug is effective when its concentration in the central compartment is greater than a minimal threshold level ($C_{effective}$). $C_{effective}$ may or may not be identical with $C_{therapeutic}$, which is the concentration to achieve a specific therapeutic effect. Drug action is maintained as long as this condition of exceeding the minimum effective concentration is fulfilled.

Useful guidelines characterizing the duration of drug action can be established on the basis of this principle. These state that **the duration of drug effects is proportional to the half-life of elimination and to the logarithm of the dose**, provided that the absorption and distribution of the drug are rapid in comparison with its elimination (including biotransformation and excretion), and that these are first-order processes.

Therefore, it is very difficult to obtain increased duration of drug action by increasing the dosage, since the latter must be raised exponentially to attain an only linear increase in the duration.

In order to demonstrate these proportionalities, let us assume one-compartmental elimination, without a distribution phase. Introducing different doses of a drug by a given route of administration, the semilogarithmic concentration-time profiles will be parallel (Fig. 5–6). Furthermore, if the ratios between the consecutively higher doses (i.e., the differences between their logarithms) are constant, then the profile curves are equally distanced. In the horizontal direction, equal distances between curves, particularly at the concentration level $C_{effective}$, imply the uniformly gradual increase in the duration of drug action (t_D). Thus, equal increments of duration are paralleled by uniform increments of the logarithm of the dose and, therefore, the two quantities are linearly related.

An important application of this rule states that **the duration of drug action is extended by one half-life when the dose is doubled.** (This conclusion can be formalized as $t_{2D_0} = t_{D_0} + t\frac{1}{2}$, and can be demonstrated by equating the threshold concentration expressed for the two conditions.)

Example: Let us assume that for the drug considered earlier, with a half-life of 4 hours and an apparent

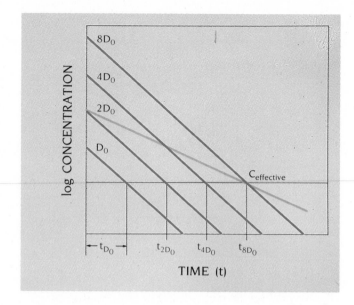

Figure 5–6 Effect of intravenously injected drug doses and biologic half-life on the duration of drug action. (*See* text for explanations.)

volume of distribution of 5 L, the therapeutically effective concentration is $C_{ther} = 5$ mg/L. We have already seen that the plasma concentration has fallen to this level 8 hours after intravenous injection of a dose of 100 mg. If the dose is doubled to 200 mg then, according to our rule, the duration of effective drug action is extended to 8 + 4 = 12 hours.

The proportionality of duration with elimination half-life can be similarly illustrated. After all, longer half-lives indicate shallower lines in the semilogarithmic plot (oblique shallow line in Fig. 5–6). Consequently, for a given intercept (initial concentration), the minimal effective concentration is reached after a longer time.

The guidelines characterizing the duration of drug action can be applied, to a very good approximation, also in the presence of fast absorption and distribution, since these alter the shape of the concentration profile only slightly. However, caution must be exercised when nonlinear kinetics or extended absorption and/or distribution causes substantial curvature in the semilogarithmic concentration-time plot.

The effect of dosage on duration can be particularly striking if absorption is not fast in comparison with elimination (Fig. 5–7). At low doses, the drug effect appears quite late and lasts only for a short time. Larger doses bring about an earlier appearance of the effects. Also, these are very substantially prolonged.

The above considerations may not be applied when the effects of a drug or chemical are not always proportional to its concentration in the central compartment. For instance, organophosphate insecticides destroy certain enzymes in the body. Consequently, their effect is prolonged well after their elimination, until the enzymes are resynthesized.

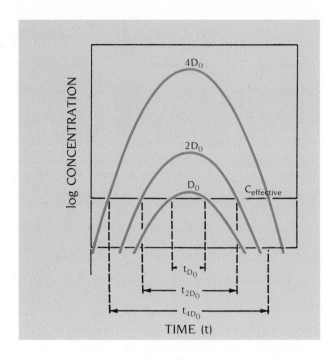

Figure 5–7 Effect of orally administered drug dosage on the duration of drug action. (*See* text for explanations.)

EXTENDING THE DURATION OF DRUG ACTION

Infusion of a Drug

If the drug is introduced at a constant rate, in the form of intravenous infusion or as a sustained-release tablet, then its concentration in the plasma increases at a gradually diminishing rate. (It may be remarked in passing that this increase can also be described by exponentials.) In the case of an infusion, after a while a fairly constant concentration level is reached. The infusion may be discontinued either before or after reaching the plateau. This is indicated by arrows in Figure 5–8, showing a curve obtained at high infusion rate that is continued to steady state at the plateau and, with identical kinetic constants, another curve that characterizes a lower-rate infusion interrupted before reaching the plateau.

After interruption of the infusion, the time course of drug concentrations follows earlier-described principles. If redistribution of the drug is essentially complete, then its elimination is characterized by a descending straight line in the semilogarithmic plot (Fig. 5–8B).

In the linear concentration-time plot (Fig. 5–8A) the accumulation curve is the inverted mirror image of the elimination pattern.

Applications of the infusion curves in clinical pharmacokinetics are described in Chapter 6.

Repeated Drug Administration; Dosage Regimens

The aim of approximately constant plasma concentration levels can be reached also by repeated application of the drug. We would like the concentration to stay above the threshold level for effective therapeutic action (C_{ther}), but safely below the toxic concentration (C_{tox}) that would begin to cause harmful side effects. This aim is achieved by gradually building up the drug level when appropriate maintenance doses are given repeatedly at the proper dosing intervals.

Figure 5–9 illustrates the time course of drug concentrations following repeated intravenous administration. A one-compartment model is assumed (rapid distribution in comparison with elimination). Thus, in the semilogarithmic plot (Fig. 5–9A) the descending segments are linear and parallel since all of them are characterized by the same elimination rate constant and half-life. In the linear concentration-time plot (Fig. 5–9B)

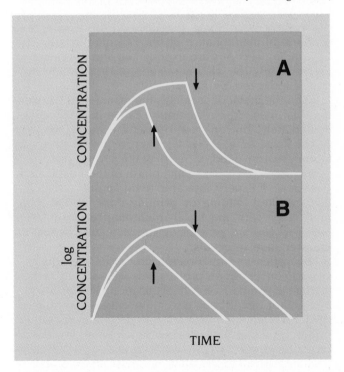

Figure 5–8 Time course of drug concentration during and following intravenous infusion. The arrows indicate the cessation of drug administration. Linear plot (*A*) and semilogarithmic plot (*B*). (*See* text for additional explanations.)

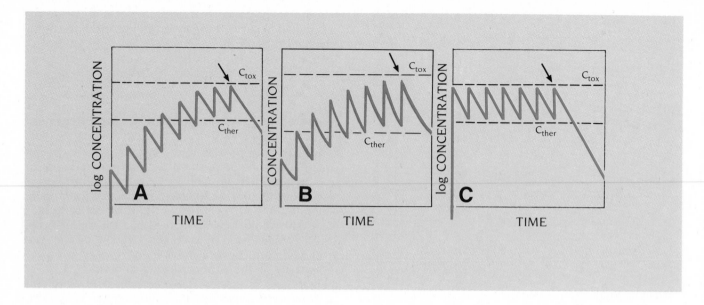

Figure 5–9 Drug concentration following repeated intravenous injections. *A* = logarithmic concentration scale; *B* = linear concentration scale; *C* = repeated injections following a loading dose, logarithmic concentration scale.

the vertical (ascending) lines are, on the assumption of identical maintenance doses, of equal length. The descending sections are exponential and not linear in Figure 5–9B. The discontinuation of drug administration is indicated by arrows.

When the initial dose equals the maintenance doses, the final, desired concentration range is reached not immediately, but only after several dosage intervals. At the same time, the patient is probably sickest and in the greatest need of reaching the proper drug concentration levels in the initial phase of the medication. Therefore, it is very desirable to administer a high initial, so-called **loading or priming dose**, and to continue later with the small **maintenance doses** (Fig. 5–9C). These are generally given at regular dosing or **maintenance intervals.**

Absorption and distribution processes alter the discussed concentration profiles only very slightly if they are fast in comparison with elimination. Slower absorption and/or distribution distort the curves in a manner similar to that seen with a single drug administration: In the semilogarithmic concentration-time plot, curvatures downward or upward, respectively, are introduced. In particular, after intramuscular or oral drug intake, the multiple peaks of the concentration profile do not rise suddenly, and are not sharp, in contrast to the ones seen in the intravenous examples.

A systematic dosage schedule involving repeated drug administration is referred to as **dosage regimen**. Its components, the loading dose, maintenance doses and dosing intervals, have been described in the preceding paragraphs. Their consideration aids the design of effective clinical drug administration. For example, in at-

tending to two patients with different elimination but identical absorption and distribution rate constants, identical minimum (threshold) plasma concentrations can be maintained if the subject having faster elimination receives the drug more frequently or if his maintenance dose is higher (or both). This is discussed in greater detail in Chapter 6.

MORE COMPLICATED MODELS

We have considered two kinds of model containing two compartments. In the one model (Model 2), elimination of the drug starts immediately after administration, even while it gets distributed between the plasma and the peripheral compartments. Thus the two processes take place simultaneously. In the other model (Model 3) a drug molecule must be absorbed into the plasma before it can be eliminated from there. The two processes must, therefore, follow each other.

These systems of parallel and consecutive processes (compartments) can of course be extended and also combined with each other. But verification of such models is substantially more difficult mathematically, and, especially, experimentally. Usually it is not sufficient to measure drug concentrations in the plasma; samples are required also from the urine and from other parts of the body. Also, the formation of metabolites should be observed.

The kinetic analysis of such models is more involved and requires the use of computers. In fact, it is advisable to evaluate the experimental results for even simpler models by computer, since this method of analysis will yield more reliable parameters.

BIOAVAILABILITY

Definitions

Bioavailability: The percentage of a drug, contained in a drug product, that enters the systemic circulation in an unchanged form after administration of the product. This concept includes not only the amount of drug that enters the body, but also the rate of entry.
Bioequivalence: Comparable bioavailability between related drugs.
Therapeutic equivalence: Comparable clinical effectiveness and safety between similar drugs.
Bioinequivalence: Statistically significant difference in bioavailability between related drugs.
Therapeutic inequivalence: Clinically important difference in bioavailability between similar drugs.

Measurements of Bioavailability

Correlation of Drug Dose with Pharmacologic Response

This is possible only for drugs with end points that can be readily measured, *e.g.*, warfarin anticoagulation. It is not a very good measure of bioavailability, since it is also affected by differences in drug-receptor combination and in intrinsic efficacy of the receptor-effector link.

Serum Concentrations

After a **single oral dose** of drug, serial measurements of serum concentrations are obtained. Three parameters of importance are derived from such a procedure (Fig. 5–10):

1. peak drug concentration,
2. time to peak concentration,
3. area under the concentration-time curve (mg-hours/L) (AUC).

The first two quantities are simple indicators for the **rate** of absorption. An increased rate is suggested by a higher peak concentration and a shorter time required to reach the peak concentration (curve Y in Fig. 5–11A). In contrast, AUC reflects the **extent** of absorption. Consequently, after oral or intramuscular administration of a drug, the bioavailability can be evaluated by comparing the measured AUC with the AUC determined

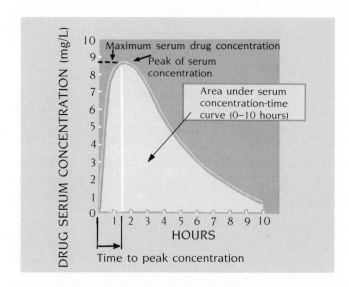

Figure 5–10 Serum concentration-time curve after oral administration of a single dose of a hypothetical drug.

after intravenous injection (*i.e.*, 100% absorption) of the same dose of the drug:

$$\text{Bioavailability} = \frac{\text{AUC (oral)}}{\text{AUC (intravenous)}}.$$

Repeated doses of most drugs result in cumulation, and the mean steady-state serum drug concentrations are a good index of drug bioavailability. Again, it is not the steady-state concentration (C_{ss}) itself, but the ratio of C_{ss} (oral) to C_{ss} (intravenous) that provides the estimate of bioavailability after oral ingestion.

Urinary Excretion

For drugs excreted predominantly unchanged in the urine, bioavailability can be determined by urine collection. For example, consider three formulations of a drug, "X", "Y" and "Z". As shown in Figure 5–11, the cumulative excretion curves reflect the plasma concentration time curves, which in turn reflect the effectiveness of absorption.

The rates of absorption of formulations X and Z are the same. However, Z has a smaller plasma AUC, lower total urinary accumulation and, consequently, lower bioavailability than preparation X. In contrast, formulations X and Y have identical plasma AUCs and cumulative urinary excretions and, therefore, their bioavailabilities are the same. However, the absorption rate of preparation Y is higher than that of formulation X.

However, this method can not be applied to the excretion curves of free drug + total metabolites of a drug that is substantially biotransformed. Any first-pass biotransformation products would appear in the urine, but they should not be included in the estimate of

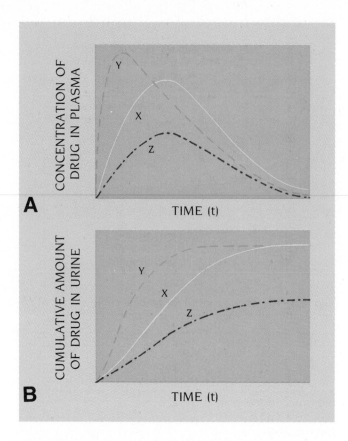

Figure 5–11 Relation between plasma concentration curves (*A*) and cumulative urinary excretion curves (*B*) for three different preparations of a drug that is excreted unchanged in the urine. Curve X = slow and complete absorption (100% bioavailability); curve Y = fast and complete absorption (100% bioavailability); curve Z = slow and incomplete absorption (<100% bioavailability).

bioavailability because they had never reached the systemic circulation in active form (*see* First-Pass Effect below).

Factors Influencing Bioavailability of Orally Administered Drugs

Formulation of the Drug Product

As was noted in Chapter 1, the first thing to happen to a drug administered by any route other than intravenous is that it must dissolve and become available for absorption. Therefore the first important influence upon bioavailability is the formulation of the tablet, capsule, suspension, or solution of the drug in the preparation that is taken by the patient.

To study bioavailability for all presently available oral medications would involve facilities, personnel, and costs too staggering to contemplate. Thus, empiric assumptions are usually made. For many drugs, tablet disintegration time or drug dissolution rate correlates

satisfactorily with their bioavailability, as in the case of digoxin. The most rapidly dissolving digoxin tablets are equivalent to digoxin solution in bioavailability, but most tablets are less effectively absorbed.

Sometimes bioavailability can be improved drastically by a simple physical change. For example, the antifungal antibiotic griseofulvin is absorbed rather poorly during its passage along the intestine. Grinding it very fine (micro-pulverization) increases the surface-to-mass ratio, speeding up the dissolution and thus enabling much more of the drug to be absorbed during the intestinal transit (Fig. 5–12).

After the patent of a drug expires, new formulations are often made available. The minimum requirement for the regulatory approval of these so-called "generic" drugs involves a demonstration that their bioavailabilities are identical to that of the original drug, *i.e.*, that they are bioequivalent. In more critical cases, the therapeutic equivalence of the two formulations must be shown.

Interaction with Other Substances in the Gastrointestinal Tract

Gastric absorption of many acidic drugs is increased if the stomach is empty. Food will slow gastric emptying and dilute the gastric and small intestinal contents. Conversely, it is possible to imagine a slowly absorbed drug for which the presence of food could result in more complete absorption.

Other substances present simultaneously in the in-

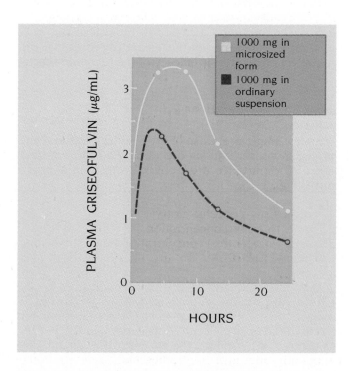

Figure 5–12 Bioavailability of griseofulvin administered orally to the same subjects as ordinary suspension and as micro-pulverized form.

testine may modify the absorption of a drug, as a result of ion neutralization, complex formation, coprecipitation, *etc.* (*see also* Chapter 11). For example, mineral oil taken as a laxative can dissolve highly lipid-soluble drugs or vitamins and impair their absorption. In contrast, alcohol weakens the barrier to the passage of iron salts and causes excessive absorption, which may cause disease due to iron-pigment accumulation in the tissues.

Biotransformation in the Intestinal Mucosa or Liver (First-Pass Effect)

The bioavailability of some drugs is low because the drug, after its absorption and transfer to the portal venous blood, is avidly extracted and biotransformed in the liver. Examples of such drugs include hydralazine, lidocaine, organic nitrates, propranolol, morphine, and nortriptyline. (*See also* Chapters 4 and 7, *Drug Biotransformation* and *Drug Clearance*.)

For some drugs, this can also occur in the intestinal mucosa, immediately after absorption and before the drug can pass into the portal venous blood. This may be an important determinant of the bioavailability of diazepam. The first-pass effect on bioavailability is illustrated in Figure 5–13.

Intramuscular Injection

Highly perfused muscle would seem to be a reasonable route for drug administration. However, the bioavailability of intramuscularly administered chlordiazepoxide, digoxin, and phenytoin is variable and low (Fig. 5–13). In part, this is because blood flow through muscle varies greatly according to the muscle chosen for the injection (deltoid > quadriceps femoris > gluteus maximus), and also according to its state of activity (blood flow can be as low as 3 mL/100 g/minute at rest, and as high as 30 mL/100 g/minute during hard work).

Therapeutic Importance of Bioavailability

Fluctuations and differences in the completeness of absorption can be of major therapeutic importance if a drug exhibits at least one of the following characteristics:
* A given (*e.g.*, two-fold) variation in the attained concentration evokes a large change in the response in the therapeutic range (*e.g.*, warfarin).
* The relationship between effect and concentration is strongly non-linear at the recommended doses

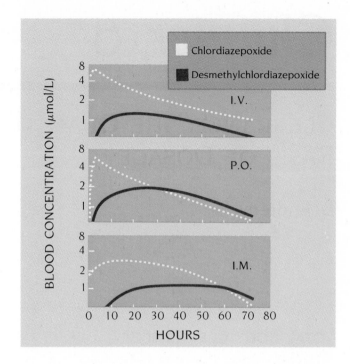

Figure 5–13 Concentration curves of precursor drug (chlordiazepoxide) and biotransformation product (desmethylchlordiazepoxide) after three different routes of administration. Intravenous injection gives 100% bioavailability; oral administration shows first-pass effect with lower precursor and higher product curves; intramuscular injection gives slow absorption relative to excretion, so that both precursor and product curves are lower.

(*e.g.*, phenylbutazone, phenytoin, salicylate in high, anti-inflammatory doses).
* The difference between concentrations eliciting therapeutic effects and those associated with toxicity is small, resulting in a narrow margin of safety (*e.g.*, digoxin); *see* Chapter 8.

SUGGESTED READING

Notari RE. Biopharmaceutics and clinical pharmacokinetics. 4th ed. New York: Marcel Dekker, 1987. [An introduction with little mathematics.]
Gibaldi M, Perrier D. Pharmacokinetics. 2nd ed. New York: Marcel Dekker, 1982. [More detailed, fairly mathematical.]

Chapter 6

CLEARANCE: THE QUANTITATIVE BASIS OF DOSAGE

L. Endrenyi

TOTAL BODY CLEARANCE

Clearance is a quantitative measure characterizing the rate of removal of endogenous or exogenous substances, including drugs, from the body or from a specific part of the body. Hepatic biotransformation, excretion by the kidney, exhalation by the lungs, and fecal excretion are the usual routes of drug elimination. The corresponding specific clearances are considered in Chapter 7. Here we shall deal with their sum, the total body clearance (TBC), measuring the overall rate of disappearance or elimination of a substance from the whole body.

Clearance is expressed as the volume of body fluid from which this substance (drug) is removed in unit time. Consequently, when concentrations are measured in the plasma, the volume of this fluid from which the drug is apparently removed (cleared) in unit time, is referred to as the plasma clearance.

In terms of kinetic parameters, *i.e.*, the first-order elimination rate constant (k) and apparent volume of distribution (V), the total body clearance can be expressed as

$$Cl = kV \quad [mL/min] = [min^{-1}] \times [mL].$$

[Dimensions of the various quantities in this and all following equations are given in square brackets.]

This simple calculation is in agreement with the definition of clearance given above since, as seen in Chapter 5, *Pharmacokinetics*, the rate constant is, numerically, the fraction of a substance eliminated (cleared) in unit time; its product with the apparent volume of distribution yields the volume from which the drug is apparently removed in unit time.

The volume defined by clearance is often measured by dividing the amount of drug removed in unit time by the concentration of the drug in the relevant body fluid. Usually, however, evaluation of the total body clearance is based on a different kinetic principle. It can be shown that clearance is inversely proportional to the area under a curve (AUC) fitted to concentration readings obtained at different times. If the drug is completely absorbed following its administration, such as after intravenous injection, then

$$Cl = D/AUC \quad [mL/min] = [mg] / [(mg/mL) \times min],$$

where D is the drug dose. When only a fraction (F) of the dose is absorbed, as is often the case following oral administration, then

$$Cl = F \cdot D/AUC.$$

For measuring the AUC, the concentrations should be plotted on a linear scale (Fig. 6–1). Also, AUC refers to the complete area under the curve evaluated between the times of zero and infinity following drug administration. Therefore, the curve fitted through observations must be extrapolated by an algebraic procedure.

The clearance of drugs is of great importance for kinetic considerations. Its magnitude is independent of modeling assumptions. This is reasonable, since the area under the curve is the same whether we hypothesize the presence of one or two or any number of compartments.

The concept of clearance is biologically meaningful and important. Its study enables pharmacologists to reach conclusions about the effect of hepatic blood flow, renal processes, and protein binding on drug elimination. This is discussed in other chapters.

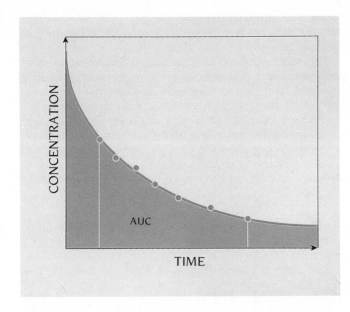

Figure 6–1 Drug concentration in plasma following a single intravenous injection. AUC = area under the curve (shaded). Borders of the experimental range are indicated.

Furthermore, the steady-state concentration of drugs, which is reached when the rate of intake equals the rate of elimination, is determined by the total body clearance. We shall now discuss this question in some detail.

DOSAGE FOR INTRAVENOUS INFUSION

Let us consider the rate of input and output processes involving the whole body.

Input could refer to the sum of endogenous production and exogenous intake of a substance. We shall be concerned mainly with the latter. Initially we shall assume that a drug is administered at a constant rate, Q (*e.g.*, by intravenous infusion). The rate is the amount administered per unit time with units of, say, mg/hour.

The amount of drug in the body is, at any time, VC, where, as before, V is the apparent volume of distribution and C the concentration in the plasma. The fraction of this that is being removed in unit time is given by the rate constant (k). Consequently, the amount eliminated per unit time is kVC.

At steady state, the rate of input is equal to the rate of elimination. Therefore,

$$Q = kVC_{ss}.$$

Thus, it is possible to calculate the rate of drug administration (Q) that is required **to maintain** a desired concentration (C_{ss}).

In terms of clearance,

$$Q = Cl \cdot C_{ss}.$$

Consequently, the steady-state concentration is

$$C_{ss} = Q/Cl \quad [mg/mL] = [mg/min] / [mL/min].$$

This is reasonable since, according to this expression, the steady-state concentration is determined by the ratio of inflow and outflow rates.

(We could consider the analogy of water in a bathtub [Fig. 6–2] in which both the faucet and the drain plug are open. The level of water finally attained depends on the rates of inflow and outflow.)

Since an immediate effect is desired, a **loading dose** of the drug is given by rapid administration (*e.g.*, by injection) to fill the body stores and establish the effective, steady-state plasma concentration. As we have seen, at steady state the amount of drug in the body is VC_{ss}. This is the amount that the loading dose (L) should introduce at once. Consequently,

$$L = VC_{ss} \quad [mg] = [L] \times [mg/L].$$

(The relationships between infusion rate, clearance, and steady-state concentration are used for the convenient evaluation of the clearance. This can be done since the infusion rate is set by the physician or the investigator, and the steady-state concentration can be easily measured. If, in addition, the elimination rate constant or the related half-life is observed, then the apparent volume of distribution can also be calculated. This is often the preferred approach.)

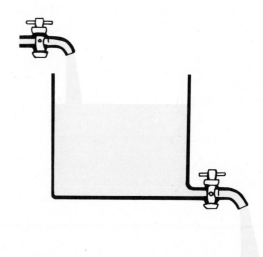

Figure 6–2 Hydrodynamic analogy for drug kinetics: Water in the bathtub.

Example: Lidocaine Infusion.

Besides being a local anaesthetic agent, lidocaine is effective in the treatment of cardiac arrhythmias. Continuous infusion is indicated in patients in whom the arrhythmia tends to recur, and to whom oral therapy cannot be given.

Let us assume the following characteristics of the drug in a 70 kg man:

C_{ther} = 2.0 mg/L (therapeutically effective plasma concentration),
$t\frac{1}{2}$ = 80 minutes (biologic half-life),
V_w = 0.70 L/kg (apparent distribution volume related to body weight).

Consequently:

k = 0.693/80 = 0.0087 min^{-1},
V = 0.70 [L/kg] × 70 [kg] = 49 L.

(Question: What is the distribution space for lidocaine?)

Therefore, the desired infusion rate is

Q = kVC_{ss}
   = 0.0087 × 49 × 2.0 = 0.85 mg/min.

Incidentally, the total body clearance is

Cl = kV
    = 0.0087 × 49 = 0.43 L/min.

The corresponding loading dose is

L = VC_{ss}
   = 49 × 2.0 = 98 mg.

In practice, a loading dose of 100 mg could be given. The steady-state infusion rate would be about 1 mg/min.

TIME TO STEADY-STATE CONCENTRATION: PLATEAU PRINCIPLE

Let us assume again that a drug follows first-order kinetics and, for now, that it is administered by continuous intravenous infusion. We have seen that the steady-state concentration (C_{ss}) depends on the rates of both administration and removal of the drug. In contrast, the rate of approach to the steady-state level depends only on the elimination rate constant. Thus, according to the so-called plateau principle, **the time to reach a given fraction of the steady-state concentration is determined only by the elimination rate constant.** (In the example of the partially filled bathtub of Figure 6–2, if, following an earlier achieved constant level [including an empty bathtub], either of the two

faucets is adjusted, the rate at which the new water level is approached depends solely on the setting of the outflow tap.)

The sense of the plateau principle can be appreciated by recalling that the plasma concentration of a drug changes at a rate determined by two simultaneously occurring processes. A constant rate of inflow is assumed by maintaining steady infusion. Thus, the rate of outflow (elimination) completely determines the overall rate of concentration change and, with it, the time course of plasma concentration. The elimination rate, in turn, is defined by the elimination rate constant.

Mathematical Derivation of the Plateau Principle

The rate of concentration change is:

dC/dt = (Rate of drug infusion) – (Rate of drug elimination),
       = (Q/V) – kC.

Integrating between the initial and the measured plasma concentrations (C_0 and C) observed at times 0 and t, and remembering that the steady-state concentration is

C_{ss} = Q/kV,

we obtain the **fractional attainment (f)** of the new steady state, defined as

$$f \equiv (C_0 - C)/(C_0 - C_{ss}) = 1 - e^{-kt}.$$

This relationship is shown in Figure 6–3 and listed in Table 6–1.

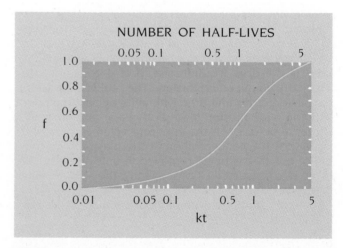

Figure 6–3 Relationship of fractional attainment of the plateau to kt. Recall that kt = 0.7 (t/t½). Consequently, the diagram depicts also the dependence of the fractional attainment on the number of half-lives elapsed.

TABLE 6–1 Relationship Between the Fractional Attainment (f) of New Plateau and kt or t/t₁/₂

kt	t/t½	f	% Fluctuation	f	kt	t/t½
0.05	0.07	0.049	5.2	0.05	0.05	0.07
0.06	0.09	0.059	6.3	0.10	0.11	0.15
0.08	0.12	0.077	8.3	0.15	0.16	0.23
				0.20	0.22	0.32
0.1	0.14	0.095	10.5	0.25	0.29	0.42
0.2	0.29	0.181	22.1			
0.3	0.43	0.259	35.0	0.30	0.36	0.52
0.4	0.58	0.330	49.3	0.35	0.43	0.62
0.5	0.72	0.394	65.0	0.40	0.51	0.74
0.6	0.87	0.451	82.1	0.45	0.60	0.86
0.8	1.15	0.551	122.7	0.50	0.69	1.00
				0.55	0.80	1.15
1.0	1.44	0.632	172			
1.5	2.16	0.777	348	0.60	0.92	1.32
2.0	2.89	0.865	641	0.65	1.05	1.51
2.5	3.61	0.918	1120	0.70	1.20	1.74
3.0	4.33	0.950	1900	0.75	1.39	2.00
4.0	5.77	0.982	5456	0.80	1.61	2.32
5.0	7.21	0.993	14200	0.85	1.90	2.74
6.0	8.66	0.998				
8.0	11.54	1.000		0.90	2.30	3.32
				0.95	3.00	4.32
				0.98	3.91	5.64

t/t½	kt	f	% Fluctuation
0.5	0.35	0.293	41
1	0.69	0.500	100
2	1.39	0.750	300
3	2.08	0.875	700
4	2.77	0.937	1500
5	3.47	0.969	3100
6	4.16	0.984	6300

Continuation of right columns:

f	kt	t/t½
0.99	4.61	6.64
0.995	5.30	7.64
0.998	6.21	8.97
0.999	6.91	9.97

% Fluctuation
$= 100 \; (C_{max} - C_{min})/C_{min}$
$= 100 \; f/(1 - f)$

The relationship displayed in Figure 6–3 is presented here in tabular form. On the left, one can obtain from the number of half-lives (t/t½) the fractional attainment (f) as well as, following repeated injections, the percentage fluctuation of the steady-state concentration. Conversely, on the right, one reads off the number of half-lives required to reach the desired fractional attainment.

Note that for the case of drug elimination $C_{ss} = 0$ and, therefore, with

$$f = (C_0 - C)/C_0$$

we get again the well-known relationship

$$C = C_0 e^{-kt}.$$

Thus, the concentration achieved depends on Q and t (k and V are usually constant for a drug in a given person). Note, in addition, that the fraction of the plateau attained (*i.e.*, time to plateau) given by $f = 1 - e^{-kt}$ is **independent** of Q.

Envisage five separate infusions of a drug at five different infusion rates Q5 > Q4 > Q3 > Q2 > Q1 (Fig. 6–4). Since the drug's half-life (or elimination rate constant) does not change, the **time** to reach a plateau will be identical for the five curves. The steady-state concentration will depend directly on the corresponding infusion rates.

Attained Fraction of Steady State

According to the plateau principle, any fraction of the steady-state concentration depends only on kt, and therefore, the time to reach this fraction depends only on the elimination rate constant, k. The principle applies to all shifts from one steady state to another.

The time to a given fractional attainment, $f = 1 - e^{-kt}$, of the steady-state level can be evaluated from the formula, or from the diagram depicting it (Fig. 6–3), or from Table 6–1.

From the graph or table, the time to reach 90% of a steady state is kt = 2.3.

But $k = 0.693 / t½$,
$t = 2.3/0.693 \times t½ = 3.3 \; t½.$

Consequently, 90% of the steady-state, plateau concentration is reached during a period of 3.3 half-lives.

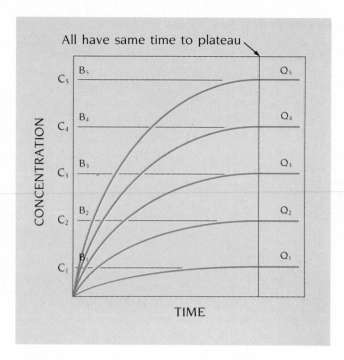

All have same time to plateau

CONCENTRATION

TIME

Figure 6–4 Illustration of the plateau principle.

Analogous calculations show:

Time to reach 95% plateau = 4.3 × t½,
99% plateau = 6.6 × t½,
99.9% plateau = 10.0 × t½.

A useful ''rule of thumb'' to remember:

For any drug, time to plateau ≃ 5 × half-life.

This approach is quite simplified but nevertheless will give a good ballpark estimate for most drugs. These calculations hold in general for drugs administered by **any route.**

Application of the Plateau Principle

1. Lidocaine is effective in the treatment of ventricular premature beats. Lidocaine t½ = 1.4 hours. If a continuous infusion was started, it would take 6.6 × t½ = 9.2 hours before plasma concentrations reach 99% of the maximum. This would explain the late appearance of toxicity to the drug.
2. Phenytoin t½ = 22 hours. Time to plateau = 110 hours (by rule of thumb).
3. For drugs administered orally, the same calculations estimate when a given proportion of maximum cumulation of drug has taken place; e.g., phenytoin p.o. will take 3 days for 90% cumulation.

It will also take this long to eliminate these drugs. (Why?) Several examples one may wish to think about are tetrahydrocannabinol t½ = 50 hours; diazepam (Valium®) t½ = 35 hours; amitriptyline (used in the treatment of depression) t½ > 24 hours; phenobarbital t½ = 3.5 days.

If the dose (or rate of administration) of a drug is changed, the time to reach the new plateau is calculated in exactly the same way as if one started from zero concentration.

DOSAGE REGIMEN FOR REPEATED INTRAVENOUS DRUG ADMINISTRATION

Fluctuation Around Average Steady-State Concentration

The principles described for continuous drug administration apply also to the situation when the drug is given intermittently. The main difference is that we cannot now **exactly** maintain the steady-state concentration. Rather, the concentration will fluctuate around an **average** value. This average concentration is brought about by the balance of the outflow rate (represented by the clearance) and the average inflow rate.

Consequently, the relationships described earlier remain applicable as long as we consider average concentrations and input rates. When **maintenance doses** of D_m are administered following each **maintenance interval** of T_m, then the average rate of drug intake is D_m/T_m. Therefore, the average steady-state concentration is

$$\overline{C}_{ss} = (D_m/T_m)/Cl.$$

Thus, in order to sustain this concentration, a maintenance dose of

$$D_m = Cl \cdot \overline{C}_{ss} \cdot T_m \text{ or}$$

$$D_m = kV\overline{C}_{ss} \cdot T_m$$

is required. The expression is useful in approximate preliminary calculations.

(Rather incidentally, it can be shown that for the calculation of total body clearance, AUC can be calculated also as the area under the plasma concentration curve segment that is obtained, at steady state, between the administration of consecutive maintenance doses [Fig. 6–5A].)

The maintenance dose is proportional to the maintenance interval. This implies that plasma concentrations show larger fluctuation when a drug is administered less frequently (see also Table 6–1).

The proportionality between maintenance dose and

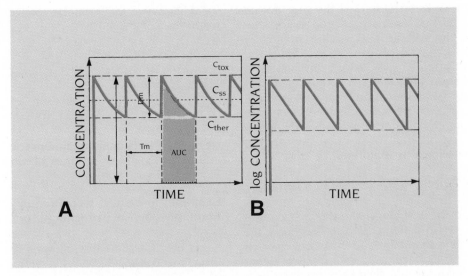

Figure 6–5 Plasma concentration following repeated intravenous injections. Linear (*A*) and logarithmic (*B*) concentrations. L = loading dose; D_m = maintenance dose; T_m = maintenance interval; C_{ther} = therapeutic concentration; C_{tox} = toxic concentration; C_{ss} = steady-state concentration; AUC = area under the curve.

maintenance interval raises an important question: How should these two quantities be chosen? The answer will be the result of a compromise between two considerations: the **safety** and the **convenience** of drug administration.

The drug concentration fluctuates around its steady-state average value proportionately to the maintenance dose (Fig. 6–5). Thus, when, following shortening of the maintenance intervals, the maintenance doses are reduced, the concentration changes also become smaller. As a result, the safety of drug administration is improved.

On the other hand, larger maintenance doses permit longer maintenance intervals, *i.e.*, less frequent administration of the drug. Beyond the obvious convenience, it may increase the probability of a patient's cooperation and compliance with the schedule.

Therefore, the balance of safety and convenience leads to the following procedure. First, an "ideal" dosage schedule is evaluated from the toxic and the therapeutically effective concentrations. Following this, the ideal dosage is adjusted on the basis of available dosage forms and convenient timing of administration.

"Ideal" Dosage Regimen

The maintenance dose keeps the plasma concentration safely between the minimum therapeutically effective (C_{ther}) and toxic (C_{tox}) concentrations. Therefore,

$$D_m = (C_{tox} - C_{ther})\ V.$$

According to Figure 6–5, the maintenance interval can be calculated by the formula

$$T_m = (\ln C_{tox} - \ln C_{ther})/k$$

$$= (2.30/k) \log (C_{tox}/C_{ther})$$

$$\simeq 10/3\ t\frac{1}{2} \log (C_{tox}/C_{ther}).$$

Here ln refers to the natural, e-based logarithm, and log to the 10-based logarithm.

An equivalent, but perhaps more convenient, procedure for the evaluation of the maintenance interval takes advantage of the definition of fractional attainment during elimination:

$$f = (C_{tox} - C_{ther})/C_{tox}.$$

The value of kT_m can be read off Figure 6–3 or Table 6–1 and, since the rate constant (k) is known, T_m can be calculated.

The **loading dose** (L) aims at reaching the maximum of the steady-state concentration range immediately following drug administration. Therefore:

$$L = VC_{tox}.$$

Two Frequently Applied Dosage Regimens

Two dosing procedures deserve particular consideration; their background is discussed in greater detail in the last section of this chapter. In the first dosing approach, maintenance doses are administered at intervals equalling the half-life ($T_m = t^{1/2}$). At steady state, the maximum plasma concentration is twice the minimum concentration ($C_{max} = 2C_{min}$); this implies a substantial fluctuation amounting to 100% (*see also* Table 6–1). It can be demonstrated (*cf.* last section) that the maximum concentration reached at steady state is twice the maximum concentration obtained after a single drug administration. It follows that **the loading dose should be twice the maintenance dose**, $L = 2D_m$.

The second interesting dosing strategy administers the drug relatively frequently, at maintenance intervals that are less than the half-life of the drug, say, by a factor of at least 3 ($T_m < t^{1/2}/3$). With this regimen, the plasma concentration at steady state shows only moderate fluctuation. These concentrations are much higher than those seen following a single administration, thereby indicating a substantial accumulation of the drug. As a result, the loading dose should substantially exceed the maintenance dose. Their relationship is approximately given by $L = 1.44\ (t^{1/2}/T_m)D_m$ (*see* last section).

Practical Dosage Regimens

The calculated ideal maintenance interval should be reduced to a practically manageable value such as 24, 12, 8, 6, or 4 hours, for giving the drug once, or two, three, four, or six times a day. The maintenance dose is adjusted correspondingly. It will be set by taking into account the available dosage forms and the desirability of staying within the toxic and therapeutically effective concentration levels (Fig. 6–5).

Thus, drugs that have long half-lives, exceeding 24 hours, will be ingested daily. Consequently, the dosing interval is less than the half-life, and the initial dose is more than double the maintenance dose.

Drugs having reasonably high safety margins and intermediate half-lives of between 6 and 24 hours could be ingested at intervals approximating their half-lives. Ideally then, the loading dose is twice the maintenance dose. With drugs having a low therapeutic index, more frequent administration of lower maintenance doses is required. Occasionally, prolonged-release formulations can be used satisfactorily.

If a drug has a half-life shorter than 6 hours, then it must have a very high safety margin if we wish to consider its repeated administration. The initial dose will equal the maintenance dose. Drugs having a low therapeutic index must be administered by continuous infusion.

The useful formulae for evaluating the practical dosage regimens are similar to those applied for calculating the "ideal" schedule. However, the maximum concentration reached (C_{max}) will now replace C_{tox}, and the minimum concentration (C_{min}) will be used instead of C_{ther}.

Additionally, C_{max} will be conveniently calculated from

$$C_{max} = D_m / Vf,$$

and C_{min} from

$$C_{min} = C_{max}e^{-kT_m} = C_{max}\ (1-f).$$

Here f, the fractional attainment for elimination (at the end of the maintenance interval) can be evaluated from Figure 6–3 or Table 6–1.

Example: Repeated Intravenous Administration of Aminophylline, a Bronchodilator.

(a)   Let us assume the following characteristics of the drug in a 50 kg, 32-year-old woman:

C_{ther} = 5 mg/L (therapeutically effective plasma concentration),
C_{tox} = 20 mg/L (toxic plasma concentration),
$\overline{C}_{ss}$ = 10 mg/L (approximate average steady-state plasma concentration),
$t^{1/2}$ = 4.5 hr (biologic half-life),
V_w = 0.56 L/kg (apparent distribution volume related to body weight).

Consequently:

k = 0.693/4.5 = 0.154 hr^{-1},
V = 0.56 × 50 = 28 L.

Therefore, to get a ballpark figure, the desired approximate rate of drug administration is

$$D_m / T_m = kV\overline{C}_{ss}$$
$$= 0.154 \times 28 \times 10 = 43.1 \text{ mg/hr},$$

where the total body clearance is

$$Cl = kV = 0.154 \times 28 = 4.31 \text{ L/hr}$$
$$= 4.31 \times 1000/60 = 72 \text{ mL/min}.$$

(b)   The dosage required for **ideal dosing** is evaluated from the toxic and therapeutically effective concentrations:

$$\mathbf{D_m} = (C_{tox} - C_{ther})\ V$$
$$= (20-5) \times 28 = \mathbf{420 \text{ mg}}.$$

The maintenance interval can be evaluated directly from

$$\mathbf{T_m} = (2.303/k)\ \log\ (C_{tox}/C_{ther})$$
$$= (2.303/0.154)\ \log\ (20/5) = \mathbf{9.0 \text{ hr}}.$$

More indirectly, but more easily,

$$f = (C_{tox} - C_{ther})/C_{tox}$$
$$= (20-5)/20 = 0.75.$$

From Table 6–1, and also from Figure 6–3, we read off

$kT_m = 1.39$.

From this

$T_m = 1.39/0.154 = $ 9.0 hr

is calculated again. (This makes sense: The time required to reduce the concentration from 20 mg/L to 5 mg/L [indicated also by $1 - f = 0.25$] is two half-lives.)

(The ideal dosage schedule corresponds to an average dosing rate of

$D_m/T_m = 420/9 = 46.7$ mg/hr,

which gives rise to an average steady-state concentration of

$\overline{C}_{ss} = (D_m/T_m)/kV$
$= 46.7/4.31 = 10.8$ mg/L,

close to the original "ballpark" figure.)

The ideal loading dose is

$L = VC_{tox}$
$= 28 \times 20 = $ **560 mg.**

(c) For a **practical dosing** schedule, the maintenance interval should be lowered from nine hours. If we choose eight hours, then the maintenance dose would be approximately

$D_m \simeq 420 \times (8/9) = 373$ mg.

However, in this example, preparations for intravenous administration are available in either 250 or 500 mg forms. Therefore, we should consider a maintenance interval of

$T_m = $ 6 hr.

This would lead to an approximate maintenance dose of

$D_m = 420 \times (6/9) = 280$ mg,

which is close to the actually available dose of

$D_m = $ 250 mg.

(Let us see what concentrations are obtained from this dosage schedule:

With $f = 0.60$ [from Fig. 6–3 or Table 6–1, based on $kT_m = 0.154 \times 6 = 0.92$] we have

$C_{max} = D_m/Vf$
$= 250/(28 \times 0.60) = 14.8$ mg/L.

The minimal concentration can be calculated by two simple methods. According to the first,

$C_{min} = C_{max} (1 - f)$
$= 14.8 \times 0.40 = 5.9$ mg/L.

The second method takes advantage of the relationship

$D_m = (C_{max} - C_{min}) V$,

from which

$C_{min} = C_{max} - D_m/V$
$= 14.8 - 250/28 = 5.9$ mg/L.

Thus, the practical dosage regimen of aminophylline restricts the concentrations to the desirable range [Fig. 6–5]. The corresponding average steady-state concentration is

$\overline{C}_{ss} = (D_m/T_m)/kV$
$= (250/6)/4.31 = 9.7$ mg/L,

again close to the originally desired value of 10 mg/L.)

The loading dose, establishing immediately the steady-state levels, is

$L = VC_{max}$
$= 28 \times 14.8 = $ **414 mg.**

In practice, therefore, a loading dose of 500 mg would be given. (This yields an initial maximum concentration of $500/28 = 17.9$ mg/L, still below the toxic level.) This would be followed by the administration, four times a day, of 250 mg of the drug in 10 mL diluent, which is injected over a 10-minute period.

Note that we have ended up with a dosage schedule in which the maintenance interval (6 hr) was somewhat higher but fairly close to the half-life of the drug (4.5 hr). As a result, the plasma concentration showed over two-fold fluctuation. The loading dose (500 mg) was twice the maintenance dose (250 mg).

REPEATED ORAL ADMINISTRATION

The expressions evaluating dosage regimens for repeated oral administration are almost the same as those discussed for repeated intravenous injections when these aim at reaching an **average** steady-state concentration. The only difference is that for oral administration, all dosing equations must be **multiplied** on the right-hand side by the **bioavailability** (F), *i.e.*, by the fraction of a drug dose reaching the systemic circulation.

If we aim again at remaining between the therapeutic and toxic concentration levels, the exact formulae for calculating dosage regimens for repeated oral administration are more complicated and require kinetic information about the relative rates of absorption and elimination.

Fortunately, in many cases it is quite sufficient to apply the expressions given for repeated intravenous administration, since the resulting loading dose and also the maintenance interval and maintenance dose are generally conservative. Indeed, we may recall the following pharmacokinetic observations:

If equivalent doses of a drug are given to a person by a single intravenous and oral administration, then the maximal concentration (C_{max}) attained by the oral route is lower, and the time taken to get down to the minimum therapeutically effective concentration (C_{ther}) is usually longer. The latter statement is equivalent to saying that, from about the time of reaching C_{max} by the oral route, the corresponding concentration remains higher than that seen following the equivalent intravenous administration.

These principles are valid also for the case of repeated drug administration. Consequently, with the oral C_{max} being lower and the C_{min} higher than the equivalent quantities calculated for repeated intravenous dosing, we maintain the plasma concentration safely within the desirable range of C_{tox} and C_{ther}.

In the case of oral administration, all dosing equations must be again **multiplied** on the right-hand side by the **bioavailability** (F). This is the reason for talking about "equivalent doses" for the two routes of drug administration.

ACCUMULATION RATIO

The fractional attainment (f) of steady state during the elimination phase provides insight into the degree of accumulation.

Recalling that the loading dose is, for repeated intravenous injections,

$$L = VC_{max}, \text{ where } C_{max} = D_m/(Vf),$$

we get

$$L/D_m = C_{max}/C_0 = 1/f = 1/(1 - e^{-kt}).$$

Here $C_0 = D_m/V$ is the (extrapolated) initial concentration after a single administration of a dose of D_m.

The ratio of C_{max}/C_0 contrasts the maximum concentrations obtained by repeated and single injections of the same dose, respectively. Therefore, $1/f$ is called the **accumulation ratio**. It characterizes also the ratios of minimum concentrations for repeated and single administrations that are observed at times T_m following the respective maxima.

A good approximation for the accumulation ratio can be obtained by noting that

$$C_{max} \simeq \bar{C}_{ss} + (1/2)(D_m/V) = \bar{C}_{ss} + C_0/2.$$

Since

$$\bar{C}_{ss} = (D_m/T_m)/kV = C_0/kT_m,$$

we have

$$\bar{C}_{ss}/C_0 = 1/kT_m = (1/\ln 2)(t_{1/2}/T_m) \simeq \mathbf{1.44(t_{1/2}/T_m)}$$

and

$$\mathbf{C_{max}/C_0 = 1/f \simeq 1.44(t^{1/2}/T_m) + 0.5.}$$

Similarly, for the minimum concentration

$$\mathbf{C_{min}/C_0 \simeq \bar{C}_{ss} - C_0/2 \simeq 1.44(t^{1/2}/T_m) - 0.5.}$$

Note that all three ratios can be approximated by

$$C/C_0 \simeq 1.5(t^{1/2}/T_m)$$

when the drug is given frequently, *i.e.*, when $t_{1/2} > T_m$. (A rule of thumb for this condition could be: $t_{1/2} > 3T_m$.) This is a useful, simple calculating formula.

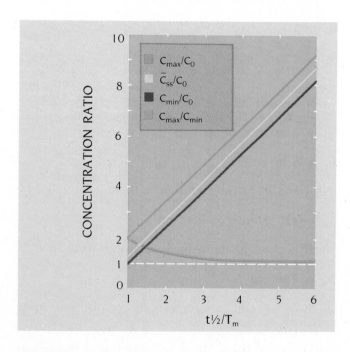

Figure 6–6 Concentration ratios characterizing repeated drug administration. (*See* text for explanation.)

With frequent dosing, the expressions characterize also the relationship between the loading and maintenance doses since, as we have seen,

$$L/D_m = C_{max}/C_0.$$

The (not approximated) ratios of C_{max}, $\overline{C}_{ss}$, and C_{min} to C_0 are shown in Figure 6–6. The diagram illustrates also

$$C_{max}/C_{min} = e^{kT_m} = 1/(1-f),$$

which measures the fluctuation of plasma concentration upon repeated drug administration. The following conclusions are worth noting:

1. In the special case of $T_m = t\frac{1}{2}$, i.e., when the maintenance interval equals the half-life, the accumulation ratio is 2. Consequently,

$$C_{max} = 2C_0, \quad L = 2D_m, \quad \text{and} \quad C_{max}/C_{min} = 2.$$

Thus, the maximal concentration reached upon repeated drug administration is double that attained by a single injection. Also, we can observe, under this condition, a two-fold fluctuation of the concentration.

2. The accumulation ratio increases and the fluctuation decreases with smaller T_m, i.e., when the drug is administered more frequently.

3. In particular, when T_m is very small, the accumulation ratio becomes very large. For instance, we can consider continuous exposure to chemicals in the environment. Even though their intake during a limited period (say, a day) is small, their accumulation could be very substantial.

SUGGESTED READING

Gibaldi M, Levy G. Pharmacokinetics in clinical practice. JAMA 1976; 235:1864–1867; 1987–1992.

Greenblatt DJ, Koch-Weser J. Clinical pharmacokinetics. N Engl J Med 1975; 293:702–705; 964–970.

Rowland M, Tozer TN. Clinical pharmacokinetics: Concepts and applications, 2nd ed. Philadelphia: Lea & Febiger, 1987.

Chapter 7

DRUG CLEARANCE BY SPECIFIC ORGANS

L. Endrenyi

ADDITIVITY OF ORGAN CLEARANCES

In Chapter 6, total body clearance was defined as the volume of body fluid (usually blood) from which the drug has been completely removed in a unit time. Similarly, **clearance by an individual organ** (e.g., the liver or kidney) **refers to the volume of body fluid from which that organ completely removes the drug in a unit time.**

The total amount of a drug eliminated from the body is the sum of the amounts eliminated by the various routes. Correspondingly, the overall rate of elimination is the sum of the specific rates of elimination of the drug through the various routes. (This is so since the rate of elimination is the amount of a drug removed in unit time.) For first-order processes, the respective specific (organ) clearances are also additive and sum up to the total body clearance (Cl or TBC, *see* Chapter 6). This can be seen from the additivity of the corresponding elimination rate constants and by noting that the clearances can be thought of as being products of the apparent volume of distribution and the respective rate constants.

As an example, let us consider a drug eliminated completely by hepatic (H) biotransformation and renal (R) excretion. Then, the total amount of the eliminated drug can be considered as a sum of its components:

Amount eliminated = Amount transformed in liver + Amount excreted in kidney.

The overall rate of elimination can be regarded in the same way:

Rate of elimination = Rate of hepatic transformation + Rate of renal excretion.

Since first-order rate constants are additive, the hepatic and renal constants sum to the elimination constant:

$$k = k_H + k_R.$$

The corresponding clearances are obtained by multiplying both sides of this expression by V (the apparent volume of distribution):

$$kV = k_H V + k_R V.$$

Consequently the equation

$$Cl = Cl_H + Cl_R$$

illustrates the additivity of the organ clearances.

In the following sections, drug elimination by various organs, and the corresponding clearances, will be considered briefly.

Organ clearance can also be obtained by dividing the amount of a drug removed by the organ during a unit time by the concentration of the drug entering the organ. This second definition is demonstrated below under *Perfusion Model*.

CLEARANCE BY THE LIVER

Perfusion Model

Consider an organ such as the liver, into which the drug enters at a concentration of C_a and from which it goes out at a smaller concentration of C_v (Fig. 7–1). The blood flow through the organ is Q mL/min. Then, at steady state during one minute:

Amount of drug entering the organ $= Q \cdot C_a$,
amount of drug leaving the organ $= Q \cdot C_v$,
amount of drug removed in the organ $= Q \cdot (C_a - C_v)$.

The fraction of drug removed or extracted by the organ from the blood is $(C_a - C_v)/C_a$. This fraction is called the (steady-state) **extraction ratio (E)**, which characterizes the effectiveness of the process of removing the drug:

$$E = (C_a - C_v)/C_a.$$

A value close to 1 (unity) suggests that most of the drug is quickly and efficiently cleared by the organ; a small extraction ratio, approaching zero, indicates a slow, ineffective process of removal.

If we multiply the blood flow (Q) by the fraction (E) of drug extracted by the organ, we should obtain the volume of blood from which the organ removes the drug. This is the organ clearance as defined earlier. As an example, the hepatic clearance is

$$Cl_H = Q \cdot E.$$

In the liver: Q = total hepatic blood flow; C_a = mixed portal venous and hepatic arterial drug concentration; C_v = hepatic venous drug concentration. Notice that hepatic clearance can be written as

$$Cl_H = Q \cdot (C_a - C_v)/C_a.$$

The numerator is the amount of drug cleared by the liver from the blood in one minute. This is divided by the concentration of the drug entering the organ. When expressed thus, the clearance is indeed calculated by following the second definition given in the previous section.

For an effectively extracted drug (E = 1), the hepatic clearance approaches the blood flow ($Cl_H \approx Q$). The liver is admirably set up for extracting large amounts of drugs because of its large size (1500 g), high blood

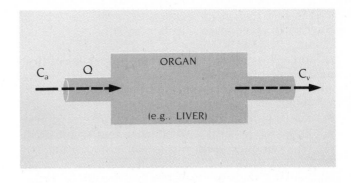

Figure 7–1 Model for organ clearance of drugs. As applied to the liver: Q = total hepatic blood flow; C_a = mixed portal venous and hepatic arterial drug concentration; C_v = hepatic venous drug concentration (*see* text).

flow (approximately 1 mL/g tissue/min), and unique architecture that brings blood into contact with many cell surfaces. It follows that the hepatic clearance of highly extracted drugs approaches 1500 mL/min. Conversely, low extraction is indicated by hepatic clearance much below 1500 mL/min.

First-Pass Effect

Following oral intake of a drug, only a fraction (F) of the administered amount may reach the systemic circulation. Losses may occur by decomposition or by biotransformation in the gastrointestinal lumen. From there, the drug passes across the membranes of the gastrointestinal tract into the portal vein, then through the liver, and finally into the general circulation. During this so-called first pass, enzymes may transform some of the drug either in the membranes and cells of the gut wall, or in the liver, or perhaps in both locations. For instance, lidocaine is extensively extracted by the liver, while salicylamide undergoes biotransformation and extraction in both intestinal wall and liver.

A substantial loss of a drug can be expected during its first pass through the liver if its hepatic biotransformation is fast and efficient, *i.e.*, if its hepatic extraction ratio is high. Generally, the availability after first passage through the liver can be obtained from

$$F_H = 1 - E.$$

For example, the hepatic extraction ratio of lidocaine, an antiarrhythmic drug, is 0.7. Consequently, the oral bioavailability of the drug is only 30%. This is an upper limit for the oral bioavailability of the drug, since losses during the first pass of the drug can occur not only by hepatic biotransformation but also by other processes.

This is one reason for administering the drug by intravenous injection or infusion.

There are a number of **important properties of first-pass drug extraction**:
- It is drug-specific, ranging from zero to complete removal.
- The first-pass effect is often saturable.
- For some drugs it is so effective that at low doses no drug may reach the systemic circulation.
- In liver disease, drugs with high first-pass extraction will become available systemically in higher than expected concentrations. This can happen as a result of either impaired function of liver parenchymal cells, or intrahepatic shunts bypassing the sinusoid and carrying blood directly from the hepatic artery and portal vein to the terminal hepatic vein. Therefore, the drug dose may need to be decreased to prevent toxicity.
- Pharmacologic effects may be markedly different after intravenous than after oral administration. For instance, if it is a drug metabolite that is active, oral administration of a drug may be more effective (or toxic) than intravenous injection of the same dose, provided that the biotransformation occurs in the liver.
- Low systemic bioavailability often indicates a first-pass effect.
- Complex and unpredictable drug kinetics can be expected as a consequence of the first-pass effect, depending on the relative contribution of intestinal or hepatic binding and/or biotransformation to the phenomenon.

Factors Affecting Hepatic Clearance

Two main factors contribute to the efficiency of hepatic drug clearance:

1. The amount extracted by the liver is expected to increase along with the blood supply, *i.e.*, when the **blood flow** (Q) is higher.

2. Transformation in the liver is assisted when the molecular relationships and conditions in that organ are favorable to biotransformation. These conditions can be characterized by a parameter that is called the **intrinsic clearance of the free (unbound) drug** ($Cl_{intr,f}$). The intrinsic clearance increases together with (1) a larger concentration and amount of the catalysing enzyme in the liver, and (2) a greater affinity between the drug molecule and the enzyme.

If one of the two components, blood flow and intrinsic clearance, is much smaller than the other, then it has controlling influence on the extraction ratio and, therefore, on the hepatic clearance. For instance, if the intrinsic clearance is much lower than the blood flow ($Cl_{intr,f} \ll Q$), then the blood supply is quite ample and its change would, in practice, not affect the hepatic extraction. Alteration of the intrinsic clearance, on the other hand, directly modifies the hepatic clearance in such cases. (Low intrinsic clearance can be a consequence of a drug entering the hepatic cells relatively slowly, by simple diffusion. Drugs with low intrinsic clearance include antipyrine and the anticoagulant warfarin.)

In the reverse condition, if the intrinsic clearance substantially exceeds the blood flow ($Cl_{intr,f} \gg Q$), the available enzymic activity is relatively in excess and does not limit the overall rate of biotransformation. Hepatic clearance is dependent now on blood flow: a change in the blood flow causes a corresponding alteration of the clearance. (Drugs having high intrinsic clearance are often concentrated in the hepatocytes and thereby allow the efficient execution of enzymatic reactions. Examples of drugs with high intrinsic clearance include acetylsalicylic acid, morphine, and propranolol.)

Thus, for drugs exhibiting a low extraction ratio, the hepatic clearance is modified by various factors that affect the intrinsic clearance of the free drug. These factors include:

- The binding of a drug to plasma proteins and other constituents in the blood. Binding reduces the concentration of the free drug and its intrinsic clearance.
- Conditions modifying the activity of the catalysing enzyme. Inhibitors reduce, and enzyme inducers increase, this activity.

These factors lose importance for drugs having a high intrinsic clearance. In fact, binding to plasma proteins may have, to some extent, an opposite effect. Since proteins efficiently carry the drug molecules within the circulation, binding to them may actually facilitate clearance. As we have already seen, drugs with strong intrinsic clearance show a substantial first-pass effect.

Table 7–1 summarizes factors involved in, and influencing, the hepatic clearance of high- and low-extraction drugs.

CLEARANCE BY THE KIDNEY

Urinary excretion is a major route for the elimination of many drugs from the body. Generally, the kidney efficiently removes polar (hydrophilic) substances, but not lipophilic drugs. Consequently, before being excreted, many of these drugs undergo either conjugation or hydroxylation reactions that yield more polar products (*see* Chapter 4).

The functional anatomic units of the kidney are the nephrons. Arterial blood passes first through the glomerulus, which filters some of the plasma water and its contents. Many, but not all, substances are also secreted in the proximal tubules. Most of the water is reabsorbed all along the nephron, in sequence, from the proximal, distal, and collecting tubules. Consequently, only 1–2 mL/min of the filtered water remains in the form of urine for elimination. Many, but not all,

TABLE 7–1 Features of, and Representative Drugs with, High and Low Hepatic Extraction

High Extraction	Low Extraction
Hepatic clearance controlled by rate of blood flow.	Hepatic clearance controlled by intrinsic clearance (hepatic biotransformation processes).
Strong first-pass effect.	Biotransformation limited by diffusion.
Plasma protein binding may facilitate clearance.	Plasma protein binding reduces clearance.
	Sensitive to enzyme inhibition, induction.
Amitriptyline, Imipramine	Antipyrine
Chlorpromazine	Diazepam
L-Dopa	Digitoxin
Lidocaine	Phenylbutazone
Morphine, Methadone, Heroin	Phenytoin
Propoxyphene	Theophylline
Propranolol, Alprenolol	Tolbutamide
Tyramine	Warfarin

substances can also be reabsorbed by the tubular epithelium and passed into the renal interstitial fluid and from there back into the plasma.

Thus, renal excretion of drugs is the result of three processes: glomerular filtration, tubular secretion, and tubular reabsorption. Therefore:

Rate of renal excretion = Rate of filtration + Rate of secretion – Rate of reabsorption.

The renal clearance of a substance can be calculated, in accordance with the definition given earlier, by measuring the amount excreted during a time period and dividing it by the length of the period and by the average plasma concentration observed during this interval:

$$Cl_R = \frac{\text{Excreted amount/Time interval}}{\text{Plasma concentration}}$$

Similarly to the rate of excretion, the clearance can be subdivided into components representing filtration, secretion, and reabsorption.

Glomerular Filtration

Glomerular filtration is limited by the size of the pores in the capillary endothelium and the ultrafiltration membrane (400–600 Å diameter). Thus, only small molecules are filtered by the glomeruli into the tubular fluid. Large macromolecules, including most proteins, can not pass

through the filter. Consequently, only free drugs, unbound to plasma proteins, can be filtered. Farther down the tubule, most of the filtered water is reabsorbed, together with variable amounts of free drug, which would reassociate with protein. The end result is that the binding equilibrium is almost unchanged.

The filtration process is passive (i.e., it proceeds in the direction of the concentration gradient) and relatively slow: it is limited by the rate of diffusion to and across the filter.

Plasma water is filtered at a rate of about 120 mL/min. This is called the glomerular filtration rate (GFR). Inulin, an exogenous polysaccharide, and creatinine, an endogenous N-containing substance, do not bind to plasma proteins and do not undergo tubular secretion or reabsorption to any significant degree. Therefore, they are widely used as indicators of the GFR. An observed inulin or creatinine clearance of substantially less than 120 mL/min suggests impairment of renal glomerular function.

The GFR of about 120 mL/min is also used as a marker of excretion processes in healthy subjects. A renal clearance in excess of 120 mL/min points to tubular secretion of a substance in addition to its glomerular filtration. A renal clearance less than 120 mL/min indicates net tubular reabsorption (following, or in addition to, filtration and secretion).

Tubular Secretion

The cells of the proximal convoluted tubules actively transport certain substances from the plasma to the tubular urine. The transfer of drugs occurs here **against the concentration gradient**: the drugs become relatively concentrated within the tubular lumen.

Active transport processes are characterized by:

1. **Energy requirement**. They do not occur if the cell metabolism is impaired. Uncouplers of oxidative phosphorylation, such as dinitrophenol, which inhibit the synthesis of ATP by the cell, block active transport.

2. **Saturation kinetics**. In most cases the process can be described by simple Michaelis-Menten type kinetics in which the combination of the molecule to be transported (D) and the carrier system (C) occurs first; CD is translocated and dissociation occurs afterwards. As in enzymatic reactions, the carrier system recognizes the transported molecules in a stereospecific fashion. When all the carrier molecules are in the CD form, maximal velocity of transport, called T_m, is attained. Since the cell membrane contains limited amounts of carrier molecules, in the presence of two substances (D_1 and D_2) transported by the same carrier, D_1 acts as an inhibitor of the transport of D_2 and vice versa. In general, the more slowly a substance is transported (i.e., the longer it occupies the carrier), the more effectively this substance inhibits the transport of another one.

Active tubular secretion is a relatively fast process

that clears practically all of the drug, bound to plasma proteins or free, from the blood. Actually only the unbound drug is transported across the tubular epithelium. However, as the free drug is removed from the plasma, its equilibrium with the protein-bound entity is disturbed, and the complex dissociates, replacing some of the unbound substance. The result is the apparent (but not physically simultaneous) removal of nearly all of the drug during the passage of the blood along the peritubular capillaries.

There are at least two transport mechanisms, one for acidic, the other one for basic substances (Table 7–2). It is the ionized molecules that are transported.

Para-aminohippuric acid (PAH), an exogenous organic acid, is virtually completely filtered and secreted, but not reabsorbed. Since, following ingestion, it is located in the plasma (partially bound to proteins), its renal excretion provides a measure of renal plasma flow. Typically it is around 600 mL/min.

Tubular Reabsorption

The importance of renal tubular reabsorption of organic substances as a homeostatic process is clear when one considers that most nutrients and vitamins present in plasma gain access to the glomerular filtrate. Consider, for example, the case of glucose. Under normal conditions virtually all the glucose filtered is reabsorbed, so that no glucose appears in the urine, unless the capacity of the transporting mechanisms is exceeded, as occurs in the advanced diabetic state or after large infusions of glucose. The fact that glucose, an uncharged substance, is reabsorbed into the blood against a large concentration gradient (tubular fluid:plasma) indicates that an **active transport process** is responsible for the absorption.

Not all the reabsorption of organic molecules is accomplished by active transport processes. Many compounds are **passively reabsorbed**. These substances leave the filtrate to enter the tubular cells and should be able to leave the cell again, in the direction of the blood. Thus, at least two lipidic cell membranes have to be crossed. As will be remembered, lipid-soluble substances are able to cross cell membranes and are thus passively reabsorbed. Charged molecules, in general, are not able to cross the tubular epithelial cell membranes and are thus excreted in the urine. (Note, however, that this does not mean that all uncharged molecules will be reabsorbed. Molecules such as sucrose, that are not charged but that are not lipid-soluble either, are not passively reabsorbed.)

Factors that have to be considered in the passive reabsorption of substances from the tubular filtrate are the volume of the filtrate formed per minute (and thus the rate of movement down the tubule and the degree of probability of contact with the membrane) and, most importantly from the clinical point of view, the pH of tubular fluid. Acidification of urine by different means results in a greater proportion of an acidic molecule A^- being in the uncharged HA form, thus increasing its passive reabsorption at the tubular level. The reverse will occur for basic molecules, which in an acid medium will tend to shift to the BH^+ (charged) form. The pK_a of the substance (i.e., the pH of the aqueous phase at which the numbers of ionized and nonionized molecules are equal) will of course determine the relative proportions of the charged and uncharged forms at any pH. Changes in the pH of the tubular fluid are known to affect markedly the urinary excretion of phenobarbital and salicylate (Table 7–3). Some types of diuretics will render the filtrate acid or alkaline (see Chapter 40). For a large variety of drugs, conjugation with strong acids occurs in the liver. Conjugates that are strong acids, such as glucuronic acid conjugates and sulfuric acid conjugates, will remain dissociated at most physiologic pHs attained in the kidney and are therefore readily excreted in the urine.

TABLE 7–2 Examples of Drugs and Drug Metabolites That Are Actively Secreted Into the Renal Tubules

Acids	Bases
Penicillin	Quaternary ammonium compounds
Chlorothiazide	(e.g., choline, tetraethylammonium,
Salicylic acid	N-methylnicotine, N-methylnicotinamide)
Phenolsulfonphthalein	Guanidine derivatives
Diodone (urographic medium)	Tolazoline
Carinamide	Quinine
Probenecid	Mepiperphenodol
Cinchophen	
p-Aminohippuric acid and other glycine conjugates	
Glucuronic acid conjugates	
Sulfuric acid conjugates	

TABLE 7–3 Effect of Degree of Ionization on Rate of Urinary Excretion of Drugs

		Urinary Clearance Ratios*	
Drug	pK$_a$	Acid Urine	Alkaline Urine
Basic Drugs		(more ionized)	(less ionized)
Quinacrine	7.7	3.0	0.5
Procaine	8.95	2.25	0.25
Mecamylamine	11.2	4.6	0.06
Acidic Drugs		(less ionized)	(more ionized)
Phenobarbital	7.4	0.1	0.7
Salicylate	3.0	0.02	1.6

* Clearance ratios are equal to $\dfrac{\text{clearance of substance}}{\text{clearance of inulin}}$.
Ratios greater than 1 imply net tubular secretion; ratios less than 1 imply net reabsorption.

Examples of Drugs Affecting Tubular Secretion and Reabsorption

Probenecid

Probenecid is a drug specifically developed in the early 1950s to prevent the rapid excretion of penicillin when this antibiotic was very scarce and expensive. Penicillin (*see* Chapter 53) is secreted in the proximal tubule by the acid-secreting system. As can be expected, probenecid is also an acid, and it thus acts by competition, inhibiting the secretion of penicillin.

As illustrated in Figure 7–2, probenecid in low concentrations also depresses the urinary excretion of uric acid by inhibiting its secretion. Nevertheless, probenecid (Benemid®) is of clinical usefulness in the treatment of gout (for which one tries to *increase* the excretion of uric acid), due to the fact that higher doses also inhibit the active reabsorption of uric acid farther down the

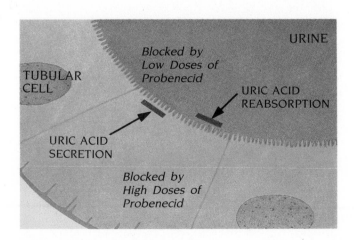

Figure 7–2 Actions of probenecid on the secretion and reabsorption of uric acid by renal tubular cells.

tubule. The reabsorption system has a greater capacity to translocate uric acid than the secretory system does. Therefore, under these conditions uric acid excretion is increased.

Sulfinpyrazone

In the process of synthesizing a uricosuric agent of the potency of phenylbutazone (*see* Chapter 33), but without its undesirable side effects, sulfinpyrazone (Anturan®) was discovered. This is a strong organic acid (pK$_a$ 2.8) that can form soluble salts.

This drug, in sufficiently high doses, is a potent inhibitor of the renal tubular reabsorption of uric acid. In low doses, however, it reduces the excretion of uric acid, presumably by inhibiting the secretory process. As described for other drugs (*e.g.*, salicylic acid) that are also transported by the acid-secretory system, the mechanism appears to be a simple competition.

BILIARY EXCRETION

Bile is formed by secretion in liver cells (*see* Chapter 62). From bile capillaries (canaliculi) located there, the bile flows into the larger bile ductules, which converge into the bile ducts. These lead into the gall bladder where the bile is stored and concentrated, and from where it is emptied into the duodenum.

The biliary excretion of substances involves two steps, (1) their transfer from the plasma across the hepatic cell membrane into parenchymal cells of the liver, and (2) their active transport across the membrane separating the liver cell from the bile canaliculus. After transient storage in the gall bladder, the compounds enter the small intestine. From here, they are either excreted into the feces or reabsorbed into the portal circulation. By returning to the plasma, they complete the **enterohepatic cycle**, which can substantially extend the duration of their presence in the body.

The active secretion of drugs into the bile takes place against a concentration gradient and results in elevation of their biliary concentration. Acids and bases have separate transport systems; two substances transferred by the same system can inhibit each other's secretion.

The biliary clearance can be calculated by dividing the amount excreted in unit time by the plasma concentration. The amount excreted in unit time is the product of the concentration in bile and of the bile flow. Hence:

$$Cl_B = \frac{\text{Concentration in bile}}{\text{Concentration in plasma}} \times \text{Bile flow.}$$

The bile flow is typically 0.5–0.8 mL/min. Consequently, biliary clearance is sizeable only when the drug concentration in the bile is much higher than that in the plasma. For example, with a concentration ratio of 1000, the biliary clearance is about 500–800 mL/min.

Generally, polar compounds are able to undergo biliary excretion. Often, such substances are formed in the liver when a drug is transformed to a polar conjugate such as a glucuronide, glycine, or sulfate conjugate. A substantial fraction of the conjugates can be hydrolysed again to re-form the original drug when reaching the gut, thus allowing it to be reabsorbed under certain conditions.

Another limitation on substances undergoing biliary excretion involves their size. Only those having molecular weights of at least 250 appear in the bile. The explanation for this phenomenon is not well understood.

SUGGESTED READING

Cafruny EL. Renal tubular handling of drugs. Am J Med 1977; 62:490–496.

Plaa GL. The enterohepatic circulation. In: Gillette JR, Mitchell JR, eds. Handbook of experimental pharmacology. Vol. 28. Berlin: Springer-Verlag, 1975:130.

Rowland M, Benet LZ, Graham GG. Clearance concepts in pharmacokinetics. J Pharmacokinet Biopharm 1973; 1:123–136.

Wilkinson GR, Shand DG. A physiological approach to drug clearance. Clin Pharmacol Ther 1975; 18:377–390.

Chapter 8

DOSE-RESPONSE RELATIONSHIPS

L. Endrenyi

LOG-DOSE–RESPONSE CURVES

A central question of drug therapy is the proper dose of the drug under consideration that produces a desired therapeutic action without harmful side effects. To clarify the problem, an analysis of the relationship between dose and response is required.

It is customary to contrast these quantities in diagrams that plot the effect of the drug against the logarithm of the corresponding dose. These diagrams yield **log-dose–response (LDR) curves**.

For example, increasing doses of histamine cause gradually increasing contraction of the guinea pig ileum. Very low doses of histamine have practically no effect, and responses can be observed only beyond a threshold dose of about 20 ng. Again, very high doses of more than about 50 μg have no additional effect and the response remains constant at this maximal level (Fig. 8–1).

The effect of using a logarithmic dose scale is very important. First, notice that in the example of the histamine response, the horizontal dose scale is indeed logarithmic since the distances between 1 and 10 μg, or 10 and 100 μg (or 20 and 200 μg, or 5 and 50 μg) are identical. Second, Figure 8–1 indicates that there are only small differences between the responses that are produced by doses of, for instance, 1.0 or 1.1 or even 1.5 μg histamine. The physician is often concerned

too much about such minute differences. Rather, one should want to know what the effects are of double, five-fold, ten-fold, *etc.* dosages.

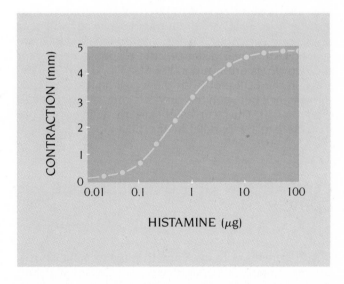

Figure 8–1 Log-dose–response relationships between doses of histamine and muscle contraction (*see* text).

PROPERTIES OF LOG-DOSE–RESPONSE CURVES

1. They describe the LDR-relationship over a wide range of doses.

2. LDR-curves are typically S-shaped or "sigmoidal." Their middle section is approximately straight: this observation facilitates their statistical analysis. This property is used to good advantage in the analysis of bioassays when drug concentrations (doses) are evaluated from the corresponding responses observed in biologic samples.

3. Frequently the same effect is produced by different drugs acting with an identical, or at least similar, mechanism. In such cases the LDR-curves of the drugs may be expected to run parallel to each other. For example, let us assume that drug A is twice as potent as drug B. Then, in comparison with A, twice as much B is needed to produce some given, identical response. This is true throughout the full range of concentrations. Consequently, in a plot contrasting a response with the corresponding dose, points on the curve characterizing drug B will always lie the same distance to the right of the curve for drug A (Fig. 8–2).

Furthermore, at a given height (*i.e.*, response) of the plot, the dose of drug B will be twice as great as that of drug A (*see* Fig. 8–2B). In the plot having the linear dose scale (when 20, 40, 60, and 80 mg/kg doses are spaced with equal distance), the response curves for the two drugs are not parallel (*see* Fig. 8–2A). In contrast, in the LDR-plot (with the logarithmic dose scale) the distance between the curves is constant and equals log 2 = 0.30. Thus, curves of similarly acting drugs are expected to be parallel in the LDR-plot.

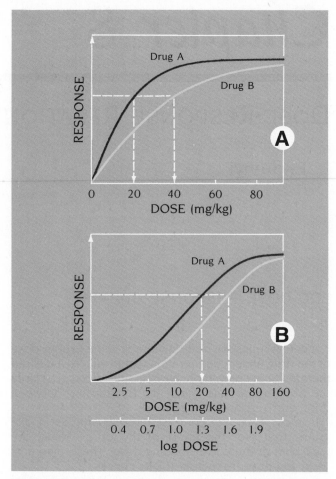

Figure 8–2   (*A*) Linear dose-response plot, and (*B*) LDR-plot of two drugs having different potencies.

COMPARISON OF DOSE-RESPONSE CURVES

The strengths of drugs A and B, in the example above, can be compared quantitatively. In this example, when the potency of drug A is double the potency of drug B, we would say that the relative potency of drug A with respect to drug B is R = 2.0. Of course, this can be stated in other ways, *e.g.*, that drug B is only one-half as potent as drug A, or that the relative potency of drug B with respect to drug A is R = 0.50.

In general, if different drugs have parallel LDR-curves (as when they act by identical mechanisms), then from their horizontal distances the relative potencies can be evaluated. This is so, since the horizontal concentration scale is logarithmic and therefore the horizontal distance between two curves equals the corresponding value of log R.

Relative potencies are customary measures for comparing relative strengths of different drugs or drug preparations. Their use implies parallelism of LDR-curves. In contrast, parallelism is not assumed when the strengths of drugs are compared on the basis of their **equipotent doses**. These are doses of the investigated drugs that give rise to the same designated response. For instance, in Figure 8–2, 20 mg/kg of drug A and 40 mg/kg of drug B are equipotent doses.

AN INTERPRETATION OF THE LDR-CURVE: RECEPTOR OCCUPANCY

According to one frequently adopted theory of drug action, the drug molecules would have to attach themselves to receptors in the body before these initiate the process of response action (*see* Chapter 9). Thus, the intensity of drug action is proportional to the occupancy of the receptors or, in other words, to the concentration of the drug-receptor complexes, [DR]:

$$Response = \alpha[DR] \,.$$

The complex is formed from its components and decomposes into them in a dynamic equilibrium:

$$D + R \underset{k_{-1}}{\overset{k_1}{\rightleftharpoons}} DR \,.$$

This picture is quite analogous to the Michaelis-Menten description of simple enzyme reactions, in which an enzyme-substrate complex is in dynamic equilibrium with its components and forms the reaction product at a rate proportional to the concentration of the complex. It is not surprising, then, that the mathematical descriptions of the two processes are also similar. The dependence of the response on the concentration of unbound drug is characterized by an expression of a hyperbola:

$$Response = \frac{\alpha[D][R]}{(K+[D])} \,,$$

where $K = k_{-1}/k_1$ is the dissociation constant of the drug-receptor complex; the square brackets imply the appropriate concentrations. This expression is analogous to the relationship between the velocity of an enzyme-catalysed reaction and the free substrate concentration. It can be converted into a straight-line expression:

$$\frac{1}{Resp} = \frac{1}{Resp_{max}} + \frac{K}{Resp_{max}} \cdot \frac{1}{[D]} \,,$$

where Resp and $Resp_{max}$ refer to the response and its maximally attainable value, respectively. Figure 8–3 illustrates the histamine data replotted in this way.

The two formulae are not important, just as the calculations shown in Figure 8–3 illustrate only the essential point: The dissociation constant and the maximal response can be evaluated from the "double reciprocal" plot (and also from some other similarly linear plots).

ALL-OR-NONE EFFECTS

The example of histamine, which we have just discussed, described a typical graded effect: a slight increase of the dose should bring about a small increase of the response. There are occasions when the available information indicates only that a given dose of a drug either has or has not evoked a certain effect

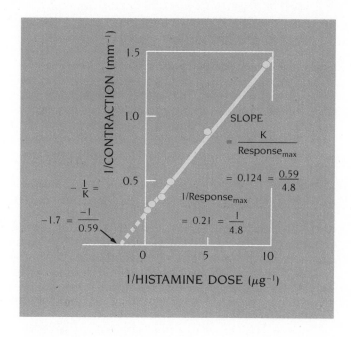

Figure 8–3 Double reciprocal plot for the effect of histamine on muscle contraction (data from Figure 8–1).

in the various subjects under investigation. Examples for such **quantal** or **all-or-none** responses are the presence or absence of convulsion, death, anaesthetic effect, improvement in a disease state, *etc*. Usually, either the proportion, the percentage, or the actual number of subjects responding to a given dose of the drug is recorded.

Thus, actually only a fraction of the subjects responds to certain drug dosages, while the remaining proportion fails to react. The reason lies in biologic variation, *i.e.*, in the diversity, the differing sensitivity of the subjects to drug action. Individuals range from the very sensitive, hyperreactive to the least sensitive, hyporeactive subjects: persons whom the drug produces its usual effect at unexpectedly low or uncommonly high doses, respectively.

HISTOGRAMS AND CUMULATIVE FREQUENCY PLOTS

When the dosage is varied, the number (or better, the fraction or the percentage) of subjects responding can be plotted against the dose or, preferably, its logarithm. Consider the following example: In each of 60 dogs an investigator gradually increased the rate of intravenous adrenaline* infusion until a 35% enhancement of the heart rate was observed. Up to 10 ng/kg/min, this endpoint was reached in one dog; between

---

* epinephrine

10 and 13 ng/kg/min in two additional dogs; between 13 and 17 ng/kg/min in six more of the animals; and so on. These data are displayed in a so-called histogram, which illustrates the distribution of sensitivities to adrenaline induction of heart rate increases in the various dogs (Fig. 8–4). The histogram is characteristically bell-shaped in similarity to curves describing the so-called **normal distribution** (*see* below).

The data can be rearranged to include the number (or fraction) of subjects responding to **all** doses that are lower or equal to the dose under investigation. For example, as before, 35% increase in the heart rate was recorded **up to** an adrenaline infusion rate of 10 ng/kg/min in one dog (1.7%); **up to** 13 ng/kg/min **in a total of** three animals (5.0%); **up to** 17 ng/kg/min **in a total of** nine dogs (15.0%); and so on. The data characterize the **cumulative distribution** of the sensitivities (Fig. 8–5). A curve fitted to them describes the cumulative rearrangement of the normal distribution, the shape of which is very similar to that of an LDR-curve.

It is important to notice that all-or-none responses are observed in individual subjects (or experimental animals) and that the recorded quantity (proportion, percentage, actual number of subjects reacting) is not identical to the response itself. On the other hand, as illustrated in the example of the response to adrenaline, graded effects (*e.g.*, increase in the heart rate) can be converted to quantal responses by selecting

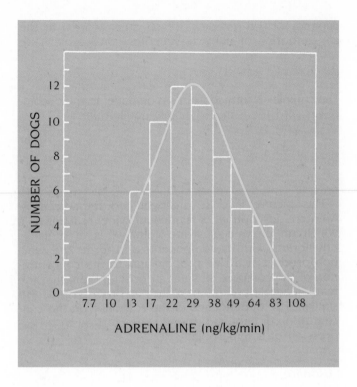

Figure 8–4 Distribution of dogs responding to various infusion rates of adrenaline. (Histogram indicating normal distribution; *see* text.)

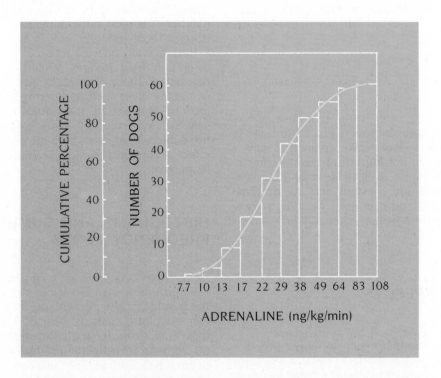

Figure 8–5 Cumulative distribution of dogs responding to various rates of adrenaline infusion. (Data from Fig. 8–4. The fitted curve describes distribution similar to an LDR-curve.)

a given level of the former (*e.g.*, 35% increase) and observing the number (or fraction, or percentage) of subjects affected to that degree by certain doses of the drug.

In the example, the doses corresponding to consecutive class limits have been increased by a constant ratio, by about 30%. Equivalently it can be said that the observations are pooled into groups (classes), which have limits with logarithmically uniform increments, *i.e.*, that the horizontal dose scale is approximately logarithmic.

MEDIAN EFFECTIVE AND MEDIAN LETHAL DOSE

It is possible to evaluate doses to which 20%, 70%, 84%, or any other percentage of the subjects responds. It is customary to calculate such **effective doses**, abbreviated as ED_{20}, ED_{70}, ED_{84}, *etc.*, and especially the **median effective dose** or **ED_{50}**, which is, of course, the dose that gives rise to a response in 50% of the subjects. When drugs have parallel LDR-curves, their potencies can be compared through their ED_{50}s; the more potent the drug, the lower is its ED_{50}.

If the response is mortality (*e.g.*, in animal experiments designed to evaluate potency or toxicity), then instead of effective doses we speak of **lethal doses**. For instance, we characterize a dose that gives rise to the death of 50% of the subjects as the **median lethal dose** or **LD_{50}**. A harmful side effect is manifested in one-half of the subjects at the **median toxic dose** or **TD_{50}**. Anaesthetists talk about anaesthetic doses or AD_{50}s, which have the same interpretation as the ED_{50}s.

The strict definition of effective doses, and specifically of the ED_{50}, involves quantal responses: The dosage is sought at which a given percentage (frequently 50%) of the subjects is affected. A looser, less rigorous definition, which is often used in the pharmacologic literature, extends the applicability to graded responses. According to this interpretation, the ED_{50} is the dose giving rise to one-half of the asymptotic, maximum (continous) effect.

LINEAR PROBIT PLOT

As seen earlier, sensitivities of various subjects responding to a given drug dosage are frequently characterized by the normal distribution. For all-or-none responses, the cumulative arrangement of this distribution takes the form of the sigmoidal log-dose–response relationship (*see* Fig. 8–5). This becomes very useful since properties of the normal distribution have been investigated in great detail.

The considerations described below suggest that straight lines are obtained if the cumulative fractions or percentages of quantal responses are plotted against the logarithm of the dose on a normal probability paper or in the probit scale. Figure 8–6 illustrates such a plot for the adrenaline data.

BASIS OF THE PROBIT PLOT

The diagram in Figure 8–7 shows the bell-shaped (theoretical) normal distribution and the corresponding cumulative curve that represents the LDR-plot. The centres of both curves (coinciding with the peak of the bell curve) occur at the mean. Fifty percent of the subjects respond at this point and the corresponding dose is the ED_{50}.

One of the characteristic features of the normal distribution curve is that two-thirds of the population under study will fall within the range of 1 standard deviation (SD) to each side of the mean or ED_{50}. In other words, the ED_{16} and ED_{84} (*i.e.*, the doses that cause the effect in 16% and 84%, respectively, of all the individuals tested) lie at equal distances of 1 standard deviation below and above the ED_{50}. The ED_{31} and ED_{69} represent 0.5 standard deviation below and above the ED_{50}; the ED_7 and ED_{93} are 1.5 standard deviations, and the $ED_{2.3}$ and $ED_{97.7}$ are 2 standard deviations to each side, and so forth (*see* Fig. 8–7).

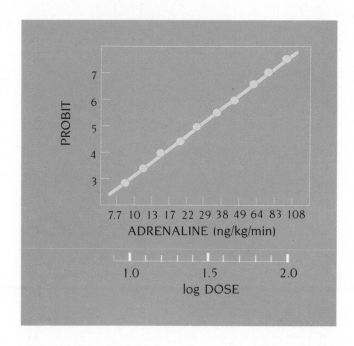

Figure 8–6   Probit plot for responses to adrenaline infusion shown in Figures 8–4 and 8–5.

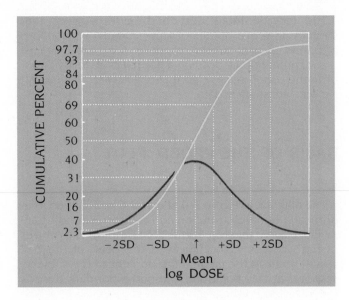

Figure 8–7 Bell-shaped, theoretical normal distribution (with arbitrary vertical scale), and corresponding cumulative curve representing the LDR-plot (actual scale).

tion units above or below the ED_{50}. The response corresponding to ED_{50} then has a value of 0, the ED_{16} is -1.0, the ED_{84} is $+1.0$, and so forth. (These values are called Normal Equivalent Deviates, or NED.) To avoid the $+$ and $-$ signs, 5 is added to every value, so that the response corresponding to ED_{16} (-1) becomes 4, at ED_{50} it is 5, at ED_{84} ($+1$) it is 6, and so on. The units in this scale are called "probability units" or **probits** (Fig. 8–8).

Special "probability papers" and "probit papers" (*i.e.*, pre-printed graph papers) are available for plotting the results in probits against the logarithms of the doses, to give a straight line. However, such plots can be constructed also without using special graph papers if the observed cumulative percentages are directly converted into probits with the help of the tabulation given in Table 8–1.

EVALUATION OF DRUG SAFETY

Therefore, one way of converting the sigmoidal LDR-curve to a straight line is to express all the values on the vertical (response) axis in terms of standard devia-

In addition to its therapeutic effect, a drug is likely to have one or more kinds of harmful side effects. Higher doses may even cause death. Each of these responses can be characterized by an LDR-curve. In general, the drug is considered to be safe if the LDR

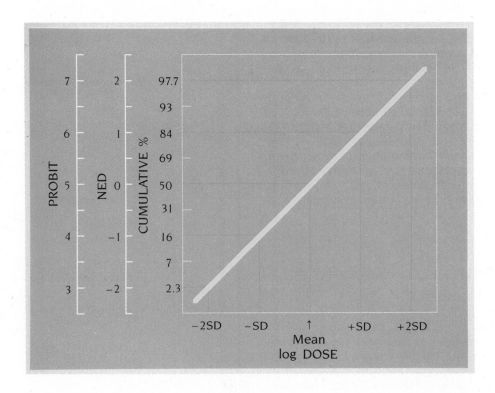

Figure 8–8 Probit plot for normal distribution (NED = Normal Equivalent Deviates).

TABLE 8–1 Conversion of Percent to Probit

%	0	1	2	3	4	5	6	7	8	9
0	—	2.67	2.95	3.12	3.25	3.36	3.45	3.52	3.59	3.66
10	3.72	3.77	3.82	3.87	3.92	3.96	4.01	4.05	4.08	4.12
20	4.16	4.19	4.23	4.26	4.29	4.33	4.36	4.39	4.42	4.45
30	4.48	4.50	4.53	4.56	4.59	4.61	4.64	4.67	4.69	4.72
40	4.75	4.77	4.80	4.82	4.85	4.87	4.90	4.92	4.95	4.97
50	5.00	5.03	5.05	5.08	5.10	5.13	5.15	5.18	5.20	5.23
60	5.25	5.28	5.31	5.33	5.36	5.39	5.41	5.44	5.47	5.50
70	5.52	5.55	5.58	5.61	5.64	5.67	5.71	5.74	5.77	5.81
80	5.84	5.88	5.92	5.95	5.99	6.04	6.08	6.13	6.18	6.23
90	6.28	6.34	6.41	6.48	6.55	6.64	6.75	6.88	7.05	7.33

region of the harmful side effects is much higher than the therapeutic dose range. This idea is expressed by the

therapeutic index: TI = TD_{50}/ED_{50} ,

which should be as high as possible for maximal safety.

However, this frequently used index does not characterize sufficiently the relative safety of different drugs. Figure 8–9 shows the therapeutic and one of the toxic all-or-none LDR-curves of two drugs, A and B. (For convenience only, the responses are illustrated in the probit scale in which straight lines are obtained. For further convenience, parallel lines for therapeutic and toxic responses are assumed. However, the following arguments could be pursued also with non-parallel responses depicted in any diagram.)

The two drugs shown in Figure 8–9 have identical ED_{50} and also TD_{50} values; consequently they have identical values for the therapeutic index. The relative safeties of the two drugs, however, are quite different: a comparatively high dose of drug B may be beneficial to many or even most patients, but it will also be toxic to some of them (indicated by solid circles in Fig. 8–9). Drug A, on the other hand, which has a steeper probit line, does not involve such risks: an almost completely curative dose has nearly none of the toxic effects (indicated by solid squares in Fig. 8–9). Such differences in drug behavior are characterized by the

certain safety factor: CSF = TD_1/ED_{99} .

It will be low for drug B and much higher for the "safer" drug A. Such quantitative considerations of drug safety apply of course equally to side effects and to lethality: In the latter case, CSF = LD_1/ED_{99}.

Two further remarks can be made: First, a drug may have several therapeutic indices and certain safety factors, one for each comparison of a toxic or lethal response with a therapeutic effect. Second, the LDR-curves for various responses to a drug, whether therapeutic, toxic, or lethal, need not be parallel. Indeed, evaluation of therapeutic indices and certain safety factors does not require any assumption of parallelism.

There is an additional complication. The therapeutic and side effect LDR-curves vary from patient to patient. So it is possible, and it occurs with alarming frequency, that a dose that is therapeutic in one patient causes ill effects in the other. The physician must be alert to such variations.

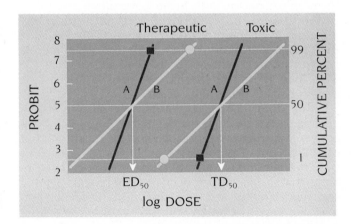

Figure 8–9 Plot illustrating the certain safety factor (*see* text).

SUGGESTED READING

Tallarida RJ, Jacob LS. The dose-response relation in pharmacology. New York/Heidelberg/Berlin: Springer-Verlag, 1979.

Chapter 9

DRUG RECEPTORS

P. Seeman

The late 1800s saw a rapid development of the synthetic pharmaceutical industry as an outgrowth of the invention of color-fast dyes. These dye-based pharmaceuticals were to become the first antibacterial agents with selective toxicity. In this intellectual climate of rapid biologic discoveries, Paul Ehrlich experimented with arsphenamine ("Salvarsan"), which he attempted to develop into a specific anti-syphilis drug. In explanation of the apparent specific drug action, Ehrlich introduced the idea that a drug might act as a "magic bullet" that went for a vulnerable "receptor." Although Ehrlich's concepts were not entirely realized, his ideas eventually led to the discovery of sulfonamides ("Prontosil") for the systemic treatment of bacterial infections by Domagk in 1935, and to the further refinement of receptor concepts as presently understood.

The direct identification (by means of ^{3}H-ligands) of receptors for drugs, hormones, neurotransmitters, *etc.*, occurred between 1965 and 1975. During this time it slowly became apparent that most of these receptors had so great an affinity for their respective "ligands" (*i.e.*, hormone, drug, or neurotransmitter) that the receptors became saturated when the ligand concentration was in the nanomolar range. Once this was realized, it became essential to prepare radioactive drugs or hormones having radioactivity sufficiently high to permit detection of very small amounts of receptors that were readily occupied and saturated at these low (nanomolar) concentrations.

A crucial step forward was made when the following simple calculation was appreciated. At 1 nM (nanomoles/L, 1 nmol = 10^{-9} moles) a typical receptor will usually be fully occupied by a radioligand. The tissue concentration of most receptors is extremely low, around 10 femtomoles (1 fmol = 10^{-15} moles) of receptor per milligram of tissue, so that 1 mg of the tissue will bind only about 10 fmol of ^{3}H-ligand at most. At the same time, the minimum radioactivity that one can decently monitor in a hospital laboratory is about 200 dpm (disintegrations per minute). All this

means, therefore, that in order to detect receptors in 1 mg of a typical tissue, one must use a radioligand that has a specific radioactivity of at least 200 dpm per 10 fmol, or 10 Curies per mmol (there are about 220 dpm in 100 picoCuries). Drugs having this high specific activity were at first difficult and expensive to make, but such compounds are now becoming much more readily available.

NATURE OF BIOLOGIC DRUG RECEPTORS

A drug receptor is any biologic component that interacts specifically with a drug molecule and that leads to an effect on the cell. If the absorption or binding of the drug to the component does not lead to any effect, as in the case of drug binding to albumin, then the component is not called receptor, but is merely referred to as a nonspecific binding site or acceptor site. Thus, there are specific and nonspecific binding sites for most drugs (Fig. 9–1).

Do **all** drugs act on receptors? The answer to this question is no, if we use the definition of receptor given above. Many drugs act through specific receptors, but others do not. The following examples serve to illustrate the enormous range of different biologic components that may serve as specific or nonspecific binding sites mediating the actions of drugs. A later section lists the differences between specific receptors and nonspecific binding and drug action.

Water as a Nonspecific Drug Target

Osmotic diuretics, such as mannitol, are not reabsorbed by the kidney and therefore retain, in the

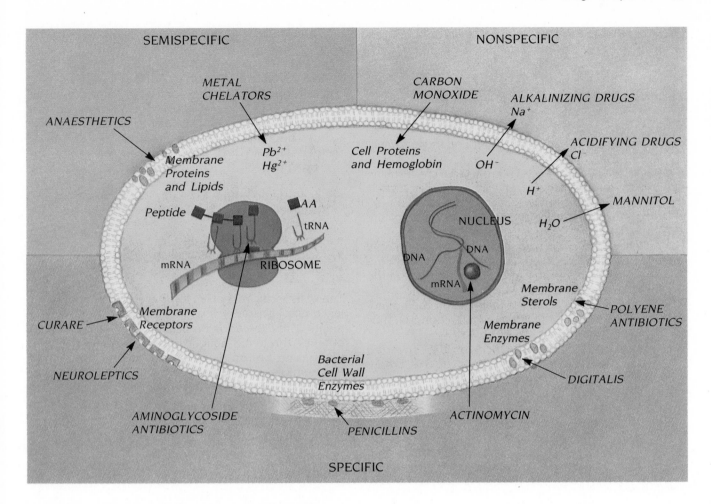

Figure 9–1 Types of specific and nonspecific receptors.

lumen of the renal tubule, water that would otherwise have been reabsorbed. Thus they "act on" body water, so to speak, in producing diuresis.

Some laxatives, such as agar or methyl cellulose, have molecules that are too large to be absorbed from the intestine. When taken by mouth, they swell by absorbing water and so retain more water in the intestinal lumen. The resulting bulk promotes intestinal motility and relieves constipation.

High-molecular-weight dextrans, when injected intravenously, cause water to enter from the tissues into the circulation and expand the blood volume.

Thus, osmotic diuretics, bulk laxatives, and plasma expanders may all be considered to be "acting" on water as the target site. In this case, however, we are not dealing with a specific receptor, since the water could be replaced by any other polar solvent.

H⁺ or OH⁻ Ions as Nonspecific Targets

A drug such as ammonium chloride is used to acidify the urine. After ingestion of NH_4Cl the liver converts

the ammonium ion to urea, and the kidney excretes the chloride ion; the Cl^-, however, takes protons (hydrogen ions) along with it, thus raising the concentration of protons (cH^+) in urine, i.e., lowering the pH. The protons, therefore, may be considered as the drug target sites in this case.

Alkalinizing drugs, such as sodium lactate and sodium bicarbonate ($NaHCO_3$), lower the urine cH^+ and stomach cH^+, respectively. The lactate ion, for example, is metabolized to CO_2, together with OH^-. The extra Na^+ is excreted in the urine, replacing some of the urine H^+, and the urine cH^+ thus falls. In this case, the H^+ might be considered as the target for the sodium lactate.

Metal Ions as Relatively Specific Receptors

Divalent metal ions may be considered as the receptors for chelating drugs, such as dimercaprol for Hg^{2+} or As^{2+} poisoning, penicillamine for Cu^{2+} in Wilson's disease, and EDTA for Pb^{2+} poisoning (see Chapter 72). Although these chelating drugs bind all divalent metal ions, they have a somewhat greater specificity or affinity for the ones for which they are used clinically.

Enzymes as Specific Drug Receptors

There are numerous examples of enzymes that are specific receptors for drugs. These include the following:

- Penicillin specifically acts on a bacterial cross-linking enzyme that connects together the polymer strands of N-acetylglucosamine-N-acetylmuramic acid pentapeptide from which the tough outer wall of the bacterial cell is built (see Chapter 53).
- Sulfonamides inhibit bacterial growth by specifically acting on a bacterial condensing enzyme that condenses p-aminobenzoic acid with a pteridine in the formation of folic acid (see Chapter 56).
- Oligomycin is an antibiotic that acts on the adenosine triphosphatase (ATPase) of mitochondria, thus depleting the bacterial cell of ATP.
- 5-Fluorouracil is an anticancer drug. It is converted to ribose and deoxyribose derivatives that are incorporated into RNA and DNA in place of the thymine analogs. Thus, cell division is stopped.
- Cyanide is a poison that specifically acts on the trivalent iron (Fe^{3+}) of cytochrome oxidase. Poisoning of this enzyme stops cell respiration.
- Digitalis increases the force of contraction of a weak heart muscle by acting on a membrane enzyme, $(Na^+ + K^+)$-ATPase (see Chapter 34).

Nucleic Acids as Specific Receptors

DNA is a receptor for the antibiotic actinomycin D. Streptomycin is an antibiotic that specifically binds between the messenger-RNA and the transfer-RNA to interfere with protein synthesis in the ribosome.

Membrane Sterols as Receptors

Polyene antibiotics (nystatin, amphotericin B; see Chapter 54) bind to ergosterol specifically, and cause leakiness or lysis of the fungal cell membrane.

DIFFERENCES BETWEEN SPECIFIC AND NONSPECIFIC DRUG RECEPTORS

The most important thing about a drug-specific receptor is that the receptor has a complex arrangement of partial binding groups to which the drug must be able to fit, if it is to produce its pharmacologic effect. This generally means that minor alterations of the drug

molecule drastically alter its potency. For example, the addition or removal of one carbon atom often alters the potency by a factor of 10 or 20, as shown in Table 9-1 for acetylcholine analogs. A different order of relative potencies for the different analogs distinguishes the muscarinic receptor (on the guinea-pig ileum smooth muscle) from the nicotinic receptor (on the frog rectus abdominis skeletal muscle).

Practically all drugs act on specific receptors, with the exception of:

- anaesthetics, and probably most hypnotics and sedatives;
- alcohols;
- osmotically-active drugs;
- acidifying and alkalinizing drugs;
- antiseptics.

The nonspecific receptors for these nonspecifically acting drugs have very low chemical structural requirements. Thus, the addition of one carbon increases the potency three-fold almost invariably, while the deletion of one carbon decreases the potency three-fold. For example, it requires about 46 g (or 1.5 oz) of pure ethanol (CH_3CH_2OH) in the body of a person of average build to produce the blood level at which driving is legally prohibited in most jurisdictions (80 mg/100 mL, or 22 mM). The same degree of impairment would be produced by 135 g of methanol (CH_3OH) or 15 g of propanol ($CH_3CH_2CH_2OH$).

Specific Receptors Are Stereoselective

The nonspecific receptors for anaesthetics do not distinguish between optical isomers of the anaesthetics. For example, levo-halothane and dextro-halothane are equipotent. There are local anaesthetics of which the levo-isomer and the dextro-isomer differ in potency about eight-fold, but this is a very small difference compared to specific receptors. For specific receptors, one optical isomer is generally 100 to 1000 times more powerful than the other isomer, as shown in Table 9-2.

The term "stereoselectivity" indicates a relative preference for one stereoisomer. The term "stereospecificity" is reserved for cases in which essentially all activity resides in a single enantiomer or in a single

TABLE 9-1 Relative Potencies of Acetylcholine Analogs

	Guinea Pig Ileum %	Frog Rectus Abdominis %
Formylcholine	25	10
Acetylcholine	100	100
Propionylcholine	5	400
Butyrylcholine	0.5	150

TABLE 9–2 Examples of Active Enantiomers: Relative Potencies

	Levo-isomer(−)	Dextro-isomer(+)
Noradrenaline	100	1
Methadone	50	1
Atropine	30	1
Tetrahydro- cannabinol	15–25	1
LSD	1	Very high
Butaclamol	1	>1000

stereoisomer. In other words, an extremely stereo-selective drug is referred to as stereospecific.

Specific Receptors Can Be Selectively Blocked by Antagonist Drugs

Selective blockade of specific receptors can be obtained with drug antagonists. Atropine, for example, can block the muscarinic receptors without affecting the nicotinic or histamine receptors.

Another example is propranolol, which can block the tissue responses to (−)-noradrenaline* but not to glucagon or another hormone.

Nonspecific receptors, on the other hand, cannot be selectively blocked by antagonists.

Specific Receptors Are Occupied at Nanomolar or Micromolar Concentrations

Nonspecific receptors, such as those for ethanol, require very high concentrations of drugs (in the millimolar or molar range). For example, in the case of ethanol, it takes about 46 g (22 mM) of pure ethanol to produce legally defined impairment of driving ability in most social drinkers. Specific receptors, on the other hand, are occupied and affected by concentrations in the micromolar or nanomolar range.

EXPERIMENTAL STUDIES OF THE BINDING BETWEEN DRUGS AND RECEPTORS

The first step in the binding between a drug and a tissue is referred to as the association step or the adsorption step. The affinity of the receptor for the drug can be precisely measured, and the index of this affinity is referred to as the association constant K_A. Some workers use the term dissociation constant (K_D),

---

* norepinephrine

which is defined as the reciprocal of the association constant ($1/K_A$). These constants are derived from the equation:

$$D + R \underset{k_{offset}}{\overset{k_{onset}}{\rightleftharpoons}} DR \text{ complex},$$

where k_{onset} is the onset constant reflecting the rate of drug attachment to the receptor site, and k_{offset} is the offset constant, which is an index of the speed of dissociation of the drug from the receptor.

$$K_A = k_{onset}/k_{offset}.$$

The dissociation constant of the drug for the receptor is the concentration of drug at which 50% of the receptors are occupied ($C_{50\% occupancy}$). The dissociation constant is equal to the ratio of the offset constant over the onset constant:

$$K_D = C_{50\% occupancy} = \frac{k_{offset}}{k_{onset}}.$$

Measurement of the Receptor's K_D for Drug

The steps in measuring the dissociation constant of any particular drug for its receptor are as follows.

Obtain ³H-Ligand with Highest Possible Radioactivity

It is almost always necessary to obtain a ligand that is sufficiently radioactive to be detectable when diluted down to the nanomolar concentration range. Hence, the specific activity of the isotope must be at least 5 Curies per mmol (see introductory paragraphs). Such high specific activity is generally feasible with tritium (³H) or with ¹²⁵I, but usually not with ¹⁴C.

Measure Binding of ³H-Ligand to Tissue Homogenate

Samples of the tissue homogenate are mixed with different concentrations of the ³H-ligand. After incubation of the mixtures for generally 30 minutes (time to reach equilibrium depends on the temperature), each one is filtered through a separate glass fibre filter; each filter is then washed very quickly with 10 to 15 mL of buffer to wash off (as much as possible) the ³H-ligand that is nonspecifically bound to the membranes (Fig. 9–2). The filters are then put in a scintillation fluid and counted.

Typical results are shown in Figure 9–3A, where it can be seen that there are always specific and non-

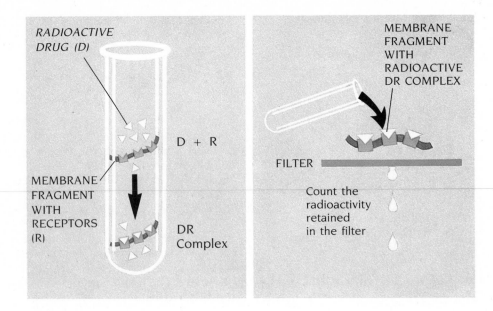

Figure 9–2   Ligand method for detecting receptors. The ligand (radioactive drug) is mixed with homogenized tissue, the mixture is filtered, and the loosely attached ligand is washed.

specific components of binding. The key problem is to distinguish between these.

Specific binding of a ^{3}H-ligand is defined as that amount of binding that can be displaced competitively by an excess of "cold" (*i.e.*, non-radioactive) ligand. Experience indicates that an "excess" is any concentration between 100 nM and 1 μM. This definition of specific binding is based on the idea that specific receptor sites are relatively few in number, and thus the ^{3}H-ligand can be displaced in competition with an excess of the cold ligand. The amount of ^{3}H-ligand remaining on the filter (in the presence of the excess cold ligand) is defined as nonspecific binding; the number of non-specific binding sites is extremely high and includes binding and adsorption to nonspecific sites with very low affinity ($K_D > 500$ μM) as well as partitioning of the ligand into the membrane.

As shown in Figure 9–3B, therefore, the amount of specific binding is obtained by simply subtracting from the total binding of ^{3}H-ligand the binding that remains in the presence of an excess of cold ligand. Figure 9–3C shows the same data graphed on linear scales, and one can see that the curve representing specific binding to a receptor is simply a rectangular hyperbola.

Obtain K_D and B_{max} by Scatchard Analysis

Since the amount of tissue applied to each filter is known (in mg of protein per filter), the data of Figure 9–3C can be regraphed in the style suggested by Scatchard, in Figure 9–3D. The intercept on the horizontal axis gives the maximum number of binding sites in the tissue (*i.e.*, the density of receptors). The K_D is measured from the slope, as shown in Figure 9–3D.

The Scatchard equation is derived from the classic Langmuir equation, and for the straight line in Figure 9–3D is:

$$\frac{\text{Amount bound}}{C_{\text{free}}} = \frac{B_{max}}{K_D} - \frac{\text{Amount bound}}{K_D}.$$

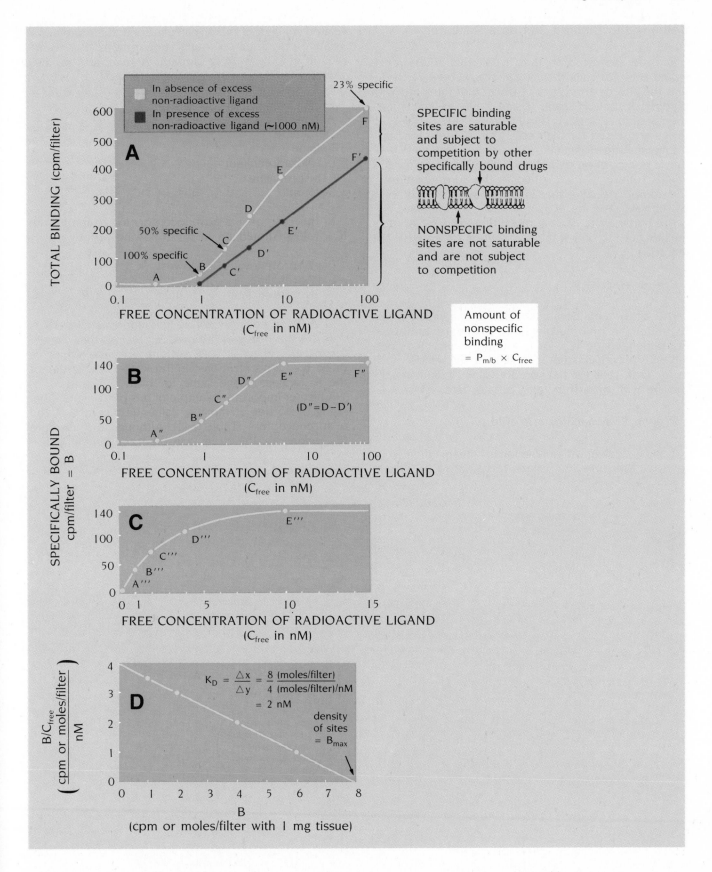

Figure 9–3   Measurement of binding of ^{3}H-ligand to tissue homogenate. *A*, Total binding. *B*, Specific binding. *C*, Linear plot of specific binding. *D*, Scatchard plot of specific binding.

Defining the Binding Site as a Receptor

In order to establish that a site that binds a ³H-ligand is biologically meaningful, it is necessary to define the site by the types of drugs that interfere with binding of that ³H-ligand. Using 2 nM ³H-ligand (*i.e.*, the conditions at point C in Figure 9–3A), a variety of drugs are tested for their ability to compete for binding *versus* the ³H-ligand; this is shown in Figure 9–4. These competition experiments result in a list of IC_{50} values, where IC_{50} is defined as the concentration of the competing drug that inhibits the specific binding of the ³H-ligand by 50%.

The binding site can be interpreted as a biologically meaningful site only if the competition data reveal the following:

Stereoselectivity

The active enantiomer should have a much lower IC_{50} than the pharmacologically inactive enantiomer. For example, the IC_{50} for (−)-noradrenaline (competing with an adrenoceptor ³H-ligand) should be much lower than that for (+)-noradrenaline, if one is truly dealing with an adrenergic receptor site.

Proper Pharmacologic Profile

If one is dealing with a functionally meaningful receptor site, then the IC_{50} values for a series of closely related congeners should correlate with their traditional relative potencies on intact preparations. For example, in the case of a dopamine receptor the IC_{50} values should be in the following order:

Bromocriptine . . . . lowest IC_{50}
Apomorphine
Dopamine
Epinine
(−)-Noradrenaline
(−)-Adrenaline*
Serotonin . . . . highest IC_{50}

In the case of a β adrenoceptor, for example, the IC_{50} values should be in the following order:

(−)-Isoproterenol . . . . . . lowest IC_{50}
(−)-Adrenaline
(−)-Noradrenaline . . . . . highest IC_{50}

In defining each receptor, it is important to stress that it is the **order** of the drug IC_{50} values that characterizes the receptor, and **not** the absolute values of these IC_{50} concentrations. In Table 9–3, the order of the IC_{50} values is the same for both ³H-ligands.

A further important example of this principle emphasizing the order of the IC_{50} values is the case of the α adrenoceptors (Table 9–4). Although the absolute IC_{50} values for the drugs are different for the differ-

---

* epinephrine

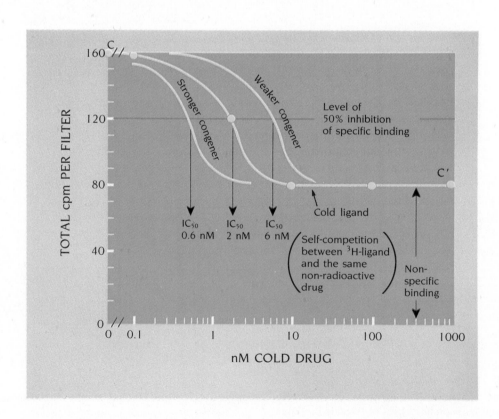

Figure 9–4 Pharmacologic characterization of sites by drug competition experiments.

TABLE 9–3 IC_{50} Values for β Adrenoceptors (Frog Erythrocyte Membranes)

Competing Cold Ligand	^{3}H-Ligand*	
	$(-)$-^{3}H-DHA	$(\pm)$-^{3}H-HBI
$(-)$-Propranolol	20 nM	15 nM
$(-)$-Isoproterenol	1500 nM	100 nM
$(-)$-Adrenaline	15,000 nM	400 nM
$(-)$-Noradrenaline	20,000 nM	20,000 nM
Dopamine	400,000 nM	100,000 nM
$(+)$-Isoproterenol	600,000 nM	300,000 nM

* DHA is dihydroalprenolol, an antagonist of β adrenoceptors; HBI is hydroxy-benzyl-isoproterenol, a potent agonist of β adrenoceptors.

TABLE 9–4 IC_{50} Values for α_1 and α_2 Adrenoceptors (Cerebral Cortex)

Competing Cold Ligand	^{3}H-Ligand	
	^{3}H-Clonidine α_2 (Pre-synaptic)	^{3}H-WB4101 α_1 (Post-synaptic)
$(-)$-Adrenaline	10 nM	860 nM
$(-)$-Noradrenaline	29 nM	1500 nM
$(+)$-Adrenaline	110 nM	41,000 nM
Dopamine	420 nM	64,000 nM
$(-)$-Isoproterenol	9,500 nM	$>10^6$ nM

TABLE 9–5 IC_{50} Values for α_1 and α_2 Adrenoceptors (Cerebral Cortex)

Competing Cold Ligand	^{3}H-Ligand	
	^{3}H-Clonidine α_2 (Pre-synaptic)	^{3}H-WB4101 α_1 (Post-synaptic)
Clonidine	9.7 nM	630 nM
α-Methylnoradrenaline	27 nM	10,000 nM
Phentolamine	37 nM	5 nM
Yohimbine	250 nM	700 nM
Prazosin	620 nM	0.6 nM

ent ^{3}H-ligands in Table 9–4, the order of the IC_{50} values is the same for each ^{3}H-ligand.

Thus, the order of the IC_{50} values for these adrenoceptor agonists correlates with their order of potencies, as originally defined by Ahlquist for action on adrenergically sensitive tissues. This significant correlation provides a meaningful interpretation of these binding sites, suggesting that they are truly the sites on which the adrenergic drugs act to produce their characteristic effects.

The fact that the absolute values of the IC_{50}s are very different for the different ^{3}H-ligands, however, suggests that there may be more than one type of α adrenoceptor. This is so, since it is known that there are both α_1 adrenoceptors and α_2 adrenoceptors (see Chapters 13 and 16). These two different α adrenoceptors have the same sensitivities to the classic drugs listed in Table 9–4, but have a different order of sensitivities to the drugs shown in Table 9–5.

It is important to note that the function of presynaptic receptors in general is the opposite of postsynaptic ones; for example, when presynaptic receptors are stimulated by their own transmitter, they reduce the further release of this transmitter.

Drugs Compete Over a 100-Fold Concentration Range

The classic Langmuir type of drug adsorption to a single site (i.e., the Law of Mass Action) indicates that the set of single sites becomes fully occupied over a 100-fold range (i.e., two decades on a logarithmic scale) of drug concentrations. This is also true for a competing drug. Hence, if any drug competes over more than a 100-fold range, it suggests that the ^{3}H-ligand may be binding to more than one set of receptors.

This is shown in Figure 9–5, where it can be seen that two receptors are clearly distinguished and resolved only if their K_D values for the competing drug differ more than 100-fold. If their K_D values differ less than 100-fold, then only the shallow slope of competition curve over three or four decades of concentrations will actually suggest that one is dealing with two receptors. The slope of the competition line under these conditions has what is known as a low Hill coefficient.

For example, a drug that competes over the standard two decades will exhibit a Hill number of about 1, while a drug that competes over three or four decades reveals a Hill number of about 0.5.

Affinity Constant

The affinity constant (K_A) between the receptor and the drug is defined as the reciprocal of the dissociation constant. For example, the dissociation constant (K_D) of the strychnine receptor complex is 4×10^{-9} M. Therefore the affinity constant of the strychnine receptor for strychnine is:

$$K_A = 1/K_D = 1/(4 \times 10^{-9} \text{ M})$$
$$= 2.5 \times 10^8 \text{ litres/mole.}$$

Since the units of K_A are rather strange at first glance, it is not a very clear way of expressing the affinity of the receptor for the ^{3}H-ligand.

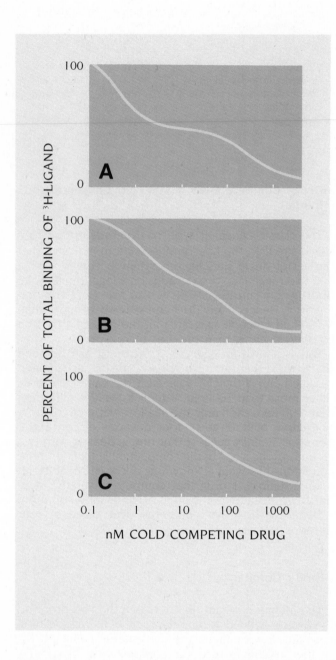

Figure 9–5   Drug competition for receptor sites. *A*, The ^{3}H-ligand binds to two receptors that have 100-fold different affinity for the competing drug. *B*, The two receptors have less than 100-fold different affinity for the competing drug. *C*, The two receptors have less than 50-fold different affinity for the competing drug.

CLINICAL SIGNIFICANCE OF RECEPTOR ASSAYS

There are a number of practical benefits that stem from the development of assays for drug receptors. These benefits are as follows.

Discovery of Endogenous Substances

Receptors are constituents of the cell, even in individuals who have never been exposed to the drug in question. There cannot have been any survival advantage from evolving receptors for drugs that did not yet exist. Therefore the primary function of the receptors must have been to bind ligands naturally present in the body. For example, the development of ^{3}H-opiate receptor assays led to the discovery of the endogenous anti-pain substances, the endorphins and enkephalins.

Screening of New Drugs

These receptor assays provide a very simple, rapid, and reliable method for screening new potential drugs. For example, a drug that displaces ^{3}H-haloperidol from its membrane receptor might be a good neuroleptic (*see* Chapter 27). The concentration at which the drug displaces ^{3}H-haloperidol is related to the clinical potency of the drug, as shown in Figures 9–6, 9–7, and 9–8.

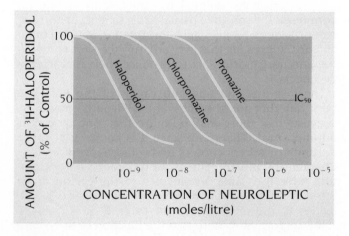

Figure 9–6   An example of how the ligand-binding method can be used to screen the potency of drugs (Fig. 9–7).

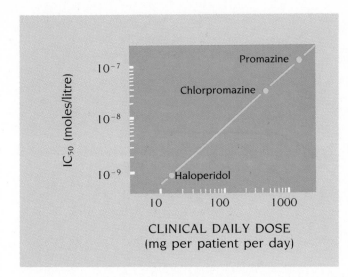

Figure 9–7 Using the screening data from Figure 9–6, it can be seen that there is a very good correlation between the IC$_{50}$ values (determined in the test tube) and the clinical potencies for neuroleptic drugs. (Neuroleptics are antagonists of dopamine receptors.)

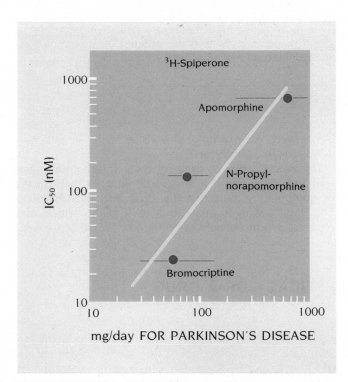

Figure 9–8 Showing that there is a fair correlation between IC$_{50}$ values for dopamine agonists and their clinical potencies.

Receptor Diseases

Abnormalities in the density of receptors (B$_{max}$) and/or in the dissociation constant (K$_D$) of tissue receptors can now be studied.

In Parkinson's disease, for example, a higher-than-normal density of dopamine receptors has been found in the putamen and the caudate nucleus; such an increase presumably reflects denervation supersensitivity following the degeneration of the dopamine-releasing nigral neurons (see Chapter 20).

In postmortem brains from patients who had schizophrenia there is also an elevation in the density of dopamine receptors (see Chapter 27).

Receptor Desensitization in Disease

In certain diseases the tissues are very unresponsive to drugs or hormones. This is sometimes synonymous with drug tolerance, drug tachyphylaxis, or drug desensitization. The basis for this may sometimes be that the receptors in the tissue have either "disappeared" or have been "occluded" into the cell. For example, in insulin-resistant diabetes, there are fewer insulin receptors on the cell membrane.

A second example is seen following the long-term administration of antidepressant drugs. These drugs act to block the uptake of noradrenaline by the nerve terminals, thus causing more noradrenaline to bombard the β adrenoceptors in the brain. After many weeks of such antidepressant therapy, the number of β adrenoceptors decreases by 50%.

In studying human tissues, therefore, it is essential to measure both the K$_D$ and the B$_{max}$ in order to determine whether the sensitivity of the tissue has changed because of different numbers of receptors or because of a genetic abnormality (different K$_D$) in the receptors (Fig. 9–9).

Receptor Auto-Immune Diseases

There may be auto-immune diseases of receptors. A possible case is that of myasthenia gravis, in which there appear to be circulating antibodies to nicotinic cholinoceptors. These antibodies can cause normal nicotinic receptors to behave abnormally. Radioreceptor assays can detect such abnormal antibodies in the serum of patients.

Measurement of Plasma Drug Levels

Finally, the development of these simple radioreceptor assays permits the ready detection and measure-

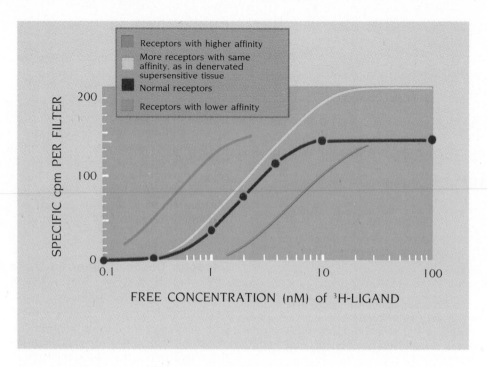

Figure 9–9 Illustrating examples of possible changes in receptors that may account for the changes in tissue sensitivity to a drug. The denervated tissue may have a higher density of receptors ("denervation supersensitivity"); this would be experimentally detected by a higher amount of specific cpm of ^{3}H-ligand bound to the tissue on the filter. A second possible explanation for a higher sensitivity of the tissue to the drug would be that the receptors have a higher affinity for the drug; this would be experimentally shown by a saturation of the receptors at lower concentrations of free ^{3}H-ligand. Finally, some tissues become desensitized; this may be reflected in either a lower density of receptors, or lower affinity of the receptors for that ^{3}H-ligand.

ment of a variety of drugs in the plasma of patients. Some drugs, for example, are particularly difficult to measure by conventional methods, such as gas chromatography / mass spectrometry (GC/MS). Neuroleptic drugs are a case in point. In principle, these drugs can be measured in the plasma of patients by the simple (and cheap) radioreceptor assay using displacement of either ^{3}H-haloperidol or ^{3}H-spiperone. However, in practice there are still many technical problems to be solved.

EFFECT OF DRUG ON RECEPTOR

It is thought that the drug changes the shape (or conformation) of the receptor, although there is no direct proof of this point. Most pharmacologists think that the drug acts only as long as it occupies the receptor; this is referred to as the **occupation theory** of drug-receptor interaction. This is analogous to a musical organ where the tone is emitted only as long as the key remains depressed. An example of a drug acting in this way is an enzyme inhibitor.

The **rate theory** of drug-receptor interaction states that the drug action is proportional only to the rate of combination between the drug and the receptor. This mechanism is analogous to a piano where the sound is produced only when the key is first depressed.

EFFICACY OF A DRUG

The efficacy of a drug is a measure of its ability to stimulate a response once it has bound to the receptor. For example, if drug A only needs to occupy at least 1000 receptors to exert a cell action, while drug B must occupy at least 10,000 receptors to exert the same amount of cell action, then the efficacy of drug A is higher than that of drug B. Perhaps this is because drug A has a more "snug" fit with the receptor and, hence, drug A is more effective per occupied receptor.

SPARE RECEPTORS AND SPARE CELLS

Not all receptors of a cell or tissue must be occupied in order to give the maximum effect of the drug. Each cell or tissue has spare receptors. At the nerve-muscle junction, for example, it is known that there are about 20,000 receptors for acetylcholine on the muscle membrane sole-plate region. It is known, however, that about one-quarter to one-half of these receptors can be blocked without affecting the full muscle twitch response. In other words, about 25–50% of these receptors are spares. This is illustrated in Figure 9–10, which shows that, as more and more acetylcholine receptors become blocked by increasing concentrations of a toxin (such as bungarotoxin, prepared from a snake venom), as much as 50% of the sole-plate receptors can become occupied by the toxin before any reduction occurs in the muscle twitch evoked by stimulating the nerve.

Since different drugs have different efficacies, the number of receptors that must be occupied to produce a maximum effect will vary from drug to drug. Thus, the number of spare receptors will also vary for each drug. A maximum response by the tissue may result from occupation of as few as 0.001% of available receptors, to as many as 100%. The height of the maximum response is **not** a measure of efficacy (see below).

It is also known that many cells of tissues such as smooth muscle are electrotonically connected to one another, making a functional syncytium (Fig. 9–11). This means that stimulation of the receptors of one cell may lead to contraction of as many as 200 cells.

ANTAGONISTS AND PARTIAL AGONISTS

If the efficacy of a drug is very low, then the stimulus exerted by occupation of 100% of the receptors will not be sufficient to produce a maximum response of the tissue. Such drugs are referred to as partial agonists. If the drug has zero efficacy, then it will occupy the receptors and produce no response, but interfere with the binding of active drugs. It is therefore referred to as an antagonist. Partial agonists may have a high affinity so that they may function as antagonists in the presence of a full agonist (e.g., nalbuphine, see Chapter 22).

NUMBER OF RECEPTORS ON ONE CELL

Considering only drug receptors on the membrane, the density of these specific receptors is between 1 and about 1000 per μm^2 of membrane; the density of nonspecific receptors for anaesthetics, however, is about 1 million per μm^2 (Table 9–6).

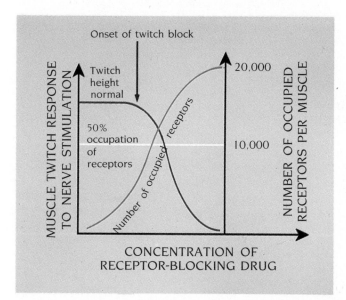

Figure 9–10 Illustrating an example of "spare receptors" for acetylcholine at the nerve-muscle junction. As more and more acetylcholine receptors are blocked by the addition of bungarotoxin to the preparation (abscissa), the amplitude of the muscle twitch in response to nerve stimulation is not diminished until at least 50% of the receptors become occupied by the toxin. This means that at least 50% of the receptors are "spares" in the sense that they were not required for a completely normal twitch.

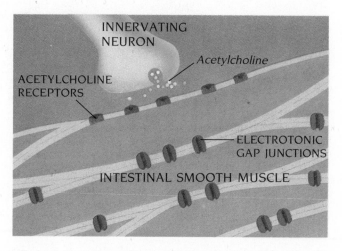

Figure 9–11 Electrotonic gap junctions causing electrical spread of a drug's action on one cell to many other cells.

TABLE 9–6   Examples of Receptor Density for Specific and Nonspecific Drug Binding

Receptor	Receptor Density (per μm^2)	No. of Sites per Cell
Digitalis	10	1300/red cell
Tetrodotoxin	27	
Noradrenaline	10	
Morphine		10^4/neuron
ACTH	0.1	
Glucagon	10	
Insulin	20	500/fat cell
Angiotensin	600	1000/fat cell
Anaesthetics	~1,000,000	

SECOND MESSENGER INTERMEDIARIES

There are many intermediate steps between the attachment of the drug to the receptor and the eventual response of the cell. The receptor on the membrane is attached to transducers, which may be enzymes or transport sites, and these ultimately lead to the response of the cell. For example, as shown in Figure 9–12, the attachment of a drug to the receptor may lead to an activation of adenylate cyclase and/or to the entry of Ca^{2+} into the cell. The Ca^{2+} and/or the cyclic AMP (second messenger) then produce four types of cell responses:

- contractile work;
- metabolic work;
- secretory work;
- electrical work.

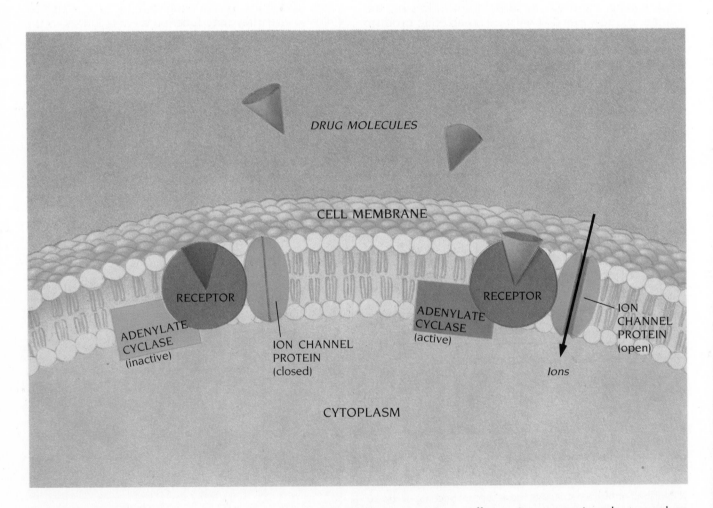

Figure 9–12   General scheme indicating how a drug or hormone exerts its primary effect on its receptor in order to produce a secondary effect on ion fluxes (such as entry of Ca^{2+}) or metabolic events in the cytoplasm (*via* stimulation or inhibition of adenylate cyclase).

DIFFERENT STATES OF A RECEPTOR

It is now clear that many, if not most, receptors have two states of existence. For example, the β adrenoceptor has a state with 100 nM affinity for noradrenaline (*i.e.*, it is half-saturated at 100 nM noradrenaline), and under different conditions this receptor can also exist in a state where it has a 10,000 nM affinity for noradrenaline. The 100 nM state is referred to as the high-affinity state, while the 10,000 nM state is termed the low-affinity state.

The following are a few examples of receptors known to have high- and low-affinity states (ranked in alphabetical order, because the relative importance of one over another is not known):

- α adrenoceptors,
- angiotensin receptors,
- benzodiazepine receptors,
- β adrenoceptors,
- dopamine receptors,
- glucagon receptors,
- insulin receptors,
- muscarinic receptors,
- nicotinic receptors,
- opiate receptors,
- prostaglandin E receptors,
- serotonin receptors.

Although there is much current research aimed at determining which of the affinity states are functional, it is established, for example, that only the high-affinity state of the dopamine receptor in the pituitary lactotroph is the functional state controlling prolactin secretion as well as cell division.

Factors that are known to convert high-affinity states of receptors to low-affinity states include sodium ions and guanosine 5'-triphosphate (GTP). Figure 9–13 illustrates typical data for the binding of ^{3}H-dihydroalprenolol (^{3}H-DHA), which is an antagonist, to β receptors of red blood cells. It can be seen that isoproterenol inhibited the binding of ^{3}H-DHA in both the high-affinity region of 100 nM and the low-affinity region of 10,000 nM. Approximately 75% of the β receptors (labelled by ^{3}H-DHA) were in the high-affinity state, while about 25% were in the low-affinity state. In the presence of GTP, however, much higher concentrations of isoproterenol were needed to inhibit the binding of ^{3}H-DHA. This indicates that most or all of the receptors had now "converted" to the low-affinity state.

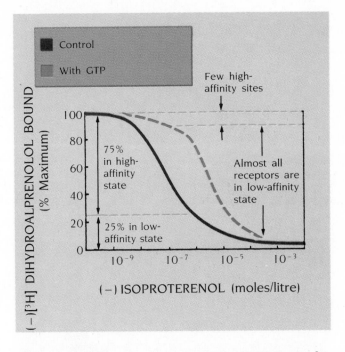

Figure 9–13 The isoproterenol agonist displaces the ^{3}H-antagonist in two phases. Low concentrations (10–100 nM) of isoproterenol displace the ^{3}H-antagonist from the high-affinity states of the receptor. High concentrations (10^{-7}–10^{-5} M) of isoproterenol displace the ^{3}H-antagonist from the low-affinity states. In the presence of GTP most of the receptors are in the low-affinity state.

REGULATION OF RECEPTORS AND ITS CLINICAL SIGNIFICANCE

The molecular explanation for the regulation of the agonist state of the receptor by GTP is that GTP attaches to a G-protein, which changes the shape of the receptor, lowering the receptor's affinity for the agonist, as shown in Figure 9–14.

The clinical significance of this is illustrated in tissues from asthmatic patients who have developed a resistance to the therapeutic effects of adrenaline or noradrenaline. Such tissues (*e.g.*, lung) now exhibit lower amounts of high-affinity state receptors, but higher amounts of low-affinity state receptors. Apparently the continued presence of the agonist leads to a change in the level of GTP and thus to changes in the predominant receptor state.

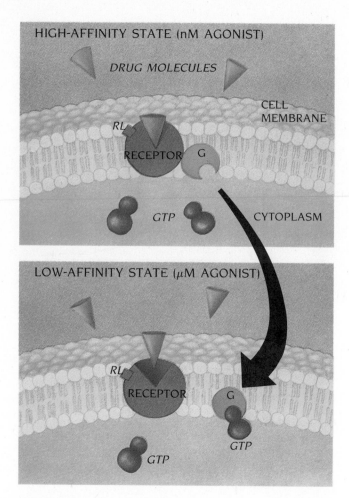

HIGH-AFFINITY STATE (nM AGONIST)

DRUG MOLECULES

CELL MEMBRANE

RL

RECEPTOR   G

GTP   CYTOPLASM

LOW-AFFINITY STATE (μM AGONIST)

RL

RECEPTOR   G

GTP

GTP

Figure 9–14   Illustrating how GTP attaches to the G-protein, which then separates from the receptor, while the receptor loses its affinity for the agonist drug. RL is the radioactive label that tags both the high-affinity state (top) and the low-affinity state (bottom) of the receptor.

OH

HO

NH₂   Dopamine

N

Br

N   R   Bromocriptine

CH₃

N

OH

NH₂   Serotonin

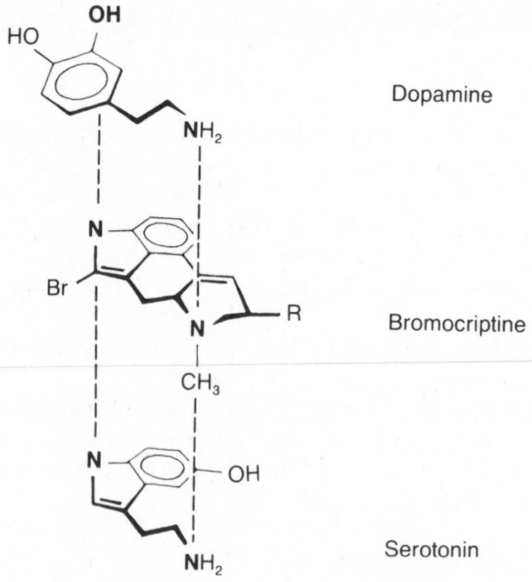

Figure 9–15   Illustrating the essential components between different molecules that are required in order to stimulate a specific receptor. The distance between the — OH group and the — NH₂ group in the dopamine molecule is identical to the distance between the two nitrogen atoms in bromocriptine. However, since there are certain structural similarities between serotonin and bromocriptine, this may account for the fact that bromocriptine has serotoninergic receptor-stimulating action as well.

DRUG BINDING TO MULTIPLE RECEPTORS

Ideally, a perfectly selective drug is one that only attaches to a single type of receptor. In practice, however, many drugs are simply not this selective, and they usually bind to several different types of receptors (*see* Chapter 10, *Specificity of Drug Action*) causing unwanted side effects. A good example of this is found in the ergot type of drugs, such as LSD or bromocriptine.

As illustrated in Figure 9–15, the chemical structure of bromocriptine contains the necessary binding groups spaced at the critical distances necessary to stimulate dopamine receptors, adrenoceptors, and serotonin receptors. Thus, although bromocriptine is primarily used to stimulate dopamine receptors in pituitary tumors, this drug has side effects directly related to its stimulation of these other receptor types found in blood vessels or the gastrointestinal tract.

SUGGESTED READING

Lamble JW, ed. More about receptors. Cambridge: Elsevier, 1982.
Lefkowitz RJ, Caron MG, Michel T, Stadel JM. Beta-adrenoceptors. Fed Proc 1982; 41:2664–2670.
Seeman P. Brain dopamine receptors. Pharmacol Rev 1980; 32:229–313.
Seeman P, Chau-Wong M, Tedesco J, Wong K. Brain receptors for antipsychotic drugs and dopamine: direct binding assays. Proc Natl Acad Sci 1975; 72:4376–4380.

The structurally specific, stereospecific, saturable binding of pepperoni to pizza

The binding of pepperoni (P) to pizza (Pizza) is well known (Doonesbury, 1982). In a recent study we have undertaken to elucidate the characteristics and mechanism of this binding. The following is a summary of the results of that study.

We have successfully demonstrated that the binding of the ligand P to Pizza is structurally specific, in that prior exposure of Pizza to various concentrations of kolbase, bratwurst or kosher salami will reduce, or in the extreme case prevent, the subsequent binding of P. This clearly demonstrates the structural specificity of the binding.

The suspected stereospecificity of the binding was confirmed when it was found that P would not bind to the underside of the Pizza. The specific receptor is presumed to be mozzarella (MMM) cheese because it had to be present for binding to occur. The binding characteristics of P to Pizza and to MMM were found to be very similar. Thus, while not absolutely certain, it does appear that it is the cheese that binds. The affinity of P for MMM was quantitatively related to the number of MMM strands appearing when separation of P from MMM was attempted. P was also shown, quite inad-

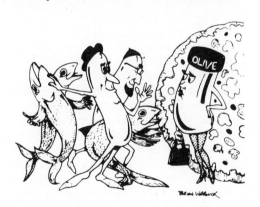

vertently, to bind (but not well) to napkins and trousers.

The binding of P to Pizza was found to be saturable, reaching satiation as an asymptomatic hyburpola. Onions and garlic both exerted alliosteric effects. Garlic's effect was potently expressed whereas onion's effect was dicey.

The structurally-specific, stereospecific, saturable binding of P to Pizza is readily

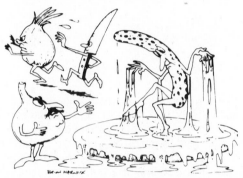

antagonized by a variety of agents, including olive oil (in excess) and anchovies. Of these, the anchovies appear to compete with P for binding sites while olive oil's antagonism is insurmountable.

The competitive antagonisms by anchovies and kosher salami each show quite different kinetics leading to the suggestion that there may be at least two different receptors for P. We have chosen to call these receptors P_1 and Poo-Poo.

Finally, it must be reported that, the above results notwithstanding, P's binding to Pizza is probably not of great functional significance and P may exert at best only a modulatory effect.

PAUL S. GUTH

Department of Pharmacology, Tulane University, New Orleans, LA 70112, U.S.A.

Reproduced from *Trends in Pharmacological Sciences (TIPS)*, December 1982, page 467, by permission of the author and the publisher, Elsevier Publications, Cambridge, U.K.

Chapter 10

SPECIFICITY OF DRUG ACTION

H. Kalant

No drug known is completely specific in the sense of acting on exclusively one type of cell or tissue, to produce only one type of effect. However, different drugs do show different degrees of specificity, and the therapeutic usefulness of a drug is usually directly related to its degree of specificity. If a substance acts on all tissues by some effect that is basic enough to affect all cell functions without any compensating advantage, it is called a **poison**. An example is **cyanide**, which combines strongly with ferric iron in various proteins including cytochrome oxidase, as shown in reaction [1] below, and prevents oxidative metabolism in the mitochondria of all tissues. This same nonspecificity also provides a method of treatment for cyanide poisoning, because cyanide can combine with Fe^{3+} in methemoglobin even more strongly than with cytochrome oxidase (*see also* Chapter 72):

[1] $CN^- + \text{cytox-Fe}^3 \rightleftarrows \text{cytox-FeCN}$

[2] $NaNO_2 + [O] + \text{HbFe}^{2+} \rightarrow \text{HbFe}^{3+} + NaNO_3$

[3] $\text{HbFe}^{3+} + \text{cytox-FeCN} \rightleftarrows \text{HbFeCN} + \text{cytox-Fe}^{3+}$

In this case, $NaNO_2$ is used to convert hemoglobin to methemoglobin (reaction [2] above), which removes the cyanide from the cytochrome oxidase (reaction [3] above), thus "poisoning" some of the O_2-carrying capacity of the blood, but gaining the compensating advantage of increasing the tissue O_2-utilizing capacity.

In contrast, **penicillin** inhibits a bacterial enzyme involved in the formation of bacterial cell walls, at concentrations that have no detectable effects on mammalian tissue enzymes. This specificity underlies its use as an antibiotic.

In between these extremes are many drugs that produce desired therapeutic effects at low doses and toxic effects at somewhat higher doses, with varying margins of safety between the two levels. For example, **methotrexate** (an anticancer drug) in doses of 2.5 to 5 mg/kg daily has been used to treat severe psoriasis by inhibiting the rapid reproduction of epithelial cells in the psoriatic plaques. At slightly higher doses it may also inhibit reproduction of mucosal cells in the intestine, leading to ulceration and diarrhea.

These examples illustrate the general principle that most, if not all, drugs act by inhibiting or interfering with one or more cellular functions. This can be regarded as toxicity; from this, it follows that useful drug actions are instances of "selective toxicity" (Adrien Albert), while "nonselective" toxicity gives rise to what we consider poisoning.

Generally, the toxic effects of a drug are separable from its therapeutically useful effects on the basis of differences in (a) their respective mechanisms of production, (b) their dose-response relationships if the mechanisms are similar, or (c) the sites at which they are produced. Therefore, attempts to increase the utility of a drug are based on either an improved **pharmacodynamic specificity** (if the mechanisms of toxic and therapeutic effects differ) or an enhanced **pharmacokinetic selectivity** of distribution to the desired target site.

PHARMACODYNAMIC SPECIFICITY

Molecular Basis of Specificity

The concept of specific drug-receptor combinations is an outgrowth of the study of the mechanism of action of acetylcholine and other neurotransmitters, and the mechanisms of reaction of substrates and inhibitors with enzymes. In the general case, the effective drug molecule is seen as having several points of attachment to corresponding points on the molecule or group of molecules making up the receptor site. The nature of these points of attachment and their relative positions and distances apart are all critical to the ability of the drug to combine with the receptor and produce a response.

This is illustrated by acetylcholine, its analogs, and its blockers (*see also* Chapters 14, 15, and 19). The molecule is often represented schematically as shown in Figure 10–1A. The points usually mentioned as being essential for its activity are the positively charged

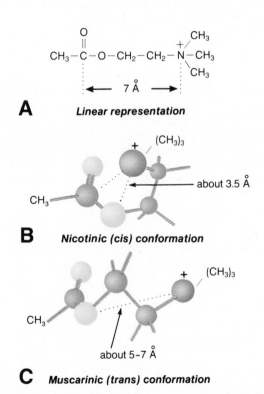

A *Linear representation*

B *Nicotinic (cis) conformation*

about 3.5 Å

C *Muscarinic (trans) conformation*

about 5-7 Å

Figure 10–1 Three representations of the molecular structure of acetylcholine. *A,* Linear representation, which shows the features essential for cholinergic activity but does not differentiate specific receptor-binding conformations. *B,* Specific conformation for nicotinic receptors: all binding groups are on the same side of the 2-carbon chain (*cis*). *C,* Specific muscarinic conformation: N and ester O are on opposite sides of the carbon chain (*trans*).

N, the three methyl groups attached to it, the ester linkage, and the spacing of 7 Å between the N and the carbonyl C.

Yet this does not explain the observation that there are two different sets of acetylcholine receptors (muscarinic and nicotinic), and some of the analogs are quite active at one set and almost inactive at the other. The acetylcholine molecule can change its shape easily because only single bonds are involved in the essential part of it, and free rotation can take place about these bonds. It appears that two different conformations of the molecule correspond to the two types of receptor sites (Fig. 10–1B and 10–1C).

In both, the ionic N^+ serves to attract the molecule toward a negatively charged site in the receptor. The total bulk of the three methyl groups on the N^+ seems necessary for proper fit in some concavity in which the receptor anionic site is located. But to complete the fit to the receptor sites, there seems to be a requirement for specific spacings between the N^+ and the ester O (hydrogen-bonding site) at muscarinic receptors. At nicotinic receptors there appears to be even greater specificity, because the distances between the N^+ and both the ester O and the carbonyl C (weak dipole) are critical. Some further modification of the steric requirements seems to differentiate nicotinic sites in ganglia from those at skeletal nerve-muscle junctions.

Unlike acetylcholine, a number of analogs, such as muscarine and nicotine (for which the receptors were named), muscarone, and various thio-substituted analogs, have large cyclic structures, bulky sidegroups, or double bonds that prevent free rotation. Such compounds are able to bind to only one or other receptor type, and thus are more specific than acetylcholine itself.

Specificity of Receptor Blockade

Blockers for these respective sites are thought to act by having enough of the necessary features to permit binding, but not all the features required to produce an acetylcholine-like effect after binding. Accordingly, they must have the specific groups and spacings to fit either the muscarinic sites (atropine), the nicotinic ganglionic sites (hexamethonium), or the nicotinic muscular sites (curare, decamethonium). Specificity is guaranteed by the fact that these blockers are not free to change conformation to fit different receptors as acetylcholine can. They have either ring structures of fixed dimensions, or chain lengths such that even free rotation only permits the N^+ groups a limited range of positions relative to each other. If this were not the case, one blocker might be active at all the sites of acetylcholine action, and the result would be biologic disaster, *i.e.,* it would be a poison rather than a useable drug.

Similar structural specificity applies to adrenergic and other receptors. Corresponding to the cholinergic division into muscarinic and nicotinic receptors, there is the division into α- and β-adrenergic receptors with their specific agonists noradrenaline* and isoproterenol respectively. Further, analogous to the subdivision of nicotinic into ganglionic and neuromuscular receptors, there is a subdivision into α_1, α_2, β_1, and β_2 receptors, each with its own specific agonists and blockers (*see* Chapters 16 and 17).

A striking current example is provided by the subdivision of opioid receptors into at least four categories designated μ, κ, σ, and δ (Chapter 22). Different opioids can be agonists at one type of receptor, antagonists at another, and partial agonists at yet another. Pure antagonists (naloxone, naltrexone) show different degrees of effectiveness as blockers at the different types of receptor.

Stereospecificity

Stereospecificity is not an obligatory feature of receptor specificity, but may add significantly to it. There are many examples of drugs having optical isomeric forms, only one of which is active. This is consistent with the type of receptor specificity mentioned above, provided that at least three points of attachment between drug and receptor are required, and that all three binding groups are chemically different and attached to either a centre or plane of asymmetry. This is illustrated schematically in Figure 10–2.

This seems to be the probable explanation for such examples as the following:

- Atropine is a mixture of d- and l-hyoscyamine, of which only the l-form is active as a muscarinic blocker.
- Morphine has d- and l-forms, of which only the l-form is active as an analgesic.
- Noradrenaline has d- and l-forms, of which only the l-form has significant potency in the elevation of blood pressure and other peripheral vascular effects.
- d-Amphetamine is a much more effective central stimulant than l-amphetamine, but they are equipotent in producing hallucinations.

Degrees of Specificity

Since drug-receptor specificity depends upon a combination of chemical groupings with different types of bonding possibilities and strengths, and arranged in specific three-dimensional patterns, it is possible to have widely differing degrees of specificity. A receptor with five critical bonding sites set at several different distances from each other will have vastly greater specificity than one with only two critical sites and one fixed distance between them.

Thus, at one extreme is tetrodotoxin, a highly specific

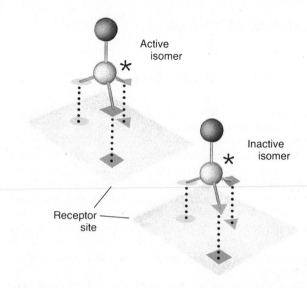

Figure 10–2 Schematic representation of complementarity of binding groups between drug and receptor, to account for activity of one optical isomer (*upper*) and inactivity of the other (*lower*). The asterisk marks the asymmetric carbon. The four different substituents are indicated by different shapes; three of these have complementary binding sites on the receptor. If there were only two binding sites, both isomers would be effective, by simply rotating the molecule.

molecule, which apparently combines only with the sodium channels in nerve cell membranes, acting to block the action potential.

In an intermediate position are drugs that have some basic parts of their molecules in common, while other parts differ. The parts in common enable them to combine with various types of receptor, but the parts that differ give them some degree of specificity. For example, the group

$$R - CH_2 - CH_2 - CH_2 - N \begin{array}{c} CH_2 - \\ \\ CH_2 - \end{array}$$

or

$$R - O - CH_2 - CH_2 - N \begin{array}{c} CH_3 \\ \\ CH_3 \end{array}$$

seems to enable a molecule to combine to some extent with receptors for histamine, acetylcholine, and possibly catecholamines, and if R is a large cyclic hydrocarbon portion, the drug can function as an antihistaminic, a local anaesthetic, a myocardial membrane stabilizer (*i.e.*, an antiarrhythmic agent), and to varying degrees also as an anticholinergic or antiadrenergic agent.

---

* norepinephrine

For example, chlorpromazine, procaine, and diphenhydramine are all good local anaesthetics, antihistaminic agents, and reducers of myocardial excitability. In addition, however, the other parts of the molecule give chlorpromazine an antiemetic effect, some minor cholinergic and adrenergic blocking action, and major tranquilizing (neuroleptic) activity. Procaine has a central stimulant action like that of cocaine in that it can act as a convulsant. Diphenhydramine is relatively more effective as an antihistaminic and also as a sedative and a cholinergic blocker (Fig. 10–3). Quinidine, propranolol, and phenytoin can be represented in the same way, with their cardiac antiarrhythmic effects as the common feature.

It is through this mixture of shared and unshared actions that many drugs have evolved into families of new drugs with preferential increase of one type of action and reduction of another. For example sulfanilamide, with a combination of antibacterial, hypoglycemic, and carbonic anhydrase-inhibitor effects, evolved into three separate families of drugs, each one relatively more specific for one or other of these effects (Fig. 10–4).

At the other extreme are drugs that are not believed to act on specific receptor sites at all. Alcohols and general anaesthetic agents act by dissolving in a large part of the lipid portion of the cell membrane and interacting with protein inclusions in the membrane. Such drugs have very little stereoselectivity, no strict molecular structural requirements for activity, and are not specific blockers or antagonists. At the same time, they act on a wide variety of different cells and tissues in a similar way, differing only in the relative concentrations needed to affect different types of cells or different functions of the same cell.

Even with such drugs, some minor degree of specificity is possible. The lipid portion of the cell membrane is not homogeneous, but in fact is quite heterogeneous with respect to the types of lipid immediately adjacent to, and interacting with, the various protein inclusions in the membrane (the "boundary lipids") and those constituting the lipid matrix of the membrane. A drug such as ethanol may interact preferentially with certain boundary lipids rather than with the bulk of the matrix lipids.

Specific Actions Versus Nonspecific Applications

Sometimes a therapeutic application of a drug does not require a particular specific mechanism of action, and a variety of drugs with different mechanisms of action may be used to achieve the same therapeutic objective(s). For example, all immune responses, involving both B and T lymphocytes, are initiated by stimuli that lead to cell proliferation (see Chapter 61). These processes, like all growth, whether normal or malignant, require production of DNA, RNA, and protein. Therefore, treatment of malignant growths, prevention of heterologous transplant rejection, treatment of autoimmune diseases, and control of severe psoriasis can all make use of the same groups of drugs. These include inhibitors of DNA synthesis, DNA inactivators (alkylating agents), and corticosteroids. Equally, the toxic effects also reflect nonspecific inhibition of growth and replication in the fastest-growing normal tissues: bone marrow suppression, loss of gastrointestinal epithelium, alopecia, and impairment of normal immune mechanisms against viral diseases and malignancies.

PHARMACOKINETIC SELECTIVITY

For those drugs that either do not act on specific receptors or act on receptors that are found on many or all tissues or cell types, some degree of selectivity of action may still exist because of either (1) selective distribution of the drug to an intended target site, or (2) metabolic differences between tissues that result in activation of a drug in one site more than another.

The difference between "specificity" and "selectivity" may be illustrated by two examples. Atropine is highly specific for muscarinic receptors, but is relatively nonselective because such receptors are found in many organs and tissues (e.g., eye, GI tract, salivary glands, bladder, or heart). In contrast, general anaesthetic

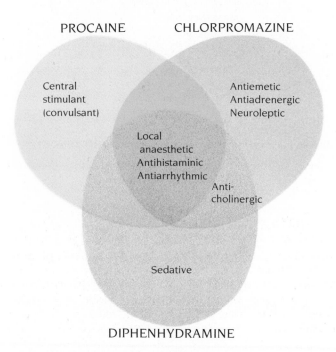

PROCAINE   CHLORPROMAZINE

Central
stimulant
(convulsant)

Antiemetic
Antiadrenergic
Neuroleptic

Local
anaesthetic
Antihistaminic
Antiarrhythmic

Anti-
cholinergic

Sedative

DIPHENHYDRAMINE

Figure 10–3 Gradations in specificity of actions of three drugs with diethylaminoethanol side-chains. All three share local anaesthetic, antihistaminic, and myocardial stabilizing actions. Two share anticholinergic action. Each has other unshared actions.

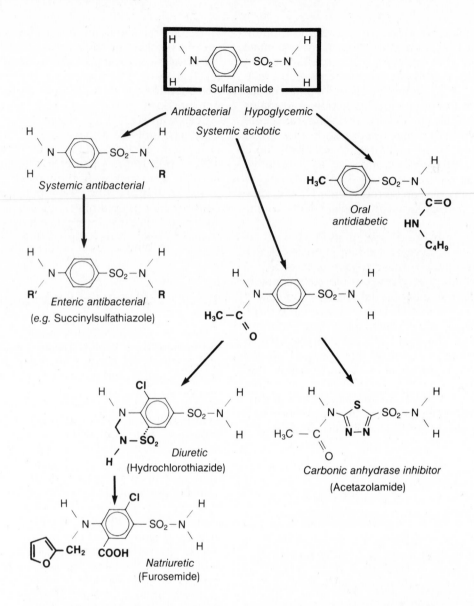

Figure l0–4 Evolution of a drug with multiple actions into separate families of drugs with more specific actions.

agents are nonspecific, but are relatively selective when administered in the usual fashion, because the circulation delivers a high initial concentration to the brain, and nerve cell function is more sensitive than are the functions of nonexcitable cells.

Selectivity Related to Drug Distribution

Topical Application

This is clearly the most selective route of drug administration. The drug is applied, in the desired concentration, directly at its intended site of action. This may be on a body surface; in the ear, eye, or nose;

by irrigation into the bladder; by insertion of suppositories into the rectum or vagina; by inhalation into the bronchi; by injection into a joint cavity, the pleural space, an abscess cavity, etc. The selectivity results from the fact that any drug absorbed from the site is diluted in such a large volume of circulating blood, and tissue fluid at other sites, that it is much less likely to have significant effects elsewhere in the body.

Intra-arterial or Portal Venous Injection

This achieves selectivity on a similar basis. Certain antitumor drugs have very little margin of safety between their effects on cancer cells and on rapidly growing normal cells such as GI epithelium. Selectivity can be achieved in some cases by injecting the drug intra-arterially, just upstream from the cancer, in a concentration that is locally active. But when the drug is diluted in the venous blood, the concentration is too low to affect the rest of the body. This method has been successfully used to treat malignant hepatoma or hepatic metastases by injection into the hepatic artery or into a tributary of the portal vein.

Selectivity by Ionization

Another example of specificity based on distribution is that of **atropine** versus **propantheline**. Both are effective blockers of muscarinic receptors, but propantheline does not readily cross the blood–brain barrier because it has a quaternary N, which is a permanent cation. Therefore, it has very little effect on cholinergic sites in the central nervous system compared to atropine when given in doses that produce equal degrees of peripheral effect.

Differential Blood Flow

Thiopental acts as a depressant on all cells with excitable membranes, including peripheral and central neurons, skeletal muscle, cardiac muscle, and smooth muscle. However, when injected intravenously it is first distributed among the various organs in proportion to their relative blood flows. Since the brain has a very high blood flow, and the drug is highly lipid-soluble, it passes rapidly into the brain and causes anaesthesia. As the drug gradually redistributes to other tissues with larger bulk but lower blood flow, the drug passes back out of the brain into the blood and thus ends its anaesthetic effect. In contrast, phenobarbital is much less lipid-soluble and does not enter the brain so readily despite the high blood flow. Therefore, it does not exert a rapid initial effect on the brain, and by the time it reaches an anaesthetic concentration in the brain it has also reached high levels in other tissues. Thus, it is not suitable for use as an anaesthetic, because an effective dose would take much too long to be eliminated.

Selective Concentration by Excretion

Many drugs are concentrated in the urine because they are filtered through the glomeruli, or actively secreted by the tubules, and poorly reabsorbed farther down. Therefore, they may reach effective concentrations in the tubule or lower urinary tract, even though the concentration in the plasma is too low to produce significant effects in the rest of the body. Examples include the use of **nitrofurantoin** as a urinary antiseptic and of **organomercurials** and **thiazides** as diuretic agents.

This same principle underlies the **selective renal toxicity** of the sulfonamides. These drugs are concentrated in the lumen of the renal tubule as described above. At the same time, the urine becomes acidified by exchange of H^+ for Na^+, and the concentrated sulfonamides crystallize out of the acid urine. The crystals may damage the tubular epithelium.

Selectivity Related to Tissue Metabolic Differences

Selective Cellular Binding

Some drugs that are capable of acting on many different types of cell, if present in high enough concentration, show selectivity at ordinary dosage by achieving the effective concentration only in certain cells in which there are binding sites with very high affinity. For example, **quinine** and many other antimalarial agents, though capable of exerting a quinidine-like effect on tissue cell membranes, have a much higher affinity for DNA inside the malarial parasites. Therefore, they can be used at plasma concentrations that are too low to produce myocardial effects, but that permit the accumulation of high enough concentrations inside the parasites to inhibit reproduction of the plasmodia. **Griseofulvin**, an antifungal antibiotic, can also be toxic to mammalian cells. However, it has selectively high binding to keratin (skin, hair, nails). When given in low doses that do not affect other tissues, it can build up a high enough concentration in keratinized structures to inhibit growth of the fungi, such as *Trichophyton rubrum*, which cause difficult infections of skin and nails.

Selective Intracellular Activation

Some drugs are not pharmacologically active in the form that is given, but are biotransformed to active metabolites. If one tissue has a particularly effective mechanism for forming the active product, it may be affected by a precursor drug concentration that is too low to affect other tissues. **Cyclophosphamide** is an inactive cyclic derivative of nitrogen mustard that is activated by hydroxylation of the cyclic amide ring, opening of the ring at the hydroxylation site, and cleavage of the opened ring to form free phosphoramide mustard, the active antitumor agent. The hydroxylation occurs in the liver, but the final cleavage seems to occur preferentially in the tumor cells. **Enteric sulfonamides**, such as phthalylsulfathiazole and succinylsulfathiazole, are not active against bacteria because their *p*-amino group is conjugated. However, bacterial hydrolases are able to split off the phthalyl or succinyl groups from the *p*-amino N, forming free sulfathiazole, which has antibacterial activity.

Selective Tissue Vulnerability

A drug may be relatively nonselective in terms of the range of tissues it acts on, yet it may have therapeutic specificity if the cellular function that it affects is more important in one tissue than in the rest. For example, the cardiac glycosides of the digitalis family inhibit the $(Na^+ + K^+)$-stimulated ATPase, which is involved in the active transport of cations across the cell membrane. This enzyme is present in many, probably all, types of cell. However, in muscle cells the levels of Na^+ and K^+ in the cells affect both the trans-membrane potential and the levels of free and membrane-bound Ca^{2+}, and thus influence both the excitability and the contractile force (see Chapter 34). The concentration of digitalis glycoside required to inhibit the enzyme is lower in heart muscle than in skeletal muscle, liver, kidney, or many other tissues.

Also, in other tissues the effect of the same degree of ATPase inhibition is not very obvious; for example, the liver does not contract, or conduct impulses, so that the consequences of digitalis action on it are not very visible. Therefore, therapeutic specificity (relatively speaking) is achieved by keeping the drug concentration finely balanced between limits that give the desired effect on contraction, or on A-V bundle conduction, but not the undesired effects on myocardial irritability, or on brain or other organs. However, when the drug concentration is a little higher, the same biochemical action in higher degree leads to the effects on myocardial excitability (ectopic foci) and on the nervous system that we recognize as toxic effects.

INDIVIDUAL AND SPECIES DIFFERENCES IN SPECIFICITY OR SELECTIVITY

In some instances a species may be unusually resistant to a drug because of a unique metabolic trait; for example, the rabbit is very resistant to procaine toxicity because of high serum esterase activity. This is merely a biologic curiosity, because procaine exposure in the rabbit is likely to be only an experimental procedure in isolated animals. In other cases, however, "selective toxicity" (i.e., useful drug action) depends upon differences between two species in the same field of drug exposure. Good examples are provided by bacterial-mammalian and insect-mammalian systems.

Inter-Species Differences

Bacteria Versus Host

The usefulness of **penicillin** as an antibiotic depends upon its structural resemblance to N-acetylmuramic acid (NAMA), with which it competes for binding to an enzyme that incorporates the NAMA-peptide into bacterial external cell walls (see Chapters 52 and 53). As the bacteria divide and grow, they must produce more cell wall to protect themselves against osmotic rupture because, like all plant cells, they have a high internal

osmotic pressure. Animal cells do not have external cell walls and do not require them because their internal osmotic pressure is kept isotonic with that of the extracellular fluid. Therefore, penicillin has little or no effect on animal cells at concentrations that are bactericidal by means of osmotic rupture.

Sulfonamides are bacteriostatic because of another species difference between bacteria and mammals. All cells require folic acid as a constituent of enzyme systems involved in methyl and formyl group transfer reactions, which are necessary for nucleic acid synthesis and hence for growth and cell reproduction. Mammalian cells require preformed folic acid, i.e., it is a vitamin for them. In contrast, many bacteria can not take up folate but require its precursors, from which they synthesize the folate intracellularly. One of the precursors is **para-aminobenzoic acid** (PABA). The para-aminobenzenesulfonic acid amides (sulfonamides) act as competitive antagonists of PABA for the bacterial enzyme systems that act on PABA (see Chapter 56). For other species of bacteria (e.g., leprosy bacilli), a similar role is played by **para-aminobenzene sulfones**.

Trimethoprim acts on a related enzyme, dihydrofolate reductase, to inhibit the conversion of dihydrofolate to tetrahydrofolate. This step occurs in mammalian cells as well as bacteria, but trimethoprim has many thousand times as great an affinity for the bacterial enzyme as for the mammalian enzyme. It is also preferentially active against the corresponding enzyme in the malaria parasite.

Insect Versus Mammal

Sometimes advantage can be taken of a similar species difference in enzyme activities to develop selectively toxic insecticides. **Malathion** is an organophosphate cholinesterase inhibitor that is metabolized in the liver to inactive products. This metabolic inactivation is more rapid in birds and mammals than in insects, so that an appropriate concentration can be selected that is toxic to insects but relatively safe for higher species.

Genetic Differences Within Species

In contrast to the preceding examples, there are instances of "selective toxicity" of a harmful type rather than a therapeutically useful one, as a result of genetic variations within species. An example is that of **primaquine** sensitivity. Primaquine gives rise to oxidized metabolites, which in turn tend to oxidize hemoglobin to methemoglobin inside the erythrocytes. Too high a concentration of methemoglobin is associated with membrane changes that lead to hemolysis. In the normal erythrocytes this is prevented by the reaction sequence shown in Figure 10–5A.

The right-hand step depends on glucose-6-phosphate dehydrogenase (G-6-PD). Various black and Mediter-

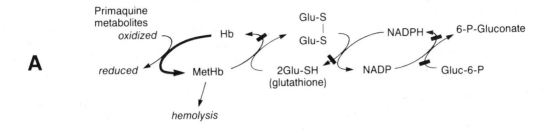

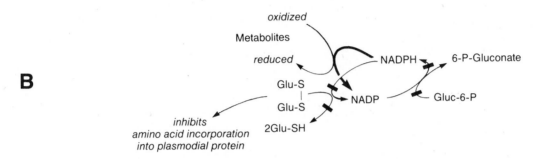

Figure 10–5 Interaction of glucose-6-phosphate dehydrogenase deficiency and primaquine metabolites in *A*, the host's erythrocytes and *B*, the host's liver and intrahepatic *Plasmodia*. Reaction steps that are impaired by G-6-PD deficiency are indicated by cross-bars. (*See* text for fuller explanation.)

ranean racial groups have a rather high frequency of hereditary deficiency of G-6-PD. The affected individuals are abnormally sensitive to hemolytic anemia that is produced by primaquine and various other drugs.

However, the same enzyme deficiency also has a selective advantage for the people affected. The oxidized metabolites of primaquine also reduce the concentrations of NADPH and reduced glutathione (Glu-SH) in the liver cells, and this is aggravated by G-6-PD deficiency. The malaria parasite draws its supply of NADPH and Glu-SH from the host cells, and too much oxidized glutathione inhibits protein synthesis in the parasites. Therefore, G-6-PD deficiency reduces the ability of the parasite to survive in the liver of the host and gives a greater therapeutic response to primaquine in the liver ("radical cure") (Fig. 10–5B).

Developmental Differences Within Individuals

Both desirable and undesirable drug effects may be selectively favored by metabolic differences found at different developmental stages in the same cell type or individual. Most of this chapter has dealt with specificity or selectivity in relation to therapeutic use of drugs. It is worthwhile to note some instances in which toxic effects are favored.

Thalidomide was formerly used widely as a sedative for pregnant women. It is metabolized by hydrolysis of the glutarimide ring, and the resulting metabolite is thought to interfere with an enzyme system that goes

through a period of maximum activity in the embryo between the 4th and 7th weeks of its development. Therefore, the drug can cause severe defects in the embryo at that time, yet is relatively harmless earlier or later (*see* Chapter 64).

Similarly, the newborn infant has a deficiency in the glucuronide conjugation system until it reaches several weeks of age (*see* Chapter 4). During the same period, it undergoes a physiologic hemolysis, from a breakdown of fetal erythrocytes during conversion to extra-uterine conditions. The excess hemolysis gives rise to more bilirubin than the conjugation system can cope with, and the extra bilirubin is carried in the plasma, bound to protein. During this period, drugs that compete either for the limited capacity of conjugation or for the protein binding sites cause overload of the bilirubin-carrying capacity, and free bilirubin passes into the brain and may cause **kernicterus**.

CONCLUSION

All therapeutically useful drug action is based on some degree of specificity or selectivity, but this may depend upon various factors related to the drug itself, the person to whom it is given, and the manner of administration. The mechanisms of the specificity or selectivity determine the margin of safety between desired and undesired effects, as well as the range of clinical applications.

SUGGESTED READING

Albert A. Selective toxicity: the physicochemical basis of therapy, 6th ed. London: Chapman and Hall, 1979.

Goldstein A, Aronow L, Kalman SM. Principles of drug action, 2nd ed. New York: Wiley Medical Publishers, 1974.

Chapter 11

DRUG INTERACTIONS

E.M. Sellers

The simultaneous use of several therapeutic agents has become commonplace. At some time during their stay in a general hospital most patients receive more than five drugs concurrently. On medical services the median number of drugs administered to patients during one hospitalization is 10 to 13, and many patients receive 20 or more drugs. Concomitant prescription of several drugs for ambulatory patients is the rule in many diseases. Furthermore, such patients commonly consume analgesics, cold remedies, and other drugs that are available without prescription. Finally, there is universal exposure to bioactive foreign chemicals in the form of food additives, insecticides, cleaning agents, cosmetics, and inhalants.

Unfortunately, it is an exceptional drug that does only "its own thing" in the body. One drug may change the effect of another by altering its metabolic fate or by enhancing or opposing its activity at the site of action. The latter type of interaction is more predictable and more generally appreciated, particularly when it is related to the expected pharmacologic actions of the drugs. There is nothing surprising about the ability of propranolol to alter the actions of isoproterenol, nor in the interactions between insulin and glucagon. Metabolic interactions between drugs are generally more subtle and are fully predictable only when the processes of absorption, distribution, binding, biotransformation, and excretion of each drug are thoroughly understood. Since this is seldom the case, the frequency of unexpected, adverse, and sometimes serious drug interactions has grown with the increasing use of potent drugs.

CLASSIFICATION

Consequence

The consequence of drug interactions can be (1) beneficial (enhancement of therapeutic effectiveness, diminution of toxicity) or (2) adverse (diminution of therapeutic effectiveness, enhancement of toxicity) (Table 11-1). The tactics of optimal, modern drug therapy often rely on the wise combination of drugs with complementary modes of action in order to reduce toxicity or enhance therapeutic efficacy. Several examples are shown in Table 11-2.

Table 11-3 illustrates the mutual enhancement of CNS-depressing effects of barbiturates and ethanol.

TABLE 11-1 Classification of Drug Interactions

Consequence
  Beneficial or adverse

Site
  External or internal

Mechanism
  Pharmacodynamic
  Pharmacokinetic
  Physiologic

TABLE 11–2 Examples of Drug–Drug Interactions and Their Consequences

Therapeutic Efficacy	Toxicity
Enhanced	
Combination drug therapy in cancer, hypertension, angina pectoris, infection, etc.	CNS depressants + ethanol (see Table 11–3)
Diminished	
Methotrexate effect negated by prior inhibition of thymidylate synthetase by 5-fluorouracil	Vasodilator + beta-blocker Naloxone + opiates Thiazides + potassium Carbidopa + L-dopa

Site of Interaction

External

Not surprisingly, there are many physicochemical incompatibilities when drugs are mixed in intravenous infusion, vials, or syringes. Precipitation or inactivation may occur. In general, it is better not to mix drugs together in the same solution. Hospital pharmacies can provide a full listing of intravenous incompatibilities when this information is needed.

Internal

This can be a body site or system (e.g., GI tract, liver) or the site of drug action (e.g., cell membrane, receptor sites, DNA-RNA, or intermediary metabolism). With respect to the latter, much of pharmacology is in fact the study of drug interactions! For example:

Cholinergic receptors: Hexamethonium competitively blocks the depolarizing action of carbachol at nicotinic synapses in ganglia; some antibiotics (e.g., kanamycin, gentamicin) potentiate the depolarizing block produced by succinylcholine at the neuromuscular junction; atropine competitively blocks pilocarpine at muscarinic receptors (see Chapters 15, 19, and 55).

Adrenergic receptors: Phentolamine, phenothiazines, and phenoxybenzamine block noradrenaline* action on α adrenoceptors in blood vessels. Metoprolol blocks β_1 (cardiac) adrenoceptor agonists, e.g., isoproterenol (see Chapters 17 and 27).

Other receptors: Morphine-induced respiratory depression is reversed by the narcotic antagonist naloxone (see Chapter 22).

---

* norepinephrine

Mechanism

Pharmacodynamic Interaction

This term refers to drug-induced changes in the effects of other drugs and needs to be distinguished from interactions based on changes in disposition (i.e., "pharmacokinetic" interaction). The barbiturate-ethanol interaction shown in Table 11–3 is a pharmacodynamic interaction. The term **physiologic interaction**, which may be encountered in some publications, refers to drug actions that are exerted at or on different sites or systems (e.g., heart and peripheral resistance vessels) but have the net effect of augmenting or offsetting each other. For example, hydralazine decreases total peripheral resistance; propranolol can block the reflex tachycardia induced by the fall in peripheral resistance, and thereby augment the antihypertensive effects of hydralazine. After reading this book, the reader should be able to think of many other examples.

With respect to quantitating the magnitude of pharmacodynamic drug interactions, several descriptive terms are encountered.

- **Additive**: The consequence (C) of an interaction is the simple sum of the separate effects of each drug (A and B); $C = A + B$.
- **Supra-additive**: $C > A + B$.
- **Infra-additive**: $C < A + B$.

These terms, though used, have very limited usefulness because they are only correct for a particular drug effect at a specified dose (more accurately, concentration), at a specified point in time, under specified conditions. These terms say nothing about mechanisms of interaction.

Pharmacokinetic Interaction

Pharmacodynamic interactions are often predictable on the basis of a full knowledge of the pharmacology

TABLE 11–3 Concentrations of Barbiturate and Ethanol in Blood Associated with Death in Various Groups of Overdose Patients

Mean *barbiturate* concentration in blood (mg/L)	
Death from barbiturate alone	3.67
Death from barbiturate + ethanol	2.55
Mean *ethanol* concentration in blood (mg/L)	
Death from ethanol alone	6500
Death from ethanol + barbiturate	1750

of the drugs in question. In contrast, the changes in the pharmacokinetics of one drug induced by another drug are often not intuitively obvious. Table 11–4 classifies pharmacokinetic interactions, to be taken up in detail in the remainder of this chapter.

PHARMACOKINETIC INTERACTIONS

Gastrointestinal Absorption

Physicochemical Interactions

The following five examples illustrate physicochemical interactions (Fig. 11–1).

- Changes in gastrointestinal pH by one drug (e.g., cimetidine, ranitidine, antacids) that affect the ionization of another drug (see Chapter 50).
- Chelation (e.g., of Ca^{2+} or Fe^{3+} by tetracycline) (see Chapter 55).
- Exchange resin binding (e.g., binding of warfarin and other drugs by cholestyramine) (see Chapter 37).
- Adsorption. Activated charcoal (AC) adsorbs many drugs. This observation is used therapeutically in drug poisonings by giving patients activated charcoal (approximately 1.5 g/kg) mixed in water. Typically a 10:1 ratio of AC to drug is desired in order to maximize gastrointestinal sequestration of the ingested drug and minimize systemic absorption (see Chapter 72).

TABLE 11–4 Pharmacokinetic Interactions

Absorption
  Physicochemical interaction
  Gastrointestinal motility
  Bacterial flora
  Mucosal function

Distribution
  Blood flow
  Serum binding
  Tissue binding
  Active transport to site of action

Biotransformation
  Hepatic
  Other sites

Excretion
  Renal
  Biliary
  Other sites

- Dissolution in non-absorbable material (e.g., of fat-soluble vitamins in mineral oil) (see Chapter 49).

Changes in Gastrointestinal Motility

Changes in gastrointestinal motility affect the rate and/or the completeness of drug absorption (i.e., absolute bioavailability). It is important to realize that absorption may be slowed, but nevertheless be complete, since absorption occurs along the whole gastrointestinal tract. The importance of such interactions depends on the rate of onset of drug action and the drug's therapeutic index.

Increased gastric emptying and intestinal motility. Metoclopramide increases the rate of gastric emptying, and hence might result in earlier and higher peak concentrations for drugs rapidly absorbed from the upper small intestine (see Chapter 14). Castor oil and other cathartics increase intestinal motility and might decrease the completeness of absorption of drugs (see Chapter 51).

Decreased gastric emptying and intestinal motility. All opioid analgesics and anticholinergic drugs decrease the rate of gastric emptying and intestinal motility (e.g., codeine, morphine, atropine, loperamide) (see Chapters 15 and 22). Decreased gastric emptying will be associated with slower absorption, lower peak drug concentrations, and later times of peak concentration.

Figure 11–2 summarizes the results of a study to determine the effects of opioids (pentazocine, meperidine, heroin) on drug absorption. Acetaminophen is used as the test drug. Note that metoclopramide does not reverse the decreased gastric emptying caused by the opioids.

Changes in Bacterial Flora

Bowel bacteria may play an important role in synthesizing vitamin K essential for normal clotting function or may reactivate some inactive drug metabolites, excreted *via* the bile, by deconjugating them. Hence, broad-spectrum antibiotics may interact with these drugs by modifying or eliminating intestinal flora (see Chapters 55 and 56). The biotransformation of digoxin within the gastrointestinal lumen is altered by antibiotic therapy.

Drug-Induced Changes in Mucosal Function

Drugs with specific gastrointestinal toxicity (e.g., colchicine) may damage the GI mucosa or block active transport (see Chaper 51). This action can, in theory, result in interactions with other drugs.

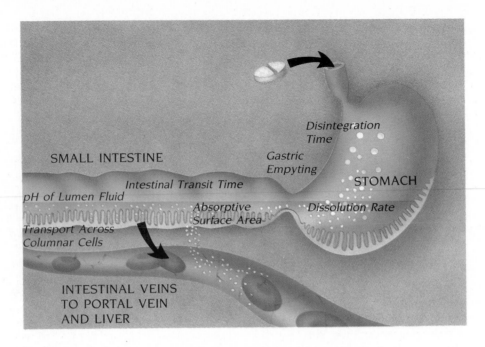

Figure 11-1 Factors involved in gastrointestinal drug interactions.

Distribution

Blood Flow

Since organ uptake and clearance of drug are ultimately dependent on blood flow, it is not surprising that some drug interactions involve alterations in such flow. For example, propranolol may produce an important decrease in cardiac output. This in turn can reduce hepatic blood flow and hepatic clearance of propranolol itself and of lidocaine and other drugs with high first-pass extraction (*see* Chapter 7).

Tissue Uptake or Binding

Many drugs localize in tissues at sites that have nothing to do with the desired therapeutic action of the drug (*e.g.*, digoxin in skeletal muscle). Tissue binding of these drugs serves as a potentially large store from which they can be displaced by other drugs.

The liver's strategic placement between the small intestine and the systemic circulation can permit important drug interactions. Recall that F (bioavailability) = 1 − E (extraction ratio). Drugs that interfere with hepatic uptake, biotransformation, intracellular binding, or biliary excretion of other drugs may markedly increase the systemic bioavailability of those with high first-pass effect during the absorptive phase. For example ethanol, administered 1 hour before amitriptyline, causes a doubling of amitriptyline concentrations during the drug's absorptive phase (Fig. 11-3). Cimetidine has similar effects on the uptake of propranolol.

Serum Protein Binding

Many drugs are highly bound to serum proteins, typically albumin. Such highly bound drugs may be dis-

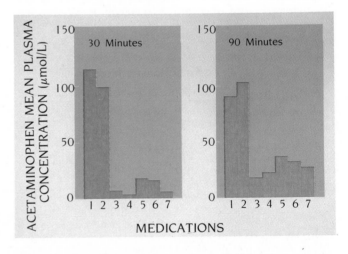

Figure 11-2 Mean plasma acetaminophen concentrations (S.E. omitted for clarity) in 46 women in labor and 10 women postpartum at 30 and 90 minutes after a single oral dose of 1.5 g, with and without administration of narcotic analgesics alone or in combination with metoclopramide. Medications: 1 = no narcotics; 2 = postpartum; 3 = pentazocine; 4 = meperidine; 5 = meperidine/metoclopramide; 6 = heroin; 7 = heroin/metoclopramide. (Modified from Prescott LF, Nimmo WS, Heading RC. Drug absorption interactions. In: Grahame-Smith DG, ed. 1977:45–51.)

placed by other highly bound drugs administered concurrently. For example, warfarin is displaced by trichloroacetic acid (a metabolite of chloral hydrate), and thus increased anticoagulation may occur. Bilirubin is displaced by some sulfonamides, and kernicterus may result (*see* Chapter 56).

The **immediate consequences** when a displacing drug is added to therapy can in theory be the appearance of toxicity or otherwise altered response (Fig. 11–4, Table 11–5). Even a small amount of displacement of a highly plasma-bound drug causes a large relative increase in the free active fraction of the drug in the serum (Fig. 11–4; in the case illustrated, an 18% displacement of bound drug causes a 100% increase in free concentration). However, the displaced drug does not remain confined in the circulation but redistributes throughout the body. After such redistribution the increase in free drug concentration in serum and extracellular fluid depends mainly on the apparent volume of distribution for the free drug. If the free drug distribution volume is large, the increase in free drug concentration will be small and probably pharmacologically unimportant.

Other processes also act to buffer the consequences of the acute changes in free concentration after a drug's partial displacement from albumin. An increase in the concentration of unbound drug in the serum also makes more drug available for glomerular filtration or hepatic biotransformation. For drugs restrictively eliminated by the liver, this displacement results in a greater elimination of the free drug (*via* first-order Michaelis-Menten kinetics), which may be reflected in temporary slight shortening of the serum half-life of total drug. At this new steady state, the total drug concentration in the serum is lower than before displacement, the serum half-life of total drug is the same, and the free drug concentration in the serum is a higher fraction of the total. Clearance of free drug will be the same as before displacement, but clearance calculated on the basis of total drug will be apparently greater.

For drugs that are removed from the circulation by high-capacity or -affinity uptake mechanisms in kidney or liver, displacement from albumin may decrease the rate at which drug is delivered to these sites of elimination. Thus, displacement of such drugs from albumin, in theory, can increase their total and free concentrations (*see* Chapter 7).

Clinically important pharmacokinetic interaction due to displacement from plasma proteins will occur only when (1) administration of the displacing drug is started in high doses during chronic therapy with the displaced drug, (2) the volume of distribution of displaced drug is small, and (3) the response to the drug occurs faster than redistribution or enhanced elimination. Maximum potentiation occurs shortly after addition of the displacing drug and reaches a maximum fairly quickly. The potentiation is usually transient.

Because the free drug level is the determinant of the

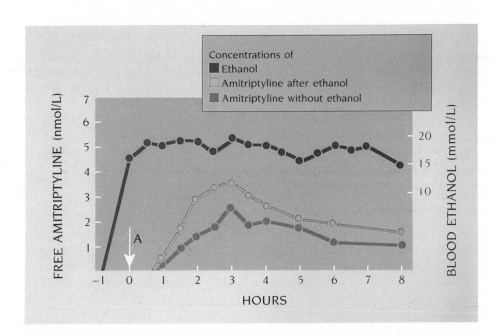

Figure 11–3 Mean plasma concentrations of free amitriptyline (nmol/L) and ethanol (mmol/L) for 5 subjects. Ethanol was administered as an oral loading dose of 0.9 g/kg lean body weight, followed by approximately 0.1 g/kg every half hour to maintain blood ethanol levels at 15–20 mmol/L. Amitriptyline 25 mg (A) was administered at time 0, with and without a preceding dose of ethanol. (Modified from Dorian P, *et al*. Amitriptyline and ethanol: pharmacokinetic and pharmacodynamic interaction. Eur J Clin Pharmacol 1983; 25:325–331.)

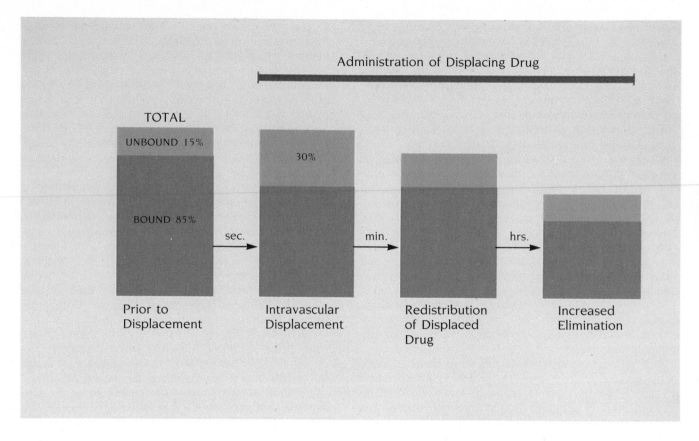

Figure 11-4 Sequence of changes in plasma drug concentrations during displacement interactions.

pharmacologic effect, changes in **total** steady-state levels may not predict a change in pharmacologic effect observed clinically, during concurrent therapy with an interacting drug. For example, inhibition of biotransformation of warfarin, coupled with its displace- ment from plasma proteins, could result in "normal" steady-state **total** drug concentration in the plasma, yet free concentrations would be markedly elevated and result in a prolonged prothrombin time (*see* Chapter 41).

TABLE 11-5   Potential Consequences of Drug Displacement from Plasma Proteins

	Immediately After Displacement*	At Steady State
Free drug fraction in serum	Increased	Increased
Free drug concentration in serum	Increased	Unchanged
Total drug concentration in serum	Unchanged	Decreased
Pharmacologic activity	Increased	Unchanged
Glomerular filtration	Increased	Unchanged
Tubular secretion	Variable	Unchanged
Diffusion into liver cells	Increased	Unchanged
Active hepatic uptake	Variable	Unchanged

* All changes are compared to those concentrations and effects immediately prior to displacement. This phase may last only a short time, because redistribution starts to occur immediately (*see also* Fig. 11-4).

Active Transport to Site of Action

A number of complex interactions involve alterations in regulation of neurotransmitters. A classical example of such an interaction is summarized in Figure 11–5. Tricyclic antidepressants block the uptake of noradrenaline, thus increasing the postsynaptic concentration of active neurotransmitters. Guanethidine decreases the release of noradrenaline and with chronic guanethidine pretreatment one can expect the postsynaptic noradrenaline receptors to be "supersensitive," in compensation for the chronically low noradrenaline level (see Chapters 16, 17, and 18). Thus, when the low synaptic level of noradrenaline is somewhat increased by desipramine it results in a significant rise in blood pressure. Desipramine decreases the pressor activity of tyramine infusions but increases the pressor action of noradrenaline. Interactions involving antihypertensives and tricyclics, L-dopa, phenothiazines, direct- and indirect-acting sympathomimetics, and amphetamine congeners often have a similar basis.

Biotransformation

Enzyme Induction

Stimulation of microsomal enzyme activity by drugs and other chemicals is an important clinical problem. Hundreds of drugs including analgesics, anticonvulsants, oral hypoglycemics, sedatives, and tranquilizers stimulate the biotransformation of either themselves or other drugs. (See Chapter 4.)

Enzyme induction:

- increases the rate of hepatic biotransformation of drug,
- increases the rate of production of metabolites,
- increases hepatic drug clearance,
- decreases serum drug half-life,
- decreases serum total and free drug concentrations,
- decreases pharmacologic effects if the metabolites are inactive.

Drugs that induce major increases of drug biotransforming enzymes in the human include barbiturates (e.g., phenobarbital), cigarette smoke hydrocarbons, carbamazepine, chronic heavy ethanol ingestion, and rifampin.

With barbiturates, approximately 4–7 days are required before any clinically significant effect occurs; enzyme induction may take 2–4 weeks to disappear. This period of offset of induction can be important. For example, phenobarbital enhances the biotransformation of the anticoagulant warfarin, and higher doses of warfarin will be needed to achieve satisfactory anticoagulation if phenobarbital is given concurrently. If the phenobarbital is discontinued and the warfarin dose is not adjusted, bleeding may result (Fig. 11–6).

Rifampin, an antibiotic, is another potent enzyme inducer. Concurrent administration with oral contraceptives can result in contraceptive failure because of increased biotransformation of the steroid. Similar increases in biotransformation after rifampin have been shown with prednisone, oral anticoagulants, and some hypoglycemics.

Enzyme Inhibition

Inhibition of microsomal enzymes:

- decreases the rate of hepatic biotransformation of drug,

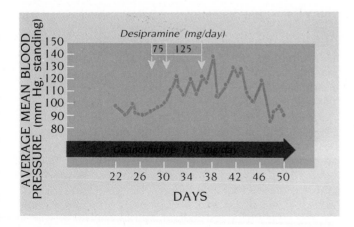

Figure 11–5 Antagonism of guanethidine by desipramine. Guanethidine was given in increasing doses until blood pressure was controlled with 150 mg daily. Desipramine was administered as indicated. See also Chapter 18, Figure 18–4 for a similar experiment.

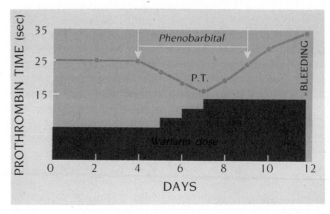

Figure 11–6 Clinical consequences of enhancement of warfarin biotransformation by phenobarbital.

- decreases the rate of production of metabolites,
- decreases total clearance,
- increases serum drug half-life,
- increases serum total and free drug concentrations,
- increases pharmacologic effects if the metabolites are inactive.

Clinically important inhibitors of drug biotransformation include acute ethanol exposure, chloramphenicol (and some other antibiotics), cimetidine, disulfiram, and propoxyphene.

Acute ethanol exposure inhibits biotransformations mediated by the mixed-function oxidase system. Inhibition of demethylation and hydroxylation of diazepam, chlordiazepoxide, propranolol, amitriptyline, propoxyphene, and others has been shown. As with other inhibitors, conjugation reactions seem to be spared.

Cimetidine (a histamine H_2-receptor blocker used to reduce gastric acid secretion; *see* Chapter 50) has been reported to inhibit the biotransformation of acetaminophen, beta-blockers, chlordiazepoxide, diazepam, digitoxin, ethanol, imipramine, phenytoin, quinidine, theophylline, and warfarin. Since cimetidine also decreases hepatic blood flow, more than one mechanism may be present. For each of these drugs affected by cimetidine, the therapeutic or toxic consequences of inhibition of biotransformation may be important and should be reviewed by the reader.

A widely used H_2-receptor blocker, ranitidine (*see* Chapter 50), has lesser effects on drug biotransformations. However, one would expect the H_2-mediated blood flow changes occurring with cimetidine to occur also with ranitidine.

Disulfiram inhibits the mitochondrial enzyme acetaldehyde dehydrogenase and causes acetaldehyde accumulation after consumption of alcohol. This is the cause of the disulfiram-alcohol reaction and is the theoretical basis for use of the drug in the treatment of alcoholism (*see* Chapter 25). However, disulfiram also inhibits microsomal enzymatic steps, including hydroxylation and demethylation, but not conjugation.

Some clinically important drug interactions that are usually attributed to changed albumin binding of one or both drugs actually involve other mechanisms as well. For example, phenylbutazone can displace both warfarin isomers from plasma albumin *in vivo* and *in vitro*, and invariably and importantly enhances the hypoprothrombinemia of patients on anticoagulant therapy with warfarin. Phenylbutazone also inhibits the biotransformation of the S-isomer while stimulating the elimination of the R-isomer of warfarin. Since the S-isomer is five times as potent as the R-isomer, potentiation of warfarin-induced hypoprothrombinemia occurs. Another example is that of sulfaphenazole, which displaces the oral hypoglycemic drug tolbutamide from albumin but also reduces its rate of hepatic oxidation, thereby preventing the compensatory increase in inactivation that usually occurs after displacement interactions. Both effects undoubtedly play a role in the potentiation of tolbutamide-induced hypoglycemia by

sulfaphenazole. In general, inhibition of drug biotransformation is the clinically most important mechanism of pharmacokinetic interactions.

Excretion

Drug interactions may theoretically alter the rates of elimination of drugs by any of the excretory routes (*e.g.*, feces, bile, sweat, tears, and lungs). However, the only drug interactions of this type that have received careful study are those involving renal excretion. The following major types have been observed:

1. Glomerular filtration of drugs is increased by displacement from albumin.
2. Tubular reabsorption of filtered drugs is decreased by:
   - diuretics (in some instances),
   - alkalinizers (*e.g.*, $NaHCO_3$, acetazolamide) for weakly acidic drugs such as salicylates and barbiturates,
   - acidifiers (*e.g.*, ascorbic acid, NH_4Cl) for weak amines such as amphetamines, methadone, quinidine and procainamide.
3. Tubular secretion of drugs is decreased by competition for active transport systems (*e.g.*, probenecid blocks secretion of penicillins), so that their half-life in the body is prolonged.

In recent years, interactions at the renal tubular site have been recognized as important and more frequent than previously thought. For example, cimetidine was studied in six healthy volunteers by comparing the single-dose pharmacokinetics of oral procainamide before and during a daily dose of cimetidine. The area under the procainamide plasma-concentration-time curve was increased by cimetidine by an average of 35%, from 27.0 ± 0.3 μg/mL·h to 36.5 ± 3.4 μg/mL·h. The elimination half-life increased from a harmonic mean of 2.92 to 3.68 h. The renal clearance of procainamide was reduced by cimetidine from 347 ± 46 mL/min to 196 ± 11 mL/min. The area under the plasma-concentration-time curve for N-acetylprocainamide (NAPA, the active metabolite of procainamide) was increased by a mean of 25% by cimetidine, because of a significant reduction in renal clearance from 258 ± 60 mL/min to 197 ± 59 mL/min. The data suggest that cimetidine inhibits the tubular secretion of both procainamide and N-acetylprocainamide. Such a renal interaction is important not only for basic drugs that are cleared by the kidney, but also for metabolites of basic drugs and endogenous substances that require active transport into the lumen of the proximal tubule of the kidney for their elimination.

Digoxin (a cardiac glycoside used to treat heart failure; *see* Chapter 34) provides another example of interactions involving renal excretion of drugs. Several reports in 1978 indicated that digoxin concentration rose almost two-fold when the antiarrhythmic drug quinidine was given concurrently and that this increase was associated with clinically important toxicity. Subsequent studies have shown similar effects with verapamil and amiodarone. Detailed studies suggest that the basis of this interaction is a fall (34%) in renal clearance of digoxin without a change in glomerular filtration, a decrease (32%) in V_d, and a fall (36%) in total body clearance. Half-life does not change greatly. Other studies suggest that quinidine may displace digoxin from tissue binding sites. The importance of renal tubular transport systems for bases and neutral compounds has become clinically apparent.

TABLE 11-6 Summary of Drugs Interacting with Warfarin

Increased Anticoagulant Effect

Displacement from Protein Binding Sites	Decreased Biotransformation	Altered Platelet Function	Direct Effect on Synthesis or Catabolism of Clotting Factors
Chloral hydrate§	Allopurinol	ASA*	ASA(>2g/day)*
Clofibrate§	Amiodarone	Dipyridamole§	Thyroid hormones
Ethacrynic acid	Chloramphenicol	Indomethacin§	
Nalidixic acid	Cimetidine‡	Other nonsteroidal anti-inflammatory agents§	
Oxyphenbutazone*	Ciprofloxacin		
Phenylbutazone*	Clofibrate		
Sulfonamides	Co-trimoxazole		
	Disopyramide		
	Disulfiram‡		
	Erythromycin		
	Ethanol		
	Influenza vaccine		
	Metronidazole		
	Oxyphenbutazone*		
	Phenylbutazone*		
	Sulfonamides		
	Sulfonylureas		

Decreased Anticoagulant Effect

Decreased Coumarin Absorption	Induced Biotransformation	Direct Effect on Clotting Factors
Cholestyramine	Barbiturates†	Oral contraceptives‡
	Carbamazepine†	
	Ethanol	
	Glutethimide†	
	Griseofulvin	
	Rifampin†	

* High probability of serious interaction, *avoid*.
† Consistent.
‡ Inconsistent interaction, consider alternative drugs.
§ Interaction unpredictable, consider alternative drugs.
The table compiles some of the drugs known to interact with coumarin anticoagulants. The mechanisms suggested are known with variable degrees of confidence. A number of drugs with unknown mechanisms of interaction are excluded. Often more than one mechanism is occurring—all such possibilities are not cross-tabulated. When interacting drugs are given together, prothrombin time should be monitored carefully. Interacting drugs may be administered concurrently when this precaution is taken. However, if possible, the use of non-interacting drugs is preferred since control of anticoagulation is often variable during concurrent therapy, and hence there is a higher risk of bleeding or inadequate anticoagulation.

CONCLUDING EXERCISE

Interactions with oral anticoagulants are of particular clinical importance. Table 11–6 will allow the reader to review the concepts in this chapter. This table demonstrates pharmacodynamic interactions alone and in various combinations. The details ("What drug is in what list") are not critical, but the answers to the following types of question could be important: "A patient on anticoagulant therapy has suddenly started to have hematuria. Could it be due to the nonsteroidal antiinflammatory drug he has just begun to take? If so, what would be the most likely mechanisms?"

SUGGESTED READING

Doering W. Quinidine-digoxin interaction. N Engl J Med 1979; 301:400–404.

Drug Interactions Update. Med Lett Drugs Ther 1984; 26(654): 11–14.

Grahame-Smith DG. Drug interactions. Baltimore: University Park Press, 1977.

Kelly LJ, Bell RG. Mechanism for potentiation of warfarin by phenylbutazone. Biochem Pharmacol 1981; 30:2443–2449.

Koch-Weser J, Sellers EM. Drug interactions with coumarin anticoagulants. N Engl J Med 1971; 285:487–498(part I); 547–558(part II).

Koch-Weser J, Sellers EM. Drug therapy: binding of drugs to serum albumin. N Engl J Med 1976; 294:311–316(part I); 526–530(part II).

Loewe S. The problem of synergism and antagonism of combined drugs. Arzneim-Forsch 1953; 3:285–290.

Medical Letter Handbook of Drug Interactions. New Rochelle (N.Y.): Medical Letter Inc., 1983.

Somogyi A, McLean A, Heinzoq B. Cimetidine-procainamide pharmacokinetic interaction in man: evidence of competition for tubular secretion of basic drugs. Eur J Clin Pharmacol 1983; 25:339–345.

Chapter 12

HUMAN PHARMACOGENETICS

W. Kalow and S. Spielberg

Pharmacogenetics deals with the influence of heredity on the response to drugs or on their fate in the body. The object of studies in pharmacogenetics is to explain and control variability in response to drugs and toxic agents. This definition of pharmacogenetics includes, for instance, heritable resistance of bacteria to antibiotics, or differences between inbred strains of mice in responding to an enzyme inducer. As the title indicates, this chapter deals exclusively with human pharmacogenetics, and it will be restricted to items of clinical relevance.

Some geneticists use the yet rare word "ecogenetics" as a term of higher order to denote the occurrence of deviant responses to any environmental chemical including drugs, foods, and vitamins. However, there are no generally recognized sharp distinctions of terminology. For instance, lactase deficiency renders milk an unsuitable nutrient to many people; some authorities may cite this as an example of pharmacogenetics, others of ecogenetics.

Pharmacogenetics is **not** genetic toxicology, a branch of science concerned with the chemical production of mutations or similar events.

Why is pharmacogenetics of special interest? First, it is a branch of pharmacology and therapeutics with a well-circumscribed core of knowledge. Second, pharmacogenetics increases the physician's awareness and anticipation of abnormal drug responses. Third, knowledge of frequently occurring genetic defects that alter drug responses will enable drug manufacturers to avoid the introduction of unreliable drugs. Fourth, genetic defects may be used as experiments of nature to help unravel some mysteries that underlie normal drug responses.

In the context of this textbook, not more than an outline can be presented. It begins with an introduction into classification systems of pharmacogenetics, and a brief survey of prime examples. This will be followed by relatively extensive coverage of a few important examples.

CORE OF PHARMACOGENETICS

The subject matter of pharmacogenetics can be subdivided and presented in different ways. For instance, a recent survey quoted some 70 items, using the following main classification:

- Disorders characterized by increased sensitivity to drugs.
- Differences resulting from increased resistance to drugs.
- Disorders exacerbated by enzyme-inducing drugs.
- Diseases to which chronic drug exposure may contribute.
- Disorders of unknown etiology.
- Disorders associated with diet.
- Reported polymorphisms; clinical disorders not yet demonstrated.

This is incongruous as a classification, but nevertheless gives an indication of the broad range of events. However, in order to develop an understanding of the underlying problems, it is advantageous to divide the field systematically by two criteria, one of them genetic, one pharmacologic. The genetic distinction is between monogenic and multigenic variations, i.e., those depending on the presence or absence of one particular kind of allelic gene, and those governed by several genes; the latter systems are usually influenced by environmental factors. The pharmacologic distinction is between alterations of a drug's fate and alterations of the dynamics of its action, i.e., between alterations of drug-metabolizing enzymes and those of drug receptors or other targets. In either case, the variation could be quantitative or qualitative.

The concept of multigenic inheritance implies that three or more kinds of genes contribute to the variability of a particular character. The characters of concern are usually quantitative entities, such as stature, IQ, plasma half-life of antipyrine, or increase of cardiac rate after phenylephrine. Since environmental factors generally contribute to such characters, the genetic component is measured in terms of heritability. Typical heritability values considered useful in animal husbandry range between 20 and 50%, crudely implying 50–80% environmental contribution to a variable ("crudely" because hereditary and environmental influences do not simply sum up if there are interaction terms). Heritability values in humans are usually derived from studies on twins; measurements of plasma half-life, clearance, or steady-state concentrations have tended to give heritability values above 50%, even as high as 98% in one set of measurements with antipyrine. The tested drugs include dicoumarol, phenylbutazone, nortriptyline, tolbutamide, and phenytoin, among others. In summary, there appears to be a substantial element of genetic control in the elimination rate of all or most drugs that have been investigated appropriately.

It would be wrong to consider the available heritability data in pharmacogenetics as biologic constants. They provide some guidance but are strictly valid only for the population in which they were determined. For instance, most differences in antipyrine metabolism between nonsmoking healthy adults of similar stock and similar eating habits are genetic, while nutrition, life style, and disease likely contribute much to the variability of antipyrine metabolism among the mixed population attending a large city practice.

By contrast, an immutable impact on pharmacology is shown by certain monogenic traits that are as purely genetic as the color of the eye, and that generally result in some biochemical or functional feature that can be counted in a population. It is important to realize that such traits are not necessarily rare. A list of prominent examples is given in Table 12–1. It is not possible here to explain all entries: the listing should leave the reader with the strong impression that there are many genetically definable causes of aberrant drug responses.

SELECTED EXAMPLES OF GENETIC INFLUENCE ON DRUG METABOLISM

Hydrolysis of Succinylcholine

A perspicuous example of genetic control of drug metabolism is provided by the cholinesterase variants in human plasma. The most frequent of these variants is called "atypical cholinesterase." The clinically significant cholinesterase variants occur in approximately 1 in 2000 subjects in Caucasian populations.

TABLE 12–1 Monogenic Traits of Pharmacologic or Toxicologic Concern

Enzymes of Drug Biotransformation

*Atypical plasma cholinesterase
Serum paraoxonase polymorphism
*Acetyltransferase deficiency
*Debrisoquine-sparteine oxidation defect
Mephenytoin hydroxylase deficiency
Acatalasemia
Deficient glucuronide conjugation
Alcohol dehydrogenase polymorphism
Aldehyde dehydrogenase deficiency
Dopamine-β-hydroxylase deficiency
Catechol-O-methyltransferase deficiency
Thiopurine methyltransferase deficiency

Genes and Drug Targets

Alterations of Enzyme Activity or of Protein Structure as a Basis for Altered Drug Responses:
*Hypoxanthine-guanine phosphoribosyltransferase (HGPRT) deficiency or defect (various forms of gout)
*Glucose-6-phosphate dehydrogenase (G-6-PD) deficiencies (hemolytic disorders)
NADH methemoglobin reductase deficiency (methemoglobinemia)
Uroporphyrinogen I synthetase deficiency (acute intermittent porphyria)
Coproporphyrinogen oxidase deficiency (hereditary coproporphyria)
δ-Aminolevulinic acid synthetase—excessive induction (variegate porphyria)
Steroid hydroxylase deficiencies (various endocrine vulnerabilities)
1_α-Hydroxylase of vitamin D precursors—enzyme absence (vitamin D-resistant rickets)
*Glutathione synthetase deficiency (hemolysis potential, drug-induced hepatotoxicity)
α_1-Antitrypsin deficiency (emphysema)
Unstable hemoglobins (various vulnerabilities)

Response Differences on a Biochemically Undefined Basis:
*Malignant hyperthermia
Electroencephalographic differences in alcohol response
Steroid-induced glaucoma
Tasting ability for a series of bitter-tasting substances
Smelling abilities for cyanide, phenylacetic acid, or blossom odors
Plasma:erythrocyte ratio of lithium
*Diminished receptor occupation of dicumarol-type anticoagulants
*Susceptibility to drug-induced hepatotoxicity demonstrable with lymphocytes *in vitro*

The purpose of this list is to show the scope of the subject of pharmacogenetics, and thereby to lend perspective to the examples (marked*) cited in the text. The porphyrias listed here may all lead to drug-induced, acute neurologic crises.

The plasma cholinesterase is capable of hydrolysing a number of drugs including cocaine and heroin, but of greatest clinical importance is its action upon the muscle relaxant succinylcholine. This drug is given intravenously, which means that it is immediately and fully exposed to plasma cholinesterase. The fate of the drug therefore depends directly on esterase action. In the presence of atypical cholinesterase, the action of an ordinary dose of succinylcholine lasts for about an hour instead of a couple of minutes (Fig. 12–1). The reason is a very low affinity between atypical esterase and the drug (*i.e.*, high K_m), so that the two do not readily combine; thus, in regard to succinylcholine, the enzyme is nonfunctional. This can be demonstrated *in vitro* by using succinylcholine as substrate (Fig. 12–2).

Since the drug paralyses respiratory as well as other muscles, the patient requires artificial respiration until the drug effect wears off. Occasionally, there are families with about three-fold higher than average esterase activity. In these cases, ordinary doses of succinylcholine have very little effect.

Isoniazid Acetylation

Genetic control has also been observed for the acetylation of isoniazid and other drugs. The capacity for rapid acetylation occurs in families as a Mendelian dominant. As a rule, one can tell without ambiguity whether a person is or is not a rapid acetylator, since the blood levels of isoniazid a few hours after intake of a standard dose are very low in rapid, and fairly

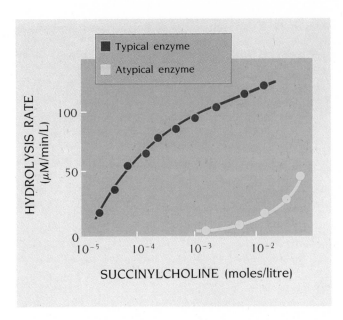

Figure 12–2 *In vitro* interactions of succinylcholine with plasma cholinesterase, showing the rate of hydrolysis of succinylcholine by human plasma containing either the usual or the atypical form of the enzyme. Note the greatly reduced affinity (high K_m) of the drug for atypical esterase. Deficient combination between succinylcholine and atypical cholinesterase explains the clinical failure of drug elimination. (Adapted from Kalow W. Pharmacogenetics: heredity and the response to drugs. Philadelphia/London: WB Saunders, 1962).

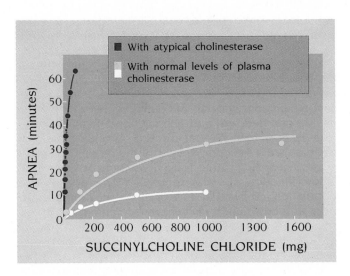

Figure 12–1 Duration of apnea (respiratory muscle paralysis) from succinylcholine administration in patients with normal and atypical plasma cholinesterase. (Adapted from Kalow W. Pharmacogenetics: heredity and the response to drugs. Philadelphia/London: WB Saunders, 1962).

high in slow, acetylators. Blood levels tend to differ by a factor of 4–6. In the populations occupying the temperate zones of the Western world (including North American Blacks), about half the subjects are slow, the other half rapid, acetylators. In Oriental populations (and the genetically related North American indigenous peoples) the proportion of fast acetylators approaches 80–90%.

The genetically variable enzyme is an N-acetyltransferase found in the soluble fraction of human liver cells. In addition to isoniazid, this enzyme catalyses the acetylation of a series of drugs (phenelzine, hydralazine, sulfadimidine, sulfapyridine, procainamide, dapsone), of drug metabolites (nitrazepam and caffeine), and of several carcinogens (benzidine, 2-aminofluorene, and 4-aminobiphenyl). The acetylation of para-aminosalicylic acid (PAS) and some antibacterial sulfonamides varies much less from person to person, as if produced by other acetyltransferases.

There are a number of adverse drug reactions, diseases, or therapeutic outcomes associated with acetylator phenotype, and these are summarized in Table 12–2. These complications are all more frequent in slow acetylators. It should be noted that some of these associations are speculative.

TABLE 12–2 Consequences of Polymorphic Acetylation

Isoniazid (INH)
  Peripheral neuropathy is more common among slow acetylators (and elderly patients).
  Slow acetylators accumulate INH, which in turn inhibits hepatic mixed-function oxidases.
  Increased phenytoin toxicity has been described in slow acetylators treated with INH and phenytoin.

Hydralazine
  Lupoid reactions are more common among slow acetylators.

Procainamide
  Slow acetylators develop lupus earlier and more frequently than fast acetylators.

Phenelzine
  Severe adverse reactions (nausea, drowsiness) are more common among slow acetylators.

Salicylazosulfapyrimidine
  Side effects of sulfapyrimidine (e.g., hemolysis) are more common among slow acetylators.

It has been suggested that a disproportionate number of patients with systemic lupus erythematosus and rheumatoid arthritis are slow acetylators.

Occupational bladder cancers in chemical workers were recently reported to have a high prevalence in slow acetylators.

Drug Oxidations

The most common forms of drug biotransformation are oxidative reactions of various kinds. Drug oxidizing enzymes include flavin-containing monooxygenases, alcohol and aldehyde dehydrogenases, xanthine oxidase, and various other oxidoreductases, but most important are the group of enzymes often referred to as mixed-function oxidases of liver microsomes (Chapter 4), which have as terminal element a cytochrome P-450, so that their reactions have some individually specific features and some characteristics that are common to all. The P-450 cytochromes are currently subject to massive investigations at the molecular level. They represent a superfamily of heme proteins consisting of many families, two of which (recommended nomenclature: P450 I and P450 II) are families of drug-metabolizing enzymes (Table 12–3). P450 II consists of ten subfamilies, some of which have their structural genes on different chromosomes, an indication that there are truly different enzymes subject to independent regulation. Some enzymes are constitutive, others are subject to induction. Nineteen P450s have been sequenced at the time of writing. Structural genetic variants (= allozymes) of three P450s are currently known and under intense investigation.

Clinically, the first evidence for a genetic control within this system of enzymes was obtained some years ago by Kutt et al., who observed that intoxication with

phenytoin occurred in members of a family that biotransformed this drug at an extraordinarily low rate. Phenytoin undergoes aromatic hydroxylation by microsomal enzymes. An equivalent observation was made by Shahidi, in a woman in whom large doses of phenacetin had led to substantial methemoglobin formation. The cause was found to be an unusual oxidation of phenacetin, yielding a methemoglobin-forming metabolite. This unusual pathway of phenacetin metabolism was due to a deficiency of the usual O-dealkylation and proved to be familial.

A widespread, monogenic defect severely affecting the fate of several drugs was discovered only a few years ago. The discovery arose from the observation of two drugs that are metabolized by the P-450 system, apparently by a single isozyme. There were two independent discoveries:

(1) Eichelbaum et al., in Germany, found in 1975 that roughly 5% of the population were incapable of metabolizing sparteine. Sparteine is an alkaloid of the broom and lupine plants, with antiarrhythmic and oxytocic properties. In non-metabolizers, sparteine had a long half-life and accumulated in the body on repeated administration.

(2) Idle, Smith, and their collaborators in England investigated, in 1977, the metabolism of debrisoquine (an antihypertensive drug of the guanethidine class) in order to explain the 30-fold dose range of the drug required by different patients during therapy. They found in about 8% of the British population a severe deficiency of formation of the main metabolite, 4-hydroxydebrisoquine. It was later shown that the failures to biotransform sparteine and debrisoquine appear to have an identical cause, which we will refer to as the SD-defect (sparteine-debrisoquine metabolizing defect). The deficiency state is inherited as a recessive genetic trait. A list of drugs affected by the SD-defect is shown in Table 12–4.

Recessive inheritance of the SD-defect means that the "poor metabolizers" have a double dose of a defective gene; therefore, the group of "extensive metabolizers" would consist partly of heterozygotes, i.e., people having one deficient and one activity-conveying gene. Homozygous extensive metabolizers would be the only people with a full complement of the metabolizing enzyme. According to the Hardy-Weinberg law of population genetics, the occurrence of 8% recessives in a population implies that 41% of the population are carriers with only half the full enzyme complement. In this sense, the 8% with the deficiency are like the tip of an iceberg.

Assignment of any given subject to the group of poor or extensive hydroxylators of debrisoquine or sparteine can be done by giving a small dose of either drug and measuring the ratio of drug and metabolite excreted in urine during the following 8 hours. The use of dextromethorphan for discrimination between the subjects is being explored.

A healthy subject with the SD-defect receiving an average dose of debrisoquine is prone to fainting from ex-

TABLE 12–3 Drug-Metabolizing Cytochromes P-450

Families	Subfamilies	Number of Enzymes	Chromosomal Location in Man	Some Characteristics	
P450 I	Nil	2	15	*Ind:*	Polycyclic aromatic hydrocarbons, Smoke
				S:	Benzo(a)pyrine, Caffeine
P450 II	A	2	?		
	B	2	19	*Ind:*	Phenobarbital
	C	10	10	*S:*	Mephenytoin (Enzyme C9)
	D	2	22	*S:*	Debrisoquine, Sparteine
	E	12	?	*Ind:* } *S:* }	Ethanol (Enzyme E1)

Ind = Inducers; *S* = Substrates.
Homologies: Less than 36% between families, 40–60% between subfamilies, more than 70% within subfamilies (= between isozymes).
Divergence: Between families 600–900 MYA, between subfamilies 150 MYA, within subfamilies 12 MYA (MYA = Million Years Ago).

TABLE 12–4 Drugs with Impaired Biotransformation in Poor Hydroxylators of Debrisoquine and/or Sparteine

With Clinical Consequences

*Debrisoquine	Orthostatic hypotension
*Sparteine	Excessive uterine contraction
*Perhexiline	Peripheral neuropathy, hepatotoxicity
*Guanoxan	Orthostatic hypotension
*Phenformin	Lactic acidosis
Metoprolol	Excessive beta-blockade; loss of cardioselectivity
Timolol	Low dose requirement
Nortriptyline	CNS toxicity
Captopril	Agranulocytosis (?)
Propafenone	CNS and cardiac toxicity

Consequences Mild or Not Established

Desipramine
Encainide
Amiflamine
Amitriptyline
Bufuralol
Alprenolol
Methoxyphenamine
Amphetamine
Dextromethorphan

*Drugs withdrawn or infrequently used.

cessive lowering of blood pressure. Two decades ago, the alkaloid sparteine became popular in North America as an oxytocic, but it fell into disuse when it was discovered that about 7% of women receiving it had severe side effects. On hindsight, these 7% must have been the ones with the SD-defect. There are also clinical consequences with other drugs.

The fate of some drugs is biochemically affected by the SD-defect, but not clinically. The reasons may vary. For instance, the beta-blocker propranolol undergoes biotransformation by several parallel pathways; only one depends on the SD-defect so that other reactions and effective renal elimination can compensate. The beta-blocker bufuralol is selectively biotransformed by the debrisoquine hydroxylase, but parent drug and metabolite have similar pharmacologic activity; hence, the clinical consequences of the deficiency are limited.

The biotransformation of quinidine is not noticeably affected by the SD-defect, but it has a very high affinity for debrisoquine hydroxylase, thereby inhibiting the enzyme ($K_I = 10^{-8}$ M). A person receiving quinidine is like a person with the SD-defect in terms of drug-metabolizing capacity. An almost equally potent inhibitor of debrisoquine hydroxylase turned out to be the hallucinogenic, neurotoxic MPTP (N-methyl-4-phenyl-1,2,3,6-tetrahydropyridine). Also, many neuroleptics cause clinically significant inhibition of debrisoquine hydroxylase. In short, the study of the SD-defect has revealed and explained several drug–drug interactions.

It has become clear recently that the SD-defect is not a uniform entity; there are different mutants leading to identical biochemical deficiency. This may also be the explanation for discrepancies between the biotransforming capacities for debrisoquine and sparteine in some African countries (*e.g.*, Ghana). The SD-defect is distinctly more rare in Oriental than in Caucasian populations.

GENES AND TARGET TISSUES

Genetic control of drug metabolism is only one genetic factor influencing drug response. Many genes confer a special vulnerability or drug resistance on a subject by causing an alteration of a target tissue of a drug. A special category consists of hereditary diseases that include, among other manifestations, altered drug effects; for example, in persons with acute intermittent porphyria, barbiturates may cause fatal paralysis or other neurologic dysfunctions; in familial dysautonomia, autonomic stimulants elicit over-responses; in sickle cell disease, anaesthesia or acidifying drugs may provoke a sickling crisis with plugging of capillaries. However, the following examples concern genes that affect drug

response and that became known only because of an abnormal drug response.

Glucose-6-Phosphate Dehydrogenase Deficiency

The most intensively investigated examples have been hemolytic drug reactions related to a deficiency of glucose-6-phosphate dehydrogenase (G-6-PD). The exact mechanism by which G-6-PD deficiency causes red cell destruction is not established; however, it appears to be related to the cell's inability to maintain the necessary concentration of glutathione in its reduced form. It has been shown that oxidant drugs form H_2O_2 in the red cell and that this oxidizes glutathione. The oxidized disulfide form of glutathione may be attached to hemoglobin. The mixed disulfide-glutathione-hemoglobin complex is unstable and results in hemoglobin changes leading to its oxidation and denaturation (Heinz bodies). These changes result in damage to the erythrocyte membrane with consequent hemolysis.

Approximately 400 million people carry the trait for G-6-PD deficiency, and approximately 300 enzymic variants are known. All of these variants are inherited as sex-linked traits; many are associated with specific biologic sequelae.

There are several variants that must be classified as "normal"; there is one variant with increased enzymatic activity, and some variants (Oklahoma, Chicago, Eyssen, *etc.*) cause such severe deficiencies of enzyme activity that they lead to hemolytic disease even in the absence of drugs. The role of drugs has been most closely investigated with respect to two G-6-PD types, one being the so-called A⁻ variant in American blacks, the second, the Mediterranean variant. The A⁻ variant is an unstable enzyme. Young erythrocytes have about the normal level of enzyme activity, but the activity diminishes more rapidly than normal during the lifespan of the red cell. Drug-induced hemolytic reactions are, therefore, self-limited and cease once the older erythrocytes have been eliminated. The Mediterranean variant conveys a low G-6-PD activity even in young erythrocytes. As a consequence, hemolytic crises when they occur are much more severe, since they do not tend to be self-limiting. A number of agents (*e.g.*, quinine, ASA) in high doses have caused hemolysis in the presence of the Mediterranean G-6-PD deficiency while they do not do so in the A⁻ variant (Table 12–5). The Canton variant has been shown to be similar to the Mediterranean variant.

The differential frequencies of G-6-PD deficiency in various populations are determined by elements of Darwinian selection. G-6-PD deficiency favors survival by increasing resistance to *P. falciparum* malaria (*see* Chapters 10 and 57), a factor beneficial only in countries where malaria occurs, so that the gene tends to accumulate in such countries. For several, but not all variants, the main lethal factor is icterus neonatorum.

TABLE 12–5 Drugs That May Cause Hemolysis in G-6-PD Deficient Subjects

Aminoquinolines
Primaquine
Pamaquin
Chloroquine
Pentaquine

Sulfones
Dapsone
Sulfoxone
Thiazosulfone

Sulfonamides
Sulfanilamide
Sulfacetamide
Sulfafurazole
Sulfisoxazole
Sulfamethoxypyridazine
Salicylazosulfapyridine

Nitrofurans
Nitrofurantoin
Furazolidine
Nitrofurazone

Analgesics
Acetylsalicylic acid
Phenacetin (Acetophenetidin)
Acetanilid

Miscellaneous Agents
Vitamin K (water-soluble analogs)
Naphthalene (moth balls)
Probenecid
Dimercaprol (BAL)
Methylene blue
Acetylphenylhydrazine
Phenylhydrazine
p-Aminosalicylic acid
Nalidixic acid
Neoarsphenamine
Quinine ⎫ Not shown to
Quinidine ⎬ be hemolytic
Chloramphenicol ⎭ in Blacks.

Glutathione Synthetase Deficiency

Glutathione synthetase deficiency is a rare autosomal recessive trait characterized by hemolytic anemia, acidosis, and abnormalities of polymorphonuclear leukocyte function. From a pharmacologic point of view, the significant consequence of the disease is a markedly decreased intracellular glutathione content. Deficiency in red blood cell glutathione predisposes the patients to drug-induced hemolytic anemia from oxidant drugs, similar to that which occurs in G-6-PD deficiency. Low glutathione content in nucleated cells, particularly in the liver, has raised the question of possible increased susceptibility to hepatotoxicity from drugs whose reactive, electrophilic metabolites are detoxified by glutathione conjugation (*see* Chapters 62 and 63). Recently, it has been possible to use lymphocytes from patients

with this disorder to assess susceptibility to such drug metabolites. Thus, cells from patients with glutathione synthetase deficiency exhibit increased damage from metabolites of drugs such as acetaminophen and nitrofurantoin. Cells from the patients can be used for *in vitro* determination of potential *in vivo* drug toxicity for the patients, as well as for establishing the role of glutathione in detoxifying potentially toxic metabolites of ''new'' compounds.

Susceptibility to Drug-Induced Hepatotoxicity Demonstrable with Lymphocytes *In Vitro*

When a patient presents with a possible idiosyncratic reaction to a drug, such as hepatotoxicity, several questions immediately arise: (1) Are the patient's symptoms indeed caused by the drug? (2) If so, what is the pathophysiology of the toxic reaction? (3) Why did this patient among thousands of exposed individuals suffer a side effect? (4) Is susceptibility to such toxicity inherited? In order to answer questions about drug toxicity experimentally in humans, it is necessary first to have a testable hypothesis for biochemical mechanisms of altered susceptibility, and then an assay for assessing individual differences in susceptibility that does not expose patients to further drug-related risk.

For example, phenytoin is associated in rare cases with a complex clinical syndrome including fever, skin rash, lymphadenopathy, and hepatotoxicity. It is postulated that the toxicity is mediated by a reactive arene oxide metabolite of this aromatic drug. Recently, it has been found that lymphocytes from patients who experienced phenytoin hepatotoxicity showed increased toxicity from arene oxide metabolites of phenytoin *in vitro*. Furthermore, cells from relatives of the patients also exhibited abnormal dose-response curves to these metabolites, with a family pattern suggestive of an autosomal recessive trait. The data suggest that susceptibility to phenytoin hepatotoxicity is based on a genetically determined deficiency in the detoxification of certain types of reactive metabolites. The biochemical basis of the defect remains to be determined. Such *in vitro* studies can help significantly in the diagnosis of idiosyncratic reactions and in determination of their pharmacogenetic basis.

Malignant Hyperthermia

A puzzling but rare reaction, that usually was fatal until recently, is called malignant hyperthermia. It is a complication of general anaesthesia and it occurs on the basis of a genetic predisposition. Failure of muscles to relax after succinylcholine, and an unexplained tachycardia, often herald the onset. There is a rise of body temperature, which rapidly can reach extreme values. In most cases, there is rigidity of some or most skeletal muscles. During the episode, muscle enzymes and proteins are released into the plasma. There is profound hypoxia and metabolic and respiratory acidosis, and the plasma potassium level rises. Early death is often due to cardiac failure, while delayed death may be due to renal failure as a consequence of myoglobinemia.

The cause of the condition is an unusual effect of halothane or other general anaesthetics on skeletal muscle. This was proven by pharmacologic tests: muscle biopsy samples obtained from survivors reveal high *in vitro* susceptibility of the muscle to caffeine contracture, and this caffeine effect is potentiated and partly mimicked by halothane (Fig. 12–3). This caffeine effect requires high concentrations that could not occur *in vivo*, and thus is strictly an investigative tool. Caffeine is known to affect intracellular calcium metabolism by enhancing the calcium-stimulated calcium release from the sarcoplasmic reticulum. The hyperthermic attack may be initiated by halothane inhibition of calcium uptake into the unusually susceptible reticulum. The increased calcium concentration in the sarcoplasm can be expected to have a number of biochemical effects, such as increasing ATPase activity by actomyosin, by the reticulum, and by the mitochondria: the muscular contracture and a hypermetabolic state are the consequences, and the resulting huge increase in heat production probably explains the sharp rise in body temperature.

Early recognition of the attack, speedy termination of surgery and anaesthesia, cooling of the patient and

correction of acidosis are among the indicated measures. The intravenous infusion of the muscle relaxant, dantrolene, has been life-saving by terminating the attack.

Hypoxanthine Guanine Phosphoribosyl Transferase Deficiency

Allopurinol, an analog of hypoxanthine, is used for the treatment of gout. It ameliorates the disease by two different biochemical mechanisms. First, it inhibits the conversion of hypoxanthine and xanthine to uric acid; and second, it decreases *de novo* purine biosynthesis. In some persons with gout, the second effect is absent, and this absence can be correlated with a deficiency of an enzyme called hypoxanthine guanine phosphoribosyl transferase (total HGPRT deficiency = Lesch-Nyhan syndrome).

Diminished Receptor Occupation of Bishydroxycoumarin-Type Anticoagulants

Another example of decreased drug effect on the basis of alteration of the drug target is the resistance to warfarin in some families. In these cases, it takes twenty times the normal dose to produce the usual therapeutic effect. The biochemical mechanism is likely a diminished affinity of the drug receptor for the anticoagulant (Fig. 12–4). An abnormally rapid metabolic inactivation of the drug is not the cause, although this could conceivably also create a similar drug resistance.

Marker Genes and Drug Response

An example of a completely different nature illustrating the interaction of genes and drugs has been established by statistical means. Jick *et al.* reported that women of blood groups A, B, or AB who take oral contraceptives are three times as likely to develop thrombosis as are women of blood group O (Table 12–6). This information has not led to any change of use of contraceptive pills. After all, even the relatively greater risk of thrombosis due to the pill associated with blood groups A, B, or AB is small compared to the risks due to pregnancy and childbirth. However, this study has led to numerous investigations that seem to yield new insights into the puzzling role of the blood groups.

It is certainly not claimed or believed that there is an immediate and direct interaction between contraceptives and blood group substances. One is much more likely dealing with a complicated series of interrelating events. The significance of this observation lies in the fact that an unexpected genetic risk factor related to a drug effect has been empirically identified and quantitatively evaluated. If numerous such risk factors were known, whether genetic, pathologic, or environmental,

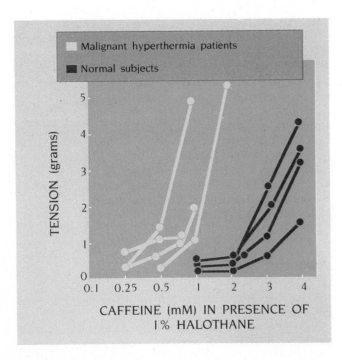

Figure 12–3 Caffeine contracture of muscles biopsied from normal subjects and from malignant hyperthermia patients. (Adapted from Kalow W *et al.* Lancet 1970; II:895.)

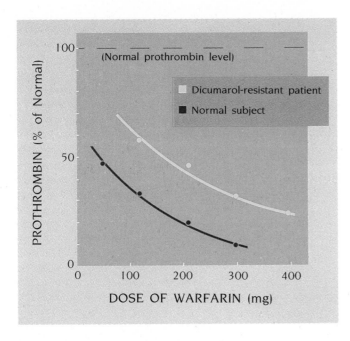

Figure 12-4 Prothrombin responses in normal and dicumarol-resistant patients. (Adapted from O'Reilly *et al*. N Engl J Med 1964; 271:809.)

TABLE 12-6 Distribution of Blood Groups, and Frequency of Thromboembolism with Oral Contraceptives

	Blood Groups	
	A+B+AB	O
Number of persons per hundred population:		
Boston	53	47
Sweden	60	40
United Kingdom	54	46
Number of women on oral contraceptives with thromboembolism:		
Boston	46	9
Sweden	49	10
United Kingdom	55	17

After Jick *et al*. Lancet 1969; I:539.

it might be possible to estimate the clinically significant risks of specific drugs for a given person and thereby improve rational drug therapy.

In conclusion, some of the specific examples that were quoted above may be rare, but abnormal drug reactions as a whole are not rare, and many must occur unrecognized. It is clear that genetic factors in such reactions are surprisingly diverse and cannot be neglected in the assessment of drug therapies and iatrogenic disease.

SUGGESTED READING

Britt BA, ed. Malignant hyperthermia. Boston: Nijhoff, 1987.

Brown SS, Kalow W, Pilz W, Whittaker M, Woronick CL. The plasma cholinesterases: a new perspective. Adv Clin Chem 1983; 22:1–123.

Calabrese EJ. Ecogenetics: genetic variation in susceptibility to environmental agents. New York: Wiley-Interscience, 1984.

Eichelbaum M. Defective oxidation of drugs: pharmacokinetic and therapeutic implications. Clin Pharmacokinet 1982; 7:1–22.

Goedde HW, Lentner C. Pharmacogenetics and ecogenetics. Basle: Geigy Scientific Tables, 8th ed., Vol.4, 1986.

Idle JR, Smith RL. Polymorphism of oxidation at carbon centers of drugs and their clinical significance. Drug Metab Rev 1979; 9:301–317.

Kalow W, Goedde HW, Agarwal DP, eds. Ethnic differences in reactions to drugs and xenobiotics. New York: Alan R. Liss, 1986.

Kutt H, Wolk M, Sherman R, McDowell F. Insufficient para-hydroxylation as a cause of diphenylhydantoin toxicity. Neurology 1964; 14:542–548.

Lockridge O, La Du BN. Amino acid sequence of the active site of human serum cholinesterase from usual, atypical, and atypical-silent genotypes. Biochem Gen 1986; 24:485–498.

Nebert DW, Gonzales FJ. P450 genes: structure, evolution, and regulation. Ann Rev Biochem 1987; 56:945–993.

Omenn GS, Gelboin HV, eds. Genetic variability in responses to chemical exposure. Banbury Report #16, Cold Spring Harbor Laboratory, 1984.

Shahidi NT. Acetophenetidin-induced methemoglobinemia. Ann NY Acad Sci 1968; 151:822–832.

Spielberg SP, Gordon GB, Blake DA, Goldstein DA, Herlong HF. Predisposition to phenytoin hepatotoxicity assessed *in vitro*. N Engl J Med 1981; 305:722–727.

Vesell ES. Pharmacogenetic perspectives: genes, drugs and disease. Hepatology 1984; 4:959–965.

AUTONOMIC NERVOUS SYSTEM AND NEUROMUSCULAR JUNCTION

———

Chapter 13

Autonomic Nervous System Neurotransmitters

K.V. Flattery and L. Spero

All efferent axons leaving the central nervous system, other than those innervating skeletal muscle, belong to the autonomic nervous system. They can regulate many physiologic activities that are mainly involuntary and not under conscious control. The autonomic nervous system plays a major role in the maintenance of homeostasis in the body, *i.e.*, it controls the steady states of the internal environment of the body by coordinating physiologic processes. It regulates the rate and force of contraction of the heart, the calibre of blood vessels, and the muscle tone in gastrointestinal and genitourinary tracts and bronchioles; it adjusts accommodation of the eye for near and distant vision, and it controls pupil size. It can also modify the secretions of both exocrine and endocrine glands.

Autonomic pharmacology can be defined as the study of those drugs that act either on the autonomic neurons or on receptors in the membranes of target organ cells that are controlled by the autonomic nervous system, such as cardiac muscle, smooth muscle, and glands. Practical applications include such examples as the pharmacotherapy of hypertension, bronchial asthma, and angina pectoris. The drugs may act directly on receptors of the system, either to excite or to inhibit; or by indirect action upon the central control or peripheral release of neurotransmitters, with corresponding results on cardiac, vascular, central nervous system, or other activity. In order to understand the selective actions of drugs on the autonomic nervous system, it is essential to have an understanding of its anatomy and physiology.

ANATOMY OF THE AUTONOMIC NERVOUS SYSTEM

The autonomic nervous system is composed of control centres located within the central nervous system (CNS) and a peripheral network of afferent and efferent nerves. The hypothalamus is the principal locus of integration of this system, but there are other important control centres, for example in the medulla oblongata, and there are the coordinating centres which form the limbic system. The various control centres are, however, not purely autonomic, and there are no important physiologic differences between visceral and somatic afferent (sensory) fibres. By convention, the term "autonomic nervous system" is used only in reference to the efferent (motor) neurons supplying the peripheral effector organs. The efferent autonomic nervous system has its origin in nerve cell bodies within the CNS, giving rise to preganglionic fibres (usually myelinated) that are outside the CNS. These synapse in peripheral ganglia with the cell bodies of the nonmyelinated postganglionic fibres that innervate the effector organs.

Structurally and functionally the autonomic nervous system is further divided into sympathetic and parasympathetic systems.

In the **sympathetic division** the cells of origin lie in the lateral horns of the thoracic and lumbar portions of the spinal cord, from T_1 to L_2–L_3. There are two major groups of sympathetic ganglia, namely the paravertebral ganglia that lie in a chain close to and on each side of the vertebral column (sympathetic trunk), and the prevertebral ganglia which lie in the abdomen at some distance from the vertebrae (e.g., the celiac ["solar plexus"] and mesenteric ganglia). The adrenal medulla resembles a sympathetic ganglion in that it is innervated by typical preganglionic fibres and is also functionally, anatomically, and embryologically related to the sympathetic ganglia.

The **parasympathetic division** comprises the craniosacral outflow of the autonomic nervous system. The cells of origin are located in the lower brain stem (midbrain and medulla oblongata) and in the sacral portion of the spinal cord from S_2 to S_4. In contrast to the sympathetic ganglia, the parasympathetic ganglia are located very close to, on, or within the innervated organs, e.g., the heart and gastrointestinal tract. The principal pathways of autonomic innervation are shown schematically in Figure 13–1.

There are important exceptions to most generalizations about autonomic innervation. Nevertheless, in general, sympathetic preganglionic fibres tend to synapse with large numbers of postganglionic fibres, parasympathetic with few. Sympathetic postganglionic fibres tend to have diffuse distributions, while parasympathetic distribution is more limited and discrete.

There is no true synapse between postganglionic autonomic nerves and their effector organs. The nerve terminals have a characteristic bead-like appearance, the beads or "varicosities" being the sites at which neurotransmitter is released. The released neurotransmitter diffuses 200–1000 Å to reach the effector cell, and effector cells may be simultaneously under the influence of neurotransmitters originating from more than one type of nerve terminal.

PHYSIOLOGY OF THE AUTONOMIC NERVOUS SYSTEM

Most organs are innervated and controlled by both sympathetic and parasympathetic nerves. There are, however, organs that are innervated and controlled by only one division of the autonomic nervous system.

In organs with both sympathetic and parasympathetic nervous control, the effects of the two divisions are usually opposite (e.g., heart, bronchi, gastrointestinal tract, bladder, eye). Thus, the level of function usually depends upon the balance between the tone of two opposing innervations. In certain organs, such as the heart and intestines, however, there is also an intrinsic control that persists even when the dual external control by the autonomic nervous system is absent. The parasympathetic and sympathetic nerves can override and adjust the activity of the organ to a level above or below that established by the intrinsic mechanisms. While many organs have dual innervation of individual cells, in some instances the opposing effects of the

sympathetic and parasympathetic divisions arise from the fact that they innervate different and functionally opposing cells. In the iris of the eye, for example, the parasympathetic fibres control mainly the circular muscles while the sympathetic fibres control mainly the radial muscles. As a result, increased parasympathetic tone causes constriction of the pupil, and increased sympathetic tone causes dilatation.

In a few organs with dual autonomic control, such as the salivary glands, the effects of the sympathetic and parasympathetic divisions are believed to be complementary.

Each division of the autonomic nervous system can exert either an inhibitory or an excitatory effect upon a given organ. The effect upon a particular organ is determined by the characteristic responses of the effector cells in that organ. In many cases, all the cells respond in the same manner; however, in the intestine the smooth muscle cells of the outer muscular layers relax in response to sympathetic impulses, whereas those of the sphincters contract. Arteriolar smooth muscle provides examples of three possible responses related to the location of the vessel. Sympathetic impulses cause constriction of the arterioles in the skin and viscera, but dilatation of some vessels in skeletal muscle, and essentially no effect on cerebral arterioles. Both systems are normally active at all times. This basal rate of activity is referred to as sympathetic tone or parasympathetic tone.

TRANSMISSION OF IMPULSES IN THE AUTONOMIC NERVOUS SYSTEM

All preganglionic fibres store and release acetylcholine (ACh) as a chemical transmitter. The postganglionic fibres store and release either acetylcholine or noradrenaline* (NA), and adrenaline† and noradrenaline are also released from chromaffin cells in the adrenal medulla. Fibres in the autonomic nervous system are therefore either cholinergic or adrenergic, depending on which transmitter is released by the particular fibre (Fig. 13–2).

Cholinergic Fibres, Releasing Acetylcholine

1. Preganglionic fibres to all ganglia in the autonomic nervous system and to the adrenal medulla.
2. Postganglionic parasympathetic fibres to effector organs.
3. Postganglionic sympathetic fibres to sweat glands, and a few sympathetic fibres to vessels in skeletal muscle.

---

* norepinephrine
† epinephrine

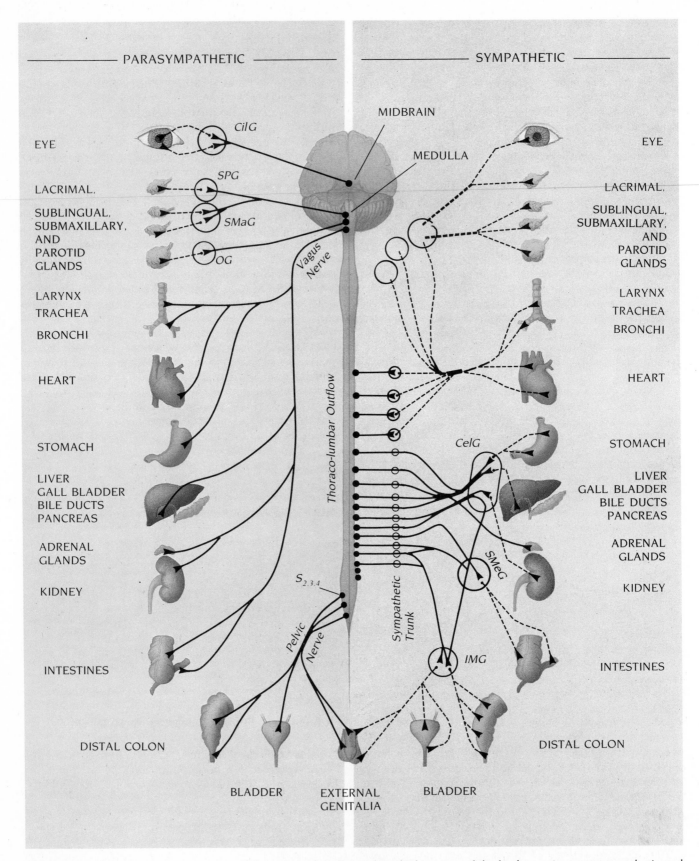

Figure 13–1 Schematic representation of the principal pathways by which organs of the body receive parasympathetic and sympathetic innervation. CelG = celiac ganglion; CilG = ciliary ganglion; IMG = inferior mesenteric ganglion; OG = otic ganglion; SMaG = submandibular ganglion; SMeG = superior mesenteric ganglion; SPG = sphenopalatine ganglion.

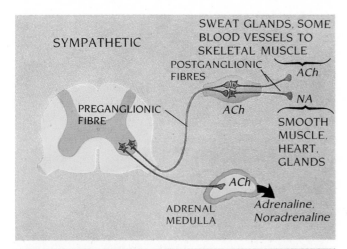

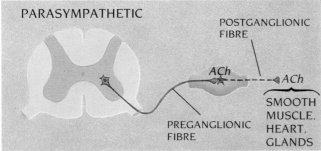

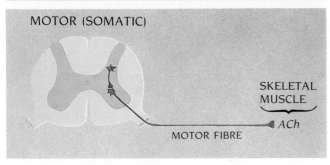

Figure 13–2 Classification of autonomic innervation, sites of impulse transmission, and type of transmitter substance. ACh = acetylcholine; NA = noradrenaline.

Adrenergic Fibres, Releasing Noradrenaline

All postganglionic sympathetic fibres to effector organs.

Autonomic Cholinergic Transmission

Biosynthesis of Acetylcholine

Acetylcholine is synthesized in the terminals of cholinergic nerves (Fig. 13–3). Acetyl coenzyme A (readily available within the cytoplasm) and choline (trans-

ported into the nerve terminal from the synapse, as well as from cytoplasmic sources) undergo an acetyl transfer reaction, catalysed by the enzyme choline acetyltransferase, to form acetylcholine, which is simultaneously transported into vesicles within the nerve terminal varicosities. Each vesicle contains approximately 10,000 molecules of acetylcholine. It is not clear whether all neuronal acetylcholine is packaged within these vesicles, but it is apparent that the acetylcholine released from the nerve terminal derives from the vesicles. When the turnover of acetylcholine is high, the transport of choline into the nerve terminal can become the rate-limiting step. Also, the most recently synthesized acetylcholine is likely to be the first to be released on stimulation. The vesicles also contain a specific protein called vesiculin, and ATP.

Release of Acetylcholine

When an action potential invades the nerve terminal, the vesicles migrate to the nerve varicosity membrane, fuse with it, and release acetylcholine. The vesicle itself is subsequently re-formed by invagination of the mem-

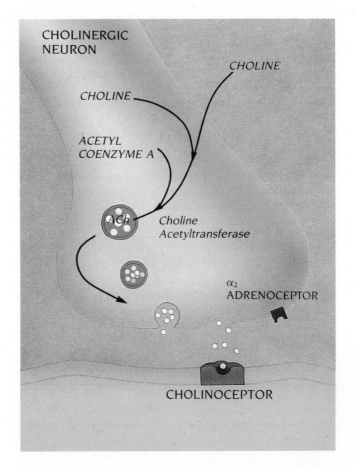

Figure 13–3 Biosynthesis of acetylcholine (ACh) in cholinergic neurons. Presynaptic α_2 adrenoceptors are found in only some cholinergic neurons (*see* Table 13–2).

brane and moves back into the nerve terminal where it can be refilled with acetylcholine.

Breakdown of Released Acetylcholine, and Choline Re-Uptake

Acetylcholine is rapidly broken down by the enzyme acetylcholinesterase, which occurs in high concentration wherever acetylcholine acts as neurotransmitter, *i.e.*, on both pre- and postganglionic membranes within autonomic ganglia, on the membranes of parasympathetic nerve terminals, and on pre- and postsynaptic membranes of neuromuscular junctions. (Low concentrations are also found in adrenergic neurons.) The action is instantaneous; as much as 90% of the released acetylcholine may be hydrolysed before it reaches the postsynaptic membrane.

The resultant acetic acid is rapidly removed into various biochemical pathways within the cytoplasm. The choline is actively transported back into the nerve terminal where it can be resynthesized to acetylcholine.

Autonomic Adrenergic Transmission

Biosynthesis of Catecholamines

The neurotransmitter in adrenergic postganglionic nerves is noradrenaline. This is also found in some areas of the brain. Dopamine, which is synthesized as a precursor of noradrenaline, is not normally present in autonomic nerve terminals, but it is a neurotransmitter in certain areas of the brain (*e.g.*, the basal ganglia and limbic cortex). Adrenaline production from noradrenaline occurs mainly in the adrenal medulla, in chromaffin tissues, and in some areas of the brain. The precursor for the catecholamine biosynthetic pathway is the amino acid L-tyrosine, which is actively transported into both adrenergic neurons and adrenal medullary chromaffin cells. In the cytoplasm of the adrenergic neuron, L-tyrosine is converted to L-dopa (dihydroxyphenylalanine) by the enzyme tyrosine hydroxylase. This is the rate-limiting step in the biosynthesis of catecholamines (Fig. 13–4).

L-Dopa is the substrate for another cytoplasmic enzyme, dopa decarboxylase (L-aromatic amino acid decarboxylase), resulting in the synthesis of dopamine (dihydroxyphenylethylamine). Dopamine is actively taken up by the storage vesicles within the neuron, and its conversion to L-noradrenaline occurs within the vesicles through the action of dopamine-β-hydroxylase (DβH) (Fig. 13–5).

Each step in the progressive conversion of L-tyrosine to L-noradrenaline may be inhibited by drugs (Table 13–1). Noradrenaline also inhibits the conversion of L-tyrosine to L-dopa by a negative feedback mechanism (so-called end product inhibition), thereby controlling the rate of its own synthesis and that of dopamine. Conversely, the synthesis of noradrenaline is enhanced

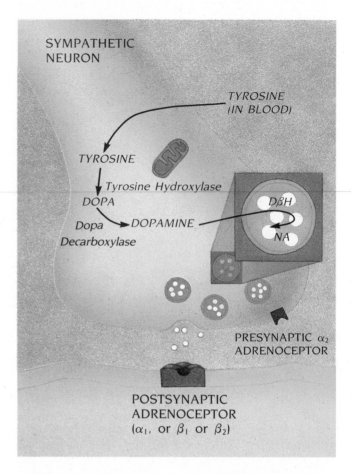

Figure 13–4 Biosynthesis of noradrenaline (NA) in sympathetic nerve terminals. DβH = dopamine-β-hydroxylase.

during increased activity of the sympathetic nerves, probably by a reduction in end product inhibition.

In the adrenal medulla noradrenaline is methylated in the cytoplasm of the cell to form the hormone adrenaline; this reaction is catalysed by the enzyme phenylethanolamine-N-methyl transferase (PNMT). The rate of synthesis of adrenaline from noradrenaline in chromaffin cells is dependent upon glucocorticoids secreted by the cortex of the adrenal gland, which are carried in high concentrations directly to the adrenal medullary chromaffin cells where they induce the synthesis of PNMT.

Storage of Noradrenaline and Adrenaline

The most important sites for the storage of noradrenaline are the granular vesicles, which are highly concentrated in the varicosities of the nerve terminals. There is evidence to suggest that storage vesicles are formed in the cell bodies of adrenergic neurons and are carried along the axons to the terminal varicosities. Identification of the storage granules was made possible

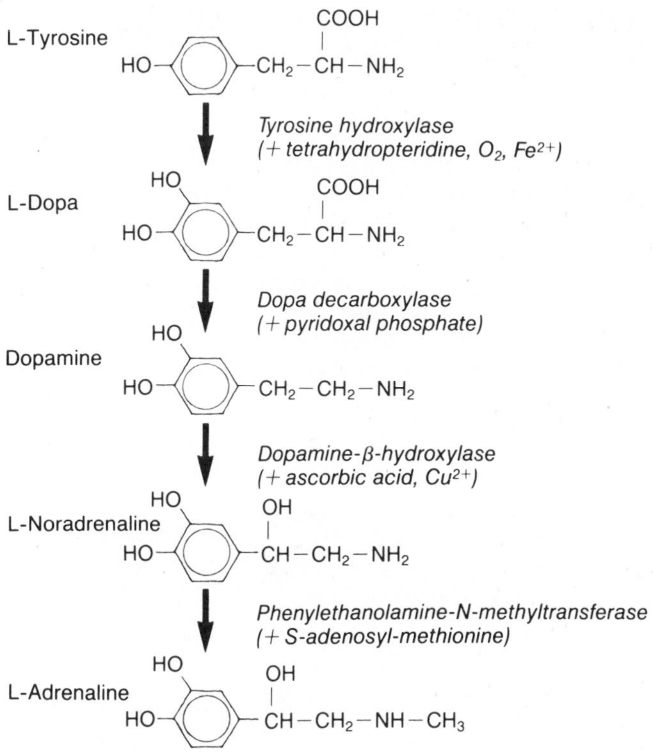

Figure 13–5 Biosynthesis of catecholamines.

by electron microscopy and other techniques, *e.g.*, immunofluorescence.

Within the storage granules noradrenaline is stored in very high concentrations in the form of a molecular complex with adenosine triphosphate (ATP). The noradrenaline : ATP ratio in the granules is 4:1. The granules also contain specific proteins (chromogranins) and the enzyme dopamine-β-hydroxylase. Noradrenaline also exists in a free unbound form within the granules, in equilibrium with the noradrenaline-ATP-protein complex. Outside the granular vesicle, noradrenaline is present in a free form. This small cytoplasmic pool probably plays some part in the regulation of synthesis of the catecholamines by means of the so-called end product inhibition of tyrosine hydroxylase.

Noradrenaline within the granules of nerve endings is present in at least two different metabolic pools, designated I and II. Pool I is conceived of as containing material with a rapid turnover; it probably functions as the sympathetic neurotransmitter. Pool II turns over slowly and contains material of limited physiologic significance; it is relatively refractory to release by sympathetic nerve stimulation. Within the granules an active transport system helps to maintain a concentration gradient of noradrenaline. This transport system can concentrate noradrenaline against a 200-fold gradient across the granular membrane, and ATP and magnesium are essential for its optimal activity. The trans-

port mechanism is sensitive to the action of certain drugs, such as reserpine, which releases noradrenaline from the vesicles into the cytoplasm.

In the adrenal medulla most of the noradrenaline leaves the granules and in the cytoplasm is methylated to adrenaline, which reenters other storage granules until released. Adrenaline accounts for approximately 80% of adrenal medullary catecholamines.

Release of Catecholamines

When a nerve impulse is propagated along the postganglionic adrenergic neuron, it releases noradrenaline from storage vesicles by exocytosis. Following fusion of the vesicular membrane with the neuronal membrane, the entire contents of the storage vesicle are discharged into the synaptic cleft. This discharge contains noradrenaline, dopamine-β-hydroxylase, chromogranin, and ATP. Calcium is also involved in the specific process of exocytosis. A similar mechanism of release occurs for adrenaline and noradrenaline in the adrenal medulla.

α_2 Adrenoceptors (*see* below), which are located at presynaptic sites (and also at some postsynaptic sites), can be activated by released noradrenaline to mediate feedback inhibition of noradrenaline release (Fig. 13–6).

Following its release, a large amount of noradrenaline is retrieved by re-uptake through an L-noradrenaline-specific active transport mechanism across the axonal membrane from the synapse to the cytoplasmic pool (*see* Fig. 13–6). Further active transport of noradrenaline occurs against a high concentration gradient from the cytoplasm to the intragranular storage pools. Thus, re-uptake is the most important mechanism by which the action of released noradrenaline is terminated. Both transport systems involved with the re-uptake of noradrenaline are susceptible to drug action.

Metabolic Degradation of Catecholamines

Two enzymes are responsible for the degradation of catecholamines: monoamine oxidase (MAO) located within the mitochondria of the nerve terminal and

TABLE 13–1 Inhibitors of Enzymes Involved in the Biosynthesis of L-Dopa, Dopamine, and Noradrenaline

Enzyme	Inhibitor
Tyrosine hydroxylase	Alpha-methyl-*p*-tyrosine Noradrenaline and dopamine (negative feedback mechanism)
L-Aromatic amino acid decarboxylase (dopa decarboxylase)	α-Methyldopa Benserazide (RO4–4602)
Dopamine-β-hydroxylase	Disulfiram (Antabuse)

catechol-O-methyl transferase (COMT) located in the synaptic cleft. Noradrenaline in the cytoplasmic pool (but not within the granules) is deaminated by MAO, as is noradrenaline entering the terminal by re-uptake. Noradrenaline within the synapse is rapidly O-methylated by COMT. Analysis of urinary metabolites of noradrenaline can provide information about neuronal turnover and the source of the parent catecholamine. Measurements of catecholamines, metanephrine, and 3-methoxy-4-hydroxymandelic acid (vanilmandelic acid or VMA) in urine are routinely used in patients suspected of having a tumor of chromaffin cells (pheochromocytoma). The enzymic degradation of catecholamines is illustrated in Figure 13–7.

RECEPTORS IN THE AUTONOMIC NERVOUS SYSTEM

To activate or inhibit the next neuron or effector cell, neurotransmitter must be released from the nerve terminal and interact with specific sites, called receptors, in the membrane of the target effector cell. When this occurs, the cell responds characteristically. The response of a gland cell may be an increase or decrease in the quantity of secretion. Likewise, a smooth muscle cell may respond by contraction or relaxation. In all cases, the response is determined by the characteris-

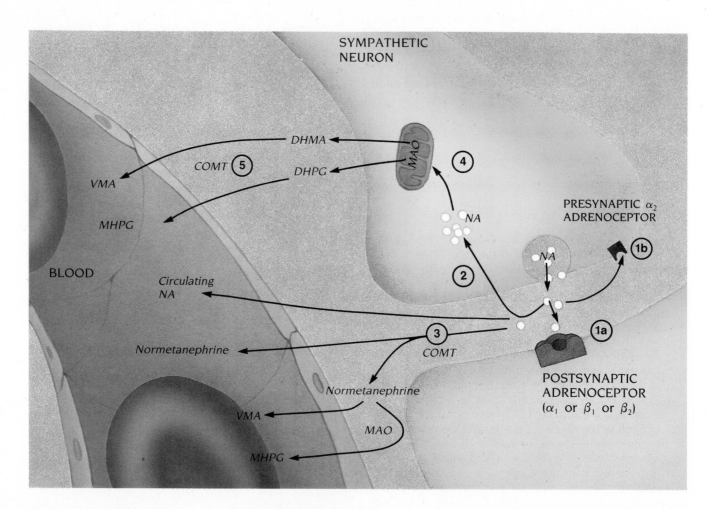

Figure 13–6 Fate of intraneuronal and extraneuronal noradrenaline (NA). COMT = catechol-O-methyl transferase; DHMA = dihydroxymandelic acid; DHPG = dihydroxyphenyl glycol; MAO = monoamine oxidase; MHPG = methoxyhydroxyphenyl glycol; VMA = vanilmandelic acid. (1) = combination with receptors; (2) = re-uptake into nerve terminal; (3) = extraneuronal metabolism by COMT, followed by MAO; (4) = intraneuronal metabolism by MAO; (5) = extraneuronal metabolism of DHMA and DHPG by COMT.

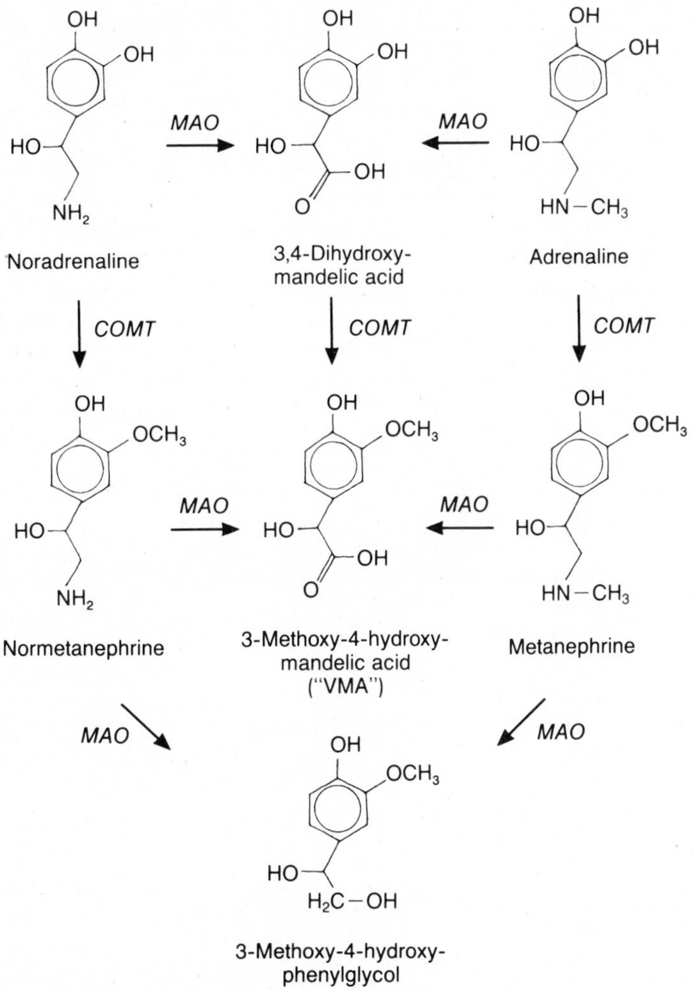

AUTONOMIC
NEUROMUSCULAR

Figure 13–7 Degradation of catecholamines by monoamine oxidase (MAO) and catechol-O-methyl transferase (COMT).

tics of the cell. This applies not only to the local response to a specific transmitter substance, but also to the response to drugs acting remotely on parts of the autonomic nervous system. These neurotransmitter receptors can be characterized by the specific agonists that will stimulate them and by the specific antagonists that block the effects of the neurotransmitter.

Cholinergic Receptors (Cholinoceptors)

Acetylcholine is the neurotransmitter at autonomic ganglia and at postganglionic parasympathetic nerve terminals, but two different classes of receptors are involved. For historical reasons they are named after the substances that were first used to study them, nicotine and muscarine.

Nicotinic (Ganglionic) Receptors

The characteristic **order of potency** for agonists at these receptors is **nicotine > carbamylcholine > acetylcholine**. These receptors are selectively blocked by drugs such as hexamethonium and other related ganglion blocking agents (*see* Chapter 15). They are located in all autonomic ganglia and are found on the cell bodies of sympathetic and parasympathetic postganglionic fibres. (There is another nicotinic cholinergic receptor type at the neuromuscular junction, described in Chapter 19, that is not blocked by ganglion blockers but is blocked by specific antagonists that have little effect at ganglia.)

Muscarinic Receptors

These receptors are located on the effector cells innervated by postganglionic parasympathetic nerves. The characteristic **order of potency** for agonists acting on them is **muscarine > acetylcholine > methacholine > carbamylcholine**. They are selectively blocked by atropine and other muscarinic antagonists (see Chapter 15). When radioreceptor experiments are carried out with unlabelled agonists that compete for binding with ^{3}H-antagonists, three separate types of binding site can be observed. These are called the very high-, high-, and low-affinity sites. Experiments with certain metals have shown that these sites can be interconverted; this suggests that they are three different states of the same receptor protein. Some agonists, such as oxotremorine, have a selective affinity for the very high-affinity site. If unlabelled antagonists compete for binding with ^{3}H-antagonists, only one site is revealed by the displacement curve. Apparently most antagonists only "see" one site. It has been reported that pirenzepine has a selective affinity for the high-affinity site, and that this confers on it a selectivity for muscarinic sites that is different from the selectivity shown by other muscarinic antagonists. Recently it has been found that the sites blocked by pirenzepine are not at the postganglionic parasympathetic synapse and it is not clear what its binding affinity represents.

Intracellular changes associated with muscarinic receptor stimulation include accumulation of guanosine 3′,5′-monophosphate (cyclic GMP), accelerated turnover of inositol phospholipids in cell membranes, and alterations in ion fluxes, e.g., increased K^+ efflux and elevated intracellular levels of Ca^{2+}. Adenylate cyclase may also be inhibited.

While muscarinic receptors in arterioles are not innervated by parasympathetic fibres, they respond to muscarinic agonists by causing a decrease in peripheral resistance and a fall in diastolic blood pressure. This effect on blood pressure depends upon the release of endothelium-derived relaxing factor (EDRF) and occurs only in the presence of intact endothelium.

Adrenergic Receptors (Adrenoceptors)

There are two main kinds of adrenergic receptor. These are called alpha (α) and beta (β) receptors.

Alpha Adrenoceptors

These are subclassified into two types, α_1 and α_2. Both types are located on postsynaptic membranes and thereby modify cell function. The α_2 subtype also includes receptors that control neurotransmitter release; they are located in the presynaptic membrane. The characteristic **order of potency** for agonists at both α_1 and α_2 receptors is **adrenaline > noradrenaline > dopamine > isoproterenol**. However, the concentrations required to stimulate α_1 and α_2 receptors are different, and this fact led to this subclassification.

α_1 Adrenoceptors are selectively blocked by prazosin, and α_2 receptors are selectively blocked by yohimbine. Other α-receptor antagonists have varying selectivity for the two subclasses of receptor.

Beta Adrenoceptors

These are also subdivided into two types, β_1 and β_2. The characteristic **order of potency** for agonists at both β_1 and β_2 receptors is **isoproterenol > adrenaline > noradrenaline > dopamine**.

β_1 Receptors are selectively blocked by metoprolol, and β_2 receptors are selectively blocked by butoxamine. Other β antagonists have varying selectivity for the two classes.

Both α and β adrenoceptors can exist in high- and low-affinity states, which can be interconverted. The conversion of high-affinity states to low-affinity states occurs in the presence of guanosine triphosphate (GTP), Mg^{2+}, and Na^+. A change in the shape of the receptor occurs when GTP binds to a regulatory protein (G protein) in the cell membrane, thus lowering the affinity of the receptor for the agonist.

Distribution of Adrenoceptors

This varies from organ to organ, as **listed in Table 13–2**. The receptor distribution determines the characteristic response, because following the endogenous release of noradrenaline (and adrenaline) all adrenoceptors are stimulated, and the effects in any given organ will depend on the balance between α and β receptors and their respective subtypes. (When noradrenaline is administered exogenously as a drug, the effects of β_2 stimulation are not observed.)

Adrenoceptors and Adenylate Cyclase

Most, if not all, of the actions of catecholamines at β-receptor sites are considered to be due to stimulation of membrane-bound adenylate cyclase, which stimulates the formation of cyclic AMP from ATP in the presence of a guanine nucleotide-binding protein (see Chapter 16). This increases the intracellular concentrations of cAMP, which acts on intracellular processes to produce the characteristic effects of the catecholamines. It has recently been found that α_2 agonists may inhibit adenylate cyclase.

Modulation of Autonomic Nervous System Activity

At central sites, e.g., the medulla oblongata, cholinergic and adrenergic systems can interact with each other by reflex mechanisms to maintain homeostasis. A drug-induced elevation of mean arterial pressure causes a

TABLE 13–2 Responses of Effector Organs to Autonomic Transmitters

Effector Organs	Adrenergic Receptors*	Adrenergic Responses	Muscarinic Cholinergic Responses
Eye			
Radial muscle of iris	α_1	Contr (mydriasis)	—
Sphincter muscle of iris		—	Contr (miosis; strong)
Ciliary muscle	β_2	Relax (slight)†	Contr (strong)‡
Heart			
Heart rate	β_1§	↑	↓
Atrial contractility/conduction	β_1	↑	↓
A-V conduction	β_1	↑	↓ (block)
Ventricular contractility/conduction	β_1	↑	↓
Blood Vessels#			
Coronary	$\alpha_1 \; \beta_2 \; \alpha_2$#	Constr; Dilat (β_2)	
Skin and mucous membranes	$\alpha_1 \; \alpha_2$	Constr (strong)	?
Skeletal muscle	$\alpha_1 \; \beta_2$	Constr; Dilat (β_2)	Dilat
Cerebral	α_1	Constr (slight)	
Pulmonary	$\alpha_1 \; \beta_2$	Constr; Dilat (β_2)	
Abdominal viscera	$\alpha_1 \; \beta_2$	Constr; Dilat (β_2)	
Lung			
Bronchial smooth muscle	β_2	Relax	Contr
Bronchial glands		Inhibition (?)	Stimulation
Stomach and Intestine			
Motility and tone	$\alpha_1 \; \beta_2 \; \alpha_2$**	↓	↑ (strong)
Sphincters	α_1	Contr (?)	Relax (usually)
Secretion		Inhibition (?)	Stimulation
Gall Bladder and Ducts		Relax	Contr
Urinary Bladder			
Detrusor muscle	β_2	Relax (usually)	Contr
Trigone and sphincter	α_1	Contr	Relax
Ureter			
Motility and tone	α_1	↑ (usually)	↑ (?)
Uterus	$\alpha_1 \; \beta_2$	α_1 = contr†† β_2 = relax	Variable
Skeletal Muscle	β_2	Increased contractility; glycogenolysis	—
Sex Organs, Male	α_1	Ejaculation	Erection
Skin			
Sweat glands	α_1	Slight secretion	Profuse secretion
Pilomotor muscles	α_1	Contr	
Spleen Capsule	$\alpha_1 \; \beta_2$	Contr (strong)	
Adrenal Medulla		—	Secretion of adrenaline and noradrenaline (*nicotinic* effect)
Pineal Gland	β	Melatonin synthesis	—
Posterior Pituitary	β_1	ADH secretion	—
Fat Cells	β_1	Lipolysis	—
Liver	$\alpha \; \beta_2$	Glycogenolysis and gluconeogenesis	Glycogen synthesis
Pancreas			
Acini	α_1	Decreased secretion	Secretion
Islet cells	$\alpha_2 \; \beta_2$	α_2 = decreased secr'n β_2 = increased secr'n	—

Continued on next page

AUTONOMIC NEUROMUSCULAR

TABLE 13–2 Responses of Effector Organs to Autonomic Transmitters (Continued)

Effector Organs	Adrenergic Receptors*	Adrenergic Responses	Muscarinic Cholinergic Responses
Salivary Glands	α_1	Potassium and water secretion (slight)	Potassium and water secretion (profuse)
Lacrimal Glands		—	Secretion (profuse)
Nasopharyngeal Glands		—	Secretion
Kidneys	$\alpha_1 \beta_1$	α_1 = ↓ renin release β_1 = ↑ renin release	—
Adrenergic Nerve Terminals	α_2 (pre-synaptic)	↓ Release of noradrenaline	
Cholinergic Nerve Terminals	α_2 (pre-synaptic)		↓ Release of acetylcholine at some sites

* Where known.
† For far vision.
‡ For near vision.
§ β_2 and α Adrenoceptors are present in the heart also, but they are less important than β_1 receptors.
\# Renal and mesenteric blood vessels have dopamine receptors, which cause dilatation when stimulated. α_2 Adrenoceptors in blood vessels cause contraction when stimulated.
** α_2 Adrenoceptors in the myenteric plexus inhibit acetylcholine release when stimulated.
†† α_1-Adrenoceptor stimulation contracts the uterus during pregnancy.
↑ = Increase; ↓ = Decrease; Constr = Constriction; Dilat = Dilatation; Contr = Contraction; Relax = Relaxation. — = No effect.

baroreceptor-mediated negative feedback response that results in marked bradycardia. This is due to increased acetylcholine release at the sinoatrial node causing a compensatory decrease in heart rate. Bradycardia occurs even when the pressor drug is a potent myocardial stimulant that normally increases the heart rate (see Chapter 16, noradrenaline). In this way the parasympathetic nervous system becomes dominant and overrides sympathomimetic effects on both the sinoatrial and atrioventricular nodes.

Control of transmitter release is another mechanism by which one system may be inhibited (or enhanced) relative to the other. Presynaptic α_2 adrenoceptors, when stimulated by released noradrenaline, exert a negative feedback control by diminishing noradrenaline release from nerve endings. Conversely, noradrenaline release can be enhanced by stimulation of β_2 adrenoceptors.

Presynaptic α_2 adrenoceptors located on parasympathetic nerve endings can also reduce the amount of acetylcholine released at certain sites. In the mesenteric plexus, for example, the release of acetylcholine is decreased to an extent that causes relaxation and reduced motility of the intestine to occur.

Other endogenous substances, e.g., prostaglandins and enkephalins, also inhibit noradrenaline release by interacting with specific presynaptic receptors. Contrasting with this is the effect of angiotensin II (see Chapter 31), which enhances the release of catecholamines.

At postsynaptic adrenoceptor sites in target organs, the response of an organ to neurotransmitters may be altered by changes in receptor numbers, e.g., desensitization due to down-regulation of receptors following periods of excessive stimulation. Up-regulation (i.e., increased receptor numbers) may occur in other circumstances, e.g., when a drug acts on neurons to inhibit transmitter release.

SUGGESTED READING

Francis GS. Modulation of peripheral sympathetic nerve transmission. J Am Coll Cardiol 1988; 12:250–254.

Iversen LL et al. Neurotransmitters and their actions [a series of articles]. Trends in Neuroscience 1983; 6:293–345.

Moreland RS, Bohr DF. Adrenergic control of coronary arteries. Fed Proc 1984; 43:2857–2861.

Starke K. Presynaptic receptors. Ann Rev Pharmacol Toxicol 1981; 21:7–30.

Chapter 14

AUTONOMIC CHOLINERGIC AGONISTS

L. Spero

ACETYLCHOLINE

As described in Chapter 13, acetylcholine acts as neurotransmitter at four distinct types of cholinergic site. The four are: preganglionic (sympathetic and parasympathetic), postganglionic parasympathetic (and some sympathetic), central, and neuromuscular, of which the neuromuscular junction will be dealt with separately in Chapter 19.

The synthesis and release of acetylcholine, and the characteristics of its receptors (two types of nicotinic receptor and the muscarinic receptor, which may also be of more than one type) are described in Chapters 13, 15, and 19.

Principal Actions

Muscarinic Actions

These are postganglionic parasympathetic actions on exocrine glands and smooth muscle, as follows.

1. Stimulation of exocrine glands such as the sweat, salivary, mucous, and lacrimal glands. Gastric, intestinal, and pancreatic secretions are also increased, although they depend only partly on parasympathetic innervation.
2. Stimulation of smooth muscle contraction in bronchi, gastrointestinal tract, gall bladder, bile duct, urinary bladder, and ureters.
3. Stimulation of the circular muscles of the iris and the muscles of accommodation so that the pupil is constricted and the lens of the eye is accommodated for near vision.
4. Relaxation of sphincters in the gastrointestinal, biliary, and urinary tracts.

5. Slowing of the heart.

Nicotinic Actions

1. Stimulation of sympathetic and parasympathetic ganglia, *i.e.*, stimulation of postsynaptic structures within the ganglia so that the postganglionic fibres release their respective transmitters at their peripheral endings.
2. Stimulation of the adrenal medulla to release adrenaline* and noradrenaline.[†]
3. Contraction of skeletal muscle.

Acetylcholine as a Drug

Acetylcholine is poorly absorbed following oral or subcutaneous administration. When it is given intravenously, very high doses are required to produce an effect because it is rapidly hydrolysed by plasma cholinesterase found in both the blood and the liver.

The pharmacologic effects of acetylcholine include: a transient fall in blood pressure; bradycardia; partial or complete heart block or cardiac arrest; flushing, sweating, salivation, lacrimation, and increased mucus secretion; and as secondary consequences nausea, coughing, and dyspnea. These are all due to muscarinic actions; no nicotinic actions are noted. The effects on skeletal muscle can be observed only after intra-arterial injection. Exogenously administered acetylcholine will not produce effects on the CNS, since the molecule is a quaternary ammonium compound that cannot cross the blood–brain barrier (Fig. 14–1).

Acetylcholine can dilate blood vessels by a direct

---

* epinephrine
† norepinephrine

141

action on smooth muscle cells even though there is no cholinergic innervation of these blood vessels.

CHOLINERGIC DRUGS

Because acetylcholine is so unsuitable as a drug, substitutes are used if parasympathetic effects need to be produced for diagnosis or therapy.

The contraindications are essentially the same for all the cholinergic drugs. They are contraindicated in patients with intestinal or urinary obstruction, and they should be used cautiously in patients with bronchial asthma.

Cholinergic drugs mimic the effects of stimulation of cholinergic nerves. They may do so either by direct action, in the same way as acetylcholine, or by inhibition of acetylcholinesterase, thereby preventing the destruction of endogenous acetylcholine. Stimulation of the mechanism for release of endogenous acetylcholine is not used therapeutically.

Directly Acting Cholinergic Agonists

Naturally Occurring Alkaloids with Direct Cholinergic Activities

Muscarine is found in the mushroom *Amanita muscaria* (Fly agaric) and related species. It was the agent used to characterize the muscarinic receptor. Its actions are solely muscarinic. Specific muscarinic antagonists (*e.g.*, atropine) are used to treat poisoning by this alkaloid.

Pilocarpine is found in the leaves of *Pilocarpus*, a South American shrub. It has both muscarinic and nicotinic actions. The effects of pilocarpine upon glands, such as the sweat and salivary glands, are particularly pronounced; therefore, it has been used to increase salivation and to induce sweating. Pilocarpine is now used mainly in ophthalmology for the treatment of glaucoma (by opening the drainage canals for the ocular fluid and thereby reducing the intraocular pressure), for producing miosis, and for counteracting the mydriatic and cycloplegic actions of drugs such as atropine and the ganglion-blocking agents.

Arecoline is derived from a seed commonly known as the "betel nut." Its peripheral actions are similar to those of methacholine. Arecoline has no therapeutic use in man, but it is of interest because the betel nut is habitually chewed by a large part of the world's population. From Africa to the East Indies, in many countries bordering the Indian and Pacific Oceans, millions of people who do not smoke tobacco show an equivalent addiction to chewing the betel nut. Presumably, arecoline has central effects that are analogous to those of nicotine.

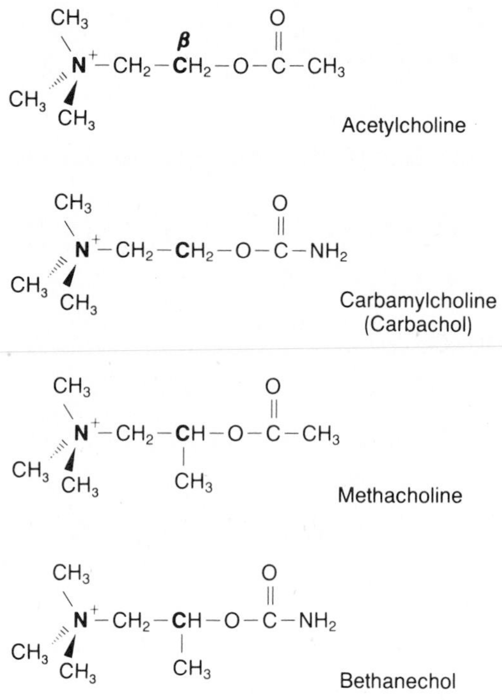

Figure 14–1   Structural formulae of acetylcholine and analogs.

Synthetic Analogs of Acetylcholine

If the acetyl group in acetylcholine is replaced by a carbamyl group, the resistance of the compound (carbamylcholine) to cholinesterase hydrolysis is greatly increased. Substitution of a methyl group at the β-carbon results in analogs (*e.g.*, methacholine) with a greater selectivity for muscarinic receptors and also somewhat reduces the susceptibility to cholinesterase hydrolysis (*see* Fig. 14–1).

Carbamylcholine (carbachol) has both muscarinic and nicotinic properties, but it is resistant to cholinesterase hydrolysis. It selectively stimulates the urinary and gastrointestinal tracts, but it is not used for this purpose because of its concomitant ganglion stimulant effects. It is available for use in ocular surgery to produce miosis, and it may also be used in certain forms of glaucoma.

Methacholine has a resistance to hydrolysis similar to that of carbachol, but because of the β-methyl group it has more selectively muscarinic activity. It is used to increase gastrointestinal motility and to overcome urinary retention consequent to anaesthesia or vagotomy.

Bethanechol may be used to test pancreatic function since it increases secretion but constricts the sphincter of Oddi. This should cause an increase in plasma amylase, since the secreted amylase is reabsorbed and passes into the blood.

Indirectly Acting Cholinergic Drugs: Cholinesterase Inhibitors

All clinically used cholinesterase blockers inhibit both acetylcholinesterase and plasma cholinesterase, although not always to the same extent. The principal pharmacologic effects are solely due to inhibition of acetylcholinesterase.

Following a lethal overdose of most acetylcholinesterase inhibitors, a characteristic sequence of reactions results from the rapid build-up of acetylcholine at receptor sites. Restlessness usually develops early and reflects the central actions of acetylcholine. This is accompanied by increasing abdominal distress, with more and more severe pain due to intestinal spasm. There is frequent, involuntary defecation and urination. The pupils of the eyes become constricted (miosis). The skeletal muscles show fasciculation, *i.e.*, small groups of muscle fibres twitch but produce no coordinated movement. The twitching muscles can not be used for voluntary coordinated contraction, so that there is virtual paralysis. Soon, there is increased glandular activity with salivation, lacrimation, sweating, and increased bronchial secretion. At the same time there is a bronchiolar constriction that, with the accumulation of bronchial secretions, results in stertorous, difficult breathing. Later, there are usually convulsions, and during the convulsions breathing ceases. The heart, although slowed, continues to beat for some time after breathing stops. Ultimately, death is due to respiratory failure.

In denervated organs in which no acetylcholine is released, inhibition of acetylcholinesterase is without pharmacologic effect. By contrast, directly acting cholinergic drugs often elicit an exaggerated response in such organs, because of denervation supersensitivity of the receptors.

Chemically, there are two main classes of compounds that inhibit acetylcholinesterase: carbamate derivatives, which are reversible inhibitors, and organophosphates, which inhibit irreversibly by forming stable complexes with acetylcholinesterase.

Acetylcholinesterase Structure

The active site of acetylcholinesterase consists of an anionic site, which interacts with the quaternary group on the choline moiety of acetylcholine, and an esteratic site, which interacts with and hydrolyses the ester grouping of acetylcholine (Fig. 14–2). A serine hydroxyl group at the esteratic site becomes acetylated and is subsequently regenerated by interaction with water.

Serum cholinesterase shows genetic variation, and some individuals have an atypical variant, which has very low hydrolytic activity. This will influence the pharmacokinetics of many drugs with ester linkages (*see* Chapter 12). Acetylcholinesterase variants have not been observed, probably because "atypical" acetylcholinesterase would be lethal in the first hours of life.

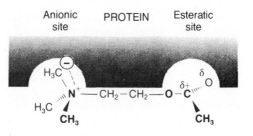

Figure 14–2 Interaction of acetylcholine and acetylcholinesterase.

Reversible Cholinesterase Inhibitors

These agents are competitive inhibitors of the cholinesterases (Fig. 14–3). They have carbamyl ester linkages that are slowly hydrolysed by the enzyme, resulting in carbamylation of the enzyme. Water can then release a carbamic acid molecule from the enzyme. These agents have mainly muscarinic side effects that can be blocked by atropine.

Physostigmine (eserine). This is an alkaloid extracted from the Calabar bean; its effects are interwoven with many African "trial-by-ordeal" ceremonies. It is

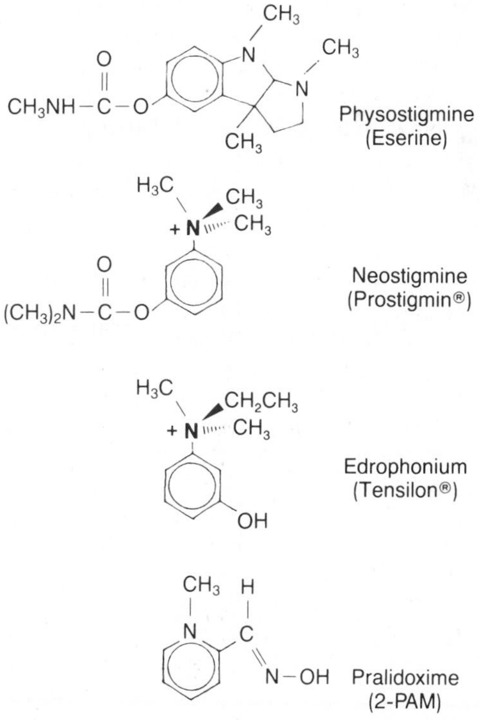

Figure 14–3 Structural formulae of reversible cholinesterase inhibitors.

lipid-soluble and can therefore cross the blood–brain barrier and produce CNS side effects. Its main use is in the treatment of glaucoma. It is absorbed readily from eye drops and, by increasing the availability of acetylcholine, reduces intraocular pressure, mainly by facilitating the outflow of aqueous humor.

Neostigmine, pyridostigmine, ambenonium. These anticholinesterases are all quaternary ammonium compounds and therefore should not cross the blood–brain barrier. They also have some direct nicotinic agonist actions in skeletal muscle, which renders them very suitable for the treatment of myasthenia gravis (*see* Chapter 19). Ambenonium has the longest duration of action, neostigmine the shortest. They are taken orally in myasthenia gravis. CNS side effects are observed with ambenonium, and it does appear to cross the blood–brain barrier slowly.

In addition to the common muscarinic side effects found with cholinesterase inhibitors, all of the reversible inhibitors described above can produce a "cholinergic crisis" as a consequence of excess acetylcholine desensitizing the nicotinic receptors at both the ganglia and, more importantly, the neuromuscular junctions. The major symptom is muscle paralysis resembling myasthenia gravis, the disease they are being used to treat.

Edrophonium. This is a short-acting reversible cholinesterase inhibitor that is used by intravenous injection to differentiate between a cholinergic crisis and myasthenia gravis itself. It has a brief duration of action (3–4 minutes); the myasthenic patient will experience transient improvement, while the cholinergic crisis will be transiently worse.

Irreversible Cholinesterase Inhibitors

This class of cholinesterase inhibitors, which consists of hundreds of active organophosphorus chemicals, is important more for toxicologic than therapeutic reasons. These agents include "nerve gases" for biologic warfare and insecticides (Fig. 14–4). They produce phosphonylation or phosphorylation of the esteratic site of acetylcholinesterase, and once this covalent interaction is complete it cannot be reversed. The reaction takes place in three stages (Fig. 14–5):

A reversible phase in which the irreversible inhibitor competes with acetylcholine for binding to the acetylcholinesterase. This stage may be symptom-free.

Phosphorylation of the serine residue in the esteratic site. At this stage the acetylcholinesterase can be reactivated by pralidoxime (2-PAM).

An "aging" process in which there is loss of an alkyl group or migration of the phosphoryl group to another amino acid residue (possibly a histidine). The enzyme is now irreversibly inhibited, and restoration of cholinesterase activity requires *de novo* synthesis of acetylcholinesterase.

Therapeutic use. Echothiophate is the only one of these compounds used in the treatment of glaucoma. It causes a reduction in the total body acetylcholinester-

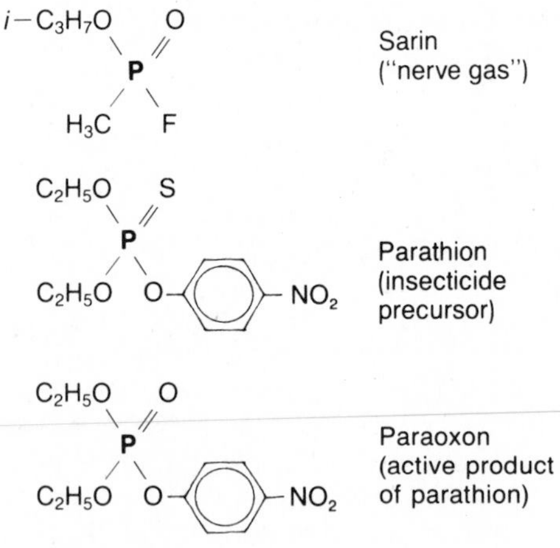

Figure 14–4   Structural formulae of irreversible cholinesterase inhibitors.

ase and should therefore not be used within 4–6 weeks of surgery because of possible complications with muscle relaxants. Muscarinic side effects can be overcome with atropine, or they may be reversed with PAM (*see* below).

Nerve gases. These inhibitors are volatile liquids that have been studied since World War II as potential chemical weapons to be used as sprays or aerosols. Being very highly lipid-soluble, they rapidly penetrate intact skin and mucous membranes, enter the circulation, and quickly reach all central and peripheral cholinergic synapses. Accidental contact with these agents has occurred through incautious handling in laboratories, storage depots, *etc.*, and during poorly controlled testing in the field. (Isolated incidents of deliberate, though brief, use as chemical weapons during armed conflicts in various parts of the world have been reported.) High concentrations kill almost instantaneously; low concentrations are more insidious because symptoms may develop slowly and resemble mental or neurologic illness. The fluorine-containing organophosphate cholinesterase inhibitors have also been shown to induce a delayed neurotoxicity even when present in trace amounts. Reactivation of the enzyme with PAM can be achieved only within the first few minutes following exposure.

Insecticides. These are organophosphate cholinesterase inhibitors that have been designed to be more toxic to insects than to mammals. They are all thiophosphates that must be converted to phosphates to become activated. This occurs very rapidly in insects but more slowly in humans. They are all designed to be readily inactivated by mammalian metabolism. However, these compounds cause human toxicity through cumulation from repeated exposure of persons handling these agents in their daily work. Mild poisoning may produce only nausea, headache, and weakness. This may lead to unusual neurologic symptoms

AUTONOMIC
NEUROMUSCULAR

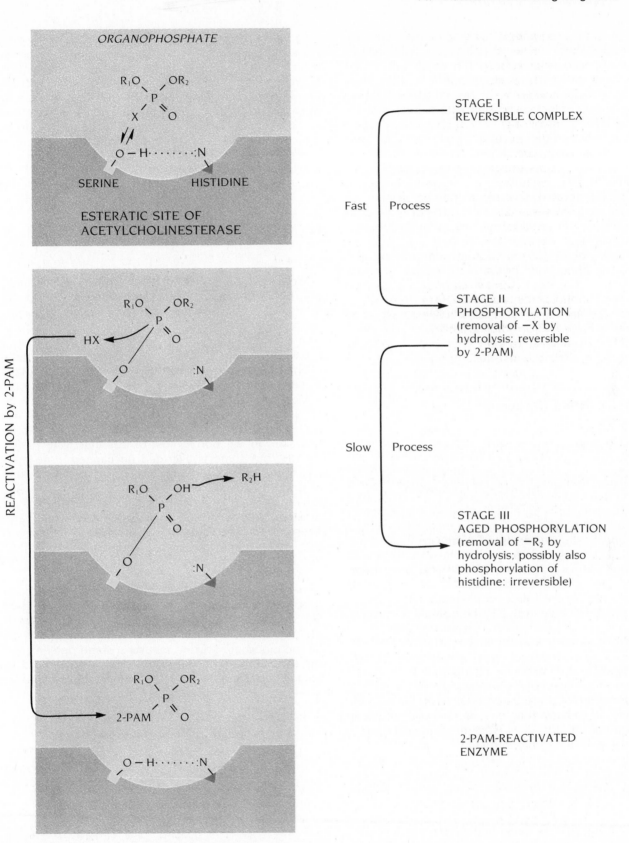

Figure 14–5 The steps of acetylcholinesterase inhibition by organophosphorus compounds, and enzyme reactivation with pralidoxime (pyridine-2-aldoxime, 2-PAM).

that may not be recognized as being due to "intoxication." Since these agents are also very lipid soluble, they may concentrate in body fat, which will form a reservoir, from which the insecticide may leak slowly into the circulation where it can be activated. Atropine can be used to block muscarinic side effects, and unless the level of inhibitor is very high, careful support of the patient and the use of artificial respiration may allow survival until *de novo* synthesis of acetylcholinesterase returns the patient to normal.

Cholinesterase reactivators. The phosphorylated acetylcholinesterase can be reactivated before the "aging" process occurs (*see* Fig. 14–5). The drug used for this purpose is pralidoxime (pyridine-2-aldoxime, 2-PAM, *see* Fig. 14–3).

The ability of PAM to reactivate the enzyme is a function of the phosphoryl group and the rate at which the "aging" process occurs, which is also a function of the organophosphate structure. PAM does not influence carbamylation of acetylcholinesterase, and because it has some anticholinesterase activity of its own, it is contraindicated in the presence of overdose of reversible cholinesterase inhibitor.

Indirectly Acting Cholinergic Drugs: Dopamine Antagonists

Incompetence of the gastroesophageal sphincter can lead to reflux of acidic gastric contents into the lower esophagus, producing irritation of the esophageal mucosa and reflux esophagitis. Cholinergic drugs can increase sphincter tone, but they also increase gastric secretion.

Metoclopramide (Fig. 14–6) increases gastroesophageal sphincter pressure, increases the force of esophageal peristalsis, increases the rate of gastric emptying without influencing the rate of acid secretion, and increases small intestinal motility. It has been shown to markedly reduce reflux esophagitis, but it has not been proved to be effective in the treatment of gastric ulcer.

Metoclopramide is a dopamine (D_2-receptor) antagonist with some neuroleptic properties; it is used extensively as a centrally acting antiemetic. Its effects on gastrointestinal motility are employed to speed up the absorption of drugs that are taken up in the lower intestine, or to hasten the passage of barium contrast medium through the small intestine. It is also used to facilitate gastrointestinal intubation.

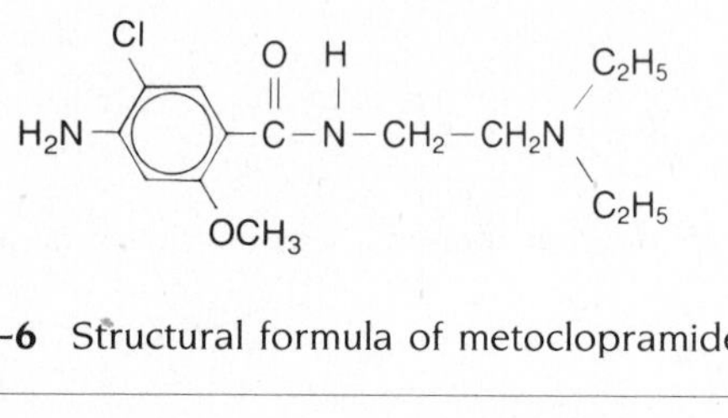

Its mode of action is not clearly understood. It may work by reducing the dopaminergic inhibitory tone on the cholinergic ganglia of the myenteric plexus. (This is analogous to the dopaminergic/cholinergic interaction in the basal ganglia—*see* Chapter 20.) It has also been reported to increase the sensitivity of intestinal smooth muscle to acetylcholine. Anticholinergic drugs diminish the effects of metoclopramide.

In spite of its structural resemblance to procainamide, metoclopramide is only a poor local anaesthetic.

NICOTINE AND LOBELINE

Nicotine (Fig. 14–7) is not used as a therapeutic agent but there are, nevertheless, three reasons for studying it. First, it is the drug that was initially used to characterize nicotinic pharmacologic responses. Second, nicotine is pharmacologically the most active ingredient of tobacco smoke. Third, nicotine is a potent and rapidly acting poison that, when used as an insecticide, occasionally takes human life.

Nicotine is an alkaloid; it is a brown liquid that is volatile and, therefore, is easily inhaled with tobacco smoke. It penetrates not only mucous membranes but also intact skin. In the body, most of it is inactivated fairly rapidly, but some is excreted unchanged.

Nicotine intake, in a dose equivalent to the smoking of one or two cigarettes (roughly 0.3–1 mg), usually causes a slight increase in heart rate, some rise of blood pressure, and a modest increase in respiratory rate. These effects are comparable to those of mild exercise. Skin temperature and cutaneous blood flow decrease. Secretion of vasopressin (antidiuretic hormone, ADH) is stimulated, with consequent suppression of diuresis, so that smoking tests have been proposed for diagnostic distinction between pituitary and other forms of diabetes insipidus. Blood sugar is likely to go up, particularly in a hungry person. Effects on the mood are hard to measure; some persons feel stimulated, others sedated. All these effects tend to be qualitatively similar whether the person is a smoker

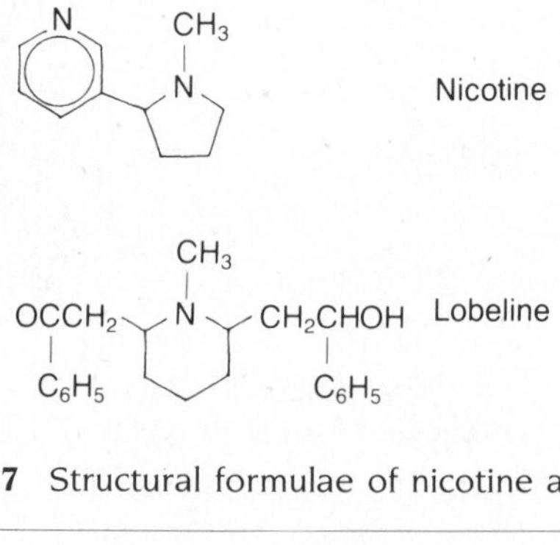

Figure 14–6 Structural formula of metoclopramide.

Figure 14–7 Structural formulae of nicotine and lobeline.

or a nonsmoker. In the latter, there may be in addition nausea and vomiting, an urge to defecate, and sometimes tremor.

The effects of small amounts of nicotine are due to the following actions. The smallest doses stimulate the chemoreceptors in the carotid and aortic bodies. This accounts primarily for the effects on respiration. The first circulatory effects are mostly due to noradrenaline released from sympathetic fibres within vascular walls and within the heart muscle. Furthermore, the adrenal medulla is stimulated to release adrenaline, and the supraoptic nucleus is stimulated to release antidiuretic hormone.

Somewhat higher doses of nicotine are necessary to act upon autonomic ganglia. With increasing dosage there is the following sequence: stimulation of sympathetic ganglia, stimulation of parasympathetic ganglia, blockade of parasympathetic ganglia. These actions account for the gastrointestinal effects and the increasing disturbance of circulation and respiration. Blockade of sympathetic ganglia requires usually very high doses and is seen only during the final stages of intoxication. Tremor and nausea are due to separate actions in the CNS. Radioreceptor assays have demonstrated the presence of nicotinic receptors in the CNS. Nicotine can cross the blood–brain barrier.

After inadvertent intake of toxic amounts, *e.g.*, an insecticide containing 40% nicotine (Black Leaf 40), dyspnea develops rapidly. Gradually, the blood pressure rises exceedingly high (250–300 mm Hg) while the pulse is very slow. There is diarrhea. Twitching and fasciculation of skeletal muscles is soon followed by paralysis. Death is due to failure of the respiratory muscles and usually occurs within 15–30 minutes of nicotine intake. This is so because, in a very high dose, nicotine behaves like a depolarizing relaxant of skeletal muscle, and paralysis is the usual cause of death in fatal poisoning (*see* Chapter 19). The emergency treatment of acute poisoning, therefore, is artificial respiration to tide the patient over the critical period.

Chronic intoxication is possible. The repeated liberation of noradrenaline in the walls of blood vessels, over long periods of time, leads to interference with circulation in susceptible vascular beds. Thus, gangrene and loss of limbs or blindness may occur in predisposed

persons. Smoking mothers often have smaller than average babies. It is not entirely clear whether this represents a retardation of growth or premature delivery, but recent animal data support the idea of growth inhibition due to nicotine.

The effects of tobacco smoke and nicotine are not completely identical. Production of cancer, allergic reactions, and smoking-related impairment of pulmonary function are probably not due to nicotine. More than 260 different chemicals have been identified in tobacco smoke and there is enough carbon monoxide, cyanide, and oxide of nitrogen for any one of these to kill the person who breathes tobacco smoke instead of air. However, the intermittent "puffing" and the dilution of smoke upon inhalation seem to reduce their acute toxicity. (Note, however, that ingestion of a whole or part of a cigarette would involve a toxic dose of nicotine—up to 22 mg. This is an additional reason for keeping cigarettes away from children.)

The alkaloid **lobeline** (*see* Fig. 14–7) is a nicotinic agonist that has been used to ameliorate nicotine withdrawal symptoms, *i.e.*, to help a person give up smoking. It also increases respiration by stimulating the carotid body, and it was at one time used as a drug for resuscitation.

SUGGESTED READING

Conti-Tranconi BM, Raftery BM. The nicotinic cholinergic receptor: correlation of molecular structure to functional properties. Annu Rev Biochem 1982; 51:491–530.

Hulme EC, Berrie CP, Birdsall NJM, Stockton JM. Regulation of muscarinic agonist binding by cations and guanine-nucleotides. Eur J Pharmacol 1983; 94:59–73.

Levitan IB. Modulation of ion channels in neurons and other cells. Annu Rev Neurosci 1988; 11:119–136.

McKinney M, Richardson E. The coupling of the neuronal muscarinic receptor to response. Annu Rev Pharmacol Toxicol 1984; 24:121–146.

Rubin LL, Anthony DT, Englander LL, et al. Neural regulation of properties of the nicotinic acetylcholine receptor. J Recept Res 1988; 8:161–181.

Chapter 15

Autonomic Cholinergic Antagonists

L. Spero

MUSCARINIC RECEPTOR ANTAGONISTS

These antagonists selectively block muscarinic receptors at parasympathetic postganglionic sites and, if they can cross the blood–brain barrier, in the CNS. They are frequently misnamed "cholinergic antagonists" or "anticholinergics" without specific reference to their selectivity for muscarinic receptors only.

Principles of Action

As described in Chapter 13, muscarinic agonists appear to bind to receptor sites with three different levels of affinity. However, the antagonists that have been examined appear to bind with equal affinity to all three types (or states?) of the receptor.

In Table 15–1 are shown the interactions of a number of muscarinic antagonists with radioactive ligands that label muscarinic receptors (see also Chapter 9). This table demonstrates that muscarinic antagonists have a similar affinity for the receptor regardless of whether it is labelled with an agonist (^{3}H-oxotremorine) or an antagonist (^{3}H-propylbenzilylcholine). These antagonist affinities are much higher (i.e., the IC_{50} values are much lower) than those of agonists (e.g., acetylcholine), even when the radiolabel is an agonist. It is also apparent that nicotinic agonists and antagonists have a very low affinity for the muscarinic receptor, as shown by the very high IC_{50} values. The radio-receptor assay may thus be used as a predictive indicator of the pharmacologic effects of muscarinic antagonists. The higher their affinity in a radioreceptor experiment, the more potent they are clinically.

Pirenzepine, a new muscarinic antagonist, was predicted to be a more selective inhibitor of gastric secretion than of gastric motility, on the basis of its unusual relative selectivity for the "high-affinity" (M_1) agonist site over the "low-affinity" (M_2) agonist site.

The blockade of muscarinic receptors by these antagonists is competitive and depends on the relative concentrations of the antagonist and acetylcholine, and their relative affinity for the receptors. As is the case with most families of antagonists, they are slightly more effective against exogenously applied agonist than against acetylcholine released endogenously as neurotransmitter. Cholinergic stimulation in the presence of a muscarinic antagonist still stimulates autonomic nicotinic ganglia, but only sympathetic effects are elicited.

Pharmacologic Effects

The effects of the prototypic muscarinic antagonist, **atropine** (Fig. 15–1), will be described.

Exocrine Glands

Salivary secretion is impaired even after very small doses of atropine. The subject experiences a dry mouth and swallowing may be very difficult.

Gastric secretion is diminished, although gastric pH is unchanged. (Therefore, its main contribution in the treatment of peptic ulcer is relief of spasm; see below.)

Bronchial secretions are suppressed, which renders atropine useful for preanaesthetic medication.

Sweating is impaired. The inability to perspire may interfere with heat regulation, which can be fatal in very hot weather.

TABLE 15-1 Muscarinic Receptor Binding. IC_{50} Values for Various Cholinergic Agonists and Antagonists Against Ligands That Label Muscarinic Cholinergic Receptors. (See Chapter 9, *Drug Receptors*.)

Competing Cold Ligand	^{3}H-Propyl-Benzilylcholine* (Antagonist)	^{3}H-Oxotremorine* (Agonist)	^{3}H-Quinuclidinyl Benzilate† (Antagonist)
Muscarinic Agonists			
Acetylcholine	3,300 nM	240 nM	3,000 nM
Oxotremorine	460 nM	38 nM	700 nM
Methacholine	2,000 nM	350 nM	2,500 nM
Muscarine	8,300 nM	—	—
Carbachol	15,000 nM	240 nM	25,000 nM
Muscarinic Antagonists			
Atropine	0.59 nM	3.0 nM	3.0 nM
Benzhexol	7.1 nM	25.0 nM	—
Methylatropine	0.35 nM	0.7 nM	0.2 nM
Nicotinic Agonists and Antagonists			
Nicotine ⎫ d-Tubocurarine ⎬ Hexamethonium ⎭	>100,000 nM	>100,000 nM	>100,000 nM

Sources: * Birdsal NJM, Burgen ASV, Hume EC. Mol Pharmacol 1978; 14:723–736.
† Yamamura HI, Snyder SH. Mol Pharmacol 1974; 10:861–867.

Smooth Muscle

Gastrointestinal tract. Atropine abolishes any excessive tone and motility of the intestinal tract, but it has relatively little effect on normal motility. It is therefore spasmolytic but not constipating. Atropine is particularly effective in relieving spasms of the cardiac sphincter of the stomach, while effects on the pyloric sphincter are less reliable.

Biliary tract. Atropine has some relaxing action and is moderately effective in relieving biliary colic. It does not influence the formation of bile.

Urinary tract. In therapeutic doses, atropine diminishes the tone of the fundus of the bladder but increases the tone of the vesical sphincter. This may cause retention of urine, which can be a serious side effect in patients after surgery and in elderly men with prostatic hypertrophy. The effect is utilized, however, to suppress the frequency and urgency of micturition in cystitis. This effect is also exploited in the control of nocturnal enuresis.

Atropine reduces tone and motility of the ureter and thus relieves attacks of renal colic.

Circulation

Large doses of atropine (2 mg) have the expected effect on heart rate, which increases by 40–50 beats/minute due to vagal blockade. Small doses of atropine (0.2 mg) decrease the heart rate by 10–15 beats/minute. This is due to a central action of atropine and has been likened to a stimulation of the "cardioinhibitory centre" in the medulla. Atropine in therapeutic doses of 0.5–1 mg in the adult has usually a dual effect, namely, first a decrease and then an increase of the heart rate.

There is no major effect on blood vessels, so that blood pressure is not affected. High doses of atropine cause selective vasodilatation, including flushing of the face.

The Eye

Atropine has two primary effects on the eye, namely mydriasis (dilatation of the pupil) and cycloplegia (paralysis of accommodation), by antagonizing acetylcholine as shown in Figure 15–2. Both effects can be produced by systemic application of atropine, but they are most prominent after local application, because local application of concentrated solutions produces much higher intraocular concentrations of atropine than is achieved by systemically tolerable oral or parenteral doses.

This combination of effects makes atropine an important drug in ophthalmology to permit precise measurements of refraction. The mydriatic effect is utilized in cases of iritis. In eyes with a narrow chamber angle (*i.e.*, the angle between iris and cornea), dilatation of the pupil may cause the iris muscle to block the canal of Schlemm and thereby to interfere with the drainage of aqueous humor; in this way atropine may produce an attack of glaucoma in predisposed persons, which may cause them to lose their eyesight. The effects of atropine applied as eyedrops may be noticeable for as long as a week.

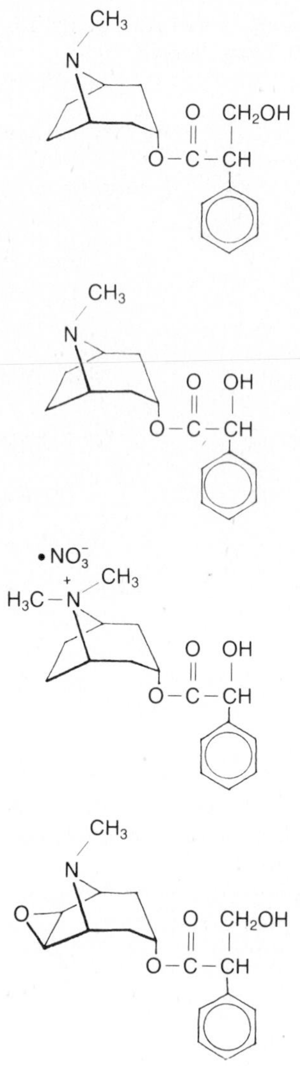

Atropine

Homatropine

Homatropine
methyl nitrate

Scopolamine

Figure 15–1   Structural formulae of natural muscarinic antagonists.

Central Nervous System

Atropine in the usual therapeutic doses has no significant effects upon the central nervous system. It has no uses in this area, except for its beneficial effects in Parkinson's disease, in which it suppresses tremor and rigidity. This is due to a central action (*see* Chapter 20), but some action upon muscle spindles may also contribute to the effect.

In high doses, atropine has complicated effects on the brain that have been broadly classified as stimulatory, but disorientation is the most characteristic feature (*see* Chapter 29, *Psychotomimetic Drugs*). After drug intake, the subject first becomes restless and quarrelsome. A state of excitation may be followed by

delirium. Usually there is recovery without recollection; only rarely will the delirium progress into coma with respiratory failure and death.

The central effects of atropine-containing plant extracts differ slightly from those of the pure alkaloid because of the admixture of scopolamine (*see* below). Belladonna alkaloids were used as medicines for many centuries, but they also found much criminal use in witchcraft and quackery. Remnants of these nonmedicinal mediaeval uses are found in the mnemonic jingle on atropine poisoning:

Dry as a Bone,
Red as a Beet,
Mad as a Hen.

Drugs in Clinical Use

Naturally Occurring Plant Alkaloids

Atropine (Fig. 15–1). Atropine is dl-hyoscyamine extracted from belladonna (deadly nightshade), hyoscyamus (henbane), or stramonium (Jimson weed) plants, all of which belong to the potato family. l-Hyoscyamine is more potent than the racemic mixture atropine, but it is less stable.

Atropine is usually given as the sulfate subcutaneously in doses of 0.5–1 mg. The effects of oral doses are less intense and occur more slowly. In the treatment of anticholinesterase poisoning, atropine may need to be given intravenously. For ophthalmic purposes, atropine is applied directly to the eye in solution or ointment. Narrow-angle glaucoma is a contraindication to its use.

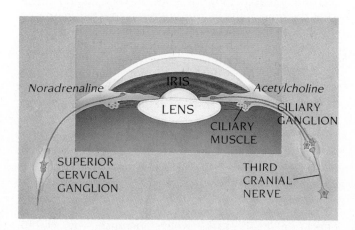

Figure 15–2   Innervation of lens and iris of the eye.

The duration of action varies depending on the dose, route of administration, and respective organ. The systemic effects of atropine, whether it is administered orally or subcutaneously, last only a few hours so that the dose must be repeated every 4–6 hours. Following local application of atropine to the eye, however, impairment of accommodation may persist for 3 or 4 days and dilatation of the pupil even for 6 or 7 days. Reversible cholinesterase inhibitors are sometimes used to overcome this problem. However, the half-life of the inhibitors is shorter than that of atropine, and the visual impairment can reappear unexpectedly.

Insofar as the cardiac and ocular effects of atropine are concerned, little or no tolerance develops. However, repeated doses of the drug produce diminishing effects upon the digestive tract and secretions. Appreciable tolerance can develop in patients receiving relatively large doses of atropine, as in the treatment of parkinsonism, so that very high doses in the order of 50 mg per day may become necessary to maintain effectiveness. Chronic use also tends to cause urinary retention.

Homatropine hydrobromide, homatropine methylbromide (*see* Fig. 15–1). These analogs of atropine have a more rapid onset and a shorter duration of action. They are, however, less potent than atropine. The hydrobromide is used solely for ophthalmic purposes. The quaternary methyl analogs of homatropine and atropine (methylatropine) are unable to cross the blood–brain barrier and, therefore, do not have the CNS effects of the parent compounds. Their main use is in the treatment of gastrointestinal disorders.

Scopolamine (*see* Fig. 15–1). Scopolamine, which has the same peripheral actions as atropine, has centrally a pronounced sedative action. For a long time it was the only drug used to subdue highly agitated mentally ill patients. However, some people get excited after scopolamine, rather than sedated.

"Twilight sleep," resulting from a combination of scopolamine and morphine, was at one time very popular in surgery and obstetrics. Its modern counterpart is neuroleptanalgesia by a combination of opioid and neuroleptic (*see* Chapter 23). In most persons, scopolamine tends to counteract the respiratory depression produced by morphine. For obscure reasons, however, this combination produces in some subjects a pronounced, and potentially fatal, respiratory depression.

Scopolamine is used prophylactically to prevent motion sickness. It is not recommended for nausea and vomiting due to nonvestibular causes.

Synthetic Muscarinic Antagonists

There are many synthetic substitutes for atropine (Fig. 15–3). Because they were developed to maximize specific actions of atropine, it makes sense to classify them according to their therapeutic use.

Suppression of gastric secretion. These agents are described in Chapter 50. They are all quaternary am-

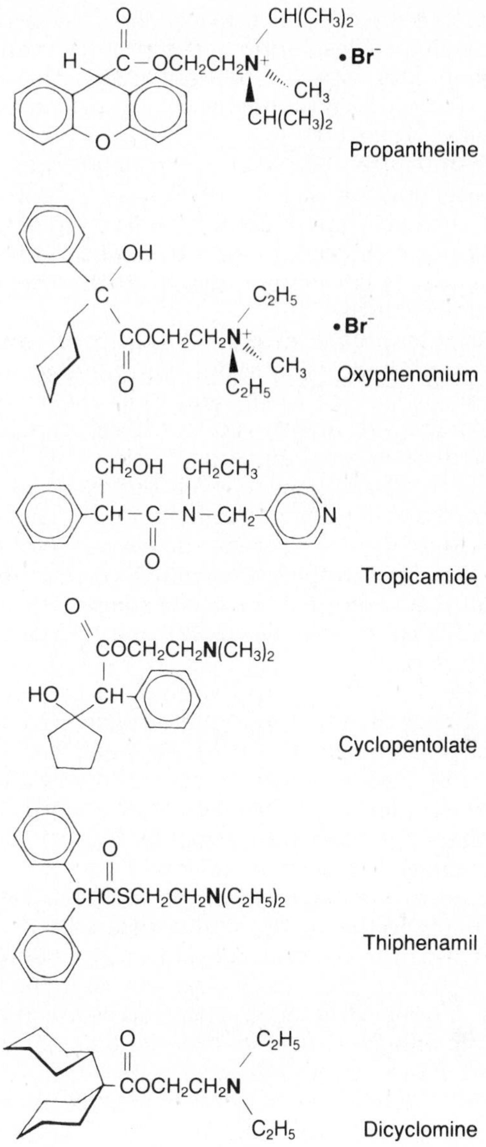

Figure 15–3 Structural formulae of some synthetic muscarinic antagonists.

monium compounds and they exist as two types: those with mixed muscarinic and ganglion-blocking properties (*e.g.*, propantheline and oxyphenonium), and pirenzepine, which is a purely muscarinic antagonist.

These antagonists all reduce gastric secretions, but the mixed antagonists reduce motility as well. The selectivity of pirenzepine for secretion makes it the muscarinic antagonist of choice in ulcer therapy. It is used only in combination with histamine H_2-receptor blockers (*e.g.*, ranitidine), antacids, or "cytoprotective" agents (carbenoxolone).

Suppression of smooth muscle spasm in gastrointestinal tract, biliary tract, and ureter. The drugs advocated for this purpose, *e.g.*, dicyclomine

(Bentylol®), have no CNS activity. They cause relaxation through their muscarinic antagonist actions as well as through a nonspecific relaxant effect on smooth muscle. They are little used in clinical practice, atropine being preferred.

Ophthalmic use. These are short-acting muscarinic antagonists that are well absorbed from eye drops instilled in the conjunctival sacs (*e.g.*, homatropine). They are tertiary amines and, therefore, can have CNS side effects including convulsions, psychotic disorders, and behavioral disturbances.

Anti-parkinsonian drugs. Parkinson's disease, described in Chapter 20, is due to an imbalance between the cholinergic activity and a chronically declining dopaminergic activity in the basal ganglia. As mentioned elsewhere, the drug of choice is L-dopa, which can restore dopamine levels but does not affect the chronically declining numbers of dopaminergic neurons. Muscarinic antagonists, such as trihexyphenidyl (Artane®) and benztropine (Cogentin®), can also restore the balance, and they may be useful adjuncts to L-dopa therapy. They are sometimes used in patients unresponsive to L-dopa.

The central effects of these synthetic drugs are relatively stronger than their peripheral cholinergic blocking actions, although the latter exist and cannot be disregarded. However, urinary retention and interference with reading ability (from cycloplegia) are usually less bothersome than with atropine.

These drugs are used for symptomatic treatment irrespective of the origin of symptoms. Thus, they are not restricted to the various parkinsonian diseases but are used also in similar disorders induced by phenothiazine neuroleptics, *etc*. The appearance of mental confusion and urinary retention usually indicates that the muscarinic antagonist has reached its limits of usefulness and should be withdrawn.

In addition to the few muscarinic antagonists in this group shown in Figure 15–3, at least 15 to 20 other muscarinic antagonists have been used for this purpose.

NICOTINIC RECEPTOR ANTAGONISTS; GANGLION BLOCKERS

These are drugs that competitively inhibit the actions of acetylcholine at autonomic ganglia. Nicotine (an agonist) in high doses can also block these receptors through a desensitization mechanism similar to that described for succinylcholine (*see* Chapter 19). There is no difference between the nicotinic receptors in sympathetic ganglia and those in parasympathetic ganglia. Any apparent selectivity in the blockade of sympathetic pathways as distinct from parasympathetic pathways results from the relative importance of the two pathways in controlling the function of a specific organ. Some differences in selectivity may be related to the anatomical location of the sympathetic ganglia a distance away from the organ involved, whereas the parasym-

pathetic ganglia are generally located within that organ. The blood flow through these two locations may be quite different.

The nicotinic receptors in autonomic ganglia are not identical to those at the neuromuscular junction. This is illustrated in Figure 15–4, which shows that the optimum chain length for ganglion blockade is not the same as for neuromuscular junction blockade. In clinical usage, drugs chosen for neuromuscular blockade will have some ganglion-blocking side effects. Historically, ganglion blockers were important in the treatment of hypertension because they lowered vascular sympathetic tone. They are no longer used for this purpose. The reasons become apparent from the description of the effects of **hexamethonium** (Fig. 15–5), a prototype of this family (*see* "hexamethonium man" below). The physiology of each organ determines its response to ganglion blockade. The wide spectrum of side effects has led to the withdrawal of these drugs from general use.

Pharmacologic Effects

What will happen to a person constantly treated with hexamethonium is illustrated by the following tongue-in-cheek description of the "**hexamethonium man**" (W.D.M. Paton: The principles of ganglionic block. In: Scientific Basis of Medicine, Vol. 2, London: Athlone Press, 1954.):

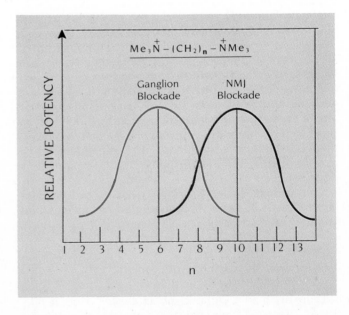

$$Me_3\overset{+}{N} - (CH_2)_n - \overset{+}{N}Me_3$$

Figure 15–4 Relative nicotinic receptor blockade as a function of optimum chain length of the onium compound for blockade of autonomic ganglia and of the neuromuscular junctions (NMJ).

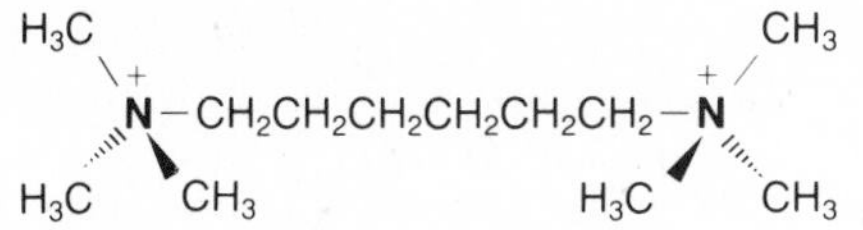

Hexamethonium

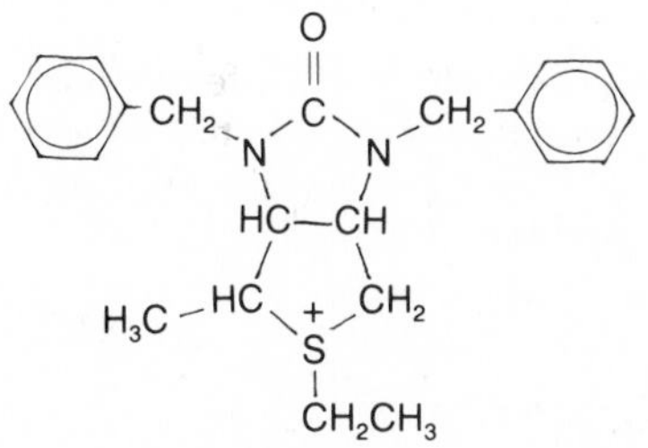

Trimethaphan

Figure 15–5 Structural formulae of ganglion blockers hexamethonium and trimethaphan.

"He is a pink complexioned person, except when he has stood in a queue for a long time, when he may get pale and faint. His handshake is warm and dry. He is a placid and relaxed companion; for instance he may laugh, but he can't cry because the tears cannot come. Your rudest story will not make him blush, and the most unpleasant circumstances will fail to make him turn pale. His collars and socks stay very clean and sweet. He wears corsets and may, if you meet him out, be rather fidgety (corsets to compress his splanchnic vascular pool, fidgety to keep the venous return going from his legs). He dislikes speaking much unless helped with something to moisten his dry mouth and throat. He is long-sighted and easily blinded by bright light. The redness of his eyeballs may suggest irregular habits and in fact his head is rather weak. But he always behaves like a gentleman and never belches nor hiccups. He tends to get cold and keeps well wrapped up. But his health is good; he does not have chilblains and those diseases of modern civilization, hypertension and peptic ulcer, pass him by. He is thin because his appetite is modest; he never feels hunger pains and his stomach never rumbles. He gets rather constipated so that his intake of liquid paraffin is high. As old age comes on, he will suffer from retention of urine and impotence, but frequency, precipitancy, and strangury will not worry him. One is uncertain how he will end, but perhaps if he is not careful, by eating less and less and getting colder and colder, he will sink into a symptomless, hypoglycemic coma and die, as was proposed for the universe, a sort of entropy death.''

The effects of ganglion blockade upon the function of the various systems depend upon the dominant tone, parasympathetic or sympathetic, for each organ. Thus, sympathetic tone predominates in the vasomotor system, and the usual response to hexamethonium is a reduction in blood pressure, particularly in hypertensive subjects. However, the most important feature is the failure of the regulating interplay of vasoconstriction and vasodilatation, which keeps the blood properly distributed in response to exertion or mere changes in posture. After hexamethonium, blood distribution becomes principally determined by gravity. The "hexamethonium man" faints when the blood accumulates in his legs after he has been standing for a while. If a person is lying down and an arm or leg is held up, the limb becomes almost bloodless. Ganglionic blockers are therefore used as an aid in special surgical procedures. The same principle is used if ganglionic blockers are employed to combat pulmonary edema.

The iris is predominantly under parasympathetic control, so the response is mydriasis. The gastrointestinal tract responds with partial or complete inhibition of gastric motility, some inhibition of salivary and gastric secretion, and disturbances of intestinal motility, usually constipation. In the respiratory tract, there is sometimes a decrease in nasopharyngeal secretion and some bronchodilatation. The skin becomes dry and flushed because of sympathetic blockade. There are no significant effects upon the central nervous system.

Ganglionic Blockers in Current Clinical Use

Trimethaphan camsylate (Arfonad®, Fig. 15–5) is given only by continuous intravenous infusion. It acts very rapidly and very briefly, so that the reduction of blood pressure can be controlled by varying the rate of infusion. Its main use is to treat hypertensive crises, to reduce blood pressure during surgery so as to minimize bleeding, and to reduce the circulating blood volume in the emergency treatment of pulmonary edema. The drug releases histamine and should be avoided if there is a history of allergy.

SUGGESTED READING

Fishman PH, Perkins JP. Receptor desensitization. Adv Second Messenger Phosphoprotein Res 1988; 21:25–32.

Nathanson NM. Binding of antagonists by muscarinic acetylcholine receptors in intact cultured heart cells. J Neurochem 1983; 41:1545–1550.

Wamsley JK, Gehlert DR, Roeske WR, Yamamura HI. Muscarinic antagonist binding site heterogeneity as evidenced by autoradiography and direct labelling with QNB and pirenzepine. Life Sci 1984; 34:1395–1402.

Chapter 16

ADRENOCEPTOR AGONISTS

K.V. Flattery

The effects of stimulation of the sympathetic nervous system can be reproduced in whole, or in part, by the administration of drugs that mimic the effects of endogenous catecholamines on effector organs. The widest spectrum of sympathomimetic activity is exhibited by the catecholamines themselves, which directly stimulate adrenoceptors when administered as drugs. However, since direct stimulation of adrenoceptors is not the only mechanism by which the action of endogenous catecholamines may be mimicked, it is essential to classify the **sympathomimetic drugs** as follows.

1. Drugs that stimulate α and/or β adrenoceptors, and/or dopamine receptors, either selectively or in combination, *e.g.*, catecholamines (Table 16–1).
2. Drugs that increase the release of noradrenaline from sympathetic nerves, sometimes with additional direct stimulation of adrenoceptors, *e.g.*, ephedrine, amphetamine.
3. Drugs that block the re-uptake of noradrenaline, *e.g.*, cocaine, imipramine.

TABLE 16–1 Classification of Adrenoceptors and Examples of Agonists (Catecholamines) and Antagonists Acting Upon Them

Receptors	Agonists	Antagonists
α_1	Noradrenaline* Adrenaline† Dopamine	Prazosin Phenoxybenzamine Phentolamine
α_2	Noradrenaline Adrenaline	Phenoxybenzamine Phentolamine
β_1	Noradrenaline Adrenaline Dopamine Isoproterenol Dobutamine	Propranolol Atenolol Metoprolol Esmolol Labetalol
β_2	Adrenaline Noradrenaline Isoproterenol	Propranolol Nadolol Labetalol Butoxamine (not used clinically)

* norepinephrine

† epinephrine

CATECHOLAMINES

Chemical Structures and Structure-Activity Relationships

Catecholamines are low-molecular-weight substances that are composed of a catechol nucleus (a phenol with two adjacent hydroxy groups) and an amine group (Figs. 16–1 and 16–2).

Phenylethylamine is the parent compound of the catecholamines, consisting of a benzene ring and an aliphatic portion, ethylamine (*see* Fig. 16–2). The structure allows substitutions to be made on the benzene ring, the α- and β-carbons, and on the terminal amino group, thus providing many sympathomimetic drugs with activity on adrenoceptors.

Maximal α- and β-adrenergic activity depends on $-$OH groups in the C-3 and C-4 positions. Absence of the $-$OH groups decreases the overall potency with a particularly marked reduction in β-receptor activity. Phenylephrine differs chemically from adrenaline in that it has no $-$OH group in the C-4 position on the benzene ring (*cf.* Fig. 16–6). It has little or no effect on β receptors but is a strong stimulant of α receptors. Nevertheless, its potency on α receptors is less than that of adrenaline and noradrenaline. Hydroxyl groups in the C-3 and C-5 positions confer β_2-receptor selectivity on compounds with large amino substituents, *e.g.*,

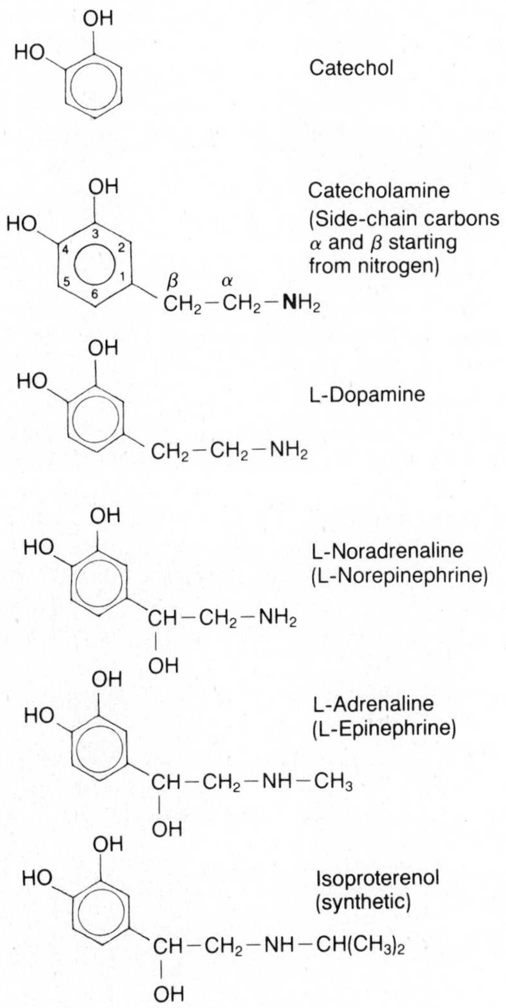

OH

HO

Catechol

OH

HO

Catecholamine
(Side-chain carbons
α and β starting
from nitrogen)

β α
$CH_2-CH_2-NH_2$

OH

HO

L-Dopamine

$CH_2-CH_2-NH_2$

OH

HO

L-Noradrenaline
(L-Norepinephrine)

$CH-CH_2-NH_2$
|
OH

OH

HO

L-Adrenaline
(L-Epinephrine)

$CH-CH_2-NH-CH_3$
|
OH

OH

HO

Isoproterenol
(synthetic)

$CH-CH_2-NH-CH(CH_3)_2$
|
OH

Figure 16–1 Chemical structures of the catecholamines.

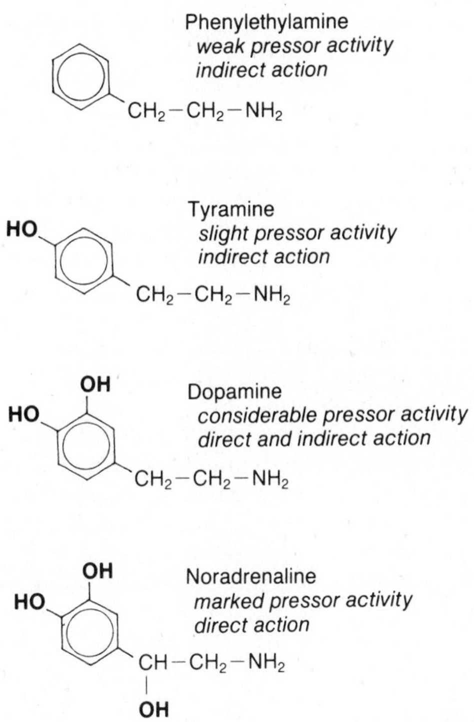

Phenylethylamine
*weak pressor activity
indirect action*

$CH_2-CH_2-NH_2$

Tyramine
*slight pressor activity
indirect action*

HO

$CH_2-CH_2-NH_2$

OH

Dopamine
*considerable pressor activity
direct and indirect action*

HO

$CH_2-CH_2-NH_2$

OH

Noradrenaline
*marked pressor activity
direct action*

HO

$CH-CH_2-NH_2$
|
OH

Figure 16–2 Effects of substituting — OH groups in the phenylethylamine molecule. Increasing the number of substitutions increases the pressor activity and introduces direct adrenoceptor-stimulant action.

metaproterenol and terbutaline. Salbutamol,* also a β_2 stimulant, has a — CH_2OH substituent on position C-3 and is an important exception to the general rule of low β activity (*cf.* Fig. 16–7).

Drugs that lack both — OH groups on the ring can produce greater CNS stimulation than adrenaline (*e.g.*, ephedrine, amphetamine, and methamphetamine). Absence of one or both — OH groups increases the effectiveness of the drug following oral administration, as well as prolonging the duration of action. Substitution on the α-carbon blocks oxidation by monoamine oxidase and therefore increases the duration of action of noncatecholamines, *e.g.*, ephedrine and amphetamine. Substitution on the β-carbon decreases CNS stimulation and increases both α- and β-adrenergic activity.

The catecholamines (noradrenaline, adrenaline, and dopamine) have a brief duration of action and are ineffective after oral administration, as they are rapidly

* albuterol

inactivated by monoamine oxidase (MAO) in the intestinal wall, or by catechol-O-methyltransferase (COMT) and MAO in the liver. Isoproterenol is also a substrate for COMT. It undergoes extensive first-pass biotransformation, probably by conjugation by a sulfotransferase in the intestinal wall.

Mechanisms of Action

The subclassification of α adrenoceptors into α_1 and α_2 receptors is based on the affinity of selective agonists and antagonists for each subtype. α_2 Receptors are also subdivided, by their localization with respect to the synapse, into presynaptic and postsynaptic or prejunctional and postjunctional receptors. Presynaptic α_2 adrenoceptors form an important part of a negative feedback loop by which noradrenaline (and other agonists) can inhibit transmitter release from sympathetic nerve terminals and some cholinergic neurons.

α_1-Adrenoceptor stimulation produces some of its effects by stimulating the metabolism of membrane phosphoinositides to produce two intracellular messengers, one of which is inositoltriphosphate (IP$_3$), which elevates intracellular Ca^{2+} levels. The other messenger is diacylglycerol (DG), which initiates the activation of protein kinase C, resulting in altered Ca^{2+} fluxes.

Postsynaptic α_2-adrenoceptor activation inhibits adenylate cyclase activity and lowers intracellular levels of cyclic adenosine monophosphate (cAMP). This may be associated with an increased influx of extracellular Ca^{2+} that interacts with calmodulin in vascular smooth muscle cells. It is possible that this may cause vasoconstriction in precapillary arterioles (resistance vessels) similar to that which occurs following α_1-receptor activation, but to a lesser extent. The mechanism by which presynaptic α_2-adrenoceptor stimulation decreases transmitter release is not yet elucidated.

When β adrenoceptors are stimulated by catecholamines (and other agonists), they react with a stimulatory guanine-nucleotide-binding regulatory protein (G_s) present in the cell membrane. G_s binds with guanosine triphosphate (GTP) to form a complex that stimulates adenylate cyclase activity and catalyses the formation of (i.e., raises the concentration of) intracellular cAMP. Cyclic AMP combines with a protein kinase that catalyses the phosphorylation of specific enzymes, the end-result of which are elevated Ca^{2+} levels in cardiac and other cells (Fig. 16–3).

The catecholamines act directly on receptors in target tissues, e.g., heart, vascular smooth muscle, glands. Sympathetic innervation is not essential for the actions or effects of synthetic catecholamines or other sympathomimetic drugs. On the contrary, denervation (or blockade of release of endogenous transmitters by drugs) enhances the receptor response to direct-acting sympathomimetics. Hence, the term "supersensitivity," which is associated with up-regulation of adrenoceptors.

Effects of Catecholamines on the Cardiovascular System

The Heart

Noradrenaline, adrenaline, and isoproterenol stimulate β_1 receptors in the heart and produce the following effects.

Tachycardia results from an increased rate of discharge of pacemaker cells in the S-A node. This increases the slope of phase 4 in the action potential, i.e., the rate of diastolic depolarization, because of altered permeability of the cell membrane, allowing a faster influx of Na^+ (and Ca^{2+}). The increase in heart rate is referred to as a positive chronotropic effect.

Noradrenaline (and adrenaline in large doses) may **increase the blood pressure** to such an extent that reflex slowing of the heart may occur, mediated by baroreceptor stimulation, which causes increased amounts of acetylcholine to be released at the S-A node. Because of reflex slowing, the cardiac output may be unchanged or decreased. The stroke volume, however, is always increased.

Automaticity of latent pacemaker cells is increased, and this may lead to arrhythmias.

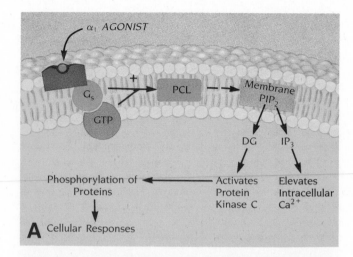

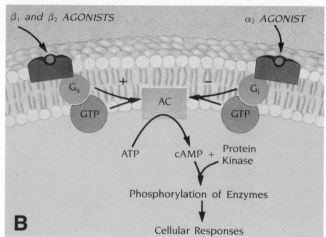

Figure 16–3 Molecular effects of (A) α-adrenoceptor agonists, and (B) α_2-, β_1-, and β_2-adrenoceptor agonists. PLC = phospholipase C; PIP_2 = phosphatidylinositol biphosphate; IP_3 = inositol triphosphate; DG = diacylglycerol; G_s = stimulatory guanine-nucleotide-binding regulatory protein; G_i = inhibitory guanine-nucleotide-binding regulatory protein; GTP = guanosine triphosphate; AC = adenylate cyclase; ATP = adenosine triphosphate; cAMP = cyclic adenosine monophosphate; + = stimulates, – = inhibits.

Shortening of the refractory period of the A-V node gives rise to acceleration of impulse conduction between atria and ventricles.

The force of contraction of the heart is increased, i.e., there is a positive inotropic effect.

Increase in stroke volume and cardiac output is accompanied by **increased oxygen consumption**. There is a decrease in efficiency of the heart, i.e., less work is done relative to the amount of oxygen consumed.

The pure β_1 effects of noradrenaline on the heart may be observed after administration of atropine or in isolated heart preparations.

Dopamine has a positive inotropic effect on the heart through stimulation of β_1 receptors. The effects of dopamine are dose-dependent. At infusion rates of 5–20 μg/kg/min, cardiac output and rate increase. Dopamine receptors in the periphery (renal and mesenteric vessels) are stimulated at doses of 1–5 μg/kg/min. High doses stimulate α receptors.

It should be noted that, while β_1 adrenoceptors are of major importance in modulating cardiac responses, there are β_2 and α_1 receptors present in the heart also. β_2 Receptors are probably stimulated by circulating adrenaline, which results in a synergistic effect with β_1-receptor stimulation in relation to increasing the heart rate. α_1 Adrenoceptors have a moderate effect on force of contraction, *i.e.*, a positive inotropic effect.

Blood Vessels

The basic difference among the catecholamines is that noradrenaline constricts all blood vessels, whereas adrenaline has mixed effects (*i.e.*, it causes vasoconstriction in some vascular beds while dilating blood vessels in skeletal muscle) and isoproterenol is a pure vasodilator. This difference is reflected in the effects of the individual drugs on heart rate.

Noradrenaline. Noradrenaline causes constriction of arterioles in the skin, skeletal muscle, mucous membranes, the kidneys, *etc*. Total peripheral resistance is therefore increased, resulting in elevated diastolic pressure. Systolic pressure is also increased. Constriction of large veins (capacitance vessels) also occurs. These vascular responses to noradrenaline are mediated through α_1-receptor stimulation.

As mentioned earlier, the pronounced increase in blood pressure slows the heart by a reflex increase in vagal tone, thus masking the β_1 effects on the heart rate. The β_1-mediated inotropic action is maintained.

Adrenaline. Adrenaline causes vasoconstriction in the skin, mucous membranes, and kidneys.

Dilatation occurs in skeletal muscle vascular beds, which contain both β_2 and α_1 receptors. The β_2 receptors in skeletal muscle arterioles are sensitive to much lower doses of adrenaline than are α_1 receptors. Decreased resistance in skeletal muscle arterioles causes a slight fall in blood pressure, and therefore tachycardia may occur rather than reflex slowing of the heart (Fig. 16–4).

Larger doses of adrenaline, however, do stimulate α_1 receptors in skeletal muscle arterioles, and the actions of adrenaline and noradrenaline become similar, resulting in reflex slowing of the heart.

Isoproterenol. Isoproterenol lowers peripheral vascular resistance (β_2 stimulation) in renal and mesenteric blood vessels and in skeletal muscle vascular beds.

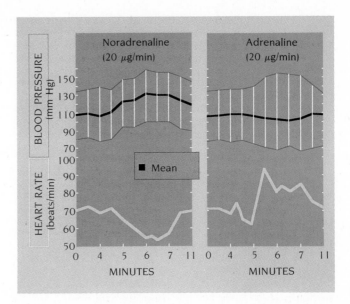

Figure 16–4   Effects of noradrenaline and adrenaline infusions on blood pressure and heart rate in man. Note the increased mean pressure and decreased heart rate following infusion of noradrenaline, and the essentially unchanged mean pressure, increased pulse pressure, and elevated heart rate following infusion of adrenaline.

Diastolic pressure falls. Cardiac output is raised because of an increase in venous return to the heart. The increase in cardiac output is enhanced by an increase in force of contraction (positive inotropic action) and tachycardia (positive chronotropic effect).

Dopamine. The effects of dopamine on peripheral vascular resistance are most pronounced when very high doses are administered, since these stimulate α receptors and cause vasoconstriction. Vasodilatation of renal and mesenteric vessels occurs following low doses of the drug, which stimulate only dopamine receptors.

The effects of catecholamines on the cardiovascular system are summarized in Table 16–2.

Effects on the Respiratory System

Activation of β_2 adrenoceptors causes relaxation of bronchiolar smooth muscle and decreased airway resistance. Antigen-induced release of asthma mediators is also inhibited.

Activation of α_1 adrenoceptors causes vasoconstriction of vessels in the upper respiratory tract mucosa;

TABLE 16–2   Effects of α- and β-Adrenoceptor Agonists on the Cardiovascular System

Receptor	Drugs	Effects
α_1	Noradrenaline Adrenaline Dopamine (higher doses) Phenylephrine Metaraminol	*Arterioles*: ↑ tone ↑ peripheral resistance ↑ diastolic pressure ↑ afterload ↓ heart rate (reflex) *Large veins*: ↑ tone ↑ venous return ↑ preload (∴ ↑ ventricular volume)
α_2	Noradrenaline Adrenaline	↑ peripheral resistance (postsynaptic α_2 receptors in some vascular smooth muscle)
β_1	Noradrenaline Adrenaline Isoproterenol Dopamine Dobutamine	↑ heart rate ↑ automaticity of all pacemaker cells (arrhythmias can occur) ↑ conduction velocity in atria, A-V node, and ventricles ↑ velocity of contraction ↑ force of contraction ↑ stroke volume ↑ cardiac output ↑ oxygen consumption ↓ diastolic time for coronary perfusion and ↓ ventricular filling (with marked tachycardia) ↓ residual (end-systolic) volume
β_2	Salbutamol (Albuterol) Terbutaline Adrenaline Isoproterenol	↓ arteriolar tone ↓ peripheral resistance ↓ diastolic pressure ↓ afterload ↑ heart rate: (1) reflex (2) β_1 stimulation with adrenaline and isoproterenol, and *high* doses of selective β_1 agonists

↑ = increased; ↓ = decreased.

this decongestant effect in nasal and bronchiolar mucosa is clinically useful.

Effects on the Gastrointestinal Tract

Stimulation of α and β adrenoceptors causes relaxation of gastrointestinal smooth muscle by different mechanisms. Noradrenaline, by stimulating presynaptic α_2 adrenoceptors on cholinergic neurons, inhibits the release of acetylcholine, causing decreased smooth muscle tone and amplitude of contractions.

Stimulation of β_2 adrenoceptors elevates cAMP, resulting in Ca^{2+} sequestration; α_1-adrenoceptor activation causes an increase in K^+ conductance and hyperpolarization.

Effects on the Uterus

Adrenaline inhibits uterine tone and contractions during the last month of pregnancy and at parturition. Based on this finding, salbutamol (a selective β_2 agonist) is occasionally used to delay premature labor.

Effects on the Eye

The radial muscle in the iris contains α_1 adrenoceptors that, when stimulated, cause mydriasis. In theory, this should tend to raise the intraocular pressure by blocking the outflow of aqueous humor. However, α_1-mediated vasoconstriction decreases the formation of aqueous humor, and this effect usually predominates, lowering the intraocular pressure. Intraocular pressure is influenced by both β and α adrenoceptors. Some β-adrenoceptor antagonists (*e.g.*, timolol) are commonly used in the treatment of glaucoma.

Metabolic Effects of Catecholamines

The important effects of catecholamines on intermediary metabolism include lipolysis, glycogenolysis, and gluconeogenesis.

Lipolysis is associated with β_1 stimulation, resulting in elevated cAMP levels. Lipase is activated and the breakdown of triglycerides to glycerol and free fatty acids is enhanced.

Glycogenolysis in the liver is increased by β_2 stimulation, which causes increased glucose release into the circulation and hyperglycemia (Fig. 16–5). α Adrenoceptors may also play a role.

Gluconeogenesis from lactate and amino acids is also stimulated. Oxygen consumption is increased by both adrenaline and noradrenaline (calorigenic effect).

Adrenaline increases plasma levels of K^+ transiently; this is followed by a more prolonged fall in K^+ plasma levels. This is a β_2-mediated effect. Adrenoceptor agonists of the β_2 type have been used in the management of hyperkalemic familial periodic paralysis, because of the ability of the drugs to increase uptake of K^+ into muscle cells.

Effects on Endocrine Glands

The release of insulin is increased by β_2-adrenoceptor stimulation and inhibited by α-receptor activation. Glucagon secretion from α cells in the pancreas is also increased. Renin release from the juxtaglomerular cells in the kidney is increased by β_1-receptor activation and inhibited by α-receptor stimulation.

Effects on the Central Nervous System

Catecholamines are potent stimulants of the central nervous system. The concentration of catecholamines in the brain is increased by cocaine (blockade of neurotransmitter re-uptake) and the amphetamines (enhanced release of transmitters). A mood-elevating (euphoriant) effect is the basis for the abuse of these drugs. Alertness and the ability to perform repetitive tasks are also enhanced by these drugs.

Effects on Skeletal Muscle

Adrenaline and other β_2 agonists facilitate the release of acetylcholine from cholinergic terminals, probably by elevating cAMP levels at presynaptic sites. Stimulation of α_2 adrenoceptors on cholinergic neurons in skeletal muscle increases the release of acetylcholine, presumably by increasing Ca^{2+} influx into the motor neurons of skeletal muscle. This contrasts with α_2-receptor stimulation on cholinergic neurons at other sites, *e.g.*, the gastrointestinal tract (*see* above), where it inhibits the release of acetylcholine. Motor power in myasthenia gravis can be increased by ephedrine and amphetamine, which increase the release of

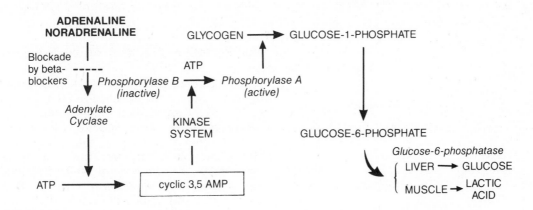

Figure 16–5 Metabolic pathways by which catecholamines stimulate glycogenolysis.

catecholamines as well as being direct adrenoceptor agonists. β_2-Adrenoceptor agonists (*e.g.*, adrenaline, salbutamol) cause muscle tremor that can be prevented by propranolol. The mechanism responsible for tremor induction is associated with β_2 adrenoceptor-mediated enhancement of muscle spindle discharge.

SELECTIVE ADRENOCEPTOR AGONISTS

α_1-Receptor Agonists

Phenylephrine

Phenylephrine (Neo-Synephrine®) (and the other drugs in this class; Fig. 16–6) is closely related chemically to adrenaline. Its actions are essentially similar to those of noradrenaline, differing in only two ways: it is less potent and it has a longer duration of action.

Phenylephrine is a powerful direct-acting α_1-receptor stimulant with little effect on the β_1 receptors of the heart. The predominant actions are on the cardiovascular system. Intravenous, subcutaneous, or oral administration all cause a rise in systolic and diastolic pressures in humans and other species. Responses are more sustained than those after noradrenaline, lasting 20 minutes after intravenous and as long as 50 minutes after subcutaneous injection. Phenylephrine is one of the more useful adrenergic agonists, as a vasoconstrictor, decongestant, mydriatic, and antiallergy agent. It is also sometimes used to treat paroxysmal atrial tachycardia.

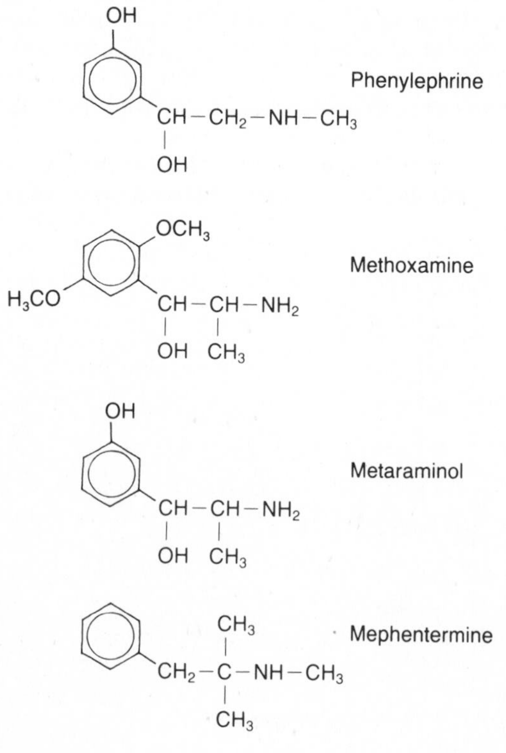

Methoxamine

Methoxamine (Vasoxyl®) is also an effective α_1-receptor stimulant used as a pressor agent. It is without effects on β_1 receptors. Reflex bradycardia follows its administration, because of increased stimulation of baroreceptors.

Metaraminol

This agent is both a direct (α_1-stimulating) and indirect sympathomimetic. It causes an increase in systolic and diastolic pressures, which is almost entirely due to peripheral vasoconstriction and is usually accompanied by vagal bradycardia. Its effects are relatively long-lasting, similar to those seen with methoxamine. Metaraminol also releases noradrenaline from sympathetic nerves and is a weak β_1 agonist.

Other selective α_1-adrenoceptor agonists include mephentermine and naphazoline.

Selective α_2-Receptor Agonists

Clonidine and α-**methyldopa** increase feedback control of noradrenaline release by stimulation of presynaptic α_2 adrenoceptors. Since they lower blood pressure primarily by this mechanism, they are described in Chapter 18, *Neuronal Blocking Drugs*.

Non-Selective β_1 and β_2 Agonist: Isoproterenol

Isoproterenol (Isuprel®) is the most potent β_1- and β_2-adrenergic agent in use. Peripheral vasodilatation, tachycardia, myocardial stimulation, and bronchial relaxation are the important effects produced. Isoproterenol is more potent than adrenaline as a bronchial dilator. It is, however, not a decongestant. The side effects of isoproterenol, which frequently may be very severe, are due primarily to its cardiac action. The tachycardia and myocardial stimulation produce signs of coronary insufficiency by increasing the amount of O_2 required by the heart.

Isoproterenol is metabolized by COMT, just as the endogenous catecholamines are, but it is unaffected by MAO.

Figure 16–6 Structural formulae of α_1-receptor agonists.

Selective β_1-Adrenoceptor Agonist: Dobutamine

This catecholamine (Fig. 16–7) is a synthetic derivative of dopamine and a selective stimulant of β_1 adrenoceptors. The action of dobutamine on the heart is unique in that it increases the force of contraction without increasing the heart rate significantly. The fact that it is possible to achieve separation of the positive inotropic and chronotropic responses to dobutamine is suggestive of subtypes of β_1 receptors in the heart.

Selective β_2-Adrenoceptor Agonists

Salbutamol (Ventolin®) and other related drugs (see Fig. 16–7) are effective bronchodilators because of their selective action on β_2 adrenoceptors in bronchiolar smooth muscle. Because they stimulate β_2 receptors preferentially, these agents lack the myocardial stimulating properties of isoproterenol. High doses of salbutamol, however, will cause β_1 receptor-mediated myocardial stimulation. Salbutamol also stimulates β_2 receptors in the smooth muscle of vessels supplying skeletal muscle, leading to a decrease in peripheral vascular resistance. Since the uterus reacts to β_2 agonists with relaxation, salbutamol can be used to delay delivery in premature labor.

Other selective β_2-adrenoceptor agonists are **terbutaline** and **orciprenaline**.*

* metaproterenol

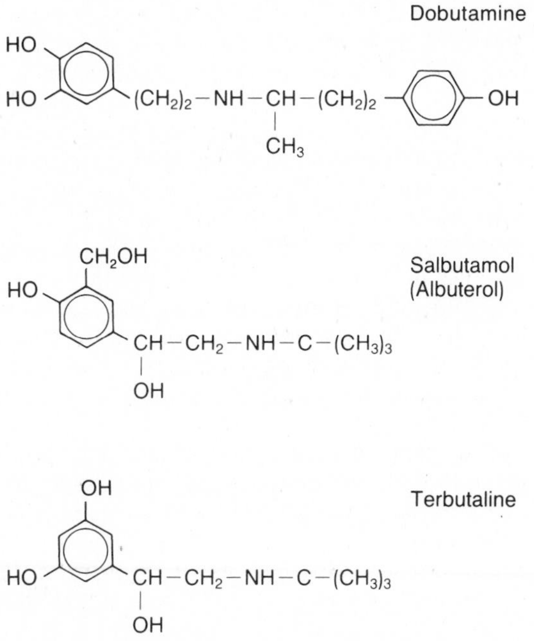

Figure 16–7 Structural formulae of selective β_1- and β_2-receptor agonists.

DRUGS THAT RELEASE NORADRENALINE FROM SYMPATHETIC NERVES

These drugs are transported across the adrenergic neuronal membrane and displace noradrenaline from storage sites within the neuron. The released noradrenaline subsequently interacts with adrenoceptors to produce characteristic responses in the effector organs, e.g., increase in heart rate and elevation of blood pressure. Additional sympathomimetic effects occur with most of these drugs, e.g., ephedrine, which not only releases noradrenaline but also stimulates adrenoceptors directly. Since this drug has indirect (noradrenaline-releasing) and direct (adrenoceptor-stimulating) effects, it is frequently classified as being a drug with "mixed" actions. (The direct stimulation of peripheral adrenoceptors by amphetamine is minimal when compared with its noradrenaline-releasing action.)

Ephedrine

Ephedrine (Fig. 16–8) is an alkaloid obtained from ma-huang (Ephedra equisedina) and has been used by the Chinese from early times. Both carbon atoms on the aliphatic side chain are asymmetric, resulting in four isomers: (+)- and (−)-ephedrine, and (+)- and (−)-pseudoephedrine. The most potent form in relation to sympathomimetic activity is (−)-ephedrine, which is used clinically.

Pharmacologically, ephedrine belongs to a special category. Its sympathomimetic effects are due to noradrenaline release from sympathetic nerves (Fig. 16–9, Table 16–3), combined with a direct effect on α_1, β_1, and β_2 adrenoceptors. Tachyphylaxis may occur with chronic administration, because of depletion of the intraneuronal pool of noradrenaline, which is susceptible to ephedrine.

The change from the phenolic structure of adrenaline to the phenyl structure of ephedrine results in a marked difference in action. Unlike adrenaline, ephedrine is effective orally, has a prolonged action, gives rise to tachyphylaxis, and is a potent central stimulant. Intravenous injection of ephedrine produces a prompt rise in blood pressure. The potency of ephedrine as a vasopressor agent is only 1/1000 to 1/100 of that of adrenaline. Its duration of action, however, is 7–10

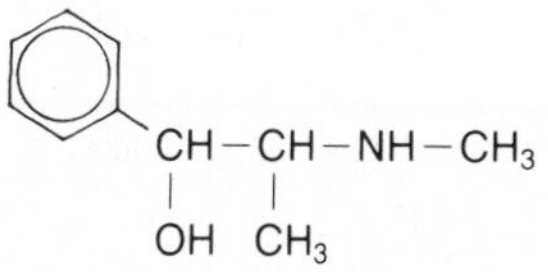

Figure 16–8 Structure of ephedrine.

times longer than that of adrenaline. The coronary vessels are dilated by ephedrine, the heart rate is increased, and the arterial blood pressure may be elevated.

Ephedrine dilates the bronchioles. Although the action of ephedrine on asthma is not as prompt or pronounced as that of adrenaline, it has the advantage of being active upon oral administration and is longer acting.

Ephedrine increases the tone of skeletal muscle, and for this reason it may be used as an adjuvant drug in the treatment of myasthenia gravis.

Pseudoephedrine is an active stereoisomer of ephedrine with similar actions and uses.

Amphetamine

This and related drugs are potent stimulants of the central nervous system; they are described in detail in Chapter 29. The peripheral cardiovascular effects caused by amphetamine are, however, an inherent part of its toxicity.

Amphetamine has a euphoriant (mood-elevating) effect, which is the basis for its inclusion in a group of drugs classified as drugs of abuse.

Methamphetamine has a higher ratio of central to peripheral effects than amphetamine.

Methylphenidate is used in the treatment of narcolepsy in adults and the hyperkinetic syndrome (attention deficit disorder with hyperactivity) in children. Its abuse potential is similar to that of amphetamine.

Other drugs of this type are **phenmetrazine** and **phentermine**. They are used occasionally as appetite suppressants, although phenmetrazine was withdrawn from the market in Canada because of the risk of abuse similar to that of amphetamine.

Tyramine

This compound has no direct adrenoceptor-agonistic activity; its effects are solely due to release of noradrenaline. It is never used clinically, but it is important as a research drug and in certain drug interactions when tyramine-containing food is consumed. Since tyramine depends entirely on the release of noradrenaline for its sympathomimetic effects, the prior administration of a drug that depletes intraneuronal stores of noradrenaline (e.g., reserpine) will abolish its effects.

DRUGS THAT BLOCK THE RE-UPTAKE OF NORADRENALINE

Cocaine, imipramine, and **amitriptyline** belong to this class of drugs. They interfere with the uptake

process that is of major importance in terminating the actions of noradrenaline, causing the concentration of noradrenaline to be elevated at adrenoceptor sites, and the responses of effector organs to be exaggerated (see Fig. 16–9). These drugs also prevent the uptake of certain other drugs into the adrenergic neuron, diminishing the responses to ephedrine and blocking the effects of tyramine.

CLINICAL USES OF α- AND β-ADRENOCEPTOR AGONISTS

Nasal Decongestants

Decongestion of nasal mucous membranes by vasoconstriction may be achieved by local application of α_1-adrenoceptor agonists. Drugs that are commonly used for this purpose are phenylephrine (Neo-Synephrine®), mephentermine (Wyamine®), and pseudoephedrine (Sudafed®). The beneficial decongestant effects of these drugs may be followed by rebound congestion.

Pressor Agents

Phenylephrine, metaraminol (Aramine®), methoxamine (Vasoxyl®), and mephentermine may be used parenterally to elevate the blood pressure (e.g., in hypotension associated with spinal anaesthesia). The stimulation of α_1 adrenoceptors leads to an increase in peripheral resistance, which increases diastolic (and systolic) pressure. The use of α_1-receptor agonists in shock is controversial, since there is already a maximal release of catecholamines causing intense vasoconstriction and resulting in decreased tissue perfusion. The microcirculation may be further impaired. Elevation of the blood pressure is of value only in the absence of hypovolemia and/or electrolyte disturbances.

In **cardiogenic shock** (myocardial infarction), noradrenaline (levarterenol, Levophed®), dopamine (Intropin®), and dobutamine (Dobutrex®) may be used. Dopamine, in contrast to noradrenaline, has a vasodilating action on splanchnic and renal vascular beds, mediated through specific dopamine receptors. The force of contraction of the heart is also increased (β_1 effects). Glomerular filtration rate and urine production are enhanced.

Dobutamine is selective as a β_1-adrenoceptor agonist that increases stroke volume at doses that do not increase heart rate.

Noradrenaline is administered intravenously in moderate doses sufficient to raise the arterial blood pressure and stimulate the heart without causing serious vasoconstriction.

Anaphylactic shock is traditionally treated with

TABLE 16–3 Types of Action of Representative Drugs at Adrenergic Neurons, Synapses, and Neuroeffector Junctions

Mechanism of Action	Drugs	Effects
Interference with synthesis of transmitter.	α-Methyl-p-tyrosine Disulfiram	Depletion of noradrenaline.
Metabolic transformation by the same pathway as precursor of transmitter.	α-Methyldopa	Displacement of noradrenaline by false transmitter (α-methyl-nor-adrenaline). Blockade of release of noradrenaline.
Blockade of transport system of axonal membrane, *i.e.*, uptake of noradrenaline.	Imipramine Amitriptyline Cocaine	Accumulation of noradrenaline at extracellular sites. Potentiation of sympathetic response.
Blockade of transport system of storage granule membrane.	Reserpine	Destruction of noradrenaline by intraneuronal MAO, and depletion of adrenergic terminals. Super-sensitivity to directly acting amines; subsensitivity to indirectly acting amines.
Displacement of transmitter from axonal terminal.	Amphetamine Tyramine Ephedrine	Sympathomimetic (indirect).
Prevention of release of transmitter.	Guanethidine Bretylium Clonidine	Antiadrenergic. Decreased release of noradrenaline.
Mimicry of transmitter at postsynaptic receptor.	Phenylephrine Isoproterenol	Sympathomimetic (direct).
Blockade of endogenous transmitter at postsynaptic receptor.	Phenoxybenzamine Propranolol Prazosin	α-Adrenoceptor antagonism. β-Adrenoceptor antagonism. Selective α_1-adrenoceptor antagonism.
Inhibition of enzymatic breakdown of transmitter.	MAO inhibitors (Pargyline, Tranylcypromine)	Accumulation of noradrenaline at certain sites; potentiation of tyramine.

AUTONOMIC NEUROMUSCULAR

adrenaline, which counteracts the bronchoconstrictor and vasodilator actions of histamine. Adrenaline is also used in urticaria, hay fever, and angioneurotic edema.

Bronchodilators

Selective β_2-adrenoceptor agonists are effective in the treatment of reversible airway obstruction associated with bronchial asthma and chronic bronchitis. They cause fewer cardiovascular side effects, such as tachycardia, than do the nonselective β-adrenoceptor agonists, such as adrenaline and isoproterenol. However, with increased dosage of β_2-selective agonists, cardiovascular side effects can occur. These drugs should be used with caution in patients who have thyrotoxicosis or cardiovascular disorders.

Salbutamol is the most widely used β_2-adreno-ceptor agonist. It can be used orally or by inhalation from aerosol containers. Terbutaline (Bricanyl®) and or-ciprenaline (Alupent®) are similar in action.

Isoproterenol is a potent nonselective bronchodilator with the disadvantage of causing excessive myocardial stimulation.

Adrenaline used in allergy-induced asthma (acute attacks) not only stimulates β_2 adrenoceptors but also α_1 adrenoceptors, which constrict bronchial mucosal vessels and thereby enhance the reduction in airway resistance.

All β_2-adrenoceptor agonists increase cAMP in bronchial muscle cells, resulting in Ca^{2+} sequestration and relaxation of the bronchiolar smooth muscle.

Cardiac Arrest and Heart Block

Isoproterenol or adrenaline may be administered in-travenously or directly into the heart in asystole.

Isoproterenol or adrenaline may be used in complete heart block with a slow ventricular response or asystole. The long-term treatment of heart block may also re-quire isoproterenol for maintenance treatment.

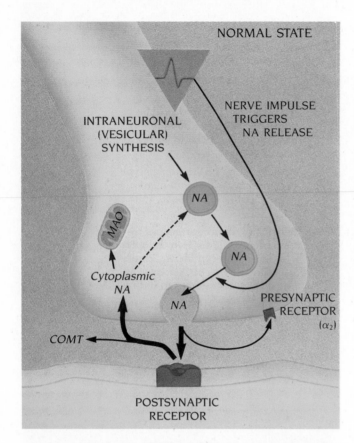

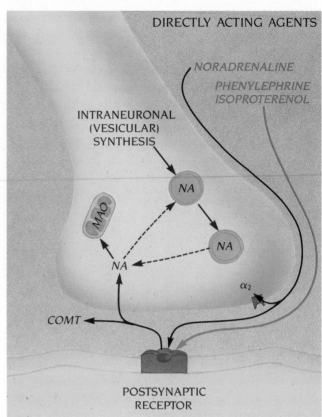

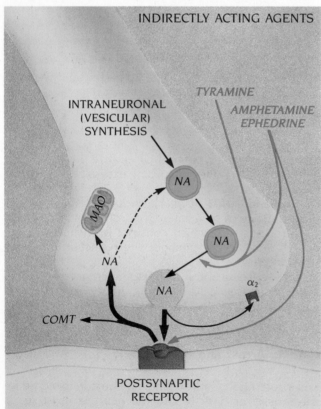

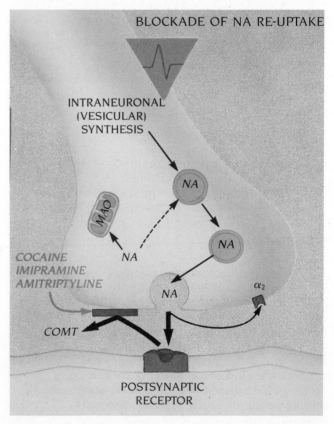

Figure 16–9   Schematic representation of various mechanisms of action of drugs on sympathetic nerve activity. NA = noradrenaline (norepinephrine); MAO = monoamine oxidase; COMT = catechol-O-methyltransferase; α-CH₃-DOPA = α-methyldopa; α-CH₃NA = α-methyl-noradrenaline. (Although not shown in the diagrams, there is a constant resting release of noradrenaline from adrenergic nerve terminals.)

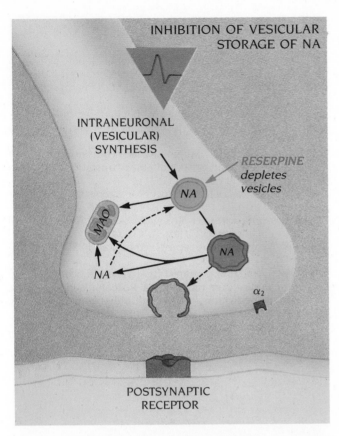

INHIBITION OF VESICULAR STORAGE OF NA

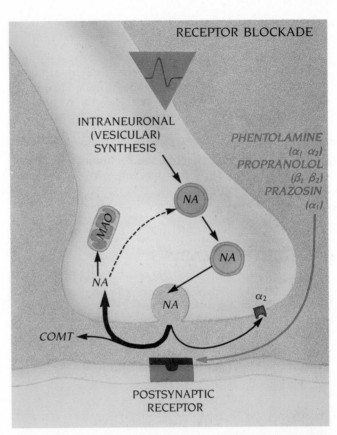

RECEPTOR BLOCKADE

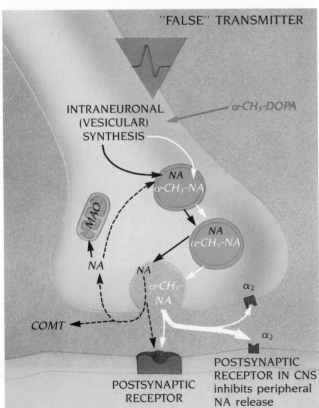

"FALSE" TRANSMITTER

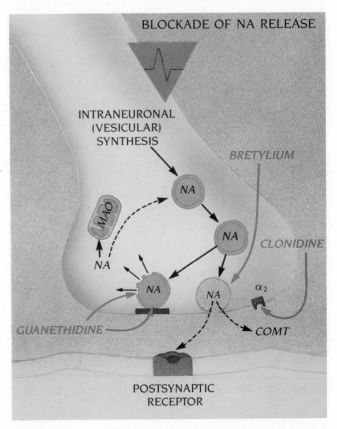

BLOCKADE OF NA RELEASE

Figure 16–9 Continued.   Schematic representation of various mechanisms of action of drugs on sympathetic nerve activity. NA = noradrenaline (norepinephrine); MAO = monoamine oxidase; COMT = catechol-O-methyltransferase; α-CH$_3$-DOPA = α-methyldopa; α-CH$_3$NA = α-methyl-noradrenaline. (Figure 16–9 and Table 16–3 are summaries of drug effects on adrenergic nerve activity, as discussed in Chapters 16, 17, and 18.)

Ophthalmic Applications

Phenylephrine and ephedrine applied topically are examples of drugs used to dilate the pupil (mydriasis), usually to permit examination of the fundus. They have the advantage of not causing paralysis of accommodation (cycloplegia). In glaucoma, phenylephrine or adrenaline may be used to decrease the intraocular pressure by their local vasoconstrictor action, which decreases the production of aqueous humor. All effects described in the eye are mediated by α_1-adrenoceptor stimulation.

SUGGESTED READING

Berridge MJ. The molecular basis of communication within the cell. Sci Am 1985; 254(4):142–152.

Brodde OE. The functional importance of β_1 and β_2 adrenoceptors in the human heart. Am J Cardiol 1988; 62:24C–29C.

Eggleston PA, Beasley PP. Bronchodilatation and inhibition of induced asthma by adrenergic agonists. Clin Pharmacol Ther 1981; 29:505–510.

Flavahan NA, McGrath JC. Alpha$_1$-adrenoreceptor activation can increase heart rate directly or decrease it indirectly through parasympathetic activation. Br J Pharmacol 1982; 77:319–328.

Lafontan M, Berlan M, Prudhon M. Beta-adrenergic agonists. Mechanism of action: lipid mobilization and anabolism. Reprod Nutr Dev 1988; 28:61–84.

Lulich KM, Goldie RG, Paterson JW. Beta-adrenoceptor function in asthmatic bronchial smooth muscle. Gen Pharmacol 1988; 19:307–311.

Seale JP. Whither beta-adrenoceptor agonists in the treatment of asthma. Progr Clin Biol Res 1988; 263;367–377.

Starke K. Alpha-adrenoceptor subclassification. Rev Physiol Biochem Pharmacol 1981; 88:199–236.

Starke K. Presynaptic receptors. Annu Rev Pharmacol Toxicol 1981; 21:7–30.

van Zwieten PA, Timmermans PB. Alpha-adrenoceptor stimulation and calcium movements. Recent advances in sympathetic neurotransmission. 6th Meeting on Adrenergic Mechanisms, Porto, Portugal, 1986. Blood Vessels 1987; 24:271–280.

Chapter 17

ADRENOCEPTOR ANTAGONISTS

K.V. Flattery

The characteristic responses of effector organs to endogenous catecholamines and sympathomimetic drugs can be selectively blocked by α- or β-adrenoceptor antagonists. The extent of the blockade obtained is related to the relative concentrations of the agonist and antagonist present at adrenoceptor sites in the effector organ cells and their relative affinities for these sites. Selectivity of the antagonist drug for α or β adrenoceptors is further enhanced by differing affinities of the drugs for α-receptor subtypes (α_1 and α_2) and for β-receptor subtypes (β_1 and β_2).

The selective inhibition of some of the physiologic effects of catecholamines was first reported in 1906 by Sir Henry Dale who demonstrated that the pressor effects of large doses of adrenaline* could be reversed to cause a fall in blood pressure by certain ergot preparations now known to have α-adrenoceptor blocking properties. Later work led to the synthesis of a large number of drugs with the ability to antagonize the effects of α-adrenoceptor stimulation.

The introduction of drugs that selectively blocked β adrenoceptors provided the final confirmation of Ahlquist's general classification of adrenoceptors into α and β types. The existence of subgroups of β adrenoceptors has also been confirmed by the quantitative difference in the responses of these receptors to agonists and antagonists.

α-ADRENOCEPTOR ANTAGONISTS

α-Adrenoceptor blocking drugs are classified as follows.

1. Irreversible noncompetitive antagonists (e.g., phenoxybenzamine). This antagonism outlasts the presence of free phenoxybenzamine, is noncom-

petitive, and its effects are not overcome by agonists such as noradrenaline.*
2. Reversible competitive antagonists that produce equilibrium blockade, i.e., the free drug and the drug-receptor complex are in equilibrium and the blockade disappears as the free drug is destroyed (phentolamine and prazosin belong to this class).

A further classification distinguishes between selective and nonselective α-receptor antagonists; e.g., phentolamine and phenoxybenzamine block both α_1 and α_2 adrenoceptors while prazosin selectively blocks α_1 receptors. Yohimbine, a plant alkaloid with prominent CNS effects, is a selective α_2 antagonist but is not used clinically as such.

Irreversible α-Adrenoceptor Antagonist

Phenoxybenzamine. The haloalkylamine phenoxybenzamine (Fig. 17–1) is closely related chemically to the nitrogen mustards. It contains a tertiary amine, which cyclizes to form a reactive ethylenimonium intermediate. The molecular configuration directly responsible for blockade is a highly reactive carbonium ion formed when the three-membered ring breaks. The persistence and completeness of the blockade produced appear to be dependent upon covalent bonding to the receptor, which is difficult to reverse. After a single dose of phenoxybenzamine, a progressively decreasing but still significant blockade persists for at least 3 or 4 days. With increasing doses of the blocking agent, the dose-response curve for an agonist is shifted progressively to the right, and the maximum possible response is reduced as the number of available receptors is reduced. Phenoxybenzamine also blocks the reuptake of noradrenaline and enhances its release from sympathetic neurons by blockade of presynaptic α_2 receptors.

---

* epinephrine

* norepinephrine

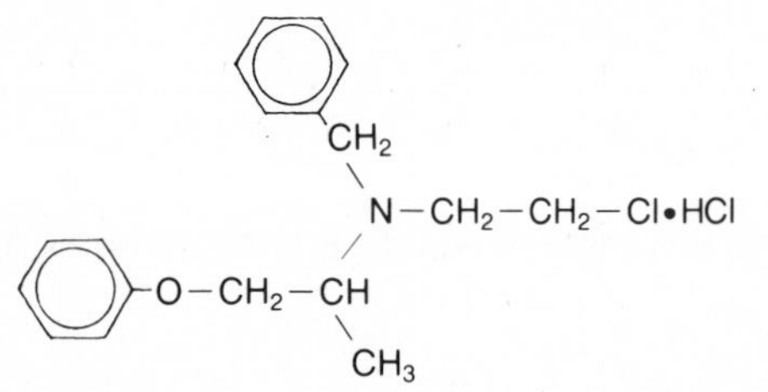

Figure 17–1 Structural formula of phenoxybenzamine HCl.

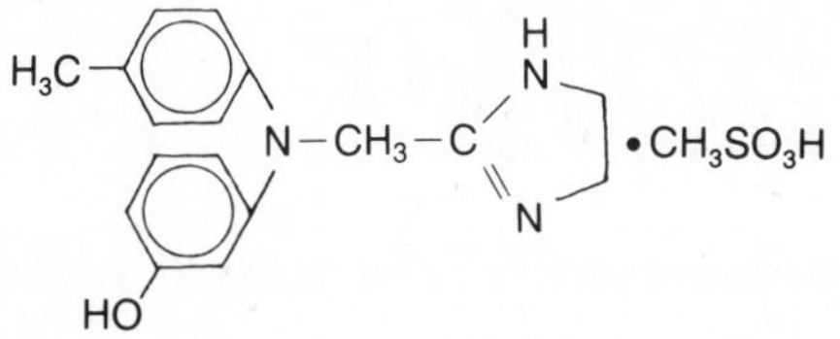

Figure 17–2 Structural formula of phentolamine mesylate.

In the **cardiovascular system**, a fall in diastolic blood pressure occurs because of decreased peripheral resistance. Systolic blood pressure drops sharply when the patient assumes an upright position (postural hypotension). Reflex tachycardia is induced when peripheral resistance is decreased and following decreased venous return to the heart. Tachycardia is also caused by blockade of presynaptic α_2 adrenoceptors, which inhibit feedback control of noradrenaline release.

Metabolic effects consist of an increase in insulin secretion because of α-receptor blockade, which prevents the inhibitory effect of endogenous catecholamines on insulin secretion, and sometimes increased lipolysis. β_2-Receptor activity of endogenous adrenaline is unmasked, which further enhances the release of insulin.

Reversible α-Adrenoceptor Blocking Drugs

Tolazoline, Phentolamine

These drugs (Fig. 17–2) have a wide range of pharmacologic actions. They are weak partial agonists at several types of receptor and also have some inhibitory effect on neurotransmitter re-uptake and inactivation. They produce a moderately effective competitive adrenoceptor blockade that is relatively transient. Responses to 5-HT (serotonin) are also inhibited. The cardiovascular effects of phentolamine are similar to those of phenoxybenzamine but are more transient. The cardiostimulating properties of nonselective α-adrenoceptor antagonists, resulting from blockade of presynaptic α_2 receptors (causing an increased release of noradrenaline from sympathetic nerve endings), can be blocked by the drug propranolol, which is an antagonist of β_1 adrenoceptors in the heart.

Prazosin

This selective α_1-adrenoceptor antagonist (Fig. 17–3) is an effective drug used clinically for the treatment of hypertension. Its very low affinity for α_2 receptors provides a distinct therapeutic advantage. The adverse effects that are characteristically observed with nonselective α-adrenoceptor antagonists (e.g., tachycardia, positive inotropy, and renin release) are uncommon with prazosin treatment.

The selectivity of prazosin for α_1 adrenoceptors allows the negative feedback loop for noradrenaline to be retained. This may prevent the tachycardia observed with the nonselective adrenoceptor antagonists. Tachycardia, mediated by reflex baroreceptor mechanisms, may occur occasionally.

Diastolic pressure falls as a result of decreased peripheral resistance and reduction of circulating blood volume (due to venous pooling of blood in the large veins), causing decreased venous return. Orthostatic hypotension occurs because of α_1-adrenoceptor blockade in the large veins. Dizziness or syncope may occur as a "first-dose phenomenon" and lead to loss of consciousness. This effect may be circumvented by starting with a low dose and increasing the dosage slowly.

The drug is well absorbed following oral administration. The plasma half-life is 3–4 hours. There is extensive protein binding (approximately 97% at therapeutic concentrations). Elimination is by biotransformation in the liver and excretion in the bile.

Therapeutic Uses of α-Adrenoceptor Blocking Drugs

α-Adrenoceptor antagonism has been employed or suggested as therapy in a wide variety of conditions, but as yet it has few established uses.

Although currently the approach to the treatment of essential hypertension is through inhibition of sympathetic vasoconstrictor tone or β_1-adrenoceptor blockade, results with α-adrenoceptor antagonists other

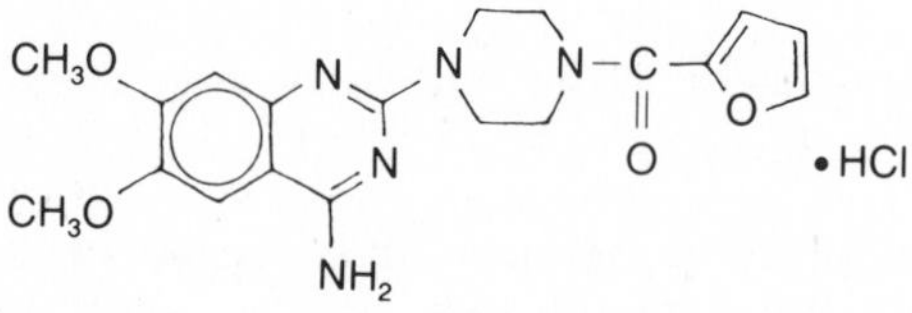

Figure 17–3 Structural formula of prazosin HCl.

than prazosin have been disappointing. An important factor in relation to nonselective α-receptor blockade is that tachycardia and palpitation are added to the other side effects associated with inhibition of sympathetic vasoconstriction. These and other unpleasant side effects prohibit the use of such drugs in the therapy of hypertension.

Formerly, an important use of adrenoceptor antagonists was in the diagnosis of pheochromocytoma, a catecholamine-secreting tumor of chromaffin tissue. Several different agents have been used for this purpose, but phentolamine was the most commonly employed. A significant fall in blood pressure within 2 minutes of administering the drug was considered to be a positive response. With the advent of chemical methods for the estimation of catecholamines and their metabolites in urine and blood, however, the phentolamine test for pheochromocytoma has declined in importance. α-Adrenoceptor blocking agents are useful in the preoperative management of cases of pheochromocytoma, for the prolonged treatment of cases not amenable to surgery, and to prevent paroxysmal hypertension during operative manipulation of the tumor.

The use of α-adrenoceptor blocking drugs in the treatment of shock is occasionally recommended, since vasoconstriction is an important feature of shock, with resultant decreased tissue perfusion. Phenoxybenzamine may be effective clinically in the treatment of Raynaud's disease, a condition characterized by vasoconstriction due to increased sympathetic nerve activity.

Prazosin is used routinely in the treatment of hypertension, sometimes in conjunction with other drugs such as propranolol and hydrochlorothiazide. The side effects of prazosin consist of the first-dose phenomenon (*see* above), orthostatic hypotension, edema, and aggravation of preexisting angina. Other occasional adverse effects are vertigo, headache, depression, vomiting, diarrhea, or constipation.

β-ADRENOCEPTOR ANTAGONISTS

The β adrenoceptors are classified as β_1 and β_2 on the basis of the finding that there are drugs that selectively stimulate or block either one or other β adrenoceptor. A subclassification of β-adrenoceptor antagonists into nonselective and selective was necessitated by the fact that drugs such as propranolol block both β_1 and β_2 receptors, while other drugs such as metoprolol selectively block the β_1 receptors with only minor effects on β_2 adrenoceptors.

β-Adrenoceptor antagonists are used extensively in the treatment of cardiovascular diseases, *e.g.*, hypertension, angina pectoris, cardiac arrhythmias, and in the secondary prevention of myocardial infarction and sudden death in patients with coronary thrombosis. While β-adrenoceptor antagonists may differ in their profile of activity, pharmacokinetics, and adverse effects, they all antagonize β adrenoceptors, some with greater selectivity for β_1 adrenoceptors in the heart. These "cardioselective" β_1 antagonists are less likely to cause the adverse effects of bronchospasm, intermittent claudication, cold hands and feet, and potentiation of insulin-induced hypoglycemia. High doses of cardioselective antagonists can also cause some degree of β_2 adrenoceptor blockade and precipitate asthma in some patients.

The membrane-stabilizing (local anaesthetic) and intrinsic sympathomimetic activities (*i.e.*, partial agonist activity) should increase the antiarrhythmic effects and reduce the cardiodepressant action. When patients are dependent on sympathetic drive because of poor cardiac reserve, a partial agonist of β_1 adrenoceptors is preferred (*e.g.*, pindolol). Conversely, a partial agonist would be less suitable in thyrotoxicosis, which is associated with excessive activity of the sympathetic nervous system.

Propranolol

This drug (Fig. 17–4) was the first beta-blocker to come into wide clinical use; it remains the most important of the β-adrenoceptor antagonists and is described here as the prototype. It is a racemic mixture of levorotatory (−) and dextrorotatory (+) propranolol. The (−) form is 100 times more potent in blocking β_1 and β_2 adrenoceptors than the (+) isomer. The two isomers are equally effective as membrane stabilizers (local anaesthetics), but this property of the drug is usually observed at higher concentrations. Propranolol is a competitive, reversible antagonist of endogenous noradrenaline and adrenaline and of all sympathomimetic drugs acting on β_1 and β_2 adrenoceptors. The dose-response curve of β-receptor agonists is shifted to the right but remains parallel to the original curve. The effects of propranolol antagonism of endogenously released catecholamines (noradrenaline and adrenaline) are dependent upon the extent of sympathetic tone in a given organ or tissue. Since cardiac function is influenced by sympathetic tone, propranolol (in effective concentrations) will cause significant alterations in cardiac activity.

Pharmacokinetics

Propranolol, because of its lipid solubility, is quickly and completely absorbed from the gastrointestinal tract. Following absorption, it undergoes first-pass metabolism in the liver to the extent that, because of hepatic extraction of the drug from blood, systemic availability of an oral dose is frequently less than 30%. (The availability of an oral dose to the cardiovascular system is therefore much less than that of an intravenously administered dose.) Since the hepatic extraction mechanisms are saturable (and vary between

Nonselective β-Adrenoceptor Antagonists

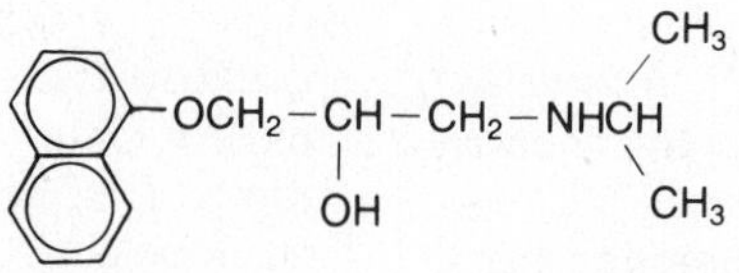

Propranolol

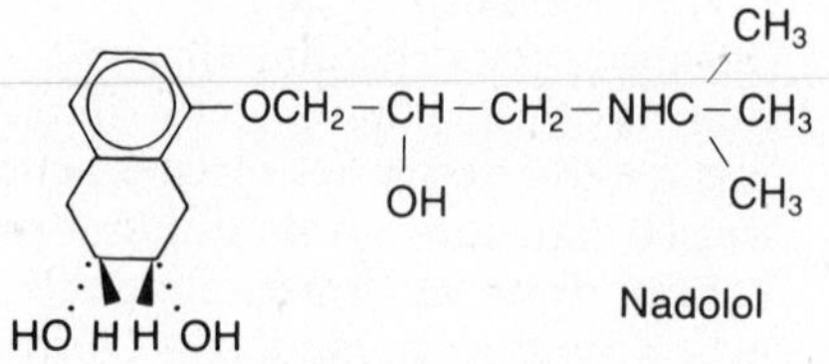

Nadolol

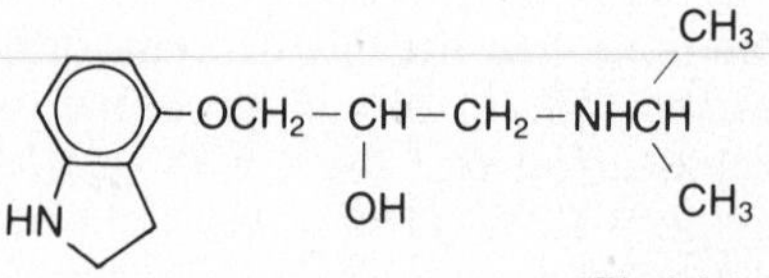

Pindolol

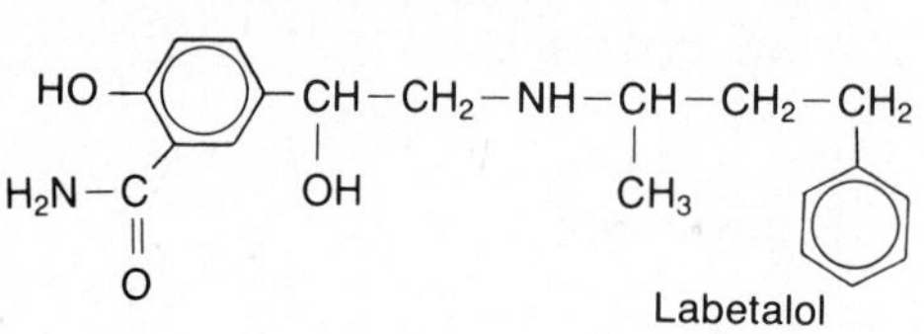

Labetalol

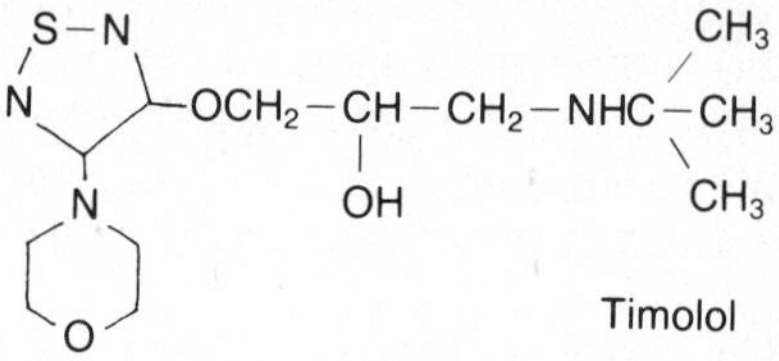

Timolol

Selective β₁-Adrenoceptor Antagonists

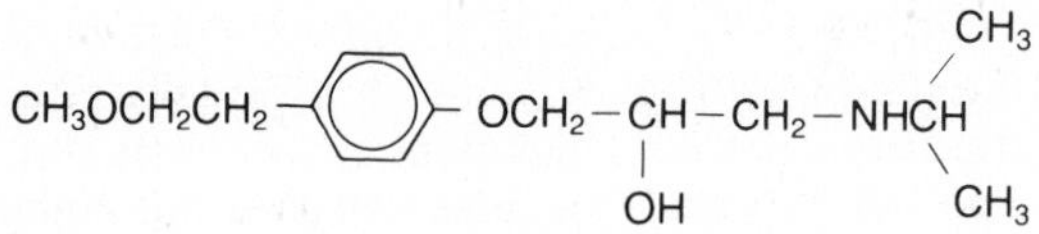

Metoprolol

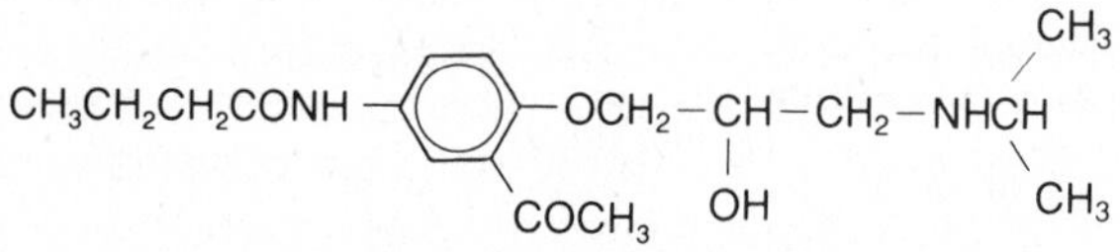

Acebutolol*

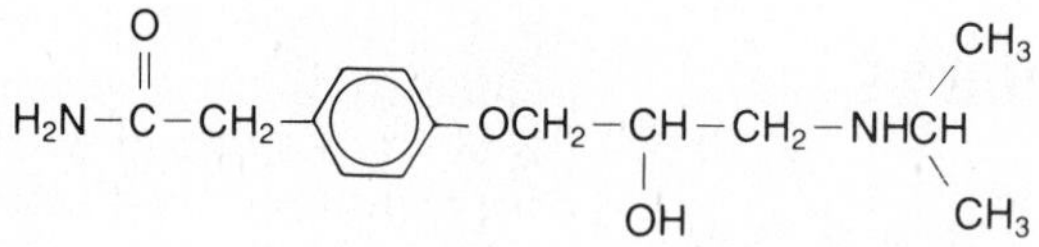

Atenolol

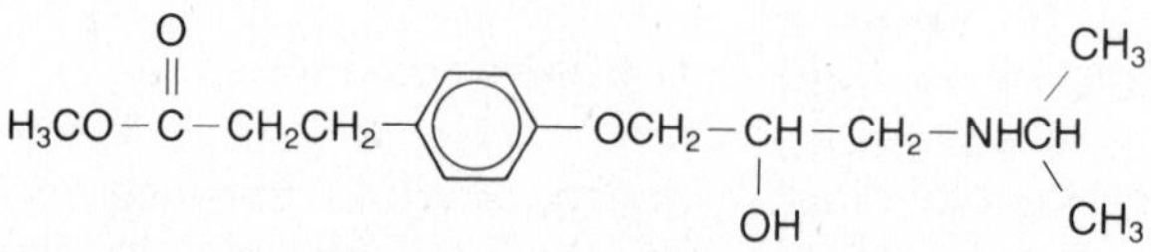

Esmolol

Figure 17-4   Structural formulae of β-adrenoceptor antagonists. (*Acebutolol is a selective antagonist—and partial agonist—that is metabolized to a nonselective antagonist.)

individuals), increasing the dose of propranolol may result in disproportionate increases in plasma levels. Hydroxylation of propranolol in the liver produces an active metabolite, 4-hydroxy-propranolol, which has a shorter half-life than the parent compound. A large proportion of circulating propranolol is bound to plasma proteins (>90%), and the plasma half-life in man is approximately 4 hours. However, the clinical effect may last longer than the period suggested by the plasma half-life because of the formation of the active metabolite (Table 17–1).

Pharmacologic Effects

Cardiovascular (Table 17–2). Propranolol exerts a negative chronotropic action on the heart, i.e., bradycardia, particularly when sympathetic discharge to the heart is high, as in exercise.

It also has a negative inotropic action, i.e., it produces a decrease in the force of contraction. The rate of rise of tension in the heart (dp/dt) and the peak force attained are decreased.

Cardiac output is decreased, i.e., the amount of blood ejected per minute is reduced.

Atrioventricular (A-V) conduction velocity is decreased, since vagal action on the A-V node becomes dominant.

Automaticity of pacemaker cells is decreased. This is the basis for its use in suppressing ectopic foci.

Oxygen consumption is decreased because of decreased work of the heart.

Peripheral vascular resistance is increased because of reflex increase in sympathetic tone, causing vasoconstriction and unopposed α-receptor stimulation by endogenous noradrenaline in arterioles that contain both α_1 and β_2 receptors (e.g., vessels to skeletal muscle). Nevertheless, hypotension occurs following chronic administration of propranolol, probably due to the decrease in cardiac output, possible central actions,

and blockade of renin release from juxtaglomerular cells in the kidneys resulting in decreased rate of formation of angiotensin II and decreased aldosterone release from the adrenal cortex (Fig. 17–5).

Bronchiolar smooth muscle. Bronchodilatation mediated by β_2-receptor stimulation is blocked by propranolol. Airway resistance is always increased to a minor extent even in normal individuals. Bronchospasm following propranolol administration can be extremely hazardous in asthmatic patients. Propranolol also potentiates bronchospasm induced by acetylcholine (or drugs that prevent the hydrolysis of acetylcholine) and histamine, particularly in asthmatic patients.

Metabolic effects. The stimulant effects of endogenous catecholamines and sympathomimetic drugs on carbohydrate and fat metabolism are believed to be mediated via β adrenoceptors, stimulation of which activates adenylate cyclase and leads to elevated levels of cyclic AMP. In humans, propranolol inhibits the increase in plasma free fatty acids induced by catecholamines.

The effects on carbohydrate metabolism are less clear; propranolol inhibits the secretion of insulin from the pancreas in response to β_2-receptor stimulants and prevents the hyperglycemic response to adrenaline. Resting plasma glucose concentrations in nondiabetic patients are usually normal. However, the rate of recovery of blood glucose levels following insulin administration may be delayed, resulting in hypoglycemia. Propranolol must therefore be used cautiously in diabetics. A cardioselective β_1-adrenoceptor antagonist (e.g., metoprolol) may be less hazardous in diabetic patients, since metabolic effects appear to be more closely associated with β_2 adrenoceptors.

Central effects. Propranolol crosses the blood–brain barrier and therefore affects central adrenoceptors. Its use in the treatment of anxiety, acute psychotic states, and schizophrenia is controversial.

Tremor due to hyperthyroidism, alcohol withdrawal,

TABLE 17–1 Pharmacokinetics of Some β-Adrenoceptor Antagonists

	Atenolol	Metoprolol	Pindolol	Propranolol	Timolol
Extent of absorption (%)	~50	>95	>90	>90	>90
Extent of bioavailability (% of Dose)	~40	~50	~90	~30	75
Interpatient variations in plasma levels	4-fold	10-fold	4-fold	20-fold	7-fold
β-Blocking plasma concentration (ng/mL)	200–500	50–100	50–100	50–100	5–10
Protein binding (%)	<5	12	57	93	~10
Lipophilicity	Low	Moderate	Moderate	High	Low
Elimination half-life (hr)	6–9	3–4	3–4	3–5	3–4
Predominant route of elimination	Renal excretion (mostly unchanged)	Hepatic biotransformation	Renal excretion (~40% unchanged) and hepatic biotransformation	Hepatic biotransformation	Renal excretion (~20% unchanged) and hepatic biotransformation
Active metabolites	No	No	No	Yes	No

TABLE 17-2 Effects of β-Adrenoceptor Antagonists

β₁-Adrenoceptor Blockade	β₂-Adrenoceptor Blockade

Cardiovascular Effects (effects on cardiac function are more prominent during exercise)
 	
Reduced heart rate.
 	
Delayed conduction velocity at the A-V node.
 	
Decreased rate of diastolic depolarization in all pacemaker cells (the basis for antiarrhythmic action).
 	
Decreased force of contraction (negative inotropy), leading to:
 	
   reduced stroke volume;
   increased residual (end-systolic) volume; and
   decreased cardiac output (decreased heart rate and
   stroke volume).
 	
Reduced velocity of contraction.
 	
Decreased cardiac O₂ consumption (decreased rate and ventricular systolic pressure and contractility).
 	
Reduced blood pressure.
 	
Inhibition of renin release from kidneys, causing subsequent lowering of angiotensin II.
 	
Edema formation due to sodium retention caused by decreased cardiac output.
 	
Other Effects
 	
  Decreased lipolysis.
	Vasoconstriction in some arterioles, *e.g.*, those supplying skeletal muscle.
	
	Increased airway resistance and precipitation of asthma.
	
	Decreased glycogenolysis and gluconeogenesis.
	
	Inhibition of insulin release.
	
	Antagonism of catecholamine-induced tremor.

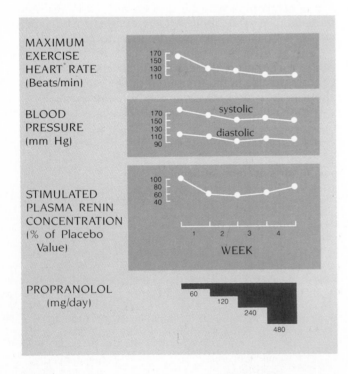

Figure 17-5 Dose-response relationships between the fall in blood pressure, the degree of cardiac blockade, and plasma renin concentration produced by propranolol. Dose increments at weekly intervals.

or nervousness responds successfully to propranolol.

The antihypertensive effect of the drug may be related in part to a central sympatholytic action, thereby enhancing vagal tone in the heart.

Toxic Effects

These are predictable on the basis of its mechanism of action in producing β-adrenoceptor blockade. Adverse effects are also widespread because of the diffuse distribution of sympathetic nerves throughout the body. Serious reactions to propranolol include:

- Severe bradycardia.
- Heart failure of the congestive type in patients with borderline failure prior to treatment with propranolol.
- Depression of A-V conduction leading to A-V dissociation, especially in patients with conduction defects or in those who are receiving digitalis.
- Bronchoconstriction; propranolol (and other beta-blockers) should be avoided in patients with obstructive airway diseases.
- Hypoglycemia, particularly following insulin administration.
- Aggravation of peripheral vascular disease, *e.g.*, intermittent claudication and Raynaud's disease, because of unopposed α₁ receptor-mediated vasoconstriction by endogenous noradrenaline.

- Abrupt cessation of propranolol treatment has been associated with fatal cardiac rhythm disturbances or severe anginal attacks. The dosage of propranolol (and other β antagonists) should therefore be reduced gradually over one or two weeks. The effects may be associated with rapid reinstallation of sympathetic drive to the heart or with increased β-adrenoceptor sensitivity.

Other Nonselective β-Adrenoceptor Antagonists

Nadolol (*see* Fig. 17–4) is the longest-acting beta-blocker, with a half-life of 14–24 hours. It is administered once daily.

Labetalol (*see* Fig. 17–4) is an antagonist of α_1, β_1, and β_2 adrenoceptors. Its β-blocking effects are predominant, with a 3:1 ratio of β:α antagonism. The drug decreases blood pressure without reflex increase in heart rate and cardiac output. For this reason, it is useful in controlling elevated blood pressure associated with pheochromocytoma or in hypertensive emergency.

Pindolol, and **acebutolol** (which is biotransformed from a selective to a nonselective antagonist; *see* Fig. 17–4), have sympathomimetic activity and are called partial agonists. The reduction in heart rate following administration of these drugs is less than that caused by propranolol, presumably because of their sympathomimetic effects, which are less than those of noradrenaline but which partially counteract the β_1-receptor blockade.

Selective Antagonists of β_1 Adrenoceptors

Metoprolol and **atenolol** (*see* Fig. 17–4) are of similar potency to propranolol in blocking cardiac β_1 receptors, but are much less active in blocking β_2 receptors in the respiratory tract and peripheral vasculature. The effects on insulin release and carbohydrate metabolism are also minimal when compared with those of propranolol. Metoprolol is used in the prophylaxis of angina pectoris and in the treatment of hypertension.

Esmolol (*see* Fig. 17–4) is a short-acting β_1 antagonist for intravenous use. It is rapidly hydrolysed by esterases in erythrocytes. The drug causes a rapid dose-related reduction in blood pressure and heart rate. Its current use is in the initial treatment of supraventricular tachyarrhythmias.

Therapeutic Uses of β-Adrenoceptor Blocking Drugs

Beta-blockers are used widely in disorders of the cardiovascular system (hypertension, angina pectoris, cardiac dysrhythmias) and in thyrotoxicosis, drug-induced tremors, *etc.* The properties and relative potencies of these drugs are shown in Table 17–3. Propranolol is also used for the prophylaxis of migraine headaches. The exact mechanism underlying the prevention of migraine is not known, but it may be associated with inhibition of β_2 receptor-mediated vasodilatation in the brain or with blockade of uptake

TABLE 17–3 Properties and Approximate Relative Potencies of Some β-Adrenoceptor Antagonists

Official Name (Trade Name)	Solubility	Membrane Stabilizing Effects	Intrinsic Sympatho-mimetic Activity	Approximate Cardiac Potency Relative to Propranolol	Hypotensive Doses Used (mg/day)
Propranolol (Inderal®)	Lipid	+ +	0	1	160–480
Alprenolol	Lipid	+	+ +	0.5	400–800
Pindolol (Visken®)	Lipid	±	+ +	10	15–45
Timolol (Blocadren®)	Aqueous	0	±	10	30–60
Atenolol (Tenormin®)	Aqueous	0	0	1	100–200

±, +, + + = relative degrees of activity; 0 = no activity.

AUTONOMIC NEUROMUSCULAR

of serotonin by platelets. This would enhance the vaso-tonic actions of serotonin on cerebral blood flow.

Timolol, propranolol, and metoprolol are used in the prevention of myocardial reinfarction. The drugs are beneficial and consistently effective regardless of age, sex, or site of infarction. Drug therapy is started between 5 and 28 days after the infarct. Timolol is also used in the treatment of glaucoma.

Some Drug Interactions

Cimetidine inhibits the hepatic enzymes associated with the first-pass metabolism of propranolol, metoprolol, and labetalol, and thus confers enhanced bioavailability to these agents. Verapamil may act synergistically to decrease conduction velocity at the A-V node and to enhance the negative inotropic effects of propranolol and other β_1 antagonists. Digoxin interacts in a similar manner. Indomethacin and salicylates may decrease the antihypertensive effects of β_1 antagonists by inhibiting the synthesis of vasodilating prostaglandins. The hypoglycemic effect of insulin may be enhanced and prolonged by nonselective β-adrenoceptor antagonists.

SUGGESTED READING

Cubeddu LX. New α_1-adrenergic receptor antagonists for the treatment of hypertension: role of vascular α receptors in the control of peripheral resistance. Am Heart J 1988; 116:133–162.

Feely J, deVane P, Maclean D. Beta blockers and sympathomimetics. Br Med J 1983; 286:1043–1047.

Frishman WH. Beta-adrenoceptor antagonists: new drugs and new indications. N Engl J Med 1981; 305:500–505.

Frishman WH. Beta-adrenergic receptor blockers. Adverse effects and drug interactions. Hypertension 1988; 11:II 21–29.

Kanto JH. Labetalol in the treatment of angina pectoris. Int J Clin Pharmacol 1987; 25(3):166–167.

Lader M. Beta-adrenoceptor antagonists in neuropsychiatry: an update. J Clin Psychiatry 1988; 49:213–223.

Lowenthal DT, Saris SD, Packer J, et al. Mechanism of action and clinical pharmacology of beta-adrenergic blocking drugs. Am J Med 1984; 77:119–127.

Prichard BN, Tomlinson B. The present—antihypertensive drugs in practice. Am Heart J 1987; 114:1030–1040.

VanZwieten PA. Antihypertensive drugs interacting with alpha- and beta-adrenoceptors. A review of basic pharmacology. Drugs 1988; 35(Suppl 6):6–19.

Walle T, Webb JG, Bagwell EE, et al. Stereoselective delivery and actions of beta receptor antagonists. Biochem Pharmacol 1988; 37:115–124.

Chapter 18

DRUGS ACTING ON ADRENERGIC NEURONS (ADRENERGIC NEURONAL BLOCKING DRUGS)

K.V. Flattery

The sympathetic nervous system participates in the regulation of arterial blood pressure in both normal and hypertensive individuals. Arteries, arterioles, and veins have direct sympathetic innervation, which, by releasing catecholamines, causes vasoconstriction. Also, the rate and force of cardiac contraction and, therefore, the cardiac output are increased by the activity of the sympathetic nervous system. The cardiovascular abnormalities found consistently in sustained hypertension are an increase in peripheral resistance and/or an increase in cardiac output. Historically, it is interesting to note that surgical sympathectomy was used for the treatment of severe hypertension. Early pharmacologic treatment was with ganglionic blocking drugs. Subsequently, newer antihypertensive drugs were developed, many of which act either on adrenergic neurons or on α or β adrenoceptors.

Drugs acting on adrenergic neurons do so by a variety of mechanisms, which include:

- inhibition of synthesis of catecholamines (e.g., α-methyl-p-tyrosine, see Chapter 13);
- interference with intraneuronal vesicular storage, resulting in depletion of catecholamines (e.g., reserpine); and
- blockade of release of noradrenaline* (e.g., guanethidine, clonidine).

Most, but not all, of these drugs act at both central and peripheral sites and cause distinctive, undesirable side effects, many of which are predictable on the basis of the mechanism and site of action of the individual drug.

---

* norepinephrine

DRUGS

Reserpine

Reserpine (Fig. 18–1) is one of the alkaloids obtained from *Rauwolfia serpentina* (Indian snake root), which grows in India, where it has been used extensively for the treatment of anxiety, insomnia, psychoses, and hypertension. It is an important tool in pharmacologic experimentation because of its action in reducing the concentration of biogenic amines at both central and peripheral sites. Clinically, reserpine is used only occasionally in the treatment of hypertension, usually in conjunction with other drugs such as hydrochlorothiazide. Related alkaloids are deserpidine and rescinnamine. Syrosingopine is a semisynthetic derivative with less effect on the central nervous system.

Mechanism of Action

Reserpine depletes central and peripheral stores of noradrenaline, 5-hydroxytryptamine, and dopamine. Chromaffin cells in the adrenal medulla are also depleted, but at a lower rate and to a lesser extent than the neurons. Reserpine is a potent inhibitor of the active transport system by which noradrenaline is taken up from the neuronal cell cytoplasm into the storage vesicles within sympathetic nerve endings (Fig. 18–2). The capacity of the storage granules to retain high concentrations of noradrenaline within the vesicles against

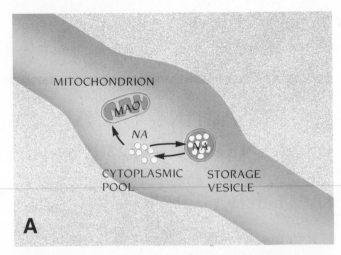

Figure 18-1   Structural formula of reserpine.

a concentration gradient is also abolished. This allows leakage of noradrenaline into the cytoplasm and from there to the mitochondria, where it is deaminated by monoamine oxidase, resulting in depletion of noradrenaline stores. The uptake of dopamine from the cytoplasm to the storage vesicle is also impaired, and synthesis of the transmitter is therefore decreased. Noradrenergic and dopaminergic neurons in the periphery and the brain are affected. The concentration of 5-hydroxytryptamine (serotonin) is significantly lowered in central serotonergic neurons, mast cells, platelets, and in the gastrointestinal tract. Decrease in catecholamine concentration occurs within an hour of reserpine administration and is maximal by 24 hours.

Effects on the Cardiovascular System

The antihypertensive actions of reserpine are probably a consequence of the reduced noradrenaline levels in peripheral sympathetic nerve endings, although a central action should not be excluded. The peripheral depletion causes an impairment of responses to sympathetic stimulation. In the vascular system, therefore, there is less transmitter available for stimulation of α_1 adrenoceptors. As a result, there is a reduction of tone in arterioles and large veins, resulting in a fall in diastolic blood pressure and venous pooling of blood. Similarly, in the heart the β_1 adrenoceptor-mediated excitatory effects of noradrenaline are reduced or abolished, allowing acetylcholine to become the dominant transmitter. This results in bradycardia and decreased cardiac output, which also contribute to the reduction in blood pressure. The blood pressure falls progressively and is dose-dependent. Since only small doses are administered in the treatment of hypertension (resulting in less depletion of noradrenaline), the side effects of severe orthostatic hypotension (decreased venous return and cardiac output) are not frequently observed.

During chronic treatment with reserpine, supersensitivity to the catecholamines (as well as to drugs with direct sympathomimetic effects) occurs. The increased sensitivity is associated with up-regulation of the receptors. In contrast, responses to indirectly-acting sympathomimetics (which normally increase the amount of

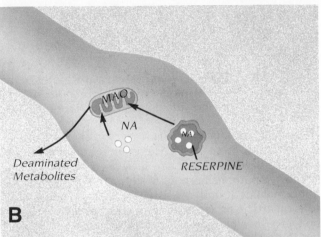

Figure 18-2   Proposed mechanism of noradrenaline depletion from a sympathetic terminal varicosity by reserpine. *A*, In the normal state noradrenaline (NA) is in equilibrium between the cytoplasm and the storage vesicles, controlled by mitochondrial monoamine oxidase (MAO). *B*, In the presence of reserpine the noradrenaline uptake into storage vesicles is prevented and noradrenaline from both cytoplasm and storage vesicles is gradually depleted by MAO metabolism.

noradrenaline released, *e.g.*, ephedrine, amphetamine, and the experimental drug tyramine) are either decreased or abolished with chronic reserpine treatment.

Adverse Reactions

In the presence of reserpine, parasympathetic activity becomes more pronounced because of loss of opposing sympathetic tone. This applies to all organs with dual innervation by both sympathetic and parasympathetic systems. Most side effects can be attributed to the unopposed activity of the parasympathetic system in many organs.

Cardiovascular.   Excessive bradycardia may occur in some patients, as do nasal congestion and flushing of the skin, as well as postural hypotension with larger doses. Nasal congestion in the newborns of mothers treated with reserpine may cause serious respiratory problems. Sodium retention and edema may occur because of decreased perfusion pressure in renal blood vessels. Rapid parenteral injection can release noradrenaline initially and cause a transient rise in blood pressure.

The most unpleasant untoward responses to reserpine (and the most important from the point of view of toxicity) are related to the CNS and the gastrointestinal tract.

Central nervous system. Decreased concentrations of dopamine in the brain may cause parkinsonism. Lethargy, sedation, nightmares, and depression (occasionally leading to suicide) also may occur. The depression of mood closely resembles the clinical condition of endogenous depression.

Gastrointestinal tract. Increase in tone and motility gives rise to abdominal cramps and diarrhea. Gastric HCl is increased, leading to reactivation or aggravation of peptic ulcer. Release of gastrin *via* a central vagal action may be responsible for the increased gastric acid secretion induced by reserpine.

Other effects. It has been claimed that long-term treatment with reserpine increases the incidence of breast carcinoma in women, but this is uncertain. The secretion of prolactin is also enhanced, probably because of decreased dopamine concentrations in the brain (*see* Chapter 27). Galactorrhea may occur occasionally.

Guanethidine

Guanethidine (Fig. 18–3) is actively transported into peripheral sympathetic nerve endings by the uptake system for noradrenaline, with which it competes, and accumulates in storage vesicles. As a result, it reduces noradrenaline concentration in the sympathetic nerve endings and produces a characteristic, prolonged decrease of noradrenaline release, which interrupts transmission of impulses between sympathetic neurons and effector organs.

Other drugs that block the neuronal uptake of noradrenaline, such as cocaine and tricyclic antidepressants, also interfere competitively with the uptake of guanethidine. This competitive interference may prevent the onset of action or reverse the neuronal blocking effects of guanethidine.

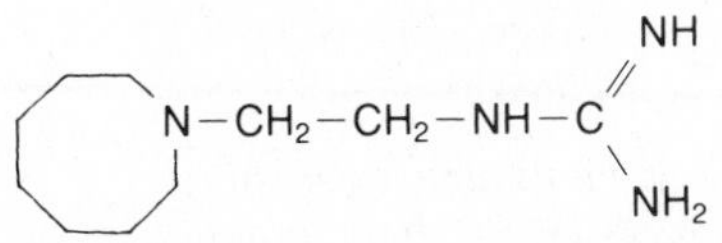

Figure 18–3 Structural formula of guanethidine.

Blockade of noradrenaline uptake by guanethidine causes partial depletion of noradrenaline stores and potentiates the actions of exogenous noradrenaline. Responses to indirect-acting sympathomimetic drugs, *e.g.*, tyramine and amphetamine, are reduced in magnitude or blocked.

Mechanism of Action

Following intraneuronal accumulation of guanethidine, noradrenaline release (which normally occurs in response to action potentials) is impaired. This effect is associated with a membrane-stabilizing (local anaesthetic) action of guanethidine. Action potentials still occur, but exocytosis is blocked at neuronal membrane sites.

Subsequent and gradual depletion of noradrenaline occurs **selectively** in peripheral sympathetic nerve endings, and is attributable to the blockade of amine uptake coupled with intraneuronal vesicular noradrenaline release and deamination by monoamine oxidase (MAO). Guanethidine effects on transmitter release and intraneuronal concentration are sometimes referred to as "drug-induced sympathectomy."

Guanethidine may also act as a false transmitter since it is released after nerve stimulation.

Effects on the Cardiovascular System

The primary mechanism by which guanethidine lowers blood pressure is the decreased release of noradrenaline, causing a reduction in sympathetic excitatory effects on the heart and vascular smooth muscle. Guanethidine causes a prolonged fall in blood pressure, particularly in hypertensive patients. The response to the drug is greater in the erect than in the supine position, so that the drug may cause postural hypotension. This is a characteristic response to drugs that block the sympathetic nervous system. The hypotension is presumably due to a reduction in the capacity of vasoconstrictor fibres to bring about the usual reflex compensations when the erect posture is assumed. This reduces venous return and cardiac output and results in hypotension. The rapid intravenous administration of a large dose of guanethidine can cause a transient increase in blood pressure attributable to a release of noradrenaline from the sympathetic nerves. This is then followed by a fall in blood pressure, which is due to blockade of release of noradrenaline, followed by subsequent depletion.

Guanethidine has little effect on the catecholamine content of the adrenal medulla and the CNS; in the latter case this is probably because the drug does not cross the blood–brain barrier.

The most important aspects of the general pharmacology of guanethidine are attributable to inhibition of responses to sympathetic nerve activity. Guanethidine is used in patients with severe hypertension. It has a very prolonged action, and the effects of a constant daily dose may continue to increase for several weeks.

Adverse Reactions

Orthostatic hypotension (postural hypotension, *see* above) is aggravated by alcohol, warm weather, and exercise.

Sodium and fluid retention may occur and lead to edema and resistance to the therapeutic effect of the drug if a diuretic is not administered concurrently.

Bradycardia, due to vagal predominance in the heart, may be a decided disadvantage, especially in older patients.

Diarrhea from unopposed activity of the vagus nerve in the gastrointestinal tract is common. Failure of ejaculation may also occur.

Severe hypertensive reactions have been reported in patients with pheochromocytoma, and are caused by supersensitivity of the adrenoceptors to catecholamines released from the tumor.

Interactions with Other Drugs

Uptake of guanethidine into sympathetic neurons is blocked by tricyclic antidepressants, cocaine, and amphetamine (Fig. 18–4). The antihypertensive action of guanethidine can be prevented by these drugs. Chronic administration of guanethidine also sensitizes effector cells to catecholamines as much as 100-fold. The fact that responses are much reduced or absent in the presence of such sensitization indicates that the amount of transmitter released must be very small indeed. The

supersensitivity of receptors reaches a maximum in 10 to 14 days and is greater for noradrenaline than for adrenaline.

Other Drugs of this Class

Bethanidine, debrisoquine, and **guanadrel** are from the same family as guanethidine, with similar mechanism of action, side effects, and interactions. The half-life of bethanidine is much shorter than that of guanethidine (7–11 hours versus 43 hours, respectively). Bethanidine is excreted unchanged in the urine, while guanethidine is both biotransformed (40%) and excreted unchanged.

α-Methyldopa

α-Methyldopa is closely related chemically to L-dopa, which is a precursor in the synthesis of dopamine, noradrenaline, and adrenaline (*see* Chapter 13).

Mechanism of Action

α-Methyldopa becomes a substrate for dopa decarboxylase (aromatic amino acid decarboxylase) within the brain and in the periphery, and is converted to α-methyldopamine. This is then converted to α-methylnoradrenaline within the vesicles by dopamine-

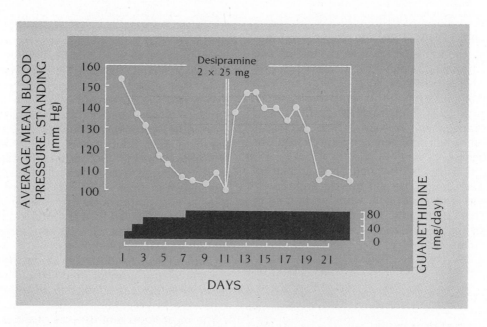

Figure 18–4 Antagonism of the antihypertensive action of guanethidine by desipramine in a hypertensive patient. The dose of guanethidine was adjusted in increments of 80 mg per day, producing a lowering of mean arterial pressure to below 100 mm Hg. Administration of 50 mg of desipramine totally reversed the guanethidine effect for approximately 1 week.

β-hydroxylase and becomes a "false" transmitter, which is responsible for the reduction of blood pressure in hypertensive patients (Fig. 18–5).

α-Methylnoradrenaline (formed from α-methyldopa) stimulates postsynaptic α_2 adrenoceptors (for which it has a high affinity) in the tractus solitarius in the medulla oblongata. This inhibits the peripheral release of noradrenaline through an inhibition of the activity of the sympathetic nervous centre.

In the peripheral nerves, α-methylnoradrenaline is stored in the vesicles and is released by nerve stimulation. It has only weak α_1-agonistic properties. The central action of α-methylnoradrenaline prevents the peripheral release of both the false transmitter and noradrenaline.

Cardiovascular Effects

α-Methyldopa produces progressive reductions in blood pressure and heart rate that are maximal in 4–6 hours. The fall in blood pressure is greater in hypertensive than in normotensive subjects; it has been reported to be due to decrease in cardiac output and peripheral resistance. The hypotension induced by α-methyldopa has not been shown to involve any major changes in distribution of blood flow. Renal blood flow and glomerular filtration are well maintained in both normotensive and hypertensive subjects.

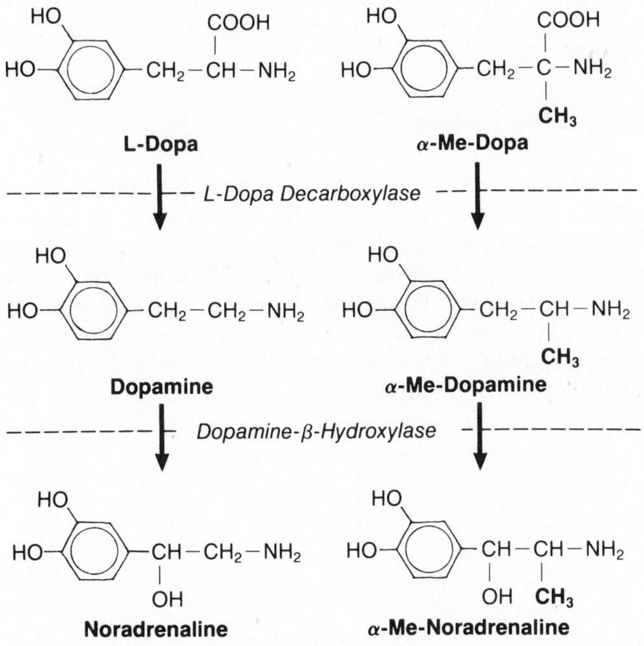

Figure 18–5 Formation of α-methylnoradrenaline from α-methyldopa.

Adverse Effects

Adverse reactions to α-methyldopa include drowsiness, psychic depression, parkinsonism, dryness of the mouth, nasal stuffiness, nausea, and gastrointestinal disturbances. Hypersensitivity reactions include jaundice, pyrexia, and rashes; occasionally hemolytic anemia may occur. Prolonged treatment may cause a positive Coombs test. Liver damage may occur in the occasional patient.

Clonidine

Clonidine (Fig. 18–6) is an imidazoline derivative chemically related to tolazoline and other α-adrenoceptor antagonists and agonists, e.g., naphazoline. Clonidine was originally developed as a nasal decongestant because of its local vasoconstrictor effects; but when tested for this purpose in humans it produced a marked reduction of blood pressure and heart rate. The α adrenoceptor-stimulant properties of clonidine result in a fall in blood pressure. Its actions in many respects resemble those of α-methyldopa. Both drugs allow vasopressor centres in the brain to retain some degree of sensitivity to baroreceptor control, thus lowering the incidence of postural hypotension.

Other drugs related to clonidine are **guanfacine** and **guanabenz**.

Mechanism of Action

Clonidine has a marked presynaptic α_2-stimulant action, which interferes with the neuronal release of noradrenaline at both central and peripheral sites. The central site of action is in the medullary area in the brain. Stimulation of α_2 (and possibly α_1) adrenoceptors in this area causes a reduction of efferent sympathetic nerve activity, which results in a fall in blood pressure and heart rate. At peripheral sites, stimulation of presynaptic α_2 receptors causes a reduction in release of noradrenaline from the terminal varicosities. The inhibitory effect of the vagus nerve on the heart is augmented probably both by increased sensitivity of the baroreceptors and by central actions.

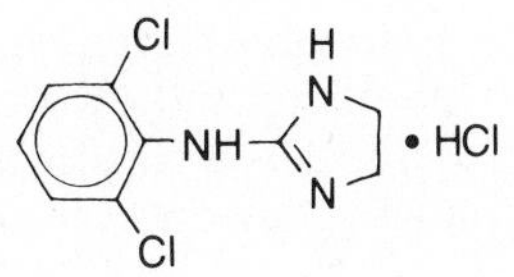

Figure 18–6 Structural formula of clonidine HCl.

Pharmacologic Effects

Intravenous administration of clonidine in humans produces an initial brief increase in blood pressure followed by a fall in blood pressure associated with bradycardia. The initial increase in blood pressure is caused by a transient stimulation of α_1 adrenoceptors.

The hemodynamic effects of clonidine include bradycardia and a reduced cardiac output, which causes a fall in blood pressure.

Following chronic administration of clonidine, peripheral resistance is also decreased. Clonidine has minor effects on reflex control of blood pressure; therefore, postural hypotension is not a common side effect. A potentially dangerous side effect of clonidine is "rebound" hypertension in patients in whom the drug has been suddenly withdrawn. Prior administration of α-adrenoceptor antagonists (e.g., phentolamine) will prevent this rebound effect. Renin release is also inhibited by clonidine.

Other Uses of Clonidine

Small doses of clonidine are effective in the prophylactic treatment of migraine by reducing the frequency and severity of the attacks. The drug has been used successfully in alleviating opiate withdrawal symptoms and also has been reported to reduce some of the symptoms of alcohol withdrawal that are attributable to adrenergic overactivity (see Chapter 22).

Adverse Effects

Sedation, dry mouth, and constipation occur frequently in the therapeutic dose range and limit the use of clonidine. It is possible that stimulation by clonidine of α_2 adrenoceptors found on cholinergic fibres innervating salivary glands and intestine may be responsible. Central mechanisms also may be involved.

The rebound hypertensive overshoot described earlier occurs only on sudden withdrawal of the drug; it is associated with overactivity of the sympathetic nervous system, as indicated by elevated plasma and urinary catecholamines. Clonidine can also potentiate insulin-induced hypoglycemia.

Interactions

Desmethylimipramine interferes with the antihypertensive action of clonidine. Other tricyclic antidepressant drugs also may block the cardiovascular responses to clonidine administration and should be used with caution.

Monoamine Oxidase Inhibitors

These drugs were introduced as antidepressants (see Chapter 28); however, like amphetamine and its derivatives, they also have important peripheral actions on the cardiovascular system. The most important pharmacologic effect is the inhibition of monoamine oxidase (MAO), which is involved in the catabolism of catecholamines intraneuronally and, therefore, in the regulation of cytoplasmic noradrenaline concentrations in sympathetic nerve terminals. Despite the elevated intraneuronal levels of noradrenaline, the release of the transmitter is impaired, resulting in orthostatic hypotension (a side effect of most MAO-inhibiting drugs). It was on the basis of this finding that the antihypertensive drug **pargyline** (Fig. 18–7) was introduced. However, tolerance to its antihypertensive actions may develop with chronic use. This fact, combined with the unpleasant side effects of dizziness, weakness (orthostatic hypotension), insomnia, headache, etc., make it unacceptable as an antihypertensive drug.

Mechanism of Action

The mechanism of the antihypertensive effects of MAO inhibitors is not clear. It is postulated that a "false" transmitter, octopamine, may be formed from tyramine following MAO inhibition (Fig. 18–8). A more recent hypothesis is that inhibition of brain MAO, leading to increased central levels of noradrenaline, may have an inhibitory effect on sympathetic outflow reminiscent of the mechanisms associated with clonidine and α-methyldopa.

Adverse Interactions

The major drawback associated with clinical use of MAO inhibitors is their interaction with tyramine-containing foods, such as aged cheese, some wines, salami, and pickled herring, to produce severe hypertensive episodes. Tyramine in such foods has the ability to release catecholamines. Since it is normally catabolized by MAO, tyramine may be absorbed into the blood stream in sufficient concentration following en-

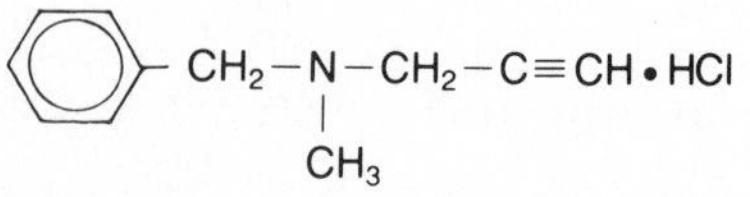

$$\text{benzene ring} - CH_2 - N - CH_2 - C \equiv CH \cdot HCl$$
$$| $$
$$CH_3$$

Figure 18–7 Structural formula of pargyline HCl.

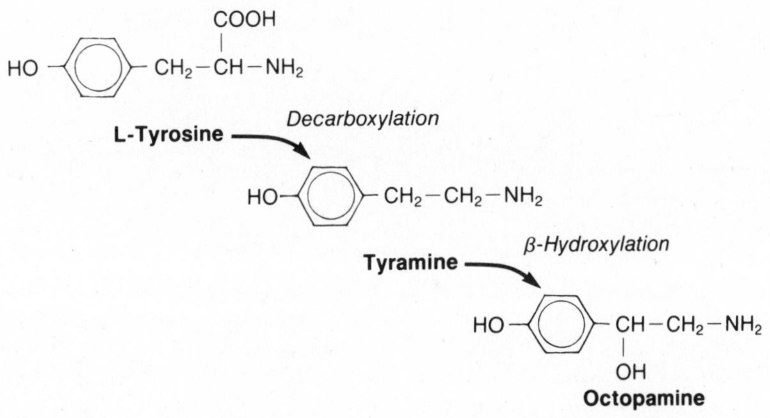

Figure 18–8 Proposed production of octopamine, a false transmitter, from tyramine. Tyramine is normally rapidly inactivated by MAO, but significant amounts of octopamine are formed when MAO is inhibited.

zyme inhibition to cause release of noradrenaline. This may result in dangerous elevation of blood pressure, often accompanied by tachycardia. This reaction, called hypertensive crisis, is illustrated in Figure 18–9.

Bretylium

Bretylium (Fig. 18–10) was first described in 1959. Like guanethidine, the drug causes inhibition of responses to adrenergic nerve stimulation and to indirectly acting sympathomimetic amines; it decreases the amount of noradrenaline released per stimulus. However, in contrast to guanethidine, a single dose of bretylium produces no detectable reduction in tissue catecholamine levels.

The major cardiovascular effects of bretylium are very similar to those of guanethidine, and at one time bretylium was used quite extensively in the treatment of hypertension. However, tolerance to its effects develops quite rapidly. It is used occasionally in the treatment of ventricular dysrhythmias.

α-Methyltyrosine

The biosynthesis of the catecholamines is inhibited at central and peripheral sites by the drug α-methyltyrosine. Chromaffin cells in the medulla of the adrenal gland are also depleted. α-Methyltyrosine is a competitive inhibitor of tyrosine hydroxylase, which catalyses the formation of L-dopa from L-tyrosine, the rate-limiting step in catecholamine synthesis. Impairment of the activity of the sympathetic nervous system occurs. α-Methyltyrosine (metyrosine) is sometimes used to treat hypertension associated with pheochromocytoma, a tumor of chromaffin cells found most commonly in the adrenal medulla. When this tumor occurs at extra-adrenal sites, it may be surgically less accessible, and therefore drug therapy may be necessary. Surgery may also be contraindicated in some patients. The effectiveness of α-methyltyrosine can be determined by measurement of blood and/or urinary catecholamines.

Adverse effects are sedation, extrapyramidal symptoms, and psychic disturbances. Severe diarrhea may also occur. The potential for urinary crystal formation requires increased water intake.

6-Hydroxydopamine

6-Hydroxydopamine is a useful research drug that has a destructive effect on sympathetic nerve endings. It does not penetrate the blood–brain barrier but can be administered intraventricularly. 6-Hydroxydopamine accumulates within the neurons following its uptake by the amine pump and causes a dramatic reduction in catecholamines. This can result in a permanent "functional sympathectomy."

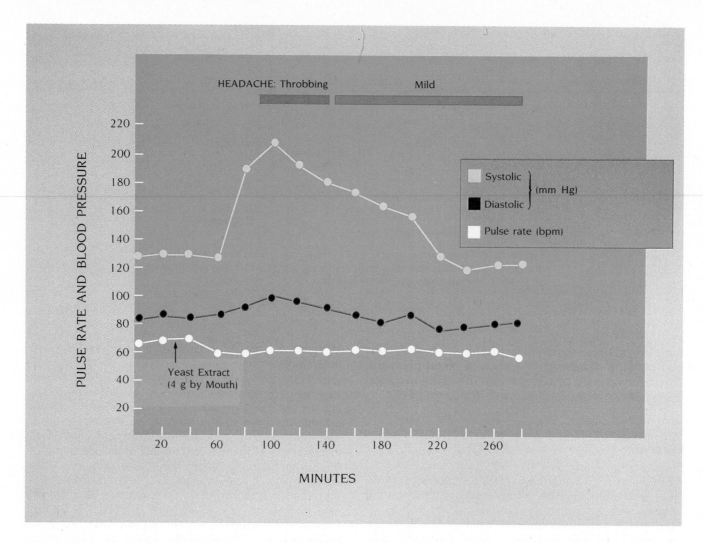

Figure 18–9 Hypertensive crisis in a woman receiving the MAO inhibitor tranylcypromine for the treatment of depression, when eating yeast extract containing tyramine.

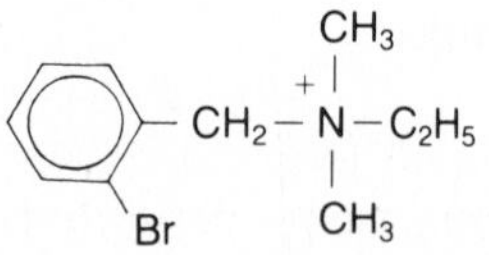

Figure 18–10 Structural formula of bretylium.

SUGGESTED READING

Davies DS, Reid JL, eds. Central action of drugs in blood pressure regulation. Baltimore: University Park Press, 1975.

Hryduk K, Bock DK, eds. Central blood pressure regulation: the role of alpha$_2$-receptor stimulation. Darmstadt: Steinkopff Verlag, 1983.

Chapter 19

NEUROMUSCULAR TRANSMISSION AND DRUGS (MUSCLE RELAXANTS)

L. Spero

The motor nerve fibres coming from the anterior horn cells of the spinal cord are myelinated up to the point where the fibres enter the muscle, after which each single nerve fibre divides into as many as 200 branches. These terminal branches are not myelinated, but they are covered by a Schwann cell. Normally, each nerve terminal branch forms a single endplate region on a single muscle fibre (Fig. 19–1).

Note that the synaptic vesicles within the nerve terminal are clustered immediately opposite the junctional folds of the sarcolemma. The acetylcholine receptors of the sarcolemma are located at the mouths of the junctional folds and constitute at least 90% of the endplate membrane.

CELLULAR EVENTS IN NERVE-MUSCLE TRANSMISSION

Impulse Invasion of the Nerve Terminal

The nerve action potential travels along the motor nerve fibre by saltatory conduction between nodes of Ranvier until it arrives at the point where the motor fibre enters the muscle. After this point the nerve fibre is not myelinated, and the action potential propagates into the terminals in the same fashion as it would in any unmyelinated fibre.

Release of Acetylcholine

The events related to the release of acetylcholine constitute a cycle that is illustrated in Figure 19–2. (For synthesis of acetylcholine see Chapter 13.) The discrete steps in this cycle are as follows.

1. As with regular action potentials, there is a small influx of Ca^{2+} associated with the action potential of the nerve terminal.

2. Since the surfaces of the membranes of the vesicles (and of the cell) are negatively charged, the entering Ca^{2+} neutralizes the charges and causes vesicles to approach the prejunctional membrane.

3. The vesicle then spontaneously fuses with the presynaptic membrane, releasing the enclosed acetylcholine by exocytosis.

4. The membrane of the vesicle, now incorporated into the presynaptic membrane, is pulled back into the cytoplasm by contractile filaments, which form a basket around the empty vesicle.

5. The basket vesicles lose their baskets and form a cistern. Within this cistern, acetylcholine is made by the action of choline acetyltransferase on choline and acetyl-CoA.

6. Vesicles containing acetylcholine then bud off from this cistern. The entire cycle from (1) to (6) is very fast and is of the order of seconds or minutes at most.

Production of Endplate Potentials

Within 0.1 millisecond the released acetylcholine diffuses across the 200 Å junctional cleft and interacts with the acetylcholine receptors on the specialized endplate region of the sarcolemma.

Each vesicle releases about 10,000 molecules of acetylcholine, which act on the nicotinic cholinergic receptors on the outside of the endplate. (Acetylcholine injected inside the muscle has no effect.)

The stimulated receptors then almost simultaneously

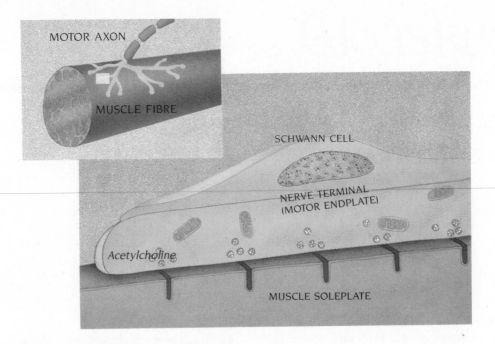

Figure 19–1 Schema of nerve-muscle junction.

open up channels for Ca^{2+}, Na^+, and K^+ in the endplate. The net result is an endplate potential. If only a single vesicle (a "quantum" of acetylcholine) is released, as occurs spontaneously at a rate of about two per second, only a miniature endplate potential (MEPP) develops, as shown in Figure 19–3. When a nerve impulse invades the nerve terminal, however, about 200 vesicles are released simultaneously, producing a normal endplate potential of 10–15 mV.

The endplate potential is a graded event and depends on the number of vesicles of acetylcholine released and the number of acetylcholine molecules interacting with the receptors. The amplitude of the endplate potential is greater with repeated stimulation of the nerve (this is called post-tetanic potentiation or PTP) and is due to an increased concentration of K^+ within the synapse, which depolarizes the nerve terminal so that an increased amount of acetylcholine is released. If the endplate potential exceeds 15 mV, the sarcolemmal membrane surrounding the endplate is raised above its threshold and an action potential is produced (Fig. 19–4). All-or-none action potentials do not originate within the endplate.

Excitation-Contraction Coupling in Muscle

The action potential travels along the surface membrane and is carried into the central portion of the muscle fibre by the transverse tubular system. The transverse tubules (T-tubules) are invaginations of the plasma membrane. They form part of the internal membrane system (also referred to as the triads). Each transverse tubule is bounded on either side by the lateral cisternae of the sarcoplasmic reticulum (thus the name triad). Electron microscopic studies have revealed a continuity (it appears as a fuzziness) between the membrane of the transverse tubules and the membrane of the lateral cisternae. This has led to the suggestion that, just as the action potential can depolarize the plasma membrane and the T-tubules, it can also pass across the junction between T-tubules and lateral cisternae and depolarize the membranes of the sarcoplasmic reticulum (Fig. 19–5). This invasion of the sarcoplasmic reticulum produces a release of Ca^{2+} from the reticulum. Normally, the Ca^{2+} concentration in the cytosol of the muscle is about 10^{-7} M or less. The Ca^{2+} released from the reticulum may bring the

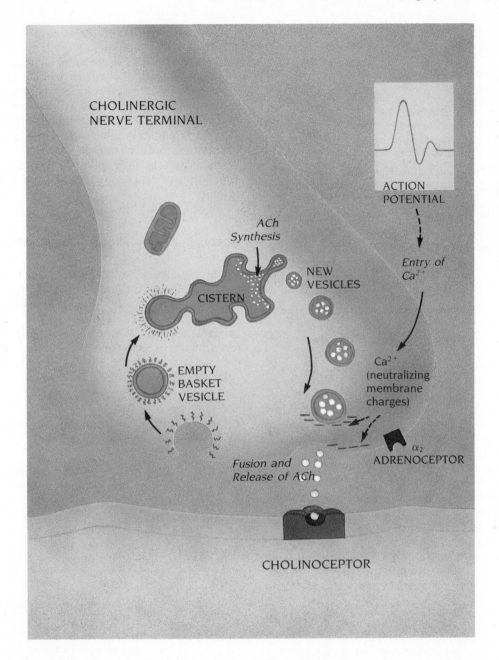

Figure 19–2 Cellular events in nerve-muscle impulse transmission.

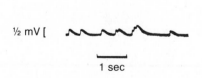

Figure 19–3 Miniature endplate potentials from the release of single vesicles of acetylcholine.

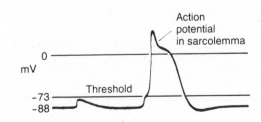

Figure 19–4 Action potential.

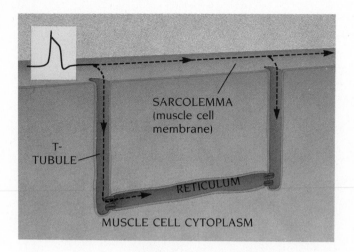

Figure 19–5 Suggested path of action potential across the internal membrane system.

cytosol Ca^{2+} level to around 10^{-6} M or so, thus triggering the troponin-actin-myosin interactions (discussed in Chapter 34).

The sarcoplasmic reticulum continuously pumps Ca^{2+} out of the cytosol, and this pump becomes more active during a contraction. Within a few milliseconds the Ca^{2+} concentration in the cytosol is reduced below 10^{-7} M and the muscle relaxes (Fig. 19–6).

The tension developed is a function of the intracellular Ca^{2+} concentration, which in turn depends on the rate of release of Ca^{2+} from the sarcoplasmic reticulum and the rate of its reabsorption into the sarcoplasmic reticulum. As the frequency of stimulation of the muscle increases, the sarcoplasmic reticulum is unable to lower the Ca^{2+} concentration below 10^{-7} M between stimuli, so that the baseline tension is elevated

and there is incomplete relaxation between twitches; this state is called clonus. When the rate of stimulation is increased further there is no significant reduction in Ca^{2+} concentration between stimuli, and a sustained tetanic contraction results. Once this frequency is reached, further increases in frequency can produce graded increases in the tetanic tension (Fig. 19–7). Tetanic stimulation, and not a single twitch, is the physiologic state of muscle contraction, and different types of muscle have different intrinsic frequencies at which they are physiologically stimulated, *i.e.*, become tetanic.

Acetylcholine Breakdown and Re-uptake of Choline

When it diffuses away from the nicotinic cholinergic receptor, acetylcholine is broken down by acetylcholinesterase to acetic acid and choline. The choline reenters the nerve terminal by an active transport process. Up to 90% of the acetylcholine released from the nerve terminal may be broken down by acetylcholinesterase in the synaptic cleft before it even reaches the receptors.

Characterization of Cholinergic Nicotinic Receptors at the Neuromuscular Junction

These nicotinic receptors are distinct from the nicotinic receptors in autonomic ganglia (*see* Chapter 13),

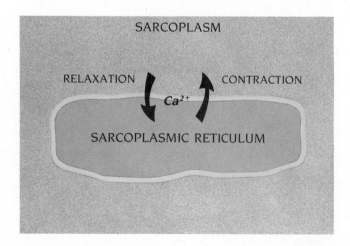

Figure 19–6 Calcium-concentration-dependent muscular contraction and relaxation.

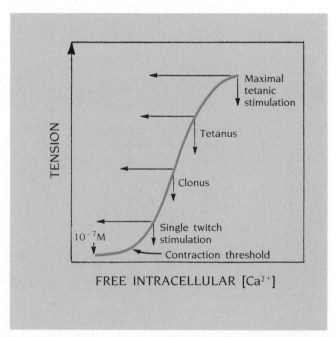

Figure 19–7 Various forms of muscle contraction dependent on baseline tension and intracellular calcium concentration.

and as can be seen in Table 19–1, they do not readily bind muscarinic cholinergic agonists or antagonists. This type of nicotinic receptor also has been found in the brain and in the electric organs (electroplax) of certain fish (torpedo) and the electric eel.

From Table 19–1 it is clear that agonists and antagonists bind to the receptor with similar affinities. This receptor does not appear to have separate subsites for agonists and antagonists. The receptor has been isolated and purified and even reconstituted into artificial membranes. The availability of antibodies to the pure receptor has been most useful in determining the level of receptors in a number of skeletal muscle diseases and in identifying the genetic determinants of receptor subtypes.

The radioreceptor binding assay with ^{131}I α-bungarotoxin can also be used to predict the potency of new nicotinic antagonists as neuromuscular blockers.

Binding of acetylcholine to this receptor leads to the influx of anions and cations through an ionophore that appears not to be ion-specific. The more receptors are occupied, the greater is the number of ionophores that are "open", and the larger are the ion fluxes down their electrochemical gradients. This is the basis for the graded endplate potential (Fig. 19–8).

Desensitization of Acetylcholine Receptors

The interaction of acetylcholine with the nicotinic receptor first leads to an "activated" state of the receptor, which goes to an inactive (desensitized) state when the acetylcholine dissociates from it. This then slowly reverts to the ground state.

Under physiologic conditions, because of the high efficacy of acetylcholine, a response can be elicited by occupying only 20–30% of the receptors; the rest constitutes a receptor reserve ("spare receptors"). This means that at any time as many as 10–20% of the receptors may be in the inactive state. A situation that would lead to an increase in the number of receptors in the inactive state can lead to blockade of the neuromuscular junction.

TABLE 19–1 Nicotinic Receptor Binding*

Competing Cold Ligand	Electroplax Receptors†	Rat Brain Receptors‡	Rat Diaphragm Receptors§
Nicotinic Agonists			
Nicotine	18.0 μM	3.1 μM	—
Acetylcholine	1.5 μM	30.0 μM	0.47 μM
Carbachol	40.0 μM	90.0 μM	3.5 μM
Nicotinic "Depolarizing"-Type Antagonists			
Decamethonium	0.8 μM	500 μM	2.1 μM
Succinylcholine	—	1,500 μM	1.33 μM
Nicotinic "Competitive"-Type Antagonists			
d-Tubocurarine	0.17 μM	1.9 μM	0.24 μM
Gallamine	0.44 μM	3.5 μM	1.7 μM
Nicotinic Ganglion Blocker			
Hexamethonium	61 μM	900 μM	118 μM
Muscarinic Agonists			
Muscarine	—	10,000 μM	—
Oxotremorine	—	2,000 μM	—
Muscarinic Antagonist			
Atropine	—	1,600 μM	—
Cholinesterase Inhibitor			
Physostigmine	—	2,000 μM	—

* IC$_{50}$ values for various cholinergic agonists and antagonists against ^{131}I α-bungarotoxin, a specific nicotinic antagonist at the neuromuscular junction, which labels nicotinic cholinergic receptors at nicotinic sites from various sources (See Chapter 9, *Drug Receptors*.) N.B. α-Bungarotoxin is a very slowly reversible ligand. These IC$_{50}$ values are therefore obtained from protection experiments and not from competition experiments. They are probably underestimates.
Sources:
† Weber M, Changeux JP. Mol Pharmacol 1974; 10:15–35.
‡ Schmidt J. Mol Pharmacol 1977; 13:283–290.
§ Colquhoun D, Rang HP. Mol Pharmacol 1976; 12:519–535.

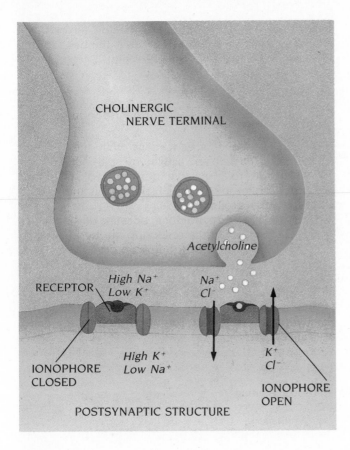

Figure 19–8 The function of ionophores in allowing ion fluxes in relation to receptor occupation by acetylcholine.

SUBSTANCES AFFECTING ACETYLCHOLINE RELEASE

Local and general anaesthetics have varying degrees of blocking action on the prejunctional nerve terminals, thus preventing nerve impulses from triggering the acetylcholine release sequence (*see* Chapter 24, *Local Anaesthetics*).

Ethanol. Ethanol at low concentrations (5–20 mM) enhances the fusion of acetylcholine vesicle membranes to the prejunctional membrane. Hence, ethanol increases the amount of acetylcholine released by an action potential. This also occurs in the spinal cord and possibly in the CNS. Higher concentrations (40–80 mM) of ethanol inhibit the release of acetylcholine. (N.B. In Canada, a person is not legally permitted to drive when the blood alcohol level is at or above 80 mg/dL; this is equivalent to about 22 mM in body water. In many American states, the corresponding levels are 100 mg/dL and 28 mM.)

Black widow spider venom. This substance causes a dramatic and almost complete release of all acetylcholine vesicles from the nerve ending. This explains why the victim of such a spider bite presents with signs of muscle and abdominal cramps. The vesicles may not subsequently be refilled, and *de novo* synthesis of vesicles is required.

Botulinum toxin. This toxin from the bacterial spores of *Clostridium botulinum* blocks the release of acetylcholine from the vesicles. It kills in very low concentrations.

Calcium. Ca^{2+} increases the release of acetylcholine, as might be reasoned.

Magnesium. Mg^{2+} decreases the release of acetylcholine.

NICOTINIC ANTAGONISTS AT THE NEUROMUSCULAR JUNCTION: MUSCLE RELAXANTS

These antagonists selectively block the nicotinic receptors at the neuromuscular junction. They do not affect motor nerves, nor do they block direct stimulation of the muscle. Side effects due to ganglion blockade are occasionally observed. These drugs are used in surgery as muscle relaxants because, while all general anaesthetics are able to cause muscle relaxation, this state is reached only during deep general anaesthesia when most other nervous functions are also severely depressed. By combining muscle relaxants and anaesthetics, one can obtain a surgically adequate skeletal muscle relaxation at relatively moderate levels of CNS depression.

Some degree of muscle relaxation can also be achieved by the blockade of interneurons with drugs of the benzodiazepine and propanediol carbamate classes (''minor tranquilizers''). These act at the level of the spinal cord. However, the muscle relaxants of this class lack some of the desirable selectivity. Their use is limited to treatment of acute muscle spasms associated with trauma and inflammation, and for certain orthopedic manipulations. (Benzodiazepines are described in Chapter 26.)

Nondepolarizing Competitive Blockers

d-Tubocurarine

The classical example of drugs acting in this manner is curare (the generic term for various South American arrow poisons). Claude Bernard demonstrated in 1856 that the site of paralytic action of curare is the synapse between nerve and skeletal muscle. The crude agent remained a pharmacologic curiosity until the 1940s, when one of the pure alkaloids, d-tubocurarine, became available for use in general anaesthesia. The designation ''tubo-'' indicates that the crude material came from Indian tribes who carried their arrow poison in hollow bamboo tubes.

The competitive nondepolarizing neuromuscular blocking agents are relatively bulky, rigid molecules with two nitrogen groups held apart at a distance of approximately 12–14 Å (Fig. 19–9). These drugs compete with acetylcholine for its receptor sites at the endplate. They have zero efficacy; there is therefore no agonist action and no depolarization, and their actions are purely competitive.

The paralytic effects of d-tubocurarine can be reversed by increasing the concentrations of acetylcholine at the neuromuscular junction through inhibition of acetylcholinesterase. The drugs used for this purpose are neostigmine and edrophonium. The characteristics of their interactions with the neuromuscular junction are illustrated in Figure 19–10.

Tubocurarine (Tubarine®) is inactive by mouth and is always administered intravenously. A typical dose is 0.3 mg/kg. It is distributed widely in body tissues but is concentrated in the neuromuscular junctions. It does not enter the CNS and does not pass the placenta. About one-third of the dose is excreted in the urine over several hours. However, the action on the neuromuscular junctions begins to wear off after about 20 minutes because of redistribution of the drug.

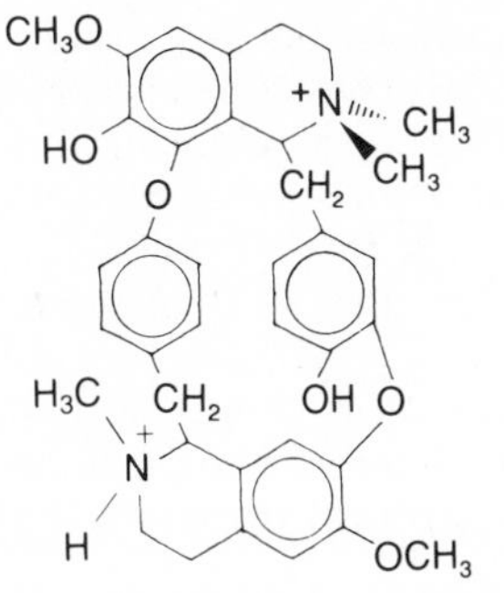

Figure 19–9 Structural formula of d-tubocurarine.

Curare causes progressive paralysis, starting with the muscles of the face, then the limbs, and finally the respiratory musculature. Cardiac and smooth muscles are not affected, but very high doses will block autonomic ganglia. Curare releases histamine, causing transient hypotension depending on the speed of administration. The drug has no analgesic properties, nor does

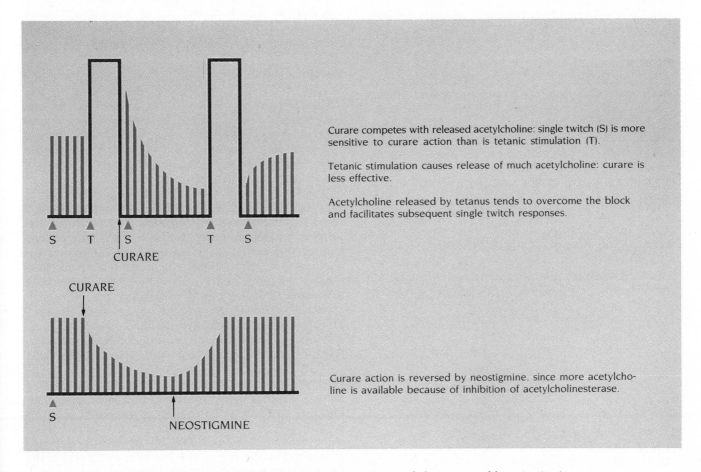

Curare competes with released acetylcholine: single twitch (S) is more sensitive to curare action than is tetanic stimulation (T).

Tetanic stimulation causes release of much acetylcholine: curare is less effective.

Acetylcholine released by tetanus tends to overcome the block and facilitates subsequent single twitch responses.

Curare action is reversed by neostigmine, since more acetylcholine is available because of inhibition of acetylcholinesterase.

Figure 19–10 The effects of curare on skeletal muscle contraction, and their reversal by neostigmine.

it affect consciousness. Since clinically useful muscle relaxation requires doses that impair or paralyse respiratory muscles, artificial respiration is necessary and must be available whenever curariform drugs are used. With artificial respiration it is possible to survive without harm doses of tubocurarine that would otherwise be fatal.

Some antibiotics (*e.g.*, aminoglycosides) potentiate curare action, and different general anaesthetics require reduction of the optimal dose of curare to different extents.

d-Tubocurarine is used in conjunction with general anaesthesia when prolonged or profound muscle relaxation is required for the purposes of surgery. The drug may have to be applied for days or weeks in cases of tetanus (*i.e.*, the disease caused by the tetanus bacillus, not the physiologic type of muscle contraction).

Pancuronium

Pancuronium (Pavulon®; Fig. 19–11) is now widely used. It is five times as potent as tubocurarine and it has a faster onset and a shorter duration of action. It does not release histamine, and in most patients it has no circulatory effects. It is used with caution in patients with impaired cardiovascular function because it can increase the blood pressure, possibly by ganglionic stimulation.

Atracurium

Atracurium (Tracrium®) is a nondepolarizing skeletal neuromuscular blocking agent that has a rapid onset and short duration of action. It is degraded nonenzymatically at pH 7.4 as well as being excreted unchanged by the kidneys. It is of particular usefulness in patients with renal failure. Cardiovascular side effects are less than with other competitive nicotinic receptor antagonists.

Desensitizing (Depolarizing) Blockers

These nicotinic receptor antagonists are noncompetitive and produce their effects by desensitizing the recep-

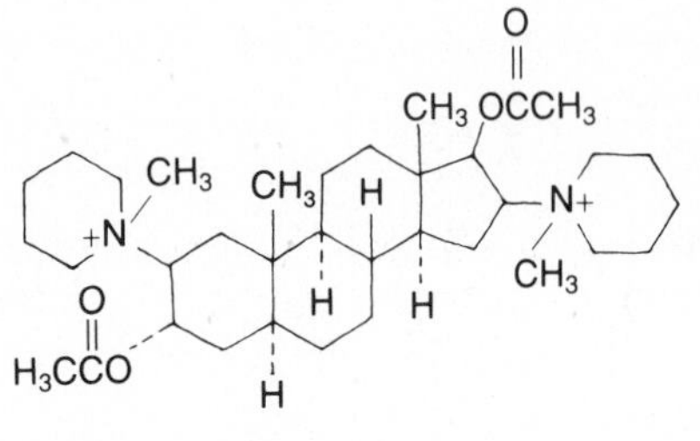

Figure 19–11 Structural formula of pancuronium.

tors in the neuromuscular junction. They act to produce effects similar to those of an excess of acetylcholine (either added exogenously or accumulated endogenously after cholinesterase inhibition). *In vitro* there is an initial stimulation of the endplate, which becomes depolarized, and the muscle contracts. Subsequently the endplate remains depolarized (for about 2–3 minutes) while the muscle relaxes. Within a further few minutes the endplate repolarizes, but the muscle is still relaxed and the endplate is unresponsive to normal acetylcholine release.

These phenomena can be explained in terms of desensitization of receptors. The depolarization occurs because these "antagonists" have both affinity and efficacy and the receptors are activated. As an excess of receptors become activated, a large fraction of the receptors are converted to the inactive state. Since the endplate membrane protein is almost solely receptor, its properties are changed, and the endplate potential no longer propagates into the sarcolemmal membrane. There are no further action potentials and the muscle relaxes. At this stage there are still sufficient "spare receptors" for the endplate potential to be maintained. As more receptors are desensitized (inactivated), the endplate potential drops, the endplate repolarizes, and the endplate is now insensitive to acetylcholine or nerve stimulation. The characteristics of the interactions of desensitizing (depolarizing) blockers in the neuromuscular junction are illustrated in Figure 19–12.

Succinylcholine

This drug (Fig. 19–13) is hydrolysed by plasma cholinesterase but not by acetylcholinesterase; it acts like an excess of acetylcholine once it reaches the neuromuscular synaptic cleft. It cannot cross the blood–brain barrier or placenta and does not release histamine.

Special features of succinylcholine (Anectine®) are its rapid onset of action (approximately one circulation time) and short duration of action (2–3 minutes). The latter is a function of the drug's hydrolysis by plasma cholinesterase. (There are rare genetic variants of this cholinesterase that do not readily hydrolyse succinylcholine, as described in Chapter 12. The duration of action may then be greatly prolonged. Therefore, succinylcholine should be used only when facilities are available for giving artificial respiration.)

The depolarizing blockade produced by succinylcholine is clinically different from nondepolarizing blockade:

1. Depolarizing blockade is preceded by muscle stimulation that takes the form of an initial, irregular, and uncoordinated contraction of muscle fibres. This state is referred to as fasciculation, it is generally of short duration (5–30 seconds), and its intensity depends somewhat on the speed of intravenous injection of the drug. Some patients have sore muscles after succinylcholine, as an untrained subject does after exercise.

2. Since depolarizing blockade is akin to having an

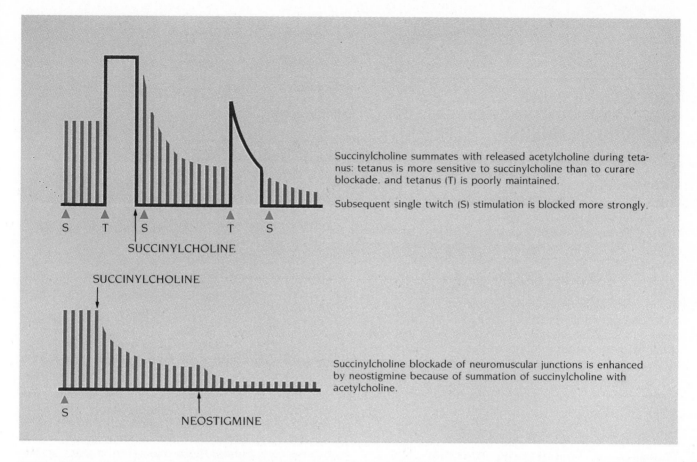

Succinylcholine summates with released acetylcholine during tetanus: tetanus is more sensitive to succinylcholine than to curare blockade, and tetanus (T) is poorly maintained.

Subsequent single twitch (S) stimulation is blocked more strongly.

Succinylcholine blockade of neuromuscular junctions is enhanced by neostigmine because of summation of succinylcholine with acetylcholine.

Figure 19–12 The effects of succinylcholine on skeletal muscle contraction (compare with Fig. 19–10).

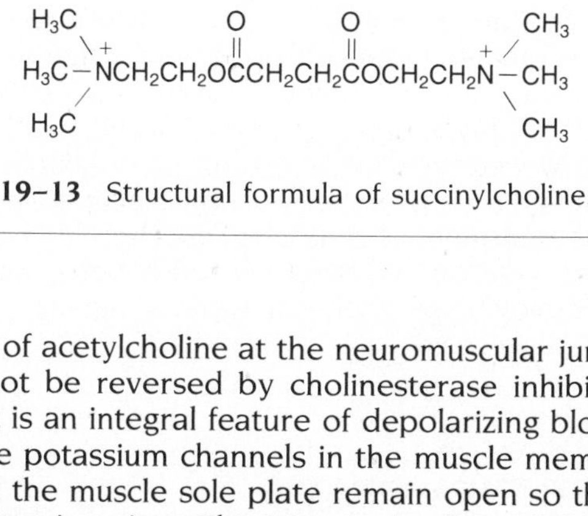

Figure 19–13 Structural formula of succinylcholine.

excess of acetylcholine at the neuromuscular junction, it cannot be reversed by cholinesterase inhibitors.

3. It is an integral feature of depolarizing blockade that the potassium channels in the muscle membrane around the muscle sole plate remain open so that serum potassium rises. This increase is often minimal and usually of no clinical significance. However, it can lead to symptoms of severe hyperkalemia with consequent cardiac arrest in patients with many freshly denervated muscles (as after spinal injury), with extensive burns, and with uremia.

The clinical use of succinylcholine takes advantage of its rapid and short action. The two main uses are, therefore, to facilitate tracheal intubation for artificial ventilation during general anaesthesia and to paralyse skeletal muscles during electroconvulsive (shock) therapy of mental disorders.

The neuromuscular effects of toxic (lethal) doses of nicotine and of anticholinesterases are similar to those of succinylcholine in principle, although not usually in the rate of development. The action of these drugs on the neuromuscular junction is also of the depolarizing type and, therefore, cannot be antagonized by pharmacologic means; survival may depend on prompt artificial ventilation.

Succinylcholine is metabolized by butyrylcholinesterase to succinylmonocholine. This metabolite is a **competitive** cholinergic nicotinic antagonist. It may accumulate during prolonged use of succinylcholine, and its effect may persist following the termination of succinylcholine administration. Competitive blockade by this metabolite can be reversed by cholinesterase inhibitors.

DRUGS ACTING ON EXCITATION-CONTRACTION COUPLING IN MUSCLE

Caffeine

Normally a muscle does not begin to contract until the membrane potential has been reduced to about -50 mV. But in the presence of caffeine (*in vitro*) the muscle begins to contract at about -65 mV.

It is thought that caffeine produces this muscle "sensitization" by releasing Ca^{2+} either from the sarcoplasmic reticulum or from the sarcolemmal membrane.

Caffeine (*in vitro*) produces contracture of muscle in the concentration range of 1–5 mM, and this may occur without depolarization of the cell membrane.

Caffeine, like theophylline, blocks the phosphodiesterase of tissues, thus enhancing the action of cyclic AMP. It may also inhibit the binding of adenosine to the adenosine receptor, which may play a role in muscle.

Dantrolene in Malignant Hyperthermia

General anaesthetics such as halothane and other uncharged anaesthetic molecules can make the muscle reticulum "leaky" to Ca^{2+}, particularly in genetically vulnerable subjects. Such patients exhibit the life-threatening syndrome of malignant hyperthermia (*see* Chapter 12). The muscles go into contracture and enormous amounts of heat are produced. This is a result of the Ca^{2+} increasing the respiratory quotient of the muscle mitochondria. The incidence of this disease is approximately 1 in 200,000.

The outcome of an attack of malignant hyperthermia is greatly improved if the patient is cooled quickly and given dantrolene (Dantrium®), a drug that increases the binding of Ca^{2+} to the sarcolemma and sarcoplasmic reticulum and can restore normal calcium movements across the membranes.

Local Anaesthetics

Procainamide and other procaine-like local anaesthetics also block the release of Ca^{2+} from muscle reticulum, inhibiting muscle contracture states. These positively charged drugs may simply stop the exit of Ca^{2+} from reticulum by "coating" the reticulum membrane with their positive charges, as in Figure 19–14.

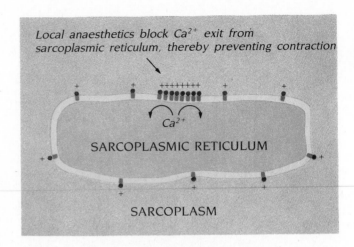

Local anaesthetics block Ca^{2+} exit from sarcoplasmic reticulum, thereby preventing contraction

Ca^{2+}

SARCOPLASMIC RETICULUM

SARCOPLASM

Figure 19–14 Effect of local anaesthetics on the movement of calcium ions across the reticulum membrane.

DRUGS ACTING ON CHOLINESTERASE

If cholinesterase is inhibited, then the effective concentration of acetylcholine in the synaptic cleft is increased. This is the essential mechanism of action of cholinesterase inhibitors. After administration of one of these compounds, the response to applied acetylcholine is increased, *i.e.*, the depolarization produced by acetylcholine is greater in the presence of a cholinesterase inhibitor.

As described in Chapter 14, cholinesterase inhibitors can be divided into two categories, reversible and irreversible. The reversible inhibitors include physostigmine, neostigmine, and edrophonium. They are used clinically for the termination of curare block and in the treatment of myasthenia gravis. Clinical use of irreversible cholinesterase inhibitors (organophosphates) is rare, though their prolonged action is occasionally useful in the treatment of glaucoma, but these compounds are used widely as insecticides and have occasionally been employed as chemical warfare agents (the so-called "nerve gases").

MYASTHENIA GRAVIS

Myasthenia gravis is a chronic disease characterized by muscular weakness of fluctuating intensity. It is aggravated by physical activity and improved by rest. The weakness is not associated with any significant atrophy of the muscles, at least in the earlier stages of the disease.

Myasthenia gravis was recognized by Erb (1879) and by Goldflam (1893), whose clinical characterization of the disorder is still valid. The symptoms are primarily due to dysfunction of the motor system. The muscles of the eyes, of the larynx, and of mastication are often affected first and most seriously. Later the muscles of the trunk and extremities may become involved (less often the symptoms of myasthenia gravis first appear in these muscles). Characteristically, an involved muscle rapidly becomes progressively weaker upon exercise. Most patients are better in the morning than in the afternoon. Remissions and relapses occur. Paralysis of the respiratory muscles may cause the death of some patients.

Noting the similarity between the symptoms shown by laboratory animals treated with curare and those of patients suffering from myasthenia gravis, Mary Walker in 1934 treated a myasthenic patient with physostigmine and observed a therapeutic effect. It became generally accepted that the clinically observed muscular weakness was caused by a neuromuscular blockade; this concept was confirmed by the supersensitivity of myasthenia gravis patients to tubocurarine (which is used as a diagnostic test).

It is now known that myasthenia gravis is an autoimmune disease in which antibodies to nicotinic receptors are produced in the thymus. The antibodies reduce the number of available receptors at the neuromuscular junction. The antibody-receptor interaction also leads to structural damage in the synaptic cleft, the postjunctional membrane loses its characteristic folds, and the cleft itself widens. The consequence of all these changes is that less acetylcholine reaches a smaller number of receptors.

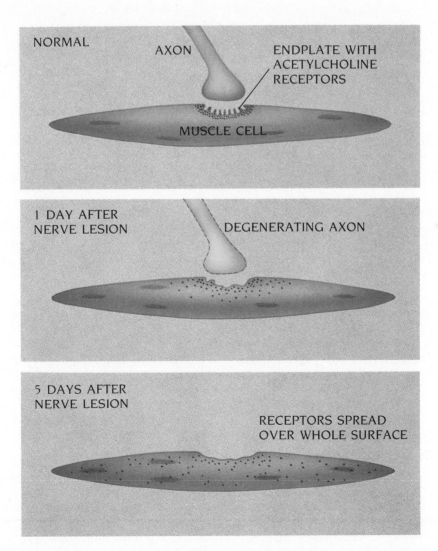

Figure 19–15 Effects of nerve lesion on acetylcholine receptor distribution. Sensitivity to acetylcholine is determined by the spread and distribution of receptors.

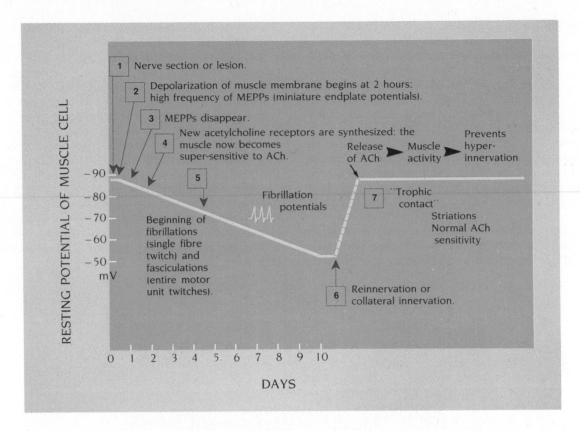

Figure 19–16 Concepts of denervation sensitivity.

Some patients respond to thymectomy, and steroids have been used to reduce the immune response. All patients are treated with neostigmine (75–300 mg orally, spaced over 24 hours as required) or a combination of neostigmine and atropine (to reduce cardiovascular complications), which increases the concentration of acetylcholine reaching the receptors. The action begins within 1–2 hours, lasting approximately 5 hours. For diagnostic purposes (myasthenic crisis versus neostigmine excess) a short-acting anticholinesterase such as edrophonium (Tensilon®) can be used; remission of symptoms during the test indicates a myasthenic crisis.

NERVE-MUSCLE EVENTS FOLLOWING NERVE SECTION OR LESION

In denervated muscles, the acetylcholine receptors are found all along the muscle membrane, not only at the endplate. This gives rise to denervation supersensitivity, and the muscle, having more receptors, is now more sensitive to exogenous acetylcholine. Inhibitors of protein synthesis can prevent the development of this supersensitivity, indicating that synthesis of receptors may be involved. Some forms of muscular dystrophy are thought to be associated with partial denervation of the muscles. Nerve fibres contain some trophic factor, not as yet isolated or identified, that acts to keep acetylcholine receptors localized to the endplate region, and that keeps the muscle fully developed. This same phenomenon is observed in reverse during the embryonic development of neuromuscular junctions. Here the muscle myotube is first covered with receptors, but as a nerve terminal makes contact with it, the receptors concentrate in the endplate region.

The spread of nicotinic receptors is accompanied by a spread of acetylcholinesterase. This is illustrated in Figure 19–15.

In the supersensitive muscle the nature of the action potentials has also changed since they can no longer be blocked by tetrodotoxin. It is as if all of the properties of the endplate (whose graded response is not blocked by tetrodotoxin) have spread out. The physiology of denervation supersensitivity is illustrated in Figure 19–16.

SUGGESTED READING

Brehm P, Henderson L. Regulation of acetylcholine receptor channel function during development of skeletal muscle. Dev Biol 1988; 129:1–11.

Lindstrom J. Using monoclonal antibodies to study acetylcholine receptors in myasthenia gravis. Neurosci Comment 1983; 1:139–157.

Stanley EF, Drachman DB. Rapid degradation of new acetylcholine receptors at the neuromuscular junction. Science 1983; 222:67–69.

Torda TA. The neuromuscular blocking drugs. Med J Aust 1988; 149:316–319.

CENTRAL NERVOUS SYSTEM

—

Chapter 20

DRUGS ACTING ON THE BASAL GANGLIA

W.M. Burnham

In mammals, the control of conscious ("voluntary") movement depends on a large number of CNS structures. The highest of these is the motor cortex. Closely allied to the motor cortex is a group of subcortical structures called the basal ganglia. While the exact function of the basal ganglia is not yet clear, pathology of these structures is known to cause a loss of control over voluntary movements. Two major types of disability are observed. In some cases, an individual loses the ability to initiate voluntary movement and freezes into immobility ("hypokinesia", "akinesia"). In other cases, "voluntary-type" movements begin to occur even when they are not wanted ("hyperkinesia", "dyskinesia"). In both cases, reflex function remains normal.

Traditionally, the prognosis for patients afflicted with hypo- or hyperkinetic syndromes was considered to be poor. During the past 20 years, however, we have begun to understand the biochemical basis of basal-ganglion dysfunction, and to evolve drugs that can alleviate (though not cure) two of the most common syndromes: Parkinson's disease and Huntington's chorea.

BASAL GANGLIA

Definitions

The term "basal ganglia" is applied to a group of forebrain structures, which includes the caudate-putamen (for physiologists, the "striatum") and the globus pallidus (the "pallidum") (Fig. 20–1). The caudate and putamen are structurally distinct in the human, but they are joined in lower mammals, and they are generally considered to function as a unit. Closely associated with the basal ganglia are two small brain-stem nuclei, the substantia nigra and the subthalamus.

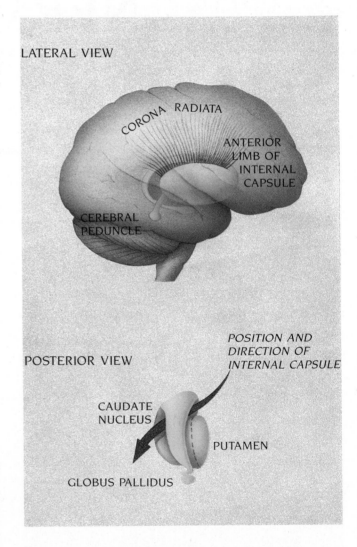

Figure 20–1 The caudate-putamen and the globus pallidus. Substantia nigra and subthalamus are not shown.

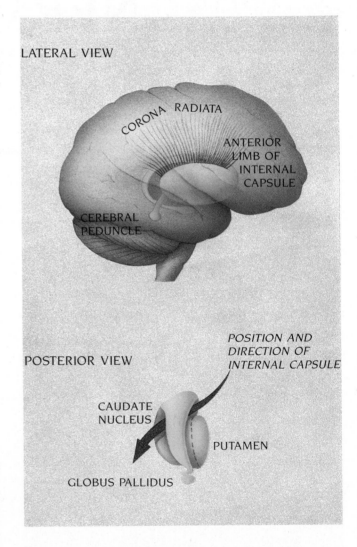

LATERAL VIEW

CORONA RADIATA

ANTERIOR LIMB OF INTERNAL CAPSULE

CEREBRAL PEDUNCLE

POSTERIOR VIEW

POSITION AND DIRECTION OF INTERNAL CAPSULE

CAUDATE NUCLEUS

PUTAMEN

GLOBUS PALLIDUS

Neural Connections

The complete connections of the basal ganglia are complex and not fully understood. Major pathways, however, are as follows (Fig. 20–2).

Through-put pathway. All parts of the neocortex project to the caudate-putamen. The caudate-putamen itself projects to the globus pallidus, which in turn projects to areas in the thalamus (VA, VL in Fig. 20–2). These connect back to the motor cortex. Thus, the major "through-put" pathway seems to be a progression from the cortex as a whole to the basal ganglia and then back to the motor cortex.

Feedback loops. In addition to the through-put pathway, there are two smaller (feedback?) loops that are important in basal-ganglion dysfunction. One of these connects the outer segment of the globus pallidus to its inner segment *via* the subthalamic nucleus. Damage to the subthalamus causes a rare hyperkinetic syndrome called hemiballismus, a condition in which the contralateral limbs make large uncontrolled swinging motions. The second loop runs from the caudate-putamen down to the substantia nigra and back. The connections from substantia nigra to caudate-putamen are called the nigrostriatal pathway. This loop is crucially involved in Parkinson's disease, a disorder involving severe hypokinesia.

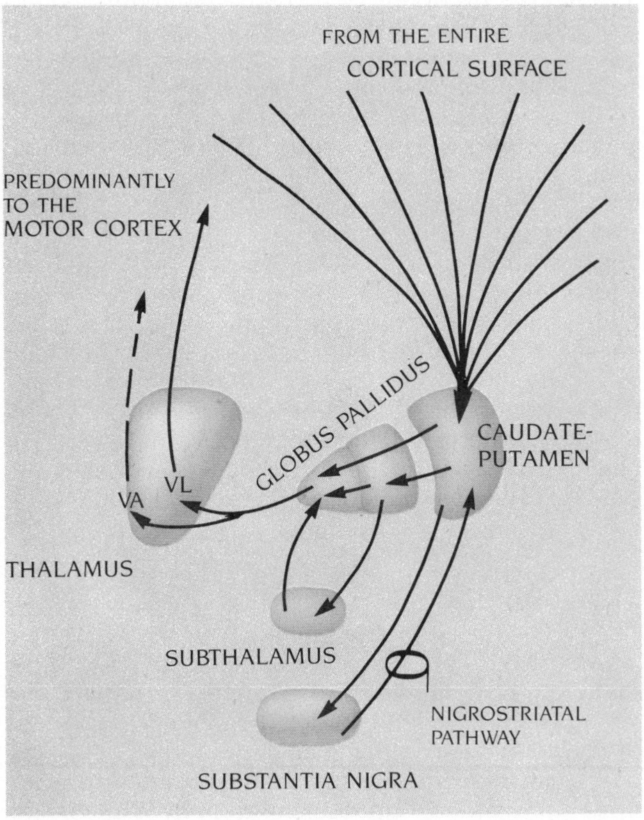

Neurotransmitters

The caudate-putamen contains a number of putative neurotransmitter substances, including noradrenaline* (NA), serotonin (5-HT), glutamate (Glu), gamma-aminobutyric acid (GABA), dopamine (DA) and acetylcholine (ACh). Figure 20–3 indicates the postulated relationship of three of these, GABA, ACh, and DA. Output pathways of the caudate-putamen, including the fibres that go to the substantia nigra, are postulated to be GABAergic. Activity in these is thought to be modulated by excitatory ACh interneurons and by inhibitory input from the substantia nigra (DA). (Note that the connections shown in Fig. 20–3 are hypothetical. The actual connections are unknown and even the excitatory/inhibitory actions of the transmitters are under debate.) Normal function of the caudate-putamen depends on the balance of these transmitters, and particularly on the balance of DA and ACh. In terms of the behavioral output, DA seems to be the "go" system, while ACh seems to be the "no go" system. An excess of DA, therefore, produces an excess of movement, while an excess of ACh produces immobility. It may seem paradoxical that an inhibitory transmitter produces movement while an excitatory transmitter produces immo-

---

* norepinephrine

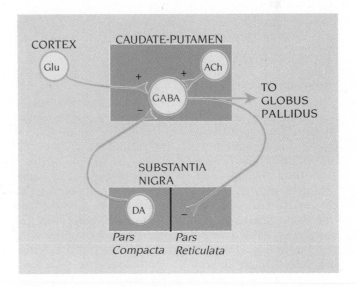

Figure 20–3 Possible (hypothetical) interrelation between transmitters in the caudate-putamen and substantia nigra (*see* text.) Glu = glutamate; ACh = acetylcholine; DA = dopamine; GABA = gamma-aminobutyric acid; (+) = excitatory; (−) = inhibitory.

Figure 20–2 Schematic, simplified representation of major connections of the basal ganglia. (VA = thalamus ventralis anterior; VL = thalamus ventralis lateralis.)

bility. It must be remembered, however, that striatal neurons are separated from the muscles by many synapses and many levels of excitation and inhibition. Inhibition and excitation in the brain can not be equated with inhibition and excitation in behavior.

PARKINSON'S DISEASE

Clinical Syndrome

Parkinson's disease is the most common of the basal-ganglion disorders, occurring in one out of every 400 people. Its cardinal symptoms are:

- Akinesia (slowness or inability to initiate voluntary movements).
- Rigidity (stiffness in the skeletal muscles).
- Tremor at rest (shaking, which ceases when the affected limb is moved, but which returns when the movement comes to an end).

The most serious symptom is the akinesia, since the patient gradually freezes into immobility and becomes dependent on others for survival. The onset of Parkinson's disease usually occurs late in life (age 50–65), and the syndrome gradually worsens until the patient becomes helpless (about ten years). The causes are varied (Parkinson's disease actually is a syndrome rather than a specific disease). The most common causes are thought to be atherosclerosis and encephalitis lethargica. Many cases, however, are idiopathic (*i.e.*, they have no known cause). It is interesting and important to note that the parkinsonian syndrome also occurs as a reversible side effect of the neuroleptic drugs (*see* Chapter 27).

Neuropathology

A number of abnormalities are found in parkinsonian brains. The crucial anatomic change, however, seems to be a progressive loss of the pigmented cells in the substantia nigra, the cells that give rise to the nigrostriatal tract. Usually 80% or more of these are gone before symptoms appear. Since these cells release DA in the caudate-putamen, their loss causes a secondary biochemical change, a reduction of DA content in the caudate-putamen (eventually to 10% or less of normal). This results in a DA/ACh imbalance, which is the actual cause of the parkinsonian syndrome. Since ACh (''no go'') predominates, immobility results.

Drug Therapy

All of the drugs used in the treatment of Parkinson's disease act to correct the DA/ACh imbalance.

L-Dopa

When it was discovered that Parkinson's disease was associated with decreased DA in the caudate-putamen, attempts were made to replace the DA. Dopamine itself does not cross the blood–brain barrier, but its precursor, L-dopa (3,4-dihydroxyphenylalanine), crosses easily. In the presence of excess precursor the surviving DA neurons are able to increase their output of DA, and parkinsonian patients quickly return towards normal mobility. L-Dopa has therefore become the mainstay therapy for Parkinson's disease.

While the introduction of L-dopa (Larodopa®, Bendopa®, and others) has greatly improved the status of parkinsonian patients, the drug has some major drawbacks.

Relief is symptomatic. L-Dopa does not replace lost neurons, it just allows the surviving cells to work with greater efficiency. Thus, relief is symptomatic and lasts only while the compound (which has a short half-life) remains in the blood stream. The patient must be dosed several times a day for the duration of therapy.

Duration of relief is limited. Most researchers believe that substantia nigra cells continue to die even in the presence of L-dopa. Eventually, perhaps due to continued cell loss, L-dopa loses its potency.

Side effects. Many of these are related to the fact that L-dopa raises DA levels all over the nervous system, not just in the caudate-putamen. In the first few months of therapy, nausea is a problem in about 80% of the patients (the effect of circulating DA on the chemoreceptor trigger zone), and cardiac arrhythmias also occur in about 30% of patients (the effect of elevated DA on β_1 adrenoceptors of the heart). Orthostatic hypotension is also seen; the mechanism is unknown. Tolerance gradually develops to these early effects. After 2–4 months, however, another set of side effects begin to develop. Paradoxically, these late effects seem to relate to the development of DA hypersensitivity. They consist of hyperkinesias (80% of patients develop this after 1 year) and psychiatric abnormalities (anxiety, agitation, psychosis, in 15% of patients). Tolerance to these late side effects does not develop, although they disappear when L-dopa is discontinued.

Carbidopa

When a dose of L-dopa is administered orally, more than 90% is metabolized to DA in the periphery and less than 5% enters the brain. The systemic dopamine produced by peripheral metabolism causes side effects, but has no therapeutic action on the parkinsonian symptoms. Carbidopa is a peripheral decarboxylase inhibitor that prevents the systemic conversion of L-dopa to DA. It has no effect in the brain, since it does not cross the blood–brain barrier. When carbidopa and L-dopa are given in combination, a much smaller dose of L-dopa is required, and systemic side effects are lessened. Combined carbidopa and L-dopa (1:10 ratio) is marketed as a standard commercial preparation (Sinemet®).

Amantadine

Amantadine (Symmetrel®) was originally developed as a synthetic antiviral agent (*see* Chapter 58); its usefulness in Parkinson's disease was later discovered by chance. Amantadine appears to work by increasing DA release from the surviving nigral neurons. If L-dopa treatment has already stimulated DA production to a maximum, amantadine will have no added effect. Amantadine alone is somewhat less effective than L-dopa, but it also has fewer side effects. Insomnia and hallucinations may occur, but only at toxic levels. Unfortunately, tolerance to its therapeutic action develops after 6–8 weeks.

Anticholinergics (Muscarinic Blockers)

An alternate way to correct the DA/ACh imbalance in Parkinson's disease is to lower ACh activity. This can be achieved with muscarinic blockers (*see* Chapter 15), atropine-like drugs such as benztropine (Cogentin®) and trihexyphenidyl (Artane®). Anticholinergic therapy is actually the historic treatment for Parkinson's disease, having been used, without theoretical basis, for more than a century. The muscarinic blockers, however, are less effective than L-dopa, and they produce a wide variety of unpleasant side effects at therapeutic dose levels, including blurred vision, dryness of the mouth, constipation, urinary retention, and ataxia (*see* Chapter 15). Since the introduction of L-dopa, anticholinergics have been relegated to secondary status. They work by a different mechanism than L-dopa, and combination with L-dopa will therefore increase the maximum effect obtained.

Therapeutic Approaches

The drugs available for Parkinson's disease may be administered in a number of different ways. One approach is to start with muscarinic blockers when the syndrome is mild, and to add L-dopa and finally carbidopa as the syndrome worsens. Other physicians prefer to use L-dopa from the start. Amantadine may be administered for short periods to help the patient over "flare-ups". Whatever the approach, a crucial aspect of therapy is to balance the therapeutic effects of L-dopa against its side effects (*e.g.*, nausea). A good plan is to start with a low initial dose of L-dopa and to increase the level gradually as tolerance develops to the side effects of the drug.

Prognosis for Drug Therapy

While impressive results can be achieved in the short term, the long-term prognosis for control of Parkinson's disease is still not good. Studies suggest that the average patient obtains relief for up to 5 years, and then reverts to pretreatment conditions, perhaps because of the continued loss of cells in the substantia nigra. Since the disease often occurs late in life, the addition of 5 "good" years may be highly significant. Nevertheless, the present drugs are far from ideal, and the search continues to produce new ones.

New Directions in Therapy

MAO-B Inhibitors

One approach is to try to raise DA levels by attacking monoamine oxidase (MAO), an enzyme that breaks down DA. Nonspecific MAO inhibitors have been available for some time, but the use of these has been associated with serious dangers to the patient (*see* Chapter 28). Recently, drugs have been developed to attack MAO-B specifically (*e.g.*, deprenyl). MAO-B is the isozyme that catabolizes dopamine. These agents elevate DA levels, but do not have the dangerous peripheral side effects associated with the traditional MAO inhibitors (*e.g.*, hypertensive crisis).

Dopamine Agonists

Another approach is to develop DA mimetics that could cross the blood–brain barrier. Since these agents would stimulate postsynaptic receptors directly, they might continue to be active even after the total degeneration of the nigrostriatal tract. At present a number of DA mimetics are known (*e.g.*, bromocriptine, apomorphine, lisuride). Bromocriptine (Parlodel®) is now available for use as an adjunct to L-dopa in the therapy of Parkinson's disease.

HUNTINGTON'S CHOREA

Clinical Syndrome

Huntington's chorea is a less common disorder of the basal ganglia, which occurs with a frequency of one in 12,000 people. The predominant symptom is not akinesia but hyperkinesia. The patient makes uncontrolled, repetitive movements, which get worse during excitement and cease only during sleep. Since these are well coordinated and **appear** to be voluntary, they give a dance-like impression (hence the name "chorea"). A separate, unrelated feature is the development of mental deterioration, which progresses to outright dementia. Huntington's chorea is an inherited disorder, transmitted by an autosomal dominant gene. Its onset is gradual, occurring in early middle age (age 30–50) after the patient may already have had children and thus transmitted the gene.

Neuropathology

Examination of the brains of Huntington's chorea victims reveals widespread alterations including degeneration of the neocortex and of the caudate-putamen. The caudate-putamen is drastically affected, often being reduced to less than half of its normal mass. The missing neurons are predominantly ACh and GABA neurons. As a result of this degeneration, ACh levels are usually low in the patient's caudate-putamen, and GABA levels are invariably low. DA levels are normal.

Drug Therapy

Barbiturates

The traditional treatment (without theoretical basis) for Huntington's chorea was barbiturate therapy. This simply served to keep the patient quiet.

Neuroleptics

The neuroleptic drugs are DA blockers that are usually used in the treatment of schizophrenia (see Chapter 27). Recently, they have also been administered to Huntington's chorea patients, on the premise that if ACh is low, DA must be predominant. Blocking DA receptors might be expected to bring the two transmitters back into balance. In line with expectations, the neuroleptics have proved to be successful at suppressing choretic movements, and neuroleptic therapy is now standard. Unfortunately, the neuroleptics do nothing to relieve the dementia that accompanies the chorea. It is suspected that this dementia relates to the degeneration of structures other than the basal ganglia, perhaps to the loss of neurons in the cortex.

New Directions in Research

Acetylcholine Enhancers

One approach has been to attempt to raise ACh levels. Dietary choline and physostigmine have been tried. So far the results have been equivocal. It seems possible that the GABA neurons normally controlled by the ACh interneurons (Fig. 20–3) have also degenerated. If so, raising ACh levels would not be effective.

Gamma-Aminobutyric Acid Agonists

A second approach has been to raise GABA activity with GABA agonist drugs. Several compounds, including imidazole acetic acid and muscimol, have been tried with ambiguous results. Currently a new GABA agonist, progabide, is being tested (see Chapter 21).

SUGGESTED READING

Current concepts and controversies in Parkinson's disease. Proceedings of a symposium held at Montebello, Québec, Oct. 21–22, 1983. Can J Neurol Sci 1984; 11:(1) (suppl).

Hayden MR. Huntington's chorea. London: Springer-Verlag, 1981.

Chapter 21

ANTISEIZURE DRUGS (ANTICONVULSANTS)

W.M. Burnham

EPILEPSY

Definitions

Epilepsy is a disorder of the central nervous system that is characterized by spontaneous, recurring seizures. It is one of the most common of the CNS disorders, occurring in one of every 200 people. In most patients, epilepsy is a permanent condition.

Seizures are self-sustaining (but self-limiting) episodes of neural hyperactivity. During a seizure, some of the neurons of the brain cease their normal activities and begin to fire in massive, synchronized bursts. Such synchronized activity produces characteristic "spike" or "spike and wave" patterns in the electroencephalogram (EEG) (Fig. 21–1). After a few seconds or minutes, the inhibitory mechanisms of the brain regain control, the seizure stops, and the person and the EEG return to normal.

Low seizure threshold. It is important to remember that seizures themselves do not equal epilepsy. Every brain contains the circuitry necessary to produce seizures, and every brain will do so if subjected to the proper stimulation (electric current, hypoxia, convulsant drugs, *etc.*). The essence of epilepsy is a **chronic low seizure threshold**, which leads to the production of **spontaneous attacks**.

Causes

Pathology Versus Biochemistry

In some cases of epilepsy, low seizure threshold is associated with obvious structural pathology in the brain (*e.g.*, an infection, a tumor, scarring due to a wound, a stroke, a birth injury). In other cases, the brain of an epileptic patient appears to be anatomically nor-mal. This suggests that the basic problem in epilepsy may be biochemical in nature—perhaps a subtle mismatch in excitatory and inhibitory transmitters. Such a mismatch might be caused by structural pathology in some patients and by genetic factors in others.

The GABA Hypothesis

Over the years, there have been a number of hypotheses concerning the biochemical flaw in epilepsy. Currently, the most popular view is based on the GABA hypothesis. This is discussed in detail in later sections of this chapter.

Seizure Types

There are a number of different types of epileptic seizures. (Because of this, some theorists prefer to talk of "the epilepsies" rather than of "epilepsy.") Pharmacologically, it is important to distinguish among the types, because they respond differently to antiseizure drugs. The wrong sort of drug may be useless, or may even exacerbate a seizure condition. Four of the commonest types of seizures are described in Table 21–1, which includes both their traditional names and their revised names under the new international seizure classification. The names and characteristics of these seizures should be learned, since misdiagnosis of seizure type is one of the most common causes of failure in drug therapy. In particular, mild complex partial seizures tend to be confused with absence attacks.

Status Epilepticus

Constantly repeating seizures of any type are called status epilepticus. This syndrome is rare, but it is life-threatening when the repeating seizures are of the tonic-

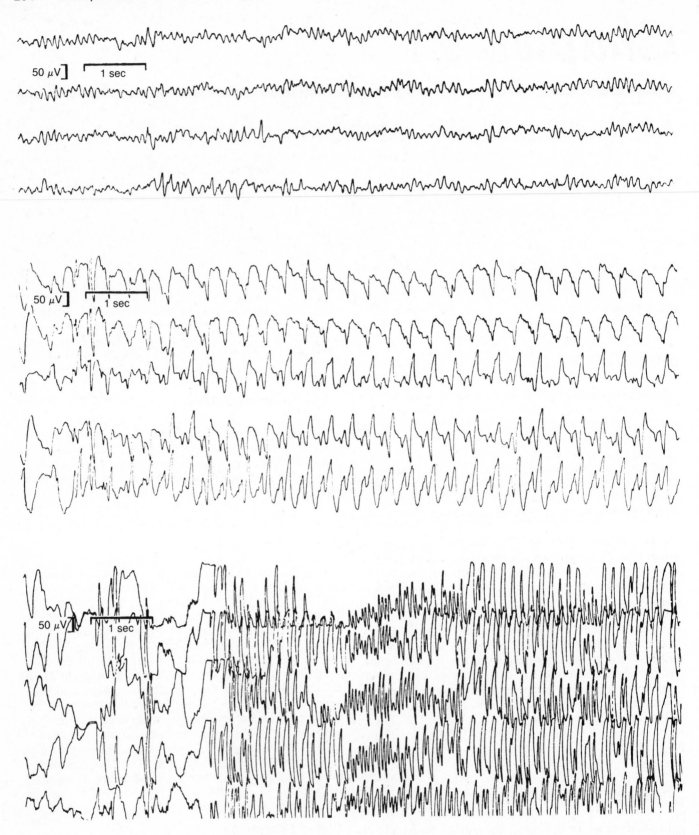

Figure 21-1   EEG patterns during seizures. *Top*: Normal during seizure-free interval. *Middle*: 3/sec spike and wave (absence). *Bottom*: "Spikes" (tonic-clonic).

TABLE 21–1 Common Seizure Types*

GENERALIZED (appear to involve the whole brain from the outset):

Absence ("Petit mal")	Attack	Brief period of unconsciousness. Patient stares blankly, eyelids may flutter.
	Duration	<30 seconds.
	EEG	3/second spike and wave during attack, whole brain.
Tonic-Clonic ("Grand mal")	Attack	Unconsciousness with dramatic tonic-clonic convulsions. May be preceded by an aura[†] and an epileptic cry, and accompanied by profuse salivation, tongue-biting, and incontinence.
	Duration	<5 minutes.
	EEG	Constant spiking, whole brain.

PARTIAL (at least initially, only part of the brain is involved):

Simple Partial ("Focal cortical")	Attack	Sensory seizure or focal motor signs (patient is conscious).
	Duration	Varies.
	EEG	Localized spiking in a neocortical area.
Complex Partial ("Psychomotor", "Temporal lobe")	Attack	May start with a simple partial attack of temporal lobe origin, *e.g.*, an olfactory aura[†], a perceptual aura[†] (déjà vu, distortion of perspective), or an emotional aura[†]. Later, the patient loses consciousness but still appears conscious. During this period motor "automatisms" may occur.
	Duration	Varies.
	EEG	Localized spiking in temporal neocortex or limbic system.

* Traditional names in parentheses.
† Any type of partial seizure may generalize to give a tonic-clonic attack with convulsions. The partial seizure is then called an "aura."

clonic variety. Tonic-clonic status is a major emergency that should be treated with great speed in a hospital setting.

THERAPY FOR EPILEPSY

In general, epileptic patients are perfectly normal between attacks, and seizures themselves are usually brief and relatively harmless. After a severe tonic-clonic attack, the patient may want to go home to rest, but will be perfectly able to work again the following day. The question arises, "Why bother to treat epilepsy?" The answer is that seizures have an impact on human life that is far out of proportion to their medical significance. Seizures look "strange," and even frightening, and the general public reacts very badly to them. Thus, epileptic patients fear having attacks in public places, and they face considerable discrimination when

they do so (such as loss of friends, jobs, housing). In addition, people with uncontrolled epilepsy are not allowed to drive. In both Canada and the United States, drivers' licences are cancelled with the first seizure, and they may be reinstated only if seizures are perfectly controlled. Naturally, patients are anxious to achieve control over their seizures.

Drug Versus Non-Drug Therapy

A number of non-drug approaches to therapy have been tried, including diet, biofeedback, cerebellar stimulation, and surgery. Of these, only surgery has gained widespread acceptance. For selected patients, neurosurgery offers a radical, but effective, cure for seizures. It is attempted, however, only when attacks arise from a clear-cut focal area, and only when they are frequent and drug resistant. Less than 10% of the epileptic population meet these criteria. Thus, for most epileptic patients, the major therapy for seizures is drug therapy.

General Principles of Drug Therapy

A large number of drugs are known to suppress seizures (*e.g.*, most sedatives); a smaller number of the safest and least toxic are used in therapy. These are called antiseizure drugs or, more commonly, anticonvulsants. ("Anticonvulsant" is not an ideal term, since many seizures do not involve convulsions.) Before individual drugs are considered, a number of general statements can be made about the class of antiseizure drugs:

- Antiseizure drugs do not cure epilepsy; they just suppress seizures on a temporary basis. Therefore, most patients must take them daily for life.
- Antiseizure drugs are fairly safe, but all of them occasionally cause life-threatening non-dose-related adverse reactions (*e.g.*, liver toxicity, suppression of bone marrow). These rare effects, some of which may relate to genetic abnormalities in the patient, are usually observed within the first months of therapy. All patients should be closely monitored during this initial period.
- Many antiseizure drugs cause rashes, stomach upsets, and/or, at higher doses, sedation. Sedation is a particular problem with the older drugs, which are chemically related to the barbiturates. Thus, antiseizure drugs are often perceived as unpleasant

to take. Compliance is a problem; abuse is not.
- The mechanisms of antiseizure drug action are not yet well understood. Hypotheses concerning mechanisms of action of specific drugs are noted below.

In the absence of definite information concerning therapeutic mechanisms, it is probably best to approach the antiseizure drugs on a practical level—to learn which drugs are available and what their uses are. Eight drugs are discussed below, categorized according to therapeutic application, and listed in the order of preference (Table 21–2 and Fig. 21–2).

Drugs for Absence Seizures

Ethosuximide

Ethosuximide is the current drug of choice for absence seizures. It has recently replaced trimethadione (Tridione®), a more toxic, less effective drug that has been withdrawn from the market.
Mechanism of action. Unknown.
Advantages. It is relatively effective, safe, and non-sedating.
Disadvantages. It may cause gastrointestinal disturbances, fatigue, photophobia, and other side effects.

TABLE 21–2 Commonly Used Antiseizure Drugs

Name (Trade Name)	Chemical Structure (see also Fig. 21–2)	Common Side Effects (At Therapeutic Blood Levels)
For *Absence Seizures* (in order of preference)		
Ethosuximide (Zarontin®)	Resembles phenobarbital	GI disturbance, fatigue, photophobia.
Valproate (Depakene®)	Novel	GI distress, initial fatigue, hair loss, weight gain, hepatotoxicity.
Clonazepam (Rivotril®)	A benzodiazepine	Sedation, personality change, paradoxical excitement. (Abrupt withdrawal is dangerous.)
For *Tonic-Clonic* and *Partial Seizures* (in order of preference for tonic-clonic seizures)		
Phenytoin (Dilantin®, *etc.*)	Resembles phenobarbital	Acne, hirsutism, gingival hyperplasia. (At toxic doses also nystagmus, ataxia.)
Carbamazepine (Tegretol®)	Resembles tricyclic antidepressants	Initial sedation, diplopia, GI disturbances, transient mild depression of leukocyte count.
Phenobarbital (Luminal®, *etc.*)	A barbiturate	Sedation, paradoxical excitement. (Abrupt withdrawal is dangerous.)
Primidone (Mysoline®)	Resembles phenobarbital	Sedation, initial GI disturbances, psychiatric disturbances.
For *Status Epilepticus*		
Diazepam (Valium®) 10–20 mg i.v., at 1 mg/min	A benzodiazepine	Not used in chronic therapy.

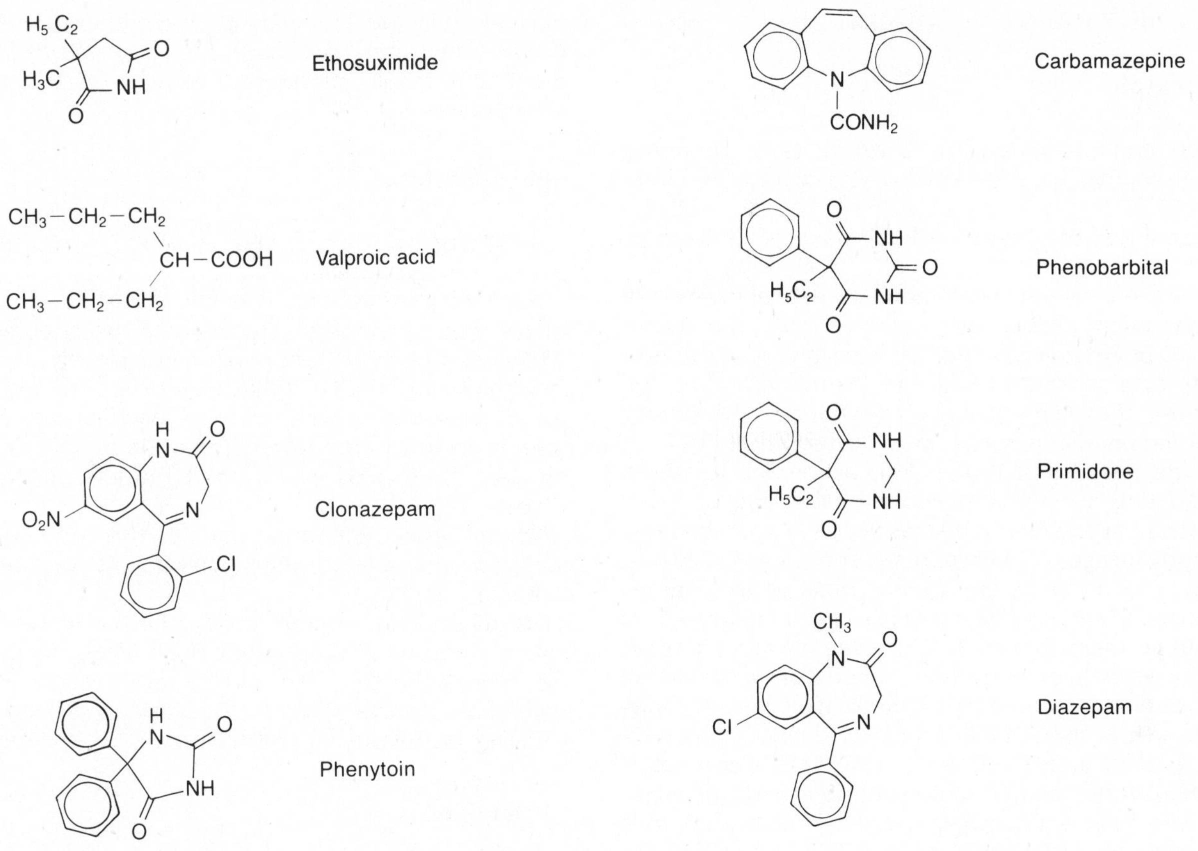

Figure 21-2 Structural formulae of antiseizure drugs.

Valproic Acid

Valproic acid (valproate) is a relatively new drug used for absence attacks.

Mechanism of action. Valproate is said to raise GABA levels by blocking GABA transaminase, the GABA degradative enzyme. This has been questioned, however.

Advantages. Effective and clearly nonsedating, valproate has some potency against both absence and tonic-clonic attacks. This is important because in some patients absence and tonic-clonic attacks occur together. Usually, these patients have to be given separate drugs for each type, but valproate alone may be sufficient.

Disadvantages. Valproate is more expensive than the older drugs, and has a short half-life, which necessitates two or more doses every day. Side effects are still being discovered. Among the known side effects are gastrointestinal disturbances (frequent in the early stage of therapy), tremor, hair loss (mild), and weight gain.

Clonazepam

Clonazepam is another of the newer drugs that may be used for absence attacks.

Mechanism of action. It binds to the benzodiazepine receptor, causing enhancement of activity in GABA synapses (*see* the last section of this chapter, as well as Chapter 26).

Advantages. There are few. It is a drug of last resort. It may, however, be useful for other, rarer forms of childhood epilepsy.

Disadvantages. This powerful benzodiazepine causes sedation or personality changes (*e.g.*, irritability, paradoxical excitement) in up to 50% of the patients who take it. It is also relatively expensive.

Drugs for Tonic-Clonic Attacks

Phenytoin

Phenytoin is an older drug (formerly called diphenyl-hydantoin) that is still the drug of choice for tonic-clonic attacks.

Mechanism of action. A large number of mechanisms have been proposed for phenytoin, most of them stressing effects on basic membrane properties (the sodium pump, ion flux, *etc.*). Very recently, the discovery of a phenytoin binding site has suggested the possibility of a specific mechanism for this drug. As yet, however, the pharmacologic relevance of the phenytoin binding site remains to be established.

Advantages. The drug is long-acting and relatively nonsedating. It replaced phenobarbital as drug of choice just before World War II because of its lack of sedation.

Disadvantages. Phenytoin has annoying side effects, which may occur at therapeutic dose levels. Among these are acne, gingival hyperplasia (excess growth of gum tissue; seen in over 30% of patients) and hirsutism (excess growth of body hair). Phenytoin also has an unusual metabolism, which complicates dosing: somewhere in the therapeutic range of plasma concentrations (10–20 μg/mL, 40–80 μmol/L), the degradative enzymes in the liver become saturated and phenytoin switches from a normal first-order metabolism to a "pseudo-zero-order" metabolism. This means that the time required to eliminate 50% of a given dose increases, and that the drug stays in the body for a much longer time. Thus, the physician who has been gradually raising the dosage may find that a moderate increase suddenly exposes the patient to phenytoin toxicity. Since phenytoin toxicity (usually ataxia and sedation) occasionally presents in an idiosyncratic form (*e.g.*, pseudo-psychosis, increased seizure frequency), monitoring of blood levels (*see* below) is particularly important when phenytoin dosage is being adjusted.

Carbamazepine

Carbamazepine (Tegretol®), like phenytoin, is now a first-line drug in the treatment of epilepsy.

Mechanism of action. Unknown; it is an adenosine receptor antagonist, but this may not explain its antiepileptic action. Its 10,11-epoxide metabolite is also active.

Advantages. Carbamazepine is as effective and usually as nonsedating as phenytoin. It does not cause acne, gum hyperplasia, or hirsutism.

Disadvantages. Carbamazepine is expensive. Its half-life can vary from 35 hours (single dose) to 10–12 hours (chronic therapy), because of auto-induction and induction by other drugs such as phenobarbital. Therefore dosage must be individually adjusted. Gastrointestinal disturbances may be observed at therapeutic doses. Though serious toxicity is infrequent, blood cell counts and liver function must be monitored carefully at the start of carbamazepine therapy. A mild depression in leukocyte count often occurs early in treatment, but usually disappears without discontinuation of therapy.

Phenobarbital

Phenobarbital, introduced in 1911, was the first modern anticonvulsant.

Mechanism of action. Recently, a barbiturate receptor has been proposed. This binding site is either the GABA-related chloride ionophore or closely associated with the ionophore. It has been proposed, although not conclusively proven, that the barbiturates act by binding to this barbiturate site and indirectly enhancing GABA-mediated inhibition at the ionophore level (Chapter 26).

Advantages. Phenobarbital is still one of the cheapest and safest anticonvulsants. Its long half-life simplifies dosing.

Disadvantages. Unfortunately, this barbiturate often causes sedation at therapeutic dose levels. Its original use, before the discovery of its anticonvulsant effects, was as a daytime sedative. Because of this effect, it is losing popularity in the treatment of epilepsy.

Primidone

Primidone is a slight variant of the phenobarbital molecule. In the body it is biotransformed into phenobarbital, and much of its therapeutic effect probably depends on the phenobarbital produced, although the parent compound may have some therapeutic effects of its own.

Mechanism of action. Primarily, conversion into phenobarbital.

Advantages. The drug is long-acting and fairly safe.

Disadvantages. Like phenobarbital, it is sedating. For this reason, it is also declining in popularity.

Drugs for Partial Seizures

The drugs used for tonic-clonic attacks are also used for partial seizures. They appear to be almost as effective against **simple** partial attacks as against tonic-clonic seizures, but they are much less effective against **complex** partial attacks. There is also a different order of preference for complex partial attacks, since carbamazepine and primidone are considered to have special efficacy against this type of seizure. The order of preference for treating complex partial attacks is: 1. carbamazepine; 2. phenytoin; 3. primidone; 4. phenobarbital; 5. valproate.

Although the same drugs are used for tonic-clonic and complex partial seizures, the fact that they have a different order of potency indicates that the two types of seizure are distinct entities. It is conceivable that we may eventually discover a new class of drugs with a special potency against complex partial attacks.

Drugs for Status Epilepticus

Benzodiazepines

Diazepam (Valium®) and **lorazepam** (Ativan®) are the drugs of choice for all varieties of status epilepticus. They are administered intravenously. The adult dose of diazepam is 10–20 mg, and the infusion rate should not exceed 1 mg/minute. If necessary, this dose may be repeated after 20–30 minutes. Lorazepam has a slower onset but a longer duration of action.

While diazepam stops status quickly, its effect wears off in time, and status may restart. To prevent this, the patient may be switched to intravenous phenytoin or phenobarbital.

Other Drugs

If tonic-clonic status resists diazepam treatment, phenytoin or phenobarbital may be administered intravenously. If these fail, paraldehyde (i.m.) or lidocaine (i.v.) may be tried. If none of these measures works, general anaesthesia will be required.

Therapeutic Approaches

The following are some rules for contemporary anticonvulsant therapy.

Whom to Treat

Before starting therapy, it is important to rule out pseudo-seizures (not uncommon), poisoning, or active pathology. If active pathology is present (*e.g.*, a tumor, an infection), this should be treated, not the seizures. Also, before initiating therapy, it is important to make sure that the seizure problem is chronic. Occasionally people have a single seizure that is never repeated.

Choice of Drug

Before therapy is started, the type of seizure must be carefully established. Different types need different drugs.

Monotherapy, Not Polypharmacy

Treatment is started with a single drug. If the drug of choice is not effective, another **single** drug is tried. Eventually, if the patient has very resistant seizures, or more than one seizure type, polypharmacy may be attempted.

Drug Interactions

If polypharmacy is attempted, two important antiseizure drug interactions should be avoided:

1. **Phenobarbital and valproate**—valproate increases phenobarbital levels by inhibiting hydroxylation, and thus may cause toxicity.
2. **Phenobarbital and primidone**—this combination produces unacceptably high phenobarbital levels.

Antiseizure drugs also interact with the drugs used for a variety of other disorders. These interactions are too numerous to discuss. Some are mentioned in Chapter 11.

Use of Blood Levels to Regulate Therapy

Therapeutic blood concentration ranges are now known for all of the common antiseizure drugs (Table 21–3), and adjustment of dosage to achieve desired blood levels has become standard practice in contemporary therapy. At the start of therapy, or when dosage is adjusted, blood samples are taken in order to help in adjusting dose levels, as well as to check for liver, kidney, and blood toxicity.

Drug "Vacations"

If a patient has had no seizures (including EEG seizures) for several years, drugs may be slowly withdrawn. This is done to see whether the seizure threshold has normalized. Patients outgrow some types of childhood attacks (*e.g.*, absence seizures) and even adults occasionally cease to have seizures. **Note**: Antiseizure drugs should not be withdrawn quickly because rebound exacerbation of seizures may occur. This is particularly true in the cases of phenobarbital and clonazepam.

Prognosis for Seizure Control

First Two Years

Table 21–4 indicates the percentages of seizure suppression that can be achieved early in therapy, assuming proper diagnosis and patient compliance. It is obvious that the drugs that are currently available work better on absence and tonic-clonic attacks than on complex partial attacks. This is unfortunate, since complex partial attacks are the most common type of seizure in adults.

Long-Term Therapy

It should be noted that the figures given in Table 21–4 apply only to the first two years of therapy. A large-

TABLE 21-3 Pharmacokinetic Parameters of Commonly Used Antiseizure Drugs

Name	Absorption	Half-Life (hours)	Therapeutic Plasma Concentration
For *Absence Seizures*			
Ethosuximide	Rapid	30–60	40–100 µg/mL (280–710 µmol/L)
Valproate	Rapid	8–15	50–100 µg/mL (350–700 µmol/L)
Clonazepam	Rapid	22–33	10–80 ng/mL (30–240 nmol/L)
For *Tonic-Clonic* and *Partial Seizures*			
Phenytoin	Slow	20–24	10–20 µg/mL (40–80 µmol/L)
Carbamazepine	Slow-moderate	12–14	4–10 µg/mL (17–42 µmol/L)
Phenobarbital	Slow-moderate	50–150	20–40 µg/mL (85–170 µmol/L)
Primidone	Slow-moderate	6–18	7–15 µg/mL (30–70 µmol/L)

scale study done in the 1960s showed some tendency for seizures to reappear as time passes.

Summary

Although the present drugs represent a great advance in the therapy of epilepsy, more and better drugs are needed. Most urgently needed are drugs that are effective against complex partial attacks. Agents with fewer side effects would also be welcome. A long-term goal is to discover drugs that cure epilepsy rather than simply suppress seizures.

NEURON-INHIBITORY AMINO ACIDS AND SEIZURES

Chemical Messengers of the CNS

As indicated in the Epilepsy section, many theorists believe that epilepsy results from the hypofunction of an inhibitory transmitter such as GABA. This section provides additional background on the inhibitory transmitters and on the GABA hypothesis of epilepsy.

Many of the chemical messengers found in the peripheral nervous system are also present in the CNS. These include acetylcholine and the monoamines serotonin, dopamine, and noradrenaline.* The **major** role in the CNS transmission, however, is played by another group of transmitters, the amino acid trans-

---

* norepinephrine

mitters. On the excitatory side, these include glutamate and aspartate, whereas on the inhibitory side, gamma-aminobutyric acid (GABA) and glycine are probably the most important.

Gamma-Aminobutyric Acid

Distribution, Synthesis, and Metabolism

GABA was formerly thought to be exclusively localized, in higher species, in the central nervous system. Although at least 90% of the GABA in the body is in the CNS, where it is the most important inhibitory transmitter of the forebrain and upper brain stem, GABA, its receptors, or its synthesizing enzyme have also been found in kidney, intestine, pancreas, and sympathetic ganglia. Within the brain, it has been estimated that at least 25% of all synapses in the neocortex and cerebellum use GABA as the neurotransmitter.

GABA, its synthetic enzyme, and its receptors are

TABLE 21-4 Success Rate of Antiseizure Drug Therapy (First 2 Years)

	Patients Showing	
Seizure Type	Total Seizure Suppression %	Significant Improvement %
Absence	50	25
Tonic-Clonic	60–65	20
Simple partial	Figures unknown—probably like tonic-clonic	
Complex partial	<30	<50

found in all brain regions examined. Some of the better identified GABAergic cells or pathways include cortical interneurons, hippocampal interneurons, a striato-pallido-nigral pathway, a habenulotectal pathway, and the cerebellar Purkinje cells.

GABA is synthesized from the excitatory amino acid, L-glutamic acid, by the specific enzyme L-glutamic acid decarboxylase (GAD), with pyridoxal phosphate as a cofactor.

The major means of removing GABA from the synapse is *via* a specific re-uptake mechanism into both nerve terminals and glia.

The breakdown of GABA is effected by the enzyme alpha-ketoglutarate-GABA transaminase (GABA-T), which also has pyridoxal phosphate as the cofactor and which regenerates glutamate (although mainly in glial cells). The metabolic sequence leads, *via* the enzyme succinic-semialdehyde dehydrogenase (SSDH), into the tricarboxylic acid cycle. This formation of succinate from glutamate *via* GABA is called the GABA shunt.

GABA Receptors

At least two GABA receptors have been identified; they are denoted as GABA$_A$ and GABA$_B$ receptors. GABA$_A$ receptors are linked to Cl$^-$ channels and are specifically blocked by bicuculline. GABA$_B$ receptors, which were only relatively recently discovered, have baclofen as a specific ligand.

The macromolecular GABA$_A$-receptor complex is one of the best studied neurotransmitter synapse mechanisms (Fig. 21–3). After GABA is synthesized and liberated into the synapse, it interacts with the GABA$_A$ receptor, resulting in the opening of a specific Cl$^-$ channel. If the GABA$_A$ receptor is located on a cell soma, this channel opening results in hyperpolarization due to increased Cl$^-$ entry; if the contact is axo-axonal, then Cl$^-$ exits from the channel and the result is a local depolarization.

It is known that in many synapses the GABA$_A$ receptor is linked in a macromolecular complex with different specific drug-recognition sites (that may in fact be receptors for as yet unknown natural ligands), which modulate the GABA-regulated Cl$^-$ channel. Thus the benzodiazepine recognition site and the recently reported barbiturate recognition site are integral parts of the complex formed by GABA, macromolecular receptor, and chloride ionophore. The natural ligands (if any) of these other recognition sites within the GABA$_A$-receptor complex are as yet unidentified.

GABA$_B$ receptors are much less well characterized. They are not linked to Cl$^-$ channels, but may well be linked to Na$^+$ channels. The pharmacologic profiles of GABA$_B$ and GABA$_A$ receptors are completely different, as discussed below.

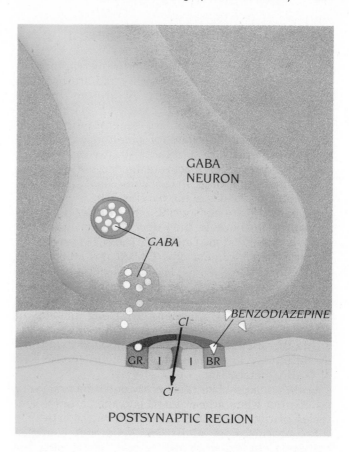

Figure 21–3 Schematic representation of the macromolecular GABA$_A$-receptor complex. I = ionophore containing the chloride channel; BR = benzodiazepine receptor; GR = GABA receptor. Note that I, BR, and GR interact biochemically to modulate each other's function. (Some investigators look upon the chloride ionophore as the receptor for barbiturates [agonists] and picrotoxinin [antagonist], as shown in Fig. 26–2.)

Physiology of GABA Receptor Function

Central GABA$_A$ synapses have a major role in the control of cerebral excitability (*see* below). In addition, GABA$_A$-synaptic function is implicated in extrapyramidal motor function, *e.g.*, in the feedback loops and output pathway of the nigro-striato-nigral circuit (*see* Chapter 20).

Central GABA$_B$-synaptic activity has been tentatively related to the control of muscle tone and reflex arcs. GABA also plays a role in pain perception, but whether GABA$_A$ and/or GABA$_B$ paths are responsible, and at what level of the neuro-axis, is as yet unclear.

The function of GABA$_A$ and/or GABA$_B$ receptors in different peripheral organs is not yet known.

Pharmacology of the GABA Synapse

GAD inhibitors, such as allylglycine or mercaptopropionic acid, are all convulsant agents and are useful in laboratory models for epilepsy. At present, they do not have any clinical uses.

GABA-T inhibitors are of two general types: chelators of pyridoxal phosphate (or inhibitors of pyridoxal kinase) and specific ''suicide-substrate'' agents (*i.e.*, agents that irreversibly inactivate the enzyme when they bind to it). Both groups are anticonvulsant agents, but the compounds acting at the pyridoxal site (*e.g.*, aminooxyacetic acid) are nonspecific and at higher doses are proconvulsant because they decrease the availability of the coenzyme at the GAD step. The suicide-substrate inhibitors (*e.g.*, gamma-vinyl GABA) are much more specific for GABA-T. Early clinical trials indicate a potential antiepileptic activity for gamma-vinyl GABA.

Valproic acid (valproate) is a clinically proven antiepileptic drug. It is a moderately strong inhibitor of GABA-T, and some investigators feel that this accounts for its therapeutic actions. This compound is also active at the succinic-semialdehyde dehydrogenase step of GABA metabolism.

GABA-uptake inhibitors generally enter the brain very poorly, but when administered into the cerebral ventricles of rats they have an anticonvulsant activity.

The pharmacology of the GABA$_A$-receptor complex has been studied in depth. Specific antagonists for either the GABA$_A$ receptor (*e.g.*, bicuculline) or the Cl$^-$ channel (*e.g.*, picrotoxin) are potent convulsants. Specific GABA$_A$-receptor agonists (*e.g.*, muscimol, tetrahydro-isoxazolo-pyridinone [THIP]) have anticonvulsant effects together with a variety of other properties (*e.g.*, analgesia, inhibition of nigrostriatal dopamine neuron activity). By definition, benzodiazepines and barbiturates interact with their specific binding sites, both of which facilitate or prolong the Cl$^-$ channel opening induced by GABA$_A$-receptor activation. Some investigators have suggested that other antiepileptic drugs, such as phenytoin, have similar actions on the GABA$_A$-linked Cl$^-$ channel, but the mechanism, and its relation to the clinical effect of the drug, are unknown.

Of the specific GABA$_A$ agonists (Fig. 21-4), muscimol is too toxic to be useful in clinical practice, but THIP is receiving trials as an analgesic and antispastic agent. The **benzodiazepines** are well known anxiolytics (with diverse other properties including antispastic and acute anticonvulsant effects) and the barbiturates are sedative-hypnotics that have been used as antiepileptics. It is not known if all the actions of benzodiazepines and barbiturates are related to their actions at the GABA$_A$-receptor complex.

Baclofen, a clinically useful antispastic agent, is a specific GABA$_B$-receptor agonist. At the present time a specific antagonist for GABA$_B$ receptors has not been identified.

Progabide is an agonist for both GABA$_A$ and GABA$_B$ receptors. In clinical trials this compound shows activity as both an antiepileptic and an antispastic agent.

The structures of some of these GABA agonists are shown in Figure 21-4.

Glycine

Glycine is the main inhibitory transmitter of the spinal cord and lower brain stem. Because this amino acid also serves a role in protein synthesis, its distribution does not parallel the sites of its neurotransmitter function. The latter has been deduced by electrophysiologic and receptor distribution studies using radioligand binding techniques.

Glycine acts at specific receptors that control (in a manner similar to GABA receptors) the opening of a Cl$^-$ channel. The glycine-receptor/Cl$^-$-channel complex is independent of the GABA$_A$-receptor/Cl$^-$-channel complex.

One of the identified roles of glycine is its function as the inhibitory neurotransmitter released by the Renshaw cell in the spinal cord, producing an inhibitory postsynaptic potential (IPSP) on the motor-neuron cell.

In addition to the brain and spinal cord, glycine receptors have also been identified in the substantia nigra and in the inferior olivary complex. In Parkinson's dis-

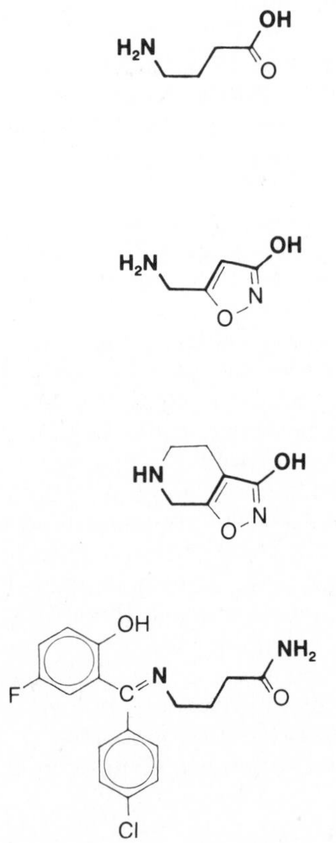

Figure 21-4   Structural formulae of clinically tested GABA agonists.

ease there is a loss of glycine receptors in the substantia nigra.

Strychnine is a specific inhibitor for glycine receptors, and is a potent convulsant compound. The mechanism for these convulsions—which are generated from the spinal cord, not the brain—is thought to be blockade of the feedback inhibition of the motor-neuron by the Renshaw cell (Fig. 21–5). ^{3}H-Strychnine is used as a pharmacologic tool for labelling glycine receptors.

In contrast to the pharmacologic agents available for the study of GABA receptors, no specific agonists exist for glycine receptors.

Inhibitory Transmitters and Seizure States: the GABA Hypothesis of Epilepsy

The normal function of the CNS depends upon a balance of excitatory and inhibitory influences. If excitation exceeds inhibition, the CNS tends to be hyperexcitable (= "low seizure threshold"). If the imbalance is severe enough, a seizure results.

An imbalance between excitation and inhibition might occur either because there was too much excitation or because there was too little inhibition. Recently, theorists have concentrated on the latter possibility, namely, that epileptic brains may have too little inhibition and, in particular, too little of the inhibition mediated by $GABA_A$ receptors. This point of view has been called the GABA hypothesis of epilepsy.

The GABA hypothesis suggests that epileptic patients have a chronic low seizure threshold because they suffer from genetic or postpathologic GABA hypofunction. A corollary of the GABA hypothesis is that pharmacologic lowering of GABA function should cause seizures, whereas pharmacologic enhancement of GABAergic activity should stop them. The evidence related to the GABA hypothesis may be considered under two general headings: pharmacologic and neurochemical.

As mentioned above, **pharmacologic** studies have shown that any agent that decreases activity in the $GABA_A$ system causes seizures. In fact, with the exception of strychnine, most of the traditional convulsant drugs have turned out to be direct or indirect GABA blockers (e.g., bicuculline, picrotoxin, mercaptopropionic acid). Conversely, many drugs that increase $GABA_A$-synaptic activity act as anticonvulsants. As noted above, several of the standard antiseizure drugs seem to act by this mechanism (e.g., phenobarbital, clonazepam, possibly valproate). Thus, the pharmacologic evidence is generally consistent with the GABA hypothesis.

Pharmacologic evidence, however, is not sufficient to prove the GABA hypothesis. Convincing proof will have to involve the **neurochemical** demonstration of a GABAergic flaw in human epileptic brains. For obvious reasons, such evidence is hard to obtain. It is known, however, that one form of childhood epilepsy, pyridoxine-dependent seizures, is due to an insufficient level of pyridoxal phosphate, a cofactor for GAD, the GABA-synthetic enzyme. Furthermore, it has been reported that a high percentage (50–65%) of patients presenting for neurosurgical treatment of intractable complex partial epilepsy appear to have deficient GAD levels in the epileptic focus. Thus, certain neurochemical data appear to support the GABA hypothesis, although far more information is required. Research in this area continues.

It is worth noting that, although the GABA hypothesis is very popular at present, there is also active research into possible epilepsy-related abnormalities in excitatory amino acids (e.g., glutamate), peptides (e.g., somatostatin), and ion fluxes (e.g., calcium).

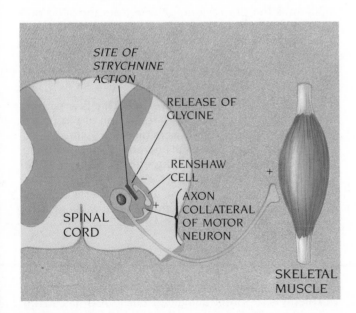

Figure 21–5 Site of action of glycine (inhibitory neurotransmitter) and of strychnine in the spinal cord.

SUGGESTED READING

Bruni J. Antiepileptic drugs. Modern Medicine of Canada 1980; 35:1377–1384.

Chapman AG, Hart GP. Anticonvulsant drug action and regional neurotransmitter amino acid changes. J Neural Transm 1988; 72:201–212.

Krogsgaard-Larsen P, Scheel-Kruger J, Kofod H, eds. GABA-neurotransmitters. New York: Academic Press, 1979.

Laidlaw J, Richens A, eds. A textbook of epilepsy. 2nd ed. London/New York: Churchill Livingstone, 1982.

Mikati MA, Browne TR. Comparative efficacy of antiepileptic drugs. Clin Neuropharmacol 1988; 11:130–140.

Okada Y, Roberts E, eds. Problems in GABA research. Amsterdam: Excerpta Medica, 1982.

Roberts E, Chase TN, Tower DB, eds. GABA in nervous system function. New York: Raven Press, 1977.

Chapter 22

OPIOID ANALGESICS AND ANTAGONISTS

H. Kalant

The opium poppy (*Papaver somniferum*) has been known and used in Asia Minor and southeastern Europe for over 2000 years. Its juice was known to contain an agent that relieved pain (= analgesic), produced sleep or drowsiness (*somniferum* = bringing sleep), relieved diarrhea, and in low doses produced a blissful or euphoric state. Only crude preparations were available for medical use until the isolation and purification of morphine by Sertürner in 1806. Other alkaloids with similar properties were isolated from crude opium over the next decades, and by the mid-19th century these pure compounds (opiates) began to replace opium in medical use. Morphine was named after Morpheus, the Greek god of sleep. The Greek word *narcosis* designates a state characterized by drowsiness, stupor, and numbness or insensitivity. Therefore these compounds, which produced drowsiness, analgesia, and a dreamy detached feeling, were called **narcotics**.

Biologists use the term to mean a substance that depresses all cellular functions, especially those involving response to a stimulus. In this sense, alcohols, anaesthetics, barbiturates, and similar drugs are also narcotics.

In the legal sense, a narcotic is any drug included under the Narcotic Control Act in Canada, or equivalent legislation in other countries. Most of these drugs are opiate analgesics or synthetic substitutes. However, the Act also covers cocaine and cannabis, which have quite different pharmacologic properties (*see* Chapter 29). To distinguish them from these other drugs, morphine and its congeners and synthetic substitutes were referred to as **narcotic analgesics**.

In recent years, the term "opioid" was introduced to include substances that are not derived from opium (hence, are not "opiates"), and do not have a morphine-like chemical structure, but do have morphine-like pharmacologic properties. The whole group, including the opiates, is now known as **opioid analgesics**. In 1973, stereospecific receptors for opioid drugs were proven to exist in the central nervous system. Since it seemed improbable that the animal brain

would have evolved receptors for a plant alkaloid to which it was never exposed, researchers postulated that these receptors must normally take up an endogenous material produced in the brain itself. In 1975, the first such materials were isolated and were found to be short peptides with morphine-like properties, which were named **enkephalins**. Soon afterward, longer peptides with similar properties (**endorphins, dynorphin**) were discovered. These are known collectively as **endogenous opioids**.

OPIUM ALKALOIDS

Opium is the dry residue of juice from the seed-pod of *Papaver somniferum*. It contains a mixture of alkaloids of two main types (Fig. 22–1).

Benzylisoquinoline Alkaloids

The main example is **papaverine**. This is a smooth muscle depressant that causes relaxation of peripheral arterioles (and therefore lowers blood pressure), coronary arteries, gastrointestinal and other smooth muscle, and has a direct quinidine-like effect on the myocardium. It has no analgesic effect. Papaverine HCl is marketed for the relief of cerebral and peripheral ischemia due to arterial spasm, but its therapeutic value in these conditions has been questioned.

Phenanthrene Alkaloids

These are mainly **morphine, codeine**, and **thebaine**. Morphine is a potent analgesic, but it also has strong excitatory effects in some tissues and some species; **thebaine** has predominantly excitatory rather than analgesic effects, and can cause convulsions.

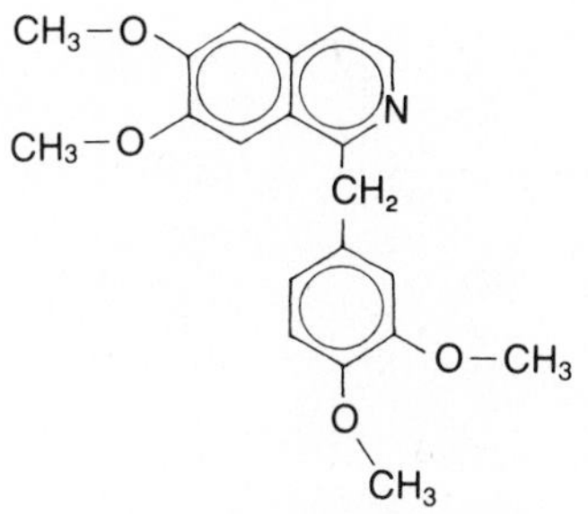

Papaverine–*a benzylisoquinoline alkaloid*

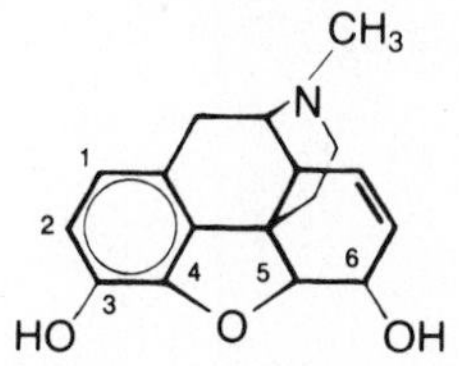

Morphine–*a phenanthrene alkaloid*

Figure 22–1 Structural formulae of the two major classes of opium alkaloid. For codeine, CH_3O- replaces $HO-$ at C-3 of morphine. Thebaine has CH_3O- groups at both C-3 and C-6 of morphine. Heroin is the 3,6-diacetate of morphine.

Note that there are **asymmetric C atoms** in the opiates. Hence, all opiates can exist in either the levo-form (l- or levorotatory form) or the dextro-form (d- or dextrorotatory form).

All morphine synthesized by opium poppy enzymes is the levorotatory or (−) isomer. The dextro- or (+) isomers of the opiates have no analgesic action, except for d-propoxyphene, a weak synthetic codeine-like analgesic.

PHARMACOLOGIC ACTIONS OF OPIOIDS

Morphine and related drugs have a large number of actions, both centrally and peripherally. Some of the actions are intimately associated with the analgesic effect, while others are not. The discovery of different classes of opioid receptor has helped to explain this dissociation of effects and the different spectra of effects shown by some of the newer synthetic opioids.

Opioid Receptors and Endogenous Opioids

Methods of Study

The binding of opioids to their receptors is studied by essentially the same techniques as those outlined

in Chapter 9. Preparations of neuronal membranes are incubated with a radioactively labelled opioid or a specific opioid receptor blocker (*see* the section on Narcotic Antagonists), and then exposed to various concentrations of the compound being studied. At each concentration, the proportion of labelled opioid or blocker that is displaced from the membranes is measured. From the displacement curve generated by these data, one can calculate the number of binding sites per gram of tissue (receptor density), and the affinity of the test compound for these sites. By preparing membrane fractions from different regions of the nervous system, one can study the opioid receptor densities and affinities in the various regions. The results of such studies generally agree well with those of autoradiographic studies of the localization of radioactivity in tissue sections after intravenous injection of ^{3}H-opioids. The receptor distribution can also be studied by incubating tissue slices in medium containing ^{3}H-opioids, then adding a large excess of unlabelled opioids to some of the slices to displace the labelled molecules. Autoradiograms of the slices with and without the displacement step are compared by video image-analysing techniques to reveal the locations and densities of the specific binding sites in different brain regions and structures at which the different opioids presumably act.

Properties of Opioid-Receptor Binding

Binding studies, of the type described above, have revealed the following properties of the binding process:

1. Structural specificity, such that small modifications of the drug molecule cause large changes in drug binding (and in drug effect *in vivo*).
2. Stereospecificity; the l (−) isomer has much higher binding affinity than the d (+) isomer, and only the l (−) isomer is active as an analgesic.
3. Competition between agonists and antagonists; drugs of partially similar structure, but lacking certain molecular features essential for opioid action, can bind to the receptor and block the binding of agonists such as morphine. (N.B.: antagonists must also be l (−) isomers; d (+) isomers do not bind to the receptor).
4. Reversibility; bound drug can be displaced from the receptors by an excess of other molecules with binding ability.
5. A good correlation between the strength of binding to the receptors and the potency of agonist or antagonist effects *in vivo* or on isolated tissues (Fig. 22–2).

Subtypes of Opioid Receptors and Ligands

The major clinical use of opioids is in the relief of pain, but all of them have numerous other effects. When they are administered in doses that produce the same degree of analgesia (= equianalgesic doses), the drugs differ with respect to the relative degrees of other effects that they produce. This observation led to the current concept of multiple receptor types mediating different effects of the opioids (Table 22–1). The opi-

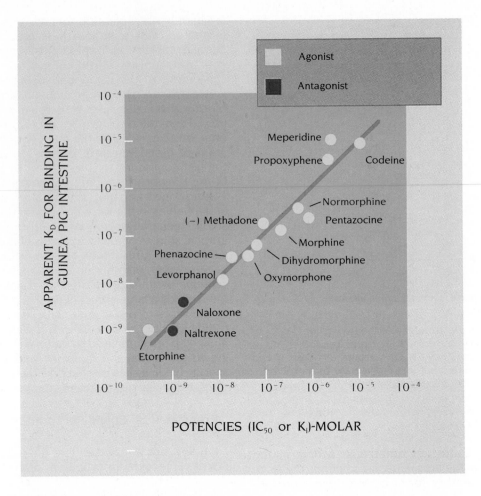

Figure 22–2 Correlation of pharmacologic potencies of opiate agonists and antagonists with their affinities for receptor binding in the guinea pig intestine. Potencies refer to IC_{50} for inhibition of electrically induced contraction of isolated gut by agonists, or to K_i for inhibition of opiate agonist activity by antagonists.

oids could then be classified according to their relative affinities and potencies at the different types of receptor. None of the drugs appear to have absolute specificity for a single receptor type; rather, each drug has a major affinity for one type, with lesser degrees of affinity for the other types (Table 22–2). Many investigators now question whether the σ receptor should be classed as an opioid receptor. Naloxone has at most a very weak blocking effect on it. Phencyclidine, a nonopioid hallucinogenic agent, was reported to bind strongly to the σ receptor, although recent evidence indicates that the σ receptor and the phencyclidine receptor are not identical (*see* Chapter 29).

Types of Endogenous Opioid Peptides

A possible explanation for the lack of strict specificity of the opiates and synthetic opioids was that the different receptor types had evolved as binding sites for specific endogenous ligands, not for exogenous drugs. To date, three groups of peptides have been discovered in the central nervous system, with properties similar to those of the opiate analgesics.

Endorphins are large peptides that are split off enzymatically from known protein hormones of the pituitary and hypothalamus. For example, β-endorphin consists of amino acids 61–91 of β-lipotropin (β-LPH).

Enkephalins are pentapeptides, and met-enkephalin (Tyr-Gly-Gly-Phe-Met) consists of amino acids 61–65 of β-LPH, *i.e.*, 1–5 of β-endorphin (Fig. 22–3). Leu-enkephalin is the same as met-enkephalin except that it has a leucine in place of methionine.

Dynorphin is an intermediate-length peptide (17 amino acids), of which the first five amino acids are the same as those constituting leu-enkephalin.

These peptides are synthesized within the brain itself as large precursor proteins, which contain the opioid peptides and other neuroendocrine peptides as parts of their amino acid sequences. The same precur-

TABLE 22-1 Postulated Types of Opioid Receptors, Their Prototypic Ligands, and Their Most Important Physiologic Effects

Receptor Type	Ligands Endogenous	Exogenous	Major Effects
μ	β-Endorphin	Morphine	Supraspinal analgesia Respiratory depression Euphoria
κ	Dynorphin ?	Ethylketo-cyclazocine	Hypothermia? Miosis Sedation Analgesia (spinal ? supraspinal ?)
σ	?	N-allyl-normetazocine	Dysphoria Hallucinations
δ	Met-Enkephalin	Etorphine	Inhibition of smooth muscle Spinal analgesia?
ε?	β-Endorphin	?	?

sor may occur at several sites in the brain, but be split by different enzymes, thus giving rise to different products at different sites. For example, the precursor protein pro-opiomelanocortin contains within itself the sequences of eight different peptide hormones or neuromodulators (*see* Fig. 22–3). However, enzymatic activity splits it primarily to β-lipotropin and ACTH in the anterior pituitary, but to β-endorphin and β-MSH in the intermediate lobe of the rat pituitary (*see also* Chapter 47).

Unfortunately, these peptides have not proven to be specific for individual types of opioid receptors. β-Endorphin, for example, is almost equally active at μ and δ receptors. Therefore, the biologic significance of

TABLE 22-2 Opioid Receptor Specificity: Agonist, Partial Agonist, and Antagonist Actions at Different Classes of Opioid Receptor

Compound	Receptor Types			
	μ	κ	σ	δ
Morphine	+ + +	+	0	+
Pentazocine	– (P?)	+	+	
Ethylketocyclazocine		+ + +		
Nalorphine	–	P	+ + +	
Met-Enkephalin	+	+	0	+ + +
Naloxone	– – –	–	–?	–
Buprenorphine	P	+ + +	0	–
Nalbuphine	–	+	0	–?

+ + + = strong agonist; + = moderate agonist.
– – – = strong antagonist; – = moderate antagonist.
P = partial agonist; 0 = no effect.
Where no symbol is shown, there is insufficient evidence to draw a conclusion.

the various categories of receptors and peptides is still under investigation.

Regional Distribution in the Nervous System

The distribution of opioid receptors and opioid peptides is not uniform throughout the nervous system. Autoradiographic and binding data, together with studies of the effects of microinjection of opioids into specific loci in the nervous system, have shown that (1) receptors mediating analgesia are concentrated mainly in the dorsal horn of the spinal cord, the periaqueductal gray matter, and the thalamus; (2) those mediating effects on respiration, cough, vomiting, and pupillary diameter are concentrated in the ventral brainstem; (3) those affecting neuroendocrine secretion are mainly in the hypothalamus; and (4) those producing effects on mood and behavior are mainly in the limbic structures (hippocampus, amygdala, *etc.*).

Within the brain, enkephalins are found in highest concentration in the striatum and nucleus accumbens, β-endorphin in the hypothalamus, pituitary, and periaqueductal gray, and dynorphin in anterior hypothalamus and substantia nigra. Lesser concentrations of all three are found in many other structures. β-Endorphin and ACTH appear to be released together from the anterior pituitary in response to stress, while dynorphin and vasopressin are co-released from the posterior pituitary by dehydration.

Opioid receptors are also found in the myenteric plexus of small intestine, the vas deferens, and possibly other peripheral tissues where opiates act. Enkephalins are found in the adrenal medulla, and in axon terminals from various parts of the spinal cord, especially in areas with high concentrations of opiate receptors. They appear to be the natural transmitter

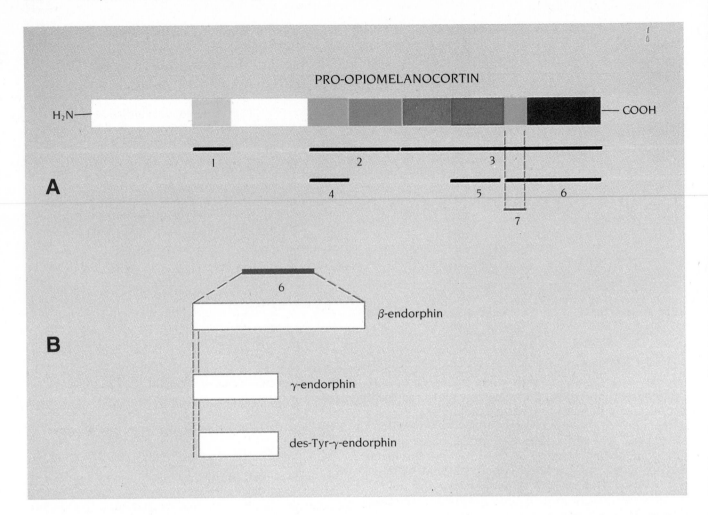

Figure 22–3 Schematic diagram of relationships among the neuropeptides derived from pro-opiomelanocortin (POMC). A, POMC contains the amino acid sequences of γ-MSH (1), ACTH (2), and β-LPH (3); ACTH contains the sequence of α-MSH (4); β-LPH contains the sequences of β-MSH (5) and β-endorphin (6); β-endorphin contains the sequence of met-enkephalin (7). All of these are marked off by pairs of basic amino acids (black bars), which theoretically can serve as points of cleavage by various peptidases. B, β-Endorphin also contains the sequences of γ-endorphin and des-tyrosine-γ-endorphin, but these are not marked by cleavage points, and are probably not formed from β-endorphin. (See also Fig. 47–3, Chapter 47.)

that binds to the receptors, inhibiting transmission of pain stimuli. Met-enkephalin is also found in the myenteric plexus, where it binds to the receptors that inhibit gut contractility by inhibiting release of acetylcholine.

At present, a great many separate facts are known about opioid peptides, their location, binding, and effects, but no clear comprehensive picture has yet emerged of their physiologic role in the nervous system. However, rapid progress is being made, and the next edition of this book may be able to offer a better integrated picture.

Major Central Effects of the Opioids

Neuronal Activity

Opioids appear to act essentially as inhibitors of neuronal electrical activity, both spontaneous and evoked, and of neurotransmitter release. For example, single-unit recordings from the neocortex show that firing rates, both spontaneous and evoked by the excitatory transmitter glutamate, are reduced after local application of met-enkephalin, β-endorphin, or morphine. The decrease is promptly abolished by naloxone, an opioid-receptor blocker. Hippocampal pyramidal cells show **increased** activity under the influence of morphine, but this is because morphine blocks the inhibitory interneurons that are activated by recurrent collaterals from the pyramidal cell axons (Fig. 22–4). A similar process occurs at the axon terminals of sensory primary afferents entering the spinal cord, where morphine may block transmitter release, and thus contribute to the analgesic effect. This locus of action is exploited in the technique of continuous epidural or intrathecal infusion of opioids for maintaining smooth, prolonged analgesia in cancer patients while minimizing effects on the brain.

Analgesia

Morphine relieves pain both by raising the threshold for pain perception and by diminishing the discomfort even if the pain is perceived, *i.e.*, **increasing the pain tolerance**. Increase in pain threshold is readily measured experimentally (radiant heat, mechanical pressure, *etc.*), but pain tolerance is greatly affected by individual temperament, setting, and other factors. Narcotic analgesics have a greater effect on pain tolerance (which possibly reflects action in the limbic system) than on pain threshold (which possibly reflects action in the spinal cord and periaqueductal gray), so that a patient can still be aware of the presence of pain but not be bothered or distressed by it. Morphine relieves all types of pain—visceral, somatic, and cutaneous. It is more

effective against dull constant pains than against sharp, severe intermittent ones.

Respiratory Depression

Opioid analgesics have pronounced respiratory depressant activity. They cause a decreased sensitivity of the respiratory centre to CO_2. The major acute toxicity from morphine is death from respiratory failure. In patients with chronic respiratory disease (*e.g.*, emphysema) morphine may be fatal. In all subjects, increased Pco_2 tends to cause cerebral vasodilatation; this leads to an increase in CSF pressure, which may be exaggerated in the presence of head injury. The respiratory depressant effect of opioids is additive with that of alcohol, barbiturates, and other CNS depressants.

Change in Mood

Part of the analgesic effect is due to a foggy, unreal feeling of being "detached" from things. For some people this is alarming or unpleasant; for others, it is a pleasant, relaxed, dreamy state (euphoria). Euphoria is a poor term because it means different things in relation to different drugs: *e.g.*, with amphetamines it means a sense of energy and exhilaration; with the opiates it means the dreamy, pleasant state just mentioned; with heroin and some other opiates it includes, in addition, an intense visceral sensation of warmth and "tingling," which may be related to the peripheral actions. Not all opiates produce euphoria in all subjects, but they all produce the clouded state.

Sedation

Not all opiates produce the same degree of sedation with equianalgesic doses, but all (especially κ agonists) produce some, and it appears to be part of the basic neurophysiologic effect. The lesser sedative effect of methadone may possibly be due to protein binding, with slower onset of action; with repeated dosage, it causes marked sedation. Even opiates with marked excitatory action may cause convulsions alternating with periods of sedation. The sedative effect of opioids is **at least** additive with that of alcohol and other CNS depressants.

Separate Central Effects

There are other actions, which are not intimately related to the analgesic action. These effects may be produced to varying degrees by nonanalgesic opiates.
Excitation. In cats, horses, pigs, cows, and a number of other species, and **in some humans, relatively low doses of morphine cause restlessness**, fright, hyperactivity, and fever. Higher doses may cause convulsions.

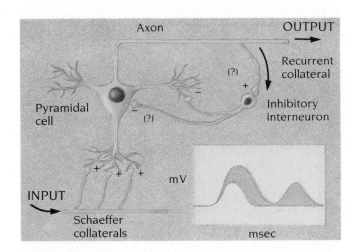

Figure 22–4 Action of morphine on hippocampal pyramidal cell activity. Inhibition of synaptic activity occurs either (?) at the excitatory synapse (+) of the recurrent collateral on the interneuron, or at the inhibitory synapse (–) on the pyramidal cell. INSET: As a result, the compound action potential (pyramidal cell output) evoked by excitatory stimulation of the Schaeffer collaterals is increased after morphine (----), compared to control conditions (——), and repetitive firing may occur.

Miosis. Miosis is seen in humans and in most species in which morphine is sedative. In species in which excitation occurs, mydriasis is noted. However, in the monkey, which is sedated by morphine, the pupils nevertheless dilate. Miosis is blocked by atropine and by decortication; therefore it is thought to be due to removal of cortical inhibitory action on the third cranial nerve nucleus. (**Meperidine**, a synthetic opioid analgesic, is an exception in not causing pupil constriction.)

Nausea and vomiting. Nausea and vomiting are due to stimulation of the chemoreceptor trigger zone. **Apomorphine, a nonanalgesic derivative, causes a much greater emetic effect** than morphine does.

Antitussive action. Direct depression of the cough centre is not related to respiratory depression. **Nonanalgesic derivatives (*e.g.*, dextromethorphan) can have antitussive action**.

Endocrine effects. Endocrine effects are produced by actions of the opioids in the thalamus and hypothalamus. These agents inhibit the release of the gonadotropin-releasing factor, LHRH (*see* Chapter 45), so that the pituitary output of luteotropin (LH) and follicle-stimulating hormone (FSH) is diminished. This in turn decreases the secretion of testosterone by the testis, and results in decreased libido, reduced volume of ejaculate, and decreased motility of sperm in males; in females, anovulatory cycles or amenorrhea occur. In contrast, serum prolactin level is raised, because the opioids inhibit the release of dopamine by hypothalamic neurons, which normally exert a tonic inhibitory influence on the prolactin secretory cells. In the past it was thought that morphine stimulates release of vasopressin from the posterior lobe of the pituitary. Recent investigations, however, indicate that the direct effect is to inhibit vasopressin secretion; the antidiuresis caused by morphine apparently results from a peripheral action on the kidney.

Poikilothermia. Most opioids inhibit the thermoregulatory mechanism centred in the preoptic anterior hypothalamic region. As a result, the ability to maintain a constant body temperature is impaired, and the direction and degree of change in body temperature depend on the ambient temperature. At normal or low room temperature, excessive heat loss to the environment occurs as a result of opioid action, and the body temperature falls.

Peripheral Effects

Histamine release. Most opioids provoke the release of histamine, causing peripheral arteriolar and venous dilatation. This results in hypotension, cutaneous flushing, and increased loss of body heat. The venous dilatation also results in a decrease in venous return to the heart. This effect made morphine very useful in the emergency treatment of acute left ventricular failure in the days before the advent of potent diuretics such as furosemide.

Contraction of smooth muscle. Contraction of smooth muscle in the biliary and bladder sphincters is stimulated by morphine and other μ agonists. The tone of the gastrointestinal and biliary tracts and of the ureter is increased, so that the intraluminal pressure in these structures increases and there may be spasm. At the same time, inhibition of acetylcholine release from the myenteric plexus causes a marked reduction in propulsive peristaltic movement, resulting in constipation. This is the basis of the antidiarrheal effect of opioids (*see* Chapter 51).

Contact dermatitis and urticaria. Contact dermatitis and urticaria occur mainly among nurses, pharmacists, *etc.*, who handle the drugs frequently.

FATE IN THE BODY

Opioids are fairly well absorbed from the gastrointestinal tract, especially the more lipid-soluble ones such as heroin, which was formerly given by mouth as a cough suppressant. Methadone is normally given by mouth in methadone maintenance therapy of opioid addicts, and codeine, d-propoxyphene, and others are given by mouth for the relief of mild or moderate pain. However, there is a significant first-pass effect in the liver, so that bioavailability is appreciably less after oral administration than after parenteral injection. The usual analgesic dose of morphine is 5–10 mg by the intravenous or the intramuscular route, but six to eight times as much may be needed by mouth, while for codeine the ratio is only 1.5 times. The advantages of oral administration are avoidance of the discomfort of injections, and a more prolonged and smooth effect; the disadvantage is slowness of onset. Oral administration is often used for continuous relief of chronic pain in cancer patients.

Morphine enters all tissues. In adults relatively little enters the brain, but in infants, whose blood–brain barrier is less effective, it enters more readily, so that infants are more susceptible to its action. Morphine also diffuses across the gastric mucosa into the lumen of the stomach, where the acidity converts it into the ionized form, which can not diffuse back across the mucosa into the blood. As a result, morphine accumulates in the lumen, a process known as "ion trapping." For this reason, gastric lavage used to be employed in the emergency treatment of morphine overdose, even when the drug had been given parenterally (*see* the question and answer at the end of Chapter 2).

Onset of analgesic action is usually quite rapid after subcutaneous or intramuscular injection, especially with the more lipid-soluble opioids. The time may range from 5–15 minutes, depending on the drug, dose, and route. After intravenous injection, the effect begins almost immediately. Continuous subcutaneous or intravenous infusion by means of a portable pump is being tested for the relief of chronic pain, especially in cancer patients. Epidural and intrathecal injections or infusion are also being studied for the same purpose.

Protein binding of opioids in the plasma varies quite

markedly from drug to drug. At therapeutic concentrations, morphine is about 30% bound, meperidine about 60%, and methadone about 85%. This difference probably contributes to the disparity of apparent half-life: e.g., 2–3 hours for morphine, and 15–22 hours for methadone. However, the dosages for the various opioids are adjusted accordingly, so that the usual duration of analgesic effect is about 4 hours for most of them.

Metabolism also varies with the drug. For morphine, biotransformation is fairly rapid and consists mostly of glucuronic acid conjugation of the phenolic hydroxyl by the hepatic smooth endoplasmic reticulum. About 90% of a dose is found as glucuronide in the urine, and 7–10% in the feces (via the bile). With other opioids, N-demethylation, hydrolysis, cyclization, and other reactions are quantitatively important, depending on the individual drug. Liver disease may reduce the rate of elimination and lead to overdose as a result of accumulation of active drug. Renal disease can lead to accumulation of normeperidine, a toxic metabolite of meperidine.

TOLERANCE AND PHYSICAL DEPENDENCE

Tolerance to the effects of morphine develops rapidly on repeated administration, and larger and larger doses are required for the same effect (see Chapter 67, *Drug Dependence*). In animal experiments, continuous slow intravenous infusion of morphine for only 4 hours can produce some tolerance. Human addicts can stand many times the normal acute lethal dose without getting respiratory arrest.

The development of tolerance is usually accompanied by the development of physical dependence. Compensatory changes in the cell are unmasked by removal of opiates and a picture of hyperexcitability is seen: restlessness, extreme anxiety, vomiting and diarrhea, runny nose, muscle twitching, chills, fever and sweating, pupillary dilatation, and sometimes circulatory collapse. This picture varies in time of onset and in severity after withdrawal of different opiates, but **can be precipitated almost immediately by opiate antagonists. It can be abolished by giving more narcotic analgesic.** (The ability of a new opiate to abolish morphine withdrawal symptoms in human volunteers is used as a method of assessing dependence liability of the new drug; see Chapter 67.)

A number of **hypothetical mechanisms** have been proposed to explain the development of opiate tolerance and physical dependence.

1. If the drug blocks release of a neurotransmitter, postsynaptic receptors for that transmitter might be induced, or their sensitivity might be increased, thereby compensating for the drug effect (i.e., tolerance). Withdrawal of the drug would allow normal release of

transmitter, but increased receptor numbers and sensitivity would cause excessive postsynaptic effects (i.e., withdrawal reaction). So far, no good evidence of supersensitivity to acetylcholine, catecholamines, or serotonin has been found in opiate-dependent subjects. However, increased sensitivity to noradrenaline* following opioid withdrawal appears to be responsible for some of the more obvious and uncomfortable withdrawal symptoms, such as anxiety, gooseflesh ("cold turkey"), intestinal cramps, and disturbances in body temperature. These symptoms can be relieved by administration of **clonidine**, a presynaptic α_2-adrenoceptor agonist (see Chapters 16 and 18) that decreases the release of catecholamines from presynaptic terminals.

2. An enzyme that is inhibited by the opiates acutely might undergo compensatory induction. There is evidence that morphine, enkephalins, and endorphins inhibit a prostaglandin-stimulated adenylate cyclase activity acutely, and reduce cAMP levels in brain cells. In tolerant animals the adenylate cyclase increases and cAMP levels return to normal; in the withdrawal reaction they are both above normal. However, there is so far no proof that changes in adenylate cyclase and cAMP **cause** the tolerance, rather than **reflect** it.

3. If the drug blocks release of a neurotransmitter, the transmitter might theoretically accumulate intracellularly until its concentration is high enough to overcome the block (tolerance). Withdrawal of the drug would allow massive release of the accumulated transmitter. However, there is no evidence for such a mechanism.

4. More than one neuronal pathway might serve the same physiologic function ("redundancy"). If the major one is inhibited by opiates and the minor one is not, the minor one might hypertrophy and compensate for the drug effect. When the drug is withdrawn, both pathways would function, causing excessive activity. Again, there is no evidence to demonstrate the importance of such a mechanism.

5. High doses of exogenous opiates would lead to a loss ("down-regulation") of their receptors, causing tolerance. At the same time, the excessive presence of exogenous opioid would cause a feedback inhibition of the biosynthesis and release of endogenous opioid peptides. Withdrawal of the opiates would leave a deficiency of the endogenous peptides and their receptors (withdrawal reaction) until readaptation occurred. A decreased rate of synthesis of β-endorphin has recently been reported in morphine-tolerant rats, but there is no evidence of change in receptors during tolerance, although there is cross-tolerance between morphine and the opioid peptides.

Tolerance and physical dependence are not the same as addiction. A normal subject can be made physically dependent, and after going through a withdrawal reaction will not resume drug-taking. Addiction

---

* norepinephrine

also involves a compulsion to take the drug again after going through withdrawal, *i.e.*, a strong psychological dependence on it. (Drug dependence is covered in greater detail in Chapter 67.)

MORPHINE CONGENERS

Codeine is a relatively weak analgesic, having one-tenth the potency of morphine, and consequently shows little respiratory depression and relatively little addiction liability. About 15% of a codeine dose is metabolically converted into morphine in the human body but, nevertheless, most effects are said to be due to codeine itself. It is used widely in combination with non-narcotic analgesics such as ASA or acetaminophen, and as a cough suppressant in doses of 10–15 mg.

Hydrocodone (Hycodan® and others), a derivative of codeine, is particularly effective as an analgesic, being as potent as morphine, and it is also commonly used as an antitussive.

Most of the **semisynthetic morphine derivatives** are fairly old. Of these, **heroin** is five to ten times as potent as morphine. The addict likes heroin because its high lipid solubility enables it to enter the brain much more rapidly than morphine, and it acts much more rapidly. Because of narcotic control regulations, heroin is no longer available for clinical use in the U.S.A. In Canada, special permission is required for its use, which is limited to the control of chronic intractable pain in terminal cancer.

Hydromorphone (Dilaudid®) has strong analgesic and antitussive activity, being more potent than morphine and codeine, respectively, on a weight basis. It is better absorbed than morphine following oral administration, with an onset of analgesic action in about 15 minutes and a duration of action of more than 5 hours. This drug can therefore be given by mouth (which is one of its advantages), as well as by subcutaneous or intramuscular injection, and as rectal suppositories.

Levorphanol (Levo-Dromoran®) is one of the more potent **synthetic analgesics** presently in wide use, being four to five times as potent as morphine. It is less constipating than morphine and is longer-acting. This drug has a levo-rotatory structure; its dextro-rotatory isomer, **dextromethorphan**, has no analgesic activity and is used only as an antitussive in doses of 10–15 mg.

Meperidine (pethidine; Demerol® and others) is the first and perhaps still most widely used **synthetic** congener. It is a relatively old preparation and has many trade names. The chemical structure resembles that of atropine as well as morphine, and it was originally believed to be an antispasmodic rather than a constrictor of smooth muscle like morphine. However, this is now known to be false; it does cause spasm. Its action is shorter than that of morphine, and it is less potent by a factor of about 10. In equianalgesic doses it causes at least as much respiratory depression as morphine.

Meperidine does not produce miosis and is, therefore, a favorite of addicted nurses and doctors (it is less likely to be detected). It is quite effective when given by mouth. Normeperidine, a metabolite of meperidine, causes CNS excitatory effects and can produce seizures.

Methadone (Dolophine®; Fig. 22–5) has about the same analgesic potency as morphine but differs from it essentially in two respects. It has a much longer duration of action because it is more slowly eliminated from the body, and in single doses it causes little sedation. The lack of sedative effect did detract from its original popularity. However, because of its much slower clearance from the body, its withdrawal effects are much milder than those of morphine. The main current use of methadone is, therefore, substitution for morphine in addicts prior to withdrawal.

In the 1960s, V. Dole and M. Nyswander began testing the use of **long-term methadone maintenance for the management of opiate addiction**. The purpose was to maintain a sufficiently high level of tolerance so that the addict's usual dose of heroin or other opiate would produce little or no "high." Rather than withdraw the patient almost immediately from methadone, they kept patients on this drug for months or years, while concentrating on psychological and social rehabilitation. Between 50% and 80% of patients in well-run methadone maintenance programs continue in treatment and hold jobs successfully. Recently, the emphasis has begun to shift towards gradual reduction in methadone dosage and eventual withdrawal, supported in some cases by use of naltrexone (*see* below) to prevent a return to heroin.

Propoxyphene (Darvon®) is a commonly used analgesic structurally related to methadone but 12 to 15 times less potent. In equianalgesic doses it has properties similar to those of the other narcotic analgesics.

Fentanyl (Sublimaze®) is chemically related to meperidine. It is about 80 times as potent an analgesic as morphine. It produces all the other effects that morphine does, in about the same ratio as the analgesia. **Sufentanil** (Sufenta®), an analog, is about 10 times as potent as fentanyl, while **alfentanil** (Alfenta®) is about one-quarter as potent. The main advantages of fentanyl are that, when given intravenously, it has an almost immediate onset of action and a short duration, the half-life of the redistribution phase being only 12.5 minutes. Therefore it lends itself very well for neuroleptanalgesia (*see* Chapter 23). It is injected intravenously

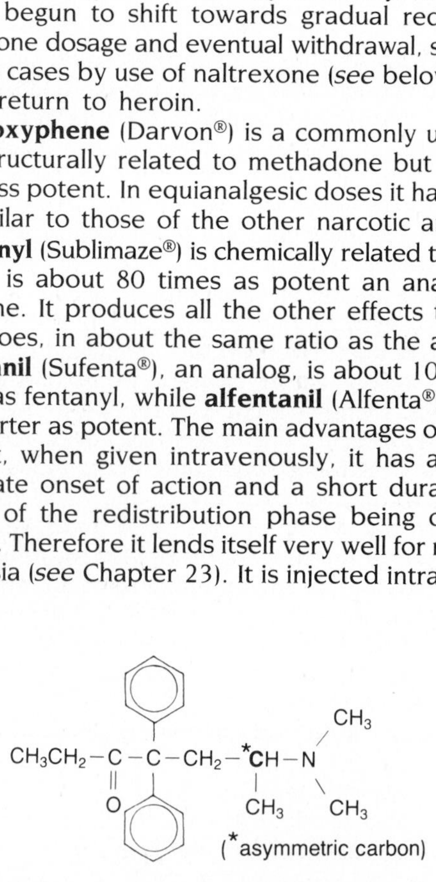

$$CH_3CH_2-\underset{\underset{O}{\|}}{C}-\underset{\underset{\bigcirc}{}}{C}-CH_2-\overset{*}{C}H-N\underset{CH_3}{\overset{CH_3}{<}}$$

(*asymmetric carbon)

Figure 22–5 Structural formula of methadone.

in a dose of 1 μg/kg, mixed with droperidol or a similar neuroleptic, and supplementary doses of 50–100 μg are given intravenously every 30–45 minutes during surgery. An important advantage is that fentanyl causes very little depression of left ventricular function, so that it carries little risk of hypotension during surgery. However, there is some danger of drug accumulation if doses are repeated too frequently. Because of the short half-life, the patient can wake up rapidly when the surgery is over, and has little difficulty with respiratory depression and constipation postoperatively. Sufentanil and alfentanyl are used for the same purpose.

High doses of fentanyl tend to produce muscular rigidity, perhaps by action at enkephalin receptors in the striatum, which may inhibit dopamine release there. The effect can be overcome by muscle relaxants, or by naloxone (*see* below).

NARCOTIC ANTAGONISTS

In the morphine molecule (*see* Fig. 22–1), the methyl group attached to the N is of critical dimensions for agonist activity when the molecule has combined with its receptor. If the CH_3 is changed to an allyl group, or if a cyclopropyl or cyclobutyl group is attached to the methyl, the molecule still binds to the receptor but no longer initiates a typical morphine response. It therefore functions as a receptor blocker, or narcotic antagonist (Fig. 22–6). Replacement of the $-OH$ at carbon 6 by a ketonic oxygen results in a highly specific and powerful blocking action.

Naloxone (Narcan®) is said to be a pure narcotic antagonist since it has no analgesic activity of its own, but has the ability to reverse or block the actions of narcotic analgesic agonists. It has the strongest affinity and blocking potency at μ receptors, where it prevents or reverses the activity not only of morphine and its congeners, but also of β-endorphin and enkephalins. It is less effective as a blocker of κ and σ receptors.

Naltrexone (Trexan®) is a related compound that is also a pure blocker, but has a much longer half-life than

naloxone, and is well absorbed when given by mouth.

When given together with morphine, these drugs antagonize many of its important actions, including analgesia, respiratory depression, euphoria, increase in CSF pressure, miosis, smooth muscle spasm, and hypotension. Their **clinical uses** are (1) to reverse the respiratory depression caused by morphine-like drugs; (2) in diagnostic tests for opioid addicts, in whom they precipitate an acute withdrawal reaction; and (3) in the treatment of addicts, **after they have been withdrawn** from opioids, to prevent the ''high'' from self-administered heroin or morphine, and thus to decrease the risk of relapse.

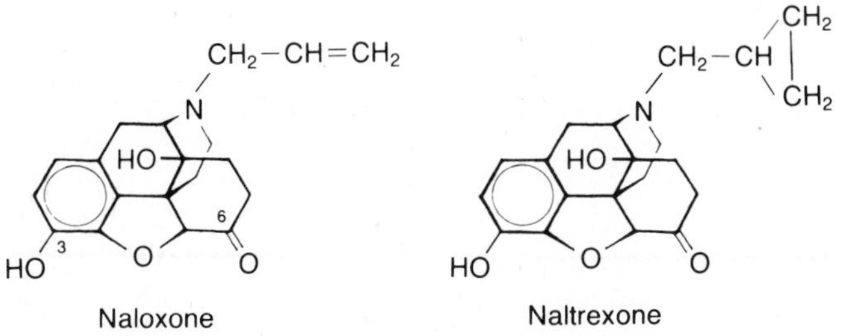

MIXED AGONIST-ANTAGONISTS AND PARTIAL AGONISTS

Opioids with allyl or 4- or 5-carbon substituents on the N, but that retain the $-OH$ group at C-6, display a mixture of agonist and antagonist properties. Examples include nalorphine and nalbuphine (Fig. 22–7). Pentazocine is a synthetic analog with similar properties.

Nalorphine (Nalline®) and **levallorphan** (Lorfan®) act as μ-receptor blockers, preventing the analgesic, respiratory depressant, and euphoriant actions of morphine. However, they are weak agonists at κ receptors, and therefore have some analgesic and sedating effects when given by themselves. They are also quite good agonists at σ receptors, and when given in larger doses they cause agitation, dysphoria, and hallucinations. Therefore, they carry a lower risk of abuse and dependence than do μ agonists.

Pentazocine (Talwin®), **cyclazocine**, and **nalbuphine** (Nubain®) are also mixed agonist-antagonists that have

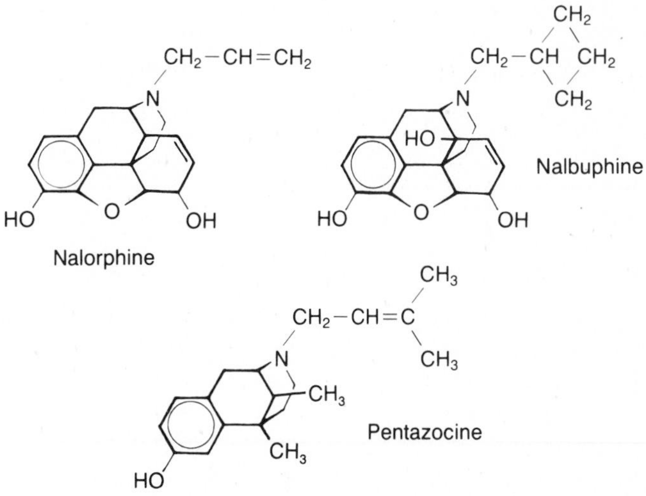

Figure 22–7 Structural formulae of some mixed agonist-antagonist opioids that act as μ-receptor blockers, but as agonists at κ and/or σ receptors.

Figure 22–6 Structural formulae of two potent narcotic antagonists. Compare these with Figure 22–1. Numbers designate the C-3 and C-6 positions mentioned in the text.

some morphine-antagonist (μ-blocking) effect but are reasonably good analgesics by themselves. Since pentazocine and cyclazocine also act at σ receptors, their mental effects seem to be intermediate between those of morphine and nalorphine. They do not cause severe mental disturbance as nalorphine does, but they are less likely than morphine to produce euphoria (*see* Table 22–2).

Buprenorphine has a cyclopropyl-methyl substituent on the N, the same as that of naltrexone, and a $-OCH_3$ group like that of codeine in place of the $-OH$ on C-6. These offset each other to some extent, so that, instead of being a μ-receptor blocker, it is a partial μ agonist. That means that it has some morphine-like action, but the maximum response attainable is considerably less than that of morphine, no matter how much the dose is increased, and by competing with morphine or heroin for μ receptors it can reduce their maximum effect. It has been suggested that this makes it less attractive to addicts, and makes it less likely to be abused.

FINAL COMMENT

The field of opioid peptides, opioid receptors, and synthetic opioids is undergoing rapid change as a result of recent research. Over the next few years there will probably be major developments permitting better separation of analgesic, euphoriant, endocrine, and other effects, and therefore better therapeutic specificity. The reader should be alert to such developments.

SUGGESTED READING

Adler MW. Multiple opiate receptors and their different ligand profiles. Ann NY Acad Sci 1982; 398:340–351.

Corrigall WA. Opiates and the hippocampus: a review of the functional and morphological evidence. Pharmacol Biochem Behav 1983; 18:255–262.

Costa E, Trabucchi M, eds. Regulatory peptides from molecular biology to function. Adv Biochem Psychopharmacol 1983; 33:1–561.

Hughes J, ed. Opioid peptides. Brit Med Bull 1983; 39(1).

Martin WR. Pharmacology of opioids. Pharmacol Rev 1983; 35:283–323.

Payne R. Role of epidural and intrathecal narcotics and peptides in the management of cancer pain. Med Clin North Am 1987; 71(2):313–327.

Portenoy RK. Continuous intravenous infusion of opioid drugs. Med Clin North Am 1987; 71(2):233–241.

Special issue: Mixed agonist-antagonist analgesics. Drug Alcohol Depend 1985; 14(3–4):221–431.

Symposium: Update on opioids, hypnotics and muscle relaxants. Anaesth Intensive Care 1987; 15(1):7–96.

Woods JH, Smith CB, Medzihradsky F, et al. Evaluation of new compounds for opioid activity: 1986 annual report. Natl Inst Drug Abuse Res Monogr Ser 1987; 76:448–484.

Chapter 23

GENERAL ANAESTHETICS

F.J. Carmichael

The proper use of anaesthesia in surgery began in the 1840s following Morton's successful demonstration of the effectiveness of ether anaesthesia in dentistry. Since that time new anaesthetic agents have been developed and introduced into clinical practice, and methods for administering these drugs have been improved. The newer agents are safer for the patient in that they are nonexplosive (compare the properties of ether to those of halothane). The improved methodology, made possible in part by technological advances, has allowed the anaesthetist to give safer anaesthesia to patients with compromised cardiovascular, respiratory, or central nervous system functions. Also, these newer agents and methods have contributed immensely to the expansion of the scope of surgery from short operative procedures limited to the extremities or abdomen to the major surgical accomplishments of the present.

DESIRABLE ACTIONS OF GENERAL ANAESTHETICS

Hypnosis (loss of consciousness). Although some surgery is conducted on the awake patient, many operative procedures are better carried out with the patient asleep. Many present-day surgical procedures are done with the patient intubated and perhaps ventilated. These latter procedures require that the patient be "asleep" or unconscious.

Analgesia (loss of pain). Surgical procedures, by their nature, are painful, and it is incumbent upon the anaesthetist to alleviate this pain whether the patient is asleep or awake.

Amnesia (loss of recall). Since surgery can be a frightening ordeal for the patient, it is desirable that there be little or no memory of the event.

Muscle relaxation. This is not always required, but many surgical procedures are made considerably easier when there is reduced muscle tone. Also, when a patient is to be intubated and ventilated there is a need for relaxation of laryngeal and respiratory muscles.

No single anaesthetic agent has yet been developed in which these properties are combined in optimal proportions; nor is it likely that any single agent could provide optimal anaesthesia for all patients and all types of procedures. Therefore a flexible approach is needed in clinical anaesthesia. Full loss of consciousness and loss of pain-induced reflexes, with good muscular relaxation but minimal disturbance of circulation, are usually obtained with a combination of light anaesthesia together with specific narcotic analgesic and muscle-relaxant drugs, a procedure known as "balanced anaesthesia."

THEORIES OF ANAESTHESIA

The mechanism by which general anaesthetics exert their effects remains uncertain, although various theories have enjoyed scientific popularity at different times. Any theory of general anaesthesia must attempt to identify a common basis of interaction between the nerve cell and drugs of quite varied physical and chemical properties to explain how such diverse substances can produce closely similar patterns of general anaesthetic effects.

Metabolic Theories

These attributed the phenomenon of anaesthesia to interference with nerve cell function by the anaesthetic agent, through depression of neuronal respiration or metabolism. Most investigators now feel that the metabolic disturbances are the result, rather than the cause, of decreased nerve cell activity.

Membrane Theories

Most theories of anaesthesia have been based on the concept that the drug interferes with changes in the cell membrane that normally occur during neuronal excitation, impulse conduction, and transmitter release.

Lipid solubility theory. The lipid solubility theory was based on the correlation between the lipid/water partition coefficients of different substances and their general anaesthetic potencies. This correlation, described by Meyer in 1899 and Overton in 1901, led to the view that the degree of anaesthesia is proportional to the concentration of anaesthetic dissolved in the lipids of the cell membrane.

Thermodynamic activity theory. In 1939, Ferguson proposed this theory to account for exceptions to the Meyer-Overton correlation. He multiplied the concentration of dissolved anaesthetic by its thermodynamic activity coefficient (TAC), which is a correction factor reflecting the degree of physicochemical interaction between the molecules of anaesthetic and those of the phase in which it is located: Thermodynamic activity = molar concentration × TAC. Ferguson claimed that equal thermodynamic activity of different anaesthetics in the cell membrane produced equal degrees of anaesthesia.

Membrane occupancy theory. Since there were still exceptions that did not fit Ferguson's theory, Mullins (1954) introduced a further correction to take account of the molecular size of the anaesthetic agent. At the same thermodynamic activity, a larger molecule would occupy a larger space within the membrane. Mullins proposed that the degree of anaesthesia is proportional to the fractional volume of the cell membrane occupied by the anaesthetic.

Membrane expansion theory. The membrane expansion theory (Eyring; Seeman; K.W. Miller) extends Mullins' theory by proposing a mechanism of action. According to this hypothesis, the anaesthetic molecules enter hydrophobic regions of the membrane (*i.e.*, in the centres of membrane proteins and between lipid molecules), distorting and expanding the membrane, as well as the proteins associated with the sodium-conductance channel (Fig. 23–1). This expansion would compress the sodium channel and thus prevent the ion flux associated with the action potential. The effect of this impairment of Na⁺ influx is seen in a slower rise of the action potential, and a correspondingly higher threshold of depolarization before the neuron responds with an action potential. All neurons would be affected in a similar way, but some are much more sensitive than others. Clinically usable anaesthesia and analgesia, without fatal respiratory depression, depends upon this difference in neuronal sensitivity to the same drug. Various investigators showed that all lipid-soluble

anaesthetics at effective anaesthetic concentration expand cell membranes by about 1%. If anaesthetized small laboratory animals, single nerve cells, or axons are subjected to 100 atmospheres of pressure so that the membranes are recompressed by about 1%, the animals wake up or nerve function returns even though the anaesthetic is still present (pressure reversal of anaesthesia).

MEMBRANE CONCENTRATION RULE OF GENERAL ANAESTHESIA

The membrane expansion theory described above, although not without its detractors, provides a qualitative explanation of the mechanisms of action of anaesthetic agents. Its quantitative aspects are stated

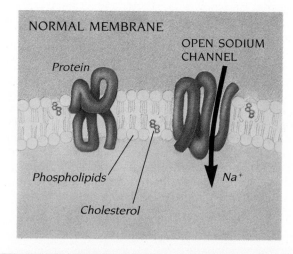

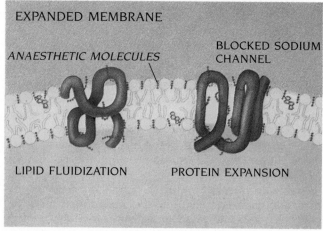

Figure 23–1 Blockade of sodium channels in excitable membranes through expansion of the membrane in the presence of anaesthetic molecules.

in the **Membrane Concentration Rule** proposed by Seeman, which can be used to predict the administered concentrations of anaesthetic agent needed to produce surgical anaesthesia. The following paragraphs show the application of this rule to clinical practice.

Membrane Rule of General Anaesthesia

The rule states that, when the membrane excitability of small neurons in the brain becomes blocked by an anaesthetic, the concentration in the membrane phase (C_{mem}) is 500 μmol per 100 mL of membrane volume. A mole of any substance contains 6×10^{23} molecules; this is known as Avogadro's number. Therefore 500 μmol contains 3×10^{20} molecules. A spherical cell of 15 μm radius would have a volume of 14,137 μm^3. If the cell membrane is 100 Å ($= 0.01$ μm) thick, the cell minus the membrane would have a radius of 14.99 μm and a volume of 14,108 μm^3, so that the volume of the membrane would be 29 μm^3. This means that at a C_{mem} of 500 μmol/100 mL, there would be 87×10^6 molecules of anaesthetic in the membrane of such a cell. Compare this with the numbers of molecules per cell needed for drugs with specific receptors (*see* Chapter 9).

Prediction of the Anaesthetic Concentration in Blood

Using halothane as an example, the required concentration of anaesthetic in the blood water can be readily predicted from the Membrane Rule, knowing only the membrane/water partition coefficient of the anaesthetic ($P_{m/w}$), which is 25 for halothane. (Note that the partition coefficient is essentially unitless. Strictly speaking, it has units of mL water/mL membrane.)

$$P_{m/w} = \frac{C_{membrane}}{C_{water}}.$$

Therefore, $C_w = \dfrac{C_{mem}}{P_{m/w}} = \dfrac{500 \ \mu mol/100 \ mL}{25}$

$$= 20 \ \mu mol/100 \ mL \ water.$$

Before surgery can proceed, therefore, the patient must have a concentration of 20 μmol of halothane per 100 mL of blood water.

Prediction of the Anaesthetic Concentration Needed in the Patient's Inspired Air

Since halothane has about the same solubility in air as in water ($P_{air/water} = 1$), the concentration in the lung alveolar air will be the same as that in the blood water, namely 20 μmol per 100 mL of air:

$$C_{air} = C_w \times P_{a/w} = 20 \ \mu mol/100 \ mL \times 1.$$

How is this halothane concentration expressed in clinical practice? In order to convert the alveolar halothane concentration into units used in the clinical setting, it is necessary to use the elementary fact that 1 mole of any gas always occupies about 25 L at body temperature. Hence,

$$C_{air} = \frac{20 \times 10^{-6}}{100 \ mL \ air} \times 25 \ L \ halothane \ (1 \ mole)$$

$$= \frac{0.5 \ mL \ halothane \ vapor}{100 \ mL \ air}.$$

Thus, the value of 20 μmol per 100 mL of alveolar air works out to be 0.5 mL of halothane vapor per 100 mL of alveolar air, or, as the anaesthetist says, 0.5%. In practice, induction of the patient starts with 2–3% halothane and the concentration is gradually lowered to 0.5–0.6% for maintenance of anaesthesia during surgery.

Prediction of Anaesthetic Equilibrium Concentrations Required in Clinical Practice

As already mentioned, to achieve a surgical level of general anaesthesia, the Membrane Rule states that the concentration of anaesthetic in the brain membranes must be 500 μmol per 100 mL of membrane. The anaesthetic concentrations used in clinical practice can thus be predicted from the partition coefficients of drugs, as shown in Table 23–1 for nitrous oxide, halothane, and ether.

Prediction of Approximate Times Needed for Anaesthetic Induction

Table 23–2 shows the calculations required to predict the speed with which particular agents induce anaesthesia. The example assumes that three subjects take a single deep breath of 5 L of nitrous oxide, halothane, or ether, respectively, each anaesthetic being at its equilibrium concentration (as described in Table 23–1).

PREMEDICATION

Before a patient undergoes a procedure requiring general anaesthesia, it is common to administer

TABLE 23–1 Calculation of Required Concentrations of Anaesthetics in Plasma and Alveolar Air

	Nitrous Oxide	Halothane	Diethyl Ether
Concentration in membrane	$\dfrac{500\ \mu\text{mol}}{100\ \text{mL membrane}}$	$\dfrac{500\ \mu\text{mol}}{100\ \text{mL membrane}}$	$\dfrac{500\ \mu\text{mol}}{100\ \text{mL membrane}}$
Membrane/water partition coefficient ($P_{m/w}$)	$\dfrac{1}{2}$	$\dfrac{25}{1}$	$\dfrac{1}{1}$
Concentration in plasma water	$\dfrac{1000\ \mu\text{mol}}{100\ \text{mL plasma}}$	$\dfrac{20\ \mu\text{mol}}{100\ \text{mL plasma}}$	$\dfrac{500\ \mu\text{mol}}{100\ \text{mL plasma}}$
Air/water partition coefficient ($P_{a/w}$)	$\dfrac{3}{1}$	$\dfrac{1}{1}$	$\dfrac{1}{10}$
Concentration in lung air (for general anaesthetics at equilibrium)	$\dfrac{3000\ \mu\text{mol}}{100\ \text{mL air}}$	$\dfrac{20\ \mu\text{mol}}{100\ \text{mL air}}$	$\dfrac{50\ \mu\text{mol}}{100\ \text{mL air}}$
	= 75%	= 0.5%	= 1%*

(% defined as mL of pure gas or vapor per mL of air)

* The value of 1% ether refers to its concentration in the alveolar air, and not the inspired air. In order for the patient to have 1% in the alveolar air at the outset, it is necessary to administer the ether at many times this concentration; this is because ether is many times more soluble in water than in air, and most of the ether molecules quickly permeate into the blood, leaving little in lung air. In clinical practice, therefore, the anaesthetist starts induction with about 30–40% ether, and reduces the inspired concentration to 5–10% before surgery.

TABLE 23–2 Relation Between Anaesthetic Concentration and Rate of Induction

	Nitrous Oxide	Halothane	Diethyl Ether
Concentration in lung air (from Table 23–1)	75% or $\dfrac{3000\ \mu\text{mol}}{100\ \text{mL air}}$	0.5% or $\dfrac{20\ \mu\text{mol}}{100\ \text{mL air}}$	1% or $\dfrac{50\ \mu\text{mol}}{100\ \text{mL air}}$
Number of μmol entering the lungs in a 5-L breath	150,000	1000	2500
Concentration in plasma water (after mixing in 5 L of air and 50 L of body water) (*value for $P_{a/w}$)	$\dfrac{150{,}000\ \mu\text{mol}}{50\ \text{L} + (5\ \text{L} \times 3^*)}$ $\simeq \dfrac{250\ \mu\text{mol}}{100\ \text{mL}}$	$\dfrac{1000\ \mu\text{mol}}{50\ \text{L} + (5\ \text{L} \times 1^*)}$ $\simeq \dfrac{2\ \mu\text{mol}}{100\ \text{mL}}$	$\dfrac{2500\ \mu\text{mol}}{50\ \text{L} + (5\ \text{L} \times .1^*)}$ $\simeq \dfrac{5\ \mu\text{mol}}{100\ \text{mL}}$
(See Table 23–1 for the needed concentration in plasma water to achieve required membrane concentrations)	This is 1/4 of that needed	This is 1/10 of that needed	This is 1/100 of that needed
Conclusion	Induction time is short	Induction time is intermediate	Induction time is long

premedication with one or more drugs in order to relieve pain and anxiety, to sedate the patient, and to block cholinergic (vagal) reflexes. The following classes of drugs are routinely employed.

Opioids. Narcotic analgesics such as morphine or its synthetic analogs offer analgesia, euphoria, and some sedation. Complicating problems can be respiratory depression, nausea and vomiting, gastric retention, and reduced sympathetic tone. For further details, *see* Chapter 22.

Benzodiazepines. Diazepam provides a reduction in the level of anxiety and some amnesia without significant effects on respiration or cardiovascular functions (*see* Chapter 26). Lorazepam and midazolam are also used for this purpose.

Belladonna alkaloids. Atropine and scopolamine will block vagal reflexes and inhibit salivary and respiratory tract secretions (*see* Chapter 15). However, the resulting dry mouth is unpleasant for the patient, and

therefore these drugs may be better used at the time of induction rather than as premedication. Scopolamine also provides some amnesia for the patient.

SIGNS AND STAGES OF GENERAL ANAESTHESIA

The classical signs of general anaesthesia with diethyl ether were described by Guedel, who divided the process into stages and planes (Fig. 23–2). These classical signs of general anaesthesia, while still essentially correct because they reflect physiologic events in response to **any** CNS-depressant agent, are no longer useful with the modern anaesthetic agents and techniques in current use. Now, depth of anaesthesia is judged by presence or absence of the eye lash reflex,

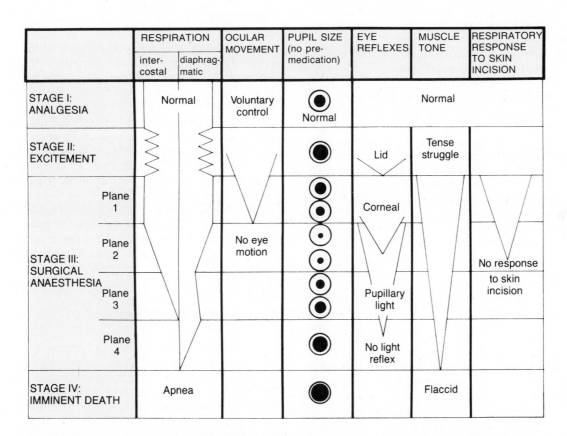

Figure 23–2 Signs and reflex reactions characterizing the stages and planes of anaesthesia (after Guedel, who devised this scheme with diethyl ether anaesthesia for the training of inexperienced medical personnel during World War I). The wedges indicate the progressive disappearance of signs and reflexes, which may vary somewhat from person to person.

rhythmic respiration, and response of the heart rate and blood pressure to surgical stimulation. However, the classical signs are given here because they draw attention to some important principles and physiologic mechanisms of general anaesthesia.

Stage I

This is the period from the beginning of anaesthetic administration to the loss of consciousness. The patient progressively loses pain sensation, but motor activity and reflexes remain normal.

Analgesia in this stage is primarily the relief of pain from cutaneous receptors. The neurons that are blocked are those in lamina 4 of the dorsal horn in the spinal cord. These are actually cells of the substantia gelatinosa, and relay onto cells that cross the midline and ascend in the spinothalamic tracts.

Stage II

This period extends from the loss of consciousness, through a stage of irregular and spastic breathing, to the reestablishment of regular breathing. The eyes still move in roving motion; the pupils are often dilated but still react to light; the eyelid reflex still occurs; and the patient may swallow, retch, vomit, or struggle intensely. It is a stage of general excitement, not without danger to the patient.

Excitement is thought to occur as a result of anaesthetic blockade of small inhibitory cells of the Golgi type II category. (As with local anaesthesia, small diameter fibres are more readily blocked than large fibres.) Consequently, excitatory effects are unmasked. A second possible reason for motor excitation is that low concentrations of anaesthetics cause a small paradoxical release of synaptic neurotransmitter, in the same way as ethanol increases the frequency of miniature endplate potentials at the neuromuscular junction (*see* Chapter 25).

Stage III

This is the stage of anaesthesia during which surgery may be performed. In Guedel's scheme it is subdivided into four planes of increasing anaesthetic depth. The movements of the eyes gradually stop; the pupils first constrict and then dilate progressively; the eyelid and then the corneal and pupillary reflexes are extinguished; swallowing, retching, and vomiting stop; skeletal muscles relax; the response of breathing to skin incision gradually fades. Respiration, which at first is deep and regular, becomes more shallow and in the deeper planes more diaphragmatic.

This stage of **surgical anaesthesia** is associated with progressive depression of the brainstem reticular systems (both activating and inhibiting pathways).

Stage IV

In this stage of **imminent death** the pupils are completely dilated and breathing stops. It is the stage of anaesthetic overdose, which is reversible if anaesthesia is discontinued and artificial respiration applied.

The spontaneous rhythmicity of the two (bilateral) respiratory centres in the medulla oblongata is reduced. Cardio-regulatory centres in the medulla are also depressed. Monosynaptic reflexes are completely abolished.

Beyond stage IV (medullary paralysis), respiratory arrest is followed by circulatory failure (paralysis of vasomotor centre) and death.

INHALATIONAL ANAESTHESIA

Technique

Anaesthetic gases (such as nitrous oxide) and vapors (such as halothane) are administered to patients at appropriate inspired concentrations, which are achieved by the use of accurate flow meters and other ancillary machinery.

The gases are supplied in compressed form and are passed through pressure reduction valves prior to the delivery of the gas through a flow meter to the patient, who is fitted with a mask over mouth and nose or a tube directly into the trachea (endotracheal tube requiring tracheal intubation).

The volatile anaesthetics are supplied as liquids that are delivered in gaseous form from thermocompensated wick vaporizers designed to deliver a precise amount (concentration) of vapor, usually as a percentage of total gas flow.

General Pharmacokinetics

Anaesthesia results when appropriate concentrations or partial pressures of anaesthetic agent are present in brain tissue. Between the anaesthetic machine and the brain exist a series of partial pressure gradients as the gas or vapor moves from the machine to the alveoli, into the blood, and finally into the body tissues including the brain.

Uptake

The rate of rise of anaesthetic concentration in the blood, and therefore tissues, is dependent upon a series of clearly defined factors:

1. The concentration of the agent in the inspired air.

2. The pulmonary ventilation, *i.e.*, delivery of the agent to the alveoli and transfer to the blood, which depends upon the solubility of the agent in blood. This is a more important limiting factor for the more blood-soluble anaesthetic agents (Fig. 23–3). Solubility, measured as the partition of the agent between blood and gas phases ($P_{b/g}$), is important: the blood tensions or partial pressures rise more rapidly with the less soluble agents such as nitrous oxide than with the more soluble ones such as methoxyflurane (*see* Fig. 23–3). The tension of the less soluble agent rises more quickly, but little of the agent has been transferred and dissolved in blood and tissue (Table 23–3). *Note:* There is virtually no barrier to the movement of anaesthetic agents between the alveoli and blood.

3. Cardiac output, to deliver the agent to the tissues. Obviously, if cardiac output is zero, uptake is zero. Uptake increases to a maximum as cardiac output increases.

4. Transfer of anaesthetic from blood into tissues, which depends upon the solubility of the agent in tissue and the concentration gradient between blood and tissue. Also blood flow, *i.e.*, rate of delivery, to the tissue is important. Brain, heart, kidneys, gut, and endocrine glands receive the highest blood flow. These are called the vessel-rich group of tissues, and reach peak levels of anaesthetic faster than tissues such as muscle or fat (Fig. 23–4).

Distribution

All anaesthetic agents have some degree of lipid solubility, so that they will cross cell membranes and distribute into the total body water. They readily cross the blood–brain barrier; otherwise they would not be able to act as general anaesthetics.

Biotransformation

Although initially it was thought that the volatile anaesthetics were chemically inert, it is now known that all are biotransformed to some degree in the liver. The proportion of anaesthetic agent taken into the body that is biotransformed ranges from as much as 50% for methoxyflurane, to 20% for halothane, 2% for enflurane, and 0.2% for isoflurane. Biotransformation may continue for a period of 4–5 days following the administration of an anaesthetic, as the drug is mobilized from muscle and fat stores.

Elimination

Recovery from a volatile anaesthetic occurs as the drug diffuses from the blood into the alveolar gas space and is exhaled. The rate of elimination from the body is dependent upon:

1. Transfer of anaesthetic from tissue into blood. This can be slow for highly lipid-soluble agents, such as methoxyflurane, coming out of adipose tissue. This accounts for the prolonged biotransformation of some drugs over 4–5 days. Transfer is, however, more rapid from the brain, so that a patient is usually awake from the inhalational agents 5–10 minutes after administration of the anaesthetic is stopped. Like uptake, elimination of an inhaled anaesthetic is more rapid for the less soluble agents such as N_2O.

2. Cardiac output, which delivers the agent to the lungs.

3. Relative solubilities of the anaesthetic in blood and in alveolar gas ($P_{b/g}$).

4. Rate of alveolar ventilation.

Figure 23–4 shows uptake and elimination phases of a relatively insoluble inhalational anaesthetic such as N_2O.

TABLE 23–3 Partition Coefficients and Minimum Alveolar Concentrations for Some Anaesthetic Gases and Vapors

Agent	$P_{b/g}$[*]	$P_{br/b}$[†]	$P_{f/b}$[‡]	MAC[§]
Nitrous oxide	0.47	1.1	2.3	105.0
Isoflurane	1.4	2.6	45	1.16
Enflurane	1.9	1.4	36	1.68
Halothane	2.3	2.3	60	0.76
Methoxyflurane	13.0	1.7	61	0.16

* Blood/gas partition coefficient.
† Brain/blood partition coefficient.
‡ Fat/blood partition coefficient.
§ Minimum alveolar concentration (μmol/100 mL) required to prevent movement of 50% of patients in response to a surgical stimulus.

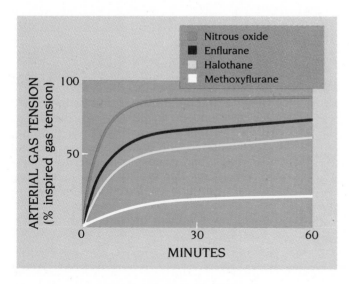

Figure 23–3 Idealized tensions of inhalational anaesthetics in blood expressed as a percent of the inspired gas tension with time. (Adapted from Eger EI, 1974.)

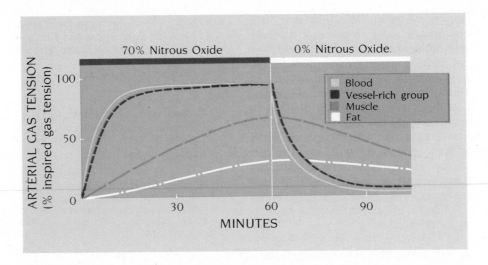

Figure 23-4   Idealized tensions of inhaled anaesthetic in blood, tissues, and fat during 60 minutes of inhaling nitrous oxide and 45 minutes of elimination. (Modified from Cowles AL, Borgsteadt HH, Gillies AJ. Anesth Analg 1968; 47:404–414.)

Minimum Alveolar Concentration

In order to compare the potencies of the various inhalational anaesthetic agents as well as give a quantitative basis for their administration, the concept of the "minimum alveolar concentration" (MAC) was developed. This is the minimal concentration of the inhalational anaesthetic agent (in percent of total gas mixture) in the alveolus at steady state that will inhibit purposeful movement of 50% of patients following surgical stimulation, such as a skin incision. Since this is measured at or near steady-state conditions, the concentration of anaesthetic agent in the brain tissue will be about 500 μmol per 100 mL of membrane volume for each inhalational anaesthetic agent used. This means that for halothane the inspired concentration must be about 0.76% (v/v) to inhibit purposeful movement by the patient, while the more lipid-soluble agent methoxyflurane will require only 0.16% (v/v).

Note that the MAC is the alveolar concentration at equilibrium and is independent of the time required to reach this (the time of induction to equilibrium depends upon the solubility of the agent; *see* above).

ANAESTHETIC GASES

Of nitrous oxide, ethylene, and cyclopropane, only N_2O is in current use. The other agents, which have explosion potential, are of historical interest and can be read about in older textbooks.

Nitrous Oxide

N_2O is a sweet-smelling, nonirritating, colorless gas. Its boiling point is $-89°C$, and its critical temperature is $36.5°C$. The critical temperature is that temperature above which a gas cannot be liquified by pressure alone. Thus, above $36.5°C$ tanks of liquid N_2O will explode unless they are equipped with pressure release valves. N_2O is nonflammable and nonexplosive but does support combustion. Its specific gravity is 1.5 times that of air. Its relevant partition coefficients are shown in Table 23-3.

Because of its low solubility in water ($P_{b/g} = 0.47$)

N$_2$O rapidly reaches its limiting concentration in the blood and tissues. It is a potent analgesic: a 50% concentration in the inspired air is equivalent to 10 mg morphine i.m. It is, however, a weak anaesthetic, the minimum alveolar concentration (MAC) for nitrous oxide being about 100%. Therefore it cannot be used as the sole agent for general anaesthesia at normal atmospheric pressures.

N$_2$O is used clinically as a supplement to other inhalational agents such as halothane or to intravenous agents such as narcotic analgesics, in concentrations up to 70% in N$_2$O:O$_2$ mixtures.

Side effects. N$_2$O augments respiratory depression caused by thiopental, opiates, and other inhalational agents. It causes some degree of cardiovascular depression, but this is small compared to that produced by other inhalational agents. Recently it has been shown that N$_2$O irreversibly oxidizes vitamin B$_{12}$, rendering it inactive as a coenzyme. This decreases DNA synthesis and may account for the teratogenic effects of N$_2$O in rats and perhaps the increased rate of spontaneous abortion seen in female operating room personnel. It will distribute into air spaces 35 times as rapidly as nitrogen will diffuse out, and this will increase the size or pressure of gas space in places such as sinuses, middle ear, and gut.

Oxygen

Although not an anaesthetic agent, oxygen is always included as part of the anaesthetic gas mixture and is considered as a drug. It is a clear, colorless, odorless gas, with a boiling point of $-182.5°C$ and critical temperature of $-118°C$. It supports combustion.

O$_2$ is normally present at a partial pressure of 159 mm Hg or 21.2 kPa in the atmosphere. Clinically it is generally used in elevated concentrations during anaesthesia and in patients in intensive care units.

When inhaled continuously for 24 hours or more in concentrations greater than 50%, O$_2$ is toxic to lung tissue. In premature infants it is also toxic to the retina.

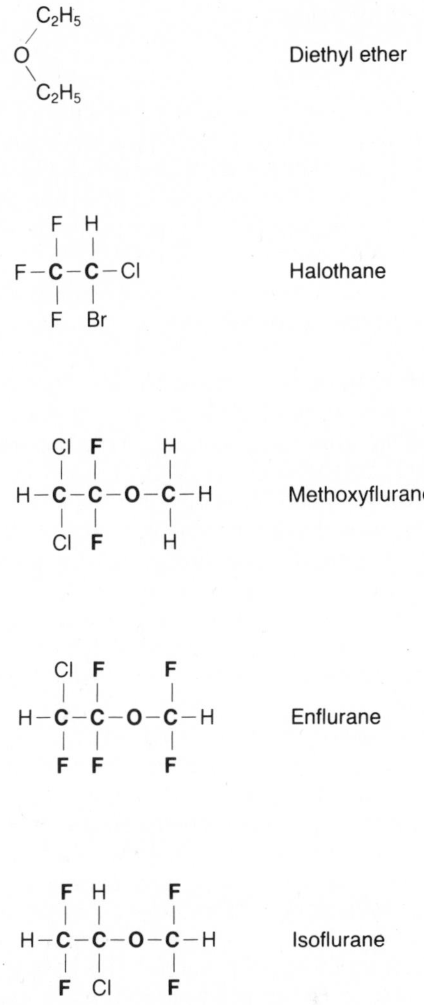

VOLATILE ANAESTHETICS

Diethyl Ether

This agent, once the most widely used, is now only of historic interest in the Western World, since it is rarely administered as an anaesthetic today. Diethyl ether (Fig. 23–5) is a potent anaesthetic agent that maintains good respiration during light anaesthesia. It maintains a

Figure 23–5 Structural formulae of some inhalational anaesthetics.

stable blood pressure by releasing endogenous catecholamines. However, this same action may give rise to cardiac arrhythmias. It is explosive.

Halothane

This volatile agent was introduced into anaesthetic practice in the late 1950s and is currently the most common agent of its class in use in North America.

Halothane (see Fig. 23–5) is a pleasant-smelling, nonirritating and nonexplosive liquid, with a boiling point of 50.2°C and a vapor pressure of 243 torr (mm Hg). It is soluble in rubber, and is therefore taken up by the tubing in anaesthetic equipment.

Pharmacokinetics

The uptake of halothane is moderately rapid (*see* Fig. 23–3), so that it can be used for inhalational induction of anaesthesia in concentrations up to about 4% (v/v). It is used for the maintenance of anaesthesia at 0.5–2% (v/v). About 20% of the inhaled dose is biotransformed in the liver, the remainder being rapidly eliminated *via* the respiratory tract.

Pharmacologic Effects

CNS. Halothane is a potent anaesthetic agent, with MAC of 0.76%. It has only a mild, clinically unsatisfactory analgesic effect, usually requiring the addition of an analgesic agent such as N_2O or a narcotic.

Respiratory. Halothane vapor does not irritate the respiratory mucosa. It produces a dose-dependent depression of minute ventilation, with increased rate of respiration but a greater reduction in tidal volume, resulting in a characteristic pattern of short, rapid breaths. There is a reduced respiratory response to CO_2 and a greatly depressed response to decreased O_2 (hypoxia).

Cardiovascular. Halothane causes a dose-dependent depression of the myocardium coupled with a relaxation of vascular smooth muscle, resulting in a fall in blood pressure. **The drug sensitizes the myocardium to catecholamines**, so that exogenous administration of these agents can produce arrhythmias.

Other. It causes dose-dependent relaxation of uterine contractility that can lead to bleeding in obstetric surgery such as caesarean sections. It also depresses motility and tone of the gut. Halothane is a poor skeletal muscle relaxant, but it will potentiate neuromuscular blocking agents, allowing for the use of less neuromuscular blocker to achieve the same degree of block.

Toxicity

Although halothane has the lowest mortality risk of any general anaesthetic, postoperative hepatitis has been described as a rare complication in about 1 in 38,000 cases of halothane anaesthesia (*see* Chapter 62). However, a cause-effect relationship is difficult to establish.

In genetically predisposed subjects, halothane (and other potent general anaesthetics) may precipitate malignant hyperthermia (*see* Chapter 12).

Methoxyflurane

This volatile anaesthetic agent was specifically designed with a high boiling point, which gave it a high solubility in blood (*see* Table 23–3), resulting in deliberately slow induction and emergence. This provided more safety because of better control during induction, but it also meant slower recovery from anaesthe-

sia. Methoxyflurane (*see* Fig. 23–5) gained some popularity in the late 1960s. However, approximately 50% of the inhaled dose is biotransformed, releasing free fluoride, which is toxic to the kidney. Therefore this agent is rarely used in North America today. It is a good analgesic and can be used for pain relief during labor or during short procedures such as wound dressing changes.

Enflurane

This is probably the second most popular volatile anaesthetic in use today in North America. Enflurane (*see* Fig. 23–5) is a pleasant-smelling, nonirritating, nonexplosive vapor. Boiling point is 56.5°C, and vapor pressure is 189 torr (mm Hg) at 20°C for this agent (*see* Table 23–3).

Pharmacokinetics

The uptake of enflurane is similar to that of halothane. The concentration used for induction of anaesthesia is usually 3–5% (v/v), and for maintenance 1–3% (v/v) in an $O_2:N_2O$ mixture. Only about 2% of the inhaled dose is biotransformed.

Pharmacologic Effects

CNS. This potent inhalational anaesthetic has mild analgesic properties. It produces CNS excitation at higher concentrations, resulting in seizure-like activity in the EEG that is manifested as twitching of the muscles. MAC is 1.68% (v/v).

Respiratory. Dose-dependent depression of minute ventilation occurs, resulting in increasing Pco_2. There is a reduced response to CO_2 and a greatly depressed response to hypoxia.

Cardiovascular. Enflurane produces dose-dependent depression of the myocardium, with a resulting fall in blood pressure. However, it does not sensitize the myocardium to catecholamines, which is one of its advantages over halothane.

Other. It produces only a mild degree of muscle relaxation, but it will potentiate neuromuscular blocking agents.

This agent will also precipitate malignant hyperthermia in genetically susceptible individuals.

Isoflurane

This isomer of enflurane (*see* Fig. 23–5) has recently been introduced into clinical practice. It has different physical and pharmacologic properties from those of enflurane, some of which are advantageous. One of these is that it tends to maintain cardiac output by dilating peripheral vascular beds and thus reducing afterload. In neurosurgery it has the advantage of not raising the intracranial pressure of ventilated patients. For surgical cases lasting more than 8 hours this agent has the advantage that only 0.2–0.3% of the inhaled dose is biotransformed. Therefore only very low levels of free fluoride are produced.

INTRAVENOUS ANAESTHETICS

Rapidly- and short-acting intravenous agents are commonly used today for the induction of anaesthesia. The most commonly used drug is thiopental. Other agents occasionally used for the same purpose, or even for prolonged procedures, include methohexital, althesin, ketamine, and a combination of agents used in a procedure referred to as neuroleptanalgesia/anaesthesia. High doses of narcotic analgesics can also be used intravenously as induction agents. The disadvantages attached to all of these are the irrevocability of intravenous administration of a potent drug and the consequent dangers of overdosing the patient.

Furthermore, while quite safe in the hands of specialists who are prepared to deal with side effects and anaesthesia accidents, the intravenous anaesthetics are very dangerous when used on an occasional basis by the inexperienced practitioner who falls prey to the temptations of convenience!

Thiopental Sodium

This thiobarbiturate is available as a pale yellow powder that is readily soluble in alkaline medium. It is usually prepared as a 2.5% aqueous solution at pH 10.5. It is a weak acid, pK_a 7.6; $P_{o/w} = 35$.

Pharmacokinetics

With rapid intravenous administration there is prompt distribution into the vessel-rich group of tissues (brain, heart, gut, endocrine glands), which induces unconsciousness in 10–15 seconds. The onset of action, therefore, is a function of the speed of injection.

The termination of action, on the other hand, is due to redistribution of the drug out of the brain and other vessel-rich tissues into less well-perfused tissues including skeletal muscle, and then into adipose tissue, where peak levels are not reached until more than 2 hours later (Fig. 23–6).

Thiopental is biotransformed in the liver by the cytochrome P-450-dependent mixed-function oxidase system, resulting in side-chain oxidation and some demethylation at carbon 5. This process, with a half-life of 6.5 hours, is much slower than the redistribution process. Because of this, with repeated doses of thiopental the various body stores begin to fill up and the drug accumulates in the body; as a result, such pa-

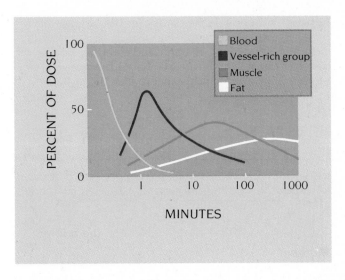

Figure 23–6 Distribution of anaesthetic agent into various compartments following intravenous administration. Note the log-scale for time.

tients might be asleep for a very long period (days). This is why thiopental is not used as the sole anaesthetic agent except for procedures of very short duration. Renal excretion is negligible.

Thiopental crosses the placenta readily, and peak fetal blood levels occur in about 3 minutes.

Pharmacologic Effects

CNS. The rapid injection of 3–5 mg/kg will produce loss of consciousness in one arm-brain circulation time. The duration of sleep is approximately 5 minutes, depending on the dose given.

Thiopental lacks analgesic activity and is a poor muscle relaxant.

It reduces brain metabolic rate and consequently brain blood flow. This will reduce intracranial pressure. Therefore thiopental is very effective for the acute treatment of raised intracranial pressure under controlled conditions.

Respiratory. It is a potent respiratory depressant, so that there is usually a period of apnea during induction of anaesthesia. This effect is enhanced by premedication with other depressant drugs. There is a dose-dependent decrease in the response of the respiratory centre to changes in P_{CO_2} and P_{O_2}.

Cardiovascular. Thiopental is a direct myocardial depressant and vascular smooth muscle relaxant, producing a dose-dependent fall in blood pressure. Accidental intraarterial injection of concentrations greater than 2.5% causes vascular spasm, primarily due to the alkalinity of thiopental solutions, which can result in tissue damage and loss of part of the limb.

Other. Clinically, thiopental is used in doses of 3–5 mg/kg in a normal patient. This dose must be reduced in hypovolemia, shock, in the elderly, and in patients with myxedema. The use of all barbiturates, including thiopental, is contraindicated in porphyria, because barbiturates cause a marked increase in porphyrin synthesis, which exacerbates the disease.

Methohexital

This is an ultra-short-acting oxybarbiturate with pharmacologic properties similar to those of thiopental. It is about three times as potent, with the usual induction dose being about 1 mg/kg i.v.

Althesin

This drug is a mixture of two steroids, alphaxolone 9 mg/mL and alphadolone acetate 3 mg/mL. At doses of 1.8 mL/kg it rapidly produces unconsciousness by the same mechanism as thiopental. There is a rapid recovery from anaesthesia, due to the redistribution of the drug out of the vessel-rich group into other tissues, and also to some degree by metabolism in the liver.

This drug produces hypersensitivity reactions in some patients on rare occasions. Partly because of this, it has been withdrawn from the market in Canada.

Ketamine

This phenylcyclohexylamine derivative can be used for rapid induction of anaesthesia by the intravenous route (1–2 mg/kg), or for longer procedures intramuscularly (5–10 mg/kg). It is a potent analgesic. It produces a state known as dissociative anaesthesia in which specific areas of the brain are anaesthetized while others are not, allowing for surgery to be conducted while muscle tone and respiration remain normal.

Ketamine stimulates the cardiovascular system so that it maintains or increases the blood pressure, cardiac output, and heart rate. Therefore this drug is useful in hypotensive patients. The use of ketamine is contraindicated in patients with cardiovascular disease or with raised intracranial pressure, since it will exacerbate their existing disease.

In subanaesthetic doses, drugs of this class can produce hallucinations and bizarre behavior (see Chapter 29).

High-Dose Narcotic Anaesthesia

This approach has proven to be highly effective in cardiovascular surgery. Although morphine was used initially, the commonly preferred drug today is **fentanyl** (see Chapter 22) at doses of up to 150 µg/kg (the usual analgesic dose is only 1 µg/kg). This is combined with a muscle relaxant, endotracheal intubation, and ventilation with 100% O_2. This technique of anaesthesia provides a high degree of stability of blood pressure and cardiac output, but because of the very large dose of fentanyl, ventilatory support is required postoperatively while the narcotic agent is being biotransformed and excreted.

Neuroleptanalgesia/Anaesthesia

This has been described as a state of depression of activity, lack of initiative, and reduced response to external stimuli. The patient has good analgesia and is sedated, yet is able to respond to simple commands.

Neuroleptanalgesia is usually produced with a combination of the phenothiazine droperidol, 2.5–5.0 mg i.v., and the narcotic analgesic fentanyl, 50–100 µg i.v., as a starting dose, with fentanyl supplements as required (see also Chapter 22). Other neuroleptic/narcotic analgesic combinations can be used. (A fixed-ratio combination drug is marketed under the name of Innovar®. Its use is considered less desirable because of its inflexibility.)

This neuroleptanalgesic state can be readily converted into unconsciousness by the addition of small doses of an induction agent such as thiopental or by the addition of a mixture of $O_2:N_2O$ or $N_2O:O_2:$halothane.

SUGGESTED READING

Dripps RD, Eckenhoff JE, Vandam CD. Introduction to anesthesia: the principles of safe practice. Philadelphia: WB Saunders, 1982.

Eger EI. Anesthetic uptake and action. Baltimore: Williams & Wilkins, 1974.

Miller RD, ed. Anesthesia. 2nd ed. New York: Churchill Livingstone, 1986.

Mori T, Matubayashi N, Ueda I. Membrane expansion and inhalation anesthetics. Mean excess volume hypothesis. Mol Pharmacol 1984; 25:123–130.

Seeman P. The membrane actions of anesthetics and tranquilizers. Pharmacol Rev 1972; 24:583–655.

Seeman P. Anesthetics and pressure reversal of anesthesia: expansion and recompression of membrane proteins, lipids and water. Anesthesiology 1977; 47:1–3.

Chapter 24

Local Anaesthetics

F.J. Carmichael

Local anaesthetics are drugs that block the generation and propagation of nerve impulses when applied locally in adequate concentrations. This block is reversible, and normal function returns to the nerve when the local anaesthetic is removed by the blood stream.

Extracts of the leaves of the Andean shrub *Erythroxylon coca* were known to confer insensitivity to delicate tissues. The active ingredient of these extracts, cocaine, had been isolated in 1860. In 1884 Koller demonstrated the local anaesthetic effects of cocaine on the conjunctiva of animals, and Hall used cocaine in dentistry. In 1885 Halstead used cocaine for nerve blocks and Corning used it for spinal anaesthesia in dogs. The first spinal anaesthetic in man was given by Bier in 1898, also using cocaine. In 1904 Einhorn synthesized procaine, and in subsequent years many new local anaesthetic agents have been synthesized and used clinically.

MECHANISM OF LOCAL ANAESTHESIA

Nerve Membrane and Action Potentials

The function of the nerve cell is to convey information from one part of the body to another. This information is passed along the axon in the form of electrical action potentials or impulses. Peripheral nerves are generally a mixed population of nerve fibres with different diameters and rates of impulse conduction. Many of the nerves are surrounded by a lamellar cylinder of myelin produced by the Schwann cell. A single nerve fibre or axon is a long cylinder of neural cytoplasm, the axoplasm, encased in a thin sheath, the plasma membrane. This membrane, 70–80 Å thick, has a framework consisting of a double layer of phospholipid molecules, with their polar head-groups oriented toward the two surfaces and their non-polar carbon chains oriented toward the middle of the membrane. Interspaced among the lipids are protein molecules. These proteins include the ion channels or ionophores, structural proteins, and enzyme systems such as $(Na^+ + K^+)$-ATPase, adenylate cyclase, protein kinase C, *etc*. The ionophores are present as gated channels for Na^+ and K^+, the control of which leads to the formation of an action potential. There are also passive ion channels for Na^+, K^+, and Cl^-, which contribute to the resting membrane potential and the leakage of ions into and out of the nerve (*see* Fig. 23–1, Chapter 23). In the resting state there is a voltage gradient across the nerve membrane of -70 mV, which is due to ionic gradients resulting from the high intracellular concentration of K^+ and high extracellular Na^+ and Cl^-. The reversal of the membrane potential during the generation or conduction of an action potential has been shown to be due to an increased permeability of the membrane for Na^+. The resultant influx of Na^+ down its electrochemical gradient (*i.e.*, the Na^+ current) and the change in membrane potential can be measured with Na^+-sensitive microelectrodes. Following the Na^+ influx there is an outflow of K^+ of a similar magnitude, which repolarizes the membrane. Studies with tetrodotoxin from the puffer fish, which specifically blocks the Na^+ channels at the outer surface of the membrane, and tetraethylammonium, which specifically blocks the K^+ channels, have demonstrated the different kinetics of Na^+ and K^+ in the nerve cell.

There are approximately 13 Na^+ channels per 100 μm^2 of nerve cell membrane. In contrast, 1×10^6 molecules of local anaesthetic per 100 μm^2 are required to give a nerve block. Also, it should be noted that the total amount of Na^+ and K^+ exchange involved in the action potential is a very small proportion of the amount of these ions outside and inside the nerve respectively. The Na^+ and K^+ that have moved across the membrane during the action potential are subsequently returned by the $(Na^+ + K^+)$-ATPase, which maintains the differential distribution of Na^+ and K^+ across the nerve cell membrane and thus

237

maintains the resting membrane potential. A nerve may be stimulated several thousand times in the presence of a (Na$^+$+K$^+$)-ATPase inhibitor without significantly changing total intracellular Na$^+$ concentrations.

Site and Mode of Action of Local Anaesthetics

Local anaesthetics exert their effect on impulse conduction through an action on the nerve membrane. In unmyelinated nerves the application of the drug to the membrane results in a dose-dependent reduction in the height of the action potential and its rate of rise. There is also an elevation of the firing threshold and a slowing of the spread of conduction down the length of the axon. With increasing local anaesthetic concentrations, the rate of rise of the action potential is progressively reduced to the point of total inhibition. Nevertheless, even when the nerve is fully blocked, the resting membrane potential remains unchanged. In myelinated nerves these phenomena occur only at the nodes of Ranvier.

Voltage clamp experiments have shown that the local anaesthetics exert their effects primarily by blocking the entry of Na$^+$ into the cell (Fig. 24–1). The effect of local anaesthetics on K$^+$ conduction is only about one-third to one-quarter that on Na$^+$ conduction.

The molecules of cationic local anaesthetics, such as cocaine and its derivatives and analogs, are thought to enter the hydrophobic regions of the nerve membrane as uncharged tertiary amines. Once the molecules have partitioned into the membrane, they can expand and distort the membrane, and thus the membrane proteins, resulting in a blockage of the Na$^+$ channel (see Fig. 23–1, Chapter 23, *General Anaesthetics*). Seeman's **Membrane Concentration Rule of Local Anaesthesia** (analogous to the rule for general

anaesthesia) states that any lipid-soluble molecule that achieves a concentration of 5000 μmol per 100 g of excitable membrane will produce local anaesthesia of that membrane. Note that this is 10 times as high as the concentration required for general anaesthesia, as described in Chapter 23. This difference suggests that general anaesthesia is produced by a similar action on especially sensitive small neurons in the brain. Any structural modification of the drug that increases its lipid solubility will increase its potency as well as the rate of onset of anaesthesia.

The charged cationic form of the local anaesthetic molecule is a more effective blocker of the nerve membrane than the uncharged free base. This can be demonstrated by altering the pH of the bathing solution in an isolated nerve preparation. Figure 24–2 shows the effect of pH on nerve blockade after the penetration of local anaesthetic into the membrane, *i.e.*, when partitioning equilibrium has been achieved. The local anaesthetic is more effective at pH 7.0 (when more of it is in the form of cation = charged) than at pH 8.0 (when more is present as free base = uncharged). Studies using permanently charged quaternary amine analogs also demonstrate that they can only block conduction when they are applied from the inside of the

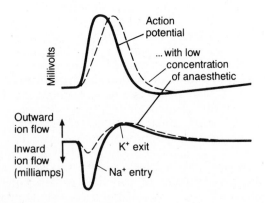

Figure 24–1 Voltage clamp experiments show that the local anaesthetics primarily block the entry of Na$^+$ without affecting the exit of K$^+$.

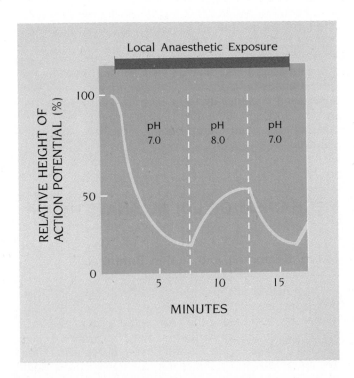

Figure 24–2 Effect of changing the pH of the internal bathing solution on the height of the action potential in the isolated giant axon of the squid while exposed to local anaesthetic action. (Adapted from Narahashi T, Frazier DT, Yamada M. J Pharmacol Exp Ther 1970; 171:32–51.)

nerve cell membrane but are ineffective when applied to the outer surface.

It appears, then, that the uncharged tertiary amine, which has some local anaesthetic activity of its own, is required to penetrate the nerve membrane. Once it has done so, the exposed amine groups can become charged, the ratio of charged to uncharged depending on the hydrogen ion concentration in the immediate vicinity. Both the charged and uncharged forms exert local anaesthetic action, but for each drug the charged form is more potent.

CHEMISTRY AND STRUCTURE–ACTIVITY RELATIONSHIPS

Most of the local anaesthetics in common use today are tertiary amines. They have in common the following fundamental structural features (Fig. 24–3):

- a lipophilic portion composed of an aromatic residue derived from para-aminobenzoic acid as in procaine, or from quinoline as in dibucaine, or from aniline as in lidocaine;
- an intermediate chain containing either an ester linkage as in procaine or an amide linkage as in lidocaine; and
- a hydrophilic portion containing either a tertiary or secondary amine group.

The physicochemical properties of some local anaesthetic agents are shown in Table 24–1.

The relative potencies of these agents, as well as their protein binding, correlate reasonably well in rank order with their lipid solubilities as measured by their partition coefficients (see Table 24–1). The increased protein binding of the more lipid-soluble compounds tends

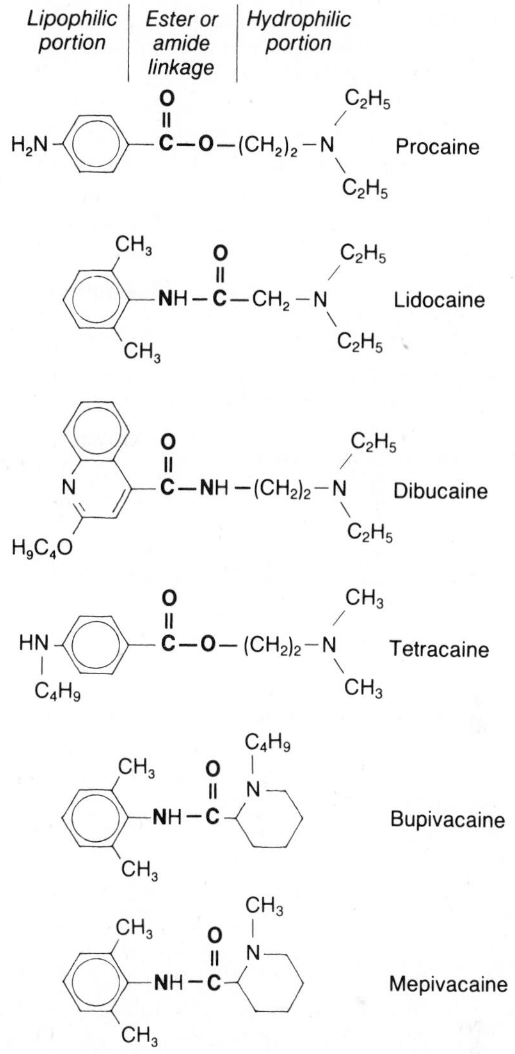

Figure 24–3 Structural formulae of local anaesthetics, illustrating common structural features (see text).

TABLE 24–1 Physical Properties, Potency, and Duration of Action of Four Representative Local Anaesthetics

Drug	$P_{o/w}$*	Relative Potency	Plasma Protein Binding[†]	pK_a	Ionized/Unionized at pH 7.4	Duration (Minutes)[‡]
Procaine	1	1	5	8.9	32/1	16
Lidocaine	4	4	55	7.9	3/1	16
Tetracaine	80	16	75	8.5	13/1	130
Bupivacaine	130	16	90	8.1	4/1	125

* $P_{o/w}$ = oil/water partition coefficient of drug.
† Plasma protein binding as percent of total drug in plasma.
‡ Duration of anaesthesia at equipotent doses.

to reduce their toxicity (*see* below). The protein binding will reduce transfer of local anaesthetics across the placenta. The more lipid-soluble agents also tend to have a longer duration of action; however, this is more dependent upon their rates of metabolism. Since the uncharged free base form of the drug penetrates the membrane and has some activity on its own, the ratio of charged to uncharged species (which depends upon the pK_a) will affect the speed of onset of action and the potency of the agent. Indeed, some local anaesthetic solutions are prepared in buffered alkaline media to promote a faster onset of action attributable to the higher proportion of uncharged molecules, which will penetrate the nerve membrane more easily. However, as noted above, most of the local anaesthetic activity is due to the charged form acting in the membrane.

FACTORS INFLUENCING LOCAL ANAESTHETIC ACTION

A prolongation of the action of local anaesthetics can be achieved by adding a vasoconstrictor such as adrenaline (epinephrine) to the drug solutions. This causes a local reduction of blood flow to the site of local anaesthetic injection, which reduces the rate of uptake and removal of the drug into the circulation and thus allows a longer exposure of the nerve to the local anaesthetic agent. At the same time, the delay in absorption reduces the plasma levels of the local anaesthetic, and thus decreases the risk of systemic toxicity. In clinical practice, adrenaline* (1 part in 200,000) or phenylephrine is used, except for nerve blocks on the extremities where vascular constriction can result in reduced blood flow and ischemic damage to the extremity.

The diameter of a nerve fibre is a most important factor in relation to the sensitivity to local anaesthetics: thicker nerves require more drug to achieve a block than do the thinner fibres. Nerve fibres have been classified by size into A ($\alpha,\beta,\gamma,\delta$), which are myelinated, with diameters ranging from 20 μm (motor α) down to 2 μm (pain δ); B (preganglionic fibres) with diameters of 3 μm; and C (nonmyelinated pain fibres) of 0.5 to 1 μm diameter. Following local anaesthetic injection, pain and temperature sensation, conducted by the small Aδ and C fibres, are lost first. Touch and pressure sensation are lost next; and finally motor function, conducted by the large Aα nerve fibres, is blocked at the highest concentrations. This phenomenon of differential block of nerve fibres reflects the difference in fibre size and allows for blocking of pain fibres with little effect on motor conduction if the appropriate anaesthetic concentration is used. There are no intrinsic differences between sensory and motor nerves; however, there are differences in fibre size and in myelination

that account for the differences observed experimentally and clinically.

Figure 24–4 represents a small and a large diameter axon, each having approximately the same density of Na$^+$ channels per unit of surface area. The nerve impulse is initially generated at the axon hillock by a strong depolarization created by a neurotransmitter or by an electrical current. The depolarized region (of the impulse) spreads electrotonically down the axon in accordance with electrical cable theory. This electrotonic spread of local electrical current extends approximately 10 mm down the large axon (because of its large cable constant), and approximately 5 mm down the small axon (which has a small cable constant). The larger fibres also conduct impulses more quickly than

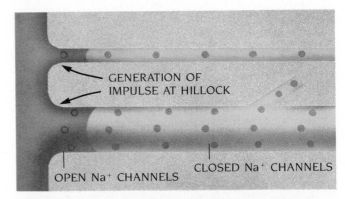

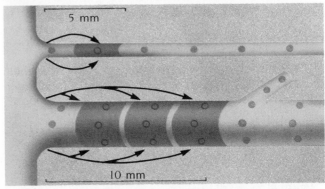

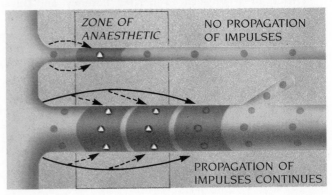

Figure 24–4 Blockade of impulse propagation in small and large diameter axons (*see* text).

---

* epinephrine

smaller fibres. These local electrical currents then trigger the opening of the Na$^+$-conductance channels (drawn as empty circles in Fig. 24–4). Thus, the large axon will have more excited channels than the small axon. Hence, when the anaesthetic is applied in a fixed concentration to a limited area of each axon, the small axon becomes completely blocked since its few excited channels are prevented from opening by the anaesthetic. The larger axon escapes blockade since more Na$^+$ channels are being excited and the limited amount of anaesthetic blocks only a portion of the channels.

The small axon collateral coming off a large axon will become blocked by anaesthetic concentrations that are insufficient to block the main trunk.

TYPES OF LOCAL ANAESTHETIC BLOCK

Topical. Local anaesthetic is applied to the surface of skin, wounds, burns, or mucous membranes.

Infiltration. Local anaesthetic is injected at one or more sites around an area to be incised or excised. This type of block is used for minor operations.

Regional nerve block. Local anaesthetic is injected in close proximity to the nerve supplying the area to be anaesthetized. This block is used for surgery and pain relief and is referred to as regional anaesthesia.

Spinal. A solution of local anaesthetic is injected into the lumbar subarachnoid space to reach the roots of the spinal nerves that supply the site of operation. Spinal block is used in surgery on the lower limbs and pelvis, and in obstetrics.

Epidural, peridural, or extradural. Local anaesthetic solution is injected into the extradural space where the drug blocks nerve roots passing through this space. Uses are the same as for spinal anaesthesia, but the advantage is that the anaesthetic agent cannot accidentally rise to a higher segment of the spinal cord than was intended.

Intravenous. Local anaesthetic is injected into the venous system of a limb in which the circulation is interrupted by a tourniquet. Intravenous block is used for surgery on that limb.

Sympathetic. Sympathetic nerve blocks can be used in the treatment of reflex sympathetic dystrophies such as causalgia and the shoulder-hand syndrome, or for the intractable pain of carcinoma of the pancreas or the upper abdomen. A diagnosis of these pain-causing conditions and their potential management is usually made with an initial block using a local anaesthetic agent. If this is successful in relieving the pain, it is followed by a phenol (7.5%) block, which destroys the sympathetic nerve tissue and results in prolonged pain relief.

UPTAKE, DISTRIBUTION, AND FATE

Local anaesthetic molecules pass into the membrane of a mixed nerve by diffusion down a concentration gradient and establish equilibrium concentrations across the neuronal membrane at rates dependent upon lipid solubility (lipid/water partition coefficient), pH (alters the ratio of charged to uncharged molecules of the local anaesthetic agent), and concentration of drug. The induction rate also depends upon the diameter of the individual fibres, small nerves being blocked more rapidly.

The duration of the block depends upon uptake by the nerve, diffusion away from the nerve into interstitial space, vascular uptake (reduced by vasoconstrictors), and metabolic inactivation.

Lipid Solubility

As noted previously (under Site and Mode of Action), local anaesthetics follow the Membrane Concentration Rule of Anaesthesia. Any structural change of the drugs that increases their lipid/water partition coefficient will increase their potency as well as the rate of onset of anaesthesia. Many drugs not usually considered to be local anaesthetics can have anaesthetic properties if they achieve the necessary concentration in the membrane, e.g., diphenhydramine (an antihistamine), anti-inflammatory steroids, and propranolol (a β-adrenoceptor blocking drug).

Hydrogen Ion Concentration

Clinically, the most useful local anaesthetics are **tertiary amines**. These can exist in the charged or uncharged form, depending on the hydrogen ion concentration of their environment. For example:

$$R-N\begin{matrix}CH_3\\\\CH_3\end{matrix} \quad + \quad H^+ \quad \rightleftharpoons \quad R-\overset{\oplus}{N}\begin{matrix}CH_3\\\\HCH_3\end{matrix}$$

In an acidic environment (low pH = high cH$^+$ or proton concentration) the anaesthetic drug will become protonated and will thus have a low lipid solubility. In a low proton concentration (more alkaline solution) the anaesthetic will be in its uncharged form and will be very lipid-soluble.

The uncharged form of the local anaesthetic will readily permeate membranes and tissue barriers. At the proton concentration in the immediate vicinity of the membrane, reequilibration takes place, generating more of the charged form that produces most of the actual blockade.

$$BH^+ \rightleftharpoons H^+ + B \quad | \quad B + H^+ \rightleftharpoons BH^+$$

Aqueous Phases | Membrane Phase

The limiting factor affecting the onset of local anaesthesia is the time needed for the drug to permeate the nerve sheath, to permeate through the myelin, and to permeate into the nerve cell membrane. Hence, it speeds up the onset of nerve blockade if there is more B or uncharged form of the drug near the nerve. For example, if one compares the speed of onset of 2% procaine applied to the nerve in solutions of two different H^+ concentrations, the speed is greatest with the lower cH^+ (higher pH) because there is more B form in that solution (Fig. 24–5). Obviously, the pK_a of a given local anaesthetic will determine the ratio of charged and uncharged forms at any given tissue proton concentration (cH^+).

Distribution and Metabolism

Being lipid-soluble, local anaesthetics in the blood readily cross cell membranes. Once absorbed from the

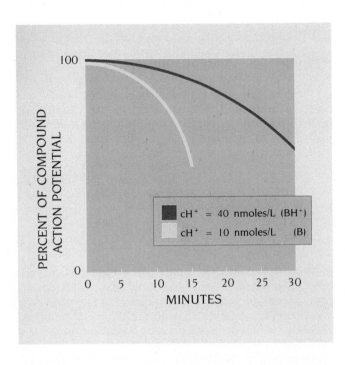

Figure 24–5 Differences in speed of onset of local anaesthesia as determined by the proton concentration (cH^+)(see text).

site of injection, these drugs distribute into total body water and are absorbed into all membranes. (This is also a cause of toxic side effects, depending upon the nature of the tissue and membrane, and the concentration of local anaesthetic in the membrane.) The agents pass rapidly across the blood–brain barrier into the central nervous system, where some of the side effects occur. They also readily cross the placenta into the fetus. The placental transfer is less for agents such as bupivacaine, which has higher maternal protein binding.

The metabolism of local anaesthetics is dependent largely upon their structure. The ester type anaesthetics, such as procaine and tetracaine, are hydrolysed by esterases in the blood and liver to yield an aromatic acid plus an amino alcohol. The amide type anaesthetics, such as lidocaine and bupivacaine, are N-dealkylated and hydrolysed by the liver mixed-function oxidase system. Reduced biotransformation, and therefore increased toxicity, will be observed in individuals with liver damage or atypical plasma cholinesterase.

A portion of the administered dose of intact local anaesthetic agents, as well as their metabolites, is excreted through the kidney.

SIDE EFFECTS AND TOXICITY

In general, the toxicity of local anaesthetics is manifested primarily in the central nervous system and the cardiovascular system. Many factors modify the toxicity, such as a raised CO_2 or H^+ level in the patient, which will increase the amount of the more active ionized form, and inadvertent intravascular injection, but the major reason for a toxic reaction is too much drug, *i.e.*, overdose, resulting in elevated blood levels.

Local anaesthetics are not selective and will act on any membrane. All local anaesthetic agents cause stimulation of the central nervous system, manifested as restlessness and tremors. With sufficiently high blood levels, the most dramatic complication is a generalized convulsion or tonic-clonic seizure, treatable with benzodiazepines (*see* Chapter 21). At even higher drug levels, local anaesthetics can depress the central nervous system, resulting in respiratory arrest and death.

Following absorption of adequate amounts, especially after intravenous administration, local anaesthetic agents affect the myocardium, where they decrease excitability, conduction rate, and force of contraction in a dose-dependent fashion. Lidocaine and procainamide, the amide derivative of procaine, have a clinically useful quinidine-like effect on the myocardium, raising the threshold for stimulation and prolonging conduction time (*see* Chapter 35). With high enough levels of local anaesthetic there can be complete asystole. Most local anaesthetics also cause a dose-dependent dilatation of the vascular bed, resulting in a further reduction in blood pressure. An exception is cocaine, which blocks the re-uptake of noradrenaline,* thus producing vasoconstriction.

On rare occasions a patient demonstrates hypersensitivity to a local anaesthetic agent, usually one of the ester types. The reaction can manifest itself as a skin rash, asthmatic attack, or most severely as an anaphylactic reaction.

These agents are devoid of direct toxicity to nerves, and nerve function recovers completely following a nerve block or spinal anaesthesia.

The use of epidural or spinal anaesthesia in obstetrics is associated with a lower incidence of neonatal depression than in general anaesthesia.

Since the major cause of systemic and central adverse reactions is a high blood concentration of the drug, the use of carefully limited doses is essential.

The safety margin for these drugs is low; however, the route of administration greatly reduces toxicity, because absorption from the site of action is slow.

COMMONLY USED LOCAL ANAESTHETICS

Cocaine

This drug is too toxic for other than topical use. Unlike other local anaesthetics, cocaine inhibits the re-uptake of catecholamines into adrenergic terminals, thus enhancing the actions of endogenous noradrenaline.

Clinically, cocaine can be used by topical application as a 2–4% solution for anaesthesia for eye surgery, or as a 5–10% solution for anaesthetizing the nasopharynx. A dose of 100 mg (1.5 mg/kg) should not be exceeded. Nonmedical use of cocaine for its psychoactive effects, and the associated risks of drug dependence and toxicity, are discussed in Chapters 29 and 67.

Procaine

This ester drug is almost without effect when applied topically, but is most effective when used for infiltrative anaesthesia or nerve blocks. It has a short duration of action because of its rapid biotransformation, which also accounts for its low toxicity. It causes vasodilatation, which increases its absorption from the site of action. This effect can be offset with adrenaline, which thus prolongs the local anaesthetic action. Concentrations of 0.25–1% are commonly used, but the total dose of procaine should not exceed 1000 mg.

Tetracaine

This ester is about 10 times as potent as procaine, with respect to its anaesthetic action and also its sys-

temic toxicity. It has a slower onset of action, taking 5 minutes or more, but has a longer duration, 2 to 3 hours.

Clinically, it can be used for topical, infiltrative, regional, epidural, or spinal anaesthesia. It is normally mixed with adrenaline and used at concentrations of 0.25–1 mg/mL; the total dose should not exceed 100 mg. For regional blocks it can be combined with lidocaine or other rapid-acting local anaesthetics for faster onset of the block.

Lidocaine

This amide anaesthetic is only slightly more toxic than procaine but is more rapid in onset, is twice as potent, and lasts longer. It is effective for all types of local anaesthetic use in concentrations up to 2%. The maximum total dose should not exceed 750 mg.

Bupivacaine

This amide is about four times as potent and toxic as lidocaine. The onset of its block is slow (5 to 20 minutes), but it has a duration of action of up to 4 to 6 hours. It exhibits a high degree of protein binding (90%). When used for epidural analgesia, this binding of the portion of the anaesthetic that is absorbed into the blood is thought to account for its wider margin of safety than that of lidocaine, as well as its reduced placental transfer and therefore greater fetal safety.

Clinically it is used for regional and spinal blocks of long duration, and it is most commonly used for continuous epidural analgesia in the management of labor and delivery. Solutions of 0.25–0.75% are used, with the maximum dose not to exceed 150 mg.

Articaine

This amide anaesthetic has gained popularity for use in dental and oral surgery. It is supplied in a 4% solution with adrenaline for injection. The total dose should not exceed 500 mg.

SUGGESTED READING

Adriani J, Naraghi M. The pharmacologic principles of regional pain relief. Annu Rev Pharmacol Toxicol 1977; 17: 223–242.

Luduena FP. Duration of local anesthetics. Annu Rev Pharmacol 1969; 9:503–520.

Miller RD, ed. Anesthesia. 2nd ed. New York: Churchill Livingstone, 1986.

Moore DC. Regional block. Springfield: CC Thomas, 1967.

Seeman P. The membrane actions of anesthetics and tranquilizers. Pharmacol Rev 1972; 24:583–655.

* norepinephrine

Chapter 25

THE ALCOHOLS

H. Kalant and J.M. Khanna

The use of ethyl alcohol dates from prehistoric times, and occurs in almost all parts of the world. Probably this is because the requirements for production of alcohol are extremely simple: some plant material containing starch or sugar, some moisture, wild yeast from the air, and a temperature high enough to permit fermentation. The earliest technologic "improvement" (still used in some primitive societies) was to chew grain or tubers to crush them and mix them with yeasts from the chewer's teeth, then spit them back into a container with water, and leave them to ferment. In ancient times, this crude method gradually evolved into fairly sophisticated methods for producing wines and beers of relatively low alcohol content. Distillation was invented by Arabic chemists, from whom it spread to Europe in the Middle Ages; this permitted the production of much more potent beverages.

In view of the very long association of alcohol with human life and culture, it is not surprising that alcohol has many religious, symbolic, social, economic, and legal roles. These are reviewed in Chapter 67. The present chapter deals primarily with pharmacologic, biochemical, and clinical aspects.

CHEMISTRY, METABOLISM, AND METABOLIC EFFECTS

Physical Chemistry

The aliphatic alcohols form a homologous series beginning with methanol:

$$CH_3 - OH \qquad \text{Methanol (wood alcohol),}$$
$$CH_3 - CH_2 - OH \qquad \text{Ethanol (grain alcohol),}$$
$$CH_3 - CH_2 - CH_2 - OH \qquad \text{n-Propanol,}$$
$$CH_3 - \underset{\underset{\textstyle OH}{|}}{CH} - CH_3 \qquad \text{Isopropanol,}$$
$$CH_3 - CH_2 - CH_2 - CH_2 - OH \qquad \text{n-Butanol, } etc.$$

The first two are completely miscible with water and have very low lipid/water partition coefficients, but water solubility decreases as chain length increases, so that octanol is virtually insoluble in water. Gram for gram, the higher alcohols are considerably more toxic than the lower ones, but because of this decrease in water solubility it is hard to achieve a toxic concentration in the body above pentanol or hexanol. All of the lower alcohols are used as solvents, but only ethanol is sufficiently nontoxic to be used as a beverage.

Absorption and Distribution

Ethanol is readily absorbed through any mucosal surface by simple diffusion. This can occur in the stomach, but is faster in the intestine, so that a delay in gastric emptying, as by food or strenuous physical activity, slows the absorption. The rate of ethanol absorption is highest with 20–30% ethanol; with very dilute solutions it is slower. More concentrated alcohol may slow absorption by causing gastric irritation and pylorospasm. Ethanol vapor can also be absorbed readily through the lung, and rats and mice can easily be made deeply intoxicated by this route.

After absorption from the GI tract, ethanol is carried to the liver and then to the systemic circulation, diffusing into all tissues and body fluids including the CSF, sweat, urine, and breath. The equilibrium partition coefficient for ethanol between blood and alveolar air in humans is approximately 2100:1. Therefore the ethanol concentration in end-expiratory air can be measured and multiplied by 2100 (*e.g.*, by the Breathalyzer machine) to provide a fairly accurate estimate of the ethanol concentration in the blood.

Since its molecular weight is only 46, ethanol moves easily through aqueous channels in cell membranes. **Therefore it distributes and equilibrates quickly throughout the entire body water**, and alcohol dilution can be used to measure total body water (*see* next section and Fig. 25–3).

However, though alcohol passes rapidly across capillary walls, differences in blood flow to different tissues result in differences in the rates at which alcohol concentrations in the various tissues and fluids come into equilibrium with the concentration in the blood. This is most marked during the phase of rapid rise of blood alcohol level. During this phase, the rapid diffusion of ethanol from capillary blood into tissue fluid causes the ethanol concentration to be lower in the venous blood leaving the tissue than in the arterial blood entering it. The smaller the volume of blood flow per gram of tissue, the larger is this early arterial–venous (A–V) difference in ethanol concentration. During this time, therefore, the concentration in a sample of blood from a hand or forearm vein is misleadingly low in comparison to the concentration reaching the brain (Fig. 25–1). Once distribution is complete, the A–V difference disappears.

Since diffusion is a first-order process, the rate at which ethanol is lost from the body in the urine, breath, and sweat is proportional to the plasma concentration of ethanol. Over the range of concentrations produced

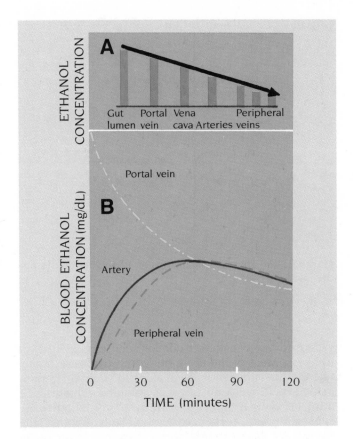

Figure 25–1 *A,* Schematic representation of the concentration gradient of ethanol from jejunal lumen to peripheral veins during the early stage of absorption and distribution. *B,* Time course of arterial–venous (A–V) differences in ethanol concentration during absorption and distribution.

by light to very heavy drinking, between 2 and 10% of the ingested dose can be lost in this way.

Biotransformation

Minute amounts of ethanol are conjugated with glucuronic or sulfuric acid (*see* Chapter 4) and excreted in the urine. By far the most important biotransformation reaction, however, is oxidation to acetaldehyde and then to acetate, primarily in the liver (Fig. 25–2).

The three principal enzymatic mechanisms that can oxidize ethanol to acetaldehyde are **alcohol dehydrogenase (ADH), catalase**, and a **microsomal ethanol-oxidizing system (MEOS)**, which is essentially part of the cytochrome P-450 system. All evidence favors the view that normally **ADH is by far the most important hepatic enzyme responsible for the *in vivo* oxidation of ethanol**. However, chronic ingestion of substantial amounts of ethanol leads to induction of a specific cytochrome, P-450$_{3a}$, which has a high substrate specificity for ethanol. This induction may be a factor in the

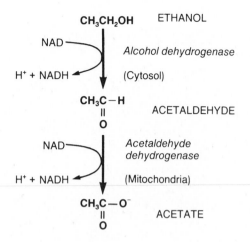

Figure 25–2 The two initial steps of ethanol metabolism in the liver.

increased rate of alcohol oxidation seen in regular heavy drinkers. Most of the acetaldehyde is oxidized to acetate by the mitochondrial acetaldehyde dehydrogenase in the liver. Small amounts of acetaldehyde that escape into the circulation are oxidized rapidly in other tissues. However, acetaldehyde is a highly reactive substance, and even transient levels in the blood can result in formation of permanent (covalently bonded) complexes with hemoglobin and plasma proteins. These complexes act as antigens, which can be measured by appropriate antibodies. Alcoholics have been found to have significantly raised plasma levels of such antigens, and this finding may give rise to a useful diagnostic or screening test.

Some of the acetate is converted to acetyl-CoA in the liver and oxidized or converted to amino acids, fatty acids, or glycogen in the same way as acetyl-CoA from other sources. However, large amounts of acetate pass into the systemic circulation and are taken up in other tissues, converted to acetyl-CoA, and oxidized to CO_2 and water *via* the Krebs cycle (tricarboxylic acid cycle) in those tissues.

The rate-limiting step in the whole process is the alcohol dehydrogenase (ADH) step. It was formerly thought that the rate of this reaction *in vivo* was determined by the availability of the cofactor NAD, which in turn depends on the rate of reoxidation of NADH. However, recent evidence suggests that in normal well-nourished individuals the rate is determined 70% by the concentration of the ADH enzyme and only 30% by the NAD concentration or NAD:NADH ratio.

There are differences between individuals, and within the same person from time to time, but **on the average a 70 kg human can oxidize about 10 g of ethanol per hour**. This means that the typical blood alcohol curve, after oral ingestion, rises to peak level in 30–90 minutes depending on the dose, followed by a steady fall at the rate of 15–20 mg/100 mL/hr until the con-

centration reaches about 25 mg/dL; below this point it falls exponentially (Fig. 25–3). Since ADH exhibits Michaelis-Menten kinetics, the apparently linear portion of the curve is really a very shallow curve, and its slope is affected by the starting concentration. Therefore the initial rate of descent is greater if the maximum concentration is higher.

If the apparently linear portion of the curve is projected back to t_0 (*see* Fig. 25–3), the intercept on the vertical axis is C_0, *i.e.*, the theoretical concentration that would have been found if all the administered dose of ethanol had been instantaneously absorbed and uniformly distributed throughout its V_d. Since ethanol is distributed almost entirely in the body water, and blood contains 80% water, then C_0 in the blood corresponds to 80% of the C_0 in the water phase, or $C_{0\ water} = 1.25 \times C_{0\ blood}$. Since $C_{0\ water}$ = dose/volume of body water, this method provides an estimate of total body water and has been used clinically for that purpose.

Since the oxidation of ethanol requires simultaneous reduction of NAD to NADH, anything that makes NAD more available by reoxidizing NADH will help to keep the rate of alcohol metabolism at the maximum permitted by the amount of ADH present. Fructose, insulin plus glucose, and other sources of pyruvate may do this. However, it is not possible to speed the process past its normal maximum by this means. Dinitrophenol can increase the rate of NADH reoxidation (and hence of ethanol oxidation) beyond the normal limit by uncoupling oxidation from phosphorylation, but it is too toxic to use clinically.

Metabolic Effects of Ethanol

The change of NAD to NADH, resulting from the metabolism of ethanol and acetaldehyde, affects other NAD-linked metabolic processes. Some of the better-studied examples are listed below.

1. Pyruvate is reduced to lactate by lactate dehydrogenase (simultaneously oxidizing NADH to NAD), causing varying degrees of **elevation of serum lactate and metabolic acidosis**. The raised lactate inhibits renal secretion of urate and thus can **precipitate attacks of gout** (Fig. 25–4).

2. Increased hepatic NADH also favors reduction of glyceraldehyde-3-phosphate to glycerol-3-phosphate and inhibits glycerophosphate dehydrogenase, leading to an elevated glycerol-3-phosphate level.

3. At the same time, the excess production of acetate from acetaldehyde, together with the raised NADH level, stimulates the synthesis of fatty acids in the liver while their oxidation *via* the tricarboxylic acid cycle is blocked.

4. The excess of glycerol-3-phosphate and of fatty acids leads to increased esterification and accumulation of neutral triglycerides in the liver.

5. The increase in NADH and decrease in pyruvate result in a reduced rate of gluconeogenesis. Therefore, if hepatic glycogen supplies are depleted by lack of

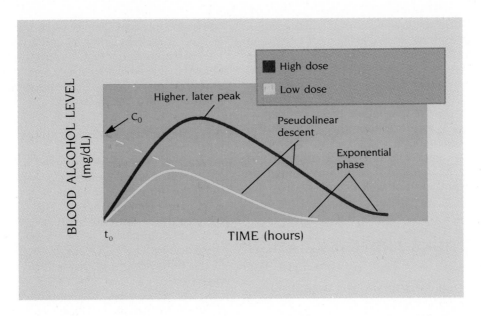

Figure 25–3 Dose-dependence of peak blood alcohol levels and rate of descent from the peak.

adequate food intake, ethanol causes hypoglycemia.

6. The raised NADH level also inhibits the enzyme systems that convert galactose to glucose and that conjugate glycine and benzoate to form hippuric acid (*see* Chapter 4), so that these liver function tests are disturbed.

These changes are all reversible when alcohol oxidation is finished.

7. However, chronic heavy ingestion of alcohol increases not only the rate of alcohol oxidation but also the rate of O_2 consumption. Consequently the risk of hypoxia in the liver is increased, especially at the hepatic

venous end of the sinusoid where the P_{O_2} is normally lowest anyway (*see* Chapter 62). This may explain why liver cell necrosis in heavy drinkers is chiefly around the collecting veins (''central veins'').

8. **In the brain**, the action of MAO on dopamine, noradrenaline,* and serotonin gives rise to aldehydes that are normally oxidized to acids (5-HIAA) or reduced to phenyl-ethyl-glycol derivatives (*see* Chapters 13 and 31). Alcohol, or acetaldehyde formed from it, can inhibit these oxidative or reductive steps, so that the levels of the intermediary aldehydes increase. These aldehydes may react with themselves, with acetalde-

---

* norepinephrine

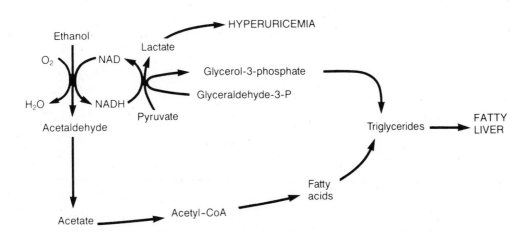

Figure 25–4 Some consequences of ethanol metabolism on intermediary metabolism of other substrates.

hyde, or with the original amines to form condensation products, as in the example shown in Figure 25–5. Some of these products have pharmacologic effects of various types, but there is no firm evidence that the levels of such compounds in the brain during the metabolism of ethanol are high enough to produce effects *in vivo*. Therefore it is not yet clear whether these condensation products play a role in either the acute or the chronic effects of alcohol.

Numerous other metabolic effects of ethanol are produced in other tissues, but their pharmacologic or pathologic significance is not well established.

ETHANOL ACTIONS AND INTOXICATION

Membrane and Cellular Effects of Ethanol

All tissues and cells can be affected by high enough concentrations of ethanol, but they differ in sensitivity. At bactericidal concentrations (about 70% or more) denaturation and precipitation of protein occurs, as in fixation of tissues for histology. In much lower concentrations (*e.g.*, less than 1%) the actions are quite different and involve a depression of cell membrane functions.

The membrane actions of ethanol are very similar to those of other general anaesthetics on excitable cell membranes (*see* Chapters 23 and 24). Ethanol elicits expansion and fluidization of the excitable membranes in accordance with the basic principles outlined for general anaesthesia. This disordering effect on membrane lipids also affects the interactions between the lipids and protein inclusions in the membranes, such as receptors, membrane-bound enzymes, and ion channels. As a consequence, a variety of membrane functions are altered in ways that tend to produce **electrical stabilization** of the excitable membrane. Among these alterations are the following.

1. At relatively low concentrations, ethanol enhances the effects of GABA on the GABA-benzodiazepine receptor-Cl^- ionophore complex (*see* Chapters 21 and 26). Under normal conditions, this results in increased Cl^- influx into the cell body and increased Cl^- efflux from axon terminals, in both cases lowering the excitability of the membrane. This action of ethanol can be blocked by Ro 15–4513, a benzodiazepine receptor "inverse agonist" (*see* Chapter 26) that also reverses some of the behavioral and physiologic signs of ethanol intoxication.

2. At somewhat higher concentrations, ethanol reduces the excitation-dependent influx of Ca^{2+}, thus diminishing Ca^{2+}-dependent cell responses such as neurotransmitter release.

3. Receptor-activated second messenger systems are also affected by ethanol. Noradrenaline-activated adenylate cyclase activity is increased by ethanol in some types of neuron, whereas noradrenaline- and acetylcholine-activated phosphoinositol turnover is inhibited. However, the pattern of changes in different parts of the nervous system is complex, and it is not yet clear what role they play in mediating the actions of ethanol.

4. At quite high ethanol concentrations, Na^+-channel opening is impaired. Therefore the rate of rise of action potentials is reduced, so that their maximum height is diminished. Nerve conduction and muscle con-

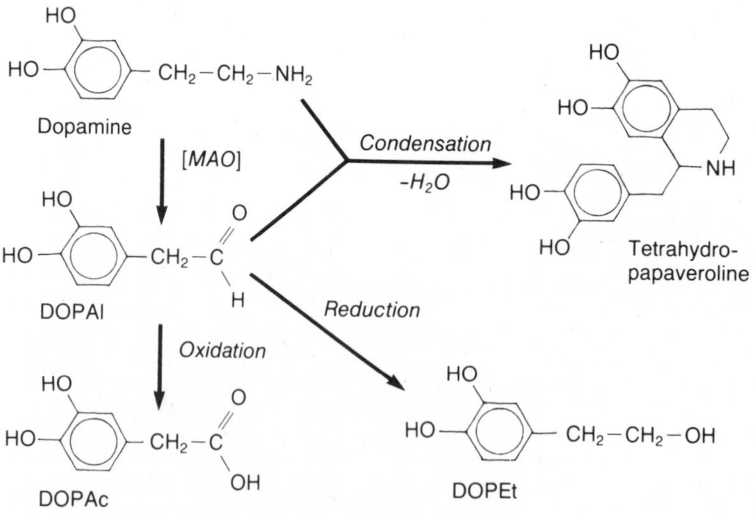

Figure 25–5 Formation of biogenic aldehyde condensation products through the action of alcohol in the brain.

traction, including myocardial contraction, are thus impaired.

5. Active transport of Na^+, K^+, and amino acids by the cell membrane $(Na^+ + K^+)$-ATPase is impaired. This may affect the resting potential of the membrane, on which maintenance of excitability depends.

6. Ethanol increases both the spontaneous and the impulse-triggered release of acetylcholine at cholinergic nerve terminals at the nerve-muscle junction and the anterior horn cell recurrent collateral. In brain slices, however, alcohol inhibits the synaptic release of acetylcholine more than that of other neurotransmitters. It is not known if the effect is exerted on the membrane of the cholinergic synapse itself or on the axons that carry the electrical impulses to the synapse. In the living organism, the overall effect of alcohol on acetylcholine release is complex, but intoxication generally reduces it in parallel with the onset of drowsiness.

While these membrane effects are most prominent in excitable tissues such as brain and muscle, they probably apply to all tissues but at different alcohol concentrations. Even in the central nervous system, some cells are more sensitive than others. In general, ethanol causes a dose-dependent reduction of both spontaneous and evoked firing rates of single units in the cerebral cortex, hippocampus, and other parts of the brain. However, depending on differences in sensitivity of small interneurons, large pyramidal or Purkinje cells, myelinated versus unmyelinated fibres, *etc.*, some units may show increased activity (disinhibition) at concentrations that decrease activity in others. Death occurs by depression of the respiratory control mechanism at blood alcohol concentrations too low to produce serious **direct** effects on most other tissues.

Effects of Ethanol on Integrated Functions of the Nervous System

Relatively low concentrations of ethanol affect the cerebral cortex, the hypothalamus, and the ascending reticular formation. One of the earliest effects produced by small doses of ethanol (10–20 g, equivalent to 1–2 oz of distilled spirits, given to an adult) is cutaneous vasodilatation of central origin. This appears to be due to disturbed functioning of the thermoregulatory centre in the preoptic area and anterior hypothalamus. The skin is flushed and warm, and there is sweating and increased heat loss from the skin. As a result, in a cool environment there may be a fall in body temperature. The vasodilatation also contributes to a fall in peripheral arteriolar resistance, tachycardia, and increased amplitude of pulse pressure.

Hypothalamic actions of ethanol also lead to increased gastric secretion of HCl and increased gastrointestinal motility.

Subjectively, such doses produce relaxation and mild sedation in an individual at rest. If alcohol is infused slowly intravenously with progressively increasing dos-

age, the sedation progresses to sleep and ultimately to anaesthesia and coma.

In the usual social setting in which alcohol is drunk, the picture is modified. At first the sedation is accompanied by loss of inhibitory control of emotions and the **subjects become talkative and emotionally labile**. This is not a unique effect of alcohol; it can be caused by many sedatives in appropriate doses, but these are not normally taken in a social setting. Small doses do not impair complex intellectual ability and may even improve it slightly in tense, nervous people. Even in high doses, the impairment stems principally from slowing and inability to concentrate, rather than from loss of actual intellectual ability. The impairment of the reticular activating system results in decreased ability to attend to incoming sensory information from several sources simultaneously, so that complex tasks requiring alertness and rapid decision-making are more easily disrupted than those in which time is not a critical factor. Sensory acuity is impaired, and at higher blood alcohol concentrations anaesthesia is produced.

Electroencephalographic (EEG) changes are not specific for ethanol, but are reflections of the state of arousal or depression. At low blood alcohol levels, during the stage of excitation and talkativeness, there is a desynchronized (aroused) EEG with an increase in the mean frequency of beta activity. At higher levels, with increasing drowsiness, there is a progressive shift toward EEG synchronization with increased amplitude and steady fall in dominant frequency toward the 1–3 Hz range. Cortical and hippocampal evoked responses at first show increased amplitude, but as severe depression develops the amplitude falls. The latency is also increased, not only in the cortex but also in the afferent paths in the brainstem; this is indicative of a fall in conduction velocity and of a delay in synaptic transmission.

The action of ethanol on the midbrain and medullary reticular formation, and on the input to cerebellar Purkinje cells, also affects descending fibres that modulate the responses of sensory organs and spinal motor synapses. Loss of descending inhibitory control at synapses in the motor pathways, together with impaired proprioceptor sensation, results in **motor ataxia, positive Romberg sign**, and **slurred speech**. Changes in reflexes vary with the complexity of the pathways. Loss of descending inhibitory influences may facilitate simple reflexes, such as tendon jerks, at low or moderate alcohol levels. In contrast, complex **polysynaptic reflexes** are impaired easily. At very high alcohol levels, even monosynaptic reflexes are blocked.

Endocrine Effects

Numerous **endocrine effects**, mediated *via* the hypothalamus, have been shown.

1. Pituitary **antidiuretic hormone secretion is inhibited** by rising blood ethanol levels, causing **diuresis**

of low specific gravity and of variable intensity and duration. This can be **abolished by the action of nicotine** on the hypothalamus. This suggests that the effect of ethanol may result from decreased neuronal input to the supraoptic and paraventricular nuclei, rather than from direct suppression of secretory cells in the neurohypophysis.

2.   Secretion of oxytocin is inhibited, and infusion of dilute ethanol intravenously was, for a time, used clinically to stop uterine contraction and prevent premature labor. This practice has been abandoned because of the risk of damage to the fetus.

3.   **Increased secretion of adrenaline,* noradrenaline**, and adrenal **corticosteroids** occurs during severe intoxication with respiratory and circulatory depression. On the other hand, small doses of ethanol diminish stress responses to a variety of stressors. This anti-stress effect includes reduction or prevention of the elevations in plasma corticosteroid and catecholamine levels. The blood ethanol level at which stress reduction is replaced by ethanol-induced stress probably varies with the person and the circumstances.

4.   **Secretion of LH** is impaired and, as a result, serum **testosterone levels** tend to fall. Another factor contributing to the reduction in testosterone output is the inhibition of steroid hydroxylation in the testis as a result of NADH accumulation caused by alcohol dehydrogenase activity in the testis itself.

Ethanol Intoxication

Signs of intoxication appear at different blood levels, depending on individual differences in tolerance and also on the speed of drinking and thus on the rate of rise of the blood ethanol level.

Mild signs appear in most people at levels below 500 mg/L (11 mmol/L, 0.05%). Frank intoxication with psychomotor impairment is present in many subjects at levels below 1000 mg/L (22 mmol/L, 0.1%), but in practically everyone at 1500 mg/L (33 mmol/L, 0.15%). Profound intoxication with anaesthesia and/or coma is likely at 2500 mg/L (54 mmol/L, 0.25%) or higher, although chronic heavy use of ethanol may increase tolerance to such a degree that some individuals are still conscious and active at blood levels of over 0.25%.

Death occurs, as a result of respiratory depression in most cases, at levels of 5000 mg/L (108 mmol/L, 0.5%) or higher. **Barbiturates and other sedatives, phenothiazines (both tranquilizers and antihistamines), rauwolfia, propanediol tranquilizers, and benzodiazepines show additive or potentiating effects with alcohols.** When such drugs are used to quiet someone who becomes "roaring drunk," great care must be taken to avoid fatal overdosage.

In many countries, it is illegal to drive a motor vehicle at blood alcohol levels specified in the traffic and criminal codes. In various European countries, this is 0.05% (500 mg/L, 11 mmol/L). In Canada and some

states of the U.S.A. it is 0.08% (800 mg/L, 17 mmol/L). In many states of the U.S.A. it is 0.1%. Note that these values do not constitute a legal definition of intoxication, because the legislators recognized that even at 0.1% some individuals with higher tolerance might not be demonstrably intoxicated. However, in Canada it was considered likely that most drivers would be impaired to varying degrees at levels of 0.08% or higher. Therefore it is an offense to drive at these levels, whether a given individual is impaired or not.

Treatment of Acute Intoxication

Treatment might theoretically be aimed at either (1) speeding the disappearance of alcohol from the body or (2) counteracting its effects. As already mentioned, metabolic disappearance can not be speeded up very much. In extreme cases, where death may occur, hemodialysis is undoubtedly rapid and effective in removing the alcohol. Usually, however, such treatment is not needed.

Pharmacologic reversal of the effects of ethanol is not usually attempted in mild intoxication. Many compounds have been tested for their claimed **amethystic** (anti-intoxicant) properties; a recent example is the antiparkinsonian agent amantadine (see Chapter 20). However, the results are not very convincing. In serious intoxication with profound coma, central nervous system stimulants (analeptics) are occasionally used, but they are not very helpful because there is a small margin between doses that are ineffective and those that are too large and cause seizures. As noted earlier in this section, the benzodiazepine receptor inverse agonist Ro 15–4513 can reverse some of the signs of alcohol intoxication, but it does not antagonize the lethal effect of ethanol overdose. The opioid antagonist naloxone has been reported to reverse alcoholic coma, but there are numerous reports that it has failed to work, and in experimental animals it works only at doses that have an analeptic effect of their own. Therefore **supportive therapy (intravenous fluids, artificial respiration, etc.) is the principal approach**. This is kept up until metabolism lowers the blood alcohol level to the point where the danger is past.

ALCOHOLISM AND RELATED PROBLEMS

Alcoholism ("Chronic Alcoholism," Alcohol Dependence, Alcohol Addiction)

Alcoholism constitutes a very complex medical and social problem. The factors involved include such things as the prevalent social attitudes towards drinking and drunkenness, parental attitudes and habits, drinking practices among certain occupational groups, personal emotional conflicts, and appropriately rewarding phar-

* epinephrine

macologic effects of ethanol. There is some evidence suggesting a congenital or hereditary predisposition. (Much research is currently being directed at a search for biochemical markers for detecting those who have a genetic predisposition, and also for biochemical tests for identifying heavy drinkers at an early stage.) In almost every case, most of these factors are involved in varying degrees, so that there is no single cause of alcoholism. This question is examined in more detail in Chapter 67.

The adverse consequences of alcoholism are also seen in many different aspects of the individual's life, including physical and mental health, family relations, work and economic performance, accidents, legal problems, and others. Most of these are beyond the scope of this chapter. Only a few of the pharmacologic problems can be covered here.

Nutritional Problems

Oxidation of ethanol yields 7 cal/g. At an average oxidation rate of 10 g/hr or 240 g daily, one could derive nearly 1700 cal/day from ethanol. In some individual cases and in regular heavy drinkers, the amount may be much higher. If the average dietary intake of a man with sedentary occupation is 2500–3000 cal/day, steady drinking can provide well over half of the total. Since alcoholic beverages contain little or no protein, vitamins, or lipotropic factors, a variety of nutritional deficiency diseases can result. **Peripheral neuropathy, Korsakoff's psychosis, Wernicke's disease, and pellagra are examples of B-vitamin deficiencies occurring in alcoholics**; they have become much less frequent since vitamin supplementation of bread and other foods became common practice. Since nutrition is frequently insufficient during drinking bouts and hepatic glycogen content is reduced, serious hypoglycemia can occur, as explained above under Metabolic Effects.

Organ Damage

Fatty liver is common among alcoholics as a result of the metabolic disturbances described earlier. **Alcoholic hepatitis** and **cirrhosis**, however, appear to result from different processes than fatty liver. As noted in the section on metabolism, chronic ingestion of large amounts of ethanol leads to increased O_2 consumption by the hepatocytes, and therefore a much lower Po_2 at the venous end of the sinusoid. Anything that reduces arterial Po_2 can therefore precipitate hypoxia in that zone, resulting in hepatocellular necrosis and a local inflammatory cell response (alcoholic hepatitis). Ethanol also reduces the hepatic level of reduced glutathione, and this effect may contribute to the production of hepatocellular necrosis (*see* Chapter 62).

Current research is also exploring the possibility that autoantibodies to acetaldehyde complexes with hepatocellular proteins may produce liver cell necrosis. Repeated episodes of necrosis lead to fibroblast response, which eventually produces portal cirrhosis (*see* Chapter 62). Even if the hepatocellular damage is reversible, the cells remain sensitive to ethanol for months after the cessation of heavy drinking: even small doses can produce a prompt rise in serum glutamic-pyruvic transaminase and gamma-glutamyl transpeptidase levels.

Another important type of organic damage in alcoholics is **cerebral cortical atrophy**, with widening of the sulci and enlargement of the ventricles. This can be revealed by computerized tomography (CT) scanning at a stage before gross neurologic or psychologic deficits are detectable clinically. This is a different type of lesion from the nutritional-deficiency effects previously noted, and may possibly reflect a direct toxic effect of ethanol itself. Fortunately, it is often reversible if drinking is stopped at an early stage.

Some alcoholics, after years of heavy drinking, show a relatively sudden "break" or loss of tolerance, becoming quite intoxicated by amounts of alcohol that previously produced only mild symptoms. This is usually the result of organic damage to either the liver or the nervous system. Liver damage, resulting in reduced ethanol-oxidizing ability, causes the same amount of ethanol to yield higher and more prolonged blood alcohol levels than previously. Brain damage, with cortical and hippocampal neuron loss, may render the nervous system more sensitive to the same blood alcohol level.

The **fetal alcohol syndrome** (FAS) is a complex picture of **irreversible** damage to the fetus and results from ingestion of alcohol by pregnant women. The complete picture includes small head, widely separated eyes with short palpebral fissures and epicanthic folds, a broad upper lip that lacks the normal midline vertical groove (the philtrum), a short nose, mental and physical retardation, often cardiac valvular defects, and continued retardation of development postnatally. Lesser degrees of FAS may lack some of these features. FAS appears to be caused by a direct toxic effect of ethanol and/or acetaldehyde, perhaps in part by impairment of placental circulation, rather than a consequence of maternal malnutrition. The severity appears to be dose-dependent, but the minimum dose required to produce it is not known. Therefore many obstetricians advise their patients not to drink alcohol at all during pregnancy.

In general, alcoholics have a higher mortality rate than the general population of the same age and sex. The "**excess mortality**" is due not only to liver cirrhosis but to many different causes including hypertensive heart disease, stroke, cancer of the pharynx and esophagus, and accidents. In contrast, there is considerable epidemiologic evidence suggesting that a low or moderate alcohol intake may reduce the risk of fatal myocardial infarction; the mechanism is not yet known.

Tolerance and Dependence

With steady intake of alcohol, tolerance develops, *i.e.*, larger amounts of alcohol are required to produce the same degree of effect. This reflects both **metabolic tolerance** produced by faster oxidation in the liver, and **functional tolerance** in the nervous system. Absorption and distribution of the alcohol are not significantly altered.

The **functional tolerance is an actual change in sensitivity of the CNS**. Two different time frames of tolerance are commonly recognized. Acute tolerance occurs within the course of a single exposure to ethanol, so that there is less intoxication at a given blood alcohol level on the descending limb of the blood alcohol curve than there was at the same level on the rising limb. Chronic tolerance is the gradual decrease in degree of intoxication at the same blood alcohol level over the course of repeated alcohol exposures. The relation between acute and chronic tolerance is not yet wholly clear. The maximum degree of tolerance to ethanol is considerably smaller than the tolerance that can develop to opiates or to benzodiazepines.

The mechanism of functional tolerance to ethanol is complex and not yet fully known, but it appears to be related to the development of physical dependence, which proceeds more or less in parallel with the growth of tolerance. Physical dependence is revealed by the occurrence of serious disturbances, referred to as **withdrawal symptoms**, when alcohol intake is reduced or stopped. (*See* Chapter 67, *Drug Abuse and Drug Dependence.*)

Ethanol Withdrawal Syndrome

Since ethanol depresses neuronal excitability and spontaneous activity in various parts of the brain, adaptation must involve some type of compensatory hyperactivity to offset the alcohol effect. This is seen as tolerance when the alcohol is present. When the alcohol is withdrawn the hyperactivity gives rise to the withdrawal symptoms. Their severity and duration depend upon the severity and duration of the preceding period of drinking.

Following a single intoxicating dose of alcohol or a single short period of drinking, *e.g.*, one evening, the only consistent physiologic change that can be correlated with ''hangover'' (and is suggestive of withdrawal effect) is some degree of **neuronal hyperexcitability** (Fig. 25–6).

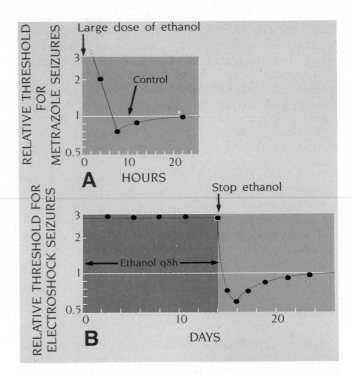

Figure 25–6 Effects of ethanol withdrawal on neuronal excitability by pentylenetetrazol (Metrazol) or electric shock. *A*, After a single large dose of ethanol at zero time. *B*, After prolonged ingestion of ethanol. Note the difference in the time scales in *A* and *B*.

After longer drinking bouts lasting several days or more, the symptoms include marked hyperirritability, exaggerated reflexes, sleeplessness, tremor, muscular tension, cold sweaty skin, nausea, and marked thirst. In severe cases there may be generalized convulsions.

After chronic drinking for many weeks or months, abrupt cessation or even some reduction of alcohol intake can precipitate a two-stage withdrawal reaction. In addition to the symptoms already described, which begin very soon after withdrawal, there can be a second stage beginning 2 or more days later. This is characterized by severe hyperactivity with delirium, hallucinations, fever, profuse sweating, intense vasodilatation, and severe tachycardia. This stage (delirium tremens) is still sometimes fatal despite the newer treatments. One hypothesis is that this picture results from rebound hypersensitivity of β-adrenergic receptors that had been suppressed during prolonged intoxication and early withdrawal.

Treatment of the withdrawal syndrome depends on the severity. **Phenothiazine neuroleptics, chlordiazepoxide, or diazepam** are usually effective in reducing the irritability, tremor, and sleeplessness. The first dose is sometimes given parenterally for rapid action (however, see Chapter 26). Phenothiazines do not prevent convulsions, and may even increase the risk, so that anticonvulsant drugs may also be necessary. For this reason, diazepam is now the preferred drug. Barbiturates, paraldehyde, etc., are useful but less safe and probably somewhat less effective than the drugs mentioned. They are now very seldom used clinically (see Chapter 26). Ethanol itself is effective, and a tapering-off treatment is preferred in some countries; however, it is hard to adhere to and is psychologically bad for the patient who wishes to stop drinking, unless it is given by a different route, e.g., intravenously, which is not associated with the stimuli that ordinarily accompany the ingestion of alcohol. Supportive therapy may include large amounts of fluid either orally or intravenously, but some patients are actually overhydrated when first seen. A high-calorie balanced diet with vitamin supplements is usually recommended.

Disulfiram and Related Drugs

Tetra-ethyl thiuram disulfide (= disulfiram, or TETD) inhibits the hepatic enzymes that oxidize acetaldehyde to acetate. Consumption of ethanol is, therefore, followed by accumulation of acetaldehyde in the blood and tissues, causing acetaldehyde poisoning. Within minutes the subject becomes hot, flushed, and cyanotic. The pulse rate, cardiac output, and respiratory rate rise. These effects are thought to result from excessive release of catecholamines from sympathetic nerve endings under the influence of acetaldehyde. However, disulfiram also inhibits dopamine-β-hydroxylase, so that the stores of catecholamines in the nerve endings are low to begin with. Therefore, after 30–60 minutes the sympathetic tone falls abruptly and there is a marked fall in blood pressure, pallor, and nausea. This reaction lasts for up to 2 hours and can be very severe and occasionally fatal. Alcoholics are often given disulfiram so that fear of a reaction will deter them from drinking. It is not a cure for alcoholism, merely a deterrent (see Chapter 67).

Disulfiram is absorbed rapidly from the GI tract, begins to act within 2–4 hours, and reaches maximum effect in 24 hours. It should not be started until 12–24 hours after the last drink of alcohol. The drug is metabolized in the body by splitting of the disulfide bond to form diethyldithiocarbamate, which may be the active form. This in turn is broken down to CS_2, which appears in the breath, and to sulfate, which is excreted slowly in the urine over the next week.

Disulfiram itself has some toxicity apart from the inhibition of dopamine-β-hydroxylase and possibly some other enzymes. Toxic symptoms may include weakness, dizziness, mental disturbances, cardiac arrhythmias, skin reactions, and impotence. It can also inhibit metabolism of other drugs by liver microsomal enzymes, thus alter-

ing the effects of these drugs. Patients using disulfiram must be monitored carefully.

Citrated calcium carbimide, developed in this department by J.K.W. Ferguson and his co-workers, also inhibits acetaldehyde dehydrogenase. However, it does not inhibit dopamine-β-hydroxylase, and its toxic effects are much less severe than those of disulfiram. It has therefore found clinical use (in Canada and some other countries, but not in the United States). The reaction to alcohol is also less severe than with disulfiram, and possibly is not so effective a deterrent to drinking.

Tolbutamide, metronidazole, and **cephalosporins** have similar interactions with alcohol. Patients being treated with these drugs should be warned not to drink alcohol. Conversely, chronic intake of alcohol may cause faster metabolism of tolbutamide, with correspondingly shorter duration of action (see Chapter 4).

METHANOL INTOXICATION

Methanol is a milder intoxicant than ethanol in that larger doses are necessary to produce the same degree of intoxication. The serious toxicity is not that of methanol itself, but of its metabolic products. It is oxidized by catalase, as well as by alcohol dehydrogenase, to **formaldehyde**, which is in turn oxidized to **formic acid**. These substances are specifically toxic to the retina and optic nerve and may produce partial or complete permanent blindness. In addition, the formic acid gives rise to severe metabolic acidosis, which may be fatal.

Treatment requires (1) vigorous measures to correct the acidosis with intravenous sodium bicarbonate solution and (2) attempts to eliminate the methanol before it can be oxidized. This is achieved by combining hemodialysis (for removing methanol) with administration of repeated doses of ethanol, which competitively inhibits oxidation of the methanol. Folate is also used, to enhance oxidation of any formate produced.

HIGHER ALCOHOLS

Propyl and isopropyl alcohols are used as antiseptics and for alcohol rubs. The higher alcohols (butyl, pentyl, etc.) are used mainly as solvents for industrial processes. They are of concern pharmacologically for two reasons. (1) Distilled beverages contain small amounts of higher alcohols and aldehydes, referred to as "congeners." There is some slight evidence that they may contribute to the toxicity of the ethanol. (2) They are often consumed by "skid row" alcoholics in the form of antifreeze, cleaning fluid, and numerous other toxic mixtures with gasoline, benzene, *etc*. The intoxicating effects are similar to those of ethanol but much more severe for the same dose. Organic toxicity, especially to the liver, kidney, and bone marrow, is also more severe with these mixtures.

Certain other higher alcohols, mainly unsaturated tertiary alcohols such as ethchlorvynol (Placidyl®) and methylpentynol (Dormison®) and certain acetaldehyde derivatives (trichloracetaldehyde hydrate, paraldehyde), were formerly used fairly widely as sedatives and hypnotics. They are still used occasionally, but have been replaced almost completely by the benzodiazepines. They are therefore no longer described in detail in this text.

SUGGESTED READING

Goldstein DB. Pharmacology of alcohol. New York: Oxford University Press, 1983.

Kalant H, LeBlanc AE, Gibbins RJ. Tolerance to, and dependence on, some non-opiate psychotropic drugs. Pharmacol Rev 1971; 23:135–191.

Kalant H, Lê AD. Effects of ethanol on thermoregulation. Pharmacol Ther 1984; 23:313–364.

Kalant H, Woo N. Electrophysiological effects of ethanol on the nervous system. Pharmacol Ther 1981; 14:431–457.

Khanna JM, Israel Y. Ethanol metabolism. In: Javitt NB, ed. Liver and biliary tract physiology I. Int Rev Physiol 21:275–315. Baltimore: University Park Press, 1980.

Majchrowicz E, Noble EP, eds. Biochemistry and pharmacology of ethanol (2 volumes). New York: Plenum Press, 1979.

McCoy GD, Koop DR. Biochemical and immunochemical evidence for the induction of an ethanol-inducible cytochrome P-450 isozyme in male Syrian golden hamsters. Biochem Pharmacol 1988; 37:1563–1568.

Naranjo CA, Sellers EM. Clinical assessment and pharmacotherapy of the alcohol withdrawal syndrome. In: Galanter M, ed. Developments in alcoholism. Vol. 4. New York: Plenum Publishing, 1986:265–281.

Sherlock S, ed. Alcohol and disease. Br Med Bull 1982; 38(1):1–114.

Smith CM. The pharmacology of sedative/hypnotics, alcohol and anaesthetics: sites and mechanisms of action. In: Martin WR, ed. Handbook of experimental pharmacology: drug addiction I. Berlin: Springer-Verlag, 1978.

Streissguth AP, Landesman-Dwyer S, Martin JC, Smith DW. Teratogenic effects of alcohol in humans and animals. Science 1980; 209:353–361.

Wallgren H, Barry H III. The actions of alcohol. Amsterdam: Elsevier Publishing Co., 1970.

Chapter 26

ANXIOLYTICS, HYPNOTICS, AND SEDATIVES

E.M. Sellers and J.M. Khanna

The anxiolytic, sedative, and hypnotic drugs constitute a large and chemically heterogeneous group (Table 26–1), which includes some drugs covered in other chapters. Benzodiazepines and barbiturates are among the most commonly prescribed or used drugs in the world. About 10% of all Canadians use a benzodiazepine each year. Between 30% and 50% of hospitalized patients receive such drugs.

The terms sedative and hypnotic are rather old and are not very precise when applied to modern therapy. When alcohol, opiates, and belladonna were the only available psychopharmacologic drugs, a wide variety of behavior disorders were managed by sedating the anxious or disturbed patient. A sedative drug decreases activity and agitation and calms the patient. With the possible exception of benzodiazepines, most modern anxiolytic drugs have sedative action such as that seen with barbiturates. Even benzodiazepines share this property when high doses are given. The term hypnotic, on the other hand, is derived from the Greek word (hypnos) for sleep and was applied to drugs used to promote sleep in any patient, not necessarily an anxious or agitated one. In fact, however, most of the drugs with sedating activity are also hypnotic, and in modern usage they are called sedative-hypnotics.

The main use of sedative-hypnotics is to promote drowsiness and facilitate the onset or maintenance of sleep, which ideally should have all the characteristics of normal sleep. Hypnotic-induced and -maintained sleep is, however, never identical to normal physiologic sleep.

Sedation

Mild suppression of arousal and behavior, with slight reduction of alertness and responses to stimuli, is called sedation and the drugs are called sedatives.

The mechanism of sedation produced by drugs is not fully known because of the complexity of their actions. Several features are important: (1) such drugs act on polysynaptic pathways; (2) they usually increase presynaptic inhibition; (3) different parts of the brain have different sensitivity towards them (i.e., regional selectivity and specificity); and (4) the drugs stimulate pre- (and occasionally post-) synaptic effects of gamma-aminobutyric acid (GABA).

TABLE 26–1 Anxiolytic, Sedative, and Hypnotic Drugs

Alcohols (see Chapter 25)*
  Ethanol
  Ethchlorvynol, Chloral hydrate

Benzodiazepines

Barbiturates

Piperidinediones *
  Glutethimide
  Methyprylon

Miscellaneous *
  Propanediol carbamates
    (e.g., meprobamate)
  Methaqualone
  Paraldehyde
  Bromides
  Monoureides
  Ethinamate
  Antihistamines (see Chapter 32)

* *Note:* These drugs, even though occasionally still used as anxiolytics, sedatives, and hypnotics, are mainly of historical interest, except for the nonmedical use of ethanol. They have been largely replaced by drugs with greater efficacy and lesser abuse and dependence liability and a wider margin of safety (e.g., benzodiazepines). The same can be said of all barbiturates except thiopental and phenobarbital.

Sleep

Further depression, by larger doses of the same drugs, causes sleep and the drugs are then called hypnotics. One can normally be roused by strong enough stimuli (*e.g.*, pain, alarm clock).

Normal sleep consists of at least two phases: (1) slow-wave sleep (SWS) (stages 3 and 4), so-called because the EEG shows predominantly high-voltage synchronous activity, but with sustained tonus of skeletal muscles; and (2) rapid-eye-movement (REM) sleep, in which the EEG shows an arousal pattern, the eyes move rapidly and irregularly, skeletal muscles relax completely, and dreaming is thought to take place. These two phases alternate throughout the total sleep period, REM sleep making up about 25% of the total. This alternation appears to depend upon a balance of 5-HT and catecholamine influences on the reticular formation. Hypnotic drugs suppress the reticular formation to different degrees.

The **sleep produced by hypnotics** differs from normal sleep, in that SWS patterns are altered and shortened by the appearance of EEG spindles, REM sleep is suppressed, and total sleep time is prolonged. Most of the benzodiazepines produce similar effects on the patterns of sleep, although to a lesser degree. With chronic use the effects tend to decrease but do not disappear. If after 3–4 weeks the drug is suddenly stopped, the amount and intensity of REM increase to levels greater than in normal sleep ("REM rebound"). This is considered by some investigators to represent a mild degree of physical dependence and withdrawal reaction (*see* the section on Adverse Effects of Barbiturates, and Chapter 67).

Anaesthesia

Deeper depression, such that even intense stimuli do not cause arousal, is called anaesthesia (*see* Chapter 23).

These three divisions are merely differences of degree and give no indication of different mechanisms. For drugs that have general CNS depressant actions, decreased anxiety, sedation, sleep, and general anaesthesia fall along a continuum of increasing CNS depression. (Note, however, that benzodiazepines are normally incapable of producing anaesthesia.)

In addition to sedation, sleep, or anaesthesia, CNS depressant drugs can depress other central states characterized by neuronal excitation. Hence, these drugs may be useful as antiepileptics or muscle relaxants.

BENZODIAZEPINES

Chlordiazepoxide was first marketed in 1960. This was followed by diazepam (1963) and oxazepam (1965), and many others since then. The popularity of these drugs is the result of a combination of their pharmacologic actions, their relative safety, and the demand for agents of this type by both physicians and patients. Benzodiazepines can be classified on the basis of their chemical structure, kinetic characteristics, and therapeutic indications.

Structural Classification

All benzodiazepines are variations upon the 5-aryl-1,4-benzodiazepine nucleus (Fig. 26–1). 1,5-Benzodiazepines also exist, but are not different in pharmacologic action. Other than the apparent requirement for the 5-aryl group, the structure-activity relationships are not stringent.

Chlordiazepoxide and diazepam are the prototypic benzodiazepines. Diazepam and many other benzodiazepines are metabolized to the active metabolite N-desmethyldiazepam, also called nordiazepam (ND). ND is marketed as a separate drug in some countries. Chlorazepate and prazepam are quite rapidly converted to ND, one by acid hydrolysis and the other by dealkylation, and owe their clinical effects to the active metabolite (*see* Fig. 26–1).

The 3-OH substituent of oxazepam and lorazepam determines that the principal metabolic pathway is conjugation rather than production of ND.

Triazolam shares with other triazolo-benzodiazepines rather rapid biotransformation without production of active metabolites.

Mechanism of Benzodiazepine Action

In 1977, specific receptors for the benzodiazepines were discovered in the nervous system. These receptors are characterized by the following properties.

Saturability

The receptors are saturable by ^{3}H-diazepam with a K_D of 3.6 nM, or by ^{3}H-flunitrazepam with a K_D of 1–3 nM.

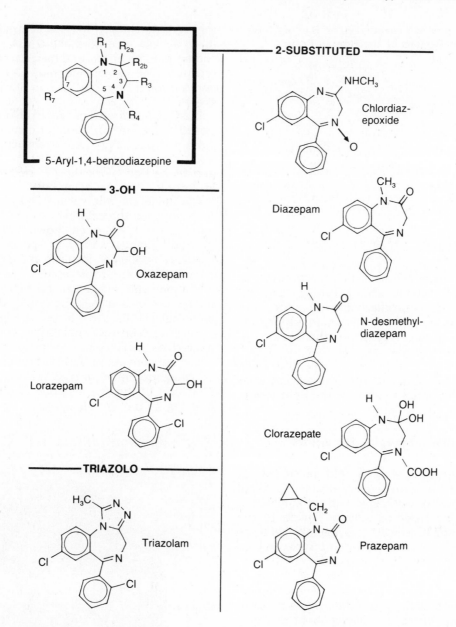

Figure 26–1 Structural formulae of several clinically significant benzodiazepines.

Stereoselectivity

The (+)-enantiomers of benzodiazepines are about 200 times more active than the (−)-enantiomers in inhibiting the specific binding of ^{3}H-diazepam.

Receptor Distribution in the CNS

The receptors are highest in density in the cerebral cortex, as shown in Table 26–2, but are also present in significant numbers in the cerebellum and parts of the limbic system.

Recently two subclasses of receptors, designated I and II, have been postulated. Type I receptors predominate in the cerebellum, and Type II receptors in cerebral cortex. Whether these "receptor types" represent distinct receptors or interconverting forms of the same receptor class is not resolved. In any case, most benzodiazepines have equal affinity for both receptors. The highly speculative view that Type I mediates the antianxiety action and Type II the sedative and other actions is not borne out in various studies.

TABLE 26–2 Density of Benzodiazepine Binding Sites in Different Regions of the Human Brain

Region	^{3}H-Diazepam B_{max} (fmoles of ^{3}H-ligand per mg protein)
Cerebral cortex	1200
Cerebellar cortex	730
Amygdala	720
Hippocampus	610
Hypothalamus	520

Endogenous Ligands

None of the common neurotransmitters compete for binding with ^{3}H-diazepam. The following have no direct effect on the benzodiazepine receptor: noradrenaline,* dopamine, GABA, glutamate, glycine, or histamine. It had once been proposed that the benzodiazepine receptor was the same as that for glycine or GABA, but this view is no longer accepted, since glycine has no effect. Current research suggests that the endogenous neurotransmitter for the benzodiazepine receptor may be a purine.

GABA-Linked Benzodiazepine Receptors

Since both GABA (at 1 μM) and muscimol (at 100 nM; muscimol is a GABA agonist) enhance the binding of ^{3}H-diazepam to its receptor, it is thought that the benzodiazepine receptor may be linked to the GABA receptor (*see* Chapter 21). It is possible that there may be a cooperative effect between the two receptors. This hypothesis would be compatible with the idea that elevated GABA levels in brain tissue are associated with stable, electrically-suppressed nervous tissue. Hence, it may be that the benzodiazepines produce their anticonvulsant effect by bringing about an elevation in the GABA levels or increasing the effect of GABA at its receptor.

GABA-Receptor/Chloride-Ionophore Complex

Postsynaptic GABA receptors are functionally linked to benzodiazepine receptors, barbiturate receptors and a Cl$^-$ channel. The collective term for these individual components is the GABA-receptor/chloride-ionophore complex. This entire complex is involved in the mediation and modulation of GABAergic inhibitory transmission. The physiologic effects of GABA are mediated by increases in chloride conductance while regulation of the chloride ionophore involves all three receptors.

Figure 26–2 is a theoretical model of the GABA-receptor/Cl$^-$-ionophore complex. This transverse two-dimensional view of the receptor complex represents the chloride channel located centrally, surrounded by three distinct receptors: the GABA receptor, the benzodiazepine receptor, and the picrotoxinin-barbiturate receptor. The ion channel may be a separate component or could be a part of one of the distinct binding sites.

The GABA-receptor-regulated chloride channel is proposed as the site of action for convulsant and anticonvulsant drugs. Thus neurotransmitters or drugs that open the Cl$^-$ channel are thought to be antiseizure, and those that block the Cl$^-$ channel are convulsant in nature.

The functional interrelationships between the three receptors and the chloride ionophore are of particular importance. It has been shown that interaction of the benzodiazepines with their specific binding sites increases chloride conductance in the presence of GABA, meaning that benzodiazepines potentiate GABAergic inhibition. This effect can be blocked by the GABA antagonist bicuculline, suggesting that a functionally meaningful GABA site is involved. Likewise, barbiturates potentiate GABAergic inhibition, and this effect is inhibited by picrotoxin. The proposed mechanism by which anticonvulsant barbiturates such as phenobarbital cause potentiation of GABAergic inhibition is prolongation of the postsynaptic action of GABA in the opening of the Cl$^-$ channels.

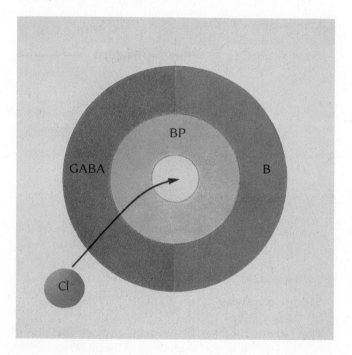

Figure 26–2 Schematic representation of the GABA-chloride ionophore receptor complex, transected in the plane of the cell membrane. (Note that this is an evolving field of investigation with at times conflicting views. *See* Chapter 21 for additional interpretations.) GABA = GABA receptor; B = benzodiazepine receptor; BP = barbiturate and picrotoxin receptor, believed to be closely associated with the chloride ionophore; Cl$^-$ = chloride channel.

* norepinephrine

In contrast to these depressant drugs, picrotoxin is a CNS-stimulatory drug that is thought to cause convulsions by blocking the Cl^- channels without affecting the binding of GABA to its receptor site.

So far, work on the linkage between the benzodiazepine receptor and the GABA-chloride-ionophore complex has offered a possible explanation of the anticonvulsant effects of benzodiazepines. It is not clear whether this linkage is related to the anxiolytic properties of these drugs.

Benzodiazepine Antagonist

The investigation of the role of the benzodiazepine receptor has been advanced by the discovery of a selective and specific antagonist, Ro 15-1788 (Ro = Hoffmann-LaRoche, the company where the drug was discovered). This substance (Fig. 26-3) blocks or reverses diazepam effects, but has no apparent intrinsic activity of its own. When given to monkeys to which diazepam has been administered chronically, the antagonist precipitates a withdrawal syndrome.

β-Carbolines

Benzodiazepine antagonistic properties have also been discovered among receptor ligands structurally different from Ro 15-1788. Various β-carboline derivatives bind specifically to the ^3H-diazepam receptors but produce effects opposite to those of benzodiazepines, *i.e.*, they show proconvulsant activity and anxiogenic effects. Therefore they have been called **inverse agonists** rather than antagonists. It has been suggested that β-carbolines produce effects opposite to those of benzodiazepines because these agents reduce the coupling of GABA receptors with the Cl^- ionophore, thereby decreasing the frequency of chloride channel opening. Interestingly, Ro 15-1788 also blocks the effect of β-carbolines, since it blocks the binding of inverse agonists as well as of agonists.

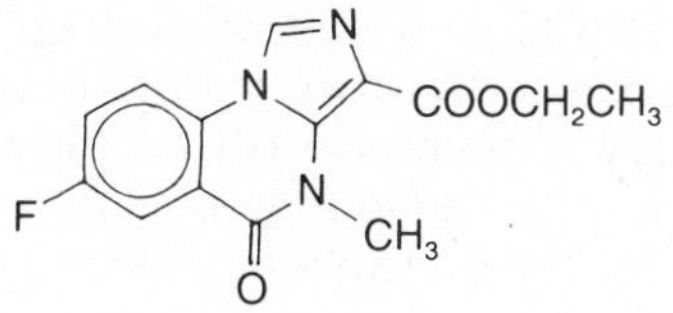

Figure 26-3 Structural formula of Ro 15-1788, a selective and specific benzodiazepine receptor antagonist.

Pharmacokinetics

Absorption

After oral administration, the absorption of diazepam, alprazolam, and triazolam is very rapid. The peak plasma concentration occurs about 1 hour after ingestion. Such rapid absorption accounts for the acute subjective "high," drowsiness, "spaced-out" feeling, or motor impairment after the drug is ingested. Diazepam has a systemic bioavailability of 100%. Oxazepam, lorazepam, and prazepam are absorbed more slowly, maximum plasma concentration occurring 2-3 hours after ingestion; the bioavailability of oxazepam taken orally is about 50-70%. Clorazepate is converted by acid hydrolysis in the stomach to its active form, desmethyldiazepam; antacids reduce the rate of conversion and decrease the drug's peak effects.

After intramuscular injection of diazepam or of chlordiazepoxide in healthy persons, chronic alcoholics, or alcoholics in withdrawal, absorption is slow (the plasma concentration peaking at 10-12 hours) and erratic, but eventually complete. As a consequence, clinical effects may be delayed and unpredictable. Therefore, these drugs should not be given intramuscularly.

Protein Binding

Most benzodiazepines are extensively bound to serum albumin (*e.g.*, diazepam is 98% bound at therapeutic concentrations). The binding decreases the concentration of free active drug in equilibrium with the sites of action and elimination, thereby decreasing the intensity of action but prolonging the effect and slowing the elimination. Glomerular filtration of many benzodiazepines is low because of their extensive serum protein binding. Conversely, in persons with cirrhosis and hypoalbuminemia the concentration of free active drug is higher and side effects such as drowsiness are more common.

Biotransformation and Disposition

All benzodiazepines undergo biotransformation in the liver, mainly by microsomal mixed-function oxidase activity or by conjugation. Rates and patterns of benzodiazepine biotransformation vary considerably among healthy and sick humans.

Figure 26-4 summarizes the typical patterns of biotransformation. Note that, even though there are many benzodiazepines, there are only a few patterns of biotransformation. Metabolites indicated with an asterisk

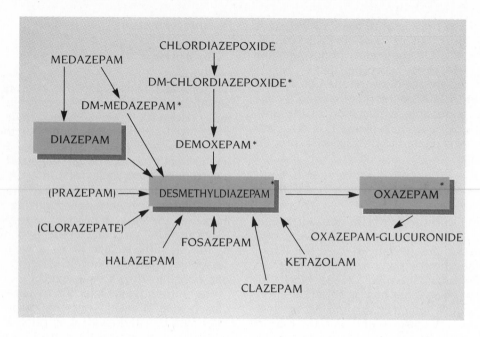

Figure 26–4 Patterns of benzodiazepine biotransformation. (DM = desmethyl, * = active metabolites.)

are active. Table 26–3 classifies the benzodiazepines on the basis of their half-lives and patterns of disposition.

Chlordiazepoxide and **diazepam** each have two major active metabolites that contribute to their clinical effects and toxicity: (1) chlordiazepoxide is converted to desmethylchlordiazepoxide and then to demoxepam; (2) diazepam is converted to desmethyldiazepam and then to oxazepam, itself a marketed benzodiazepine.

Desmethyldiazepam has a longer mean half-life than the parent drug (50.9 ± 6.2 hours versus 32.6 ± 11.3 hours). By coincidence, the half-life of diazepam in hours is about equal to the patient's age in years; however, there are many exceptions to this rule. Little diazepam is excreted in the bile, and enterohepatic recirculation is not responsible for the slow elimination.

These long half-lives and the extent of variation between patients make prediction of the time of maximum clinical effect or toxicity very difficult, but during long-term therapy cumulative and long-lasting effects can be expected for those benzodiazepines with long half-lives. On average, the time for cumulation to peak concentration during long-term oral administration is approximately five times the half-life of the drug, i.e., for chlordiazepoxide 3 days, diazepam 7 days, and desmethyldiazepam 10 days. The slow cumulation of drug means that the full therapeutic effect or toxicity cannot be determined for a considerable time, and that the dosage should not be adjusted until cumulation is maximal. Conversely, elimination of the drug is slow and the offset of drug effect may be delayed.

Because of the long half-lives of chlordiazepoxide and diazepam, multiple daily doses may in theory be unnecessary. However, if the entire 24-hour dosage is given as a single dose, it may cause extreme sedation. Because of this sedating action, it is best to give most of the daily dose at bedtime.

The biotransformation of chlordiazepoxide, diazepam, and desmethyldiazepam is impaired in patients with severe liver disease, and the half-life may increase up to six-fold. The biotransformation of chlordiazepoxide and diazepam is inhibited by concurrent administration of disulfiram or ethanol.

Lorazepam, a more potent benzodiazepine, is similar to **oxazepam** in structure and pattern of disposition, and its intramuscular bioavailability is complete. Unlike chlordiazepoxide and diazepam, these drugs are biotransformed simply by glucuronide conjugation to inactive metabolites. Furthermore, since the mean half-life of oxazepam is 7 hours, cumulation is minor and a full therapeutic response occurs after a few doses. Similarly, excessive sedation rapidly disappears. On the other hand, for the therapeutic effect to be maintained the drug should be given three times a day. Neither liver disease nor advanced age alters the half-life of oxazepam or lorazepam. Oxazepam or lorazepam may be preferable for treating acute anxiety disorder, when dose titration is required and hangover or day-time lethargy are particularly to be avoided. The slower absorption of oxazepam and lorazepam, however, somewhat detracts from their usefulness as hypnotics.

Triazolam is well absorbed, is rapidly metabolized, and has no active metabolites.

Flurazepam, though marketed as a hypnotic, has few

TABLE 26-3   Kinetic Classification of Some Benzodiazepines by Half-Life

Drug	Maximum Recommended Daily Dose (mg)	Time to Peak Effect (hr)	Half-Life (hr)	Therapeutic Indications	Active Metabolites (half-life in hr)
Long half-life, rapid pro-drug conversion					
Chlorazepate*	60	1–2	1	Anxiety	DM diazepam (30–200)
Flurazepam*	30	1	1.5	Insomnia	Desalkylflurazepam (40–250)
Slow pro-drug conversion					
Chlordiazepoxide*	100	2–4	130	Anxiety	DM diazepam (30–200)
Diazepam*	40	1–2	20–100	Anxiety	DM diazepam (30–200) Oxazepam (5–15)
Flunitrazepam*	0.5–1.0	1–2	2	Insomnia	DM diazepam (30–200)
Prazepam*	60	3	3	Anxiety	DM diazepam (30–200)
Intermediate half-life					
Alprazolam	3	1–2	6–20	Anxiety/ Depression	
Lorazepam	6	1–6	10–20	Anxiety	
Nitrazepam	10	2	15–40	Insomnia	
Oxazepam	120	1–4	5–15	Anxiety	
Temazepam	30	0.8–1.4	10–20	Insomnia	
Short half-life					
Brotizolam	0.125–0.5	1–2	2–7	Insomnia	
Midazolam	7.5–15	0.25–0.5	1.5–5	Sedation	
Triazolam	0.5	1–2	1.5–5	Insomnia	

* Biotransformation results in desmethyl (DM) derivative, which has long half-life as indicated.

properties to qualify it as such. The cumulation of the slowly eliminated active metabolite, desalkylflurazepam, over 7–10 days results in slow onset of the hypnotic effect and causes drowsiness as a side effect during long-term use. Older patients are particularly likely to experience toxic effects because they are more sensitive to various psychoactive drugs and may have altered biotransformation of the drug.

Distribution

Benzodiazepines are distributed widely in the body; tissue concentrations in brain, liver, and spleen exceed those of unbound drug in the serum. Diazepam is more lipophilic than chlordiazepoxide and has a larger apparent volume of distribution in the body. The volume of distribution of benzodiazepines correlates well with *in vitro* measures of lipid solubility; hence, the volumes of distribution of chlordiazepoxide and diazepam are larger in females than in males and in elderly patients (over 70 years of age) than in younger ones. The larger volume of distribution accounts in part for the prolonged half-life in older patients (*see* Chapters 5 and 69). Chlor-

diazepoxide, diazepam, and desmethyldiazepam enter the CNS at rates proportional to their lipid solubility, while steady-state concentrations in cerebrospinal fluid are determined by the degree of serum protein binding of the drugs. Chlordiazepoxide and diazepam cross the placenta and appear in small amounts in breast milk.

Pharmacologic Actions and Therapeutic Uses

Behavioral Effects

Antianxiety action. The effects of the benzodiazepines in the relief of anxiety can be demonstrated readily in experimental animals. In conflict punishment procedures (*see* Chapter 66), benzodiazepines greatly reduce the suppressive effects of punishment. In such models, animals will continue to seek food or water despite the concurrent presence of electrical shock. While other drugs such as barbiturates may show similar effects, these actions with benzodiazepines occur without sedation or alteration of other animal behaviors. The majority of the benzodiazepines have been approved for use in acute anxiety disorders. Although most of these drugs are also used for chronic anxiety states, the efficacy of these compounds decreases somewhat after a few weeks and, thus, there is less indication for the drugs to be used for chronic anxiety.

These antianxiety drugs have no antidepressant and no antischizophrenic (neuroleptic) actions. Recently alprazolam has been shown to have some activity in depression.

No benzodiazepine has been shown to be superior in efficacy to chlordiazepoxide for the treatment of acute anxiety disorder or chronic anxiety states.

Anticonvulsant activity. Benzodiazepines are potent anticonvulsants (*see* the earlier section on GABA-receptor/Cl⁻-ionophore complex for the mechanism; *see also* Chapter 21) and have been shown to prevent or abolish seizures in various animal models of epilepsy. These drugs are very potent in preventing pentylenetetrazole-induced seizures, but are less potent in electroshock-induced seizures. Although very effective in the treatment of status epilepticus (*e.g.*, with diazepam), absence attacks, and other types of childhood seizures (*e.g.*, with clonazepam), oral benzodiazepines have only a limited role in the long-term management of seizure disorders because of the development of tolerance to their anticonvulsant effect.

Alcohol withdrawal. Most benzodiazepines are effective in the treatment of alcohol withdrawal syndrome (*see* Chapter 25). The kinetic properties of longer-acting benzodiazepines, such as chlordiazepoxide or diazepam, seem to result in more effective treatment of the alcohol withdrawal syndrome than shorter-acting benzodiazepines can provide.

Muscle relaxant effects. Benzodiazepines reduce elevated skeletal muscle tone and are effective in various neuromuscular disorders including cerebral palsy, tetanus, and "stiff-man syndrome." They are frequently used in a variety of problems for which the efficacy of benzodiazepines is unproven, such as backache and muscle trauma.

Sedation. The wide margin of safety of benzodiazepines permits their use in a variety of clinical situations in which the objective is simply to produce sedation or amnesia (*e.g.*, endoscopy, bronchoscopy, preanaesthetic sedation and anaesthesia induction, cardioversion, and delivery). In these situations diazepam is the most commonly used benzodiazepine and is given intravenously; it is at least as effective as and safer than barbiturates but is probably not superior to other parenterally administered benzodiazepines. Midazolam, a benzodiazepine with very rapid elimination, is available for induction of anaesthesia or acute sedation.

These drugs should be chosen with consideration of the desired duration of action (*see* Table 26–3).

Insomnia. Insomnia is best classified under three headings—transient, short-term, and long-term (chronic).

Transient insomnia occurs in those who normally sleep well and is usually due to an alteration in the conditions which surround sleep, *e.g.*, noise, shiftwork, or intercontinental travel. A hypnotic may or may not be needed.

Short-term insomnia is usually related to an emotional problem or to a serious medical illness. It may last a few weeks and may recur. Good management is needed to avoid long-term problems. A hypnotic is likely to be useful, but it should not be prescribed for more than three weeks, preferably for only a week or so. Intermittent use is desirable, with skipping of some nightly doses after the first few nights of good sleep.

There is considerable controversy over the use of hypnotics in chronic insomnia. One-third to one-half of all patients with chronic insomnia have an underlying psychiatric disorder, most commonly depression, that will require specific treatment. Another group of patients that suffer from chronic insomnia includes those who abuse drugs or alcohol. Still another group who suffer chronic insomnia are those patients with specific sleep disorders, such as sleep apnea, in whom hypnotics would be absolutely contraindicated.

Finally, there is a large group of patients with chronic insomnia in whom no apparent cause can be established. For this group of patients the recommended treatment consists of exercise, controlled curtailment of sleep, reduction in stress, restriction of caffeine and alcohol, and intermittent use of a hypnotic for one night in three, for a one-month period. If, after a month, such treatment is unsuccessful, a trial of a sedative antidepressant for another month is proposed.

Responsiveness

Dose requirements for patients vary greatly. For example, the diazepam concentration required to produce sufficient sedation and relaxation to permit passage of a gastroscope varies 22-fold; hence, there must be such differences in receptor sensitivity that it is virtually impossible to predict a clinical response at a particular dose in a particular patient. Sensitivity to benzodiazepines increases with age and liver disease, and decreases with smoking and recent use of benzodiazepines, alcohol, or other drugs that produce cross-tolerance to benzodiazepines.

As a rule of thumb the initial dose of benzodiazepine should be reduced by 50% in the elderly (>65 years), patients with liver disease, or patients concurrently receiving other CNS depressants.

Relation of Drug Concentration and Effect

Single measurements of the concentration of chlordiazepoxide or diazepam in whole blood or plasma do not correlate closely with the therapeutic or toxic effects because of the presence of active metabolites, the variation between patients in the concentration of free drug, the development of tolerance, and the inaccurate quantitation of the response. These drugs are slowly eliminated from the body; hence metabolites may be detected in plasma or urine for weeks after administration of a single dose, even though clinically significant effects are no longer present.

Tolerance, Dependence, and Withdrawal

Acute, subacute, and chronic tolerance to benzodiazepines have been demonstrated in studies with animals and humans (*see also* Chapter 67). During long-term administration, tolerance commonly manifests itself as a decrease in side effects or a need to increase the dose to induce sleep or maintain symptomatic improvement.

Tolerance to benzodiazepines appears to be primarily functional in nature. Tolerance to the sedative, anticonvulsant, and muscle relaxant effects of benzodiazepines has been shown. There appears to be some disagreement concerning development of tolerance to their anxiolytic effects. Physical dependence may develop in patients taking large amounts of diazepam (more than 40 mg/day) or chlordiazepoxide (more than 200 mg/day), and the consequent signs and symptoms of withdrawal may be seen when use of the drug is stopped. However, elimination of diazepam and chlordiazepoxide (and their metabolites) is slow enough that the withdrawal reaction is often mild. When it occurs, anxiety, hand tremor, insomnia, disorders of perception, and, rarely, seizures are the clinical features. More rapidly eliminated benzodiazepines may produce a more severe clinical withdrawal syndrome. The reason for this is that, after termination of treatment with a short-acting benzodiazepine, the tissue levels of drug decline rapidly, "uncovering" the causing rapid onset of the withdrawal reaction before there has been any return toward normal sensitivity. In contrast, sudden abstinence from a long-acting benzodiazepine results in a delayed and attenuated withdrawal reaction because tissue levels of benzodiazepine decline slowly and the receptors have more chance to return to a normal state (this is equivalent to "tapering"). Just as with opiates, the precipitated withdrawal reaction induced with a benzodiazepine antagonist may not be identical to the withdrawal reaction resulting from cessation of drug administration.

Psychologic dependence can occur at any dose, and the resultant signs and symptoms are difficult to distinguish from those of withdrawal reaction and from anxiety. Patients who have taken therapeutic doses of benzodiazepines for a long time frequently experience severe anxiety when an attempt is made to discontinue the drug. Recent reports indicate that some of these patients, in fact, are experiencing drug withdrawal effects. The risk of physical dependence can be minimized by avoiding long-term (more than 6 weeks) therapy. For most conditions for which efficacy of benzodiazepine therapy has been proven, only 2–4 weeks of therapy is required, and such short-term therapy will ordinarily not give rise to clinically important withdrawal symptoms. Sometimes the diagnosis is not clear and a trial of therapy with a benzodiazepine is reasonable. At the commencement of such a trial, the desired therapeutic goal and the duration of therapy should be specified.

Drug Interactions

Benzodiazepines interact with many psychoactive drugs. The combination of ethyl alcohol and benzodiazepines can impair driving skills to a degree greater than that caused by the same amount of either drug alone. This fact is of significant forensic importance and physicians should warn their patients about the hazards of drinking alcohol when they are taking benzodiazepines. Interactions among benzodiazepines, analgesics, antihistamines, phenothiazines, and tricyclic antidepressants are also well documented. A list of such proven interactions is not helpful, and patients must always be cautioned when taking other psychoactive agents together with benzodiazepines, against driving a car or engaging in other activities in which there is risk to themselves or others.

Benzodiazepines do not induce the synthesis of drug-biotransforming enzymes, have less risk of interaction with coumarin anticoagulants than barbiturates do, and are safer to use in combination with anticoagulants, antiarrhythmics, antineoplastic agents, and antiepileptic drugs, with which metabolic interactions are most common during barbiturate therapy.

Adverse Reactions

Orally administered benzodiazepines cause side effects, which are not life-threatening, in less than 10% of hospitalized patients who receive them. The common adverse effects of benzodiazepines are direct extensions of their pharmacologic actions, namely drowsiness, lethargy, and rarely coma. However, paradoxical excitation may on occasion be observed. Benzodiazepines may interfere with memory acquisition, consolidation, and recall; hence, using them in situations such as studying for examinations requires a balancing of benefits and risks. Such use is not advised.

The frequency of side effects of chlordiazepoxide and diazepam therapy increases with age, dose, duration of therapy, and presence of liver disease and hypoalbuminemia.

Hematologic, renal, and hepatic toxicity have seldom been reported for benzodiazepines. Various unusual responses have been observed, including nightmares, paradoxical delirium and confusion, depression, aggression, and hostile behavior. Rarely patients experience a dry mouth, a metallic taste, or headaches. Awareness of the sometimes bizarre effects of these drugs is important.

Uncommon but important acute adverse effects after **intravenous** administration include respiratory or cardiac arrest or both, hypotension, and phlebitis at the site of injection. Life-threatening adverse reactions occur with a frequency of 1.7% after rapid intravenous administration of diazepam. Patients particularly at risk often have coexisting severe pulmonary or cardiac disease or have concurrently received cardiorespiratory-depressant medications. Whenever possible and practical, the rate of injection should be less than 12.5 mg/min for chlordiazepoxide and less than 2.5 mg/min for diazepam. Phlebitis is most common after repeated injections at the same site and can be minimized by flushing the vein with 50 mL of saline after each injection.

Since the administration of benzodiazepines to pregnant women has not been proven to be safe for the fetus, these drugs should be prescribed in such cases only when their use is mandatory, and then for the shortest time possible.

An **overdose** of benzodiazepines alone is never fatal. On the basis of this wide margin of safety alone, benzodiazepines should replace barbiturates. However, since 35% of drug overdoses involve more than one drug, combinations of benzodiazepines and more dangerous drugs, such as alcohol, are common and may cause death.

BARBITURATES

The uses of barbiturates are very limited in modern therapeutics. These drugs have largely been replaced by the benzodiazepines that are, on balance, safer.

Chemical Structure

A barbiturate results from the condensation of malonic acid and urea, as shown in Figure 26–5. Barbituric acid itself has no sedative effect, but if the two hydrogen atoms on C-5 are replaced by ethyl (C_2H_5)

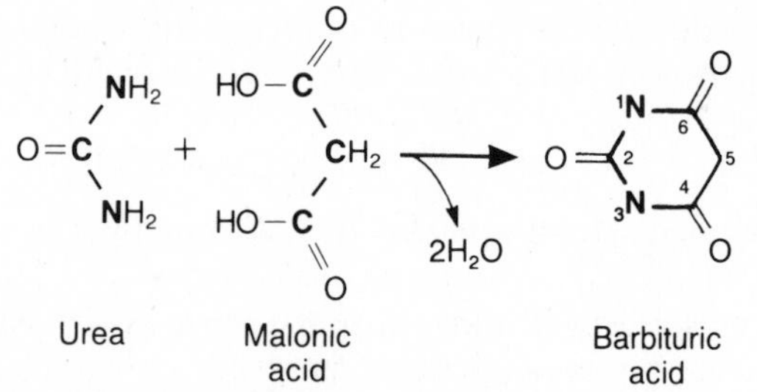

Figure 26–5 Schematic representation of the production of barbituric acid, the parent compound of barbiturates.

or larger hydrocarbon groups, the resulting products are pharmacologically active. Drugs in which the oxygen on C-2 is replaced by sulphur are called thiobarbiturates; e.g., the thio equivalent of pentobarbital is called thiopental. Such compounds are extremely rapid- and short-acting when injected intravenously, and they are used exclusively in this way as general anaesthetics (see Chapter 23). There are differences in British and U.S. pharmacopoeial nomenclature for these drugs, the British names ending in "-itone," the American in "-ital."

Pharmacokinetics

Factors determining speed of onset and duration of barbiturate action include the following.

Lipid Solubility

In general, the speed of onset and duration of action both depend on the relative lipid solubility, as reflected by the membrane/water partition coefficient. As Table 26–4 indicates, the barbiturate derivatives with higher lipid solubility have a more rapid onset but a shorter duration of action. Thiopental and other ultrashort-acting barbiturates are very highly lipid-soluble and enter the brain very quickly, producing anaesthesia almost instantaneously. However, within a few

TABLE 26–4 Characteristics of Some Barbiturates

C-5 Substituents	Nonproprietary Name	Duration (half-life)	Membrane/Buffer Partition Coefficient ($P_{m/b}$)
Phenyl and ethyl	Phenobarbital	Long (35–150 hr)	9
Isopentyl and ethyl	Amobarbital	Intermediate (8–42 hr)	11
Methylbutyl and ethyl	Pentobarbital	Intermediate (15–48 hr)	11
Methyl and cyclohexenyl	Hexobarbital	Ultrashort (2.7–7 hr)	36

minutes they get widely distributed throughout the body, with the result that the concentration in brain decreases and, therefore, central depression decreases (*see* Chapter 23 and Fig. 26–6).

Barbiturates with a more prolonged duration of action (pentobarbital and secobarbital) enter the brain less readily than thiopental and become widely distributed in the body before peak concentration is achieved in the central nervous system. Therefore extensive redistribution of the drugs from the brain to other tissues is obviated. Recovery from pentobarbital and secobarbital, therefore, depends more on biotransformation of the drug than on redistribution.

Ionization

Barbiturates are weak acids. For some, the pK_a is such that urinary excretion can be increased by alkalinization of the urine. This applies, for example, to phenobarbital, which has a pK_a of 7.2 (*see* Chapter 7).

Biotransformation

Most barbiturates are biotransformed extensively, by the drug hydroxylating system located in the smooth endoplasmic reticulum, to inactive metabolites (*see* Chapter 4, *Drug Biotransformation*). Some barbiturates are biotransformed slowly. In humans, about 20% of a sedative dose of phenobarbital is converted to *p*-hydroxyphenobarbital and excreted in the urine over a 5-day period; 15–20% is eliminated unchanged in the same period. The mean plasma half-life of unchanged phenobarbital is about 86 hours. With barbital, up to 90% is eliminated unchanged.

Recently, other pathways of barbiturate metabolism have been discovered, including N-glucosylation. Oriental populations show much more glucosylation relative to hydroxylation of barbiturates than occidental populations do. However, the clinical significance of this difference is not yet clear, and it does not affect the overall elimination half-life of the drug.

Clinical Uses

There are few recommended uses of barbiturates today. Some barbiturates (*e.g.*, phenobarbital) are anticonvulsants and may be employed clinically to reduce the frequency and severity of seizures in epileptics (*see* Chapter 21).

Other uses are in anaesthesia induction (*e.g.*, thiopental) referred to above and in Chapter 23, in special neuropsychiatric investigations, and to reduce cerebral edema (potentially effective).

Barbiturates are no longer considered appropriate for the treatment of anxiety or insomnia. Though they are still used to some extent as hypnotics, they have largely been replaced for this purpose by short-acting benzodiazepines.

Adverse Effects of Barbiturates

1. In very low doses, instead of sedation the barbiturates may occasionally produce uncontrolled **hyperactivity of the cortex**. The patient may be euphoric, excited, restless, agitated, or violent. This resembles early alcohol intoxication, or the early stage of ether anaesthesia (*see* Chapter 23). In chronic users who have developed some tolerance, an otherwise normal hypnotic dose may produce these effects.

2. With large doses of barbiturate, depression may persist for longer than intended, and the patient feels **groggy and "doped"** the next day. This is the result of the relatively long half-lives of the drugs used as hypnotics (*e.g.*, pentobarbital and secobarbital) with continuation of drug action into the following day.

3. Chronic use of barbiturates, especially as day-time sedatives in repeated doses, may lead to **tolerance**, **dependence**, and the risk of a **withdrawal syndrome**. Tolerance is in part metabolic, by induction of the drug-biotransforming enzyme system contained in the hepatic smooth endoplasmic reticulum. To be effective as an inducer, the drug must be present for a suffi-

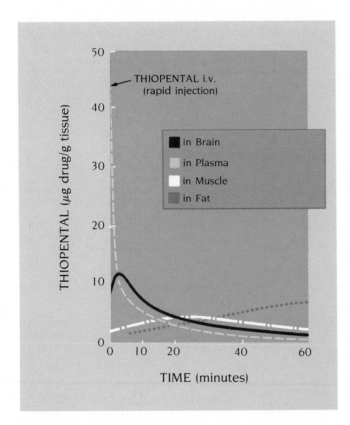

Figure 26–6 Calculated time courses of thiopental concentration in human tissues.

ciently long uninterrupted period. Therefore, the long-acting (*i.e.*, slowly eliminated) barbiturates such as barbital and phenobarbital are the best inducers of the biotransformation of other drugs; however, they do not induce their own biotransformation. Short-acting barbiturates act as inducers only if repeated doses are given at short intervals so as to maintain an appreciable blood level for some time. When induction does occur, drug metabolism can be greatly speeded up, not only for most barbiturates themselves but also for a whole range of other drugs (*see* Chapter 4, *Drug Biotransformation*).

The other major component of tolerance is an adaptive change in the nervous system itself, which compensates for the drug effect by an increase in neuronal excitability. When the drug is withdrawn, a barbiturate abstinence syndrome occurs that is very similar to an alcohol withdrawal syndrome in an alcoholic patient (*see* Chapters 25 and 67).

4. In **congenital porphyria**, barbiturates can precipitate or aggravate attacks by increasing the production of porphyrins in the liver.

5. With severe **overdose**, depression extends to the hypothalamus and the medullary centres for cardiovascular and respiratory control. Respiration is slow and shallow.

6. **Death from overdose**: Barbiturates are encountered in about 12% of acute drug ingestions (toxic overdoses). Alone or in combination with other drugs such as alcohol they can cause death, frequently due to respiratory failure. **Treatment of overdose** consists of support of cardiovascular and respiratory function, removal of drug by gastric lavage, and occasionally forced diuresis and alkalinization of the urine (*see* Chapter 72).

OTHER NONBARBITURATE HYPNOTICS AND SEDATIVES

Table 26–1 lists several other classes of hypnotic drugs, including some that are related to alcohols or

to acetaldehyde (paraldehyde), or that are chemical analogs of barbiturates (methyprylon, glutethimide). All of these drugs are still available commercially, and are still described in many textbooks of pharmacology and therapeutics. However, they now account for only a very small fraction of the total amount of hypnotics prescribed each year, and the fraction is decreasing steadily. Like the barbiturates, they have largely been replaced by the benzodiazepines, which have greater efficacy, less abuse potential and dependence liability, and a wider margin of safety. Therefore these older drugs are not described in detail in the present edition of this textbook.

SUGGESTED READING

Bowery NG, ed. Actions and interactions of GABA and benzodiazepines. New York: Raven Press, 1984.

Busto U, Sellers EM, Naranjo CA, *et al.* Withdrawal reaction after long-term therapeutic use of benzodiazepines. N Engl J Med 1986; 315:854–859.

Greenblatt DJ, Shader RI. Pharmacokinetics of antianxiety agents. In: Meltzer HY, ed. Psychopharmacology: the third generation of progress. New York: Raven Press, 1987: 1377–1386.

Griffiths RR, Sannerud CA. Abuse of and dependence on benzodiazepines and other anxiolytic/sedative drugs. Ibid, 1987:1535–1541.

Hommer DW, Skolnick P, Paul SM. The benzodiazepine/GABA receptor complex and anxiety. Ibid, 1987:977–983.

Nicholson AN. Hypnotics: their place in therapeutics. Drugs 1986;31:164–176.

Smith DE, Wesson DR, eds. The benzodiazepines: current standards for medical practice. Lancaster, England: MTP Press, 1985.

Chapter 27

NEUROLEPTICS (ANTIPSYCHOTICS)

P. Seeman

In 1949, Laborit, a surgeon in Paris, was testing various antihistamine drugs, such as promethazine, to prevent postoperative surgical shock. He noted that these drugs calmed the patients postoperatively, producing almost a euphoric indifference in the patient. He felt that this was not sedation, but was a form of "autonomic stabilization." In 1950, Charpentier synthesized the chemically related compound chlorpromazine. When used in anaesthesia, this drug reduced the amount of surgical anaesthetic required, as well as reducing the patient's anxiety. Laborit noted a resemblance between the deconditioning effect of chlorpromazine and Pavlovian deconditioning therapy in psychiatry. He urged psychiatrists to test the drug because of its strong central actions, and the first psychotic patient was treated in January 1952 with great success.

Since the introduction of these drugs (now called "neuroleptics") in 1952 by Laborit, psychiatric wards have been miraculously transformed. Rarely does one see patients who are unkempt, violent, incontinent, catatonic, or actively hallucinating. The neuroleptics improve 95% of such acutely ill psychotic patients.

Neuroleptics keep psychotic patients out of hospital and reduce symptoms (Figs. 27–1 and 27–2). They do not eliminate the fundamental disorder of thinking, nor do they reverse all social or work-related problems.

MECHANISMS OF NEUROLEPTIC ACTIONS

Classification of Neuroleptic Agents

All of the neuroleptics in current clinical use are either phenothiazines or butyrophenones, or derivatives of these. The molecular formulae of chlorpromazine (a

phenothiazine) and haloperidol (a butyrophenone) are shown in Figure 27–3. Incorporation of the phenothiazine sidechain $-N(CH_3)_2$ into a ring structure and replacement of the Cl on the benzene nucleus by other groups give rise to a variety of other phenothiazines including thioridazine, trifluoperazine, and fluphenazine. Replacement of the N in the phenothiazine nucleus, by a C doubly-bonded to the side chain, yields thioxanthene derivatives such as thiothixene. Similar substitu-

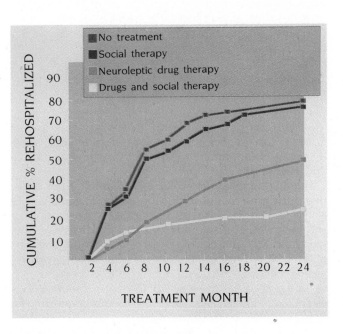

Figure 27–1 Rehospitalization rates of schizophrenic patients. After being discharged from hospital after a 2-month stay, patients taking neuroleptic medication were much less likely to be rehospitalized. (Adapted from Hogarty GE *et al.*, Arch Gen Psychiatr 1974.)

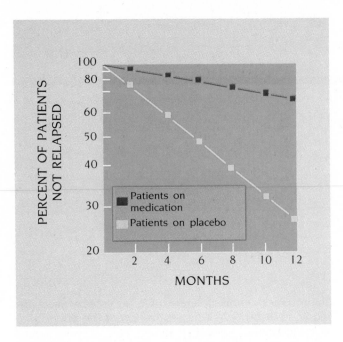

Figure 27-2 Effect of neuroleptic medication on relapse rate of schizophrenic patients. (Adapted from Davis JM, Arch Gen Psychiatr 1976.)

tions in the haloperidol structure give rise to a variety of derivatives including droperidol, penfluridol, spiperone, fluspirilene, and pimozide. Domperidone, another derivative of the butyrophenones, is not a neuroleptic because it is too polar to enter the brain readily.

Molecular Mechanism of Action

All present-day neuroleptic drugs, at their lowest doses or lowest concentrations that elicit effects, selectively act on dopamine receptors throughout the brain and the body.

The fundamental molecular explanation for the selective dopamine receptor-blocking action of neuroleptics is that all these drugs can adopt a conformation or shape in which certain portions and dimensions of the molecule are identical to the corresponding features of dopamine. For example, haloperidol and chlorpromazine are neuroleptics with very different structure; yet, these neuroleptics overlap with the dopamine molecule, as shown in Figure 27-3, and thus readily compete with dopamine for its receptor sites.

This dopamine-receptor explanation of neuroleptic action is consistent with the fact that reserpine, which depletes the brain of dopamine and noradrenaline* (see Chapter 18), also has a neuroleptic effect, though it is no longer used clinically for this purpose.

Because of this fundamental dopamine receptor-blocking action of neuroleptics, the neuroleptics also

* norepinephrine

block the actions of other dopamine-type agonist drugs such as apomorphine or bromocriptine. Figure 27-4 indicates how these molecules overlap with dopamine.

Cell Mechanisms of Neuroleptic Actions

The main actions, as well as the side effects, of the neuroleptics are compatible with the hypothesis that these drugs block dopaminergic transmission in the central nervous system. Dopamine-containing neurons include:

- nigro-caudate and nigro-putamen fibres;
- nigro-cortical fibres;
- arcuate neurons in hypothalamus;

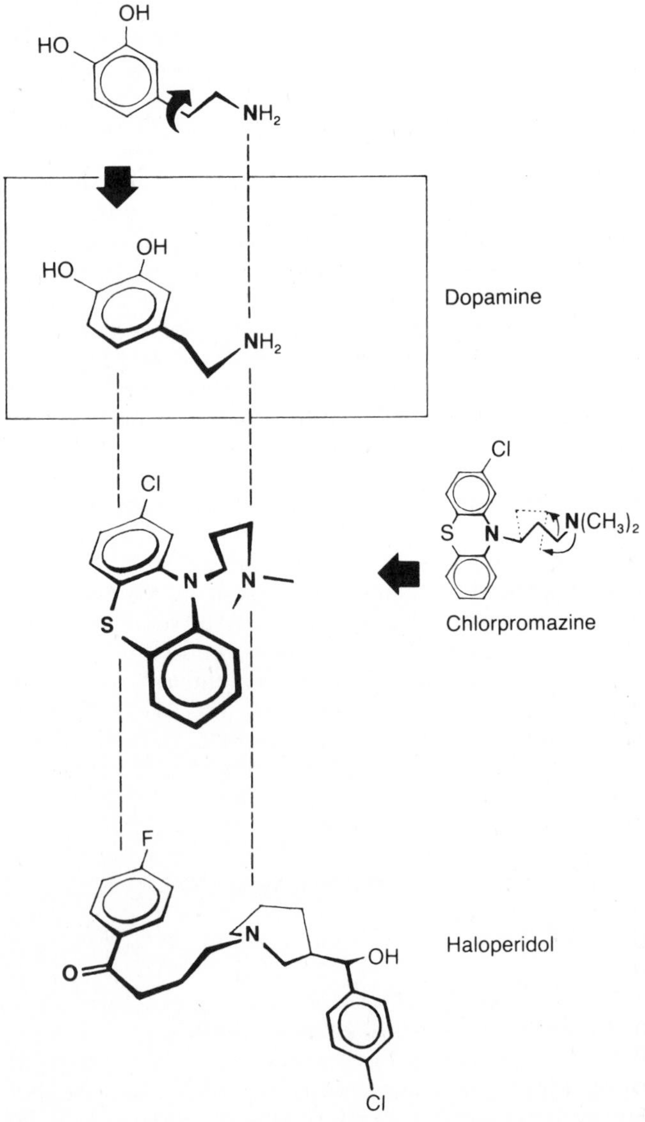

Figure 27-3 Structural overlap (benzene rings and nitrogen atoms; dotted lines) of dopamine and neuroleptics.

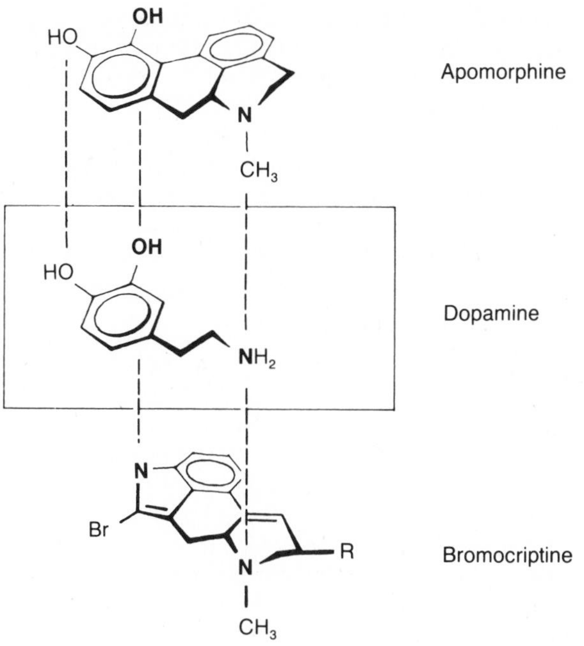

Apomorphine

Dopamine

Bromocriptine

Figure 27–4 Structural fit of dopamine and anti-Parkinson drugs.

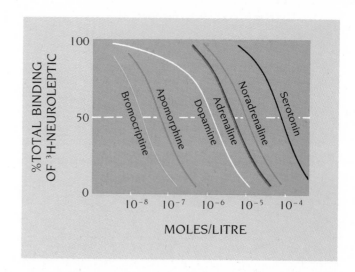

Figure 27–5 Displacement curves showing the comparative potencies of various neurotransmitters and related compounds in displacing ^{3}H-haloperidol from its binding sites on brain membranes.

- mesolimbic fibres;
- neurons in the floor of the IVth ventricle (near the vomiting centre).

The blockade of receptors acted on by each of these neurons will lead to different effects and side effects (*see* the relevant sections on adverse effects and side effects). The antipsychotic action is thought to stem from the effect on the cortical and limbic dopaminergic fibres, but there is no direct evidence of this. The main evidence for the antidopaminergic action of neuroleptics is as follows.

1. Of all the endogenous neurotransmitters, dopamine is the most effective in inhibiting the specific binding of ^{3}H-neuroleptics to dopamine-containing tissues in the brain (Fig. 27–5 and Table 27–1). Figure 27–5 shows that the IC_{50} values (*i.e.*, the concentrations of drugs that inhibit the binding of radioactive ligands by 50%) for blockade of ^{3}H-haloperidol binding are as listed in Table 27–1.

2. Neuroleptics block the psychotomimetic actions of amphetamine, which are thought to be caused by the release of dopamine from the vesicles in the nerve terminal.

3. Neuroleptics block the peripheral and central actions of L-dopa, apomorphine, and bromocriptine. (For example, motor dyskinesias, which can be caused by L-dopa, are suppressed by neuroleptic drugs.) Furthermore, the actions of apomorphine, such as apomorphine-induced stereotyped behavior, are all blocked by neuroleptic drugs.

4. Low doses of neuroleptics selectively accelerate the turnover of dopamine in the caudate nucleus and putamen.

5. The clinical side effects of neuroleptics simulate such "hypodopaminergic" syndromes as parkinsonism, breast-swelling and galactorrhea.

Cellular Events in Neuroleptic Action

1. Neuroleptics selectively block the D_2 type of dopamine receptors in brain and pituitary (Fig. 27–6). There are at least two types of dopamine receptors (Table 27–2). The D_1 receptor is defined as that which stimulates the formation of cyclic AMP (cAMP). Since the D_1 receptors can be blocked only by high (*i.e.*, micromolar) concentrations of neuroleptics, they are not blocked at ordinary doses that patients take.

TABLE 27–1 IC_{50} Values for Various Transmitters and Analogs in the Displacement of ^{3}H-Haloperidol from Brain Membranes

	IC_{50} (nM)
Dopamine (high state)	10
Bromocriptine	20
Apomorphine	50
Dopamine (low state)	2000
(−)-Adrenaline*	5000
(−)-Noradrenaline	10,000
Serotonin	100,000

* epinephrine

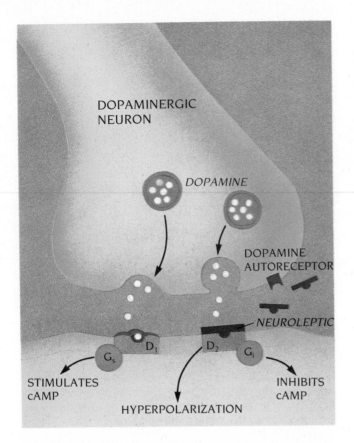

Figure 27–6 Dopamine receptor block by neuroleptics. Hyperpolarization, and inhibition of cAMP synthesis, are effects of D_2 receptor activation by dopamine, and are blocked by the neuroleptics. D = dopamine receptors; G = G-proteins.

The D_2 type, on the other hand, is defined as the dopamine receptor that is sensitive to nanomolar concentrations of neuroleptics.

There are important clinical implications to the fact that the D_2 receptor exists in two states: a high-affinity state (termed D_{2high}), which is very sensitive to nanomolar concentrations of dopamine; and a low-affinity state, which is only affected by micromolar concentrations of dopamine. Both states are readily

blocked by nanomolar concentrations of neuroleptics. The D_2 receptor interferes with the synthesis of cAMP in both brain and pituitary. The D_2 receptor hyperpolarizes the cell. There is as yet no known functional correlate for the D_1 receptor site.

Of the two different states for the D_2 receptor, it is now clear that in the anterior pituitary gland the D_{2high} state is that which responds to bromocriptine or to the dopamine released by fibres from the median eminence of the brain. The D_{2low} state may be a desensitized form of the D_2 receptor.

2. Since dopamine generally inhibits the neuron, neuroleptics disinhibit the neuron. This eventually results in a feedback activation of the presynaptic dopamine neuron, such that the presynaptic cell fires more frequently (*i.e.*, trying to overcome the postsynaptic blocking action of the neuroleptic).

3. Finally, the increased frequency of impulses activates tyrosine hydroxylase, which then synthesizes more dopamine; thus, dopamine turnover is increased by neuroleptics. In clinical practice this accelerated turnover of dopamine can be detected by measuring the amount of DOPAC released into the cerebrospinal fluid or into the plasma, and the amount of HVA released into the CSF (Fig. 27–7).

FUNCTIONAL EFFECTS OF THE NEUROLEPTIC DRUGS

Neurolepsis

The neuroleptics cause psychomotor slowing and affective indifference, these two features constituting the neuroleptic syndrome. As Delay and Deniker stated in 1952 about chlorpromazine:

"The apparent indifference or the slowing of responses to external stimuli, the diminution of initiative and of anxiety without a change in the state of waking and consciousness or of intellectual faculties constitute the psychological syndrome attributable to the drug."

Sedation is not essential for antipsychotic action, since

TABLE 27–2 Binding Properties of Dopamine Receptor Types

	D_1 Receptor	D_2 Receptor $D_{2high} \rightleftharpoons D_{2low}$		Autoreceptor
Sensitivity to Dopamine	μM	nM	μM	nM
Sensitivity to Neuroleptics	μM	nM		nM
Formation of cAMP	stimulates	interferes		?
^{3}H-Ligand	^{3}H-flupenthixol	^{3}H-haloperidol		?

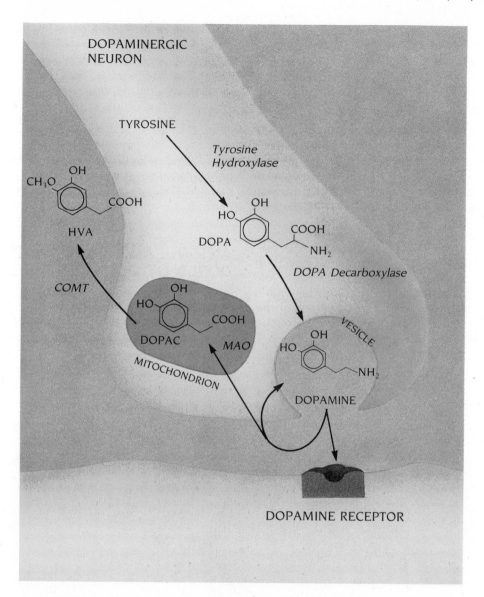

Figure 27–7   Metabolism of dopamine in the terminal of a dopamine neuron. DOPA = dihydroxyphenylalanine; DOPAC = dihydroxyphenylacetic acid; MAO = monoamine oxidase; COMT = catechol-O-methyl transferase; HVA = homovanillic acid.

the sedative effect of chlorpromazine is seldom seen with the butyrophenone neuroleptics.

The sedation by the phenothiazines differs from barbiturate or anaesthetic sedation in that there is minimal motor incoordination, and the patient may be easily aroused. The reason for calling the drugs "tranquilizers" is that they are calming and reduce agitation and hyperactivity without impairing wakefulness.

Neuroleptics selectively block or attenuate the response-eliciting properties of peripheral stimuli, thus abolishing conditioned responses. For example, the animal trained to avoid shock when a buzzer sounds, under neuroleptics ignores the warning buzz but escapes when it feels the shock applied. Thus, the condi-

tioned avoidance response is a good screening procedure for testing new tranquilizing drugs. (This applies also to anxiolytic drugs and to sedative-hypnotic drugs in certain dose ranges. Therefore, it is a screening procedure for tranquilization, but not specifically for neuroleptic action.)

Many of the original studies on neuroleptic action were done with chlorpromazine, the oldest, "classical" drug of this class. The following four sites of chlorpromazine action are thought to be the basis for induced "indifference" in the patient.

1.   Chlorpromazine reduces activity in the ascending reticular formation (reticular activating system) in the brain stem, so that external stimuli are less effective

in eliciting the normal arousal pattern (Fig. 27–8). (Note that this action is probably not dopaminergic and is not shared by the newer neuroleptics.)

2. Chlorpromazine also depresses the arousal response of the limbic system.

3. Chlorpromazine depresses the hypothalamus, as indicated by its ability to produce poikilothermia (i.e., hypothermia at low, and hyperthermia at high ambient temperature). This effect is useful in heart and brain surgery. Chlorpromazine action on the hypothalamus is also indicated by the fact that the drug stimulates the patient's appetite, so that many patients complain of markedly increased weight. Chlorpromazine also has an antipyretic effect.

4. The indifference to pain that some patients report ("Oh yes, doctor, that tumor pain is just as bad, but it doesn't bother me much since you started giving me those pills") can be explained on the basis that chlorpromazine affects dopamine neurons in the limbic regions (as well as acting on small interneurons in the reticular formation, which receives about 80% of the fibre input of the spino-thalamic tracts).

Anti-Nausea and Anti-Vomiting Action

The chemoreceptor trigger zone in the reticular formation of the medulla has D_2 receptors that are blocked by neuroleptics. The neuroleptics effectively reduce nausea produced by other drugs, pregnancy, radiation sickness, cancer, etc., but not the nausea secondary to bowel obstruction or to motion sickness. Only particular phenothiazines are effective in motion sickness (such as thiethylperazine). These compounds localize in high concentrations in the vestibular nucleus. The phenothiazines also suppress hiccups.

ANTI-DOPAMINERGIC ACTION OF LOW DOSES OF DOPAMINE-LIKE DRUGS

It has been known for many years that low doses of amphetamine, methylphenidate (Ritalin®), and apomorphine tend to cause a brief sedative-like, hypo-

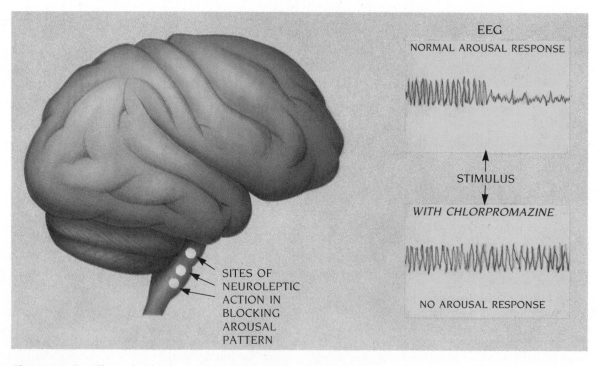

Figure 27–8 Effect of chlorpromazine on the EEG arousal response.

locomotor action. For example, methylphenidate or amphetamine is used clinically at between 10 mg and 40 mg per day for the childhood Attention Deficit Disorder (with hyperactivity) so that the child can pay attention to schoolwork. In addition, under certain circumstances, 50% of adults surprisingly feel drowsy within the first hour after taking 10–15 mg amphetamine, before psychomotor stimulation and euphoria begin.

These antidopaminergic actions stem from the fact that the dopamine-containing neuron itself has presynaptic dopamine receptors, which are extremely sensitive to dopamine (at about 10 nM). When these presynaptic dopamine receptors are stimulated by dopamine, they cause less dopamine to be released.

Thus, low doses of L-dopa, amphetamine, methylphenidate, or apomorphine may have a weak "neuroleptic-like" action. In fact, it is known that very low doses of L-dopa (about 300–600 mg/day) exert a significant antipsychotic or neuroleptic-like action. Higher doses of L-dopa, however, cause stimulation of the postsynaptic dopamine receptors and aggravate the schizophrenic symptoms.

PHARMACOKINETICS AND DOSAGE

Absorption, Biotransformation, and Elimination

The commonly used neuroleptics show quite variable bioavailability, despite their lipid solubility. This may indicate a large and variable first-pass effect in the gastrointestinal mucosa or the liver. Bioavailability (see Chapter 5) is increased as much as ten-fold by intramuscular injection. Most of these drugs show a high degree of serum protein binding, and also accumulate in tissues with a high blood supply, such as brain, lung, and kidney. They also cross the placenta into the fetal circulation quite readily.

The kinetics of elimination are complex, because these drugs follow multiple pathways of biotransformation, with different rate and affinity constants. Sulfoxidation, N-dealkylation, ring hydroxylation, and glucuronide conjugation are among the more important reactions, and each parent compound may have a large number of different metabolites, most of them inactive. Prolonged administration may cause some induction of hepatic microsomal enzymes, since the plasma concentrations of the drugs tend to fall gradually, despite a constant level of dosage. Excretion occurs into the urine (the more polar metabolites) and into the bile.

Most of these agents show plasma elimination half-lives in the range of 10–20 hours. However, if body fat has accumulated a large store of drug, traces of the drug and its metabolites may continue to appear in the urine for many weeks or months after the last dose. This may account for the observation that after chronic treatment of a psychotic patient there may be no relapse for months after the drug is stopped.

Onset of action is difficult to interpret. The typical physiologic effects (e.g., on circulation, arousal, emesis, thermoregulation) appear rapidly, as one would expect from the high lipid solubility, and they last for about 24 hours. In contrast, the antipsychotic effects usually take several weeks to occur, and may not be maximal until after several months of treatment. This suggests that the antipsychotic action is complex, and that the change in thinking and behavior is the end result of a long sequence of alterations that is started by the drug.

Therapeutic Concentrations of Neuroleptics

The therapeutic concentrations of three neuroleptics in plasma water are shown in Table 27–3. Figure 27–9 shows that the IC_{50} values (with respect to the inhibition of ^3H-haloperidol binding) for various neuroleptics all correlate with their clinical potencies. Equally important is the fact that the IC_{50} values happen to be similar to the therapeutic concentrations of neuroleptics in the plasma water (Table 27–3).

Lipid Solubility and Drug Dosage

A very important factor is that the association between a drug and its receptor is favored by a higher lipid solubility of the drug. This is true even if the receptor is on the outside surface of the cell membrane. In other words, drugs with high lipid solubilities generally have very low dissociation constants or K_D values. The reason for this is that once the lipid-soluble drug attaches to the receptor, the lipid solubility greatly reduces the dissociation of the drug from the receptor. That is, the drug "sticks" to the receptor. In terms of the oral dose in milligrams, therefore, the lipid-soluble drug is more potent.

Lipid solubility also plays a role in the absorption of orally administered drugs, and their ability to cross the blood–brain barrier. It is reasonable to expect that the more lipid-soluble neuroleptics permeate more

TABLE 27–3 Order of Magnitude for Therapeutic Concentrations of Neuroleptics

	Average Concentration in Plasma (ng/mL)	Bound to Plasma Proteins (%)	Concentration in Plasma Water (nM)
Chlorpromazine	250	95	30
Thioridazine	100	95	15
Haloperidol	5–10	92	1.5

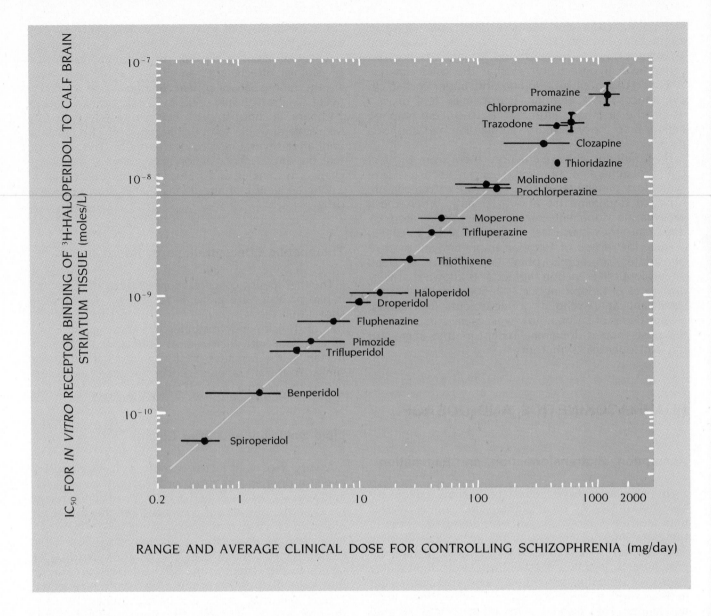

Figure 27–9 Relation between doses of neuroleptics to control schizophrenia and their respective receptor-binding potencies.

readily, reach their target tissues more rapidly, and thus may require lower doses for equi-neuroleptic action.

Domperidone (Fig. 27–10) is a special case since it is not sufficiently lipid-soluble to permeate across the blood–brain barrier into the brain. Thus, domperidone is not a "neuroleptic" because it cannot enter the brain. It does, however, block all the actions of dopamine and dopamine-like drugs on the peripheral tissues of the body. For example, when one is treating Parkinson's disease or galactorrhea with high doses of the dopamine receptor agonist bromocriptine (80 or 90 mg/day p.o.), there are undesirable side effects on the dopamine-sensitive tissues (vasodilatation, flushing, or hypotension). These side effects of bromocriptine are readily blocked by domperidone, so that the dosage

of bromocriptine can be doubled without incurring side effects due either to bromocriptine or to the usual central actions seen with typical neuroleptics.

Depot Injections of Neuroleptics

Fluphenazine has an alcohol substituent (− OH) attached to the end of the molecule, so that an ester can be formed by linking it to such fatty acids as enanthic or decanoic acid. When injected intramuscularly, the fatty esters (Fig. 27–11) remain as an oil drop within the muscle tissue, diffusing out slowly because the fluphenazine ester is poorly soluble in the tissue

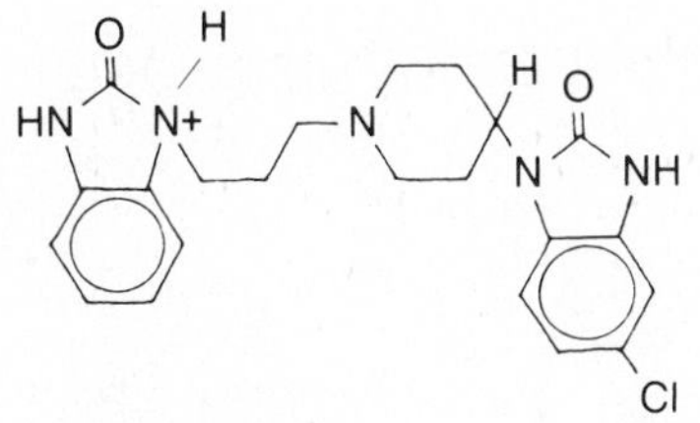

Figure 27–10 Domperidone, a peripheral dopamine receptor blocker, is a positively charged molecule and does not readily enter the brain.

and plasma water. When the fluphenazine ester does diffuse into plasma, the plasma esterases immediately split off the fatty acid, freeing the fluphenazine to act directly on the brain. Note that decanoic acid contains 10 carbon atoms and so is much more lipid-soluble than enanthic acid, which contains only seven carbon atoms; thus, a single injection of the enanthate lasts for only about 2 weeks while the decanoate lasts for 3 weeks.

ADVERSE EFFECTS OF NEUROLEPTICS

Side effects or adverse effects of neuroleptic medication occur in practically all of the patients treated with these drugs. In about 10–20% of patients these side effects are minimal. In the remaining 80% of patients the side effects are sufficiently significant that they should be watched and treated if necessary. Some of these effects (neuroleptic-induced parkinsonism, neuroleptic dyskinesias and dystonias, and neuroleptic-induced akathisia) appear within days or weeks of initiation of therapy, others (*e.g.*, tardive dyskinesia) require months or years to develop.

Neuroleptic-Induced Parkinsonism

In 75–80% of patients the neuroleptics cause extrapyramidal signs that mimic Parkinson's disease (Fig. 27–12). These signs include the following.

Akinesia. The patient has shorter steps, reduced arm swing, and cramped handwriting. The patient has difficulty initiating motion, such as slightly more difficulty in getting up from a chair.

Rigidity. The patient will complain of ''feeling stiff.'' Often the extent of ''cogwheel rigidity'' may be minimal, but the patient still finds the feeling to be restricting.

Tremor. This tremor is similar to the ''pill-rolling'' tremor seen in Parkinson's disease.

A rare but very severe (and sometimes fatal) form of parkinsonism, accompanied by marked autonomic disturbances, stupor, and myoglobinemia, is called **neuroleptic malignant syndrome**.

Neuroleptic Dyskinesias and Dystonias

Acute dyskinesia may set in within 1–3 days of neuroleptic therapy and consists of involuntary motions of the lips, jaw, and tongue; the patient may grimace, chew, or have difficulty speaking.

Acute dystonias consist of twisting motion of the neck, the pelvis, and of the eyes (oculogyric crises).

Neuroleptic-Induced Akathisia

Akathisia or restlessness is a common side effect of neuroleptic therapy. Despite the fact that the patient is feeling rigid or stiff and has difficulty initiating motion, there is a tremendous urge to keep walking and moving around.

Mechanism and Treatment of Neuroleptic-Induced Parkinsonism, Dystonias, and Akathisia

As shown in Figure 27–12, and discussed in greater detail in Chapter 20, there is normally a balance between the cholinergic and dopaminergic inputs into the neurons in the striatum (caudate and putamen). When a neuroleptic blocks the dopamine receptors, then the cholinergic influence becomes relatively excessive. This

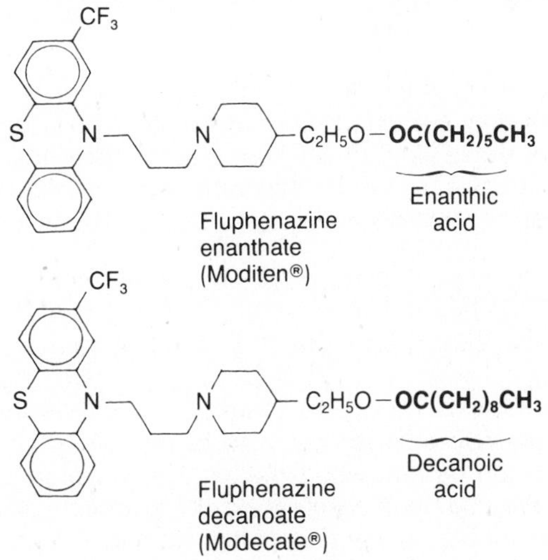

Figure 27–11 Fluphenazine enanthate (Moditen®) is slightly less lipid-soluble and so is injected i.m. (25 mg) once every 2 weeks. The more lipid-soluble decanoate ester needs to be injected only once every 3 weeks on the average.

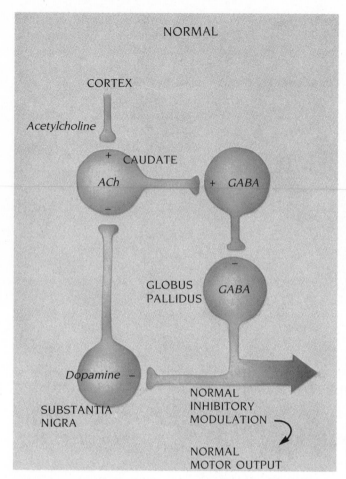

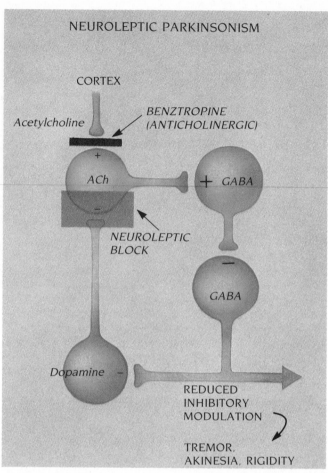

Figure 27-12 Production by neuroleptics of extrapyramidal signs resembling those of parkinsonism. (The exact relationships in the caudate are not yet fully elucidated; *see also* Fig. 20-3, Chapter 20.)

relative dominance of the cholinergic system results in parkinsonian signs and acute dystonias. Thus, the treatment of these side effects is to restore the cholinergic-dopaminergic balance, which is best done by administering an anticholinergic drug such as

benztropine (Cogentin®):   1–2 mg p.o.
trihexyphenidyl (Artane®):   2–5 mg p.o.
procyclidine (Kemadrin®):   2.5 mg t.i.d., p.o.

In principle, a restoration of the cholinergic-dopaminergic balance can also be made by giving L-dopa to the patient who is taking the neuroleptic. This would, of course, be defeating the purpose of giving the neuroleptic in the first place, since the high doses of L-dopa that would be required to restore the chemical balance would simply antagonize the action of the neuroleptic, and the patient's psychosis would reappear.

Some physicians have routinely prescribed the anticholinergic medication together with the neuroleptic from the very beginning of therapy. This is good practice when dealing with children who have childhood

autism or schizophrenia-like symptoms, because children are particularly sensitive to neuroleptics and readily develop dystonic reactions. Such reactions can be fatal when the tongue goes into spasm, occluding the respiratory passages.

In the majority of adult cases the neuroleptic is administered first, and after 1 or 2 weeks the anticholinergic drug is added if this is warranted. After about 1 or 2 months of neuroleptic therapy, most patients develop tolerance to the ''stiffness''-producing side effect of the neuroleptic, and the anticholinergic drug is no longer needed. However, about 25% of patients will continue to require anticholinergic therapy together with the neuroleptic drug for an indefinite period.

Development and Treatment of Tardive Dyskinesia

After many months or years of neuroleptic therapy, the patient may develop tardive dyskinesia. The signs are the same as those sometimes seen in acute dyskinesia, namely, involuntary oro-buccal-lingual motion (as if the patient were chewing gum). Also seen sometimes are dystonic motions of the neck, chest, and trunk.

The biologic basis for tardive dyskinesia is as follows. During the course of the long-term dopamine receptor blockade by the neuroleptic drug, the striatal nerve cells synthesize more dopamine receptors, thus making the cells supersensitive to the small amounts of dopamine still getting through the neuroleptic blockade. This supersensitive state causes the dopaminergic input to outweigh the cholinergic input, and the patient exhibits the aforementioned excessive movement, which is diametrically opposite to parkinsonism.

The treatment of tardive dyskinesia, once again, is a matter of restoring the dopaminergic-cholinergic balance. Because the dopamine system has become dominant here, it makes no sense to add an anti-cholinergic drug, since such a drug actually aggravates tardive dyskinesia. Thus, benztropine is contraindicated in tardive dyskinesia. The treatment of tardive dyskinesia, therefore, involves one of the following approaches.

Increasing the blockade of dopamine receptors. This can be done by raising the dose of the neuroleptic. Since it was the neuroleptic that produced the dopaminergic supersensitive state, however, it means that there is a vicious cycle. In other words, raising the neuroleptic dose masks the signs of dyskinesia by producing signs of parkinsonism; however, this will ultimately lead to more supersensitivity.

Depletion of dopamine with reserpine. Although in principle this should work, in practice the doses of reserpine required (2 mg/patient) are rather high and cause hypotension.

Elevation of acetylcholine levels. This can be done in principle with such drugs as deanol or lecithin. The doses required, however, are many grams per day, and the results obtained are no better than 20% successful.

Neuroleptic drug holidays. Prolonged holidays from neuroleptics are the ideal way to manage tardive dyskinesia, since in most instances the dyskinesia will diminish or disappear within 3 months. Some dyskinesias persist for as long as a year, but these, too, diminish in intensity. The younger the patient, the sooner tardive dyskinesia disappears. The difficulty with drug holidays is that one runs the risk of relapse of the schizophrenia.

Current clinical opinion is to treat the first two episodes of schizophrenia with neuroleptics for as long as is necessary (months), and then to forego long-term maintenance therapy. If, however, the patient develops a final profound episode of psychosis within the next year, it would be best to keep the patient on long-term neuroleptic therapy despite the risk of tardive dyskinesia.

Jaundice

Phenothiazine-induced jaundice occurs in 3% of patients. It is of the obstructive type with elevated plasma bilirubin but without fever, liver tenderness, or pruritus. It is thought to be a hypersensitivity reaction since there is eosinophilia, and the severity of the jaundice is not related to the neuroleptic dose.

Dermatitis and Photosensitivity

This occurs in 4% of patients. Patients are sensitive to sunlight, and they develop exaggerated sunburn. They should be warned about this. Ultraviolet light readily oxidizes chlorpromazine, forming a pigment that accumulates in melanin-containing tissues such as the eye, the skin, and the substantia nigra.

Pseudopregnancy

The dopamine neurons in the hypothalamus (arcuate cells) release dopamine, which then travels *via* the hypophyseal portal blood vessels down to the pituitary to inhibit the release of prolactin from the mammotroph cells (Fig. 27–13). Neuroleptics will block the dopamine receptors on these mammotrophs, resulting in a release of prolactin. At the same time, the neuroleptics block the release of FSH and LH. Thus, the woman does not ovulate, does not menstruate, has hyperprolactinemia with swollen breasts and possibly

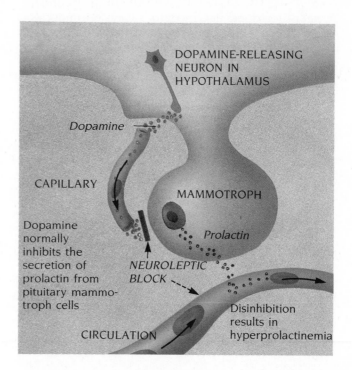

Figure 27–13 Mechanism of production of hyperprolactinemia by neuroleptics.

galactorrhea, the whole picture simulating pregnancy. Breast swelling and galactorrhea can occur in men as well.

Neuroleptic Hypotension

The phenothiazine neuroleptics depress blood pressure by dilating the arterioles by a direct action as well as *via* the CNS. The patients thus show orthostatic hypotension, which clears up after about 4 weeks.

Seizures

Since high doses of neuroleptics decrease the seizure threshold, they can produce seizures. Susceptible patients may be epileptics or have another predisposing cause.

MOLECULAR BASIS OF SEPARATION BETWEEN NEUROLEPTIC EFFECTS AND SIDE EFFECTS

In order to understand how the primary effects and side effects arise clinically, it is instructive to examine Table 27–4. The degree of specificity of the neuroleptic agent for dopamine receptors plays an important role. Spiperone, for example, is very potent, blocking the ³H-neuroleptic/dopamine receptors at very low concentrations but requiring very high concentrations (40 nM) to block the adrenergic receptors. Thus, spiperone selectively acts to block dopamine receptors

without causing the sedation associated with the blockade of adrenergic sites. Droperidol, on the other hand, readily blocks not only dopamine receptors (at 0.09 nM), but also α adrenoceptors at low concentrations (1 nM). Droperidol, therefore, is strongly sedating and is not used for schizophrenia, but is quite convenient for inducing surgical anaesthesia (*see* Chapter 23, *General Anaesthetics*).

Note also that there is a 25-fold difference between the concentration at which haloperidol blocks the dopaminergic and α-adrenergic receptors. Thus, haloperidol does not cause sedation in the usual dose range.

Chlorpromazine and thioridazine, on the other hand, exhibit only a small difference between the concentrations that block dopaminergic and α-adrenergic receptors. Thus, these drugs are rather strongly sedating in the usual doses, and are less selective than haloperidol.

Note that all the neuroleptics, except thioridazine, require extremely high concentrations to block the cholinergic receptors. Thus, all except thioridazine elicit parkinsonism by blocking dopamine receptors in most patients (about 75%). The molecular structure of thioridazine, however, is such that it has some anticholinergic action of its own; hence one sees very little neuroleptic-induced parkinsonism with this drug (only about 5%), and in some hospitals thioridazine is very popular for this reason.

THERAPEUTIC INDICATIONS AND USE

The neuroleptics are used primarily for treating different types of psychosis. The compounds are therefore also referred to as antipsychotic drugs. The psychoses include (with their respective disease/disorder classification numbers from the Diagnostic and Statistical

TABLE 27–4   Relationship Between Neuroleptic Side Effects and IC$_{50}$ Values on Receptors

Receptor Type:	IC$_{50}$ Values (nM)		Hypotension and Sedation	IC$_{50}$ Values (nM)	Extra-pyramidal Signs (% of patients)
	Dopaminergic	α-Adrenergic		Cholinergic (Muscarinic)	
³H-Ligand Used:	³H-Haloperidol	³H-WB-4101		³H-PrBCM or ³H-QNB	
Reference:	1	2		3	
Spiperone	0.07	~40	+	~10,000	75
Droperidol	0.09	~ 1	+ + +	~ 5,000	75
Haloperidol	1.2	~25	+	~ 5,000	75
Chlorpromazine	30	~10	+ + + +	~ 300	75
Thioridazine	12	~10	+ + + +	~ 30	5

References: (1) Seeman P *et al.* Nature 1976; (2) Snyder SH. Am J Psychiat 1976; (3) Miller RJ, Hiley CR. Nature 1974.

Manual of Mental Disorders, 3rd Edition [DSM-III] of the American Psychiatric Association):

1. The **schizophrenias** (DSM-III: 295), characterized by disturbances of:
- association of thoughts;
- affect (dissociation of feeling, or affect, from thought);
- autism (or withdrawal behavior);
- ambivalence (conflicting thoughts and feelings).

There is little agreement on a simple definition of schizophrenia, but there is reasonably good agreement between psychiatrists on the diagnosis of schizophrenia. The prevalence of these psychoses is 1% of the general population.

2. The **organic psychoses**, such as:
- toxic psychosis (drug-induced delusions; DSM-III: 292.11);
- infectious psychosis (delirium; DSM-III: 293.00);

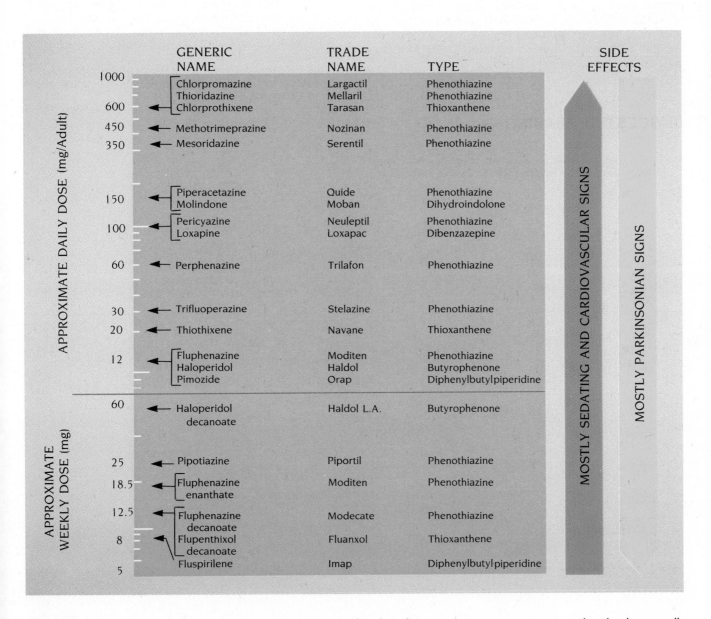

Figure 27–14 Approximate doses of various neuroleptics used in clinical practice. It is important to stress that the dose usually varies from about half to double that shown. The intensity of side effects is shown on the right. It is best to stick to one neuroleptic and adjust the dose according to the response of the particular patient. (Adapted from Seeman MV. Can Med Assoc J 1981.)

- alcoholic psychosis (alcoholic hallucinosis; DSM-III: 291.30);
- senile psychosis (organic hallucinosis; DSM-III: 293.82).

It is recommended that the physician be familiar with three neuroleptics: haloperidol, chlorpromazine, and depot fluphenazine. Almost all psychotic patients, if they respond to medication, will respond to one of these neuroleptics if the physician adjusts the dose appropriately, and adds benztropine to counteract the parkinsonian side effects, if necessary. There should be no need for switching a patient from one neuroleptic to another. Since the choice of neuroleptics varies from hospital to hospital, a more complete listing of drugs and dosages is given in Figure 27-14.

SUGGESTED READING

Davis JM. Comparative doses and costs of antipsychotic medication. Arch Gen Psychiatr 1976; 33:858–861.

Gunnet JW, Moore KE. Neuroleptics and neuroendocrine function. Annu Rev Pharmacol Toxicol 1988; 28:347–366.

Hogarty GE, Goldberg SC, Schooler NR, Ulrich R. Drug and sociotherapy in the aftercare of schizophrenic patients. Arch Gen Psychiatr 1974; 31:603–608.

Miller RJ, Hiley CR. Anti-muscarinic properties of neuroleptics and drug-induced parkinsonism. Nature 1974; 248:596–597.

Seeman MV. Pharmacologic features and effects of neuroleptics. Can Med Assoc J 1981; 125:821–826.

Seeman P. Brain dopamine receptors. Pharmacol Rev 1980; 32:229–313.

Seeman P. Dopamine receptors and the dopamine hypothesis of schizophrenia. Synapse 1987; 1:133–152.

Seeman P, Lee T, Chau-Wong M, Wong K. Antipsychotic drug doses and neuroleptic/dopamine receptors. Nature 1976; 261:717–719.

Snyder SH. The dopamine hypothesis of schizophrenia: focus on the dopamine receptor. Am J Psychiat 1976; 133:197–202.

Chapter 28

ANTIDEPRESSANTS AND LITHIUM

J.M. Khanna

Antidepressants and lithium salts are used in the treatment of major affective disorders. These disorders include bipolar disorder (*i.e.*, manic-depressive) and major depression (without manic episodes). While the etiology of the major affective disorders is still unknown, research on antidepressant drugs has led to the "monoamine hypothesis"—that manic and depressive symptoms are caused by disturbances in the metabolism of central catecholamines or indoleamines (5-HT), or both.

There were no effective treatments for the major affective disorders until the antimanic property of lithium was first recognized by Cade in 1949. It is now the treatment of choice for bipolar affective disorder (manic-depressive psychoses).

There are two main groups of antidepressant drugs, the tricyclic antidepressants (TCAs) and the monoamine oxidase inhibitors (MAOIs), which were both introduced into the clinical therapy of affective disorders in the late 1950s and are still used for the treatment of major depression (*i.e.*, without manic episodes). However, both of these groups have numerous side effects, and both are quite slow in onset of their antidepressant action.

The demand for antidepressant drugs with fewer side effects (especially less anticholinergic effect) and faster onset of action, together with the observation that tricyclic antidepressants block the neuronal re-uptake of noradrenaline* (NA) and/or serotonin (5-HT), have led to the synthesis of a plethora of antidepressant compounds, which are sometimes termed the "second-generation antidepressants." Some of these antidepressants do not inhibit MAO and have little or no effect on the amine re-uptake process.

---

* norepinephrine

TRICYCLIC ANTIDEPRESSANTS

These drugs, of which there are several types, were developed by modification of the central ring of the phenothiazine molecule (Fig. 28–1). The iminodibenzyl type, including imipramine and related drugs, has a $-C-C-$ bridge in place of the S atom. This is also true of the dibenzocycloheptene type (*e.g.*, amitriptyline), which in addition has the N atom of the phenothiazine ring replaced by a doubly-bonded C. Additional modifications gave rise to the dibenzoxazepine and dibenzoxepine types (*see* Fig. 28–1). Although many of the original compounds of this class, including imipramine and amitriptyline, were synthesized as potential antipsychotic agents, they were found to be ineffective in quieting agitated psychiatric patients, but proved to be effective in typical endogenous depression.

Pharmacologic Properties

Actions on Central Nervous System and Behavior

Tricyclic antidepressants do not elevate the mood or the level of arousal in normal persons. In fact, they tend to produce drowsiness and fatigue in humans. In depressed patients, however, they cause a gradual rise of mood and activity, which develops gradually over a period of 2–3 weeks.

In laboratory animals, these drugs prolong hexo-

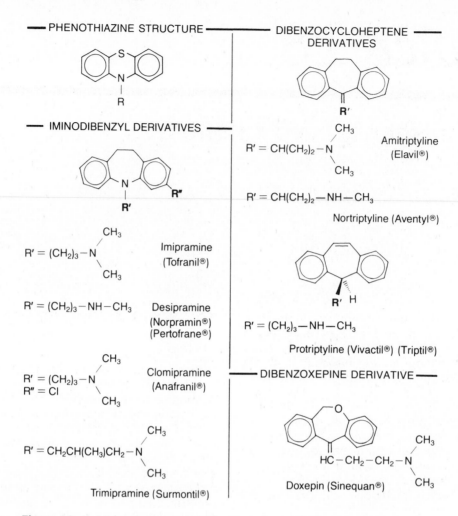

Figure 28–1   Molecular structures of commonly used tricyclic antidepressants.

barbital-induced sleep, and impair both learning and performance of various behaviors, such as conditioned avoidance responses. These sedative-like effects are accompanied by slowing and synchronization of the EEG, as seen with barbiturates or other sedatives. Only at high doses do the tricyclics produce EEG signs of stimulation, such as an increase in fast beta-wave activity, and seizure activity.

Inhibition of Noradrenaline and Serotonin Re-uptake

Tricyclic antidepressants (Table 28–1 and Fig. 28–1) are potent inhibitors of the neuronal re-uptake of NA and 5-HT. Generally speaking, tricyclic secondary amines (e.g., desipramine, nortriptyline) are more potent than the corresponding tertiary amines in inhibiting NA re-uptake. On the other hand, tricyclic tertiary amines (e.g., imipramine, amitriptyline) are more potent inhibitors of 5-HT re-uptake than the corresponding secondary amines. In humans, tertiary amine tricyclics are metabolized into demethylated derivatives (the

secondary amine tricyclics), many of which have antidepressant activity, e.g., desipramine and nortriptyline (the demethylated metabolites of imipramine and amitriptyline respectively).

The mechanism of antidepressant action of these drugs is not clear. Although it is generally believed that their antidepressant effect is related to the actions on re-uptake of NA and 5-HT, this has been questioned for several reasons. First, effects on amine re-uptake are seen rapidly, whereas the therapeutic benefit develops gradually over several weeks after initiation of therapy. Secondly, some of the second-generation antidepressant drugs (iprindole, alprazolam, and bupropion) do not inhibit the uptake of NA or 5-HT, nor do they inhibit MAO. Recent work seems to implicate down-regulation of β-adrenergic receptors in the mechanism of action of antidepressants (Fig. 28–2). β-Adrenergic receptors are down-regulated not only by different types of antidepressant drugs (TCAs, MAOIs, and some second-generation antidepressants), but also by electroconvulsive therapy (ECT), which also has anti-depressant effects in many patients.

TABLE 28–1 **Relative Effects of Tricyclic and Second-Generation Antidepressants on Uptake of Various Neurotransmitters, and Other Pharmacologic Actions**

Drug	Re-uptake Inhibition			Sedation	Anticholinergic Effect	Cardiotoxicity
	NA	5-HT	DA			
Imipramine	+ +	+ + +	−	+ +	+ +	+ + +
Amitriptyline	±	+ + +	−	+ + +	+ + +	+ + +
Desipramine	+ + +	−	−	+	+	+ + +
Nortriptyline	+ +	−	−	+ +	+ +	+ + +
Amoxapine	+ + +	−	+ +	+ +	+	+ +
Maprotiline	+ + +	−	−	+ +	+	+
Mianserin	±	−	−	+ + +	−	−
Zimelidine	−	+ + +	−	−	−	−
Nomifensine	+ + +	−	+ + +	−	−	−
Trazodone	−	+	−	+ + +	−	−

NA: Noradrenaline; 5-HT: Serotonin; DA: Dopamine; − : Weak or no response; +, ++, +++ : Increasing intensity of response.

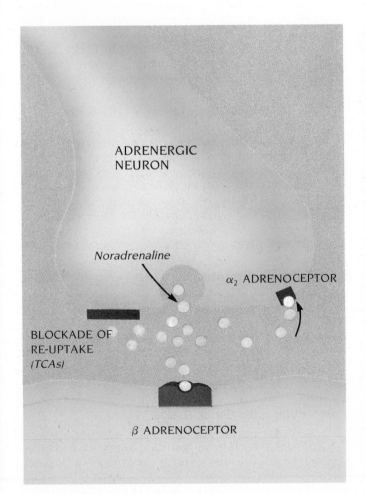
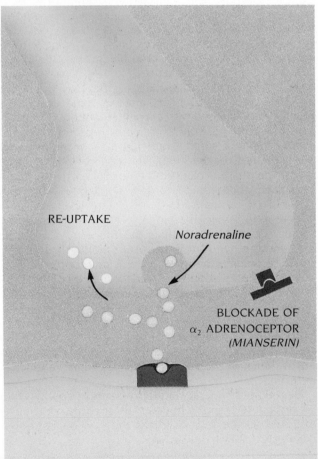

Figure 28–2 Mechanisms by which tricyclic antidepressants (TCAs, *left*) and a second-generation antidepressant (mianserin, *right*) increase the concentration of noradrenaline at the postsynaptic β adrenoceptor. TCAs block noradrenaline re-uptake, while mianserin blocks presynaptic α₂ adrenoceptors. Both processes increase the amounts of neurotransmitter available at postsynaptic receptors.

Anticholinergic and Antihistaminic Effects

The tricyclic antidepressants, like many phenothiazines, possess strong anticholinergic properties. Thus, their side effects include blurred vision, dryness of the mouth, constipation, and urinary retention. They are also potent antihistamines. The feelings of sedation and fatigue observed with tricyclic antidepressants are related to their antihistaminic action.

Absorption, Plasma Level, Biotransformation, and Excretion

Absorption of tricyclic antidepressants from the gastrointestinal tract is essentially complete. Patients treated with identical doses show great inter-individual differences in their steady-state plasma concentrations. The differences may be related to inter-individual variation in hepatic blood flow, resulting in differences in the amount of drug being biotransformed on the first pass through the liver. Clinical improvement has been shown to correlate well with plasma drug levels of some tricyclic antidepressants.

The slow onset of antidepressant action may be related to the time required for the changes in central 5-HT or NA pathways to take place (*e.g.*, receptor desensitization). The half-life of unchanged tricyclics in humans ranges from 9 to 20 hours after multiple doses (the half-life is prolonged with chronic treatment; a half-life of more than 48 hours has been reported in some studies), and a steady-state plasma concentration is generally not reached until the second week of treatment. The pharmacokinetics of the many active metabolites have not been thoroughly studied.

In elderly patients, the steady-state levels of tricyclics tend to be higher than in younger subjects on the same dose. This may explain the increased risk of toxicity and the need for lower doses in elderly subjects.

The biotransformation of tricyclic antidepressants involves demethylation, hydroxylation, and conjugation. Many of the metabolites have antidepressant action themselves. In patients receiving the tertiary amine tricyclic antidepressants, the ratio between the plasma concentrations of the tertiary amine and its secondary amine metabolite shows great inter-individual differences. Much of the variation appears to be genetically determined.

Excretion of tricyclic antidepressants is slow (40% in 24 hours, 70% in 72 hours). The greatest portion is excreted as the N-oxide or as the nonconjugated or conjugated 2-OH derivative.

Adverse Effects

Pronounced Anticholinergic Activity (Atropinic Effects)

Blurring of vision, dryness of the mouth, urinary retention, and constipation are regularly observed. There is a danger of acute glaucoma, and tricyclic antidepressants must be prescribed with caution to patients with narrow-angle glaucoma or prostatic hypertrophy.

Cardiovascular System

Tricyclic antidepressants have potent and complex effects on the cardiovascular system related in part to their anticholinergic property and to inhibition of catecholamine uptake. The tricyclic antidepressants also have direct toxic effects on cardiac muscle, and may contribute to cardiomyopathies. Side effects include postural hypotension, tachycardia, hypertension, ECG changes (T-wave abnormalities, arrhythmias, impaired conduction), and congestive heart failure. These reactions are more likely to occur in the presence of existing cardiovascular disease and with high doses. The risk of heart block by tricyclic antidepressants is directly related to their plasma concentration.

CNS Effects

Drowsiness is very common. A fine rapid tremor, especially in the upper extremities, occurs in about 10% of elderly patients; it may be treated with propranolol, 40 mg b.i.d. Tricyclic antidepressants lower the seizure threshold, as phenothiazines do, and may produce tonic-clonic seizures in high doses. Psychotoxic side effects vary from faulty memory to delirium. Transition from depression to hypomania or mania may also occur.

Withdrawal Symptoms

These usually start within 4 days following abrupt discontinuation, in patients receiving more than 150 mg imipramine or its equivalent daily for more than two months. Symptoms consist of gastrointestinal disturbances, anxiety, and insomnia.

Interaction with Other Drugs

Hypertension and hyperpyrexia may result when tricyclic antidepressants are given in combination with MAO inhibitors, because both drugs tend to increase the amounts of biogenic amines available to act at post-synaptic receptors.

Concurrent administration of tricyclic antidepressants and sympathomimetic amines can augment the amine pressor effects to the point of a hypertensive crisis. The drugs can interfere with the therapeutic effects of certain antihypertensive agents (e.g., guanethidine, clonidine, see Chapter 18).

In epileptic patients maintained on anticonvulsant drugs, reduction of the seizure threshold by the tricyclics could be clinically important.

Tricyclic antidepressants tend to enhance the effects of all oral hypoglycemic agents.

Overdosage

The clinical picture of overdosage is dominated by marked anticholinergic activity (see above). In severe cases, coma, myoclonic seizures, hyperpyrexia, hypotension, impaired cardiac conduction and contractility, and ventricular arrhythmias may occur.

In addition to routine life-support measures and gastric lavage, the majority of severe overdose cases have been successfully managed with neostigmine methyl-sulfate (1–2 mg by slow i.v. injection, repeated at 20–30 minute intervals as necessary). Close monitoring of cardiac function is also critical in the early stage of treatment with tricyclic antidepressants.

The Choice Among Tricyclic Antidepressants

Although conclusive evidence for differential clinical therapeutic effects of tricyclic antidepressants is lacking, clinical impressions (including Kuhn's original observation in 1958) suggest that some are more potent in their anxiolytic and sedative properties (e.g., doxepin, amitriptyline) and others are more selective in counteracting motor retardation (e.g., imipramine, desipramine; see Fig. 28–1).

As mentioned before, tertiary amine tricyclic antidepressants such as amitriptyline and chlorimipramine are generally potent inhibitors of serotonin re-uptake, secondary amine tricyclics such as desipramine and protriptyline are generally potent inhibitors of noradrenaline re-uptake, and some tricyclic antidepressants possess both properties. When a tertiary amine tricyclic antidepressant fails to work in a particular patient, it is the empiric practice of some psychiatrists to switch to a secondary amine tricyclic, and vice versa.

(Some studies suggest that the levels of certain biogenic amine metabolites, especially urinary methoxy-hydroxyphenyl glycol (MHPG) and CSF levels of 5-hydroxyindoleacetic acid (5-HIAA), may serve as indicators for choosing the correct tricyclic agent for a given patient.)

Certain tricyclic antidepressants may also be chosen for their strong sedating properties (e.g., amitriptyline)

when insomnia or excitation is present. It is important to point out that there is, so far, no conclusive evidence that any one tricyclic antidepressant drug is superior to another as far as antidepressant action is concerned. The choice in clinical practice depends largely on the individual patient's tolerance of an antidepressant's side effects. There is growing evidence that tricyclics can be cardiotoxic even when given in normal doses. Some of the new antidepressants (Second-Generation Antidepressants discussed below) should be considered for those patients who are particularly predisposed to the cardiotoxic properties of the tricyclics.

MONOAMINE OXIDASE INHIBITORS

Iproniazid (an isopropyl derivative of isoniazid, an antitubercular drug) was synthesized in 1951 in a search for a better chemotherapeutic agent for tuberculosis. When this drug was given to the patients, it was observed that they became cheerful and energetic, and showed marked improvement in their outlook. Yet there was no change in their lung pathology. In 1952, Zeller and co-workers discovered that iproniazid inhibits the enzyme monoamine oxidase (MAO). Iproniazid was introduced for treatment of depression in 1957, but was abandoned because of its hepatotoxicity. However, its effects on mood spurred pharmaceutical chemists to synthesize other monoamine oxidase inhibitors (MAOIs) in a search for less toxic ones. The structures of some of the MAOIs used clinically are shown in Figure 28–3.

Monoamine oxidase exists in two forms, MAO-A for which 5-HT is the most specific substrate, and MAO-B for which phenylethylamine is the specific substrate. Noradrenaline, dopamine, and other monoamines are oxidized equally well by the A and B forms. In the human brain MAO-B is the predominant form, but it is mostly extracellular. The intracellular enzyme is mainly MAO-A. It is not yet clear whether inhibition of the A or the B form is the more important for antidepressant effect.

Pharmacologic Properties

MAOIs induce appreciable euphoria initially, but their prolonged administration provokes agitation, hostility and aggressiveness, and renders normal subjects insomniac and unmanageable. However, these drugs increase the activity of chronically or acutely depressed, apathetic, and withdrawn subjects. These patients gradually become more alert and less irritable.

MAOIs inhibit not only the enzyme MAO but also many other enzymes. The antidepressant action, however, is considered to be related to the inhibition of MAO. Following inhibition of MAO, concentrations of serotonin, dopamine, and noradrenaline are markedly

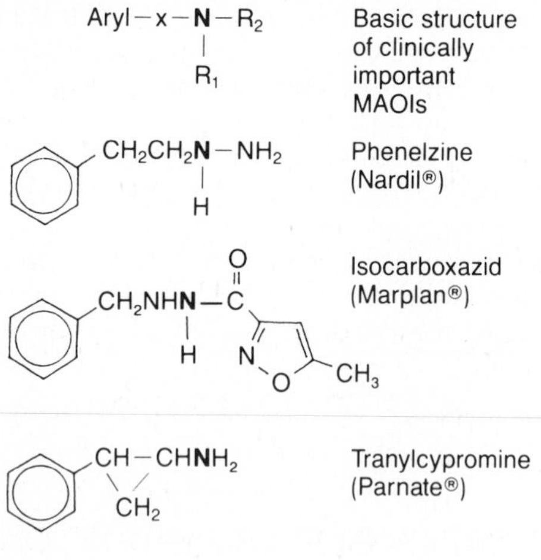

Aryl—x—**N**—R₂   Basic structure
of clinically
important
MAOIs

CH₂CH₂**N**—NH₂   Phenelzine
(Nardil®)

CH₂NHN—C   Isocarboxazid
(Marplan®)

CH—CHNH₂   Tranylcypromine
(Parnate®)

Figure 28–3 Examples of monoamine oxidase inhibitors (*see* text).

elevated in the body. Increased availability of these monoamines in the brain was thought to be responsible for the antidepressant effect, but this hypothesis is now questioned.

MAO inhibitors lower blood pressure, but it is uncertain whether this action is related to MAO inhibition.

Some MAOIs (*e.g.*, phenelzine, tranylcypromine) also have sympathomimetic activity similar to that of amphetamine, *i.e.*, releasing stored noradrenaline.

The currently available MAOIs are readily absorbed when given by mouth, but excretion is slow. The onset of antidepressant action is slow, but because the drugs inhibit MAO irreversibly, their effects are long-lasting. Termination of drug effects depends upon synthesis of fresh enzyme, a process taking more than a week.

Adverse Properties

Because MAO is widely distributed throughout the body and present in many different cell types, diverse pharmacologic effects can be expected to occur after the administration of MAOIs.

Side Effects

MAOIs cause insomnia, and therefore evening and night doses should be avoided (unlike some tricyclics, of which the whole dose is sometimes administered at night for its beneficial effect on sleep).

Other side effects are similar to those of the tricyclic antidepressants. They may be grouped as (1) signs of excessive central nervous system stimulation, including insomnia, irritability, ataxia, and seizures; (2) peripheral vascular effects, including orthostatic hypotension and dizziness; and (3) atropine-like effects such as dry mouth, impotence, urinary retention, con-

stipation, and other gastrointestinal disturbances that probably reflect imbalance between sympathetic and vagal tone.

Conversion of depression to mania is a potential danger in patients with personal or family histories of bipolar depression.

Interactions with Other Drugs

Because MAOIs inhibit catecholamine breakdown, coadministration of other substances that contain or release catecholamines may result in marked increase in adrenergic activity with such consequences as hypertension, tachycardia, agitation, occipital headache, and occasionally intracranial bleeding (secondary to increase in blood pressure, *see* Chapter 18). Drugs that may interact in this way with MAOIs include tricyclic antidepressants, reserpine, and L-dopa. Foods containing tyramine, dopa, or serotonin include cheese (especially if well matured), bananas, beer, wine, yeast products, yogurt, and meat extracts (*e.g.*, Bovril). Patients being treated with MAO inhibitors must be warned not to use over-the-counter medication of any kind (especially medicines for coughs and colds, many of which contain sympathomimetic amines) and must receive detailed instructions about their diet. Hypertensive crisis resulting from such interactions can be treated with short-acting α-adrenoceptor blockers (*e.g.*, phentolamine).

Enzyme inhibition by MAOIs may result in potentiation of the effects of other drugs, including alcohol, sedative-hypnotics, general anaesthetics, analgesics, and narcotics. After the discontinuation of MAOIs, MAO-inhibiting action will continue for about a week. Therefore, it is recommended that, if tricyclic antidepressants or another MAOI are to be substituted for an MAOI that is being discontinued, an interval of 7–10 days be left before the new drug is started. Treatment with MAOIs should also be discontinued at least 7 days prior to elective surgery, in order to avoid possible interactions with the anaesthetic or the pre-anaesthetic medications. Similarly, allow a medication-free interval of at least 7 days before initiating MAOI treatment, in order to avoid interaction with drugs that may have been used previously.

Overdosage

The clinical picture of MAOI overdosage consists of hyperpyrexia, hypertension, hyperreflexia, involuntary movements, agitation, hallucinations, and coma. These signs and symptoms closely resemble those of major overdosage with amphetamines or atropine-like drugs (*see* Chapters 15 and 29), which also results in excessive central and peripheral catecholaminergic activity. Hypotension may sometimes occur, probably as a result of a different type of pharmacologic action.

There is an initial asymptomatic period (up to 12 hours after drug ingestion) during which manifestations of overdosage may not be apparent.

Utmost care is recommended in the management of overdosed patients. Many drugs tend to be potentiated by MAO inhibitors (*e.g.*, sympathomimetics, barbiturates), as noted above, and should be used only under expert guidance.

Indications for MAO Inhibitors

Most studies suggest that MAOIs are indicated for "atypical depressions" characterized by chronic fatigue, oversleeping, phobic anxiety, anhedonia, and somatic complaints. The drugs are also used in the treatment of phobic anxiety syndromes, and to treat nonresponders to therapy with tricyclic antidepressants.

Dosage

The initial doses for phenelzine and tranylcypromine range from 30 to 90 mg and 20 to 60 mg respectively. The dosage is usually reduced for maintenance therapy. Because insomnia is not uncommon during treatment with MAOIs, they are usually given in divided doses.

SECOND-GENERATION ANTIDEPRESSANTS

The introduction of TCAs and MAOIs in the late 1950s revolutionized the treatment of affective disorders. However, the tricyclics produce troublesome anticholinergic and cardiovascular effects in a significant percentage of patients receiving these drugs. Similarly, MAOIs pose potentially dangerous diet– and drug–drug interactions. Therefore, there was a need for new compounds with less anticholinergic and cardiotoxic effects. This led to the development of a number of new antidepressants, the so-called "second-generation antidepressants." Many of these are not tricyclic, and they have structures and pharmacologic effects quite distinct from those of the typical tricyclic drugs (Fig. 28–4). Many of these antidepressants appear as effective as TCAs in treating depression. However, the efficacy and comparative evaluation remain to be established. A brief description of some of the compounds follows (*see also* Table 28–1).

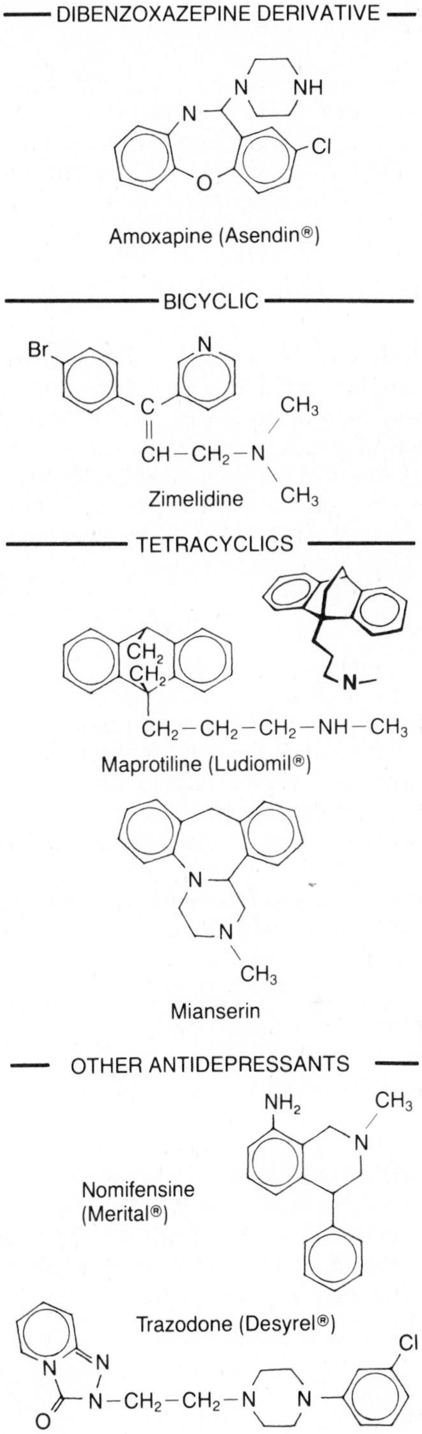

Amoxapine

In addition to being a strong inhibitor of NA re-uptake, amoxapine (Asendin®) has strong dopamine-blocking activity. It has no significant effect on 5-HT re-uptake and its anticholinergic activity is weak. Although its

antidopaminergic activity is theoretically useful for some patients, it has many side effects (orthostatic hypotension) similar to those of TCAs, and of neuroleptics (*see* Chapter 27).

Figure 28–4 Molecular structures of bicyclic and tetracyclic antidepressants and other new antidepressants.

Maprotiline

Maprotiline (Ludiomil®) strongly inhibits NA re-uptake but does not block 5-HT re-uptake. It has a strong antihistaminic and a weak anticholinergic action. There is a lower incidence of cardiovascular complications associated with its use than with that of the TCAs.

Mianserin

Mianserin has only weak effects in blocking monoamine re-uptake, but it blocks presynaptic α_2 receptors, thereby increasing NA turnover. In addition, its independent strong sedative and anxiolytic properties are useful for some patients. Mianserin, like maprotiline, shows no significant anticholinergic effects and is much less cardiotoxic than TCAs in therapeutic doses.

Zimelidine

Zimelidine is a strong 5-HT re-uptake inhibitor and until recently was one of the most popular antidepressant compounds. It is virtually free of cardiotoxicity, anticholinergic or sedative effects. This drug has now been withdrawn from the market because of suspected hepato- and neurotoxicity. **Fluoxetine**, another blocker of 5-HT re-uptake, is also being used as an antidepressant, but it is still too early to assess its relative effectiveness and safety.

Nomifensine

Nomifensine (Merital®) is an antidepressant with a novel tricyclic structure, and it inhibits both NA and dopamine (DA) re-uptake. It also releases DA. Its hydroxylated metabolite has direct agonist actions on DA receptors. This action on the DA system may explain its beneficial effect in patients showing severe motor retardation. The drug is nonsedative, and its anticholinergic effect is very weak. There is also an absence of cardiovascular effects.

Trazodone

A relatively selective but weak inhibitor of 5-HT re-uptake, trazodone (Desyrel®) also has weak anticholinergic and cardiovascular effects. It does, however, produce sedation.

LITHIUM

Lithium differs from other psychotropic drugs in that it does not produce obvious depressant or euphoriant effects in normal individuals. Therefore it stabilizes mood in the manic patient without producing drowsiness or motor incoordination. Just as with the antidepressants discussed above, the full effects of lithium are not obtained until 2–3 weeks after initiation of treatment. For this reason, lithium is usually given initially together with an anxiolytic or antipsychotic drug in order to provide immediate relief of symptoms. Once the patient is stabilized, the tranquilizing medication is withdrawn and lithium treatment is maintained.

Mechanisms of Action

It is not clear how lithium works in mania or in bipolar affective disorder, but recent work suggests an important action of lithium on the phosphoinositide (PI) system, which is a prominent second messenger system for neurotransmitters. Evidence has been obtained that lithium at therapeutic concentrations (0.5–1.0 mmol/L) blocks the enzymatic hydrolysis of inositol monophosphate, resulting in alterations of PI signal transduction by limiting the regeneration of inositol, an essential precursor in PI synthesis. Inhibitory effects of lithium have also been noted on the synthesis of cyclic AMP in several tissues. Although lithium does not inhibit adenylate cyclase activity directly, it does inhibit hormonal responses that are mediated by adenylate cyclase (*e.g.*, thyrotropin activation of thyroid adenylate cyclase, and antidiuretic hormone activation of renal adenylate cyclase). Lithium has also been reported to accelerate the uptake of NA by synaptosomes. Lithium is also an inhibitor of the cell membrane $(Na^+ + K^+)$-ATPase activity, but it is not clear whether this action contributes to its therapeutic effect.

Absorption, Excretion, and Doses

Lithium absorption from the gastrointestinal tract is rapid, with peak blood levels occurring about 2–4 hours following a single oral dose. The serum half-life is approximately 24 hours. However, it has been reported that the half-life of lithium increases with continuous lithium therapy, and a mean half-life of 57.6 hours has been demonstrated in patients who had been on lithium for more than a year.

Lithium is not protein-bound. The optimal serum lithium concentration for control of manic symptoms is 0.7–1.4 mmol/L 12 hours after the most recent dose. A daily dose of 1200–2100 mg, depending on the patient's weight and age, will generally provide serum lithium levels within the therapeutic range.

There is a competitive interaction between sodium and lithium ions in the renal tubule. An increase in sodium intake decreases renal reabsorption of lithium and thus lowers the serum lithium level slightly, while reduced sodium intake elevates it. Thus, patients on a sodium-restricted diet or on diuretics are at risk of lithium intoxication. As lithium is excreted mainly by the kidney, patients with impaired renal function are also at great risk of lithium accumulation and lithium intoxication. In pregnancy and after childbirth, as renal lithium clearance increases and decreases respectively, the plasma lithium level must be monitored carefully.

Side Effects and Toxicity

Gastrointestinal disturbances, polyuria and polydipsia, fatigue, dizziness, muscle hyperirritability (fasciculation and twitching), and fine tremor of the hands may occur at serum lithium levels within the therapeutic range.

Severe poisoning (serum lithium above 2 mmol/L) primarily affects the central nervous system. Disturbances in higher cortical functions, motor incoordination, slurred speech, and coma may develop.

Endocrine and metabolic effects may occur during lithium therapy. These include hypothyroidism and goitre, alterations in carbohydrate and steroid metabolism, and pitressin-resistant diabetes-insipidus-like syndromes.

Some patients show leukocytosis during long-term lithium therapy, which is reversible when therapy is stopped.

ECG changes (especially T-wave depression), arrhythmias, and peripheral circulatory disturbances have been observed.

The key measure to avoid toxicity is the monitoring of serum lithium levels and the avoidance of tissue accumulation. Lithium therapy is generally not recommended for patients with renal and cardiovascular diseases.

SUGGESTED READING

Coccaro EF, Siever LJ. Second-generation antidepressants: a comparative review. J Clin Pharmacol 1985;25:241–260.

Frazer A, Conway P. Pharmacologic mechanisms of action of antidepressants. In: Lake CR, ed. Psychiatric Clinics of North America, Symposium on clinical psychopharmacology I. Philadelphia: WB Saunders, 1984; 7(3): 575–586.

Garattini S, Samanin R. Drugs: guide and caveats to explanatory and descriptive approaches—I. A critical evaluation of the current status of antidepressant drugs. J Psychiatr Res 1984; 18:373–390.

McDaniel KD. Clinical pharmacology of monoamine oxidase inhibitors. Clin Neuropharmacol 1986; 9:207–234.

Rudorfer MV, Golden RN, Potter WZ. Second-generation antidepressants. In: Lake CR, ed. Psychiatric Clinics of North America, Symposium on clinical psychopharmacology I. Philadelphia: WB Saunders, 1984; 7(3):519–534.

Chapter 29

HALLUCINOGENS AND PSYCHOTOMIMETICS

H. Kalant

These are drugs that produce distortions of perception, sometimes giving rise to hallucinations and behavior such as may be seen in psychotic patients. They are variously called **hallucinogens** or **psychotomimetics**. In some people the experience may trigger a panic state or a true psychosis, so that the drugs are also called **psychodysleptics** and **psychotogens**.

All these names are inappropriate because each emphasizes one effect, rather than the common underlying actions. A further problem is that the drugs are not all identical in their mechanisms and consequences of action. Amphetamines and cocaine do produce a psychotic state that has frequently been mistaken for paranoid schizophrenia; therefore the term "psychotomimetic" is appropriate. In contrast, the pictures produced by LSD, mescaline, and similar drugs may contain elements reminiscent of true psychoses, but they are seldom mistaken for psychoses, and the user can generally recognize that the symptoms are due to the drug. Therefore, "hallucinogens" is a more applicable term for such drugs.

DRUGS AND METHODS OF STUDY

The two main groups of drugs to be considered in this chapter are indolealkylamine derivatives related chemically to serotonin (5-hydroxytryptamine), and phenylethylamine derivatives related chemically to noradrenaline.* The chemical structures of a number of drugs in each group are shown in Figures 29–1 and 29–2.

In addition to these major groups, drugs related pharmacologically to atropine and drugs derived from cannabis can sometimes produce hallucinations when given in high dose or under certain circumstances.

Therefore they are also reviewed here in relation to their perceptual and behavioral effects.

Unfortunately, this division into families does not correspond to a clear-cut separation of their pharmacologic effects. The mescaline-like drugs shown in the lower half of Figure 29–2 are closely similar in actions and effects to the LSD-like drugs shown in Figure 29–1, even though they are chemically related to amphetamine. Therefore a meaningful classification must be based on a functional approach, and two complementary techniques have been used to generate a functional classification.

The first technique is that of **receptor-binding studies**. LSD is extremely potent: a hallucinogenic dose in an adult human can be as little as 2 $\mu g/kg$ (150 μg total dose). Moreover, it is highly stereospecific, only the d-form having activity. For these two reasons, it is virtually certain that LSD acts through specific receptors. Because of the indole nucleus in LSD and related compounds (see Fig. 29–1), various theories have been based on the idea that these substances act as either agonists or antagonists at 5-hydroxytryptamine (5-HT) receptors. These hypotheses were supported by neurophysiologic findings such as the fact that LSD and related hallucinogens, when applied by micro-iontophoresis directly to serotonergic neurons in the raphe nuclei, produced a very marked suppression of spontaneous firing by these neurons. However, the molecular structure of LSD and similar compounds also contains a portion corresponding to the structure of dopamine (see Fig. 29–1), and binding to dopamine receptors might also occur. Conversely, the amphetamine and mescaline families are generally believed to act at catecholamine receptors, yet they also overlap with essential parts of the 5-HT structure (see Fig. 29–2) and might be acting at 5-HT receptors. Therefore recent investigations have involved systematic comparison of the in vitro binding affinities of all of these compounds at both 5-HT and dopamine receptors, by the techniques described in Chapter 9. The results confirm the exten-

---

* norepinephrine

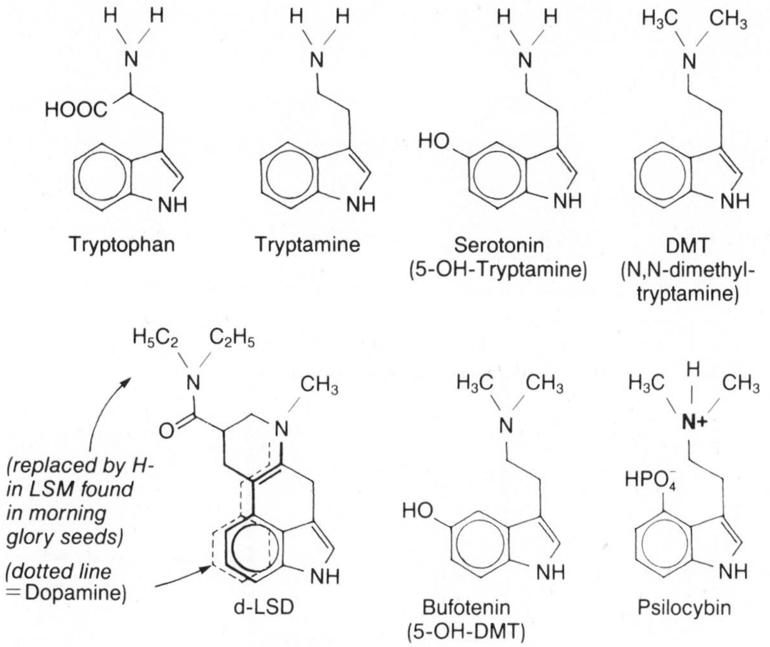

Figure 29–1 Chemical structures of some representative members of the lysergic acid and psilocybin families of hallucinogenic substances.

sive overlap of binding patterns, as schematically shown in Figure 29–3.

However, recent work has revealed clearly that 5-HT receptors are of several different types, including 5-HT$_{1A}$, 5-HT$_{1B}$, 5-HT$_{1C}$, 5-HT$_2$, and 5-HT$_3$. Highly specific agonists and antagonists are available for several of these types, so that receptor-binding studies can now be much more selective and discriminating. Use of these newer methods has shown that LSD and related hallucinogens have a much higher affinity for 5-HT$_2$ receptors than for other serotonin or dopamine receptors. Recently a specific subset of 5-HT$_2$ receptors (high-affinity state, guanylate-sensitive), anatomically localized to the cerebral cortex and some limbic structures, has been reported as the preferential binding site for LSD and several mescaline-like hallucinogens.

The second technique is the *in vivo* study of **discriminative stimulus generalization** (*see* Chapter 66). Rats are trained to press one lever for food reward while under the influence of a certain drug, and a second lever while under placebo. They are then tested under a different drug, and the relative numbers of responses they make on the training drug lever and on the placebo lever indicate whether they perceive the subjective effects of the test drug to be more like those of the training drug or more different from them. Again, the results indicate a considerable overlap of subjective effects. When compared against the training drugs quipazine (predominantly a 5-HT agonist), 5-methoxy-DMT (a pure 5-HT agonist), and amphetamine (predominantly a catecholamine receptor agonist), most of the drugs of both the indoleamine

and phenylethylamine groups show varying degrees of cross-generalization.

In general, the results of the receptor-binding studies are in agreement with those of the discriminative stimulus generalization studies. A drug with a very high affinity for 5-HT$_1$ receptors is likely to show high generalization to 5-methoxy-DMT training stimuli and little or none to amphetamine stimuli. A drug with lower receptor specificity will show more cross-generalization. There appears to be a continuum of gradation between the two "pure" pictures. Therefore the spectrum of subjective and objective effects contains similar elements for the two families, but in different proportions. The typical pictures for the various drug groups are subsequently described.

LSD SYNDROME

Typical Sequence

The typical sequence of effects of LSD and similarly acting drugs includes three phases.

Somatic Symptoms

The first phase, beginning within minutes of the administration of an effective dose, includes a variety of subjective symptoms such as dizziness, weakness,

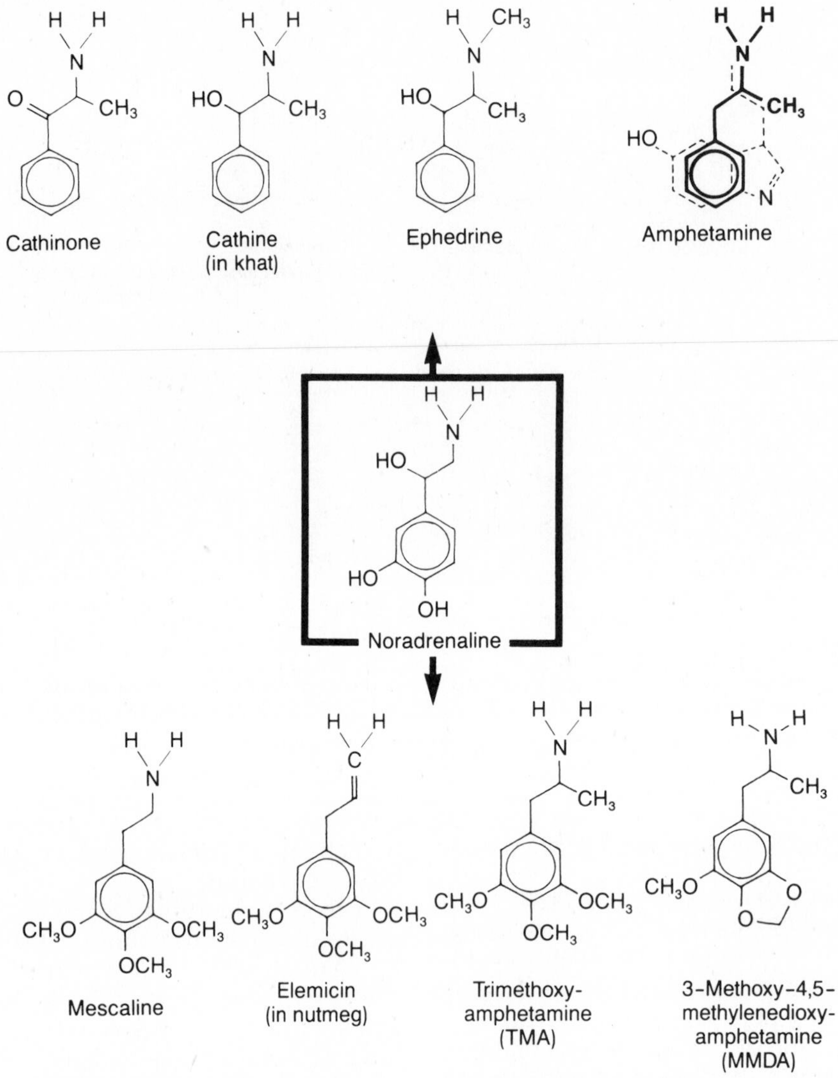

Figure 29–2 Chemical structures of noradrenaline and some representative members of the phenylethylamine group of hallucinogens. *Upper row*: members of the amphetamine family; *lower row*: mescaline and related compounds. Superimposed on the amphetamine formula are the main features of the 5-hydroxytryptamine molecule.

tremors, nausea, sleeplessness, restlessness, and paresthesias, indicative of strong central stimulant action. Muscle tension and hyperreflexia result in some degree of incoordination. Centrally produced sympathomimetic effects include pupillary dilatation, blurred vision, hyperthermia in some species, tachycardia, hyperglycemia, piloerection, and dry mouth. There is also a direct stimulatory effect on uterine muscle, reflecting the relation between LSD and the ergot alkaloids (*see* Chapter 43).

Perceptual Symptoms

These begin about an hour after ingestion of the drug, and tend to be mainly visual. The first effect is fluctuation in the perceived brightness of illumination. Shapes become distorted, undulating; colors become brilliant, constantly varying in tone and intensity; and objects appear surrounded by colored halos or rainbows. Distances between objects become confused. The body image becomes distorted, hands and feet may feel enor-

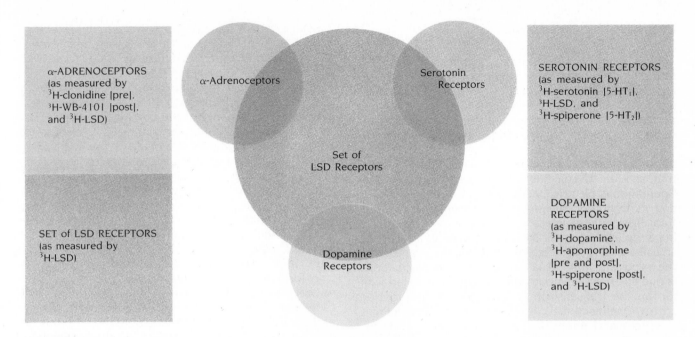

Figure 29-3 Possible receptor interactions of LSD, serotonin, dopamine, and α-adrenoceptor agonists, as revealed by *in vitro* receptor binding assays; [pre] indicates presynaptic receptors; [post] indicates postsynaptic receptors; [5-HT₁] indicates high-affinity postsynaptic receptors; [5-HT₂] indicates low-affinity (presynaptic?) receptors.

mous, or the whole body may seem to be shrinking away. Sense of hearing is sharpened, and occasionally senses become fused (synesthesia), *e.g.*, "the noise of water gushing from the faucet was transformed into optical illusions," or colors appear to have specific smells, *etc*. With mescaline there is a tendency to see geometric patterns, even with the eyes closed. The preponderance of visual phenomena, rather than auditory, tactile, or olfactory ones, has been attributed by some investigators to an action of LSD and mescaline in the lateral geniculate. The sense of time may become distorted; things seem to hang in suspended animation for a long time that, to an observer, is really only a few seconds. During this stage there are often rapid mood changes, the subject being happy, sad, irritable, meditative, or frightened at various times during the same drug experience; some degree of anxiety is almost universal.

Psychic Symptoms

At the peak of the experience, about 2 hours or more after ingestion of the drug, there is marked difficulty in expression of thoughts, dream-like feeling, and difficulty in concentration on voluntary thought. At the same time, there is a tendency to fixation on specific stimuli, and difficulty in moving the attention away from them. The visual illusions may lead into actual hallucinations. Depersonalization is common; the subject feels that the mind has left the body and is looking down on it from a distance. In this state, the subject may

feel that he is freed from his body and is becoming united with the whole universe, in much the same manner as in a religious ecstasy without drugs. In contrast, the same feeling of drifting away from one's concrete self may prove terrifying and give rise to panic or an acute psychosis. **The emotional reaction is strongly influenced by the setting and by other people present**, as well as by the user's previous drug experience, expectations, and emotional state at the time of taking the drug.

Psychological Effects

As with all hallucinogenic drugs, the content and nature of the experience depend strongly on the individual user. The neurologic and perceptual phenomena are probably the same in all subjects, but the way in which these effects are subjectively perceived differs widely. Aesthetically sensitive people place great emphasis on the beauty of the experience, while insensitive people experience mainly the mood changes. Artists refer to the effect of these drugs on creativity, but their artistic skills actually deteriorate badly during the drug effect, so that it is the memory or insight retained **after** the drug experience that may be relevant. This memory tends to be selective, most subjects remembering only pleasant or beneficial aspects of the drug experience, while jitteriness, depression, hostility, auditory hallucinations, and paranoid delusions tend to be forgotten.

Pharmacologic Mechanisms

Small doses of LSD, mescaline, *etc.*, cause increased frequency and desynchronization of the EEG, and they reduce the stimulation threshold of the midbrain reticular formation. This hyper-arousal state resembles that produced by amphetamines and suggests to some investigators that sensory overload plays a role in the hallucinogenic effect. With larger doses, the EEG shows intermittent bursts of slow-wave high-voltage activity that appear to coincide with hallucinatory periods. Spontaneous electrical activity of the retina increases and its excitation threshold is lowered, but synaptic transmission in the lateral geniculate nucleus is partially impaired and the cortical evoked potentials after visual stimuli are markedly altered. These findings suggest that the predominantly visual nature of the hallucinations is due to excessive input from the retina, coupled with incomplete transmission to the optic and association cortex. One functional consequence is that after-images are prolonged, intensified, and fused. Possibly this factor contributes to the production of visual hallucinations. Effects on spinal reflexes are variable, but small doses tend to facilitate tendon reflexes and to inhibit polysynaptic reflexes.

Molecular Mechanisms

As noted earlier, there is evidence to suggest that LSD acts primarily at 5-HT receptors, but also to some extent at dopamine receptors. However, the nature of the actions at these receptors is not at all clear. There is some evidence to support the view that LSD acts as an agonist at both types of receptor, and other evidence to support an antagonist action. For example, LSD decreases the turnover of both 5-HT and dopamine in some parts of the brain and increases it in others, but the nonhallucinogenic analog lisuride has the same effects. Another analog, 2-brom-LSD, inhibits the activity of 5-HT-containing neurons in the midbrain raphe nuclei, and pretreatment with 2-brom-LSD blocks the action of LSD, yet 2-brom-LSD has no hallucinogenic effect of its own. LSD stimulates dopamine receptors in the striatum, and this effect (as well as the hallucinogenic effect) is blocked by chlorpromazine; yet depletion of brain catecholamines does not block the effect of LSD and may even enhance it. These examples illustrate the complexity of interaction of the 5-HT and dopamine systems in the brain, and underline the fact that the mechanism of action of LSD is not yet understood.

Absorption, Distribution, and Biotransformation

All the commonly used drugs in this group are readily absorbed by mouth, except DMT, which must be injected. Effective doses vary widely, *e.g.*, for LSD 2 μg/kg is usually quite potent in humans, while equivalent doses are 150 μg/kg for psilocybin and 5 mg/kg for mescaline. In part, this difference is due to distribution differences: mescaline is tightly bound to plasma proteins, and only a small proportion is free to diffuse into the tissues. In contrast, LSD is also largely protein-bound in the plasma, but the binding is loose and the drug passes rapidly into the tissues. This also affects duration of action: the half-life of LSD in humans is about 3 hours, while that of mescaline is about 6 hours. With all of these drugs, the bulk of a given dose is found in the liver, spleen, kidneys, and adrenals, and only a minute fraction in the brain. However, LSD enters the brain rapidly, possibly by active transport. Within the brain the highest concentrations are found in the pituitary, pineal gland (relation to 5-HT?), hypothalamus, limbic system, and visual and auditory relays. Biotransformation occurs in the liver by routes that differ for each drug. LSD is converted chiefly (almost 90%) to its glucuronide, which is excreted mainly in the bile and a little in the urine; the remainder (10–12%) is oxidized to 2-oxy-LSD and a variety of other oxygenated or hydroxylated derivatives. Mescaline undergoes oxidative deamination to 3,4,5-trimethoxyphenylacetic acid. Psilocybin is dephosphorylated to psilocin, which is also active, but is in turn N-demethylated and oxidized to a hydroxyindole acetic acid.

Relation to Other Drugs

The most commonly used antidote for all these drugs was formerly chlorpromazine, but now it has been replaced by diazepam as the preferred symptomatic treatment. Reserpine enhances the effects of all these drugs.

Tolerance develops rapidly to LSD on repeated use if the drug is taken at too short intervals. This is apparently more a form of tachyphylaxis than tolerance of the usual type, and no withdrawal reaction has been reported. Cross-tolerance is then found to the other drugs in this group, but not to cannabis or amphetamine.

LSD Toxicity

LSD has a very large margin of safety: no human fatality due to direct toxicity of the drug has been reported. The few known deaths were the result of accidents (falls, jumps, *etc.*) occurring during the hallucinated state.

The commonest ill effects are psychological: "bad trips" or panic states, arising from the loss of contact with reality, may trigger serious psychotic breakdown in people with chronic emotional problems. "Flashbacks" are spontaneous (and usually frightening) sensations of being under the influence of LSD even though the person has taken none. They occur in regular users and can be triggered by cannabis in former LSD users. It is not known whether they are really a form of drug toxicity, or a conditioned behavioral response to subjective stimuli formerly experienced under the effects of the drug.

Chromosome damage, leukemia, and teratogenic effects have been reported in humans and other species exposed to LSD, but there are many contradictory reports, and the question is not settled. Women using LSD appear to have a higher proportion of spontaneous abortions, and their offspring have more chromosome breaks and more congenital anomalies than nonusers. But the role of LSD is not clear, since other drugs, viral infections, and other incidental factors may have been important causative or contributing factors.

AMPHETAMINES AND COCAINE

Pharmacology of Amphetamines

The amphetamines and related compounds are strong central nervous system stimulants that are related, both chemically and pharmacologically, to noradrenaline (*see* Fig. 29–2).

Amphetamine has an asymmetric carbon, so that optical isomers, d- and l-forms, exist (Fig. 29–4). While both forms are active peripherally, only the d-form is a central stimulant. Therefore the racemic (d,l) mixture (Benzedrine®) has only half as much central action as an equal weight of the d-form (Dexedrine®).

These drugs are sympathomimetics, and they produce peripheral effects on blood pressure, GI motility, vasoconstriction, pupillary dilatation, *etc.*, similar to those of ephedrine and other sympathomimetic drugs (*see also* Chapter 16). They do so primarily by causing release of noradrenaline from its storage sites in adrenergic nerve terminals. However, amphetamine also appears to have some direct agonist effect on postsynaptic adrenoceptors, and it is also a weak inhibitor of monoamine oxidase.

In the central nervous system, d-amphetamine also causes the release of catecholamines from nerve endings, but this effect is important at both noradrenergic and dopaminergic synapses, which consequently show a higher turnover rate and a reduced content of their respective neurotransmitters. The resulting noradrenergic hyperactivity is probably responsible for the marked increase in wakefulness, alertness, speed of response, and amount of voluntary activity. In normal individuals, this often leads to feelings of well-being or even euphoria, and of increased energy and capacity for work. With overdose, however, mental processes are speeded up so much that the subject becomes submerged in a flood of thought associations, and the attention jumps rapidly and ineffectually from one thought to another, as in a manic psychosis.

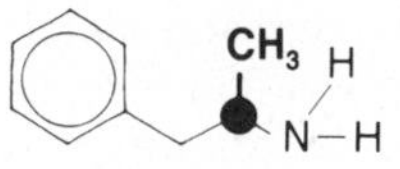

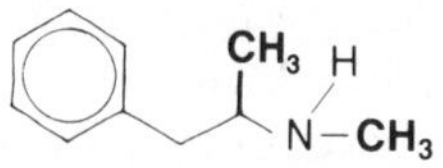

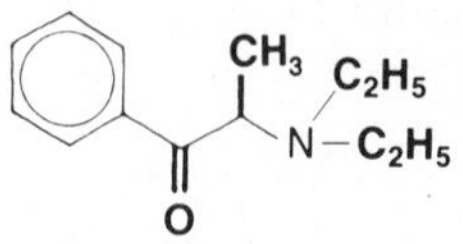

Figure 29–4 Structural formulae of amphetamines and related compounds.

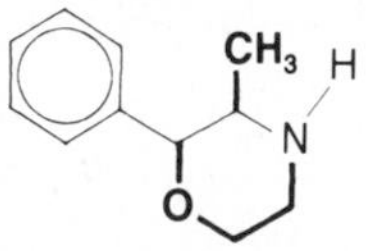

Dopaminergic hyperactivity is believed to be responsible for a different set of effects, including stereotypy (continuously repeated, purposeless movements), paranoid ideas, and hallucinations. All of these effects have been produced experimentally in human volunteers by the administration of large doses of amphetamine, and were blocked by phenothiazine or butyrophenone neuroleptics. The picture is easily mistaken for paranoid schizophrenia.

Medical and Other Uses of Amphetamines

Amphetamine was originally developed as a substitute for ephedrine to raise the blood pressure if hypotension occurred during surgical anaesthesia. Its vasoconstrictor properties also led to its use as a nasal decongestant. For both of these uses it has been replaced by newer sympathomimetics with less central effect.

In many activities, amphetamines will delay the onset of mental and physical fatigue, and they are sometimes used to **enhance performance**, for example, by soldiers on forced marches, by truck drivers on long overnight drives, by students "cramming" for examinations, by athletes striving for peak performance, *etc.* In rare situations, such as a temporary emergency, this use may be justified, but in the other cases mentioned it can be very dangerous. It maintains performance not only by maintaining wakefulness, but also by diminishing the **awareness** of fatigue, which normally warns a person that he is near the end of his reserve strength. Therefore, the subject may push his exertion to the point of serious damage or even death.

In neurology, the main use of the amphetamines is for treatment of **narcolepsy**, a disease of unknown cause characterized by sudden attacks of sleep occurring in completely inappropriate situations. Large doses of amphetamine, as much as 30 to 200 mg a day, depending on the frequency of attacks, are quite effective. Because of its dopamine-releasing action, which occurs in the striatum as well as in other locations, am-

phetamine is also useful as a supplementary therapy in some cases of Parkinson's disease (*see* Chapter 20). The relation between some of the therapeutic uses of amphetamines and the postulated psychotomimetic mechanisms is shown in Figure 29–5.

Amphetamine-type drugs, especially methylphenidate, are also widely used in the treatment of behavioral disorders in children. They reduce the restlessness and hyperactivity in **hyperkinetic children** (attention deficit disorder with hyperactivity). There is no adequate explanation for this apparently paradoxical effect of these drugs. However, barbiturates are also known to produce an opposite effect in these children (*i.e.,* hyperactivity rather than sedation) and further aggravate the

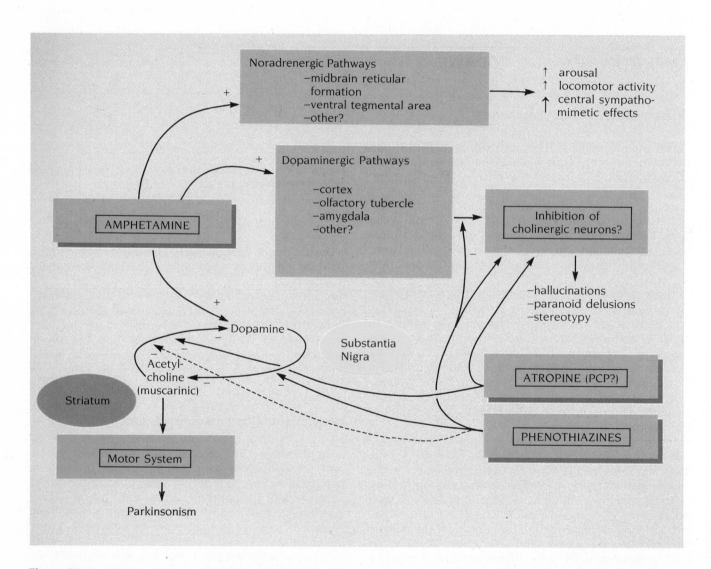

Figure 29–5   Schematic outline of postulated relations among amphetamine-like drugs, atropinic agents, and phenothiazines. (+) indicates stimulatory action, (−) indicates inhibition. For example, amphetamine stimulates dopamine release by the substantia nigra neurons, which inhibits the striatal cholinergic neurons and relieves parkinsonism; atropine inhibits the cholinergic neurons, removing the reciprocal inhibitory effect on the dopamine neurons and also relieving parkinsonism, but at the same time causing hallucinations at other loci. Phenothiazines block dopamine receptors at those loci and alleviate endogenous and amphetamine-induced psychosis, but cause parkinsonism unless they also have anticholinergic effects in the striatum (*broken line*).

condition. It has been reported that all children show sedation with amphetamines, but that the effect is more obvious in hyperkinetic children. There is now considerable argument about the long-term value of amphetamine-like drugs in the treatment of hyperkinetic children.

In psychiatry, the drugs are sometimes used to **raise the mood and activity** of certain depressed lethargic patients. However, stimulation of the reticular activating system only guarantees an increase in mental activity, not necessarily a change in mood, and cases have been recorded of depressed inert patients who were roused by amphetamines to the point that, instead of remaining inert, they committed suicide. Atypical reactions are by no means rare—some patients become acutely anxious and irritable, some become relaxed and drowsy. Therefore these drugs should be used only under close supervision.

By far the commonest use was formerly as an aid in losing weight. Amphetamines cause anorexia by some central nervous action that is not understood. Thus it helps people to adhere to a reducing diet. Amphetamine itself is no longer permitted to be used for this purpose. It was replaced by newer drugs such as **diethylpropion** and **phenmetrazine** (*see* Fig. 29–4). Although these are merely modifications of amphetamine, they have somewhat less peripheral sympathomimetic action. But they are basically similar and have the same dangers (for this reason, phenmetrazine was withdrawn from the market in Canada and some European countries). Therefore they too have largely been replaced by **chlorphentermine**, which produces drowsiness and some lowering of mood, rather than wakefulness and euphoria, when given acutely. Because of these properties, chlorphentermine is much less likely to cause dependence. However, it is still too early to tell whether chronic use will be free of the risks encountered with amphetamine use.

Absorption, Distribution, and Elimination

Amphetamines are readily absorbed from the gastrointestinal tract, so that they can be administered orally as well as parenterally. They are sufficiently lipid-soluble (in the nonionized form) to cross cell membranes readily, including the blood–brain barrier, so that they distribute rapidly to all tissues. Biotransformation occurs almost entirely in the liver, and several different pathways are involved: hydroxylation of the phenyl ring, N-demethylation (in the case of methamphetamine), deamination, and conjugation reactions. The metabolites, as well as an appreciable fraction of the unchanged drug, are excreted in the urine. Because of the numerous different reactions involved, the half-life of drug in the plasma shows considerable individual variation, but it is usually in the range of 12–18 hours.

Side Effects and Toxicity

When these drugs are given for one purpose, the other usual actions constitute the principal side effects; *e.g.*, when they are given as a mental stimulant, anorexia is a side effect, and *vice versa*.

When death occurs from poisoning, it is by excessive sympathomimetic activity, resulting in hypertension, severe tachycardia and collapse, hyperpyrexia, delirium, and convulsions.

The two main nonlethal risks are (1) psychic dependence and tolerance, and (2) psychotic episodes. Dependence is much more common than is usually realized; one British study indicated that the commonest victims were housewives taking amphetamines either to lose weight or to get a "lift" in energy and spirits. Psychotic episodes usually occur after continued intake of large amounts, and they closely resemble paranoid schizophrenia, for which they are often mistaken. Tolerance may be very marked, some addicts taking hundreds of milligrams daily (the normal dose is 5 mg of d-amphetamine, two to three times daily). The drug is largely excreted in the urine for a day to a week or more after the last ingestion, depending on the amount taken. Disappearance from the body is thus gradual, and withdrawal symptoms are relatively mild, consisting of profound sleepiness and depression and a huge rebound in appetite.

Amphetamine Syndrome

In high doses, amphetamines give rise to an acute psychotic picture with hyperactivity, anxiety, paranoid delusions, and auditory and tactile hallucinations, but with clear consciousness and little or no disorientation. This last point differentiates the picture from that of the delirium produced by atropine-like drugs (described in the following section). The picture is differentiated from that of the LSD group by the prominence of paranoid ideas and the predominance of auditory and tactile rather than visual hallucinations. Moreover, amphetamine-induced hallucinations are more a matter of misinterpretation than of distorted perception. Stereotyped behavior is a common finding, and is probably related to dopamine release by amphetamine.

Intravenous injection ("speed") greatly increases the rate of onset and intensity of effects. Experiments in human volunteers produced typical amphetamine psychoses in 2 to 3 days, as compared to months with oral use.

After the drug is stopped, the psychotic picture usually clears rapidly, at a rate that depends directly upon the speed of elimination of the drug from the body. The rate can be increased by acidification of the urine, which increases the degree of ionization of the N and thus reduces the reabsorption of amphetamine in the renal tubule. However, in some instances a frank schizophrenic state was precipitated by the drug use in persons already close to clinical breakdown, and in such cases the symptoms may continue even after the drug is totally eliminated.

In addition to the amphetamine toxicity already mentioned, death also may result from complications of intravenous injection, such as viral hepatitis, necrotizing angiitis, acquired immune deficiency syndrome (AIDS), or septicemia. However, most deaths in amphetamine users are due to violence: accident, suicide, or murder related to aggressiveness and abnormal behavior while "high."

Cocaine

Cocaine was isolated from coca leaves in the 1850s, but clinical interest in it did not arise until 1884, when both its central stimulant and local anaesthetic actions were reported. It was at first recommended for the treatment of depression and of morphine and alcohol dependence, but within a few years it was recognized to give rise to dependence itself. It rapidly became popular among drug addicts (see Chapter 67), and eventually came under strict legal controls in most countries.

The pharmacology of cocaine is discussed in Chapter 24, *Local Anaesthetics*. The main points in the present context are that it is absorbed rapidly through the nasal mucosa, enters the central nervous system rapidly, inhibits the re-uptake of noradrenaline and dopamine by catecholaminergic axon terminals, and thus gives rise to intense central stimulation. Cocaine is **almost identical to amphetamine** in its acute effects and its patterns of toxicity. "Double-blind" experiments in humans have shown that even experienced cocaine users have great difficulty in distinguishing between the two drugs after intravenous injection. The **main differences** are:

- a shorter duration of effect for cocaine;
- lower incidence of complications associated with intravenous use, since cocaine is usually sniffed; instead, rhinitis and perforated nasal septum can occur;
- evidence about tolerance to cocaine is ambiguous; tolerance occurs to some effects, such as anorexia, but it is not clear whether there is any tolerance to the hallucinatory and stereotypy effects, and there may even be sensitization.

In recent years there has been a rapid increase, in North America, of a crudely prepared (and therefore inexpensive) cocaine in the free base form, popularly known as "crack." This form, unlike the salts of cocaine, is volatile when heated. It is mixed with tobacco in a cigarette and, as the cigarette burns, the free cocaine base volatilizes as the heat of the combustion zone approaches. The cocaine vapor can be inhaled, and is absorbed rapidly into the pulmonary circulation, so that its central effects are experienced more rapidly.

This is entirely analogous to the amphetamine free base that, being volatile, could be used in nasal inhalers and had a very rapid onset of effect, whereas the hydrochloride or sulfate salts are nonvolatile, must be taken orally or by injection, and have much slower onset of action when swallowed.

ATROPINE SYNDROME

The pharmacology of anticholinergic drugs is described in Chapter 15. In the present context, the important point is that antimuscarinic agents that can cross the blood–brain barrier induce a toxic delirium, which is deliberately sought by some people as another form of drug "high" and can be mistaken for the effects of LSD-type drugs. The drugs include atropine, scopolamine, benactyzine, piperidyl benzylate esters (e.g., Ditran®), and a variety of crude belladonna preparations. The main features of the atropine syndrome are:

- strong peripheral antimuscarinic effects;
- much more severe disruption of thought processes than with LSD-type drugs;
- confusion, disorientation, and memory loss (this was the basis of the former use of these drugs in the so-called "twilight sleep" analgesia in obstetrics);
- tactile, auditory, and visual hallucinations, including microhallucinations;
- somnolence combined with restlessness, incoordination, and hyperreflexia;
- hyperthermia, with dry hot skin and flushing.

The full-blown drug state may last for well over 24 hours, with residual effects for several days. Chlorpromazine does not relieve the symptoms and may even make them worse, because phenothiazines and tricyclic antidepressants have some degree of atropine-like effect of their own. Treatment is usually symptomatic, using diazepam or some other sedative.

PHENYLCYCLOHEXYLAMINE DERIVATIVES

These compounds, of which phencyclidine (PCP) was the first example, produce a mental state somewhat similar to that caused by the atropine group. However, there are enough differences to warrant treating them as a separate class of hallucinogens. They are chemically and pharmacologically related to the dissociative anaesthetic, ketamine (Fig. 29–6).

The peripheral autonomic effects of these drugs are less marked than those of atropine, and also differ somewhat in pattern. Although they are predominant-

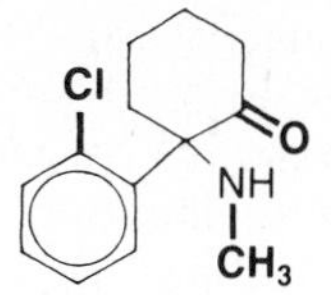

Ketamine

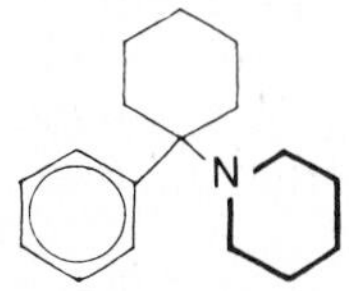

Phenylcyclohexyl-
piperidine
(PCP)
(Phencyclidine)

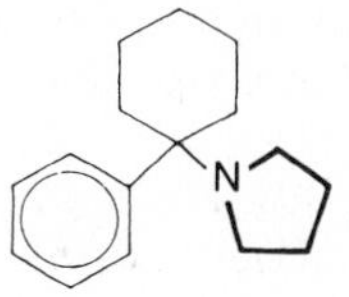

Phenylcyclohexyl-
pyrrolidine
(PHP)

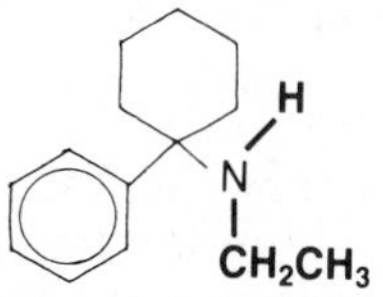

Phenylcyclohexyl-
ethylamine
(PCE)

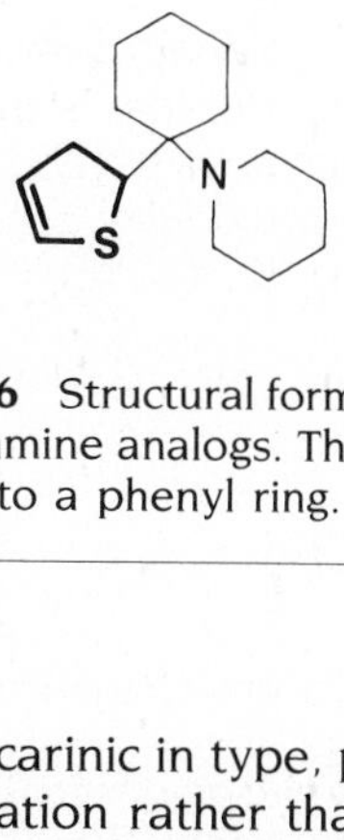

Thienylcyclohexyl-
piperidine
(TCP)

Figure 29–6 Structural formulae of ketamine and its phenylcyclohexylamine analogs. The thienyl ring in TCP is sterically equivalent to a phenyl ring.

ly antimuscarinic in type, phencyclidine tends to cause hypersalivation rather than the dryness of the mouth that is typical of atropine action. In addition, phenylcyclohexylamines have some direct sympathomimetic action, *e.g.*, they enhance the effect of noradrenaline on isolated gut preparations. They cause tachycardia, hypertension, and hyperthermia, as amphetamine does in high doses, and these effects can be life-threatening. Muscle tone is increased, sometimes to the point of rigidity, and the resulting heat production may contribute to the hyperthermia. At higher doses the drugs cause hyperreflexia and seizures. The EEG shows rhythmic spontaneous discharges in the parietal cortex, and increased amplitude of sensory evoked responses.

The behavioral effects of PCP and its congeners are characterized by restless, bizarre repetitive movements (stereotypy), as well as by the analgesia and anaesthesia for which the drugs were introduced clinically. Ataxia and dysarthria are common, and the person appears drunk. Excitement, agitation, depression, euphoria, and dysphoria may alternate rapidly or even coexist. After a large dose, the person may not return to normal for up to 2 weeks.

Like the indolealkylamines, the phenylcyclohexylamines interact with multiple neurotransmitters. They inhibit dopamine uptake in the striatum and noradrenaline uptake in the hypothalamus, but in addition they are much more potent inhibitors of 5-HT uptake. The stereotypy is reversed or prevented by dopamine blockers such as haloperidol, but many of the other effects are not. It has also been suggested that the PCP receptor is identical to the σ-opioid receptor (*see* Chapter 22). Recently, however, an irreversible photoaffinity label was developed for σ receptors, and was found to have no effect on PCP receptor-binding. This suggests that PCP receptors are separate from σ receptors.

PCP undergoes hydroxylation of the cyclohexyl ring in humans, and of all three rings in the rat. The 4-hydroxy derivatives are pharmacologically active. However, the hydroxy derivatives undergo subsequent conjugation reactions that inactivate them and allow them to be excreted in the urine. PCP itself is highly lipid-soluble and accumulates in brain and fat, where it persists for days or weeks. This may account for the slow return to normal after a large dose.

CANNABIS

The hemp plant (*Cannabis sativa*) produces a series of related compounds called "cannabinoids," of which l-Δ^9-tetrahydrocannabinol (THC) is the main active ingredient. It is a constituent of the resinous material that coats the immature flowering tops and also occurs at lower concentration in the leaves at a certain stage during the life of the plant. The dried leaf material is variously known as "marijuana," "bhang," "ganja," "maconha," *etc.*, in different parts of the world. The resinous material is known as "hashish," "kif," "charas," *etc.*, and is five to ten times as potent as marijuana in terms of THC content.

Pharmacologic Effects of Cannabis

At doses normally used by humans, cannabis produces rather trivial physiologic effects. The most consistent are a dose-dependent increase in heart rate and congestion of the conjunctival blood vessels. The EEG shows somewhat more persistent alpha rhythm of slightly lower frequency than normal. No neurologic impairment is found. Sensory acuity may be sharpened slightly. However, thinking is slowed and less accurate, and emotional reactions are more labile. There is usually mild euphoria, talkativeness, laughter, and a subjective feeling of relaxation. These changes are very similar to those found with mild alcohol intoxication. Driving skills are impaired, and the effect is synergistic with that of alcohol. In the early stages of cannabis action there may be synergism with amphetamine, but later there is usually drowsiness and synergism with barbiturates. Part of this effect may be due to cannabidiol (rather than THC itself), which can impair the biotransformation of barbiturates and other drugs by microsomal enzymes in the liver.

After very high doses of THC (e.g., 400 μg/kg or more in humans), there are effects similar to those of mescaline and LSD, including marked distortion of time and space perception, altered body image, depersonalization, auditory and visual hallucinations, transcendental or panic reactions, and even acute psychotic episodes. Visual hallucinations tend to be more of the reverie or day-dream type, rather than abstract forms and colors. Ataxia can occur, with selective impairment of polysynaptic reflexes.

The mechanism of action is unknown, and there is neither discriminative stimulus generalization from, nor cross-tolerance with, either the LSD-like or the amphetamine-like drugs. Experimental evidence indicates that some tolerance develops on regular use of high doses of cannabis, but not uniformly to all its effects.

THC is highly lipid-soluble and is absorbed rapidly across the alveolar and capillary membranes when the smoke is inhaled, so that the onset of drug action is rapid. It is less well absorbed by mouth, and equivalent effects require about three times as large an oral dose as an inhaled one. THC is converted rapidly to 11-hydroxy-THC, but this is also pharmacologically active, so that the drug effect outlasts measurable THC levels in the blood. Because of the lipid solubility, measurable amounts of THC persist in body fat for days after a single dose. This slow phase of elimination has a half-life of about 56 hours in humans.

Chronic Toxicity of Cannabis

The best-documented adverse effect of chronic heavy use of cannabis by humans is bronchopulmonary irritation. Cannabis smoke has a much higher tar content than most tobacco smoke, and the tar contains a higher percentage of known irritants and procarcinogens. Chronic heavy smokers of cannabis, therefore, have a high incidence of **chronic bronchitis**, and precancerous changes have been found in bronchiolar epithelium after only a few years of daily smoking of hashish. Since most cannabis users are also tobacco smokers, the observed effects are probably the result of additive action of the two substances.

Clinical observers have often described a condition of mental slowing, loss of memory, difficulty with abstract thinking, loss of drive, and emotional flatness in chronic heavy users of cannabis. This picture has been called the "**amotivational syndrome**." It probably represents a chronic intoxication state, and in most cases it clears gradually when use of the drug stops. In some cases, however, the symptoms remain long afterwards, and resemble those of organic brain damage, such as is seen in severe alcoholics. It is possible that malnutrition, injury, infections, or concurrent use of other drugs may contribute to this picture. However, experimental studies in rats have shown that daily administration of cannabis alone, in moderately heavy doses for 3 months, does not impair general health, but causes long-lasting or permanent impairment of learning, of a type resembling that caused by hippocampal damage.

Studies in experimental animals and in humans have shown decreased output of gonadotropic hormones, reduced serum testosterone level and low sperm count in males, and anovulatory cycles in females, as a result of chronic use of cannabis. However, there are also contradictory reports.

Chromosomal damage has also been reported in leukocyte cultures from regular cannabis users. As in the case of LSD, the information is so far inconclusive. This also applies to reports of **impaired immune responses** in cannabis users, although experimental studies in animals have confirmed that cannabis does indeed depress T-lymphocyte function.

Psychiatric problems, other than the "amotivational syndrome," consist mainly of short-duration **psychotic episodes** characterized by severe anxiety, or panic provoked by high-dose effects on perception. These usually respond rapidly to reassurance and sedation with benzodiazepines, although they occasionally last for several days or weeks. A more serious problem is the precipitation of a relapse of true endogenous psychosis (schizophrenia) in patients who were previously compensated or borderline.

SUGGESTED READING

Dewey WL. Cannabinoid pharmacology. Pharmacol Rev 1986; 38:151–178.

Fehr KO, Kalant H, eds. Cannabis and health hazards. Toronto: Addiction Research Foundation, 1983.

Heym J, Jacobs BL. Serotonergic mechanisms of hallucinogenic drug effects. In: Marwah J, ed. Neurobiology of drug abuse. Monogr Neural Sci. Vol 13. Basel: Karger, 1987:55–81.

Kalant OJ. The amphetamines—toxicity and addiction. 2nd ed. Toronto: University of Toronto Press, 1973.

Murphree HB. The pharmacology of hallucinogens. In: Smart RG, et al., eds. Research advances in alcohol and drug problems. Vol 7. New York: Plenum Press, 1983:175–205.

Pieri L, Pieri M, Haefely W. LSD as an agonist of dopamine receptors in the striatum. Nature 1974; 252:586–588.

Schultes RE. Hallucinogens of plant origin. Science 1969; 163:245–254.

Symposium on mechanisms of hallucinogenic drug action. Neurosci Biobehav Rev 1982; 6:481–536.

Washton AM, Gold MS, eds. Cocaine—a clinician's handbook. Chichester: John Wiley & Sons, 1987.

AUTACOIDS AND MEDIATORS/ MODIFIERS OF TISSUE RESPONSES

——

Chapter 30

THE EICOSANOIDS

C.R. Pace-Asciak

The eicosanoids constitute families of oxygenated products derived from 20-carbon-atom polyunsaturated fatty acids in which successive double bonds are

Some of the material in this chapter is retained from Chapter 31 (Autacoids) in the 4th edition, by A. Pilc and K.G. Lloyd.

separated by methylene groups. They are formed *via* three main oxidative pathways that utilize molecular oxygen as cosubstrate (Fig. 30–1). Products in these pathways possess a variety of biologic activities and are believed to act as "local hormones" since they are rapidly inactivated in the circulation.

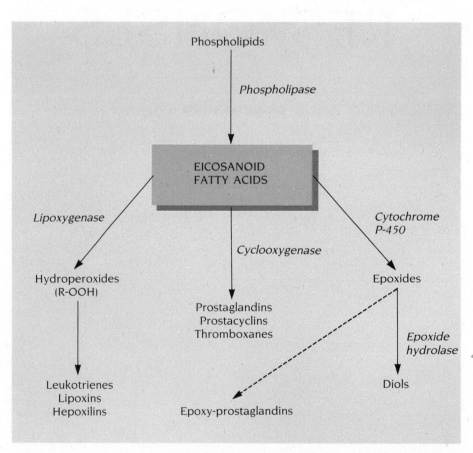

Figure 30–1 Three major pathways identified for the biologic oxidation of arachidonic acid.

THE CYCLOOXYGENASE PATHWAY

Synthesis and Metabolism of Prostaglandins, Prostacyclin, and Thromboxane

Since their discovery in the early 1930s and their chemical identification in the early 1960s, considerable effort has been made to study the biologic properties and cellular importance of the products derived from the cyclooxygenase pathway (Fig. 30–2). The prostaglandins were once believed to be the most potent pharmacologically active compounds known; however, in 1973, the thermolabile prostaglandin endoperoxides (half-life = 5 minutes) were isolated and shown to be 50–200 times more potent than the

prostaglandins in certain test systems. In 1975 another unstable compound (half-life = 30 seconds) derived from the endoperoxides was isolated from human platelets and termed thromboxane A_2. This compound possesses 1000-fold greater potency than the prostaglandins in inducing platelet aggregation and contracting the isolated rabbit aorta. Another product was isolated during the reaction of the rat stomach fundus or the vascular endothelium with the prostaglandin endoperoxides; this product was found to oppose the actions of thromboxane A_2. Its structure was elucidated and the substance was termed prostacyclin (prostaglandin I_2) (see Fig. 30–2).

The **prostaglandins (PG)** constitute a family of naturally occurring cyclopentane-containing straight-chain C-20 carboxylic acids of varying degrees of unsatura-

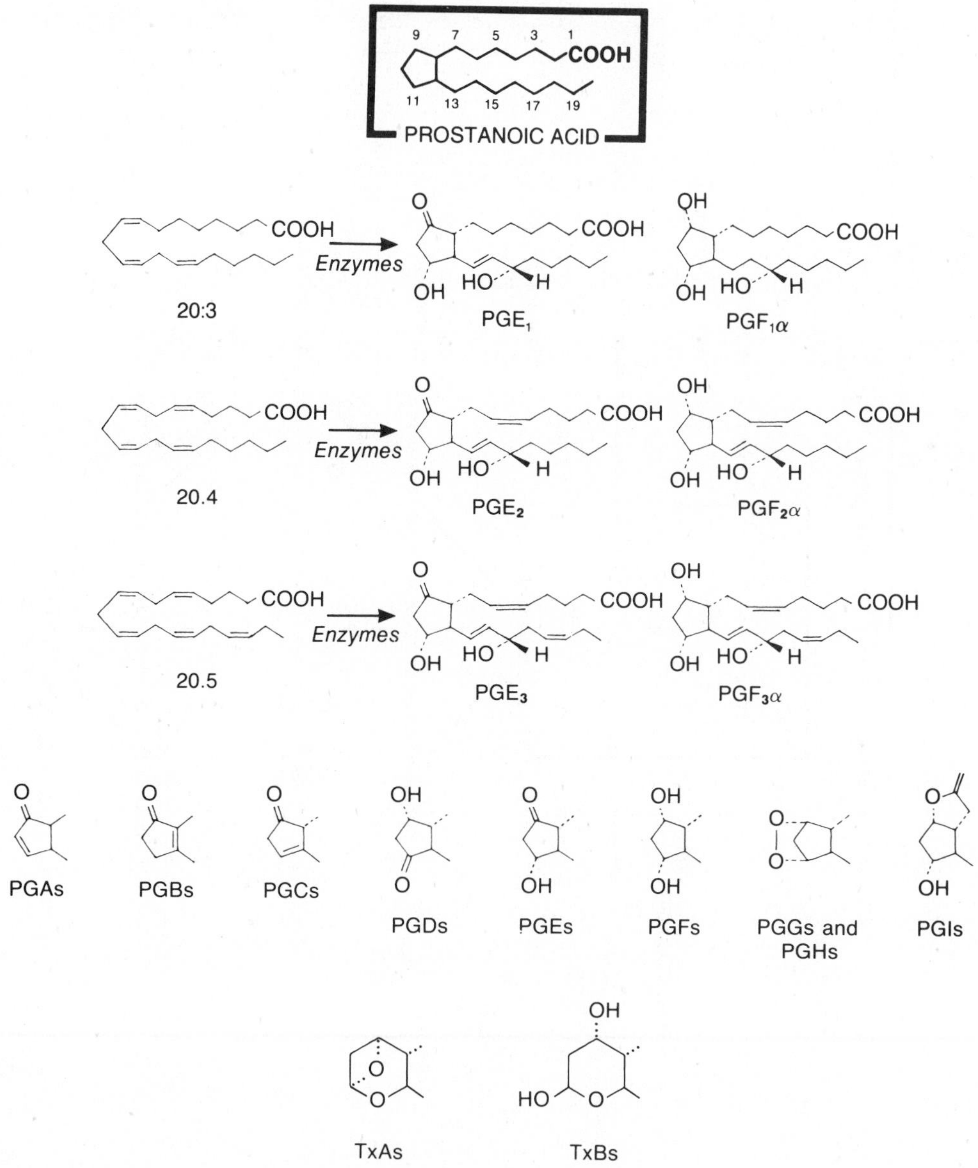

Figure 30–2 General structures of prostaglandins and thromboxanes.

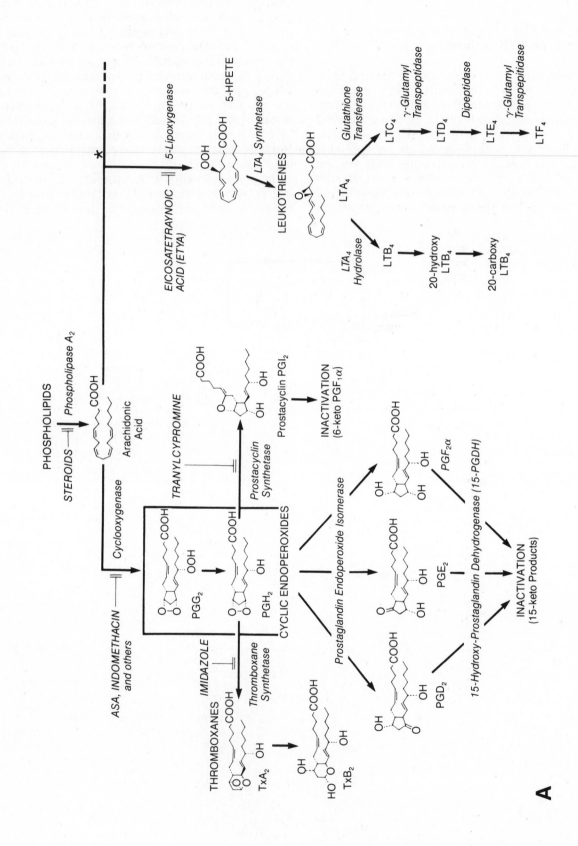

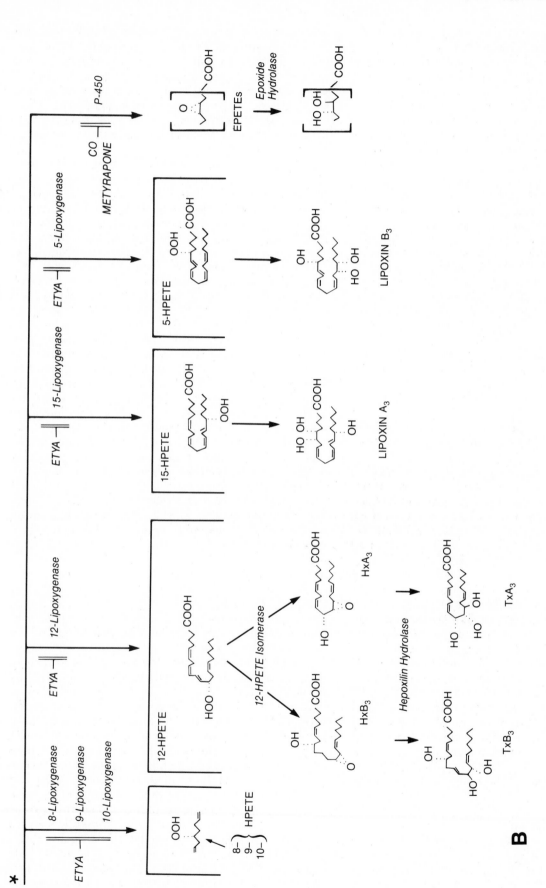

Figure 30–3 A and B, Pathways in the arachidonic acid cascade (simplified). Some sites of inhibition by selected pharmacologic agents are indicated by ‖. At (*) originate other lipoxygenase pathways leading to several hydroxyperoxyeicosatetraenoic acid products. (See text for abbreviations.)

AUTACOIDS

tion. All "primary" prostaglandins contain the same carbon skeleton conveniently termed "**prostanoic acid**," from which stems the systematic numbering and naming of structures of biologic origin and those derived through chemical synthesis. There are five classes of compounds, four named in terms of prostanoic acid, i.e., E, D, F, and I, while the fifth class, i.e., thromboxane, is unrelated to the prostanoic acid skeleton. The E and F classes are named according to whether a keto or a hydroxyl group is present in the cyclopentane ring at the 9-position; the D class is distinguished from the E class in that the former has a keto group at the 11-position instead of the 9-position. The degree of unsaturation in the alkyl side chains distinguishes members within each class (see Fig. 30–2). There are three subclasses, A, B, and C, which are formed chemically from the E compounds by either mild mineral acid or alkali dehydration respectively.

All of the prostaglandins and related substances can be produced from arachidonic acid, which is released from tissue phospholipids by the enzyme phospholipase A_2. The activity of this enzyme is inhibited by several adrenal steroids. For leukotriene formation, arachidonic acid is converted to 5-hydroperoxy-eicosatetraenoic acid by an enzyme, lipoxygenase, and further enzymatically transformed to the leukotrienes A_4, B_4, C_4, D_4, and E_4 (Fig. 30–3).

The other essential enzyme in the synthesis of prostaglandins, prostacyclin, and thromboxanes is **cyclooxygenase**, which is sensitive to inhibition by nonsteroidal anti-inflammatory drugs such as acetylsalicylic acid or indomethacin. Cyclooxygenase converts arachidonic acid to unstable cyclic peroxides (PGG_2 and PGH_2, also collectively called **prostaglandin endoperoxides**). From these cyclic peroxides the prostaglandins PGD_2, PGE_2, and $PGF_{2\alpha}$ are formed by the enzyme **prostaglandin endoperoxide isomerase**. Thromboxane A_2 (TXA_2) is formed by the enzyme **thromboxane synthetase**, and prostacyclin (PGI_2) by **prostacyclin synthetase** (see Fig. 30–3A). All these enzymes together are referred to as the "**prostaglandin synthetase complex**," which is bound to the plasma membrane and/or endoplasmic reticulum of many types of cells.

Although the prostaglandin synthetase complex is quite ubiquitous, there is a considerable degree of specificity (reasons unknown) for the occurrence of each of the pathways. For example, human platelets convert the endoperoxides into thromboxane A_2 (TXA_2), the factor responsible for initiation of the "release reaction" and aggregation of platelets (see Chapter 41). This enzyme is also abundant (although not exclusively) in lung, spleen, and brain, yet it is almost undetectable in many other organs including heart, stomach, and liver. The main pathway for the catabolism of the endoperoxides by the stomach and blood vessels is the prostacyclin (PGI_2) or 6-keto $PGF_{1\alpha}$ pathway. Prostaglandin I_2 is believed to be the biologically active factor in this pathway, with properties opposing those of thromboxane A_2, i.e., it inhibits platelet aggregation and is very potent in lowering systemic arterial blood pressure. On the other hand, the kidney appears to contain enzymes that specifically convert the endoperoxides into PGD_2, PGE_2, and $PGF_{2\alpha}$. It is not yet known what endogenous factors channel the enzymatic activities to favor one pathway or another, but it should be quite possible to manipulate these transformations in the future with drugs that act specifically to block or activate one or several of these related and competing pathways. 6-Keto $PGF_{1\alpha}$ and thromboxane B_2 are inactive hydration (nonenzymatic) products of the thermally- and pH-unstable intermediates PGI_2 and thromboxane A_2 respectively.

The whole prostaglandin sequence is dependent on the availability of the precursor fatty acid in the free form, since phospholipid-bound fatty acid or the methyl ester derivatives are not converted into prostaglandins. At the opposite end of the sequence, although PGI_2 and thromboxane A_2 possess "built-in" controls of their biologic potency through their chemical instability under physiologic conditions, PGE_2, $PGF_{2\alpha}$, and PGD_2 require specific enzymes for their inactivation. The primary enzyme responsible for the major inactivation of these products is 15-hydroxy-prostaglandin dehydrogenase (15-PGDH), which is abundant in all tissues investigated. This inactivation is rapid and extensive; for example, a single passage through the lungs inactivates over 90% of PGE_2. The metabolic products are then excreted into the urine.

As can be seen in Figure 30–3A, there are at least four stages at which drugs can influence the tissue levels of products of the arachidonic acid cascade:

1. Phospholipase step—liberation of the fatty acid precursor from phospholipids.

2. Cyclooxygenase and lipoxygenase steps—conversion of fatty acid into the prostaglandin endoperoxides or HPETE precursors of leukotrienes, hepoxilins, and lipoxins.

3. Prostaglandin endoperoxide catabolic step—channelling of the endoperoxides to any of TXA_2, $PGF_{2\alpha}$, PGD_2, PGE_2, PGI_2.

4. Catabolic step—termination of the biologic activity of prostaglandins, prostacyclin, thromboxanes, and leukotrienes.

The corticosteroids are believed to inhibit the arachidonic acid cascade by an inhibitory action at the phospholipase step, i.e., they limit the availability of precursor fatty acid. On the other hand, vasoactive peptides such as bradykinin and angiotensin II apparently activate the release of fatty acid, resulting in an enhancement of prostaglandin biosynthesis. The site of action of nonsteroidal anti-inflammatory drugs, such as indomethacin, the fenamates, salicylates, etc., is believed to be at the cyclooxygenase step. Acetylsalicylic acid is known to inactivate the cyclooxygenase by irreversible acetylation of the enzyme. Imidazole and substituted derivates inhibit at the thromboxane step, although the drug BW-755C is reported to inhibit both the cyclooxygenase and lipoxygenase steps. The prostacyclin step is extremely sensitive to hydroperoxides and tranylcypromine (an MAO inhibitor). Interestingly, although the prostacyclin synthetase is sensitive to destruction by hydroperoxides, the cyclooxygenase is activated by the presence of hydroperoxide. Phenylbutazone appears to block (although not very selectively) the prostaglandin endoperoxide isomerases. It is quite obvious that drugs with a great deal of specificity for the individual pathways will be of immense benefit to the understanding of the functional importance of each of the pathways.

Intravenously administered prostaglandins are rapidly inactivated in the lung by the specific NAD-dependent dehydrogenase, 15-PGDH. This metabolizing enzyme is found in most mammalian organs. Besides 15-PGDH, numerous other enzymes are present in many tissues to transform the prostaglandin molecule before final excretion into the urine. Figure 30–4 illustrates some of these pathways. In humans the major urinary product of PGE$_2$ is the 16-carbon dicarboxylic acid shown. These pathways are tissue- and species-specific, and the activity of several of these enzymes has been shown to change with age.

THE LIPOXYGENASE PATHWAY

Synthesis and Metabolism of the HPETEs

The lipoxygenase pathway involves the addition of molecular oxygen at one or other of the double bonds of the polyunsaturated fatty acid *via* different site-specific enzymes (*see* Fig. 30–3). Six different lipoxygenases have been described according to the site of entry of molecular oxygen into the arachidonic acid molecule. These are: 5-, 8-, 9-, 11-, 12-, and 15-LOX (lipoxygenases). The product of each LOX reaction is a hydroperoxide (termed HPETE = **h**ydro**p**eroxy-**e**icosa**t**etra**e**noic acid), which is not stable *in vivo*. Each HPETE is either degraded into the corresponding hydroxy derivative (HETE) through glutathione peroxidases present in the body, or is converted into a variety of other biologically potent compounds. For instance, 5-HPETE is the precursor of the leukotrienes (LT). The

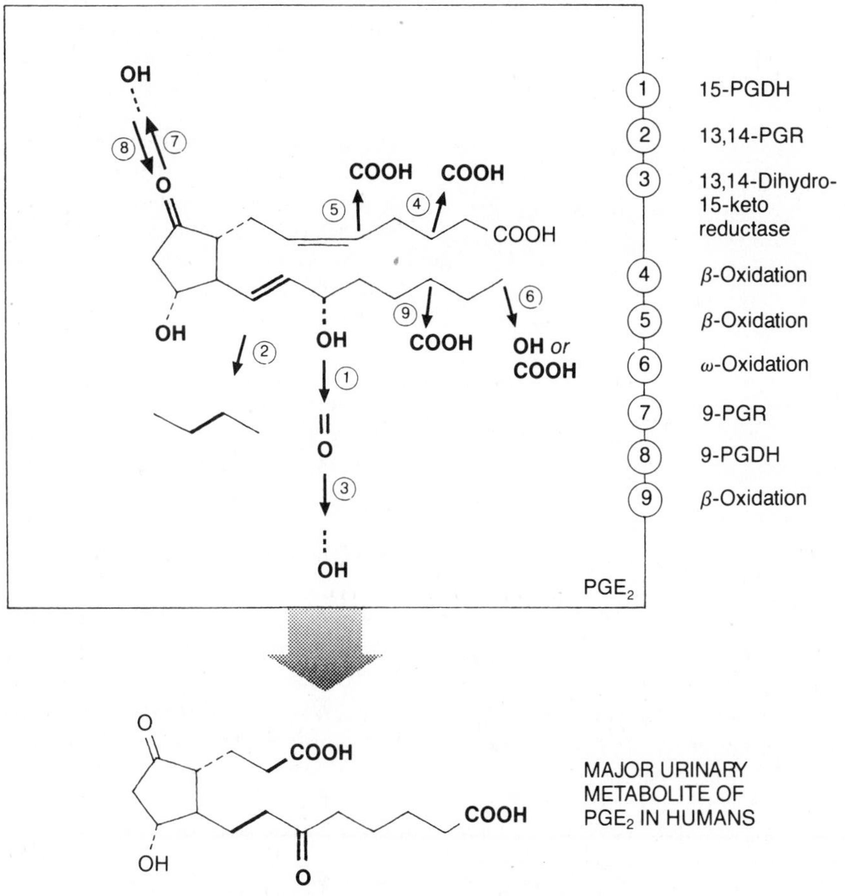

Figure 30–4 Pathways of prostaglandin catabolism. (*See* text for abbreviations.)

transformation steps into the leukotriene family, beginning with the conjugated unstable triene, LTA_4, are shown in Figure 30–3A. They involve enzymatic hydration (LTB_4), or enzymatic glutathione conjugation (LTC_4) followed by various transpeptidations (LTD_4, LTE_4, LTF_4).

Metabolites of 12-HPETE that have been identified are the hepoxilins, products formed *via* a unique intramolecular rearrangement of the hydroperoxy group to form a hydroxy epoxide (*see* Fig. 30–3B). The position of the hydroxyl group determines whether the product is referred to as hepoxilin A (hydroxyl at position 8) or hepoxilin B (hydroxyl at position 10), the epoxide group being at positions 11,12 in both products. These products are inactivated *via* specific epoxide hydrolases to the corresponding inactive trihydroxy derivatives.

Metabolites of the 15-HPETE with biologic activity relate to the lipoxins, products that possess three hydroxyl groups at positions 5, 6, and 15 (lipoxin A) and positions 5, 14, and 15 (lipoxin B). No metabolites of the 8-, 9-, and 11-HPETEs have been described to date.

THE EPOXYGENASE PATHWAY

Synthesis and Metabolism of the EPETEs

A cytochrome P-450 monooxygenase system has been described that epoxidizes the double bonds of arachidonic acid to the corresponding mono-epoxide derivatives of the fatty acid (EPETEs). Specific enzymes that catalyse site-specific formation of epoxides have not been described (*see* Fig. 30–3B). The epoxide products are transformed into the corresponding dihydroxy derivatives through the action of epoxide hydrolases (xenobiotic).

BIOLOGIC EFFECTS

The eicosanoids are formed when an activation of the phospholipase or other lipases takes place in a tissue. This activation can result from the action of a physiologic stimulus (*e.g.*, exercise, pregnancy, age), a pharmacologic stimulus (*e.g.*, angiotensin, bradykinin, noradrenaline*), or a pathologic stimulus (tissue injury or disease). Once the substrate is released from its esterified membrane stores, it is then transformed into the spectrum of products guided by the specific enzymes it is exposed to. Thus, although the cyclooxygenase and the lipoxygenases in general are ubiquitous, there is considerable tissue specificity in the types of products that are formed. For example, blood plate-

---

* norepinephrine

lets contain both a cyclooxygenase and a lipoxygenase, but the main products expressed by this tissue are thromboxane A_2 and 12-HPETE. The main products expressed by the renal papilla are PGE_2 and $PGF_{2\alpha}$. Because prostaglandins and lipoxygenase products are formed ubiquitously, and because they exhibit considerable biologic potency in test systems, yet are inactivated in one or two passes in the circulation, several physiologic roles as local hormones have been proposed, some of which are outlined below.

Prostaglandins, Prostacyclin, and Thromboxane

Cardiovascular System

In most species and vascular beds, prostaglandins E_2 and I_2 (prostacyclin) evoke vasodilatation and increase blood flow; cardiac output is increased; blood pressure generally falls. $PGF_{2\alpha}$ is generally a vasoconstrictor, albeit a weak one. **Thromboxane A_2**, previously termed rabbit aorta contracting substance, is a potent vasoconstrictor. In certain vessels such as in the nasal mucosa, prostaglandins evoke a vasoconstrictor effect and have been proposed as nasal decongestants. Thromboxane A_2 is a powerful initiator of platelet aggregation; conversely, **prostacyclin (PGI_2)** opposes this aggregation through elevation of cyclic AMP levels within the platelet. PGI_2 is further capable of reversing platelet aggregation by dissolving platelet clumps. It inhibits thrombus formation and is regarded as one of the cooperative factors responsible for the maintenance of hemofluidity. The opposing properties of thromboxane A_2 and prostacyclin on platelet function provide an interesting concept of regulation of hemostatic function; thus, an imbalance of the TXA_2:PGI_2 ratio might provide an explanation of some pathologic states of thrombus formation and inflammation. In experimental models, prostacyclin reduces the size of myocardial infarcts, reduces hypoxic damage in the isolated perfused cat liver, and reduces ischemic damage during kidney transplantation in the dog.

Smooth Muscle

Smooth muscle can be either contracted or relaxed by prostaglandins, depending on the organ studied, the species, and the prostaglandin. **Bronchial muscles** are relaxed in humans and most other species by PGE_2, although they are contracted by thromboxane. **Human uterine muscle** is always contracted *in vivo* by PGE_1, PGE_2, and $PGF_{2\alpha}$; hence these compounds induce abortion.

Gastrointestinal Tract

Prostaglandins **inhibit** the secretion of **gastric acid.** Also, the volume of secretion and the pepsin content are reduced. The secretion of pancreatic enzymes and mucus from the small intestine is increased. Prostaglandins also induce the movement of water and electrolytes into the intestinal lumen; therefore they can **produce diarrhea** in humans and animals. While prostaglandins and prostacylin are cytoprotective, thromboxane A_2 is pro-ulcerogenic in the dog and can exert cytolytic effects in myocardial and hepatic tissues.

Renal System

Prostaglandins increase urine formation, natriuresis, and kaliuresis. PGE_2 and PGI_2 are active in stimulating renin release.

Nervous System

After intracerebroventricular injection, prostaglandins cause catatonia and sedation. More importantly, PGE_2 induces a **hyperthermic** response that may be related to pyrogen-induced fever, and the antipyretic action of acetylsalicylic acid and similar drugs may result from their interference with cyclooxygenase activity. In humans, prostaglandins **cause pain** when injected intradermally and are known to sensitize the nerve ending towards the pain caused by histamine or bradykinin.

Endocrine Systems

Different prostaglandins can stimulate the release of ACTH, growth hormone, prolactin, gonadotropin, thyrotropin, and luteinizing hormone. In several mammals $PGF_{2\alpha}$ can evoke regression of the corpus luteum, which interrupts early pregnancy in these animals; however, this effect has not been observed in human females.

Possible Role in Physiology and Pathology

Prostaglandins have been implicated in the function of almost all physiologic systems, as enumerated individually above, e.g., in the control of kidney function, vascular and pulmonary smooth muscles, and endocrine and reproductive systems. One of the roles of prostaglandins is the support of renal perfusion in many diseases associated with decreased effective circulation volume. However, as acetylsalicylic acid (an inhibitor of prostaglandin synthesis) does not influence most of these physiologic systems, the relative role of prostaglandins is questionable. Stronger evidence exists for a role of prostaglandins in tissue inflammation and injury. Prostaglandins act synergistically with agents producing pain, possibly via sensitization of pain receptors (e.g., potentiating the pain induced by histamine or bradykinin). As PGE_1, PGE_2, and prostacyclin are also potent vasodilatory substances, they potentiate the abilities of histamine, bradykinin, and leukotrienes D_4 and B_4 to produce edema. The inhibition of cyclooxygenase may be the basis of the analgesic and anti-edema actions of nonsteroidal anti-inflammatory

compounds (e.g., indomethacin, ibuprofen). Prostaglandins may play a further role in chronic inflammatory joint diseases, inducing destruction of cartilage and resorption of bone (see also Chapters 32, 33).

Therapeutic Uses

Prostin® $F_{2\alpha}$, containing prostaglandin $F_{2\alpha}$ (5 mg/mL in 4- and 8-mL ampuls), is given by intra-amniotic administration to induce abortion and labor. Prostin® E_2 (dinoprostone), in vaginal suppositories containing 20 mg of PGE_2, is also used to induce abortion and labor. The side effects of these prostaglandin preparations are nausea, vomiting, and diarrhea. The drug Prostin® VR is used to maintain temporary patency of the ductus arteriosus in newborns who depend on an open ductus for survival. Misoprostol (Cytotec®) is a synthetic PGE_1 analog used in the treatment of duodenal ulcer (see Chapter 50). Other potential therapeutic uses of prostaglandins exist also for asthma.

Prostacyclin is a valuable addition to the therapy of patients with extracorporeal circulation. It has been applied with limited success in peripheral vascular disease and in angina pectoris. Disadvantages are its short duration of action (it must be administered in continuous infusion) and side effects such as headache, nausea, abdominal cramps, and collapse due to vagal activation after high doses. The drug has recently become available for clinical use in Europe under the generic name epoprostenol.

Leukotrienes

These compounds are now believed to be the biologically active constituents in previously discovered slow-reacting substances of anaphylaxis; for example, the slow-reacting substance from murine mastocytoma cells is identical with LTC_4. Leukotrienes are formed from arachidonic acid by 5-lipoxygenase. This enzyme can be inhibited by the irreversible inhibitor eicosatetraynoic acid. The leukotrienes LTB_4, LTC_4, and LTD_4 can be produced in human, rabbit, and rat polymorphonuclear leukocytes. Upon immunologic challenge, they are released from human or guinea pig lungs.

Leukotrienes (LTC_4, LTD_4, LTE_4, LTF_4) possess potent vasoconstrictor activity (e.g., in the coronary arteries) and cause constriction of small airways. Tracheal mucus secretion is also increased. Leukotrienes increase vascular wall permeability, evoking leakage from postcapillary venules and causing edema. These actions are potentiated by prostaglandins.

Leukotrienes may play an important role in immediate hypersensitivity responses as mediators of allergic bronchoconstriction and vascular permeability. The ability of corticosteroids to reduce the production of leukotrienes, by decreasing the release of arachidonic acid, might explain the antiallergic, anti-inflammatory, and antiasthmatic activity of the corticosteroids. Acetylsalicylic acid, which does not influence leukotriene production, is devoid of antiallergic and antiasthmatic properties. In fact, ASA-induced asthma might be brought on by a redirection of the substrate fatty acids into the leukotriene synthesis pathway.

Leukotriene B_4 (LTB_4), which can be produced by human polymorphonuclear leukocytes, is a potent chemokinetic, chemotactic, and aggregating agent in many types of cells. It may have a role in inflammation and tissue damage. LTB_4 has been found to induce accumulation of polymorphonuclear leukocytes in joint diseases such as gout and arthritis, as well as in skin lesions of patients with psoriasis.

HPETEs

The HPETEs have been shown to possess a variety of biologic effects in *in vitro* systems. These effects include such diverse actions as their ability to relax vascular smooth muscle of the isolated rat and rabbit stomach previously contracted with noradrenaline, the effects of 12-HPETE on the release of insulin from perfused rat islets of Langerhans, the modulation (inhibition) of the effects of prostacyclin on the release of renin, and the recently described neuromodulatory role in signal transduction in the sensory neurons of Aplysia. The effects could be produced by the HPETEs themselves or, since they are rapidly transformed into other products (*see* above), their effects may be due to their conversion into the leukotrienes, lipoxins, or hepoxilins.

EPETEs

Few studies have concentrated on the biologic role of the EPETEs. These products have been shown to possess marginal activity (10^{-6} M) on the release of calcium from liver microsomes and on the release of pituitary hormones from the hypothalamus.

Future developments of site-specific drugs that are capable of selective inhibition of the synthesis or action of the leukotrienes as well as thromboxane A_2, and of the redirection of the pathway of fatty acid metabolism towards formation of PGE_2, PGI_2, and the hepoxilins, should be found useful in the management of disease.

SUGGESTED READING

Karim SMM, ed. Advances in prostaglandin research. Lancaster (UK): MTP Press, 1975–1979.

McGiff JC. Prostaglandins, prostacyclin and thromboxanes. Annu Rev Pharmacol Toxicol 1981;21:479–509.

Moncada S, ed. Prostacyclin, thromboxane and leukotrienes. Br Med Bull 1983;39(3):209–300.

Pace-Asciak CR, Asotra S. Biosynthesis, catabolism and biological properties of HPETEs. In: Pryor WA. Free radical biology and medicine. Toronto: Pergamon Press, in press.

Pace-Asciak CR, Granstrom E, eds. Prostaglandins and related substances. Vol. 5. Amsterdam: Elsevier Publications, 1983.

Samuelsson B, Paoletti R, eds. Advances in prostaglandin and thromboxane research. New York: Raven Press, 1987.

Chapter 31

AUTACOIDS

D. Kadar

ANGIOTENSINS AND ANGIOTENSIN CONVERTING ENZYME (ACE) INHIBITORS

Occurrence and Synthesis of Angiotensins

The angiotensins are peptides of known amino acid composition and structure and are derived from angiotensinogen, a plasma α_2 globulin. Angiotensinogen is converted to the decapeptide angiotensin I by the enzyme renin, which is released by the kidneys. Peptidyl dipeptidase (angiotensin converting enzyme, ACE), which is localized in the endothelium of the blood vessels of kidneys, lungs, and other organs, converts angiotensin I (inactive) to angiotensin II (an octapeptide), the biologically most active form. Angiotensin II circulates in blood and is further catabolized to a less active heptapeptide (angiotensin III) or to inactive fragments (Fig. 31-1).

Angiotensin II has a powerful vasoconstrictor action, 40 times more powerful than that of adrenaline*. Angiotensin II releases aldosterone from the adrenal cortex, promoting sodium retention, but also has a direct inhibitory action on the reabsorption of sodium by the distal tubule. However, normally it has an antidiuretic action due to the constriction of renal vessels and the consequent reduction in blood flow and glomerular filtration.

Renin release can be induced by a decrease in blood pressure or blood volume, renal ischemia, or by the depletion of sodium ions. The induction of renin release by any of these stimuli and the subsequent production of angiotensin II increases blood pressure and induces the retention of sodium; this acts as a feedback to decrease the release of renin and bring about a return to homeostasis.

Some of the material in this chapter is retained from Chapter 31 (Autacoids) in the 4th edition, by A. Pilc and K.G. Lloyd.
*epinephrine

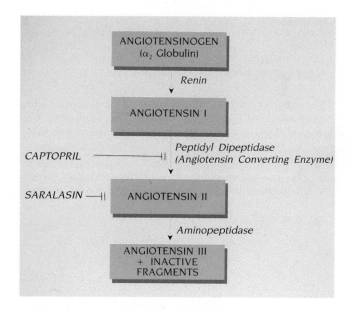

Figure 31-1 Pathway of angiotensin formation and degradation, and drugs acting on it. ‖ indicates blockade of the step shown.

The vasoconstrictor action of angiotensin II is mediated through specific angiotensin receptors located on vascular smooth muscle cells. The most strongly affected are the vessels of the skin, splanchnic region, and kidney. The vessels of brain and skeletal muscle are less contracted. Angiotensin II has no important direct effects on the heart; however, due to the elevation of systemic blood pressure, the work of the heart may increase.

The angiotensin preparation used clinically in some parts of the world is angiotensin amide (hypertensin). This must be given by slow intravenous infusion with the simultaneous measurement of blood pressure. This compound may be used to restore blood pressure if the hypotension is not due to loss of blood.

More importantly, **antagonists** of the renin-angiotensin system have a wide use as **antihypertensive agents**. The first group of antagonists were angiotensin analogs (*e.g.*, saralasin), which block angiotensin receptors. However, saralasin is a partial agonist and may sometimes induce dangerous pressor responses; moreover, as saralasin is a peptide, it is unstable and must be given *via* intravenous infusion.

A more useful group of compounds are the inhibitors of peptidyl dipeptidase (angiotensin converting enzyme), the enzyme that forms angiotensin II from angiotensin I.

Captopril

Captopril (Capoten®, Fig. 31–2) was the first clinically useful, orally administered peptidyl dipeptidase inhibitor.

Mechanism and Site of Action

The primary effect of captopril is the competitive inhibition of ACE (*see* Fig. 31–1). The inhibition was demonstrated in experimental animals and humans by blocking the conversion of intravenously administered angiotensin I. This action is specific because the pressor response to exogenously administered angiotensin II or noradrenaline* is not influenced by captopril.

*norepinephrine

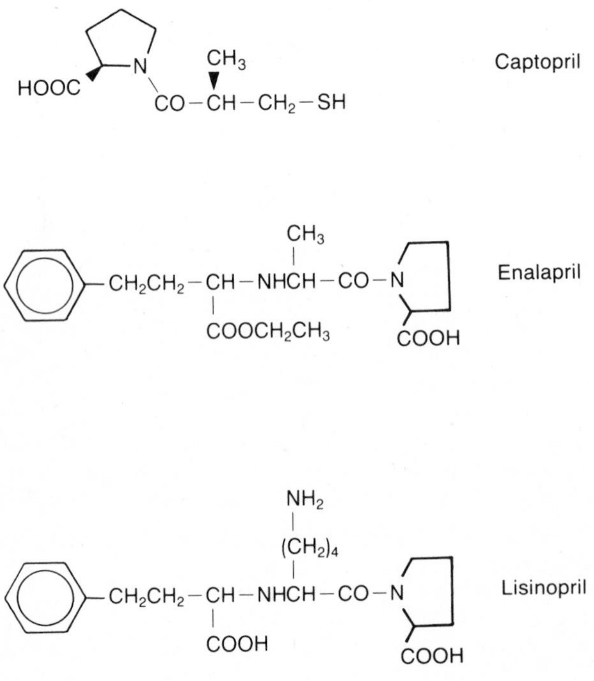

Figure 31–2 Structural formulae of ACE inhibitors.

ACE is identical to the enzyme responsible for the breakdown of bradykinin. ACE inhibition, therefore, causes accumulation of kinins, vasodilatation, and lowering of blood pressure. Some of the dermatologic side effects, such as flush and itching, can be attributed in part to kinins.

Angiotensin II stimulates the release of aldosterone to increase sodium–potassium exchange in the distal convoluted tubules. The reduced angiotensin II formation during captopril therapy may lead to a significant reduction of aldosterone release with subsequent increase in serum potassium.

Pharmacokinetics

Captopril is absorbed rapidly after oral administration, reaching peak blood levels in about 1 hour. The drug should be administered 1 hour before meals because the presence of food in the stomach reduces its bioavailability. Less than 30% of the circulating drug is bound to plasma proteins. It is unevenly distributed in total body water. A minor amount crosses the blood–brain barrier in experimental animals, but it freely crosses the human placenta. The estimated serum half-life is about 2 hours. The antihypertensive effect is much longer than the demonstrable inhibition of the circulating ACE, perhaps because the ACE present in vascular endothelium is inhibited by extremely low serum concentrations. About half the absorbed dose is excreted in the urine unchanged, the rest as the disulfide dimer of captopril and captopril-cysteine disulfide.

Pharmacologic Effects

In hypertensive patients, captopril reduces blood pressure by reducing peripheral arterial resistance, with no change, or slight increase, in cardiac output. The renal blood flow is increased, but the glomerular filtration rate remains the same. The reduction in blood pressure and the duration of effect are dose-related, with a maximum blood pressure fall about 90 minutes after oral administration. Optimal blood pressure control occurs after several weeks of continuous administration. The blood pressure-reducing effects of captopril and thiazide diuretics are additive. Orthostatic hypotension and tachycardia are rare. In heart failure, captopril reduces blood pressure, peripheral resistance, pulmonary capillary wedge pressure, and pulmonary vascular resistance, but increases cardiac output and exercise tolerance.

Additional and Adverse Effects

In the presence of renal artery stenosis, captopril may cause significant reduction in renal perfusion, resulting in increased BUN and serum creatinine. Significant increases in serum potassium may occur in patients with renal impairment, or those receiving captopril together with K⁺-sparing diuretics. Captopril may cause a false positive urine test for acetone.

Toxicity

Proteinuria during captopril therapy occurs primarily in patients with preexisting renal disease or in those who receive high doses of the drug. Neutropenia or agranulocytosis should be suspected in patients who unexpectedly develop systemic or oral cavity infections during therapy. WBC and differential counts should be performed, especially during the early stages of captopril administration. In animal tests captopril was found to have no effect on the developing fetus, but there is only limited information available on pregnant women. Dermatologic reactions, such as transient rash or pruritus with fever, arthralgia, and eosinophilia may occur during the first 4 weeks of therapy. Administration of captopril should be discontinued if laryngeal edema or angioedema occurs. Dysgeusia (i.e., perverted taste sensation) may occur, accompanied by loss of weight; the taste impairment is usually transient.

Therapeutic Applications

Captopril alone, or in combination with thiazide diuretics or other antihypertensive agents, is used for the treatment of hypertension. It is also useful for the treatment of heart failure in patients who do not respond adequately to digitalis and diuretics. Consideration should always be given to the risk of neutropenia, agranulocytosis, or laryngeal edema.

Enalapril Maleate

The intensive search for clinically useful angiotensin converting enzyme inhibitors produced a number of other potentially useful agents. Enalapril maleate (Vasotec®) is the maleic acid salt of enalapril (see Fig. 31-2), the ethyl ester of enalaprilic acid, which is a prodrug of enalaprilat.

Pharmacokinetics

About 60% of the orally administered enalapril is absorbed into the systemic circulation, with maximum serum concentration in 60 minutes. Food does not affect the bioavailability. It is hydrolysed to enalaprilat, which is much more potent than the parent drug. Peak serum concentrations of enalaprilat occur 4–5 hours after administration of enalapril. The drug is not biotransformed further, and 94% of the dose is excreted in urine and feces as enalapril and enalaprilat. There is a prolonged terminal phase in the serum concentration profile of enalaprilat that represents the ACE-bound drug. The effective serum half-life of enalaprilat is about 11 hours. Neither the drug nor its active metabolite crosses the blood–brain barrier in experimental animals, but it freely crosses the placenta.

Pharmacologic Effects

The effects of enalapril are similar to those of captopril, except that maximum antihypertensive effects occur after 4–5 hours and persist in most patients for up to 24 hours. Optimal blood pressure control may require several weeks of continuous therapy.

Adverse Effects and Toxicity

Toxicity and adverse effects of enalapril are reported to be similar to those of captopril. The risk of agranulocytosis and neutropenia attributable to the treatment with enalapril, particularly in patients with renal impairment or collagen vascular disease, is not known. The drug may cause angioedema and excessive hypotension, especially in combination with diuretics or in patients with significantly reduced renal function. The clinical indications and precautions for enalapril are similar to those for captopril.

Lisinopril

Lisinopril (Zestril®, Prinivil®; see Fig. 31-2), the most recently introduced ACE inhibitor, is an analog of enalaprilat, with lysine replacing proline. Bioavailability following oral administration is 25%, and peak serum concentration occurs after 6–8 hours. Bioavailability is not affected by food, age, or coadministration of hydrochlorothiazide, propranolol, digoxin, or glibenclamide. Lisinopril is not a prodrug like enalapril, it is not bound to serum proteins, and it is excreted unchanged in the urine. Steady-state plasma concentration is achieved after 3 days of administration, and accumulation occurs in patients with severe renal impairment. The effective serum half-life is about 13 hours, but significant blood pressure reduction continues for more than 24 hours. The pharmacologic properties are similar to those of captopril and enalapril.

Adverse and toxic effects of lisinopril are similar to those of the other ACE inhibitors, although neutropenia and agranulocytosis have not yet been reported. The occurrence of angioedema would require the immediate cessation of administration.

KININS

Kinins are a separate class of peptides that are formed from kininogen precursors (α_2 globulins) by the proteolytic enzymes, kallikreins, and some nonspecific enzymes such as trypsin (Fig. 31-3). In plasma the nonapeptide bradykinin (named for its slow contraction of the gut) is formed. In tissues, the initial product is kallidin, a decapeptide that can be converted to bradykinin by an aminopeptidase that removes a lysine residue. Bradykinin has a very short half-life (15 sec) and is inactivated by kininases. Kininase II is identical with peptidyl dipeptidase (the enzyme that converts angiotensin I to angiotensin II, *see* above), and can thus be blocked by captopril and other ACE inhibitors.

Kinins are potent vasodilators in most vascular beds, being more potent than histamine. In addition to vasodilatation, kinins also cause increased vascular permeability and edema. Bronchoconstriction induced by kinins is selectively antagonized by acetylsalicylic acid and similar analgesics. In asthmatics, kinins may cause respiratory distress. In addition, kinins are potent pain-inducing agents. The hyperalgesia, edema formation, and vasodilatation associated with the kinins are due at least partially to an interaction with prostaglandins.

At present the kinins have no therapeutic use. However, the inhibition of peptidyl dipeptidase by ACE inhibitors may contribute to the antihypertensive effects of these agents (*see* above). There are no known specific antagonists of kinins, although these might be of therapeutic value if they were available.

Aprotinin (Trasylol®) is an inhibitor of the enzyme kallikrein, probably identical with the pancreatic trypsin inhibitor of Kunitz, and is used in acute pancreatitis, in the carcinoid syndrome, and in states of hyperfibrinolysis, where it acts as an inhibitor of trypsin, kallikrein, and plasmin.

NONOPIOID PEPTIDES OF BRAIN AND GASTROINTESTINAL TRACT

Substance P

Substance P is an undecapeptide, first extracted 50 years ago from intestine. It is also found in brain and in primary afferent neurons. It is proposed to be a sensory transmitter associated with pain transmission. Substance P induces vasodilatation and contracts smooth muscles of the gut. The functions of substance P in the brain are not yet fully identified, although a cotransmitter role in some serotonin neurons has been postulated. Participation of substance P neurons in extrapyramidal motor control has also been proposed. Antagonists of substance P are not known at present.

Cholecystokinin (CCK)

This is a peptide composed of 33 amino acids; however, a shorter (eight amino-acid) fragment of CCK also has full biologic activity. CCK is localized in the brain and gastrointestinal tract. When injected into the brain, CCK causes anorectic reactions and may be a factor that triggers peripheral satiety mechanisms.

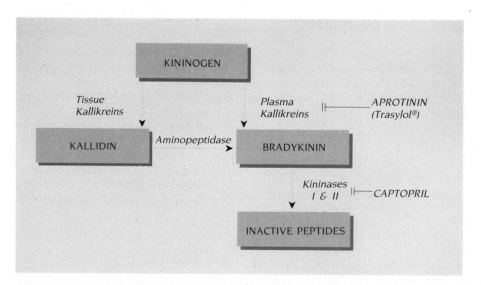

Figure 31–3   Pathways of formation and inactivation of bradykinin. ‖ indicates blockade at the point shown.

Neurotensin

This tridecapeptide was found originally in the brain and subsequently in the intestinal mucosa. Systemic administration of neurotensin causes vasodilatation, hypotension, and increased vascular permeability. These actions may be due at least in part to histamine release.

Vasoactive Intestinal Polypeptide (VIP)

VIP consists of 28 amino acids. It is present in intestinal neurons and is also found in the brain (including coexistence in some dopamine neurons). The neurons containing VIP in the intestine may be involved in reflexes facilitating intestinal transport. VIP also causes relaxation of tracheal smooth muscles.

The central roles of the above peptides are largely unknown at present. They coexist in neurons together with classical central transmitters. They seem to act through specific individual receptors, and play either a neuroregulator or a neurotransmitter role.

In the intestine, these neuropeptides likely are important in regulating intestinal motility, blood flow, and mucosal transport. The discovery in the future of specific antagonists for the individual peptides may some day greatly assist in clarifying their roles.

5-HYDROXYTRYPTAMINE (SEROTONIN)

Synthesis and Metabolism

5-Hydroxytryptamine (5-HT, serotonin) is formed from the dietary essential amino acid L-tryptophan by the sequential action of (1) the specific enzyme tryptophan hydroxylase, which converts it to 5-hydroxytryptophan (5-HTP), and (2) aromatic L-amino acid decarboxylase, which decarboxylates the 5-HTP to serotonin (Fig. 31–4).

Serotonin is catabolized by monoamine oxidase. The main end metabolite is 5-hydroxyindoleacetic acid (5-HIAA), which can be measured in body fluids.

About 90% of body serotonin is found in enterochromaffin cells of the gastrointestinal tract. The remainder is localized in platelets and in specific neurons in the central nervous system.

Physiology and Pharmacology

Role of Endogenous Serotonin

In the central nervous system serotonin (5-HT) is localized in neurons originating in the raphe nuclei and dis-

tributed throughout the brain. 5-HT generally acts as an inhibitory neurotransmitter. Its central functions likely relate to regulation of mood, food intake, and sleep. Serotonin may also participate in the regulation of adenohypophysial secretions, stimulating the release of ACTH, growth hormone, and prolactin, and inhibiting the release of luteinizing hormone (LH), follicle stimulating hormone (FSH), and thyroid stimulating hormone (TSH). In the pineal gland 5-HT serves as the precursor of the hormone melatonin.

The role of 5-HT localized in platelets is not yet understood. Enterochromaffin cell tumors (carcinoid tumors) release large amounts of serotonin, which is responsible for most of the cardiovascular, intestinal, bronchial, and other symptoms associated with these tumors (see below). 5-HT is also involved in the pathology of migraine.

Exogenously Administered Serotonin

The pharmacologic effects of exogenous serotonin are exerted through specific 5-HT receptors. In the cardiovascular system, 5-HT contracts most of the cutaneous, visceral, and cerebral blood vessels, while the blood vessels of skeletal muscles are dilated. By a direct action on the heart, serotonin induces tachycardia, and the force of contraction is increased (positive chronotropic and inotropic effects). Occasionally, by reflex action, it may cause bradycardia and hypotension, leading to vasovagal syncope.

Serotonin stimulates autonomic efferent nerve endings and thus causes the release of acetylcholine and noradrenaline. This action might participate in some

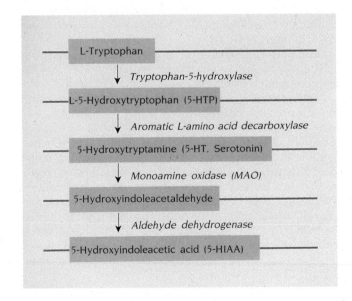

Figure 31–4 Biosynthetic pathway and metabolism of serotonin.

of the responses to 5-HT. Direct actions of 5-HT on bronchial, gastrointestinal, and other smooth muscle can be either stimulatory or inhibitory, depending on the organ, the dose, and the species.

When administered systemically, serotonin does not cross the blood–brain barrier. However, its precursors, tryptophan and 5-hydroxytryptophan, enter the brain fairly readily by active transport.

Drugs Influencing Endogenous Serotonin

Since tryptophan hydroxylase, the rate-limiting enzyme in 5-HT formation, is not saturated with its substrate, the administration of tryptophan can increase the levels of serotonin. In this manner, tryptophan may be of value in phenylketonuria. The effect of tryptophan or 5-hydroxytryptophan in depressed patients is controversial; however, monoamine oxidase inhibitors and serotonin uptake inhibitors (certain tricyclic antidepressants and new atypical antidepressants) are effective therapeutic agents in depression (*see* Chapter 28).

The compounds that lower brain serotonin levels, such as parachlorophenylalanine (an inhibitor of tryptophan hydroxylase) or 5,7-dihydroxytryptamine (which destroys serotoninergic neurons) have no clinical use at present. Reserpine, a drug that depletes serotonin storage sites (but also those of other monoamines), has been used in the treatment of hypertension and psychosis. These effects are presumably exerted not *via* the serotoninergic system, but rather *via* the analogous effects of reserpine on noradrenergic and/or dopaminergic neurons.

Lysergic acid (LSD) and other hallucinogens selectively antagonize many peripheral actions of 5-HT. A similar antagonism of 5-HT actions in the brain has been suggested as the basis of the hallucinogenic effects of LSD, but this is not proven (*see* Chapter 29). Morphine partially blocks 5-HT action on the intestine.

Compounds that were designed and synthesized specifically to block the peripheral actions of 5-HT include methysergide, pizotyline, and cyproheptadine.

Methysergide, a congener of LSD, is recommended for the prophylactic treatment of migraine. It takes 1–2 days to develop its full effect, and therapy should not be initiated during an acute attack. Continuous administration should not exceed 6 months without a drug-free interval of 3–4 weeks. Patients should be carefully monitored for side effects such as retroperitoneal or pleuropulmonary fibrosis, fibrotic changes in aortic and mitral valves, gastrointestinal disturbances, insomnia or mild euphoria, weight gain, dermatologic and hematologic manifestations, peripheral edema, and alope-

cia. The dose should be decreased gradually over 2–3 weeks before complete discontinuation in order to avoid ''headache rebound.''

Pizotyline was introduced for the prophylactic treatment of migraine headache. It is effective in reducing the frequency or severity of attacks. Since it is a potent serotonin and histamine antagonist and also has anticholinergic and sedative effects, the drug should be administered with caution, and drug-free intervals of 3–4 weeks should follow every 6 months of continuous therapy. The initial dose is 0.5 mg at bedtime; this is usually increased to 0.5 mg or more, three times a day, but the total dose should not exceed 6 mg per 24 hours. Unpleasant side effects are drowsiness, potentiation of CNS depressants (alcohol, antihistamines, *etc.*), headache, edema, dry mouth, and impotence. Hepatotoxic effects might occur after prolonged use.

Cyproheptadine is a potent 5-HT and histamine antagonist with mild anticholinergic and CNS-depressant properties. It is used primarily as an antipruritic agent when itching is caused by the release of 5-HT or histamine. It may cause weight gain and increased growth rate in children. The CNS-depressant effects of other drugs may be potentiated if these are taken concomitantly with cyproheptadine. The usual adult dose is 4 mg, three to four times a day.

Ketanserin, a 5-HT$_2$ receptor blocker, relaxes vascular and tracheal smooth muscle and has been studied as a possible antihypertensive agent. It also blocks α_1 adrenoceptors, H$_1$ histamine receptors, and dopamine receptors. It has not yet had wide clinical use.

SUGGESTED READING

Antonaccio MJ. Angiotensin converting enzyme (ACE) inhibitors. Annu Rev Pharmacol Toxicol 1982; 22:57–87.

Case DB. Angiotensin-converting enzyme inhibitors: are they all alike? J Clin Hypertens 1987; 3(3):243–256.

Gregory RA, ed. Regulatory peptides of gut and brain. Br Med Bull 1982; 38(3):219–313.

MacKenzie ET, Scatton B. Cerebral circulatory and metabolic effects of perivascular neurotransmitters. CRC Crit Rev Clin Neurobiol 1987; 2(4):357–419.

Nathan C, Rolland Y. Pharmacological treatments that affect CNS activity: serotonin. Ann NY Acad Sci 1987; 499: 277–296.

Serotonin in cardiovascular regulation. Satellite symposium to the 11th meeting of the International Society of Hypertension (several papers). J Cardiovasc Pharmacol 1987; 10 Suppl 3.

Von Euler US, Pernow B, eds. Substance P. New York: Raven Press, 1977.

Zusman RM. Effects of converting-enzyme inhibitors on the renin-angiotensin-aldosterone, bradykinin and arachidonic acid-prostaglandin systems: correlation of chemical structure and biologic activity. Am J Kidney Dis 1987; 10 Suppl 1:13–23.

Chapter 32

HISTAMINE AND ANTIHISTAMINES

D. Kadar

HISTAMINE AND ALLERGIC PHENOMENA

Histamine is widely distributed in nature. It occurs in practically all mammalian tissues and body fluids in varying concentrations.

Histamine is an amine formed by decarboxylation of the amino acid histidine (Fig. 32–1). Decarboxylation occurs in the same tissues in which histamine is stored, chiefly the lungs, skin, and gastrointestinal mucosa. In these tissues, histamine is present in the mast cells as small dense granules of an inactive histamine-anionic polymer (heparin) complex. It is also present in blood platelets and basophilic leukocytes, as well as in the CNS and fetal liver. Histamine in tissues not containing mast cells is of lesser importance than in the mast cells and has a rapid turnover because of lack of a storage mechanism.

Histamine is released from tissues in free, active form by:

1. destruction of cells, *e.g.*, bee sting venom, bacterial toxins, cold, injury;

2. dissolution of cytoplasmic granules, *e.g.*, by surfactants, radiation;

3. histamine liberators, *e.g.*, drugs (d-tubocurarine, morphine), foreign proteins, dextran, x-ray contrast media.

Despite its wide distribution and potent pharmacologic actions, the physiologic role of histamine is not yet clear. The effects are mediated through special histamine receptors that are designated as H_1 and H_2 types. A number of structural analogs of histamine have been synthesized, and specific agonists have been iden-

tified for H_1 (2-methylhistamine) and H_2 (4-methylhistamine) receptors.

Mechanism of Action

Both histamine H_1 and H_2 receptors are located on the cell surface, and the stimulus–response coupling is mediated through increased Ca^{2+} flow into the cell or increased utilization of intracellular calcium. In general, H_1-receptor stimulation resulting in contraction of the organ gives rise to cyclic GMP accumulation, which can be a direct effect of histamine or secondary to increased Ca^{2+} inflow. H_2-receptor stimulation involving gastric acid secretion, stimulation of neuronal tissue, or smooth muscle relaxation is accompanied by cyclic AMP accumulation in the responding cell. In addition, H_2 receptors appear to have an autoregulatory role since their stimulation by histamine prevents further histamine release in some experimental preparations.

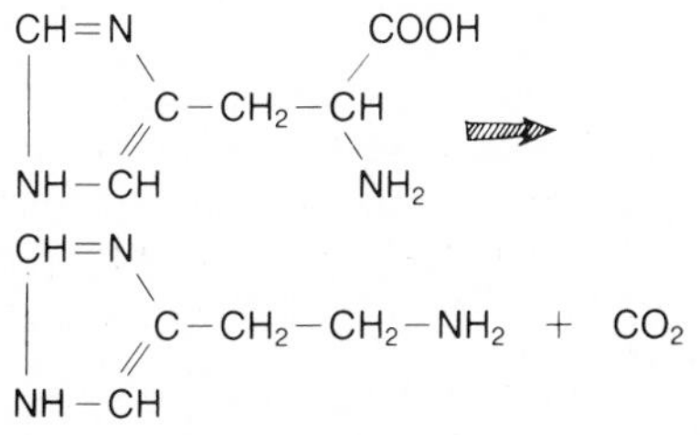

Figure 32–1 Formation of histamine from histidine.

Pharmacologic Effects

Combination of histamine with both H_1 and H_2 receptors leads to capillary dilatation and greatly increased permeability, with leakage and accumulation of plasma proteins and fluid in extracellular spaces. In the skin this gives rise to the classical "triple response" to local injury: local reddening, wheal formation, and flare ("halo"). Urticaria is the cutaneous reaction to systemic histamine release or to allergens.

The heart responds to medium-high systemic doses of histamine with positive chronotropism (H_2 receptors) and positive inotropism (H_1 and H_2 receptors).

Histamine stimulates smooth muscle (H_1 receptors), e.g., bronchioles (causing asthma) and intestine (causing cramps and diarrhea).

In humans, stimulation of H_1 and H_2 receptors usually lowers the systemic blood pressure by reducing peripheral resistance.

Histamine stimulates exocrine secretions (H_1 receptors), e.g., nasal and bronchial mucus. The stimulation of gastric HCl secretion is mediated by H_2 receptors (see Chapter 50).

Histamine stimulation of chromaffin cells causes the release of adrenaline* from the adrenal medulla.

Stimulation of sensory nerve endings by histamine produces itch and pain (mainly H_1 receptors).

Histamine appears to play an important role in the production of certain types of migraine (vascular) headaches.

Histamine seems to have some as yet poorly understood neurotransmitter function in the CNS; both H_1 and H_2 receptors appear to be involved.

Biotransformation

The inactivation of histamine occurs in many tissues by N-methylation or oxidative deamination (Fig. 32–2). Methylhistamine and imidazole acetic acid (ImAA) are converted further to a number of other derivatives.

Allergy and Anaphylaxis

There is a marked similarity between the symptoms elicited by intravenous injection of histamine and those of anaphylactic shock and allergic reactions. In both conditions contraction of smooth muscle, dilatation and increased permeability of capillaries, stimulation of secretions, and action on sensory nerve endings occur. It is generally felt, although without complete agreement, that allergic and anaphylactic reactions are due to the release from storage sites of mediators of anaphylaxis such as histamine, 5-hydroxytryptamine, leukotrienes (SRS-A), and eosinophil chemotactic factor of anaphylaxis (ECFA). The differences between

*epinephrine

localized allergic reactions (e.g., cutaneous, respiratory) and anaphylactic reactions presumably depend upon the sites and rates of mediator release.

If localized release of histamine is slow enough to permit inactivation of any that gets into the blood stream, only a local allergic reaction is presumed to occur. However, if the release is too rapid and explosive for inactivation to keep pace, the reaction will be of the anaphylactic type.

Drug-induced histamine release can be triggered by antigen–antibody reactions, but most often the presence of circulating (IgG) or cell-bound (IgE) antibodies cannot be detected. X-ray contrast media in the absence of antibodies may liberate massive amounts of histamine, causing anaphylactoid reactions, often with fatal outcome.

Therapeutic measures for the control of allergy and anaphylaxis may be specific or symptomatic, depending on their locus of action.

- Specific therapy would be the avoidance or elimination of offending antigens, or the desensitization of the sensitive individual.

- Prophylactic treatment of asthma and certain allergic conditions with sodium cromoglycate hinders the release of histamine and other autacoids. In serious cases beclomethasone by inhalation or nasal spray for localized effects can be as effective as systemic glucocorticoid therapy.

- Administration of H_1-receptor blockers ("antihistamines") will prevent the effects of histamine release, as in hay fever.

- If H_1-receptor blockade is not effective or not practical, physiologic antagonists such as adrenaline, specific β_2-adrenoceptor stimulants, or theophylline can be used.

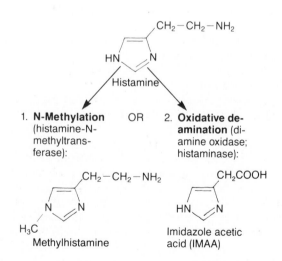

Figure 32–2 Biotransformation of histamine.

Clinical Uses

Histamine was used in the past to assess the ability of the stomach to secrete acid. Later it was replaced by betazole, an analog of histamine with preferential effects on gastric secretion. Pentagastrin, a synthetic analog of gastrin, is now preferred for stimulation of gastric HCl secretion; it has fewer unwanted effects than either histamine or betazole.

Histamine can be used to test the integrity of sensory nerves and as a provocative agent for the diagnosis of pheochromocytoma.

HISTAMINE H₁-RECEPTOR BLOCKERS

In 1937 Bovet and Staub detected histamine-blocking activity in one of a series of amines with a phenolic ether function, synthesized by Fourneau. This substance (2-isopropyl-5-methylphenoxyethyldiethylamine) protected guinea pigs against lethal doses of histamine, antagonized histamine-induced spasms of smooth muscle, and lessened the symptoms of anaphylactic shock (these are now known to be H₁ receptor-mediated reactions).

This compound was too weak and too toxic for therapeutic use, but the synthesis of related substances resulted, in 1942, in the first clinically employed antihistamine, phenbenzamine (Antergan®). Other highly effective histamine antagonists followed rapidly.

Classification

All antihistamines have the same basic structure, as shown in Figure 32–3. In addition, the terminal dimethylamine group may be incorporated into a ring structure, as in chlorcyclizine (Figs. 32–3 and 32–4).

From all these possible constituents, a tremendous number of combinations can be made. There have been more than 4000 such compounds synthesized and tested, and several dozen are in clinical use. However, none of these will inhibit the histamine-induced stimulation of gastric acid secretion, an H₂ receptor-mediated reaction. Table 32–1 lists the most often used histamine H₁-receptor blockers, of which some examples are shown in Figure 32–4.

Mechanism and Site of Action

The mechanism and site of action are virtually identical for all H₁-receptor blockers. The basic structure of conventional antihistamines is very similar to the essential structure of histamine itself. This similarity is sufficient to permit the antihistamines to compete for the

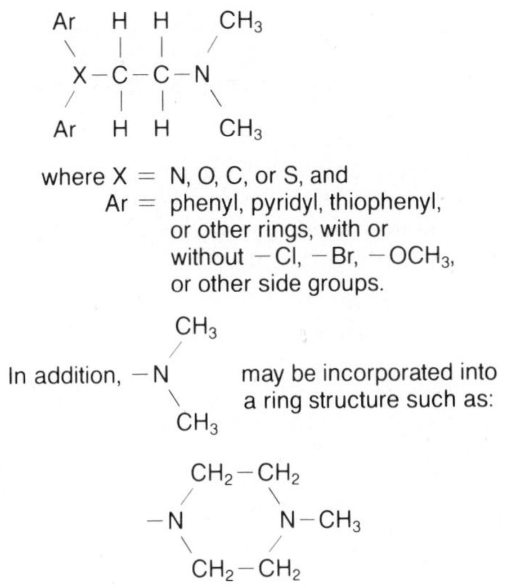

Figure 32–3 Basic structure of antihistamines.

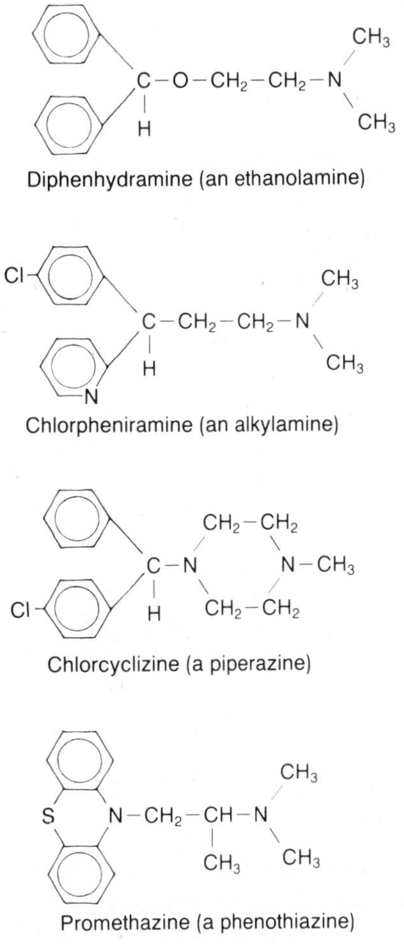

Figure 32–4 Examples of antihistamines.

TABLE 32–1   Most Often Used Antihistamines (H₁-Receptor Blocking Agents) by Class, Nonproprietary Name, Brand Name, Routes of Administration

Ethanolamines
  Diphenhydramine (Benadryl®)
    oral, parenteral
  Dimenhydrinate (Dramamine®, Gravol®)
    oral, rectal, parenteral

Ethylenediamines
  Tripelennamine (Pyribenzamine®)
    oral, topical
  Antazoline (Antistine®)
    oral
  Naphazoline (Privine®)
    nasal

Alkylamines
  Chlorpheniramine (Chlor-Tripolon®)
    oral, parenteral
  Brompheniramine (Dimetane®)
    oral

Piperazines
  Cyclizine (Marzine®)
    oral, rectal, parenteral
  Meclizine (Antivert®, Bonamine®)
    oral

Phenothiazine
  Promethazine (Phenergan®)
    oral, rectal, parenteral

Piperidine
  Astemizole (Hismanal®)
    oral
  Loratadine (Claridin®)
    oral
  Terfenadine (Seldane®)
    oral

histamine receptor sites on target cells, while the differences are such as to render them inactive as histamine substitutes, *i.e.*, they are competitive blockers of histamine. This can be demonstrated with isolated tissues *in vitro*.

In vivo, conventional antihistamines, *i.e.*, H₁-receptor blockers, antagonize all the actions of histamine, except the stimulation of HCl secretion in the stomach and that part of the vasodilatation that is mediated by H₂ receptors.

Pharmacokinetics

All H₁-receptor blockers are well absorbed following oral administration, and maximum serum levels are achieved within 1–2 hours. The bioavailability is high, except that of rectally administered preparations, which depend on too many variables to be predictably absorbed. They are distributed in all tissues including the CNS. Plasma protein binding is variable. The major site

of biotransformation of all antihistaminic drugs is the liver, and minute amounts of the unchanged drugs and most of the metabolites are excreted in the urine. The average plasma half-life is 4–6 hours, except that of meclizine, which is 12–24 hours.

Pharmacologic Effects

Antihistamines offer almost complete protection against the effects of injected histamine, but their effectiveness is less complete against endogenously liberated histamine. The histamine-induced contraction of gastrointestinal or respiratory smooth muscle is diminished or abolished both *in vivo* and *in vitro*. The H₁ receptor-mediated component of increased capillary permeability and vasodilatation is inhibited, especially if the antihistamine is administered before liberation of, or exposure to, histamine. (Full clinical effects of astemizole develop only after 2–3 days of medication.) Salivary, lacrimal, and bronchial secretions are reduced or arrested if the activity of the glands was due to excessive histamine stimulation.

The H₁-receptor blockers have limited effectiveness in severe allergic or anaphylactic reactions. In serious cases, or in the presence of laryngeal edema, adrenaline remains the drug of choice.

The effects of H₁-receptor blockers on the CNS are unpredictable. Most often they cause CNS depression, but in some patients agitation or restlessness may occur. The pharmacologic effect involved in the prevention of motion sickness is not fully understood, and not all H₁ blockers are equally effective against motion sickness.

Additional and Adverse Effects

With the exception of astemizole, loratadine, and terfenadine, all antihistamines have some **CNS depressant** effects. Some are good sedatives or hypnotics (*e.g.*, promethazine, which has a phenothiazine nucleus). Others have antitussive properties (*e.g.*, diphenhydramine). The relative prominence of these effects varies from one antihistamine to another.

All antihistamines have **local anaesthetic** activity, and some are quite potent in this respect. The dimethylaminoethanol group, either in ester or ether linkage, is common to the local anaesthetics and to many antihistamines (*see* Chapter 10).

Like the local anaesthetics, and like deanol (diethylaminoethanol), the antihistamines in high doses cause central stimulation and may cause convulsions, as may sometimes be observed in attempted suicide with antihistamines.

Also like the local anaesthetics, and like procainamide and quinidine (which also share the dialkylamino ethyl group), the antihistamines are cardiac depressants when given in high dosage.

Some of the antihistamines, and especially those in which X = O (*see* Fig. 32–3), are potent **anticholinergics**. If the acetyl group in acetylcholine is replaced by progressively larger groups, the acetylcholine-like action becomes less and less, and it is finally converted into an anticholinergic effect. Benzilic acid esters of choline (*e.g.*, oxyphenonium) are good examples. Oxygen-containing antihistamines have a chemical resemblance to these choline esters, which suggests a basis for this anticholinergic activity.

Some antihistamines, especially the phenothiazine derivatives, are adrenergic blockers, while others have a weak ganglioplegic effect.

Thus, all antihistaminic drugs have adverse effects to some degree. It is obvious that the side effects differ for different drugs, because they derive from chemical features other than those responsible for antihistaminic action. It is also worth noting that the incidence and severity of side effects varies greatly between individual subjects. Therefore, in prescribing a given antihistamine, it is essential to know the particular constellation of side effects for that drug, and to expect that about one person in four will experience some bothersome reaction during antihistamine therapy.

The most frequently observed side effect common to all histamine antagonists is **sedation**. Other untoward reactions, including dizziness, tinnitus, lassitude, incoordination, fatigue, blurred vision, and tremors, are referable to central actions of the antihistamines. Some side effects involve the digestive tract (loss of appetite, nausea), and these drugs may cause dryness of the mouth (atropine-like effect). All of these troublesome symptoms may or may not disappear with continued therapy.

The most recently introduced antihistaminic drugs, astemizole, loratadine, and terfenadine are claimed to be free from CNS-related or other side effects. In addition, they do not appear to intensify the CNS-depressant effects of other drugs or alcohol.

The antihistamines can themselves evoke allergic reactions, presumably by acting as haptens that combine with some tissue protein to form antigen complexes. The usual drug allergies, including agranulocytosis and chronic dermatoses, are thus occasionally produced by these drugs, especially if used topically or intermittently, as against the common cold, in which they have relatively little beneficial effect.

Interactions of antihistamines with other drugs can have serious consequences. They potentiate the central effects of all other CNS depressant drugs including alcohol. Patients taking antihistamines, even if one dose only, should be warned not to drink alcohol, or to drive, or to operate dangerous machinery while under the influence of the drug. The use of antihistamines, as in cough and cold preparations, is generally not a mitigating factor in impaired driving charges.

Acute Poisoning

Although the margin of safety of antihistamines is relatively high, and chronic toxicity is rare, acute poisoning with these drugs is not uncommon, especially in young children.

In acute poisoning, central effects predominate and are the greatest danger. The syndrome includes hallucinations, excitement, ataxia, and convulsions. The latter are difficult to control. In the child, the picture includes fixed dilated pupils with a flushed face and fever, and is remarkably similar to that of atropine poisoning. If untreated, deepening coma and cardiorespiratory collapse may lead to death within a few hours. In the adult, fever and flushing are less severe, and drowsiness and coma often precede the excitatory (convulsive) phase. Since there is no specific therapy for antihistamine poisoning, treatment is generally symptomatic and supportive.

Therapeutic Applications

Suppression of Allergic Phenomena

Antihistamines give good results in nasal allergies (hay fever), acute skin reactions (urticaria, drug rashes), and systemic allergic reactions (serum sickness, transfusion reactions, *etc.*), but they are almost without effect against asthma and chronic skin allergies. Perhaps it is a matter of the ability of these drugs to penetrate to the sites of endogenous release of histamine and other "autacoids" (5-HT, prostaglandins, *etc.*). It is also conceivable that different and as yet unrecognized receptor variants are involved.

Antiparkinsonian Use

Atropine and various synthetic atropine-like drugs have an antiparkinsonian effect that generally parallels their anticholinergic activity. The oxygen-containing antihistamines, which have anticholinergic side effects as already noted, also have useful antiparkinsonian properties. Orphenadrine is used almost exclusively for this purpose. It is more useful, possibly, in the short-term treatment of parkinsonian symptoms that may occur as a side effect of phenothiazine neuroleptic therapy, than in the long-term treatment of postencephalitic parkinsonism, because the drug tends to lose its effectiveness after a few months.

Anti-Motion-Sickness Use

Nausea and vomiting can result from several different types of stimuli. The phenothiazine neuroleptics are effective suppressants of the chemoreceptor trigger zone, but they do not block the effects of vestibular stimuli. Some, but not all, antihistamines do prevent or diminish nausea and vomiting mediated by both the vestibular and the chemoreceptor pathways. Among the most effective ones are promethazine, cyclizine, meclizine, and dimenhydrinate. These are different chemical types, with different side effects, so that the antiemetic action appears to be independent of the antihistaminic and other actions mentioned before. More recent preparations, including trimethobenzamide and diphenidol, are claimed to be highly effective against emesis due to both vestibular and chemoreceptor stimuli, yet with negligible antihistaminic, sedative, and anticholinergic properties.

Most recent approaches to the control of hyperemesis of multifactorial origin also employ other agents. Nabilone (Cesamet®), a cannabinoid antiemetic used in cancer chemotherapy to control nausea and vomiting, affects the cerebral cortex and has sedative and psychotropic properties. Transderm-V®, a thin multilayer circular film containing 1.5 mg scopolamine, is applied to the skin behind the ear approximately 12 hours before an antiemetic effect is required. There is a sustained absorption of scopolamine for about 3 days while the tape is in contact with the skin. Scopolamine produces all the side effects of atropine (see Chapter 15).

HISTAMINE H$_2$-RECEPTOR BLOCKERS

The chemical structure for some of the H$_2$-receptor blocking agents is very closely related to that of histamine. They have very little if any affinity for H$_1$ receptors. Unfortunately, the first two agents (burimamide and metiamide) that were found to be clinically effective in blocking the stimulatory effects of histamine and of pentagastrin on gastric HCl secretion may cause agranulocytosis; therefore their use has been discontinued. However, safer new drugs are now in use.

Cimetidine

Mechanism of Action

This drug acts on H$_2$ receptors located in stomach, blood vessels, and other sites in the body. It is a competitive antagonist of histamine, and its effect is fully reversible. It has no affinity for H$_1$ or other known receptors.

Cimetidine (Tagamet®, Peptol®) (Fig. 32–5) completely inhibits gastric acid secretion induced by histamine, gastrin, or pentagastrin; that induced by acetylcholine or bethanechol is only partly inhibited. In therapeutic concentrations it inhibits gastric HCl secretion in all phases following solid, liquid, or sham food feeding, or after insulin and caffeine administration. Extremely

high doses paradoxically facilitate histamine release by blocking the H$_2$ receptor-mediated negative feedback mechanism.

Pharmacokinetics

Close to 80% of an orally administered dose is absorbed, and maximum blood concentrations appear in 1–1.5 hours. The therapeutic plasma concentration is about 2 μmol/L. It is unevenly distributed in the various organs of the body, it crosses the placental barrier, but it does not cross the blood–brain barrier easily because of its high water solubility. It can be found in the CSF in concentrations about 30% of those in plasma. Less than 25% is bound to plasma proteins. Cimetidine has two major metabolites, which are excreted in urine together with about 50% of unchanged drug. The serum half-life is short, about 1–1.5 hours, but longer in renal failure.

Adverse Effects

The adverse effects of cimetidine are usually minor and are mainly associated with the reduced gastric juice production. Confusion, hallucinations, dizziness, or other CNS-related side effects may occur primarily in the elderly or following prolonged administration, as for Zollinger-Ellison syndrome, a chronic gastric hypersecretory state. Endocrinologic side effects include gyne-

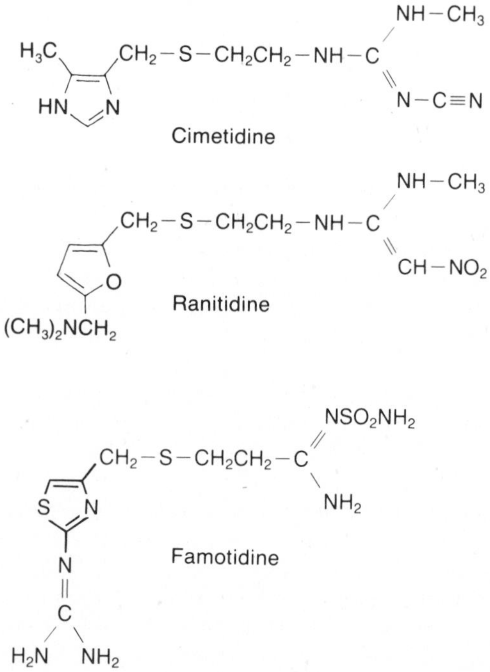

Figure 32–5 Structural formulae of cimetidine, ranitidine, and famotidine.

comastia, galactorrhea, and reduced sperm count. Cimetidine is practically nontoxic, even following accidental overdose of 10 g or so. The heart rate may be increased, probably as a reflex response to mild reductions in blood pressure. Cimetidine reduces the rate of hepatic cytochrome P-450-dependent biotransformation of a number of drugs. It also may competitively inhibit the renal tubular secretion of other organic bases (e.g., procainamide). The circulating gastrin concentration is elevated during cimetidine administration.

Ranitidine

Ranitidine (Zantac®) is a very potent H_2-receptor blocker, but its chemical structure is different from that of histamine or other antihistamines; the imidazole ring is replaced by a furan ring (see Fig. 32-5).

Mechanism of Action; Pharmacokinetics

The mechanism and site of action, as well as the pharmacologic effects, of ranitidine are similar to those of cimetidine, but ranitidine is 5–10 times more potent. Only 50% of an orally administered dose is absorbed and maximum plasma concentration occurs 1–2 hours later. The plasma half-life is 2 hours. The distribution and plasma protein binding are similar to those of cimetidine. Ranitidine has two minor metabolites, which are excreted in urine, but most of the drug is eliminated unchanged.

Adverse Effects

Adverse effects of ranitidine can not yet be fully evaluated because of the newness of the drug, but early reports indicate that gastrointestinal complaints are few and that CNS side effects are rare. Drug interactions at the renal or hepatic level are less frequent than with cimetidine. Endocrine-related symptoms have not been reported. Ranitidine is considered to be practically nontoxic.

Famotidine

Famotidine (Pepcid®), another member of the group of very potent H_2-receptor blockers, has a thiazole ring in place of the imidazole (see Fig. 32-5).

Mechanism of Action; Pharmacokinetics

The mechanism of action, pharmacologic effects, site of action, indications, and clinical use are the same as for the other H_2-receptor antagonists. Famotidine is 3–20 times as potent as ranitidine. Less than 45% of an oral dose is absorbed, with maximum plasma concentration occurring 1–3 hours later. The plasma half-

life is 2.5–3.5 hours in patients with normal kidney function; but with creatinine clearance of less than 10 mL/min the elimination half-life can be 12 hours or longer, and 20 hours or more in anuric patients. About 30% of an oral dose and 65–70% of an intravenous dose is eliminated in the urine unchanged, and the rest is eliminated as an S-oxide metabolite. The recommended single daily dose of 20–40 mg at bedtime inhibits up to 94% of nocturnal gastric acid secretion, and 25–30% for another 8–10 hours later. The nocturnal intragastric pH is between 5.0 and 6.4.

Adverse Effects

Adverse effects of famotidine observed during controlled clinical trials were few and of minor importance. The frequency of these reactions was similar to those recorded in the placebo group, and a causal relationship could not be established. Most often observed were headache, dizziness, constipation, and diarrhea. Treatment of accidental or intentional overdosage should be symptomatic and supportive. Daily doses of up to 640 mg, administered to patients with pathologic hypersecretory conditions, had no serious adverse effects. With chronic treatment, gastric emptying and exocrine pancreatic functions are not affected, but an increase in gastric bacterial flora may occur. Because adverse effects can emerge after years of extensive clinical use of new drugs, careful observation of patients treated with famotidine is advised.

Nizatidine

Nizatidine (Axid®) is the most recently approved H_2-receptor blocker for the treatment of acute duodenal and benign gastric ulcers. It is absorbed rapidly after oral administration, reaching peak serum concentrations in 0.5–3 hours. Food has no significant effect on bioavailability. About 35% is protein-bound, mainly to α_1-glycoprotein. The volume of distribution is between 0.8 and 1.5 L/kg, plasma half-life is 1–2 hours, and 60% of the dose is excreted in the urine as unchanged drug. The average plasma clearance is about 50 L/hr, which can be reduced to 7–14 L/hr in anephric patients with creatinine clearance of 10 mL/min or less, giving rise to a plasma half-life of 4–11 hours. An oral dose of 300 mg at bedtime can suppress gastric acid secretion for 10–12 hours.

In short-term trials nizatidine was found to be free of hormonal interference and had no effect on the drug-metabolizing P-450 enzymes. In clinical trials the frequency of observed side effects such as headache, somnolence, and pruritus was somewhat higher than in the placebo group, but a relationship to nizatidine administration could not be established. Serum cholesterol, serum uric acid, serum creatinine, and platelet and WBC counts showed statistically significant differences from the placebo group, but the clinical importance of these changes is not clear.

AUTACOIDS

Clinical Uses of H$_2$-Receptor Blockers

Therapeutic applications of these agents are identical. H$_2$-receptor blockers are useful in the treatment of conditions that require a reduction of gastric acid secretion, such as treatment of duodenal ulcer, nonmalignant gastric ulcer, gastroesophageal reflux disease, pathologic hypersecretion states associated with Zollinger-Ellison syndrome, systemic mastocytosis, and multiple endocrine adenomas. They are also described in this specific context in Chapter 50.

Tiotidine and oxmetidine, the most recently introduced histamine H$_2$-receptor blockers, are at present in the clinical trial phase; they are expected to be released shortly for general use.

SUGGESTED READING

Ash ASF, Schild HI. Receptors mediating some actions of histamine. Br J Pharmacol Chemother 1966; 27:427–439.

Beaven MA. Histamine. N Engl J Med 1976; 294:30–36, 320–325.

Black JW. Definition and antagonism of histamine H$_2$ receptors. Nature (Lond) 1972; 236:385–390.

Brimblecombe RW, Duncan WAM, Durant GJ, et al. Cimetidine—A non-thiourea H$_2$-receptor antagonist. J Int Med Res 1975; 3:86–92.

Dobrilla G, Vallaperta P, Amplatz S. Influence of ulcer healing agents on ulcer relapse after discontinuation of acute treatment: a pooled estimate of controlled clinical trials. Gut 1988; 29:181–187.

Green JP, Prell GD, Khandelwal JK, Blandina P. Aspects of histamine metabolism. Agents Actions 1987; 22(1-2):1–15.

Guttmann RD, ed. Immunology. A Scope® publication. Kalamazoo, Michigan: The Upjohn Company, 1981.

Ostro MJ. Pharmacodynamics and pharmacokinetics of parenteral histamine (H$_2$)-receptor antagonists. Am J Med 1983; 74(6A):15–22 (and 5 additional articles).

Owen DA. Inflammation: histamine and 5-hydroxytryptamine. Br Med Bull 1987; 43:256–269.

Riley AJ, Salmon PR, eds. Ranitidine. Proceedings of an international symposium held in the context of the Seventh World Congress of Gastroenterology, Stockholm, 1982. Amsterdam/Oxford/Princeton: Excerpta Medica, 1982.

Rocha e Silva M, ed. Histamine: its chemistry, metabolism and physiological and pharmacological actions. Handbook of Experimental Pharmacology, Vol. 18, pt 1. Berlin: Springer-Verlag, 1966.

Rocha E, Silva M, ed. Histamine II and anti-histaminics: chemistry, metabolism and physiological and pharmacological actions. Handbook of Experimental Pharmacology, Vol. 18; pt 2. Berlin: Springer-Verlag, 1978.

Chapter 33

Anti-Inflammatory Analgesics

D. Kadar

(**N.B.** Other designations for this group of drugs are: antipyretic-analgesics, anti-inflammatory agents, nonsteroidal anti-inflammatory drugs [NSAIDs], nonnarcotic analgesics.)

The beneficial effect of willow bark extract in fever and pain was known to ancient civilizations, but the first reliable description of its antipyretic effect is attributed to Rev. Edmund Stone, who was searching for an inexpensive substitute for cinchona bark in the 18th century. The active ingredient, salicin, a bitter glycoside, was isolated in 1827, and various derivatives were later found in other plants. Acetylsalicylic acid (ASA or Aspirin®) was synthesized by the Bayer Pharmaceutical Company and introduced into medicine by Dreser in 1899.

The sharp increase in the number of anti-inflammatory drugs released for medicinal use during the last 15 years can be attributed to the ease and reliability of modern *in vitro* and *in vivo* testing for the desired pharmacologic action. All of these drugs inhibit prostaglandin synthesis and prevent the development of carrageenan-induced rat paw edema (Table 33–1). With these two rather simple experimental models, hundreds of chemicals can be screened in relatively short time. Since prostaglandin synthesis is tissue- and species-specific, however, the final evaluation of the beneficial and toxic properties of such drugs requires extensive long-term experience in human subjects.

Pain is essential for survival. It can serve as a warning of impending or actual tissue or organ injury. Humans usually do not "adapt" to pain. The sensation originates from stimulation of naked nerve endings found in all parts of the body. When first-order sensory neurons from a diseased organ and from another area of the body synapse on the same second-order neurons in the spinal cord, pain actually originating in the diseased organ may be perceived as coming from the other area; this is known as "referred pain." The pain receptors (nociceptors) can be stimulated by mechanical or chemical means. Pain-producing substances such as histamine or kinins stimulate the naked nerve endings directly, while prostaglandins lower the pain threshold by increasing the sensitivity of the receptors to the stimulus.

The sensation of pain is transmitted from the periphery through the spinal cord to higher integrative centres in the CNS by "fast" myelinated Aδ fibres at 10–30 m/sec, and by nonmyelinated "slow" C fibres

TABLE 33–1 Comparison of Prostaglandin Synthetase Inhibitory Activity and Anti-inflammatory Potency of Selected Non-narcotic Analgesics

Drug	Inhibition (ID_{50}) of Prostaglandin Synthetase (μg/mL)	Reduction (ED_{50}) of Carrageenan-Induced Rat Paw Edema (mg/kg)
Indomethacin	0.06	6.5
Piroxicam	0.06	4.0
Mefenamic acid	0.17	55.0
Phenylbutazone	2.23	100.0
ASA	6.62	150.0
Acetaminophen	100	inactive

at 0.5–2 m/sec. The intensity of the sensation can be influenced by distraction (*e.g.*, "white noise"), hypnosis, placebo or suggestion, acupuncture, local anaesthetics, nerve section, or analgesic drugs. Anxiolytics and neuroleptics may interfere with the emotional response to pain through action on the limbic system and hypothalamus. Morphine and other narcotic analgesics act on opiate receptors in the gray matter around the cerebral aqueduct and adjacent to the third and fourth ventricles.

Fever is the body's response to exogenous or endogenous substances called pyrogens. Bacteria, moulds, yeasts, and viruses elaborate high-molecular-weight lipopolysaccharides capable of stimulating the release of a lipid-polypeptide complex ("pyrogen") from polymorphonuclear leukocytes and monocytes. This pyrogen acts on the hypothalamic thermoreceptive region to release arachidonic acid or stimulate prostaglandin synthesis (*see* Chapter 30) and raise the set-point of the temperature-regulating centre, which in turn will lead to vasoconstriction in the skin and increased body temperature. Fever arising from extensive tissue damage, autoimmune disease, neoplasia, or following thromboembolism is thought to be due to the release of a leukocyte-like pyrogen from the involved tissue. Antipyretic drugs appear to act by inhibiting prostaglandin synthesis or release in the thermoregulatory centre. The cerebroventricular administration of type E prostaglandin causes fever in experimental animals.

The **inflammatory process** can be initiated by invading microorganisms, immunologic reactions, tissue decay, and many other less known phenomena. Mediators of inflammation are thought to cause increased release of fatty acid precursors of prostaglandin synthesis and to increase the rate of prostaglandin synthesis. Prostaglandins may cause inflammation on their own, or they may aggravate a preexisting inflammatory condition. Endogenous mediators of inflammation may originate from plasma (bradykinin, C_3 and C_5 fragments, $C_{\overline{567}}$ complex, fibrinopeptides, fibrin degradation products) and from tissues (histamine, 5-HT, leukotrienes [SRS-A], prostaglandins, lysosomal proteases, migration inhibitory factor, chemotactic factors, lymphotoxin, skin reactive factors, mitogenic factors, lymph node permeability factor). Endogenous pyrogens and leukocytosis factors may be liberated, causing redness and swelling, with heat and pain and disturbed function of the involved organ. Practically every part of the body may suffer damage as the result of an inflammatory process. Drugs do not reverse the damage, but they may arrest the process or slow its progress. In addition, the intensity of the pain may be significantly reduced or eliminated. Most prostaglandins are known to cause peripheral vasodilatation with local redness and edema formation. Anti-inflammatory drugs reduce pain and tissue damage by inhibiting prostaglandin synthesis (*see* Table 33–1). In addition, these drugs may inhibit or slow down the phagocytic activity of poly-

morphonuclear leukocytes and stabilize lysosomal membranes. The composition, biosynthesis, or metabolism of connective tissue mucopolysaccharides can also be affected.

The suppression of antigen-antibody reactions by anti-inflammatory drugs may be due to depressed antibody production, interference with antigen-antibody reactions, reduced histamine release, or membrane stabilization.

SALICYLATES

Acetylsalicylic acid (ASA; Aspirin® is a proprietary name in Canada, but aspirin is nonproprietary elsewhere) is the most often used member of this class of drug. The others are salicylic acid, sodium salicylate, choline salicylate, choline magnesium salicylate, salicylamide, methylsalicylate, and diflunisal. The chemical structures of salicylic acid, ASA, and diflunisal are shown in Figure 33–1.

Mechanism and Site of Action

The analgesic, antipyretic, and anti-inflammatory actions of salicylates are attributed primarily to their ability to inhibit prostaglandin synthesis in the periphery and at the thermoregulatory centre. In addition, salicylates may inhibit plasmin, and thereby bradykinin, formation. Chemoreceptors that are stimulated by kinins to produce pain are blocked by salicylates.

Pharmacokinetics

Orally administered ASA is absorbed by passive diffusion, partly in the stomach but to a large extent also

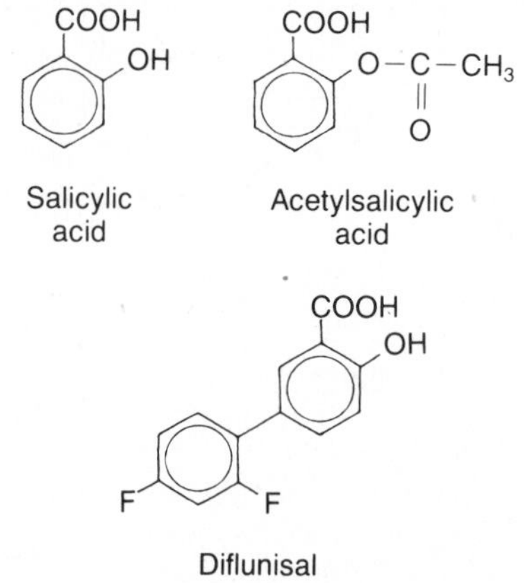

Figure 33–1 Structural formulae of salicylates.

in the small intestine. The absorption of all acidic drugs including the salicylates is influenced by the pH of the aqueous layer near the mucous membrane. In the stomach, at low pH, absorption is enhanced because the uncharged molecules of weakly acidic drugs are able to penetrate lipid membranes with relative ease. In the intestines, at almost neutral pH, the greater solubility in water aids in the dispersal of these drugs on the absorbing surface, thereby enhancing absorption. (Frequently observed gastric mucosal cell erosion could be due in part to intracellular trapping of the ionized salicylate at intracellular pH.) Rectal absorption is slow and unreliable. Salicylates, especially methylsalicylate, are absorbed through the intact skin.

After oral administration of the usual therapeutic doses, absorption is estimated to be better than 90%. Enteric-coated preparations are designed to release the drug at the pH of the small intestine. Occasionally the acid-resistant coating fails to dissolve and the intact tablet is found in the feces. The amount of drug available for absorption from delayed-release preparations is greatly influenced by gastrointestinal motility.

Salicylates are unevenly distributed in the body. High levels of ASA are found in organs of the central compartment, such as blood, renal cortex, and liver, and considerably less (one-sixth to one-tenth that of the plasma concentration) in other sites, such as brain, spinal fluid, muscle, intestine, aqueous humor, lens, and semen. The synovial fluid taken from an inflamed joint contains about five times the plasma concentration of free ASA, and the half-life of the drug is considerably longer in synovial fluid. Salicylates cross the placenta and appear in the milk, including cow milk. Salicylate competes with other drugs and bilirubin for serum albumin binding sites.

The liver is the principal site of salicylate biotransformation by the microsomal and mitochondrial enzymes. ASA is first hydrolysed to salicylic acid and then converted to salicyluric acid, salicylic phenolic glucuronide, acyl glucuronide, and gentisic acid. The biotransformation process is saturable when toxic amounts are present.

The metabolites, along with a fraction of the unchanged salicylic acid, are excreted in the urine. Excretion of the unchanged drug is enhanced by sodium bicarbonate administration, because at alkaline pH the ionized drug cannot back-diffuse from the renal tubules. This procedure is especially useful to hasten excretion after an overdose.

The plasma half-life of ASA is about 15 minutes. That of salicylic acid is longer and dose-dependent, being about 2–3 hours after a 600-mg dose and 6–12 hours after larger doses. At therapeutic doses the elimination follows first-order kinetics, but after toxic doses the elimination follows a mixed order because of enzyme saturation, and the plasma half-life may increase to 15–30 hours.

Diflunisal, the most recently introduced substituted salicylic acid derivative, has powerful analgesic and anti-inflammatory activity (by inhibition of prostaglandin synthesis), but mild and unreliable antipyretic properties. It is completely absorbed after oral administration and distributed similarly to ASA, and has a plasma half-life of 8–12 hours. Diflunisal has dose-dependent pharmacokinetics, and doubling the dose more than doubles the plasma concentration. Steady state is achieved only after several days of administration. More than 99% is bound to plasma proteins, and up to 7% of the total plasma concentration may appear in human milk. Most of the drug is conjugated with glucuronic acid in the liver before excretion in the urine. (The pharmacokinetics of salicylates are summarized in Table 33–2.)

Pharmacologic Effects

Analgesia

Low-intensity pain, such as headache, myalgia, arthralgia, and other pain arising from integumental structures rather than from viscera, is alleviated by salicylates. Part of the analgesia arises from actions on subcortical sites of the CNS, probably the hypothalamus, because at therapeutic concentrations mental function or alertness is not affected. In contrast to the narcotic analgesics, these drugs do not produce tolerance or physical dependence (see Chapter 22) during chronic administration. In addition, salicylates act on peripheral chemoreceptors and alleviate the pain induced by exogenously administered bradykinin. Prostaglandin synthesis is blocked because of cyclooxygenase inhibition; therefore the sensitivity of the receptors to pain-producing substances is greatly reduced. Paradoxically, salicylates cause headache in toxic overdose. ASA is frequently combined with codeine or other narcotic analgesics and sedatives; such combinations are claimed to give more pain relief with less toxicity than any of the ingredients given alone in effective doses, although this claim has not been clearly proven yet. The analgesic dose range is between 0.3 and 1 g, three or four times a day.

Antipyresis

Salicylates lower the body temperature in febrile patients by a direct action on the hypothalamic thermoreceptive region and the temperature-regulating centre concerned with heat production and heat loss. Normal body temperature is not affected by therapeutic doses. The increased heat loss produced in febrile patients is due to peripheral vasodilatation, especially in cutaneous areas, and to increased sweating. Sweating is important but not essential in this process, because the administration of atropine (which prevents sweating; see Chapter 15) does not prevent salicylates from lowering the elevated temperature. Heat production is not inhibited, and toxic doses of salicylates actually produce fever. The mechanism of antipyretic action is not known for certain, but it appears that antipyret-

TABLE 33–2 Recommended Dosages and Known Pharmacokinetic Data for the Described Anti-inflammatory Analgesics

Generic Name	Trade Name	Recommended Daily Dose (mg)	Serum Half-Life (hours)	Protein Binding (%)	V_d (L/kg)	Biotransformation	Excretion
Salicylates							
Acetylsalicylic acid (ASA)	Aspirin*, etc.	325–10³	0.2†	80	0.1–0.35	Hyd Con Oxi	Ren
Sodium salicylate		350–10³	2–30	80	0.1–0.35	Con Oxi	Ren
Choline salicylate	Arthropan	1000–7000	2–30	80	0.1–0.35	Con Oxi	Ren
Choline magnesium salicylate	Trilisate	1000–3000	2–30	80	0.1–0.35	Con Oxi	Ren
Salicylamide	In mixtures	200–1000	2			Con Oxi	Ren
Diflunisal	Dolobid	500–1000	8–12	99	0.09	Con	Ren
Para-aminophenol							
Acetaminophen	Tylenol, etc.	325–3900	1–5	10	1.0	Con Oxi	Ren
Pyrazolones							
Phenylbutazone	Butazolidin	300–800	36–168	98	0.08	Oxi Con	Ren Bil
Oxyphenbutazone	Tandearil	50–200	24–72	98	0.08	Con	Ren Bil
Sulfinpyrazone	Anturan	200–800	3–8	98	0.16	Oxi Con	Ren
Indoles							
Indomethacin	Indocid, Indocin	50–200	6–12	90	1.0	Oxi Con	Ren Bil
Sulindac (Indene)	Clinoril	150–400	7†	93†	Not avail.	Oxi Red	Ren Bil
Phenylpropionic acids							
Fenoprofen	Nalfon	900–2400	2.5	99	0.08	Oxi Con	Ren
Flurbiprofen	Ansaid	150–200	4	99	0.1	Oxi Con	Ren
Ibuprofen	Motrin, Rufen	600–2400	2	99	0.12	Oxi Con	Ren Bil
Ketoprofen	Orudis	100–200	1–35	94	0.1	Oxi Con	Ren
Tiaprofenic acid	Surgam	600–1800	1.7	99	0.1	Unchanged	Ren
Naphthylpropionic acids							
Naproxen	Naprosyn	500–1000 }	12–15	99	0.1–0.35	Dem	Ren
Naproxen sodium	Anaprox	825–1375 }					
Anthranilic acids							
Meclofenamate	Meclomen	300–600	4	99	Not avail.	Oxi Con	Ren Bil
Mefenamic acid	Ponstan	1000	4	99	Not avail.	Oxi Hyx	Ren Bil
Floctafenine	Idarac	600–1200	8	99	Not avail.	Oxi Con	Ren Bil
Pyrrole-acetic acid							
Tolmetin	Tolectin	600–1800	1–6	99	0.1	Con Hyx	Ren
Phenyl-acetic acid							
Diclofenac sodium	Voltaren	75–150	1–2	99	0.13	Con	Ren Bil
Oxicam							
Piroxicam	Feldene	20	35–45	99	0.12	Hyx Con Hyd	Ren

* In Canada only.

† See text for variations.

Abbreviations: Con = conjugation; Dem = demethylation; Hyd = hydrolysis; Hyx = hydroxylation; Oxi = oxidation; Red = reduction; Ren = renal; Bil = biliary.

ics block pyrogen-induced prostaglandin synthesis. The antipyretic dose range is similar to analgesic doses.

Effects on Rheumatic, Inflammatory, and Immunologic Processes

Salicylates in large doses (5–8 g daily) are used for the treatment of rheumatoid diseases and other inflammatory conditions. The increased capillary permeability during inflammation is reduced by salicylates, thereby preventing edema formation, cellular exudation, and pain. One or all of the following may contribute to this effect: (1) inhibition of prostaglandin biosynthesis (there is a fair correlation between the *in vitro* prostaglandin synthetase inhibition and anti-inflammatory potency); (2) inhibition of leukocyte migration and phagocytosis, during which histamine, 5-HT, and other substances (autacoids), may often be released; (3) stabilization of lysosomal membranes, thus preventing the escape of lysosomal enzymes into the cytoplasm, and damage to cell structures; and (4) inhibition of plasmin, a plasma proteolytic enzyme, which may activate kinin formation.

Uricosuric Effect

Salicylates in doses of 0.5 g inhibit both the tubular secretion of uric acid and the uricosuric effect of probenecid and sulfinpyrazone by competition for the same tubular transport systems. In large doses of 5–10 g daily, however, the tubular reabsorption of uric acid is also inhibited by competition with uric acid for more distal active transport sites in the tubule. The net effect of the larger doses is that most of the uric acid filtered by the glomeruli is excreted and the uric acid concentration in the blood is lowered. When this happens, the urate crystals already deposited in joints (in cases of gout) are slowly eliminated.

Additional and Adverse Effects

Respiration

Salicylates in medium or large therapeutic doses directly stimulate the respiratory centre, leading to respiratory alkalosis that is normally compensated by increased urinary bicarbonate elimination. In toxic doses salicylates cause respiratory depression and a combination of uncompensated respiratory and metabolic acidosis.

Gastrointestinal

Epigastric distress, nausea, and vomiting are quite common. Exacerbation of peptic ulcer symptoms, gastrointestinal hemorrhage, and blood loss occur in overly sensitive patients on prolonged salicylate therapy. Pain of gastritis (e.g., from alcohol excess) should not be treated with salicylates because of the danger of bleeding. Microscopic bleeding is almost universal in patients receiving salicylates. All anti-inflammatory drugs have the potential to cause damage to the gastrointestinal tract. Weakly acidic drugs, for which salicylate is a prototype, may be trapped intracellularly in high concentrations because at intracellular pH the ionized form predominates. This is similar to gastritis following excessive vinegar consumption. Also, because prostaglandins are essential to maintain cellular integrity in the gastrointestinal tract, inhibition of prostaglandin synthesis may lead to damage of gastrointestinal epithelium. (Corticosteroids, which are powerful anti-inflammatory drugs but are not acidic and do not inhibit prostaglandin synthesis, also cause gastric ulceration on long-term use for different reasons, possibly related to their protein antianabolic action.)

Blood

Large doses of salicylates administered over a prolonged period of time shorten erythrocyte survival and interfere with iron metabolism. In addition, the plasma prothrombin level is reduced, and anticoagulants may have to be given in reduced dosage during salicy-late therapy. Since ASA acetylates the active site of cyclooxygenase responsible for prostaglandin endoperoxide synthesis and subsequent thromboxane synthesis in platelets, platelet aggregation is inhibited and the bleeding time is prolonged. Platelets cannot synthesize protein; therefore this action is irreversible.

Metabolic Processes

Oxidative phosphorylation is inhibited by large doses of salicylates, and the energy normally used for ATP production is dissipated as heat. This explains the pyretic effect of toxic overdose. The occasionally observed hyperglycemia may be the result of increased adrenaline* release through activation of central sympathetic centres, and increased glucose-6-phosphatase activity. Salicylates are also known to cause hypoglycemia, probably by increased utilization of glucose and inhibition of gluconeogenesis.

Endocrine Functions

In addition to stimulating adrenaline release, ASA increases plasma adrenocorticosteroid levels by stimulating the hypothalamus to increase the release of ACTH. It also interferes with the binding of thyroid hormones by competition for binding sites on plasma proteins. This effect leads to higher tissue uptake of thyroxine and triiodothyronine, which may contribute to the higher metabolic rate seen with overdoses of salicylates.

Pregnancy

ASA may cause a variety of sometimes serious difficulties if ingested in large enough dosage during critical periods of early gestation. Some data show a strong correlation between consumption of large doses of ASA during the first 16 weeks of pregnancy and the incidence of fetal malformations. If taken regularly during the last trimester it may contribute to prolonged gestation, prolonged labor, and increased maternal blood loss during delivery. There is no evidence, however, that occasional use of small doses of ASA during pregnancy is harmful.

Hypersensitivity

The incidence is about 5%. True allergy is estimated at less than 1%. It is usually manifested as bronchoconstriction, urticaria, or angioneurotic edema; fatal anaphylactic shock is rare. Many patients sensitive to salicylates also may be sensitive to the other anti-inflammatory drugs and tartrazine, a yellow dye used in numerous pharmaceutical preparations. Some foods and beverages containing salicylate, such as curry powder, paprika, licorice, Benedictine liqueur, prunes, raisins, gherkins, and tea, may contribute to allergic reactions.

---

* epinephrine

AUTACOIDS

Drug Interactions

The combination of salicylates with oral anticoagulants or heparin can lead to hemorrhage for reasons already mentioned.

Absorbed ASA is hydrolysed to salicylic acid, and about 80% is bound to serum albumin. Other drugs that are also bound to albumin, such as sulfonamides, can be displaced by salicylates, increasing the concentration of free drug in the plasma and therefore the toxicity. For the same reason, infants with incompletely developed bilirubin-conjugating enzyme systems may develop kernicterus after salicylate administration (see Chapter 4).

The toxicity of methotrexate, a cancer chemotherapeutic agent, is increased by salicylates because they inhibit the active renal tubular secretion of methotrexate and displace the antineoplastic compound from plasma protein binding sites.

Interaction with the uricosuric effects of probenecid and sulfinpyrazone may effectively cancel urate excretion, but this risk is very small with the occasional use of ASA for headache, etc.

Increased gastrointestinal blood loss following simultaneous ingestion of alcohol and ASA is probably due to additive but independent effects of the two agents on the gastric mucosa.

Ammonium chloride, acid sodium phosphate, and ascorbic acid may acidify the urine and increase the reabsorption of salicylic acid. The resultant cumulation can be hazardous with large ASA doses.

Antacids may reduce the rate of ASA absorption from the stomach by increasing the pH of the gastric juice, but the increased gastric emptying may make more drug available for intestinal absorption.

The interaction of oral hypoglycemic agents and ASA is complex; the plasma concentration of both drugs may increase through competition for plasma protein binding sites and interference with urinary elimination.

ASA increases the plasma half-life of penicillin because it competes with penicillin for the active transport (secretory) mechanism in the renal tubules.

Toxicity

Children are particularly prone to salicylate intoxication. Salicylism, a mild form of intoxication, is characterized by headache, dizziness, mental confusion, tinnitus, nausea, and vomiting. Marked hyperventilation is also present, resulting from the direct stimulatory effect of salicylates on the respiratory centre. Prolonged hyperventilation leads to respiratory alkalosis, but compensatory increases in sodium and potassium bicarbonate excretion may produce a slight improvement in the condition of the patient. The improvement is only temporary if a large dose was ingested. Serum salicylate concentration and pH should be measured to indicate the type of procedure required for further treatment.

If the dose is large enough, and the condition remains untreated, the preceding symptoms are followed by respiratory and metabolic acidosis, restlessness, delirium, hallucinations, convulsions, coma, and death from respiratory failure. The respiratory acidosis is caused by respiratory depression and subsequent CO_2 accumulation. The metabolic acidosis is caused by reduction of bicarbonate (salicylates are acidic) and derangement of carbohydrate metabolism.

Symptomatic treatment is sufficient in mild cases of poisoning. Increasing the pH of the urine will enhance salicylate elimination. In serious cases intravenous administration of fluids, frequent measurement and correction of acid-base and electrolyte imbalance, and hemodialysis or peritoneal dialysis are mandatory.

The occurrence of nephropathy following long-term analgesic therapy is not rare, and many patients who suffer from analgesic-induced nephropathy may go on to require long-term hemodialysis. The mechanism for the development of this toxicity is not clear. The formation of a reactive metabolite that depletes glutathione and binds to cellular macromolecules in the renal tubules may only partly explain the observed cell damage. ASA may cause transient shedding of renal tubular cells, alteration in excretion, and reduced glomerular filtration with subsequent water, sodium, and potassium retention. Patients with active systemic lupus erythematosus, advanced liver cirrhosis, and chronic renal insufficiency appear to be most at risk. Prostaglandins have an important role in the maintenance of cellular integrity and renal blood circulation. Inhibition of prostaglandin synthesis may cause renal vascular constriction and alteration in vasomotion. Most patients with analgesic nephropathy are middle-aged women with histories of peptic ulcer, anemia, psychiatric disorders, headaches, and arthralgias. If the renal abnormalities are diagnosed early, the condition may stabilize or improve after drug withdrawal.

The recently observed increase in the number of infants and young children suffering from Reye's syndrome (an often fatal fulminating hepatitis with cerebral edema following a prodromal viral infection) has been attributed to the indiscriminate use of antipyretic medication. Although other factors also have been implicated, this highlights some of the risks of prescribing antipyretics, especially for children.

Therapeutic Applications

Sodium salicylate, choline salicylate (available in liquid formulation), choline magnesium salicylate, and ASA are used as antipyretics, analgesics, and for the treatment of gout, acute rheumatic fever, and rheumatic arthritis. ASA also inhibits platelet aggregation irreversibly. Salicylic acid is used topically as a keratolytic agent (corns and calluses) and for the treatment of epidermophytosis and hyperhidrosis. Salicylamide is included in a number of over-the-counter analgesic and sedative preparations, but its effect is not reliable.

Methylsalicylate is a colorless or yellowish liquid used in liniments for cutaneous counterirritation. It is the most toxic salicylate; one teaspoonful (4 g) may cause death in children.

Extensive clinical trials involving several thousands of patients were carried out to determine the beneficial effect of ASA, administered alone or in combination with dipyridamole, for the prevention or treatment (secondary prevention) of cerebral thrombosis (which causes strokes) and coronary thrombosis (which causes heart attacks). In most cases the results showed that the mortality rates of the treated and placebo groups were not significantly different, but that the rate of re-infarction was significantly reduced by drug treatment. The inability to define precisely the etiology of the disorders is seen to be partly responsible for the equivocal results and interpretation. On the other hand, ASA administration was found to be beneficial in the prevention of strokes in patients who experience transient ischemic attacks and visual disturbances prior to fully developed strokes (*see also* Chapter 41).

Diflunisal is recommended for the relief of mild to moderate pain accompanied by inflammation in conditions such as musculoskeletal trauma, pain after dental extraction, postepisiotomy pain, and osteoarthritis. It has a slow onset (2–4 hours for maximum analgesia) and long duration of action (8–12 hours). Only large doses inhibit platelet function, and the inhibition is reversible. Diflunisal in daily doses of 500 mg or more increases uric acid elimination, but on prolonged use it may cause serious fluid retention. Drug interactions may occur with oral anticoagulants, tolbutamide, diuretics, and other anti-inflammatory drugs. The most often reported side effects are gastrointestinal complaints, headache, drowsiness, cholestatic jaundice, skin eruptions, and confusion. The drug is not recommended during pregnancy or breast feeding, it should not be administered to patients with ASA hypersensitivity or allergy, and upward dose adjustments should not be made without proper instructions to the patient.

PARA-AMINOPHENOLS

The antipyretic analgesic action of **acetanilid** was discovered by accidental mixup in compounding a prescription. The drug was introduced into medicine in 1886 but abandoned several decades later because of its toxicity. **Acetaminophen** and **phenacetin** are congeners of acetanilid, with analgesic and antipyretic effects similar to those of ASA, but they have no therapeutically significant anti-inflammatory or anti-rheumatic properties. (Acetanilid and phenacetin are not used in Canada because of their toxic side effects.)

Acetaminophen

Mechanism and Site of Action

Acetaminophen (Fig. 33–2) is similar to ASA except that it is a very weak prostaglandin synthetase inhibitor *in vitro*. On the other hand, it is quite possible that the sensitivity of the enzyme is different in various parts of the body, and that significant inhibition does occur to produce analgesia and to reduce fever. In fetal lamb tissue, acetaminophen has a potency similar to that of ASA for the inhibition of prostacyclin (PGI_2) synthesis.

Pharmacokinetics

Acetaminophen is rapidly absorbed from the gastrointestinal tract, and peak plasma levels are reached in 30–60 minutes. The bioavailability is influenced by the rate of absorption, because significant first-pass biotransformation takes place in the luminal cells of the intestine and in the hepatocytes. From ordinary doses of less than 1 g, only 60% of the drug will reach the central compartment in active form. From doses greater than 1 g, up to 90% or more is available for distribution after absorption. The drug diffuses quickly into most tissues and concentrates mainly in the liver. The volume of distribution is 1 L/kg, and less than 10% is bound to plasma proteins (*see* Table 33–2).

Acetaminophen is conjugated in the liver to form inactive metabolites. Following ordinary clinical doses, 54% is conjugated with glucuronic acid, 33% with sulfuric acid, 4% with cysteine, and 5% as a mercapturic acid (*see* Chapter 4). A minor amount of acetaminophen is converted in the hepatocytes (and probably in other organs with significant cytochrome P-450 activity) to a chemically reactive intermediary metabolite. Under normal circumstances the active metabolite reacts with glutathione to form a harmless end product. Following the consumption of large doses, glutathione is depleted and the active metabolite will attach covalently to macromolecules that have an essential role in the normal biochemical processes of the cell. In some individuals this leads to liver cell death, which constitutes a very serious and life-threatening toxicity (*see* Chap-

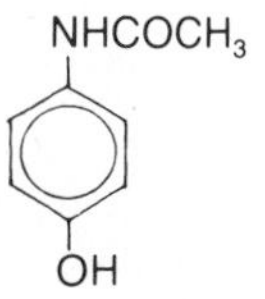

NHCOCH₃

OH

Figure 33–2 Structural formula of acetaminophen.

ter 62). Mild or moderately severe liver disease does not affect the biotransformation.

The plasma half-life of acetaminophen depends on the dose, rate of absorption, and biotransformation. The average normal half-life is 1–2 hours, which may increase to 4–5 hours following large doses or in severe hepatic insufficiency. About 2–5% of the dose is eliminated unchanged in the urine, the rest as metabolites.

Pharmacologic Effects

The antipyretic and analgesic properties of acetaminophen are very similar to those of ASA, but the duration of action is slightly shorter. The usual doses are also similar, between 0.3 and 1 g three to four times a day. It is an ideal drug for patients who suffer from gastric complaints or who cannot tolerate ASA.

Adverse Effects and Toxicity

At ordinary dosage, acetaminophen is virtually free of any significant adverse effects and has no known properties that would lead to noticeable drug interactions.

Skin rash or other minor allergic reactions occur infrequently, and minor alterations in the leukocyte count are transient. Renal tubular necrosis and hypoglycemic coma are rare complications of prolonged large-dose therapy. Renal damage is independent of hepatic toxicity. Potentially fatal hepatic necrosis may occur from overdose of 10 g or more for an adult. The reactive metabolite formed in the liver can easily deplete the normal glutathione supply and cause irreversible cell damage. In this case the administration of N-acetylcysteine can be life-saving if administered within 12–20 hours (see Chapter 62). Currently available N-acetylcysteine preparations are administered orally, but they are just as effective when administered intravenously.

Phenacetin is still marketed in a number of countries as a substitute for acetaminophen. Its pharmacologic and toxicologic properties are similar to those of acetaminophen, but in addition it may cause hemolytic anemia, methemoglobinemia, and in toxic overdose cyanosis, respiratory depression, and cardiac arrest.

PYRAZOLONES

Antipyrine and **aminopyrine** have been used extensively in the past for the treatment of rheumatic fever. In hypersensitive patients agranulocytosis occurs after aminopyrine administration; therefore its use is restricted.

Phenylbutazone and Oxyphenbutazone

Phenylbutazone (Fig. 33–3) is an antipyrine congener. Oxyphenbutazone is one of the active metabolites of phenylbutazone with all the same properties as the parent compound. They are discussed together.

Mechanism and Site of Action

Phenylbutazone inhibits prostaglandin synthesis *in vitro* and *in vivo*. In addition it stabilizes lysosomal membranes, thereby reducing the release of ribonuclease and acid phosphatase enzymes. The uricosuric effect produced by large doses is due primarily to the inhibition of uric acid reabsorption in the proximal convoluted tubules by hydroxyphenylbutazone, a metabolite of phenylbutazone.

Pharmacokinetics

Phenylbutazone is completely absorbed after oral or rectal administration, and peak plasma levels are reached after 2 hours. Due to the relatively slow biotransformation, all of the absorbed drug is available for distribution. Phenylbutazone penetrates into the synovial fluid and is distributed unevenly in body water.

Phenylbutazone is converted slowly to hydroxyphenylbutazone and oxyphenbutazone, both of which are active. The metabolites are further conjugated with glucuronic acid. The plasma half-life of phenylbutazone may vary from 36 to 168 hours in humans. In dogs and horses, elimination is much faster.

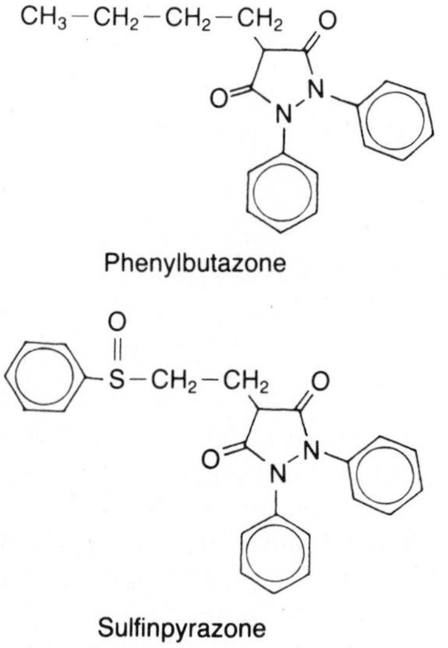

Figure 33–3 Structural formulae of pyrazolones.

Pharmacologic Effects

Phenylbutazone has powerful anti-inflammatory effects, which are comparable in magnitude to those of the adrenocorticosteroids. It is used primarily for the treatment of rheumatoid arthritis, acute gout, ankylosing spondylitis, and related disorders. The uricosuric action is due mainly to the hydroxyphenylbutazone metabolite. The analgesic and antipyretic effects are relatively weak, and the drug should not be used for these purposes because of the potential side effects. The usual daily dose is 300–800 mg.

Adverse Effects

These are primarily gastrointestinal, such as ulcerative esophagitis, acute and reactivated gastric and duodenal ulcers, ulceration of the bowel, nausea, and vomiting. Fluid and electrolyte disturbances (sodium, chloride, and water retention), allergic reactions, and renal and cardiovascular disturbances have been noted. Hearing and vision may be adversely affected in some individuals, and agitation, confusional states, and lethargy also have been reported.

Drug Interactions

These can be significant with any drug that may be displaced from binding to plasma proteins, such as other anti-inflammatory agents, oral anticoagulants, oral hypoglycemics, and sulfonamides. Phenylbutazone may cause induction of hepatic microsomal drug-metabolizing enzymes.

Toxicity

The most serious but infrequent toxic effects are fatal aplastic anemia and agranulocytosis. These may occur at any time during treatment, or when treatment is resumed after a drug-free period. Patients taking phenylbutazone should be supervised closely and should have frequent blood examinations.

Sulfinpyrazone

Sulfinpyrazone (*see* Fig. 33–3) is a phenylbutazone derivative without antirheumatic, antipyretic, analgesic, or sodium-retaining activity. It is a powerful uricosuric agent used for the treatment of chronic gout. The drug is also used to inhibit platelet aggregation in the treatment of transient ischemic attacks, thromboembolism associated with vascular or cardiac prostheses, recurrent venous thrombosis, and arteriovenous shunt thrombosis. The side effects and toxic effects of sulfinpyrazone are similar to those of phenylbutazone, the most frequent being gastrointestinal complaints. Concurrent salicylate therapy is not recommended because salicy-

lates and citrates antagonize the uricosuric effect of sulfinpyrazone, and ASA may prolong bleeding time.

Apazone

Apazone is the most recent pyrazolone derivative with analgesic, antipyretic, and anti-inflammatory properties similar to those of phenylbutazone. It is a powerful uricosuric agent with various side effects. The drug is not yet available in North America.

INDOLES

From the many compounds containing an indole group that have been tested for antipyretic, analgesic, and anti-inflammatory actions, only **indomethacin** was found to be clinically useful. **Sulindac** is an indene, chemically related to indomethacin but lacking the indole N (*see* Fig. 33–4).

Indomethacin

The analgesic, antipyretic, and anti-inflammatory actions of indomethacin are similar to those of the salicylates. It is a very potent inhibitor of prostaglandin syn-

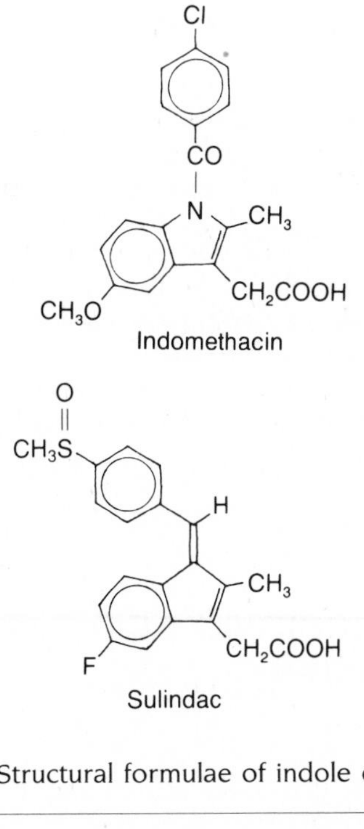

Figure 33–4 Structural formulae of indole compounds.

thetase. It also uncouples oxidative phosphorylation, depresses the biosynthesis of mucopolysaccharides, and inhibits the motility of polymorphonuclear leukocytes.

Indomethacin is rapidly and nearly completely absorbed from the upper small intestine following oral administration. Maximum plasma concentration occurs after 3 hours. It is unevenly distributed in body water (1 L/kg), and 90% is protein-bound in plasma. The drug is O-demethylated and conjugated with glucuronic acid by hepatic microsomal enzymes. The elimination is relatively fast, the plasma half-life being 4–12 hours. Unchanged drug and metabolites are excreted in urine, bile, and feces.

Indomethacin is a very potent anti-inflammatory agent. Although it has antipyretic and analgesic properties, the drug should be used only for the treatment of rheumatoid arthritis, ankylosing spondylitis, osteoarthrosis, and acute gout, and for the control of pain in uveitis and postoperative ophthalmic pain. The usual dose is 25 mg two or three times daily; total dose should not exceed 200 mg a day.

Adverse effects are present in 35–50% of patients. Gastrointestinal complaints are the most frequent, with nausea, vomiting, diarrhea, and occasional ulceration predominating. Skin hypersensitivity and adverse effects on hematopoiesis also have been reported. However, interactions between indomethacin and other drugs appear to be of no significant consequence. Drug toxicity such as hepatocellular damage, fatal hepatitis, and jaundice is very rare.

Sulindac

Sulindac (*see* Fig. 33–4), which is closely related to indomethacin, requires *in vivo* transformation to become active. Hepatic microsomal enzymes oxidize the molecule to a sulfone, and reduce it to a sulfide, which is the active form of sulindac. It inhibits prostaglandin synthesis and is about half as potent as indomethacin. The absorption, distribution, and plasma protein binding are also similar to those of indomethacin. The plasma half-life of sulindac is about 7 hours, but for the sulfide metabolite it is about 18 hours. Sulindac, the sulfone, and their conjugates are excreted in urine and feces. It has therapeutic uses similar to those of indomethacin, and the side effects and toxicity are also similar but less frequent. It has a renal sparing effect because it does not appear to affect renal PGI_2 synthesis.

PHENYLPROPIONIC ACID DERIVATIVES AND ANALOGS

This group of drugs, which is listed in Figure 33–5, has many pharmacologic and toxicologic properties in

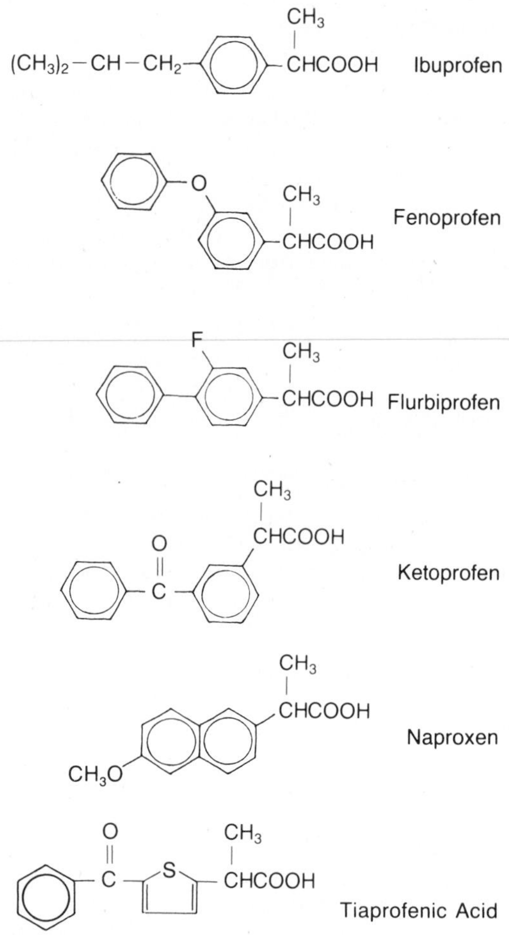

Figure 33–5 Structural formulae of propionic acid derivatives.

common. The drugs are all substituted phenyl-, naphthyl-, or thienyl-propionic acids, which are chemically and pharmacologically analogous.

Mechanism and Site of Action

These drugs inhibit prostaglandin biosynthesis *in vitro* and *in vivo* with some variation in their potency, which is reflected in the dose required to produce analgesia, reduce fever, and inhibit inflammatory responses.

Pharmacokinetics

Table 33–2 summarizes the pharmacokinetics of this group of drugs.

Ibuprofen is probably the best tolerated on long-term use, even by patients who cannot tolerate ASA because of gastric complaints. Absorption is complete after oral administration, and peak plasma levels occur after 1 or 2 hours. Rectal absorption is slower. The drug is distributed unevenly in body water and can be found in synovial fluid.

Fenoprofen is less popular than the other members of this group, probably because of less intensive commercial promotion of the drug. Absorption is fast but not complete after oral administration because food retards absorption. It is distributed unevenly in body water.

Ketoprofen is absorbed rapidly and completely after oral administration, but it is also distributed unevenly in body water. The plasma half-life may vary between 1 and 35 hours; the causes of this variability are unknown.

Flurbiprofen is completely absorbed after oral administration, and peak plasma levels occur after 1–2 hours. Not all patients treated with flurbiprofen can tolerate its side effects, which consist mainly of diarrhea, nausea, dizziness, or upset stomach.

Naproxen is well tolerated and completely absorbed after oral or rectal administration. Antacids containing magnesium oxide or aluminum hydroxide reduce the rate of absorption.

Tiaprofenic acid is one of the most recently introduced members of this group. It is rapidly absorbed from the stomach and duodenojejunal area and distributed unevenly in total body water. The plasma half-life is 1.7 hours, but it can be detected in synovial fluid for up to 11 hours. It is extensively plasma protein-bound (98%). Over 90% of the dose is excreted unchanged in the urine, indicating that the dose should be reduced for patients with impaired renal function. Tiaprofenic acid is indicated for the relief of signs and symptoms of rheumatoid arthritis and osteoarthritis. It has many side effects including GI irritation, reversible reduction of platelet adhesiveness, disturbed renal function, and possible cross-reaction in ASA-sensitive patients.

Pharmacologic Effects

These are all effective anti-inflammatory drugs used extensively for the treatment of rheumatic disorders, osteoarthritis, ankylosing spondylitis, and other inflammatory conditions. In addition, they are very effective analgesics to relieve postpartum pain, and following oral, ophthalmic, or other types of surgery. They are also effective for dysmenorrheal pain, especially if medication is started at least a day before the expected menstrual period. Personal preference by the practitioner or the patient, and tolerance, are the main criteria for selecting one or other of these similar drugs.

Adverse Effects and Toxicity

These are more or less the same as those observed following ASA administration, but probably are less frequently encountered and of reduced intensity. Gastro-intestinal complaints including nausea, vomiting, epigastric pain, reactivation of peptic ulcer, and other disturbances are common to all members of this group. CNS-related effects, such as dizziness, drowsiness, headache, and fatigue, also may occur.

Drug interactions are not many, but since these drugs are very highly protein-bound, competition for binding sites could present a problem with oral anticoagulants or other highly protein-bound drugs. Toxicity is related primarily to the gastrointestinal tract, where ulceration and bleeding can be a problem.

ANTHRANILIC ACIDS

Mefenamic acid (Fig. 33–6 and Table 33–2), like salicylates, inhibits prostaglandin synthesis. In addition it appears to inhibit the action of $PGF_{2\alpha}$ on isolated bronchial smooth muscle. It is rapidly and completely absorbed after oral administration, and maximum plasma concentration is reached in 2 hours. It is unevenly distributed in body water, and it has several metabolites that are eliminated in urine along with the unchanged drug. The plasma half-life is about 4 hours. Mefenamic acid has analgesic, antipyretic, and anti-inflammatory properties, but because of gastrointestinal side effects, including occasionally severe diarrhea, it is used for analgesia only. It is recommended especially for dysmenorrhea.

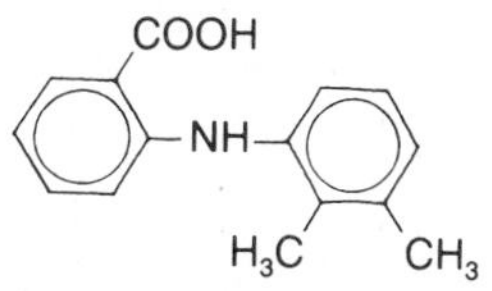

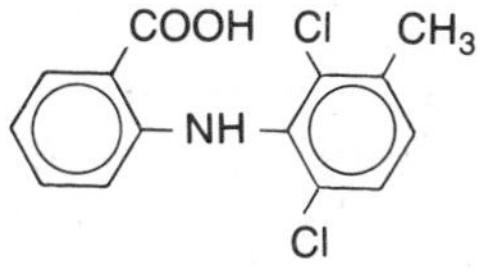

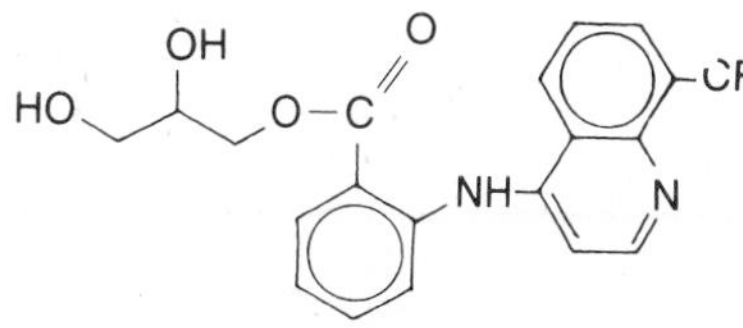

Figure 33–6 Structural formulae of anthranilic acids.

Meclofenamate sodium (*see* Fig. 33–6 and Table 33–2) acts similarly to mefenamic acid. It is rapidly and completely absorbed and has significant analgesic effects after 30 minutes. The drug is recommended primarily for the treatment of signs and symptoms of inflammatory pain and osteoarthritis. Gastrointestinal complaints are frequent during therapy.

Floctafenine (*see* Fig. 33–6 and Table 33–2) is another of the recently introduced anti-inflammatory analgesic drugs that act by inhibition of prostaglandin synthesis. The absorption following oral administration is complete, with peak plasma levels attained in 1–2 hours. The initial plasma half-life (α phase) is 1 hour, and the β phase is 8 hours. The drug is recommended primarily for the short-term treatment of mild to moderately severe pain. It has the same gastrointestinal and CNS-related side effects as other drugs in this category.

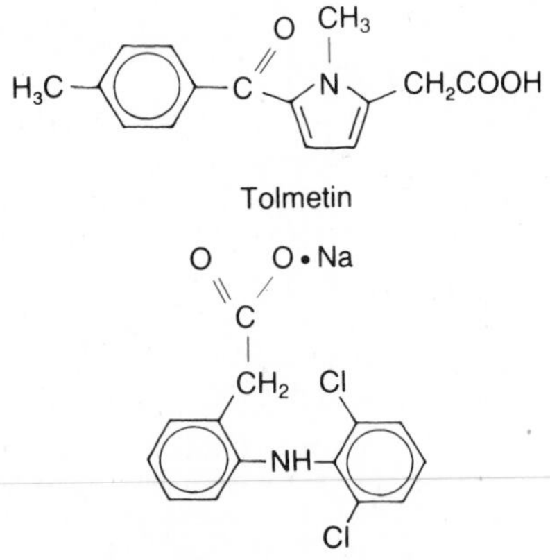

PYRROLE-ACETIC ACID AND PHENYL-ACETIC ACID DERIVATIVES

Tolmetin (a substituted pyrrole-acetic acid derivative; Fig. 33–7 and Table 33–2) has analgesic, antipyretic, and anti-inflammatory properties similar to those of ASA. It is rapidly and completely absorbed following oral administration. Peak plasma concentration is achieved after 60 minutes. Tolmetin is recommended as an anti-inflammatory drug, but many patients cannot tolerate the side effects. It may cause gastric erosion, ulceration, bleeding, and CNS-related side effects such as nervousness, insomnia, and drowsiness.

Diclofenac sodium (a substituted phenyl-acetic acid derivative; *see* Fig. 33–7 and Table 33–2), a potent prostaglandin synthesis inhibitor *in vitro* and *in vivo*, has analgesic, antipyretic, and anti-inflammatory properties that are similar to those of ASA. It is recommended for the treatment of rheumatoid arthritis and severe osteoarthritis, including degenerative joint disease of the hip. It has many side effects commonly encountered with this group of drugs, and the most serious are gastrointestinal bleeding, cardiac arrhythmias, water retention, and reversible depression of the blood-forming organs. Enteric-coated tablets are recommended for oral administration to reduce gastric irritation.

OXICAM

Piroxicam (Fig. 33–8 and Table 33–2) is an amphoteric compound and may behave either as a weak acid or a weak base. Like most other drugs in this class, piroxicam is a potent prostaglandin synthesis inhibitor.

Figure 33–7   Structural formulae of pyrrole- and phenyl-acetic acid derivatives.

It is absorbed slowly after oral administration, peak plasma levels from single doses are achieved after 4 hours. Because of its long half-life (about 45 hours), with daily doses of 20 mg the plasma levels rise for about 5–7 days to reach a steady state. Food in the stomach does not influence bioavailability. Piroxicam is recommended primarily as an analgesic for the symptomatic treatment of rheumatoid arthritis, osteoarthritis, and ankylosing spondylitis. The drug's potential side effects include gastrointestinal ulceration, disturbed hemostasis, and CNS disturbances. Caution is required when the drug is administered to patients with impaired hepatic or renal function, because of its potential for cumulation.

GOLD COMPOUNDS

Gold compounds, such as **auranofin** (Ridaura®), **aurothioglucose** (Solganal®), and **sodium aurothiomalate** (Myochrysine®), are strictly reserved for the treatment of patients with rapidly progressive rheumatoid arthritis who respond poorly to conventional drug treatment. Reliable results are obtained after intramuscular administration of a solution or oily suspension of the gold compound at weekly or longer time intervals. The

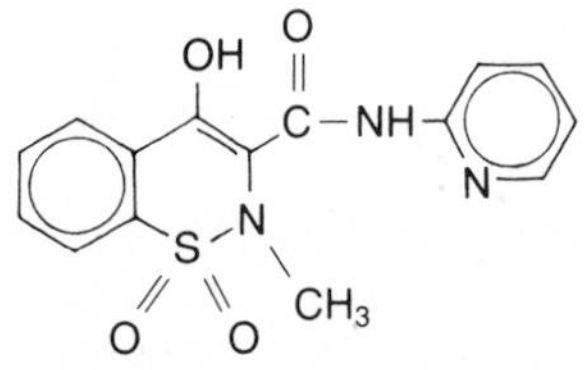

Figure 33–8   Structural formula of piroxicam.

bioavailability of orally administered preparations is low but suitable for maintenance therapy. Clinically significant improvements may take months to develop and may last for a year after discontinuation. The distribution of gold in the body is unpredictable; it tends to accumulate in inflamed tissues and joints. After termination of treatment the concentration in blood will continue to diminish over 2–3 months, but significant amounts are excreted in the urine for a year or longer. The mechanism of action is uncertain, the most acceptable theory being that gold compounds suppress immune responsiveness by inhibition of mononuclear phagocyte function. There are numerous side effects including dermatitis, proximal tubular damage, blood dyscrasias, and encephalitis.

DRUGS USED IN THE TREATMENT OF GOUT

A variety of analgesics, uricosuric agents (probenecid and sulfinpyrazone), and corticosteroids are used in the symptomatic or specific treatment of gout. They are described elsewhere (*see* Chapter 47). The acute attack responds well to colchicine, and the chronic form of gout may be controlled by reducing plasma uric acid with allopurinol.

Colchicine is an alkaloid obtained from the autumn crocus. It is used as an anti-inflammatory drug in the prevention and treatment of acute gouty arthritis. It causes the disappearance of the fibrillar microtubules in granulocytes and leukocytes, thereby preventing their mobilization to the site of inflammation. It inhibits the release of histamine and the secretion of insulin, and it arrests cell division in metaphase. It may cause nausea, vomiting, hemorrhagic gastroenteritis, and, following chronic administration, agranulocytosis, aplastic anemia, and alopecia. The usual oral adult dose is about 1 mg initially, but not more than 3 mg in 24 hours.

Allopurinol and its primary metabolite, alloxanthine, reduce plasma uric acid concentration by inhibiting xanthine oxidase, the enzyme catalysing the final steps of uric acid synthesis. Thus, hyperuricemia of almost any cause, including that induced by other drugs, is normalized. This facilitates the dissolution of tophi and prevents the development or progression of chronic gouty arthritis. Allopurinol and its metabolites are excreted in dose-dependent fashion by glomerular filtration, but there is significant tubular reabsorption, which is sensitive to probenecid inhibition. The drug is well tolerated, but hypersensitivity reactions may occur even after months or years of continuous medication. The usual dose is 100 mg, which may be increased to 300 mg/day.

SUGGESTED READING

Aspirin and acetaminophen. Arch Intern Med 1981; 141(3) (Feb. 23) (26 articles).

Brogden RN, Heel RC, Speicht TM, Avery GS. Piroxicam: a review of its pharmacological properties and therapeutic efficacy. Drugs 1981; 22:165–187.

Chaffman M, Brogden RN, Heel RC, et al. Auranofin: a preliminary review of its pharmacological properties and therapeutic use in rheumatoid arthritis. Drugs 1984; 27:378–424.

Flower JR, Vane JR. Inhibition of prostaglandin biosynthesis. Biochem Pharmacol 1974; 23:1439–1450.

Fowler PD. Aspirin, paracetamol and nonsteroidal anti-inflammatory drugs. A comparative review of side effects. Med Toxicol Adverse Drug Exp 1987; 2:338–366.

New perspectives on aspirin therapy. Am J Med 1983; 74:(6A) (17 articles).

Smith MJH, Smith PK, eds. The salicylates: a critical bibliographic review. New York: Wiley, 1966.

AUTACOIDS

CARDIOVASCULAR SYSTEM

___

Chapter 34

DIGITALIS GLYCOSIDES

F.A. Sunahara and W.A. Mahon

The drugs included under the generic term, digitalis (or cardiac) glycosides, are used primarily in the treatment of cardiac failure. A large number of extracts from plants containing cardiac glycosides have been used at various times in different parts of the world. Digitalis, which is extracted from the foxglove plant, was used prior to 1785 in folk medicine, but in that year William Withering published his celebrated book, *An Account of the Foxglove and Some of its Medical Uses: with Practical Remarks on Dropsy, and Other Diseases.* Withering thought that the drug was a diuretic, but recognized that the heart was affected, and he appreciated that it produced cardiac slowing in patients with generalized edema (dropsy).

Digitalis is extracted from the dried leaf of the foxglove plant, *Digitalis purpurea.* Seeds and leaves of a number of other digitalis species also contain active cardiac drugs. *Digitalis lanata* was also used, and a variety of other plants also contain cardiac glycosides.

Although the beneficial clinical effects of these agents have been known empirically for two centuries, their mechanisms of action have not been well understood until recently. It is now generally acknowledged that their principal clinically significant direct action is augmentation of contraction of the atrial and ventricular myocardium. A good understanding of the pharmacology of these agents is important because they are widely used, and the digitalis glycosides have a narrow margin of safety, *i.e.,* there is very little difference between the therapeutically effective dose and the toxic or fatal dose. Several studies have indicated that approximately 20% of patients taking digitalis show some form of drug-induced toxicity. These toxic manifestations are more pronounced in elderly patients: the incidence is 24% for those over 60 years of age as compared to 14% for those under 60.

PHYSIOLOGY OF MUSCLE CONTRACTION AND HEART FAILURE

Muscle Contraction

All types of muscle, including the myocardium and vascular smooth muscle, respond to effective stimuli with the same sequence of events beginning with membrane depolarization, reaching a peak in shortening of the contractile proteins actin and myosin, and ending with relaxation and return to the resting state. These events are described in some detail below, in relation to each of the three phases.

Sodium and Calcium Influx

Application of an effective stimulus—whether by neurotransmitter from an excitatory nerve terminal, by spread of an impulse from a spontaneous pacemaker cell, or by application of an electrical stimulus—causes sudden and rapid changes in membrane permeability, that lead to membrane depolarization and initiation of an action potential. The first change (phase 0 of the cardiac action potential) is an opening of Na^+ channels, the so-called fast channels, resulting in the fast inward current of Na^+ across the cell membrane. This current is dependent on extracellular Na^+ and can be blocked by tetrodotoxin and antiarrhythmic agents such as quinidine (*see* Chapter 35). When the cell has been depolarized from approximately -90 mV to -40 mV, the voltage change opens a second type of channel, and a second inward current develops that contributes to the plateau phase (phase 2) of the cardiac action potential. Since this is a much slower current than the fast Na$^+$ current, it has been termed the slow current. It has been estimated that the membrane channels carrying this current are 100 times more selective for Ca^{2+} than for Na$^+$; this justifies the term **calcium channel** (*see* Fig. 36–3).

Action potentials from contracting cells in the atria and ventricles, from the distal A-V node, and from the conducting system depend on both fast and slow inward currents. Pacemaker cells in the S-A node have slowly rising action potentials and a reduced rate of conduction and are largely activated by the slow inward current (Fig. 34–1).

In the relaxed state, the concentration of Ca^{2+} in the myocardial cytoplasm is several orders of magnitude lower than the extracellular concentration. This concentration gradient is what drives the slow inward Ca^{2+} current.

After activation, the Na$^+$ and Ca^{2+} channels remain open for only a short time (measured in milliseconds) and then close spontaneously. As a result, the inward Na$^+$ and Ca^{2+} currents are inactivated, but a K$^+$ channel opens and an outward K$^+$ current occurs, in keeping with the K$^+$ concentration gradient across the membrane (high intracellular, low extracellular K$^+$). This K$^+$ current is largely responsible for restoring the membrane potential to its normal value of -90mV, but the end result is a net gain of intracellular Na$^+$ and a net loss of K$^+$ during the entire action potential. This imbalance is corrected by the sarcolemmal (Na$^+$+K$^+$)-ATPase, which uses the energy from the splitting of ATP to transport Na$^+$ back out of the cell and K$^+$ back in.

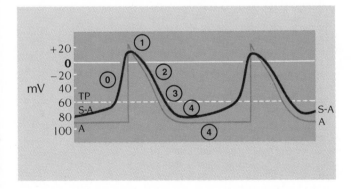

Figure 34–1 Comparison of action potentials of an atrial muscle cell (A) and a cell from the sinoatrial (S-A) node: depolarization (phase 0), repolarization (phases 1, 2, 3), resting membrane potential/diastolic depolarization (phase 4). Differences in amplitude, duration, and general configuration in the two tissue types can be seen. The slow depolarization (phase 4) of the S-A fibre diminishes its membrane potential (towards 0 mV) to reach the threshold potential (TP), and thus initiates spontaneous firing. (Adapted from Hoffmann BF, Singer DH. Prog Cardiovasc Dis 1964; 7:226–260.)

The initial influx of Na$^+$ and Ca^{2+} triggers a further massive entry of Ca^{2+} into the sarcoplasm by two mechanisms: (1) There is a bidirectional Na$^+$–Ca^{2+} exchange system that mediates the movement of calcium across the sarcolemma. The direction of this exchange is dependent upon the relative concentrations of extracellular and intracellular Na$^+$ and Ca^{2+}. In most circumstances, the result is an efflux of Na$^+$ and an influx of Ca^{2+}. (2) The Ca^{2+} that has already entered the cell triggers a further influx of Ca^{2+} from its storage site in the sarcoplasmic reticulum.

Contraction

Actin is a globular protein that forms a double helical filament, the thin filament. Myosin is a hexamere, with one pair of heavy chains and two pairs of light chains arranged in parallel, and forms the thick filament. Thick and thin filaments alternate with each other in parallel arrays. Muscular contraction is an energy-requiring cyclic process in which cross-linkages between specific portions of the actin and myosin filaments are formed and then broken, in response to changes in intracellular Ca^{2+} concentration. During the marked rise of intracellular (sarcoplasmic) Ca^{2+} that occurs as a result of membrane depolarization and the subsequent steps mentioned above, Ca^{2+} binds to a specific subunit of the actin filament, known as troponin C. This in turn activates an adjacent subunit, tropomyosin, so that in the presence of ATP as an energy source it forms a cross-linkage between the myosin and actin, generating a force that pulls the thin filament towards the centre of the sarcomere, with consequent myocardial shortening or tension development, or both (Fig. 34–2).

There are important differences between the contraction of the myocardium and that of vascular smooth muscle, such as in the coronary vasculature and systemic arterioles. In the vessels, the process that regulates contraction results from a cascade of reactions, the first of which involves a small (15,000 dalton) calcium-binding protein, calmodulin. When the Ca^{2+} concentration in the vascular smooth muscle rises to approximately 10^{-6} M, Ca^{2+} binds to calmodulin and this complex activates the enzyme myosin kinase; this in turn phosphorylates the light chain of myosin and permits myosin to interact with actin, leading to contraction of the smooth muscle cell. However, in both myocardium and vascular smooth muscle, it is the influx of Ca^{2+} that activates the contractile process, and contraction is proportional to the Ca^{2+} influx.

Relaxation

Heart muscle contains several hundred times more Ca^{2+} than is required for activation, but the Ca^{2+} is bound to, or sequestered within, many intracellular structures such as the inner layer of the cell membrane (the sarcolemma) and its invaginations (the transverse tubular system), the mitochondria and, in particular,

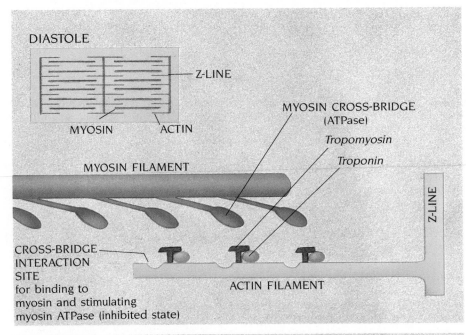

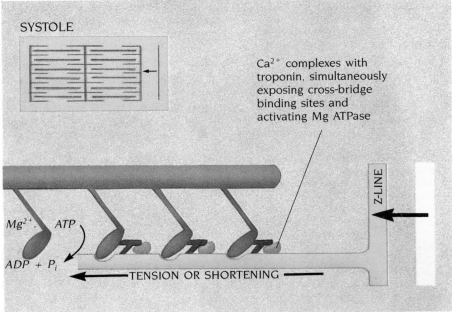

Figure 34–2   The relaxed (diastolic) and contracted (systolic) states of a myofibril, showing the sliding of actin filaments into the channels between myosin filaments. In the diastolic state, in the absence of calcium, the modulatory proteins, tropomyosin and troponin, inhibit the interaction between the contractile proteins, actin and myosin. During the systolic state, the presence of calcium abolishes the prevention of actin-myosin interaction by the tropomyosin-troponin complex. Removal of the inhibitory action of the modulatory proteins permits both the ATPase-stimulating and physicochemical interactions between actin and myosin to proceed, thereby establishing the active state and permitting the muscle to shorten and do work.

the sarcoplasmic reticulum. Although the quantity of Ca^{2+} that enters the cell from the extracellular space at the time of electrical depolarization is insufficient to activate the contractile apparatus fully, it triggers the release of a much larger quantity of Ca^{2+} from the sarcoplasmic reticulum (as noted above), resulting in activation. Relaxation results from cessation of the influx of Ca^{2+} into the cell, coupled with ATP-dependent active re-uptake of Ca^{2+} by the Mg^{2+}-ATPase of the sarcoplasmic reticulum, and extrusion of Ca^{2+} from the cell by the sarcolemmal Ca^{2+}-ATPase. Ca^{2+} is also taken up again by the mitochondria, especially when the intracellular Ca^{2+} content is very high, as it may be during ischemia or severe hypoxia. When the intracellular concentration of Ca^{2+} declines below a critical level, Ca^{2+} dissociates from troponin, and the

dissociation results in a breakage of actin-myosin cross-links, allowing relaxation to occur.

Heart Failure

The basic cause of cardiac failure is a decrease in the force of contraction of myocardial fibres, which results in slower pressure rise within the ventricle during the isovolumic phase of the contraction (dP/dt), a lower peak systolic pressure, an enlarged diastolic size, and a higher filling pressure. The sequence of events resulting from the failing heart is illustrated in Figure 34–3.

Compensatory mechanisms available to the failing heart are an increase in ventricular end-diastolic pres-

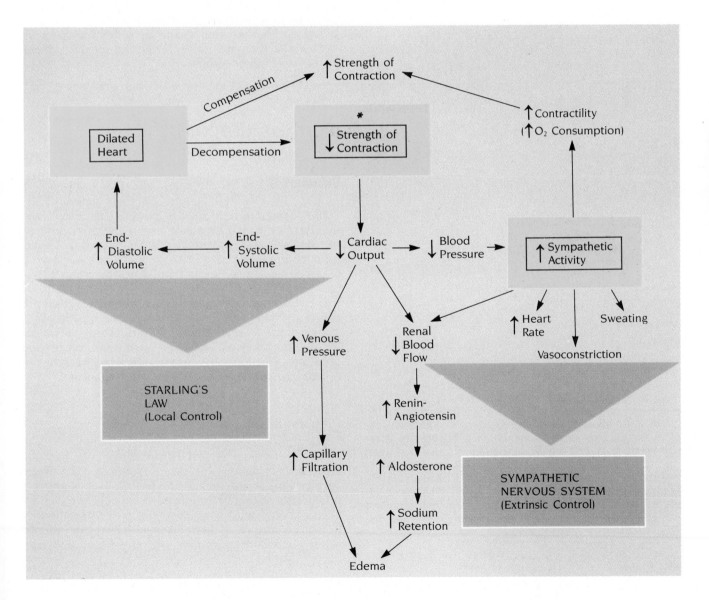

Figure 34–3 Sequence of events resulting from the failing heart (starts at *; ↑ increase, ↓ decrease).

sure that enhances cardiac output (Starling's law of the heart), myocardial hypertrophy, and increased sympathetic activity.

In conditions where these mechanisms can cope to produce adequate cardiac output, the heart failure is said to be compensated. Starling's curve (Fig. 34–4) shows that, at similar end-diastolic pressure, the cardiac output is lower in the failing heart than in the normal heart. Consequently, the heart enlarges to maintain cardiac output, and the heart rate increases to compensate for the poor cardiac function. In the decompensated heart, compensatory mechanisms fail to maintain cardiac output.

Administration of digitalis improves the cardiac performance, shifting the cardiac function curve to the left so that it approximates the normal curve. By increasing the force of myocardial contraction, digitalis reduces the diastolic pressure, and consequently the diastolic volume. This decrease in ventricular volume increases the efficiency of contraction. Digitalis thus reduces the ratio of myocardial oxygen consumption to contractile force. The effect is largely due to decreased myocardial fibre length and diastolic wall tension. Because of the improvement in circulation, sympathetic activity is reduced, which in turn reduces arterial resistance and venous tone. The former changes the afterload on the left ventricle and permits further improvement of heart function. The reduced heart rate is attributed to both direct and indirect effects on the heart. Digitalis not only reduces sympathetic tone by reflex mechanisms, but also stimulates the vagus by sensitizing the baroreceptors and/or the afferent nerve activity.

In contrast to the action of digitalis in the failing heart, in the normal heart its positive inotropic effect is negated by compensatory autonomic reflexes. Digitalis also elicits peripheral vasoconstriction, therefore causing the blood pressure to rise. Again by reflex mechanisms, the myocardial activity and cardiac output are reduced in the normal individual.

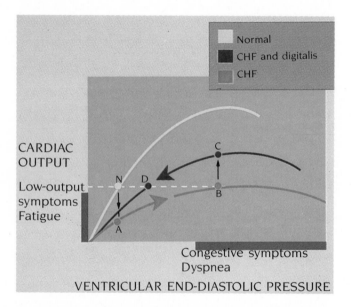

Figure 34–4 Ventricular function curves in the normal heart, in congestive heart failure (CHF), and in CHF with digitalis, showing the operation of the Frank-Starling mechanism in the preload compensation for heart failure. Points N through D indicate, in sequence, depression of contractility with decompensated heart failure (A), Frank-Starling compensation (B), increase in contractility with digitalis (C), and reduction in use of Frank-Starling preload compensation, which digitalis allows (D). Points N, D, and B indicate the same cardiac output on the vertical axis, but each point is at a different end-diastolic pressure on the horizontal axis. The excessive end-diastolic pressures causing congestive symptoms and the lowered levels of cardiac performance resulting in low-output symptoms are indicated by bars on the respective axis. (From Mason DT. Am J Cardiol 1973; 32:437–448.)

DIGITALIS GLYCOSIDES

Structure

The digitalis glycosides are complex chemicals derived mainly from plant material (*e.g.*, *Digitalis purpurea* or foxglove). All of these glycosides have three structural components (Fig. 34–5): a steroid nucleus, a series of sugar residues in the C-3 position, and a five- or six-membered lactone ring in the C-17 position.

The steroid nucleus and the lactone ring together are called a genin or aglycone. This aglycone moiety elicits the cardiotonic effects, which are qualitatively similar for all the aglycones. However, absorption, onset, and duration of action vary among different glycosides in relation to the sugar portion of the molecule.

Preparations

Several compounds with digitalis-like activity are commercially available. However, only a few enjoy widespread clinical use and confidence, and it is entirely reasonable to practice medicine using only one digitalis preparation, digoxin. At least 90% of digitalis therapy in North America is carried out with digoxin, but two other digitalis preparations are official and one may

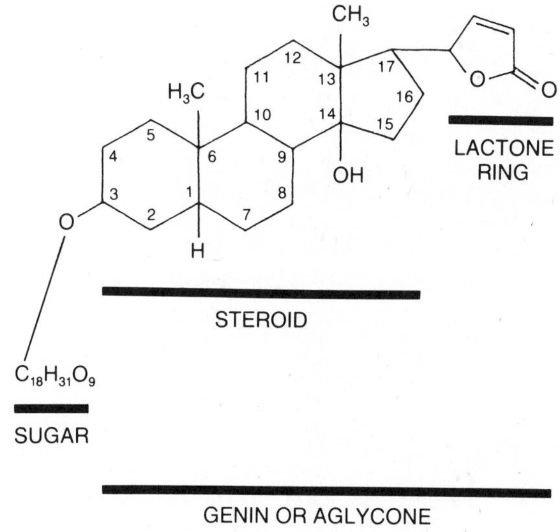

Figure 34–5 Structural formula of digitoxin. The structure of digoxin is similar except that there is an OH group on the C-12 position.

encounter patients receiving these drugs. Table 34–1 summarizes the pharmacokinetic data for three digitalis preparations, deslanoside, digoxin, and digitoxin. It is important to recognize that the values in Table 34–1 are averages, and that variations in measurements such as half-life are substantial even in normal subjects.

Mechanism of Action

Positive Inotropic Effects

The fundamental mechanisms by which digitalis glycosides stimulate the contractile forces within the cardiac cell have been widely debated. Present evidence suggests that this action is mediated through potentiation of the process of coupling electrical excitation and mechanical contraction (excitation-contraction coupling).

There is at present a consensus that the inotropic effects of cardiac glycosides result from binding of the glycoside to a subunit of the sarcolemmal $(Na^+ + K^+)$-ATPase. This causes a partial inhibition of the enzyme, impairing active transport of Na^+ and K^+ across the membrane as long as the cardiac glycoside molecule remains associated with the site. This is the only site in cardiac tissue with the binding properties required of a "digitalis receptor." Since the glycosides have no primary effects on cyclic AMP, myocardial contractile proteins, or intermediary metabolism, the inhibition of $(Na^+ + K^+)$-ATPase must be seen as the means whereby these drugs may alter Ca^{2+} movement and hence contraction.

Cardiac glycosides, by inhibiting $(Na^+ + K^+)$-ATPase activity, increase the intracellular sodium concentration. As a result, there is more Na^+ to be exchanged for Ca^{2+} by the sodium-calcium exchanger. The small increase in intracellular Ca^{2+} concentration acts as a positive feedback signal to increase Ca^{2+} entry through Ca^{2+} channels. This sequence of events leads to a greater increase of intracellular Ca^{2+} when cardiac glycosides are present (Fig. 34–6) and underlies the inotropic response to digitalis.

Electrophysiologic Effects

Some of the therapeutic and most of the serious toxic effects of digitalis can be related to its action on the electrophysiologic properties of the heart. The drug acts directly and indirectly on automaticity, conduction velocity, and effective refractory period of cardiac tissues. Also, digitalis indirectly increases cholinergic (vagal) tone in normal persons and decreases adrenergic nerve action on the failing heart. As mentioned above, $(Na^+ + K^+)$-ATPase is inhibited and there is a resultant decrease in intracellular K^+. This effect is dose-related. An increasing body concentration of digitalis ultimately leads to toxicity manifested by cardiac dysrhythmias. The decrease in intracellular K^+ leads to an increase in the slope of phase 4 depolariza-

TABLE 34–1 Cardiac Glycoside Preparations

	Deslanoside	Digoxin	Digitoxin
Gastrointestinal absorption	unreliable	60–85%	90–100%
Onset of action (minutes)	10–30	15–30	25–120
Peak effect (hours)	1–2	1.5–5	4–12
Average half-life	33 hours	36 hours	4–6 days
Principal metabolic and/or excretory pathway	renal excretion	renal; some GI excretion	hepatic biotransformation; renal excretion of metabolites
Protein binding at therapeutic concentration	—	25%	90%
Average digitalizing dose, oral	—	1.25–1.5 mg	0.7–1.2 mg
intravenous	0.8 mg	0.75–1.0 mg	1.0 mg
Usual daily oral maintenance dose	—	0.25–0.5 mg	0.1 mg

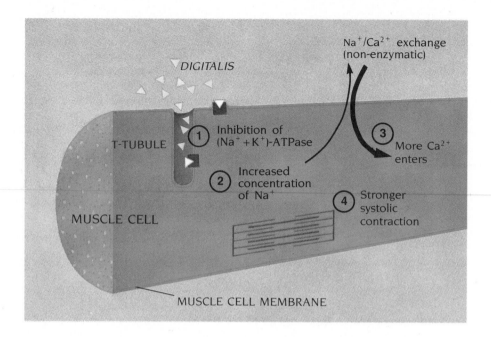

Figure 34–6   Inhibitory action of digitalis glycoside on $(Na^+ + K^+)$-ATPase.

tion and a decrease in maximal diastolic membrane potential (closer to zero membrane potential). This phenomenon leads to increased automaticity and development of ectopic rhythm. Not only are many of the electrophysiologic and dysrhythmic effects of digitalis related to intracellular K^+ depletion, but it also appears that K^+ and digitalis compete for binding sites on myocardial $(Na^+ + K^+)$-ATPase. K^+ is relatively loosely bound to the enzyme, but it delays subsequent digitalis binding. Once digitalis is bound, however, K^+ does not increase its rate of dissociation.

The various phases of the action potential recorded from the sinoatrial node and the atrium are shown in Figure 34–1. The frequency of firing of the pacemaker cell can be altered by (1) altering the threshold potential while maintaining a constant rate of depolarization, (2) altering the rate of depolarization while maintaining the threshold potential, or (3) increasing the maximal diastolic potential of the pacemaker (Fig. 34–7).

The action of digitalis on **automaticity**, *i.e.*, the property by which a single cell spontaneously depolarizes without outside influences, is dose-dependent. In therapeutic concentrations, digitalis has little effect. In toxic concentrations, the slope of phase 4 diastolic depolarization is increased in all cardiac tissues, and ectopic foci of impulse formation may develop. Indirectly, *via* the vagus, digitalis causes decreased impulse formation in the S-A node.

Conduction velocity, *i.e.*, the rate at which an impulse is conducted through cardiac tissue, is a function of the amplitude of the action potential and its rate of rise (phase 0). Both of these variables are related to the resting membrane potential present at the onset

of the action potential; the more negative the membrane potential, the steeper the slope of phase 0. All concentrations of digitalis diminish conduction velocity, but different parts of the heart respond to different degrees. The A-V node is most sensitive, followed in descending order by atrial muscle, the Purkinje sys-

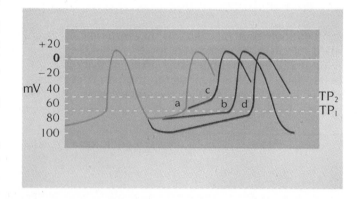

Figure 34–7   Diagrammatic representation of several mechanisms that may change the frequency of firing of a pacemaker cell. With a constant rate of depolarization during phase 4, the cell will fire at (a) or (c) depending upon the level of the threshold potential (TP_1 and TP_2). If the level of the threshold potential is fixed, firing may be delayed from (a) to (b) if the slope of phase 4 depolarization is decreased, or to (d) if the maximum potential of the pacemaker is increased. (After Hoffmann BF, Singer DH. Prog Cardiovasc Dis 1964; 7:226–260.)

tem, and ventricular muscle. The effect on the A-V node is partly direct and partly indirect. It is most prominent when the initial vagal tone is low and adrenergic tone is high, as in congestive heart failure. It should be noted that the direct effect of digitalis on atrial muscle (i.e., decreased conduction velocity) predominates over its indirect vagotonic effect (i.e., increased conduction).

The **refractory period**, phases 1, 2, and 3 in the transmembrane potential recording (see Fig. 34–1 and also Fig. 35–1), includes the periods in which a cell is inexcitable (effective refractory period, ERP) and poorly excitable (relative refractory period, RRP; see definitions in Chapter 35). The digitalis-induced increase in vagal activity shortens the ERP in the atria, causing greater discharge frequency of fibrillating atria (or it may convert atrial flutter to fibrillation). However, while the A-V node is bombarded with higher-frequency impulses, its conduction velocity is reduced and the ERP is prolonged, which in turn causes a lowering of the ventricular rate. This prolongation of the ERP of the A-V node is the main beneficial effect of cardiac glycosides when used for the treatment of atrial flutter or fibrillation.

The effects of digitalis on the electrophysiology of the heart are summarized in Table 34–2. These are the basis for slowing of the compensatory tachycardia of congestive heart failure, decreasing the ventricular rate during atrial dysrhythmias, and conversion of supraventricular dysrhythmias to normal sinus rhythm.

The tendency of digitalis glycosides to cause cardiac dysrhythmia may be related to the depletion of intracellular K^+. As intracellular K^+ falls, the resting membrane potential is reduced in magnitude, i.e., it moves toward zero. The cell now undergoes depolarization more readily as the resting membrane potential comes closer to the depolarization threshold, resulting in greater likelihood of susceptibility to dysrhythmia.

Neural Effects

Many of the electrophysiologic effects of digitalis may be related to neural actions rather than direct effects on the myocardium. For example, it has been shown that the denervated heart after cardiac transplantation does not respond to digitalis with an increase in A-V nodal effective refractory period (ERP), as the normal heart does. This suggests that intact innervation is necessary for this effect. The three most important neural effects of digitalis glycosides are increased **vagal activity** (that can be blocked by atropine), sensitization of carotid sinus **baroreceptors**, and increased **sympathetic outflow** from CNS at high doses.

Extracardiac Hemodynamic Effects

While the direct cardiac actions of digitalis are the most apparent, there are also important extracardiac effects. Cardiac glycosides constrict arterial and venous segments in isolated preparations, and arteriolar and venous constriction has been demonstrated in intact animals. Total systemic arteriolar resistance is also elevated in normal human subjects. Recent evidence indicates that these effects are mediated both by the local (direct) action of digitalis on vascular smooth muscle and indirectly through the central nervous system (see above).

Digitalis inhibits renal tubular reabsorption of Na^+. Direct infusion of a digitalis glycoside (ouabain) into the renal artery produces substantial inhibition of renal $(Na^+ + K^+)$-ATPase and impairment of both concentrating and diluting ability. However, relatively large doses of digitalis are needed to demonstrate these effects, and it is unlikely that a direct renal action of digitalis plays an important part in the diuresis that occurs in the treatment of congestive heart failure.

Pharmacokinetics

The pharmacokinetics of digoxin have been extensively studied. In tablet preparations, 60–80% of the digoxin content is absorbed from the gastrointestinal tract; an encapsulated gel is available that has improved bioavailability (90–100%). The major site of absorption appears to be in the small intestine. There is some enterohepatic circulation of digoxin (Fig. 34–8). Intramus-

TABLE 34–2   Electrophysiologic Effects of Digitalis

	Automaticity		Conduction Velocity		Effective Refractory Period (ERP)	
	Direct	*Indirect*	*Direct*	*Indirect*	*Direct*	*Indirect*
S-A node	↑*	↓				
Atrium	↑		↓*	↑	↑	
A-V node			↓↓	↓↓	↑↑	↑↑
Purkinje system	↑		↓		↓	↑
Ventricles	↑*		↑ ↓*		↓↓	

* At high or toxic doses; ↑ = increase; ↓ = decrease; ↑↑ or ↓↓ denotes therapeutically important effects.

cular injection of digoxin should be avoided because it produces severe pain.

The bioavailability of digoxin in tablet form varies widely between commercial preparations. In addition, even well standardized preparations show variable absorption within and between patients. Diarrhea, malabsorption syndromes, or food in the stomach may also influence absorption significantly.

Digoxin is excreted principally in an unchanged form in the urine; it is apparent, therefore, that renal insufficiency will delay excretion and thereby influence digoxin half-life. There is an almost linear relationship between the clearance of digoxin and the clearance of creatinine in human subjects. Similarly, an elevated blood urea nitrogen (BUN) is associated with diminished clearance of digoxin (Fig. 34–9), and it is possible to extrapolate from the BUN to an appropriate digoxin dosage.

About 25% of digoxin is bound to plasma albumin, compared to more than 90% for digitoxin (*see* Table 34–1). This difference in binding contributes to the

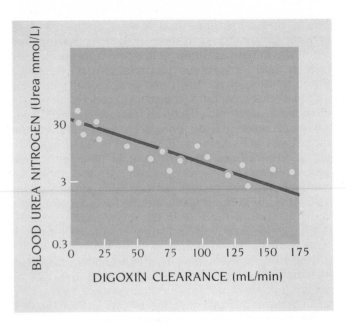

Figure 34–9 Relationship between clearance of digoxin and blood urea nitrogen in human subjects.

difference in speed of onset and duration of action of the two drugs. Digitoxin is biotransformed in the liver and its metabolites are excreted by the kidneys.

Therapeutic Applications

Cardiac glycosides have been shown to be effective in the treatment of patients with congestive heart failure whose state is complicated by the presence of atrial fibrillation. However, in the absence of supraventricular tachycardia, it is not so clear that the patient with congestive heart failure and sinus rhythm benefits from cardiac glycosides. Patients with dilated failing hearts and impaired systolic function have subjective and objective improvement after receiving digitalis, whereas patients with elevated filling pressures due to reduced ventricular compliance, but with preserved systolic function, may not benefit from digitalis therapy unless supraventricular tachycardia coexists.

Drug Interactions

Digitalis action may be **enhanced** by substances that (1) slow gastrointestinal motility and thereby increase gastrointestinal absorption of slowly absorbed preparations (*e.g.*, antispasmodics, such as atropine-like agents); (2) disturb body electrolytes by lowering plasma potassium levels, eliciting hypomagnesemia and hypercalcemia (*e.g.*, diuretics, amphotericin B, glucose by the oral or parenteral route); (3) change renal clearance and/or alter plasma protein binding (*e.g.*, quinidine,

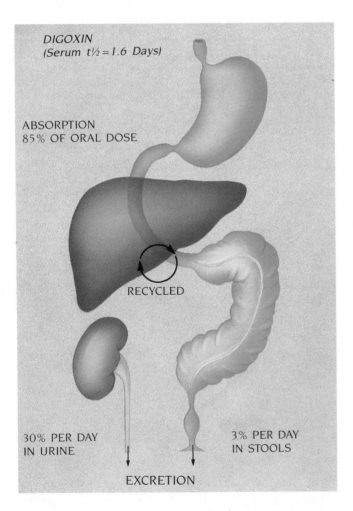

Figure 34–8 Digoxin absorption and turnover. The percentage values are calculated in terms of any given oral dose.

verapamil, amiodarone); (4) stimulate β adrenoceptors and cause cardiac dysrhythmias (e.g., adrenaline*, ephedrine); and (5) elicit cardiac dysrhythmias by unknown mechanisms (e.g., succinylcholine, anticholinesterases).

Digitalis action may be **reduced** by substances that (1) reduce gastrointestinal absorption (e.g., kaolin-pectin, antacids); (2) increase gastrointestinal motility (e.g., metoclopramide); and (3) stimulate hepatic microsomal enzymes and thus enhance the biotransformation of digitoxin (e.g., spironolactone, phenytoin, phenylbutazone, barbiturates).

Side Effects and Toxicity

The toxic manifestations of digitalis may be divided into cardiac and extracardiac. The prime danger is dose-related progressively more severe **dysrhythmia** terminating in ventricular fibrillation. The common predisposing factor is a decrease in intracellular K^+. Potassium depletion may be hastened by concurrent treatment with certain diuretics or corticosteroids, or by conditions such as extensive vomiting and diarrhea. Cardiac irregularities such as coupled beats (bigeminy) are usually signals for a reduction in digitalis dosage. Such irregularities are a sign not only that toxicity is imminent but also that the upper limit of attainable inotropic effect has been reached. Other cardiac manifestations of digitalis toxicity are premature ventricular contractions, premature atrial contractions, atrioventricular block, paroxysmal atrial tachycardia with block, paroxysmal atrial tachycardia, and ventricular tachycardia.

The principal **extracardiac** manifestations of digitalis toxicity are gastrointestinal. Vomiting is caused by stimulation of the chemoreceptor trigger zone. Diarrhea results from activation of the dorsal motor nucleus of the vagal nerve, increasing gastrointestinal motility.

A variety of central nervous system side effects occur, including anorexia, weakness, lethargy and fatigue, and visual complaints. The visual disturbances include hazy vision, difficulty in reading, various types of scotoma, altered or disturbed color perception, and photophobia. Other neurologic symptoms of digitalis toxicity include dizziness, headache, paresthesias and, with massive overdose, convulsions, delusions, stupor, and coma.

Treatment of Digitalis Toxicity

Digitalis must be discontinued immediately if toxic manifestations occur. Often these symptoms may persist for some time because of slow elimination of the drug. Since there is usually a loss of K^+ from the myocardium during treatment with digitalis glycosides, and since this loss of K^+ is the probable cause of dysrhyth-mias, immediate relief is often obtained from the intravenous administration of potassium salts. This measure raises the extracellular K^+ concentration and thus decreases the slope of phase 4 depolarization, so that problems due to excessive automaticity are diminished. There are, however, hazards associated with potassium administration when there is depressed automaticity or decreased conduction, because this may lead to complete A-V block. Digitalis-induced second- or third-degree heart block is the only type of dysrhythmia in which potassium is contraindicated. In addition to potassium, digitalis-induced cardiac dysrhythmias usually respond to drugs such as lidocaine or phenytoin.

Life-threatening arrhythmias and heart block produced by digoxin or digitoxin can be safely treated with digoxin-specific Fab fragments that have been purified from antibodies raised in sheep by immunization against digoxin. The crude antiserum from sheep is fractionated to separate the IgG fraction, which is cleaved into Fab and Fc fragments by papain digestion. The Fab fragments are not antigenic and complement-binding. They are excreted fairly rapidly by the kidney as a digoxin-bound complex. In patients who have life-threatening arrhythmias and are treated with digoxin-specific Fab fragments, the arrhythmias rapidly disappear.

Measurement of Serum Concentration of Digoxin; Digoxin Dosage

In recent years, a sensitive radioimmunoassay for digoxin has been developed with which nanomolar concentrations of digoxin can be measured in a patient's serum or in tissues post mortem. Using this technique, it has been found that the ratio of myocardial tissue concentration to serum concentration is extremely variable, but typically about 30:1. Figure 34–10 is a plot of the serum levels of digoxin in 100 consecutive patients, subdivided into a group with and a group without clinical signs of toxicity. In the majority of patients serum levels of more than 3.8 nmol/L produced clinical toxicity. However, there is considerable overlap: some patients with levels of more than 3.8 nmol/L were not adversely affected, and in some, levels as low as 2.3 nmol/L seemed to be toxic. It must be appreciated that toxicity may occur with normal serum levels in some situations such as following myocardial infarction or in association with hypoxemia, hypokalemia, or hypomagnesemia. People with hypothyroidism (myxedema) are particularly prone to develop digitalis toxicity.

The therapeutic index for digitalis is low; consequently dosage must be carefully controlled for each individual. It may be difficult to estimate the initial and maintenance doses because it would depend very much on the clinical condition of the patient, in particular the hepatic and renal function.

If no emergency exists, the daily maintenance dose may be given by mouth; steady-state concentration and therapeutic effect are reached in approximately five elimination half-lives. The dose may be adjusted at appropriate intervals. If emergency exists and the patient

---

* epinephrine

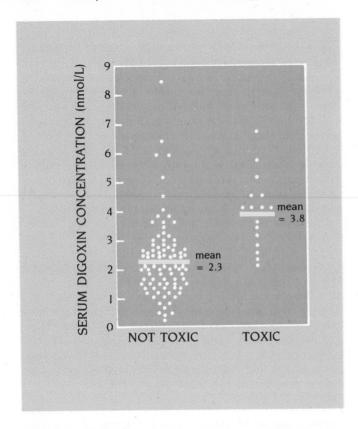

Figure 34–10   Results of 100 serum digoxin radioimmunoassay measurements. Sixteen patients were believed to show clinical toxicity; their mean serum level was 3.8 nmol/L (*right*). Of the patients without clinical toxicity (*left*), seven also had serum levels of more than 3.8 nmol/L (3 ng/mL). Overlap of normal and toxic values does occur; therefore, judgement must be used when evaluating results.

must be digitalized promptly, an initial loading dose may be given by mouth or by slow intravenous infusion. The total body content of drug (0.7–1.2 mg) should be administered in three doses at 6-hour intervals; then the patient is started on daily maintenance doses. Maintenance doses for digoxin for an individual with normal renal function would be approximately 0.25 mg daily.

OTHER CARDIOTONIC AGENTS

It is generally accepted that the cardiac glycosides are the most important cardiotonic agents for the treatment of congestive heart failure with or without atrial dysrhythmia. However, other types of cardiotonics are also sometimes employed. Among these, the sympathomimetic agents, dopamine and dobutamine, have a place in the treatment of heart failure under certain circumstances.

SUGGESTED READING

Hoffmann BF, Singer DH. Effects of digitalis on electrical activity of cardiac fibers. Prog Cardiovasc Dis 1964; 7:226–260.

Kim R-SS, Labella FS. Endogenous ligands and modulators of the digitalis receptor: some candidates. Pharmacol Ther 1981; 14:391–409.

Langer GA. Effects of digitalis on myocardial ionic exchange. Circulation 1972; 46:180–187.

Mason DT. Regulation of cardiac performance in clinical heart disease: interactions between contractile state mechanical abnormalities and ventricular compensatory mechanisms. Am J Cardiol 1973; 32:437–448.

Smith TW. Digitalis: mechanisms of action and clinical use. N Engl J Med 1987; 318:358–365.

Chapter 35

ANTIARRHYTHMIC DRUGS

P. Dorian and M.G. Myers

The management of cardiac arrhythmias is primarily concerned with restoring or maintaining sinus rhythm and abolishing or reducing the frequency of ectopic beats, with a minimum of adverse effects. It is important to understand both the electrophysiologic basis of the arrhythmia and the mechanism of action of the drug if the treatment is to be more than just empirical. Recent advances in antiarrhythmic therapy have led to the introduction of drugs with new and different electrophysiologic effects. This chapter reviews current concepts of arrhythmia formation and describes the actions of both traditional and new drugs commonly used in the clinical setting.

DEFINITIONS

Resting membrane potential: Potential difference across the cell membrane in the resting state; equal to -80 to -90 mV.

Threshold potential: Level of membrane potential at which depolarization will occur.

Automaticity: Ability to generate an action potential spontaneously. This is seen normally in pacemaker cells, but not in myocardial cells. When it occurs in myocardial cells as a consequence of cell damage or biochemical disturbance, it is considered abnormal automaticity.

Absolute refractory period: Follows initiation of depolarization; the cell is completely refractory to any stimulus regardless of its strength.

Relative refractory period: Latter part of repolarization; a stronger than normal stimulus can produce depolarization.

Effective refractory period: The shortest interval between two stimuli of equal strength that permits production of a propagated response. The ERP can be determined clinically during electrophysiologic testing: Using an intra-cardiac electrode, an electrical stimulus is applied at shorter and shorter intervals following a propagated beat. The longest coupling interval that fails to result in a propagated response to the stimulus is the ERP.

Excitability: The likelihood of a cell being depolarized. It is measured by the current intensity needed to cause excitation of a cardiac cell.

THE CARDIAC ACTION POTENTIAL

In both cardiac and skeletal muscle there is a difference in electrical potential across the cell membrane. This difference is primarily achieved through a differential distribution of the cations sodium and potassium between the exterior and interior of the cell such that the transmembrane potential difference in the resting state is maintained at -80 to -90 mV, inside negative with respect to outside. Upon excitation, the intracellular potential loses its negativity and a positive current is created by Na^+ moving into the cell. This current is achieved by an increase in the conductivity of the cell membrane to Na^+, by opening of Na^+ channels. The net result is the rapid upstroke of the myocardial action potential (phase 0, Figure 35–1).

In addition to this rapid inward movement of Na^+, there is also an inward flow of Ca^{2+} during the latter part of phase 0 of the action potential (see Chapter 36 for a more complete description of the role of Ca^{2+}). It has been suggested that the rapid movement of Na^+ into the cell reduces the potential difference across the cell membrane to a point at which a Ca^{2+} current is activated. Unlike the rapid Na^+ current, the inward Ca^{2+} flow continues into the plateau phase of early repolarization (phase 2). The plateau phase is followed by a slow repolarization process (phase 3) until the resting potential of -80 to -90 mV is restored within the myocardial cell. To attain this negative intra-

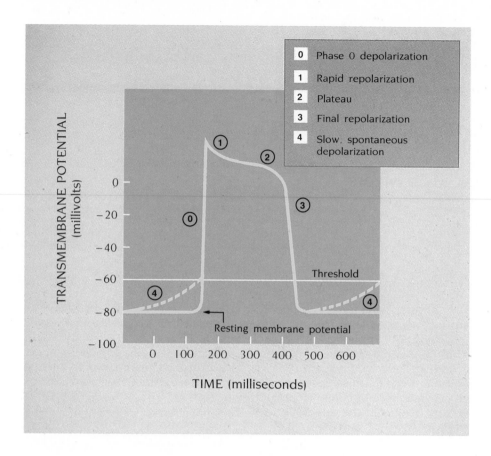

Figure 35–1 Schematic representation of the action potential of the myocardial cell. Note that the resting membrane potential of atrial and ventricular myocardial cells is replaced by slow spontaneous depolarization (phase 4) in pacemaker cells.

cellular potential, positive ions must leave the cell, and thus there is an outward positive current, carried in this instance mainly by K^+. Following a return to the resting state, the $(Na^+ + K^+)$-ATPase pump will restore the intra- and extracellular concentrations of these cations to their pre-excitation levels.

Pacemaker cells exhibit automaticity (the ability to generate spontaneous action potentials) and differ from atrial and ventricular myocardial cells in that they exhibit slow spontaneous depolarization (phase 4) during diastole. The cell membrane is never in a resting state, and it is not possible to measure a resting membrane potential for pacemaker cells. Phase 4 spontaneous depolarization is the result of an inward positive current carried by Na^+. The phase 0 depolarization in these cells is different from that for myocardial cells. It is largely caused by Ca^{2+} influx, resulting in a slower rise of phase 0 than for myocardial cells. The anatomic location of pacemaker cells correlates with the slope of phase 4 diastolic depolarization. The cells situated more proximally (e.g., sinus node) have a steeper slope and thus an inherently higher discharge rate than more distally located pacemaker cells; consequently, when

the proximal cells are in control, there is a higher heart rate.

Once depolarization begins, the cell becomes refractory to other stimuli. Initially, the cell will be totally refractory irrespective of the strength of the stimulus (**absolute refractory period**), but during the latter part of the action potential depolarization can be induced in response to a stronger than normal stimulus (**relative refractory period**). Because excitation and recovery do not occur simultaneously in all cardiac cells, asynchrony of repolarization may occur. This results in a vulnerable period during which the heart is susceptible to the induction of arrhythmias since some cells will be able to conduct impulses whereas others will not, thus allowing for the possible occurrence of reentry phenomena, as described in the following section. The application of a single stimulus at this time may elicit an abnormal response such as ventricular fibrillation. This vulnerable period corresponds approximately to the latter part of the T wave on the electrocardiogram. Antiarrhythmic drugs may alter the duration of the vulnerable period, thus altering the likelihood of an arrhythmia developing in response to a given stimulus.

MECHANISMS OF ARRHYTHMOGENESIS AND THE EFFECTS OF ANTIARRHYTHMIC INTERVENTION

There are two putative causes of arrhythmias: alterations in impulse formation leading to **enhanced or abnormal automaticity**, and alterations in impulse conduction resulting in the **reentry phenomenon**.

Effect of Antiarrhythmic Agents on Automaticity

Spontaneous phase 4 depolarization (*i.e.*, absence of a measurable resting membrane potential) is a property of the sinus node, A-V node, His-Purkinje system, and certain specialized atrial fibres. The ability of these cells to depolarize spontaneously is called **normal automaticity**. Arrhythmias caused by alterations in automaticity are thought to arise from **enhanced normal automaticity** at any one of these sites other than the sinus node. It should be noted that normal myocardial cells do not depolarize spontaneously and, therefore, arrhythmias due to enhanced normal automaticity cannot originate in these cells.

Damaged myocardial cells often remain partially depolarized, and this failure to reach maximum negative diastolic potential may induce abnormal automatic discharges. Unlike enhanced normal automaticity, arrhythmias due to **abnormal automaticity** can occur in myocardial cells as well as in specialized conduction tissue. In the presence of myocardial cell necrosis, hypoxia, or potassium imbalance, the cell fails to repolarize fully and the resting potential only reaches -30 to -40 mV; in digitalis toxicity, in the presence of potassium loss, the resting potential reaches -70 to -85 mV.

Most antiarrhythmic agents suppress automaticity by decreasing the slope of phase 4 spontaneous depolarization and/or shifting the voltage threshold to a less negative level (see Fig. 35–1). Although this effect also decreases the frequency of discharge of normal pacemaker cells (*e.g.*, the sinus node), it has a more pronounced action on ectopic pacemaker activity. The relatively selective suppression of ectopic pacemaker foci may abolish an arrhythmia due to automaticity at doses of a drug that have little effect on normal sinus node function. However, in states where the sinus node or conducting tissue exhibits impaired function (*e.g.*, sick sinus syndrome), suppression of phase 4 depolarization may result in a reduction of the heart rate or possible asystole.

Effect of Antiarrhythmic Agents on Reentry

Reentry depends upon the existence of two anatomically or physiologically distinct pathways as shown in

Figure 35–2. Normally, impulses from higher centres in the conducting system (*e.g.*, the A-V node) will be conducted in the same direction down both pathways, bifurcating to cover the entire ventricular surface. However, should there be a unidirectional block (*e.g.*, due to myocardial injury or prolonged refractoriness) in pathway 2, the impulse may only be conducted down pathway 1. If the block in pathway 2 is in the forward direction only, it may be possible for the impulse to return in a retrograde fashion through this pathway, reaching the initial point of bifurcation, provided that the refractory period in the circuit is not exceeded. Under these circumstances, reexcitation of the myocardium may occur *via* this short-circuiting of the conducting tissue, thus causing a ventricular premature contraction. If this reentry mechanism becomes repetitive, a sustained ventricular arrhythmia such as ventricular

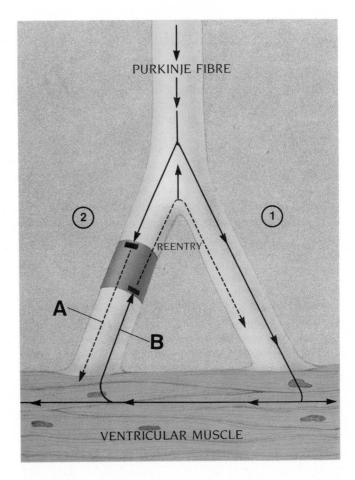

Figure 35–2 Mechanism of reentry and effect of antiarrhythmic intervention. The impulse is conducted unimpeded down pathway 1 but encounters an area of anatomic or functional block in pathway 2. The impulse can then be conducted retrogradely through pathway 2, and reentry into pathway 1 may be established. Drugs can abolish the arrhythmia by improving forward conduction (A) or by preventing retrograde conduction (B).

CARDIOVASCULAR SYSTEM

tachycardia occurs. Similar reentry mechanisms have been proposed in the atria as a common cause of atrial flutter, and in the A-V node as a cause of paroxysmal atrial tachycardia.

Antiarrhythmic agents can abolish reentry by one of two mechanisms: (1) They can improve conduction in the abnormal pathway, converting a unidirectional block to normal forward conduction. (2) They may further depress membrane responsiveness, resulting in slowed conduction and/or increased refractoriness. This results in the normal pathway becoming more resistant to early depolarization by the reentrant stimulus, or in further impairment of conduction in the area of unidirectional block, thus preventing passage of the retrograde impulse.

Most antiarrhythmic drugs appear to act by slowing conduction and/or increasing refractoriness, converting unidirectional into bidirectional block.

ANTIARRHYTHMIC DRUGS

The most widely accepted classification of antiarrhythmic drug action was initially proposed by Vaughan Williams (and later modified), who separated the various agents according to their predominant electrophysiologic effects on the action potential. It is important to understand that this classification is descriptive and its clinical relevance has not yet been clarified. Many of the antiarrhythmic drugs shown in Figure 35–3 have actions relating to more than one class or subclass in the classification. Moreover, many antiarrhythmic drugs have active metabolites with a different class of action than that of the parent drug. The classification in Table 35–1 is used in the following paragraphs.

Class I antiarrhythmic drugs, of which quinidine is the prototype, slow the rate of rise of phase 0 (V_{max}) of the action potential, by blocking membrane sodium channels and thus decreasing the rate of entry of Na^+. These drugs have little or no effect on the resting membrane potential in doses used in clinical practice. They cause a decrease in excitability and conduction velocity; some also prolong the effective refractory period, and may decrease the slope of phase 4 spontaneous depolarization in pacemaker cells. Quinidine, procainamide and lidocaine also exhibit local anaesthetic activity on the myocardial membrane.

Class II agents include the β-adrenoceptor antagonists. These drugs depress phase 4 depolarization and exert their antiarrhythmic effects through competitive inhibition of the β-adrenoceptor site. In high concentrations, many of these agents also show local anaesthetic properties, but this action is not usually seen in clinical practice.

Class III agents prolong the duration of the action potential with a consequent increase in the absolute and effective refractory period. Some of these agents (e.g., bretylium) have no significant effect on phase 4

depolarization, whereas others (e.g., amiodarone) may depress it.

Class IV agents decrease the amount of calcium available for displacement from the cell membrane and correspondingly decrease the inward current carried by calcium. The net result is a decrease in the rate of rise (slope) of phase 4 spontaneous depolarization and slowed conduction in tissues dependent on calcium currents (e.g., A-V node).

The pharmacokinetics of antiarrhythmic drugs are summarized in Table 35–2. Table 35–3 lists the important pharmacodynamic mechanisms, properties, and toxicities of the agents discussed in the following paragraphs.

Class Ia Drugs

Quinidine

Pharmacokinetics. Quinidine sulfate is rapidly and nearly completely absorbed after oral administration; the gluconate salt is absorbed more slowly and less completely. An intravenous preparation is available but can cause severe hypotension and must be administered with extreme caution. Approximately 80% of a quinidine dose is hydroxylated in the liver, but the cardioactivity of the metabolites has not been confirmed. The remainder of the drug is excreted unchanged by the kidney.

Antiarrhythmic effects. As already described, quinidine slows the rapid sodium current, thereby

TABLE 35–1 Classification of Antiarrhythmic Drug Action

Class	Predominant Action	Drugs
Ia	Slowing of rate of rise of phase 0, slowing of conduction, prolongation of refractoriness.	Quinidine Procainamide Disopyramide
Ib	Slight slowing of conduction, no change in refractoriness.	Lidocaine Mexiletine Tocainide Phenytoin
Ic	Marked slowing of conduction, little or modest prolongation of refractoriness.	Flecainide Encainide Propafenone
II	β-Adrenoceptor antagonism.	Beta-blockers (e.g., propranolol)
III	Prolongation of action potential duration, and of refractoriness.	Bretylium Amiodarone Sotalol
IV	Blockade of calcium entry, decrease of slope of phase 4.	Verapamil Diltiazem

Modified from Vaughan Williams EM. Pharmacol Ther 1975.

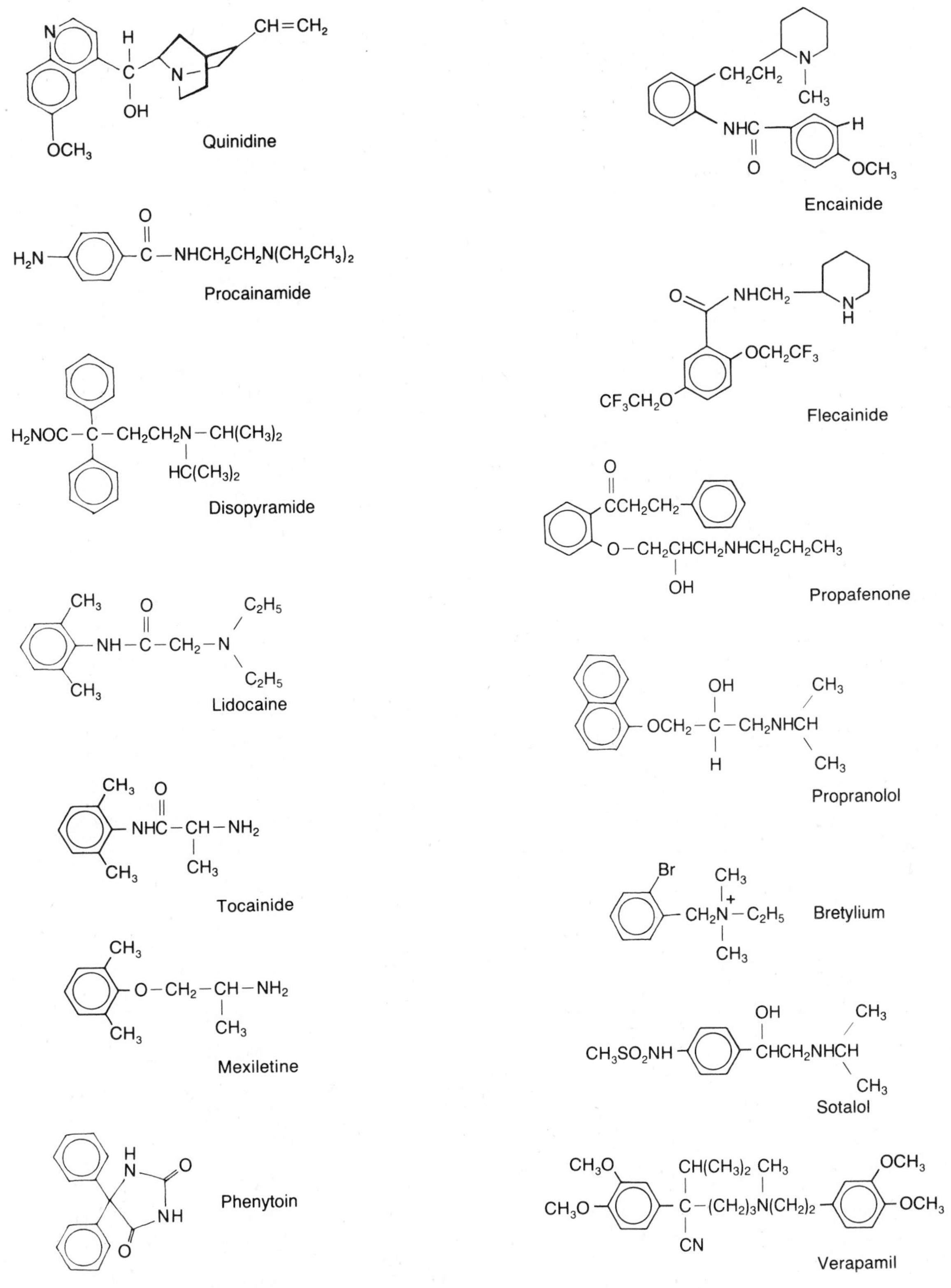

Figure 35–3 Antiarrhythmic drugs in current clinical use.

CARDIOVASCULAR SYSTEM

TABLE 35-2 Pharmacokinetics of Antiarrhythmic Drugs

Drug	Bioavailability (%)	V_d (L/kg)	Protein Binding (%)	Half-Life (h)	Therapeutic Range	Biotransformation and Excretion	Metabolites
Quinidine	75	2–3	75–90	4–8	2–6 µg/mL (7.3–21.9 µmol/L)	Liver: 80% Kidney: 10–20% unchanged	Hydroxyquinidine, slight activity
Procainamide	75–95	1.5–2.5	15–25	2–4	4–10 µg/mL (17–42.5 µmol/L)	Liver: Acetylation Kidney: 60% unchanged	N-acetylprocainamide (NAPA): Class III activity
Disopyramide	90	0.5–1.5	35–95	6–9	2–5 µg/mL	Liver: 25–35% inactive compound Kidney: 50% unchanged	N-dealkyl disopyramide, less active than parent compound
Lidocaine	—	1–2	65–75	0.3–2	1.5–5 µg/mL (5.7–21.3 µmol/L)	Liver: 90% dealkylated	Monoethylglycyl-xylidine (MEGX), glycine xylidine (GX): relatively inactive
Mexiletine	90	5–9	75	9–12	0.5–2 µg/mL	Liver: 90% Kidney: 10% unchanged (↑ with acid urine)	Inactive
Tocainide	100	2–3	2–22	11–15	4–10 µg/mL	Liver: 60% Kidney: 40% unchanged	Inactive
Phenytoin	Variable	0.5–1	90	18–36	10–20 µg/mL (39.6–79.2 µmol/L)	Liver: 95% hydroxylated to inactive compound	Inactive
Flecainide	95	9	50	14–50	200–1000 ng/mL (0.42–2.11 µmol/L)	Liver: >95%	Inactive
Encainide	7–82 dose-dependent	2.7	70	3	250–1400 ng/mL (in absence of metabolites)	Liver: >99% except in poor metabolizers	O-demethyl encainide (ODE), methyl-O-demethyl encainide (MODE): very active
Propafenone	5–12 dose-dependent	3	>95	3–5	500–1000 ng/mL	Liver: >99% genetic variation in biotransformation	5-OH propafenone: active
Propranolol	25–50	3–4	85–95	3–6	50–100 ng/mL (192.8–385.5 nmol/L)	Liver: High first-pass extraction	4-OH propranolol: slight activity
Bretylium	15–30	5–6	<10	6–10	0.5–1.5 µg/mL	Kidney: 80% unchanged	None
Amiodarone	20–50	Very large	Probably high	20–50 days	0.5–3 µg/mL	Liver: De-ethylation	Desethyl amiodarone (DEA): probably active
Sotalol	>95	1.5	Negligible	13	1–2 µg/mL (3.7–7.4 µmol/L)	Kidney: 100% unchanged	None
Verapamil	15–30	4–5	90	3–7	≈100 ng/mL	Liver: High first-pass extraction	Norverapamil: moderately active

TABLE 35-3 Pharmacologic Mechanisms, Effects, and Toxicity of Antiarrhythmic Agents

Drug	Antiarrhythmic Effects	ECG	Hemodynamic Properties	Toxicity

Quinidine		↑ HR
		↑ PR ↑ QRS
		↑ QT
			Minimal:
			  Negative inotropism
			  Vasodilatation
			  Decreased blood pressure
				Impaired conduction/asystole
				Ventricular arrhythmias
				Gastrointestinal intolerance
				Cinchonism
				Thrombocytopenia
				Drug fever

	↓ Rate of rise, phase 0
	  (V_{max})
	↓ Slope, phase 4
	Prolong ERP, but
	  modest effect on APD			

Procainamide	Abolish normal
	  automaticity
	Abolish reentry by
	  producing bidirectional
	  block
		↑ HR
		↑ PR ↑ QRS
		↑ QT
			Minimal:
			  Negative inotropism
			  Vasodilatation
				Impaired conduction and
				  ventricular arrhythmias
				Gastrointestinal intolerance
				Agranulocytosis
				Drug-induced systemic lupus
				  erythematosus

Disopyramide		↑ HR
		↑ PR ↑ QRS
		↑ QT
			Marked negative
			  inotropism
			Vasoconstriction
				Anticholinergic effects:
				  dry mouth, constipation,
				  urinary retention, blurred
				  vision
				Ventricular arrhythmias

Lidocaine		±↓ QT	No impairment of normal contractility	Drowsiness Respiratory arrest Convulsions
	↓Rate of rise, phase 0 ↓ Slope, phase 4 Shorten APD and ERP			

Mexiletine	Abolish abnormal
	  automaticity
		QT←→	Minimal or no
			  impairment of
			  contractility
				Gastrointestinal disturbance
				Dizziness, ataxia, tremor

Tocainide	Abolish reentry by producing bidirectional	↓ QT		

Phenytoin	block, removing uni-
	  directional block
		↓ QT	Decreased blood pressure
			  on i.v. administration
				Nystagmus, ataxia
				Lethargy
				Gastrointestinal intolerance

Flecainide	Marked ↓$\dot V_{max}$	↑ PR
		↑ QRS
			Moderate
			  depression of
			  contractility
				Weakness
				Dizziness
				Proarrhythmia

Encainide	Marked ↓$\dot V_{max}$
	↑ ERP
		↑ PR
		↑ QRS
		↑→QT
			Minimal
			  depression of
			  contractility
				Dizziness
				Proarrhythmia

Propafenone	Marked ↓$\dot V_{max}$
	↑ ERP
		↑ PR
		↑ QRS
		↑→ QT
			Moderate
			  depression of
			  contractility
				Dizziness
				Altered taste
				Proarrhythmia

Propranolol	↓ Slope, phase 4
	Competitive
	  β-adrenoceptor
	  blockade
	Abolishes catechol-
	  amine-dependent
	  arrhythmias
		↓ HR	Negative inotropism
			Decreased blood pressure
				Impaired A-V conduction/
				  asystole
				Bronchospasm
				Nightmares, insomnia

APD = action potential duration; ERP = effective refractory period; HR = heart rate; PR, QRS, QT = respective ECG intervals; ↑/↓ = increase/decrease.

Table continues next page

TABLE 35–3 Pharmacologic Mechanisms, Effects, and Toxicity of Antiarrhythmic Agents (Continued)

Drug	Antiarrhythmic Effects	ECG	Hemodynamic Properties	Toxicity
Bretylium	Prolongs APD Little effect on normal automaticity	↓ HR ↑ QT	Decreased blood pressure	Gastrointestinal disturbance Parotid swelling
Amiodarone	Prolongs APD and ERP Noncompetitive β-adrenoceptor blockade Abolishes normal automaticity Abolishes reentry by producing bidirectional blockade	↓ HR ↑ QT	No impairment of normal contractility Decreased blood pressure and increased coronary blood flow on i.v. administration	Photosensitivity Skin pigmentation changes Thyroid function abnormalities Corneal microdeposits
Sotalol	↓ Slope, phase 4 β-Adrenoceptor blockade ↑ APD, ↑ ERP	↓ HR ↑ QT	Negative inotropism Decreased blood pressure	Fatigue, lethargy Proarrhythmia (torsade de pointes)
Verapamil	↓ Slope, phase 4 ↑ Refractoriness of A-V node Abolishes normal automaticity Abolishes reentry by producing bidirectional blockade	↑ PR	Negative inotropism Vasodilatation Decreased blood pressure	Impaired conduction/asystole Gastrointestinal intolerance Constipation

APD = action potential duration; ERP = effective refractory period; HR = heart rate; PR, QRS, QT = respective ECG intervals; ↑/↓ = increase/decrease.

decreasing the rate of rise of phase 0 of the action potential (V_{max}). It also decreases the slope of phase 4 spontaneous depolarization, thus tending to inhibit ectopic rhythms due to automaticity. Although quinidine suppresses ventricular arrhythmias caused by increased normal automaticity, it has little effect on abnormal automaticity. Quinidine may also abolish reentrant arrhythmias: it produces bidirectional block (Fig. 35–2, example B) by depressing membrane responsiveness and prolonging the effective refractory period.

In the presence of an intact autonomic nervous system, quinidine may cause an increase in heart rate either by a reflex increase in sympathetic activity or by a decrease in vagal tone. In patients with sick sinus syndrome, severe sinus node depression may occur, causing an aggravation of bradycardia.

Quinidine is useful in the treatment of a wide variety of arrhythmias including atrial, A-V junctional, and ventricular tachyarrhythmias.

Effect on the electrocardiogram. Quinidine may increase the rate of discharge of the sinus node. In therapeutic concentrations there is little effect on the P–R interval, but prolongation of the QRS complex and Q–Tc (Q–T interval corrected for heart rate) occurs. These effects become more pronounced with increasing plasma concentrations.

Cardiovascular and hemodynamic effects. Quinidine decreases myocardial contractility (negative inotropic effect). However, therapeutic concentrations of quinidine do not usually impair myocardial performance since the negative inotropism is minimal. If administered intravenously (rarely done), quinidine may produce vasodilatation and marked hypotension.

Cautions and toxicity. With increasing plasma levels, the risk of S-A and A-V block or asystole increases, while toxic concentrations may induce abnormal automaticity and ventricular tachycardia. Another ventricular arrhythmia may be observed in patients who exhibit excessive Q–T prolongation; this is known as "torsade de pointes" polymorphic ventricular tachycardia and may occur at therapeutic plasma concentrations of quinidine.

When administered to patients in atrial fibrillation or flutter, quinidine may occasionally cause a paradoxic increase in the ventricular rate. This is because the drug may decrease the number of atrial impulses reaching the A-V node to such an extent that 1:1 conduction through the A-V node becomes possible, and may hasten A-V conduction through its anticholinergic effect. In clinical practice, most patients receive digitalis preparations before quinidine is administered in order to avoid this phenomenon.

It is important to note that quinidine can interact with other drugs. In particular, it will cause a two-fold increase in serum digoxin concentration in patients at steady state, as a result of decreased renal and non-renal clearance of digoxin and the displacement of digoxin from tissue binding sites by the quinidine molecule.

Gastrointestinal intolerance (nausea and diarrhea) is common, while large doses of the drug may produce cinchonism, which is characterized by a spectrum of symptoms including blurred vision, tinnitus, headache, and gastrointestinal upset. Drug fever and rare idiosyncratic reactions, such as thrombocytopenia secondary to antiplatelet antibodies, have also been reported.

Procainamide

Pharmacokinetics. Procainamide (Procan®, Pronestyl®) is more than 75% bioavailable after oral administration. The intravenous preparation is relatively frequently used but can cause hypotension if rapidly administered. Procainamide has a relatively short half-life of 2–3 hours.

A variable proportion of the drug is acetylated in the liver to N-acetylprocainamide (NAPA). NAPA, unlike the parent drug, has little effect on V_{max} of Purkinje fibres but prolongs action potential duration, thus having the properties of Class III drug action. The concentration-response relationship for NAPA is different from that for procainamide; it is therefore not useful to add the concentrations of the parent drug and its metabolite when using plasma level monitoring to estimate drug effect.

The NAPA metabolite is eliminated primarily *via* the kidneys. Hence the patient's acetylation status (*see* Chapter 12) and renal function will be important in determining the plasma concentration at steady state, and dosages will need to be adjusted in renal failure.

Antiarrhythmic effects. The antiarrhythmic properties of procainamide are similar to those of quinidine; it has comparable effects on automaticity, excitability, responsiveness, and conduction. This results in **similar electrocardiographic features** at therapeutic and toxic plasma concentrations.

Hemodynamic properties. Procainamide is comparable to quinidine in its minor negative inotropic effects at usual oral clinical doses. Intravenous administration may produce vasodilatation and hypotension in addition to more marked negative inotropism.

Cautions and toxicity. Excessive concentrations of procainamide impair conduction and may cause asystole or the induction of ventricular arrhythmias. Central nervous system side effects include depression, hallucinations and psychosis, but gastrointestinal intolerance is less frequent than with quinidine. Hypersensitivity reactions include occasional drug fever and, rarely, agranulocytosis. A more troublesome reaction is the development of a syndrome resembling systemic lupus erythematosus (SLE), which presents with arthralgia, fever, and pleural-pericardial inflammation. The drug-induced SLE may be accompanied by LE cells in the blood smear. An anti-nuclear factor is often present in the blood of patients receiving procainamide and is not by itself diagnostic of the SLE syndrome. This syndrome usually disappears on withdrawal of the drug, although cases of persistent SLE have been reported following procainamide therapy. The SLE phenomenon is dose- and time-related and is more likely to occur in patients who exhibit slow hepatic acetylation resulting in higher plasma drug concentrations of the parent compound.

Disopyramide

Pharmacokinetics. As 50% or more of orally ingested disopyramide is excreted unchanged by the kidneys, the dosage will require adjustment downwards in renal insufficiency. Approximately 30% of the drug is converted by the liver to the less active mono-N-dealkylated metabolite.

Antiarrhythmic effects. Disopyramide (Norpace®, Rythmodan®) has properties similar to those of quinidine, in that it slows the rate of rise of phase 0 (V_{max}) of the action potential and causes a concentration-dependent decrease in the slope of phase 4 depolarization. Disopyramide also slows the rate of discharge of the sinus node and may cause serious bradyarrhythmias in patients with preexisting sinus node dysfunction. The **electrocardiographic** features are similar to those of quinidine and procainamide.

Hemodynamic effects. In comparison with quinidine and procainamide, disopyramide exerts a marked negative inotropic effect and may produce clinically important decreases in myocardial contractility and cardiac output in patients with preexisting impairment of left ventricular function. This property limits the usefulness of the agent in patients with a history of congestive heart failure.

Cautions and toxicity. Most of the side effects seen with disopyramide relate to its anticholinergic activity (*e.g.*, dry mouth, urinary hesitancy or retention, blurred vision, and constipation). As with quinidine, patients who demonstrate an excessively prolonged Q–T interval with disopyramide are at risk of developing ventricular arrhythmias related to the therapy itself. In addition, when disopyramide is used as the sole agent in the management of atrial fibrillation it may produce an increase in the ventricular rate by a mechanism similar to that described for quinidine.

Class Ib Drugs

Lidocaine

Pharmacokinetics. Lidocaine is given intravenously because extensive first-pass transformation by the liver prevents the attainment of clinically effective plasma concentrations by the oral route. The drug is dealkylated and eliminated almost entirely by the liver, so that dosage adjustments are necessary in the presence of hepatic disease or dysfunction.

Antiarrhythmic effects. Lidocaine (Xylocard®) causes a reduction in V_{max} (phase 0) of the action potential. It also shortens the duration of the action potential and the effective refractory period of normal Purkinje fibres and ventricular myocardial cells. The shortening effect on the action potential is greater than that on the effective refractory period, and thus the effective refractory period is lengthened relative to the action potential duration. Lidocaine has little activity on the action potential duration in atrial tissue.

Sinus node function is not altered in normal subjects but may occasionally be depressed in patients with preexisting sinus node dysfunction. Unlike quinidine, lidocaine is capable of suppressing abnormal automaticity in conditions such as digitalis excess. Lidocaine abolishes ventricular reentry by a mechanism similar to that for quinidine (see Fig. 35–2, example B). The drug slows conduction most in diseased tissues (hypoxic, ischemic) and at high rates of stimulation ("use-" or frequency-dependent effect). Lidocaine is especially useful in treating ventricular arrhythmias arising during myocardial ischemia, such as during myocardial infarction. It has little effect on atrial or A-V junctional arrhythmias.

Electrocardiogram. Lidocaine has minimal effects on the ECG, although shortening of the Q–T interval is occasionally seen.

Hemodynamic effects. In clinical practice, lidocaine does not impair left ventricular function and has little or no negative inotropic effect. Unlike Class Ia drugs, lidocaine does not alter autonomic function.

Toxicity. Central nervous system side effects predominate, with drowsiness, slurred speech, paresthesias, agitation, and confusion being the most common. These symptoms may progress to convulsions and respiratory arrest (compare with cocaine, Chapter 24) if higher plasma concentrations of the drug develop.

Mexiletine

Pharmacokinetics. Mexiletine (Mexitil®) is an orally effective structural analog of lidocaine. It is well absorbed and biotransformed by the liver to inactive metabolites; the half-life is relatively long (about 12 hours).

Antiarrhythmic effects. The drug has electrophysiologic effects similar to those of lidocaine, shortening the action potential duration in normal tissues but slowing conduction, especially in diseased tissues. Mexiletine also suppresses abnormal automaticity in Purkinje fibres. Like lidocaine, it is effective in the treatment of ventricular arrhythmias and relatively ineffective for atrial or A-V junctional arrhythmias.

Electrocardiogram. Mexiletine has minimal effects on the ECG.

Hemodynamics. Very little negative inotropic effect

is seen, and the drug can be given to patients with significant left ventricular dysfunction.

Toxicity. Gastrointestinal (nausea, anorexia) and CNS side effects (tremor, ataxia, dizziness, diplopia, insomnia, confusion) are common and respond to a decrease in dose. As with lidocaine, drug-induced arrhythmias are uncommon.

Tocainide

Tocainide (Tonocard®) is another oral analog of lidocaine with a very similar electrophysiologic and chemical efficacy profile to that of lidocaine.

It is well absorbed and has high systemic bioavailability, with a half-life of approximately 12 hours.

Side effects are similar to those of lidocaine and mexiletine, but the drug can on rare occasions cause **agranulocytosis**. It is recommended by the manufacturer for use only when other antiarrhythmic agents are ineffective.

Phenytoin

This drug is described in greater detail as an antiepileptic agent in Chapter 21 (see also Table 35–2).

Antiarrhythmic effects and electrocardiogram. The antiarrhythmic properties of phenytoin generally resemble those of lidocaine. This drug is rarely used as an antiarrhythmic agent, with the possible exception of the treatment of rhythm disturbances secondary to digitalis overdose. It is more often used in children with ventricular arrhythmias. Phenytoin shortens the Q–T interval in the ECG.

Hemodynamic effects. As with lidocaine, clinically useful doses of phenytoin produce little or no alteration in left ventricular function.

Class Ic Drugs

Flecainide

Pharmacokinetics. Flecainide (Tambocor®) has a long half-life of 16–20 hours after oral administration; it undergoes minimal biotransformation to inactive metabolites.

Antiarrhythmic effects. The drug is a potent suppressant of V_{max} in Purkinje and myocardial fibres, causing marked slowing of conduction in all cardiac tissues with relatively small and variable effects on action potential duration and refractoriness. Automaticity is reduced by an elevation in threshold potential rather than a decrease in the slope of phase 4 depolarization. Like other Class Ic agents, the drug is effective in a wide variety of atrial, A-V nodal, and ventricular arrhythmias. It is a particularly potent suppressant of premature ventricular contractions ("PVC killer") and is highly effective in slowing conduction over accessory atrioventricular bypass tracts in the Wolff-Parkinson-White syndrome.

Electrocardiogram. Flecainide causes a dose-dependent increase in P–R, QRS, and Q–T intervals; Q–Tc intervals are little changed. QRS intervals may increase by up to 50%, and excessive increases appear to be associated with drug toxicity.

Hemodynamic effects. Flecainide has negative inotropic effects and can cause worsening of congestive heart failure, especially in patients with severe preexisting left ventricular dysfunction.

Toxicity. The most common side effects include dizziness, blurred vision, headache, and nausea. Like other drugs with Class Ic action, flecainide can cause a severe worsening of preexisting arrhythmias or **de novo appearance of life-threatening ventricular tachycardia resistant to treatment**.

Encainide

Encainide (Enkaid®) has an electrophysiologic profile similar to that of flecainide. It has two potent metabolites with somewhat different spectra of action than the parent drug. The clinical uses and toxicity are similar to those of flecainide. (At the time of writing, the drug is available for use in the United States, but is still investigational in Canada.)

Propafenone

Pharmacokinetics. Propafenone (Rythmol®) undergoes extensive first-pass transformation to a hydroxylated metabolite with reduced electrophysiological effects. The clearance is dose-dependent, with higher doses exhibiting lower clearance and prolonged half-life; clearance is impaired in patients with liver disease.

Antiarrhythmic effects. Propafenone, like flecainide and encainide, markedly slows conduction in all cardiac tissues. It also prolongs action potential duration in atrial and ventricular tissues, thus also prolonging refractoriness. It decreases the slope of phase 4 in Purkinje fibres but has little effect on sinus node automaticity. Like flecainide and encainide, propafenone is a ''broad-spectrum'' antiarrhythmic effective in a wide variety of arrhythmias.

Electrocardiogram. The drug causes an increase in all ECG intervals, including P–R, QRS, Q–T, and Q–Tc duration.

Hemodynamic effects. Negative inotropism with worsening of congestive failure is occasionally seen.

Toxicity. Propafenone is usually well tolerated, but can cause nausea, weakness, and a metallic taste. It may also have severe **proarrhythmic effects**, similar to those of the other agents with Class Ic properties.

Class II Drugs

Propranolol

Although propranolol is not a potent suppressant of premature ventricular contractions, it has been shown to reduce the incidence of sudden, presumably arrhythmic, death following myocardial infarction. As with metoprolol and timolol, this effect may be a direct antiarrhythmic and/or an indirect anti-ischemic effect of chronic β-adrenoceptor blockade.

This drug, and other β-adrenoceptor antagonists like it, are described in greater detail in Chapter 17 (*see also* Table 35–2).

Antiarrhythmic effects. Propranolol exerts its major antiarrhythmic effect through competitive inhibition of β adrenoceptors, which also results in a relative excess of vagal effects on the heart. Although the drug also possesses a local anaesthetic action, this property does not contribute to its role as an antiarrhythmic agent in therapeutic doses. Propranolol decreases the slope of phase 4 depolarization of the sinus node. This action characteristically results in sinus bradycardia. In conditions in which catecholamine excess is responsible for generating autonomous ectopic rhythm disturbances (*e.g.*, pheochromocytoma, exercise-induced ventricular tachycardia) propranolol is useful in abolishing the arrhythmia.

Hemodynamic and adverse effects. Other properties of propranolol, its hemodynamic effects and its toxicity, are discussed in Chapter 17. In brief, the adverse cardiac effects of propranolol are generally predictable, the most important being left ventricular failure, hypotension, bradycardia and, rarely, A-V block.

Class III Drugs

Bretylium

Pharmacokinetics. Bretylium (Bretylate®) is poorly absorbed from the gastrointestinal tract and is therefore generally administered parenterally. The drug is excreted unchanged in the urine and dosage adjustment is required in the presence of renal failure.

Antiarrhythmic effects. Bretylium differs from Class I antiarrhythmic agents in that it does not slow the rise of phase 0 (V_{max}) of the cardiac action potential, and does not reduce the slope of phase 4 depolarization. Furthermore, therapeutic serum concentrations do not alter membrane responsiveness appreciably. The drug does, however, prolong both the duration of the action potential and the effective refractory period in Purkinje fibres.

Bretylium is generally reserved for use in life-threatening ventricular arrhythmias, especially recurrent ventricular fibrillation.

Electrocardiogram.   The drug reduces the sinus rate and prolongs the Q–T interval.

Hemodynamic effects.   Bretylium initially displaces catecholamines from sympathetic terminals but then usually causes hypotension as a result of its adrenergic neuron blocking action (*see* Chapter 18). Severe postural hypotension can be seen after prolonged administration, most commonly in patients with preexisting impairment of left ventricular function.

Toxicity.   Nausea and vomiting may occur with rapid intravenous administration, and long-term oral therapy has been reported to produce painful parotid gland enlargement.

Amiodarone

Amiodarone (Cordarone®) is a very complex and incompletely understood drug originally introduced as an antianginal agent.

Pharmacokinetics.   Amiodarone is incompletely absorbed after oral administration. It is very extensively taken up by tissues, especially fatty tissues, and has a half-life of up to 60 days after long-term administration. The drug is extensively de-ethylated in the liver to N-desethyl amiodarone, which has significant electrophysiologic effects. Full clinical effects may not be achieved for up to 6 weeks after initiation of treatment, with a slower onset for some effects (increases in refractoriness) than others (slowing of A-V nodal conduction).

Antiarrhythmic effects.   The drug has complex effects and possesses Class I, II, III, and IV actions. Its dominant effect is probably through prolongation of action potential duration and refractoriness. It also slows cardiac conduction, acts as a calcium-channel blocker, as a weak β-adrenoceptor blocker, and it may have central antiadrenergic effects. The high iodine content of amiodarone exerts an antithyroid action, which may in itself have antiarrhythmic effects. Amiodarone can be used in the treatment of virtually any clinical tachyarrhythmia.

Electrocardiogram.   Amiodarone causes an increase in the Q–T interval and smaller increases in P–R and QRS intervals. Sinus bradycardia can occur.

Hemodynamic effects.   The drug is a vasodilator and an effective antianginal agent. Although it has modest negative inotropic properties, clinically evident hemodynamic compromise is rarely seen, even in patients with severe left ventricular dysfunction.

Toxicity.   Amiodarone has a very wide spectrum of toxic effects. After long-term use of several years' duration, more than 50% of patients will suffer limiting side effects, often requiring drug discontinuation. Some of the more common effects include GI intolerance, tremor, ataxia, dizziness, hyper- or hypothyroidism, corneal microdeposits (invariable) with disturbance of night vision (occasional), liver toxicity, photosensitivity, slate-gray facial discoloration, neuropathy, muscle weakness, weight loss, symptomatic bradycardia, and proarrhythmia (rare). The most dangerous side effect is pulmonary fibrosis, which occurs in 5–15% of patients.

Sotalol

Sotalol (Sotacor®) is a β-adrenoceptor blocker that also prolongs action potential duration and refractoriness in all cardiac tissues.

Pharmacokinetics.   Sotalol has a half-life of about 12 hours after oral administration. It is eliminated largely by the kidneys and doses need to be lowered substantially in patients with renal dysfunction.

Electrocardiogram.   Sotalol prolongs the Q–T interval and causes sinus bradycardia.

Antiarrhythmic effects.   The drug suppresses phase 4 spontaneous depolarization, and may produce severe sinus bradycardia. It also slows A-V nodal conduction. The combination of β-adrenoceptor blockade and prolongation of action potential duration may be especially effective in the prevention of sustained ventricular tachycardia.

Hemodynamic effects.   Significant left ventricular dysfunction can occur when sotalol is administered, especially in patients with previous left ventricular enlargement and congestive heart failure.

Toxicity.   Fatigue, dizziness, and insomnia can occur. Drug-induced polymorphic ventricular tachycardia can develop in patients with excessive Q–T prolongation, especially if hypokalemia is present.

Class IV Drugs

Verapamil, Diltiazem

These drugs are described in greater detail in Chapter 36, *Calcium-Channel Blockers* (*see also* Table 35–2).

Antiarrhythmic effects.   Verapamil (Isoptin®) and diltiazem (Cardizem®) block the inward current carried by Ca^{2+}, and exert their main antiarrhythmic action by slowing A-V node conduction and prolonging its effective refractory period; they thus slow the ventricular response to atrial fibrillation. Phase 0 of the action potential is not altered, and neither is the duration of the action potential. The slope of phase 4 depolarization is decreased, and heart rate is slightly reduced. Verapamil, when given intravenously, abolishes reentry rhythms involving the A-V node, such as A-V nodal reentrant tachycardia.

Electrocardiogram.   The P–R interval may increase, but QRS duration and the Q–T interval are not altered.

Hemodynamic effects.   Verapamil, and to a lesser extent diltiazem, have negative inotropic properties and may impair left ventricular performance in patients with preexisting myocardial dysfunction. The drugs also cause peripheral vasodilatation with a resultant fall in blood pressure.

Cautions and toxicity.   Both verapamil and diltiazem may cause bradycardia, and asystole has been reported, particularly if the drugs are used in combination with a beta-blocker. Side effects include gastrointestinal intolerance and constipation. Diltiazem on rare occasions may cause headache, flushing, and ankle swelling.

Digoxin

Although extensively described in Chapter 34, some aspects of digoxin are worthy of consideration in the management of arrhythmias. Digoxin prolongs the effective refractory period and diminishes conduction velocity in Purkinje fibres while conversely shortening the refractory period in atrial and ventricular myocardial cells. Prolongation of the effective refractory period of the A-V node causes P–R interval prolongation in the presence of sinus rhythm and permits digoxin to control the ventricular response rate in atrial fibrillation and flutter, its most important antiarrhythmic action. Digoxin also increases vagal activity and thus reduces the rate of discharge of the S-A node. If present in toxic serum concentrations, digoxin causes increased abnormal automaticity with resulting ventricular rhythm disturbance, which may be potentiated by hypokalemia. This arrhythmia has traditionally been treated with lidocaine or phenytoin.

CLINICAL MANAGEMENT OF ARRHYTHMIAS

Atrial Premature Beats

These generally do not require treatment. However, if they are symptomatic or responsible for initiating paroxysmal atrial arrhythmias, they can be suppressed with quinidine or other Class I agents (*see* Table 35–4).

Atrial Fibrillation and Flutter

In the acute state, sinus rhythm can be restored by means of electrical cardioversion. Alternatively, it may be desirable to use pharmacotherapy. Class I, II, and III drugs may terminate the arrhythmia. Drugs that slow conduction through the A-V node, such as digoxin, verapamil, propranolol, and amiodarone, will tend to control the ventricular response, and thus reduce the heart rate (*see* Table 35–4).

Paroxysmal Atrial Tachycardia

This often arises *via* a reentry phenomenon in the A-V node. Accordingly, drugs with A-V nodal blocking

TABLE 35–4   Therapeutic Choices for the Management of Common Arrhythmias

| Arrhythmia | Acute | | Chronic | |
	First Line	Alternatives	First Line	Alternatives
Atrial premature beats	Usually do not require treatment		Quinidine	Disopyramide Procainamide
Atrial flutter/fibrillation	DC-cardioversion Digitalis	Verapamil Propranolol	Digitalis + Quinidine	Propranolol Flecainide Amiodarone
Paroxysmal atrial tachycardia	Verapamil	Digitalis Propranolol	Digitalis Sotalol	Quinidine Propranolol Amiodarone
Ventricular premature beats	Lidocaine	Procainamide Quinidine Disopyramide	Quinidine	Procainamide Mexiletine Propafenone Flecainide
Ventricular tachycardia	DC-cardioversion	Lidocaine Procainamide Quinidine Amiodarone Bretylium	Procainamide Quinidine Sotalol	Amiodarone Propafenone Flecainide

properties (*e.g.*, verapamil) will often terminate this arrhythmia. Quinidine and amiodarone have been used on a chronic basis for prophylaxis of arrhythmias (*see* Table 35–4).

Ventricular Premature Beats

In the acute situation (*e.g.*, myocardial infarction), these are usually controlled by intravenous lidocaine. Alternative therapy includes intravenous procainamide or oral quinidine. The usefulness of long-term suppression of ventricular premature beats with any one specific agent has not been established; any of the Class I and III drugs may be effective (*see* Table 35–4).

Ventricular Tachycardia

If this arrhythmia occurs acutely with circulatory collapse it is treated by DC-cardioversion. In less severe cases, reversion to sinus rhythm may be accomplished by means of intravenous lidocaine or possibly other Class I agents. All of the Class I and III agents listed have been used for long-term control and suppression of this arrhythmia (*see* Table 35–4).

SUGGESTED READING

Gallagher J. Management of arrhythmias and conduction abnormalities. In: Hurst JW, ed. The heart, arteries and veins. New York: McGraw-Hill, 1982.

Karagueuzian HS. Antiarrhythmic drugs. In: Mandel WJ, ed. Cardiac arrhythmias. 2nd ed. Philadelphia: JB Lippincott, 1987.

Keefe DLD, Kates RE, Harrison DS. New antiarrhythmic drugs: their place in therapy. Drugs 1981; 22:363–400.

Nayler WG. The cellular basis of antiarrhythmic therapy. In: Krikler DM, Goodwin JF, eds. Cardiac arrhythmias: the modern electrophysiological approach. London: WB Saunders, 1975.

Singh BN, Collett JT, Chew CYC. New perspectives in the pharmacologic therapy of cardiac arrhythmias. Prog Cardiovasc Dis 1980; 22:243–301.

Zipes DP. Management of arrhythmias. In: Braunwald E, ed. Heart disease. 2nd ed. Philadelphia: WB Saunders, 1984.

Vaughan Williams EM. Classification of antiarrhythmic drugs. Pharmacol Ther 1975; 1:115–138.

Chapter 36

Vasodilators, Antianginal Drugs, and Calcium-Channel Blockers

W.A. Mahon

Narrowing of blood vessels, either by spasm or by atherosclerosis, is an element common to many important clinical problems. For example, excessive vasoconstrictor tone raises the peripheral resistance and thus contributes to hypertension; atherosclerotic obstruction of coronary or cerebral arteries reduces blood flow to the heart or brain respectively, and can give rise to angina pectoris or impaired cerebral function; atherosclerotic lesions or excessive vasoconstriction in peripheral arteries of the extremities can cause a variety of symptoms ranging from intermittent hypoperfusion (e.g., claudication) to severe ischemia (e.g., gangrene). Spasm and atherosclerosis can coexist in varying degrees in the same patient.

The drugs that are used to treat these problems are of several types, differing widely from each other in chemical and pharmacologic properties.

Vasodilatation may be produced by various types of pharmacologic agents, including pre- or postganglionic blockers of the sympathetic nervous system, α-adrenoceptor blockers, stimulators of β_2-adrenergic, histaminergic, or dopaminergic receptors in the vessels, blockers of calcium channels in the muscle cell membrane, angiotensin converting enzyme inhibitors, and drugs that relax vascular smooth muscle directly without acting on a specific receptor.

As this list implies, the drugs differ widely in chemical structure, in specificity of action, and in primary clinical application. The three main clinical indications for the use of vasodilators are angina pectoris, hypertension, and refractory heart failure. Nitrites are used primarily for angina pectoris; hydralazine, diazoxide, sodium nitroprusside, and minoxidil are used chiefly for treatment of hypertension; calcium-channel blockers are used for both purposes; and various other

agents are useful in the treatment of heart failure that is refractory to conventional treatment.

Many other drugs, including papaverine, nicotinic acid, ethanol, cyclandelate, guancycline, and theophylline and related compounds, have been used in the past as direct-acting vasodilators, for the treatment of peripheral or cerebral vascular obstructive diseases. However, these are no longer considered valid indications. If blood flow in a peripheral artery is diminished because of partial or complete obstruction of a vessel, these drugs will be of no value. Indeed, they may further impair the perfusion in an ischemic area by diverting blood to areas supplied by healthy vessels. Therefore a number of drugs have been developed to deal with the problem of vascular obstructive disease by altering the metabolism of lipids, which form the atheromatous plaques in the walls of the blood vessels (see Chapter 37).

For purposes of discussion, the drugs in current clinical use will be divided, for convenience, into three sections dealing respectively with vasodilators, antianginal drugs, and calcium-channel blockers.

VASODILATORS

Characteristics of Drug-Induced Vasodilatation

Relaxation of smooth muscle is a basic action of all direct-acting vasodilators, but there are considerable differences among them with respect to their relative effects in various tissues and also on different segments within the same vascular bed. The difference in their action on **arteries versus veins** is of particular importance in the therapeutic application of these drugs. Nitrites and nitrates have a pronounced effect on the veins, whereas sodium nitroprusside acts both on arteries (arterioles) and on veins, and hydralazine and diazoxide act mainly on arteries. The reason for this interesting difference in vasodilatory effects on arteries and on veins is not known.

In addition, vasodilators can differ in their action in various vascular areas, *i.e.*, some will increase blood flow mainly in the coronary arteries while others act chiefly in the renal, mesenteric, or skin vessels. The cause of such regional differences of action is probably complex. One factor is the relative effect of the various vasodilators on cardiac function. Blood flow in all tissues depends on the balance between vascular resistance (regulated by local factors such as adrenergic innervation, metabolites, *etc.*) and cardiac output. The relative contribution of cardiac and local factors to the regulation of blood flow is quite different in various tissues. Hence, it is easy to understand that a vasodilator that increases cardiac output (directly, through baroreceptor reflexes, or by enhancing venous return to the heart) may increase blood flow more in a particular vascular area in which perfusion depends mainly on the cardiac output, than another vasodilator that is without such cardiac effect.

The extent of vasodilatation also depends a great deal on the preexisting state of the vessels. Drug-induced relaxation in *in vitro* experiments can be best demonstrated in vessels that have been previously contracted, and will not be demonstrable in those already relaxed. This property of the vasodilators has important consequences in clinical use.

Clinical Indications for the Use of Vasodilators

Hypertension

This is the main indication for the use of vascular smooth muscle relaxants other than the nitrites. The last decade brought an upsurge of interest in these drugs for the treatment of arterial hypertension. Diastolic hypertension is consequent to increased peripheral resistance, and therefore, the rationale for lowering arterial pressure by drugs that relax vascular smooth muscle is obvious. Previously their use was limited because they tended to cause tachycardia and increased cardiac contractility due to activation of baroreceptor reflexes. These compensatory changes counterbalance the antihypertensive effect of the vasodilators. Since the discovery of β-adrenoceptor blocking drugs, however, the reflex tachycardia and the increase in cardiac output can be counteracted. Today vasodilators are used, as a rule, together with beta-blockers to treat hypertension.

The antihypertensive effect of vasodilators is enhanced by the concomitant use of diuretics. Oral diuretics have become the mainstay of antihypertensive therapy and can by themselves effectively control blood pressure in at least one-third of hypertensive patients. In more severe hypertension, diuretics are used in combination with β-adrenoceptor blocking drugs, vasodilators, or some other drugs acting on the sympathetic nervous system (*see* Chapter 38). Diuretics decrease extracellular and plasma volume; this action and their vascular effects enhance the lowering of blood pressure caused by vasodilators. In addition, diuretics prevent retention of salt and water, which is a frequent consequence of the excessive capillary permeability to Na^+ that is caused by vasodilators.

Refractory Heart Failure

Recently, vasodilators have been used with good results in patients with severe chronic heart failure refractory to digitalis and diuretics. This use of vasodilators is based on the concept that the clinical features of heart failure are related not only to severe impairment of myocardial contractile function, but also to excessive peripheral vasoconstriction, which further impairs myocardial performance. Vasodilators are used to overcome the vasoconstriction, and thus diminish the myocardial work load and oxygen requirement. Heart rate (unlike that in hypertensive patients) is not increased in these patients, because blood pressure does not fall and therefore baroreceptor reflexes are not activated. Impressive results have been reported to follow the use of angiotensin converting enzyme (ACE) inhibitors, sodium nitroprusside, isosorbide dinitrate, or prazosin, a postsynaptic α-adrenoceptor blocker. ACE inhibitors are the drugs of choice because they lower the mortality in refractory heart failure.

Vasodilators in Clinical Use

Hydralazine

Hydralazine (Apresoline®) has been widely used for many years to treat moderate or severe hypertension, although seldom as the sole antihypertensive agent. It lowers blood pressure by relaxing vascular smooth muscle and decreasing peripheral resistance, without exerting any central action such as had been proposed in earlier times. It has little effect on veins; therefore orthostatic hypotension is rarely a problem with this drug. Hydralazine reduces renal vascular resistance and tends to maintain renal blood flow. It is well absorbed from the gastrointestinal tract and, interestingly, it yields higher blood levels when given after meals. Termination of its effect is mainly by acetylation, with a higher rate of disappearance in patients who are fast acetylators (*see* Chapters 4 and 12).

Hydralazine is suitable for prolonged treatment of hypertension, particularly in combination with β-adrenoceptor blocking agents and diuretics.

Adverse effects include headache, gastrointestinal complaints, palpitation, arrhythmia, precipitation of angina, and other consequences of vasodilatation. In addition, when given in large doses (at or above 200 mg per day) hydralazine can cause lupus syndrome, particularly in patients of the slow acetylator phenotype.

Diazoxide

Diazoxide (Hyperstat®) is a nondiuretic congener of the thiazide diuretics. Its absorption from the gastrointestinal tract is unreliable and today it is given only by the intravenous route. When given intravenously, diazoxide has a powerful and prolonged blood pressure-lowering effect in the majority of hypertensive patients. The maximal hypotensive effect develops within 10 minutes, making the drug of particular value in the treatment of hypertensive emergencies. The duration of its action is variable; it lasts for 8–12 hours or longer.

Reflex tachycardia and increase in cardiac output can be prevented by β-adrenergic blockade. Salt and water retention is another consequence of diazoxide that may interfere with its hypotensive effect, but that can be controlled by the simultaneous administration of a diuretic. Hyperglycemia is rarely severe enough to cause problems during short-term therapy with diazoxide.

Sodium Nitroprusside

Sodium nitroprusside (Nipride®) is a very potent vasodilator acting directly on vascular smooth muscle. Like diazoxide, it has to be given intravenously and is used mainly for treatment of hypertensive emergencies. Unlike diazoxide, it acts also on the veins and can reduce cardiac preload. Its effect begins almost immediately after the start of an intravenous infusion, but it ends less than 10 minutes after the infusion is stopped. The dose of sodium nitroprusside required to decrease arterial pressure is quite variable, and therefore, its administration requires careful supervision and adjustment of the infusion rate.

Because of its vasodilator action, sodium nitroprusside has been given with good results to patients with low cardiac output following myocardial infarction, and also to patients with chronic refractory heart failure. It was shown to reduce right atrial, pulmonary arterial, and capillary pressure, decrease left ventricular end-diastolic pressure, and increase cardiac output. Heart rate is not altered significantly by sodium nitroprusside in patients with cardiac failure when baroreceptor reflexes are already activated.

Most of the **adverse effects** of sodium nitroprusside are relatively minor ones, such as nasal stuffiness, nausea, vomiting, and headache. The ferrous iron in the nitroprusside molecule reacts with sulfhydryl components in the red cells, permitting the formation of cyanide ion from other parts of the molecule. The cyanide is reduced in the liver to thiocyanate, which is excreted by the kidneys. There is, however, a potential danger of lethal cyanide poisoning in subjects with rhodanese deficiency. Thiocyanate may accumulate in renal failure and cause seizures and coma.

Minoxidil

Minoxidil (Loniten®) has a powerful blood-pressure-lowering effect with long duration of action. As a "last resort," it is given orally (together with a beta-blocker and a diuretic) to control severe hypertension refractory to other antihypertensive drugs.

Unfortunately, the good qualities of minoxidil are associated with frequent side effects. In most patients it causes hypertrichosis, fatigue, marked fluid retention, and often pericardial effusion. In animals, large doses of minoxidil cause subendocardial and subepicardial degenerative lesions with hemorrhage.

The production of hypertrichosis as a side effect of systemic minoxidil therapy was the stimulus to its recent use as a topical solution applied to the scalp to encourage hair growth in some types of baldness. Vasodilatation of vessels supplying the hair follicles has been suggested as the mechanism of its claimed hair growth-promoting effect. The long-term value of this treatment is not yet clear. Enough percutaneous absorption of minoxidil can occur to cause systemic side effects in some cases.

Prazosin

This drug previously was classified as a direct-acting vasodilator. Although it does inhibit phosphodiesterase, its main action is through blockade of postsynaptic α_1 adrenoceptors (see Chapter 17). Since it does not block presynaptic α_2 receptors, noradrenaline* feedback remains intact and no increase in sympathetic drive occurs (in contrast to pre- and postsynaptic α-adrenoceptor blockers such as phenoxybenzamine and phentolamine). Therefore, tachycardia and increased renin release do not occur.

The drug is well absorbed following oral administration. Serum half-life is 3–4 hours, with antihypertensive effects lasting for up to 12 hours. There is extensive protein binding (up to 97%). Elimination is via hepatic biotransformation and excretion in the bile.

Prazosin (Minipress®) is moderately effective in hypertension, to about the same degree as hydralazine. When combined with a diuretic, it has been used in patients with impaired left ventricular function.

Adverse effects may consist of orthostatic hypotension (in less than 15% of patients), especially in a hot environment or after exercise. Another possible adverse reaction is the "first-dose phenomenon"; about 30–60 minutes after the first dose, or after a significant increase in dose, postural hypotension occurs, together

---

*norepinephrine

with transient faintness, dizziness, and palpitations (up to syncope!), especially in patients who have been depleted of salt and water. The cause is not defined, but it may be related to an abrupt change in the role of sympathetic activity in the maintenance of blood pressure. Therefore, the first dose should be given at bedtime, and treatment should be started with low doses.

Captopril and Other ACE Inhibitors

These drugs prevent the conversion of angiotensin I to angiotensin II by inhibiting the angiotensin converting enzyme (ACE), a peptidyl dipeptidase (see Chapter 31). ACE inhibitors cause a reduction in peripheral arterial resistance with consequent lowering of blood pressure. Because ACE (albeit under another name) is also the enzyme that breaks down bradykinin, the vasodepressor effects of elevated bradykinin levels in the presence of ACE inhibitors may contribute to the overall picture of peripheral vasodilatation.

There is little change in cardiac output, and baroreceptor reflexes are not compromised. In patients with heart failure, ACE inhibitors reduce preload, afterload, and pulmonary vascular resistance, and they increase cardiac output. As noted above, they reduce mortality.

Captopril (Capoten®) is given orally before meals for maximum bioavailability. It has a relatively short half-life of about 2 hours, being eliminated almost totally in the urine, about half as unchanged drug and half as metabolites. The drug may be combined cautiously with other antihypertensive agents such as diuretics and β-adrenoceptor blockers. Because of its primary excretion by the kidneys, appropriate dose reductions apply in cases of renal impairment. The newer ACE inhibitors **enalapril** (Vasotec®) and **lisinopril** (Zestril®) have longer half-lives and can be given once daily.

Adverse effects consist of exaggerated therapeutic effects (hypotension) if ACE inhibitors are combined indiscriminately with other antihypertensive agents and vasodilators. Also, all agents that affect the neuronal or humoral control of vascular tone have the potential for functional drug interactions with ACE inhibitors. Elevations in BUN and serum creatinine may occur in volume-depleted patients or those with renovascular hypertension.

Adverse Effects of Vasodilators

As with other drugs, the therapeutic value of vasodilators is limited by the frequency and severity of adverse effects. All vasodilators can cause fluid and salt retention consequent to altered capillary permeability or increased renal tubular reabsorption. Another adverse effect common to all the drugs mentioned (except prazosin and ACE inhibitors) is the reflex increase in cardiac rate and contraction. This effect, together with a sudden decrease in blood pressure caused by

large doses, can precipitate angina pectoris, coronary insufficiency, and even myocardial infarction in patients with coronary heart disease in whom the coronary perfusion is already compromised. Some more specific adverse effects are shown in Table 36–1.

ANTIANGINAL DRUGS

Nature of the Problem

Angina pectoris is a characteristic chest pain occurring because of an imbalance between oxygen delivery to, and utilization by, the myocardium. The imbalance can result from spasm of the vascular smooth muscle of the coronary arteries, so that they do not dilate adequately in response to increased myocardial work. It also can result from atheroma of the coronary arteries, which narrows the lumen and restricts blood flow. As noted earlier, both spasm and atheroma may be present in varying degrees. The strategy for relief of angina is to produce either redistribution of blood flow to or within the heart muscle, relaxation of the coronary arteries, or a decrease in the oxygen demand of the heart.

Drugs that decrease coronary vasoconstriction or spasm are of two types: the classical "antianginal drugs" covered in this section, and the newer calcium-channel blockers described in the next section.

Because the presenting manifestation is a symptom, and that symptom is pain, there is significant variation in individual response and reaction, and emotional factors and expectations may play a large role in the apparent effect of treatment. One of the great difficulties in assessing drugs in angina is the high rate of response occurring with placebo. Controlled clinical trials that include placebo as well as an active drug have found that 30–50% of patients with angina pectoris respond favorably to placebo. It may be difficult to determine, therefore, whether a supposedly active drug is really more effective than a placebo.

The first pharmacologic observations on organic nitrates were made in the mid 1800s, but it was not until 1857 that an English physician, Brunton, administered amyl nitrite by inhalation and noted that anginal pain was relieved within 30–60 seconds. However, that particular nitrite was difficult to administer, and it was not until 1880 that nitroglycerin was administered sublingually for the relief of acute angina.

More recently, in the 1960s, James Black, a British pharmacologist, synthesized propranolol and other β-adrenoceptor blockers and demonstrated that reducing cardiac work by slowing the heart rate and reducing contractility in response to exercise was also an effective method to prevent angina.

Calcium-channel-blocking drugs became known even

TABLE 36–1 Some Properties and Adverse Effects of Clinically Used Vasodilators

Drug	Route of Administration	Main Indication	Veno-dilatation	Cardiac Output	Adverse Effects
Nitrites	Sublingual, oral, cutaneous	Angina pectoris, refractory heart failure	Yes	↑↓	Headache
Hydralazine	Oral (i.m.)	Hypertension	No	↑	Lupus syndrome
Diazoxide	Intravenous	Hypertensive emergency	No	↑	Hyperglycemia
Sodium nitroprusside	Intravenous	Hypertensive emergency	Yes	(↑)*	Cyanide poisoning (potential danger)
Minoxidil	Oral	Severe hypertension	No	↑	Hypertrichosis, fluid retention
Calcium antagonists	Oral (Verapamil also intravenous)	Angina pectoris, hypertension, arrhythmia	No	↑↓	Headache

* Only in congestive heart failure. ↑ = increase; ↑↓ = varies with drug, dose, method of administration.

more recently in the 1970s when Fleckenstein, in Germany, described the action of verapamil as that of relaxing vascular smooth muscle; subsequently, calcium-channel blockers have been shown to be effective agents for the treatment of angina.

Nitrites and Nitrates

These drugs (see Fig. 36–1), which are marketed under a variety of brand names, have been used for many decades in the treatment of angina.

Chemistry

Nitrates and nitrites are simple nitric and nitrous acid esters of mono- or polyalcohols. They vary from extremely volatile liquids (amyl nitrate) to moderately volatile liquids (nitroglycerin, considered the prototype of the group). The formulations of nitroglycerin used in medicine are not explosive. The conventional sublingual tablet form of nitroglycerin may lose potency during storage as a result of volatilization and adsorption to plastic surfaces.

Structure-activity studies indicate that all therapeutically active agents in this group are capable of releasing nitrite ion in vascular smooth muscle target tissues. Unfortunately, they all also appear to be capable of inducing cross-tolerance when given in large doses.

Absorption and Metabolism

Organic nitrate esters are quite lipid-soluble, and therefore are readily absorbed through the well-vascularized sublingual mucosa. They are hydrolysed by hepatic enzymes that convert the organic nitrate esters into water-soluble partially denitrated metabolites and inorganic nitrite. These are considerably less potent vasodilators; they continue to be found in the blood for several hours after a dose of nitroglycerin, but are eventually excreted in the urine.

Pharmacokinetics

The effectiveness of organic nitrates is strongly influenced by the existence of a high-capacity hepatic organic nitrate reductase that inactivates the drug. Therefore, bioavailability of all orally administered organic nitrates is very low (typically less than 10%). Consequently, the sublingual route is preferred for achieving a therapeutic blood level rapidly. Nitroglycerin and isosorbide dinitrate are both absorbed efficiently by this route and reach therapeutic blood levels within a few minutes. However, the total dose administered by this route must be limited to avoid excessive effects; therefore, the total duration of effect is brief, typically 15–30 minutes. When much longer duration of action is needed, oral preparations are available that contain an amount of drug sufficient to result in sustained systemic blood levels of drug or active metabolites despite the high first-pass effect in the liver. Other routes of nitroglycerin administration include transdermal absorption when applied to the skin as an ointment, and buccal absorption from slow-release buccal preparations.

Pharmacologic Effects

In normal individuals, the exact mechanism whereby these drugs produce vascular relaxation is unknown. Low concentrations of nitroglycerin produce venodilatation, which predominates over arteriolar dilatation.

CARDIOVASCULAR SYSTEM

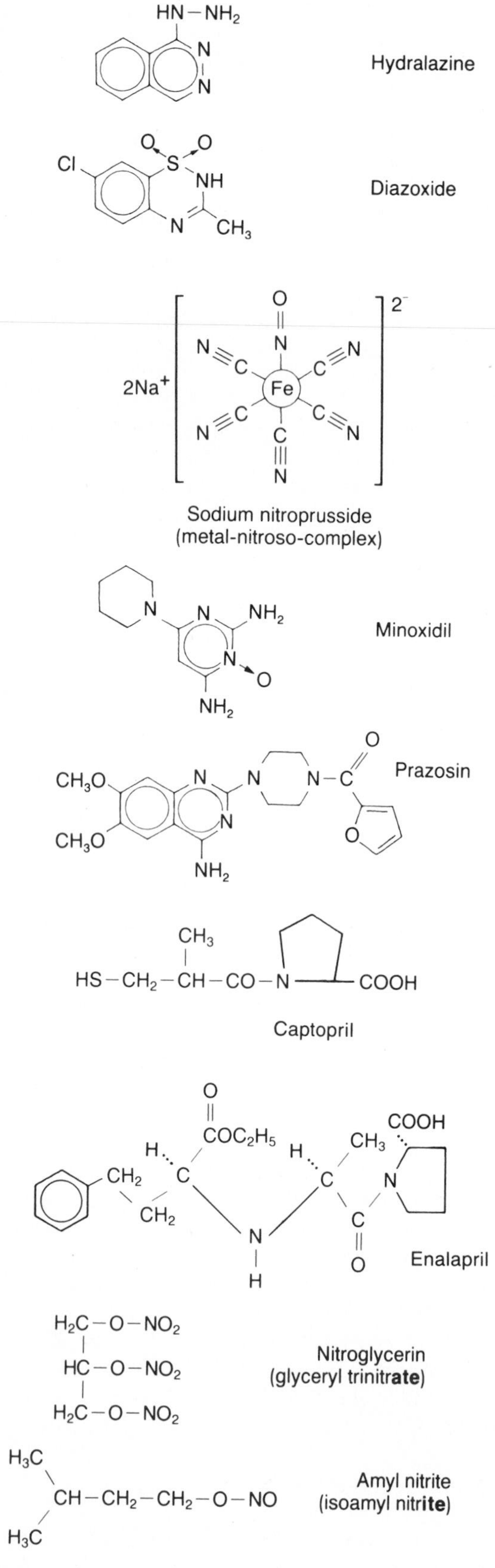

Figure 36–1 Structural formulae of vasodilators in current clinical use.

As a direct consequence of venodilatation, there is a decreased venous return, with immediate fall in left and right ventricular end-diastolic pressure. This is greater on a percentage basis than the reduction of afterload that follows the fall in systemic arterial pressure. Heart rate increases, but the systemic pressure declines, and pulmonary vascular resistance is reduced. There is a decrease in cardiac output. The effects are readily visible, because there is facial flushing due to arteriolar dilatation in the face and neck, and in normal individuals headache is a very common symptom.

High intravenous or oral doses of nitrates or nitrites decrease systolic and diastolic blood pressure and cause a fall in cardiac output, with resultant hypotension and dizziness, and activation of compensatory sympathetic responses including tachycardia. Coronary blood flow increases transiently because of direct vasodilatation in the coronary vascular bed; but if a significant decline in arterial blood pressure results, there is a reduction in coronary blood flow. The effects are particularly evident when the individual is in the upright position.

A demand for increased oxygen delivery to the heart is normally met by increasing the blood flow rather than by more complete extraction of oxygen, because the myocardial oxygen extraction is almost complete. Ischemia is the major stimulus for coronary vasodilatation and it is believed that regional blood flow is adjusted by autoregulatory mechanisms.

In patients with organic stenosis of the coronary artery, nitrates may not increase total coronary blood flow but may alter the distribution in favor of more hypoxic regions. It is believed that nitrates cause redistribution of coronary blood flow to the ischemic subendocardial areas by selective vasodilatation of the large epicardial vessels.

Whatever the exact mechanism or combination of mechanisms of action, nitrates cause a rapid reduction in myocardial oxygen demand and rapid relief of angina.

Tolerance to Nitrates

With continuous exposure to nitrates, isolated smooth muscle may develop complete tachyphylaxis (tolerance), and the intact human becomes at least partially tolerant. Continuous exposure to high levels of nitrates can occur in the chemical industry, especially where explosives are manufactured. When contamination of the workplace with volatile organic nitrate compounds is severe, workers find that, upon starting their work week (Monday), they suffer headache and transient dizziness. After a day or so, these symptoms disappear because of the development of tolerance.

Nitroglycerin is probably denitrated in the smooth muscle cell. The resulting nitric oxide (NO) is thought to react with a specific receptor. The latter appears to include sulfhydryl (–SH) groups, since tolerance to nitrite involves a decrease in tissue sulfhydryl groups, and tolerance can be reversed with sulfhydryl-regenerating agents such as dithiothreitol or N-acetylcysteine. Little is known of the steps linking receptor binding of nitric oxide and relaxation of smooth muscle. Some evidence suggests that an increase in cGMP is the first link. Other studies implicate the production of prostaglandin E or prostacyclin (PGI$_2$) as an important intermediate step. There is no evidence that autonomic receptors are involved in the primary nitrate response (although autonomic reflex responses are evoked when hypotensive doses are given).

CALCIUM-CHANNEL BLOCKERS (Calcium Entry Blockers or Calcium Antagonists)

Mechanism of Action

As described in detail in Chapter 34, the application of an effective stimulus to a muscle cell results in the influx of Ca^{2+}, which in turn triggers the intracellular events leading to muscle contraction (*see* Fig. 34–2).

Several different types of antagonist can block this sequence of Ca^{2+}-dependent steps.

Several inorganic cations, such as manganese, cobalt, and lanthanum, can function as general calcium antagonists. They probably substitute for calcium at a variety of binding sites and either block Ca^{2+} channels or actually enter the cell where they substitute for Ca^{2+} at intracellular Ca^{2+} receptors. Of much greater importance from a clinical viewpoint, however, are the organic calcium-channel blockers nifedipine, nicardipine, verapamil, and diltiazem (Fig. 36–2). Since these agents exert their actions at low (nanomolar) concentrations and exhibit stereospecificity, it appears likely that they are recognized by specific structures in the Ca^{2+} channel (Fig. 36–3). However, the great diversity of molecular structure of the calcium-channel blockers is consistent with different mechanisms and sites of action. It seems likely that nifedipine acts at a different site in the Ca^{2+} channel than verapamil and diltiazem, although their therapeutic effect is the same.

Electrophysiologic evidence based on patch-clamp studies indicates that there are at least three different

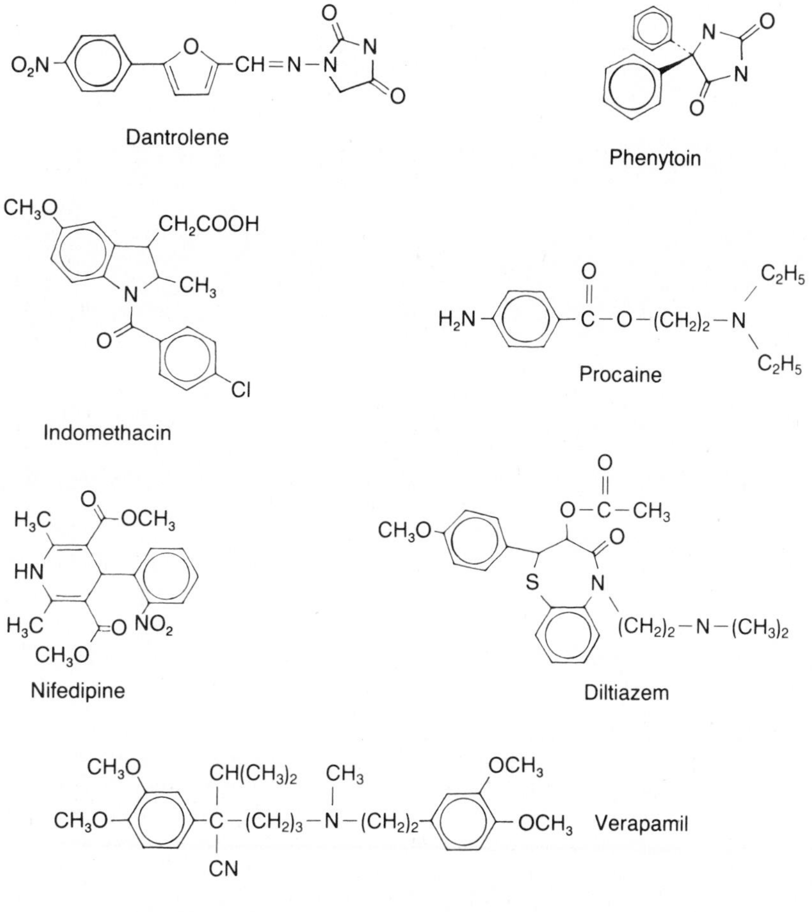

ALSO: Diazoxide and Sodium Nitroprusside (Fig. 36–1)

Figure 36–2 Structural formulae of drugs having calcium-channel blocking properties.

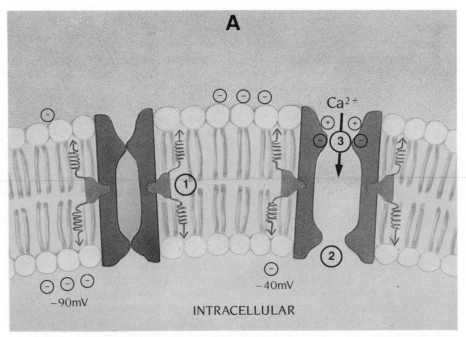

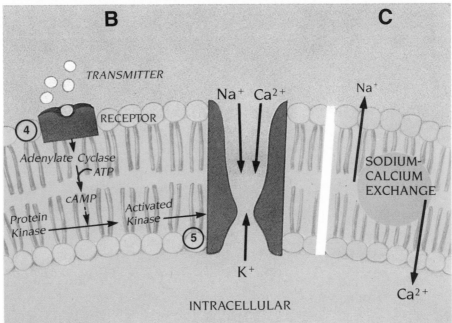

Figure 36–3 Simplified, schematic representation of Ca^{2+} movement (*via* calcium channels) across sarcolemmal membranes and sites of action of calcium-channel blockers. *A*, Voltage-dependent calcium channel with closed and open gate. Electrochemical gradients during depolarization of the cell by a "fast" Na^+ current are detected by "voltage sensors" (1), causing the voltage-dependent gate to open (2). The channel is capable of distinguishing between cations (3), making it *highly selective for* Ca^{2+}, which enters the cell with a "slow" current. The therapeutic calcium-channel-blocking drugs *nifedipine, verapamil, and diltiazem act specifically on the voltage-dependent gate* (2). The phosphorylation-dependent gate, *B*, responds to membrane receptor activation (4) and is opened by an energy-dependent process (5). It is of *low specificity*, not selective for Ca^{2+}. Also shown is the Na^+–Ca^{2+} exchanger, *C*, that mediates additional movement of Ca^{2+} across the sarcolemma, dependent on the relative concentrations of extra- and intracellular Na^+ and Ca^{2+}, causing mostly an influx of Ca^{2+}.

types of voltage-activated calcium channel: the best-studied types are designated T, L, and N channels. They are activated at different degrees of membrane depolarization, the T channels at voltages positive to -70 mV and the L channels at voltages positive to -10 mV. Only the L channels are inhibited by nifedipine and other dihydropyridine-type blockers. The different types of Ca^{2+} channels are distributed differentially. L channels are found in all neurons, gland cells, and muscle cells examined, and are the type involved in excitation-contraction coupling. N channels appear to be limited to neuronal membranes, especially at axon terminals where they mediate the Ca^{2+} influx that triggers neurotransmitter release; this process is not sensitive to dihydropyridine-type blockers.

The smooth muscle of the arterioles is far more sensitive than that of the veins to the action of calcium-channel blockers. Therefore these drugs are predominantly arterial dilators, especially of the coronary arterial bed. On an equimolar basis, nifedipine is the most active of the three compounds.

Hemodynamic Effects

Nifedipine (Adalat®; Procardia®) at an oral dose of 20 mg causes a reduction of systemic vascular resistance and therefore a fall in blood pressure. This leads to a reflex rise in heart rate and a consequent rise in cardiac output. The fall in blood pressure is directly related to the preexisting pressure; the higher the initial pressure, the greater the fall. Other dihydropyridines have similar, but not identical, effects.

Verapamil HCl (Isoptin®), in contrast to nifedipine, in a dose of 160 mg produces a lesser fall in blood pressure, some reduction in heart rate and cardiac output, but virtually no change in systemic vascular resistance.

Diltiazem HCl (Cardizem®) in a dose of 120 mg given by mouth produces a slow, progressive decline in heart rate and blood pressure and a fall in cardiac output.

Present Therapeutic Uses

Chronic Stable Angina

A variety of controlled studies have shown that nifedipine, diltiazem, and to a lesser extent verapamil, are effective in this disorder. The mechanism is probably a reduction in myocardial oxygen requirement produced by reduction of the heart rate with verapamil and diltiazem, systemic vasodilatation produced by nifedipine and diltiazem, and negative inotropism particularly with verapamil. Coronary vasodilatation also occurs, and therefore coronary blood flow increases.

In double-blind studies in which a placebo was compared with verapamil, nifedipine, or diltiazem, these agents have been shown to reduce the frequency of anginal attacks, the consumption of nitroglycerin, and

the frequency of deviations of the S–T segment in the electrocardiogram.

Unstable Angina

This is a form of angina occurring at rest, not relieved by simple measures, and requiring hospitalization. Verapamil, diltiazem, and nifedipine all have been shown to be effective in unstable angina. This is probably due to their suppression of coronary vasospasm.

Variant Angina (Prinzmetal's Angina)

This is another type of angina unrelated to exercise; it occurs at rest, often during the night. It is thought to be caused by coronary artery spasm.

Nifedipine produces benefit in over 85% of patients with variant angina. The side effects are mild but relatively frequent, ranging between 15% and 20% in different studies. They consist of facial flushing, hypotension, palpitations, and peripheral edema, which is sometimes quite marked but can usually be reversed by diuretics. Nifedipine is contraindicated when severe fixed coronary artery stenosis exists. The fall in blood pressure may result in a decline in blood flow through the stenotic artery, where flow is dependent on pressure difference.

Diltiazem produces benefit in over 70% of patients with variant angina. It has a low frequency (10%) of side effects, which include facial flushing and headache, as well as bradycardia and abdominal discomfort.

Verapamil produces benefit in 70% of patients with variant angina. Side effects occur in 10–20% of cases, and consist of constipation, nausea, facial flushing, and headache. This drug is contraindicated in the presence of congestive heart failure and in the presence of conduction abnormalities.

Hypertension

Nifedipine and diltiazem are potent hypotensive drugs (*see* Chapter 38). They relax vascular smooth muscle and produce a rapid fall in blood pressure. There are many other drugs available to treat hypertension, and at present the calcium-channel blockers cannot be regarded as first-line drugs for this purpose. However, sublingual and oral nifedipine can produce a dramatic decline in blood pressure in the emergency treatment of severe hypertension. Although it is common practice to use intravenous drugs under these circumstances, the effect of sublingual nifedipine is almost as potent and rapid as that of intravenous nitroprusside, diazoxide, or hydralazine.

Congestive Heart Failure

Nifedipine produces a reduction in afterload. It is not clear at present whether nifedipine offers a more predictable benefit than other drugs such as hydralazine, prazosin, or captopril for afterload reduction in the treatment of congestive heart failure.

Hypertrophic Cardiomyopathy

Verapamil has been shown to alleviate the ECG abnormalities in patients with cardiomyopathy. In one series it also reduced the abnormalities seen in myocardial relaxation. However, the long-term benefits remain to be explored.

SUGGESTED READING

Braunwald E. Mechanism of action of calcium-channel-blocking agents. N Engl J Med 1982; 307:1618–1627.

Brogden RN, Heel RC, Streight TM, Avery GS. Prazosin, a review of its pharmacological properties and therapeutic efficacy in hypertension. Drugs 1977; 14:163–197.

Chatterjee K, Parmley WW. Vasodilator treatment for acute and chronic heart failure. Br Heart J 1977; 39:706–720.

Flaim SF, Zelis R, eds. Calcium blockers: mechanisms of action and clinical applications. Baltimore: Urban and Schwarzenberg, 1982.

Fleckenstein A. Specific pharmacology of calcium in myocardium, cardiac pacemakers, and vascular smooth muscle. Ann Rev Pharmacol Toxicol 1977; 17:149–166.

Hurwitz L. Pharmacology of calcium channels and smooth muscle. Idem 1986; 26:225–258.

Janis RA, Silver PJ, Triggle DJ. Drug action and cellular calcium regulation. Adv Drug Res 1987; 16:309–591.

Koch-Weser J. Vasodilator drugs in the treatment of hypertension. Arch Intern Med 1974; 133:1017–1032.

Koch-Weser J. Diazoxide. N Engl J Med 1976; 294:1271–1274.

Schwartz A, Triggle DJ. Cellular action of calcium-channel blocking drugs. Ann Rev Med 1984; 35:325–339.

Triggle DJ, Janis RA. Calcium channel ligands. Ann Rev Pharmacol Toxicol 1987; 27:347–369.

Chapter 37

HYPERLIPOPROTEINEMIAS AND ANTIHYPERLIPIDEMIC DRUGS

C. Forster

The hyperlipoproteinemias are conditions characterized by lipoprotein disorders in which the plasma concentrations of cholesterol- or triglyceride-carrying lipoproteins are at the upper 5% of the distribution curve for the general population. Clinical observation has revealed that increased concentration of lipoproteins can accelerate the development of atherosclerosis, and both dietary and pharmacologic measures now are used in efforts to reduce lipoprotein levels.

Hypertriglyceridemia and hypercholesterolemia are defined in terms of the specific lipoproteins that are elevated. Such analytical information is necessary if an accurate diagnosis is to be made and the most appropriate therapy instituted.

LIPOPROTEIN TRANSPORT

Cholesterol and triglycerides are transported in the plasma in the form of lipoproteins, of which there are six classes differing in size, density, lipid composition, and the nature of the apoprotein moieties. These different classes are found in a sequence of progressively smaller and denser particles, from the initial absorption of fats in the intestine to their final disposition in the tissues (Fig. 37–1).

Triglycerides and cholesterol in the food are incorporated, in the small intestine, into large-diameter low-density lipoprotein micelles called **chylomicrons**, which are absorbed by pinocytosis and released into the circulating blood. In the capillaries of muscle and adipose tissue, the endothelial lipoprotein lipase hydrolyses some of the triglyceride content of the chylomicrons, releasing free fatty acids. These enter the muscle or adipose tissue cells and are either oxidized for energy or re-esterified for storage. The smaller, denser **chylomicron remnants** are taken up into the liver and cleaved by lysosomal hydrolytic enzymes.

The liver then secretes triglycerides and cholesterol into the plasma, for redistribution to other tissues, in the form of **very-low-density lipoproteins (VLDL)**, which are smaller than chylomicrons and have less triglyceride and more cholesterol and protein (Fig. 37–2). The lipoprotein lipase removes progressively more of the triglyceride, liberating free fatty acids that are taken up by the tissue, and leaving in the circulation the progressively smaller and denser residual particles known as **intermediate-density lipoproteins (IDL)** and **low-density lipoproteins (LDL)**. Both IDL and LDL can be taken up into the liver or other tissues, and can provide cholesterol for the synthesis of new cell membranes, steroid hormones, and bile acids. The uptake is mediated by specific LDL receptors on the cell membrane that have a high affinity for the apoprotein E on the surface of the IDL particle and a lesser affinity for the apoprotein β-100 remaining on the LDL particle. After binding to the receptor, the lipoprotein particles are taken into the cell by pinocytosis and are degraded by lysosomal enzymes. The excess free cholesterol, thus released inside the cell, exerts negative feedback control on the synthesis of new LDL receptors. The number of LDL receptors in the body can be estimated by injecting radioactively labelled LDL intravenously and measuring its disappearance half-life.

Finally, free cholesterol that is released by cell death or membrane turnover is adsorbed onto **high-density lipoproteins (HDL)** and esterified with a long-chain fatty acid by the action of a plasma lecithin:cholesterol acyltransferase (see Fig. 37–1). A specific transfer protein then transfers the cholesteryl esters to new VLDL or LDL particles, completing the plasma-tissue-plasma cycle of cholesterol turnover. Generally, up to 75% of the total plasma cholesterol is carried in VLDL and LDL,

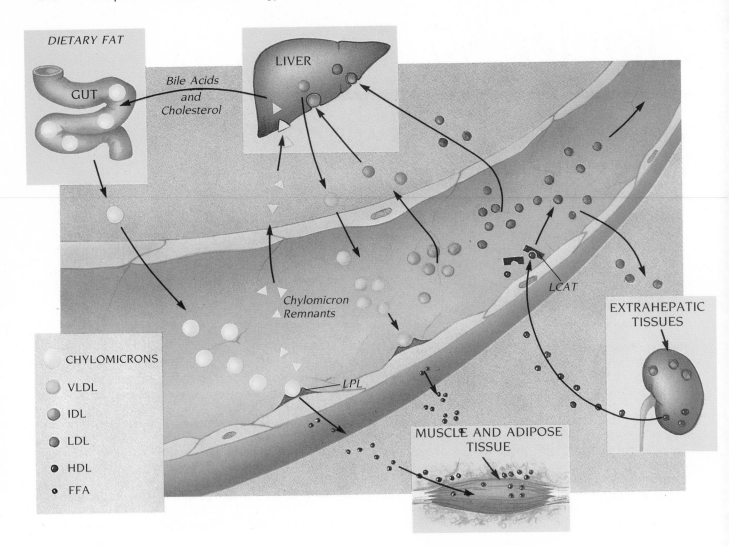

Figure 37-1 Schematic overview of lipoprotein transport and turnover. VLDL = very-low-density lipoproteins; IDL = intermediate-density lipoproteins; LDL = low-density lipoproteins; HDL = high-density lipoproteins; FFA = free fatty acids; LPL = lipoprotein lipase; LCAT = lecithin:cholesterol acyltransferase.

and 25% in HDL. When the plasma concentration of lipoprotein rises too much, because of excessive dietary intake, excessive synthesis, or impaired tissue uptake and utilization, the normal cycle can not handle it all and some is degraded by other pathways in macrophages, which deposit the cholesterol in atheromatous plaques and xanthomas.

HYPERLIPOPROTEINEMIAS

A hyperlipoproteinemia is present when plasma cholesterol and/or triglyceride levels exceed the 95th percentile values for the patient's age and sex group in the comparable general population.

Hypertriglyceridemia

Normal mean plasma triglyceride levels for each decade of life in white males and females are shown in Table 37-1. In males, the values rise steadily with age, reaching a maximum between 40 and 50 years. In females, the rise is much slower, and in middle life men tend to have higher triglyceride levels than women. Table 37-1 also shows the 95th percentile level for each age group. Individuals whose triglyceride levels exceed the 95th percentile values should be examined further to determine whether they have an associated elevation in LDL, reduction in HDL, or dysbetalipoproteinemia (abnormal cholesterol-rich VLDL). All three conditions are associated with increased incidence of cardiovascular disease.

In addition, triglyceride levels above 500 mg/dL

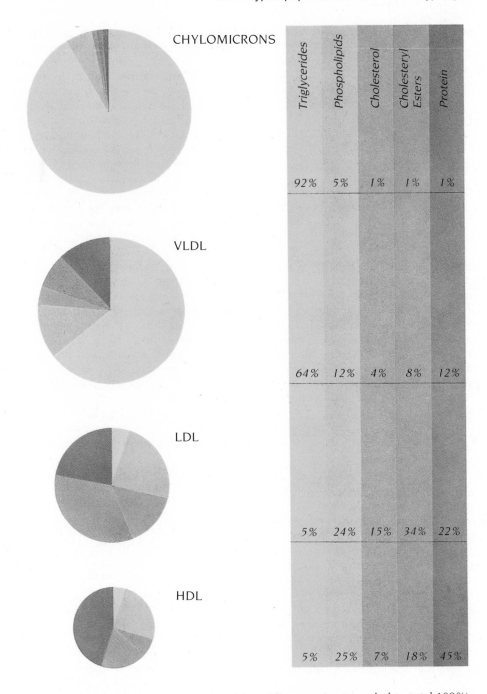

Figure 37–2 Approximate composition of lipoproteins (rounded to total 100%).

(5.65 mmol/L) may imply the presence of **hyperchylo-micronemic syndrome** or other disease processes, including hepatic disease, diabetes mellitus, and alcoholism.

Hypercholesterolemia

Normally, plasma cholesterol levels remain stable during the first two decades of life, and then gradually rise, reaching peak values in the sixth decade in both males and females. However, the rise in males is more pronounced during the fourth and early fifth decades; hence males are generally exposed to elevated cholesterol over a greater extent of adult life than females are. Of greater significance than total cholesterol, however, is the relative contribution of LDL- and HDL-cholesterol. Table 37–2 shows LDL- and HDL-cholesterol levels (mean and 95th percentile values) in males and females for each decade of life. LDL levels tend to be slightly higher in males than in females over

TABLE 37-1 Plasma Triglyceride Levels in White Men and Women

Age (Years)	Males (mmol/L) Mean	Males (mmol/L) 95th Percentile	Females (mmol/L) Mean	Females (mmol/L) 95th Percentile
<10	0.56	1.02	0.73	1.47
10–19	0.79	1.52	0.79	1.41
20–29	1.13	2.09	0.96	1.86
30–39	1.47	3.22	1.02	2.09
40–49	1.69	3.50	1.18	2.31
50–59	1.64	3.33	1.41	2.88
60–69	1.52	2.88	1.52	2.99

the 30–60 year age range. In contrast, HDL-cholesterol levels, which are similar in boys and girls, fall an average of 10–15 mg/dL in males after puberty, and remain lower than in females over the whole adult life span. It must be emphasized that, although hypercholesterolemia is defined by the presence of plasma cholesterol levels at or above the 95th percentile value, this does not mean that values below the 95th percentile are "safe." The risk of cardiovascular disease rises progressively with increasing cholesterol level throughout the distribution curve range.

Varieties of Hyperlipoproteinemia

Table 37–3 shows some of the main features of the most common classes of hypertriglyceridemia and hypercholesterolemia encountered clinically. All of them can occur as primary disturbances with familial inheritance patterns, or as secondary disturbances associated with diabetes mellitus, liver disease, and other disorders. Primary **endogenous hypertriglyceridemia** is a common disorder, affecting about 2% of the total population. Possibly 10–20% of middle-aged subjects have triglyceride levels which, though below the 95th percentile, may be associated with increased risk of heart disease.

Primary hypercholesterolemia is usually due to elevation of LDL-cholesterol, and rarely of HDL-cholesterol. A variety of genetic defects could be responsible for elevation of LDL-cholesterol, the best understood being the **monogenic** defect in synthesis of the LDL (β-100 apoprotein) receptor, seen in **familial hypercholesterolemia.** The homozygous form is rare (1 per 10^6 persons in North America), and most die of cardiovascular disease before the age of 30. However, the heterozygous form is common (1 in 500 persons) and is a major contributory factor in heart attacks during middle age. There are also **polygenic** forms of LDL elevation in which no specific inheritance pattern can be defined. LDL may also be increased in association with a rare disorder known as **sitosterolemia.**

In most conditions characterized by raised LDL levels, there is increased risk of arteriosclerotic cardiovascular disease, with earlier onset and more rapid progression of the disease. Other clinical signs caused by elevated LDL levels include corneal arcus and xanthelasma or xanthomas of the skin and tendons.

Most disorders associated with raised LDL-cholesterol levels are caused by a group of polygenic factors, superimposed upon which are exacerbating environmental influences. The most important of these is a habitual diet containing excess calories, saturated fat, and cholesterol.

Elevation of HDL levels is often familial, and appears as a result of an autosomal dominant trait (**familial hyperalphalipoproteinemia**). More often, though, mild elevations in HDL are due to polygenic and sporadic disorders. However, it appears that significant protection from arteriosclerotic lesions may be the result of such elevations. It is extremely important, therefore, to identify these patients in whom HDL elevations are the source of hypercholesterolemia, to avoid inappropriate therapy such as lipid-lowering drugs.

LIPOPROTEINS AND VASCULAR DISEASE

Table 37–3 indicates that severe lipoprotein abnormalities often lead to cardiovascular disease. A num-

TABLE 37-2 Plasma LDL- and HDL-Cholesterol Levels in White Men and Women

Age (Years)	LDL-Cholesterol (mmol/L) Males Mean	LDL-Cholesterol (mmol/L) Males 95th Percentile	LDL-Cholesterol (mmol/L) Females Mean	LDL-Cholesterol (mmol/L) Females 95th Percentile	HDL-Cholesterol (mmol/L) Males Mean	HDL-Cholesterol (mmol/L) Males 95th Percentile	HDL-Cholesterol (mmol/L) Females Mean	HDL-Cholesterol (mmol/L) Females 95th Percentile
<10	2.46	3.49	2.59	3.62	1.42	1.94	1.42	1.94
10–19	2.46	3.36	2.46	3.62	1.29	1.94	1.29	1.94
20–29	2.84	4.27	2.84	4.27	1.16	1.68	1.42	2.07
30–39	3.36	4.91	2.97	4.27	1.16	1.68	1.42	2.07
40–49	3.62	5.04	3.23	4.65	1.16	1.68	1.55	2.33
50–59	3.75	5.17	3.62	5.43	1.16	1.68	1.55	2.46
60–69	3.88	5.43	3.88	5.82	1.29	2.07	1.68	2.46

TABLE 37-3 Classes of Hyperlipoproteinemia and Their Main Features

Type	Clinical Designation	Plasma Lipid Changes	Primary Defect	Other Causes	Cardiac Risk
I	Familial hyperchylomicronemia	↑↑ chylomicrons (↑↑ TG, ↑ cholesterol)	Lipoprotein lipase deficiency, apoprotein CII deficiency	Diabetes mellitus	—
IIa	Familial hypercholesterolemia (homozygous)	↑ LDL-cholesterol	LDL receptor deficiency	Hypothyroidism, nephrotic syndrome	↑
IIb	Combined hyperlipoproteinemia	↑ VLDL, ↑ LDL* (HDL may be ↓)	LDL receptor deficiency, ↑ production of VLDL		↑
III	Familial hyperlipidemia	↑ IDL, ↑ β-lipoproteins (LDL) (↑ cholesterol, ↑ TG)	Apoprotein E deficiency	Hypothyroidism	↑
IV	Familial hypertriglyceridemia	↑ VLDL (↑ TG, ↑ or normal cholesterol) ↓ HDL	?	Diabetes mellitus, nephrotic syndrome, obstructive jaundice	↑(?)
V	Mixed hypertriglyceridemia	↑↑ chylomicrons, ↑↑ VLDL	?	Diabetes mellitus, obstructive jaundice, pancreatitis	↑(?)
VI	Familial hyperalphalipo-proteinemia	↑ HDL	?		↓
—	Dysbetalipoproteinemia	↑ VLDL (↑ cholesterol) ↑ IDL with β- rather than pre-β-electrophoretic mobility	Atypical form of apolipoprotein E, causing poor uptake of IDL by the liver		↑

* In Type IIb, the relative proportions of VLDL and LDL may change gradually, the LDL increase becoming the more prominent feature.
(↑ = increased; ↓ = decreased)

ber of studies have shown a strong relationship between total plasma cholesterol and coronary heart disease, and recent data from the Multiple Risk Factor Intervention Trial (MRFIT) indicate a progressive increase in risk as cholesterol increases. One of the difficulties in demonstrating a close correlation between total cholesterol and risk may relate to the opposing effects of LDL and HDL values.

Figure 37–3 shows that (1) with increases in LDL-cholesterol, risk increased in a linear manner; (2) in the same group a marked fall in risk occurred as HDL levels rose; and (3) predicted risk increased with increasing LDL:HDL ratios, over the entire range of ratio found in the population (Framingham Study).

The presence of high LDL- and/or low HDL-cholesterol ultimately causes damage to specific organs. This damage results from a progressive obstruction of the large arteries by atherosclerosis. A high concentration of LDL-cholesterol can directly damage the endothelial surface, resulting in the accumulation, within the intima, of foam cells filled with cholesteryl esters. If the insult with LDL-cholesterol is continuous or repeated, marked cellular proliferation occurs, together with increasing frequency of cell death. A marked thickening of the vascular wall slowly develops, caused by increased collagen and other substances.

The correlation between LDL levels and cardiovascular disease is satisfactory for large populations, but the correlation is less satisfactory in individual patients, since HDL and LDL are independently variable. This has led to greater awareness of the importance of LDL:HDL ratio. Thus, a person with a very high LDL and a very low HDL has a markedly amplified predicted risk, but the same high LDL together with a high HDL might place the risk of an individual somewhere in the middle of the range.

Evidence has accumulated to suggest that treatment to lower the LDL level and raise the HDL level will diminish or prevent arteriosclerotic lesions and reduce the risk of coronary heart disease (Lipid Research Clinics Program, 1984). Nevertheless, treatment of these disorders remains controversial.

NONPHARMACOLOGIC (DIETARY) INTERVENTION

The first approach to lowering cholesterol levels should be by diet. Dietary emphasis will vary, depend-

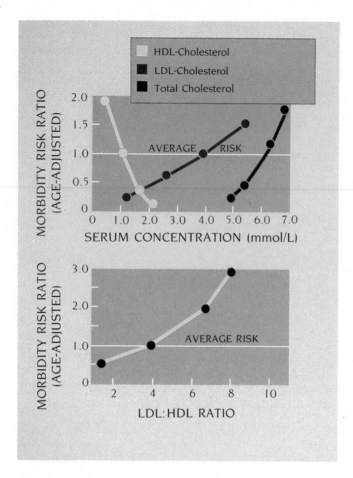

Figure 37–3 Various cholesterol fractions as related to risk (male subjects in Framingham study).

DRUG THERAPY

In general, the use of lipid-lowering drugs is recommended only in cases that do not show an adequate response to a careful test of dietary management.

Even in such cases, indications for drug use vary with the patient's age and clinical diagnosis. The long-term safety of lipid-lowering drugs in children is still under investigation. Some clinicians favor their use at a very early age in order to prevent coronary artery disease later in life, but most physicians feel that these drugs should be avoided in children, except in extreme circumstances such as homozygous familial hypercholesterolemia. At the opposite extreme, the use of these drugs in an elderly person with life-threatening disease due to some other cause would obviously be totally inappropriate. The major indications for use of cholesterol-lowering agents are in young and middle-aged adults. For example, aggressive therapy might be indicated in a young person with already diagnosed coronary artery disease. Drug therapy may also be necessary for a middle-aged person who does not yet show evidence of coronary disease, but who has an LDL-cholesterol level greater than 175 mg/dL (4.5 mmol/L) and an LDL:HDL ratio greater than 3.0.

Drugs can lower cholesterol either by decreasing production of lipoproteins or by increasing the efficiency of their removal. Six groups of such drugs are currently available and a seventh group, the 3-hydroxy-3-methylglutaryl-coenzyme A (HMg-CoA) reductase inhibitors, was recently introduced and appears promising. These different groups are described below, in relation to their different sites of action (Fig. 37–4).

ing on the diagnosis. When the VLDL triglycerides are elevated, the most effective treatment is reduced caloric intake and increased exercise. When chylomicrons are present, reduction of dietary fat is indicated. Elevated LDL level indicates a need for reduction in dietary intake of saturated fats and cholesterol, and then a reduction in body fat. Other factors such as carbohydrate sources and fibre content of the diet must also be considered. Table 37–4 outlines the dietary guidelines according to the American Heart Association. If, after 3–6 months of dietary intervention, an adequate reduction in LDL-cholesterol has not been achieved, then drug therapy may be initiated.

When the elevation of LDL is a secondary consequence of alcoholism, diabetes, hypothyroidism, or other diseases, therapy should be directed toward proper management of the primary disease, rather than specifically toward reduction of LDL level.

TABLE 37–4   Dietary Guidelines for Treatment of Hyperlipidemias

Fat	Not to exceed 30% of daily caloric intake; saturated fat and polyunsaturated fat each limited to not more than ⅓ of total fat
Cholesterol	<100 mg per 1000 kcal (the desirable therapeutic plasma target level in adult males = <6.6 mmol/L)
Calories	Initially reduce calories to bring obese individuals down to desirable body weight
	Then adjust caloric intake to the amount necessary to maintain ideal body weight

Data from Grundy SM. Arteriosclerosis 1984; 4:445A–468A.

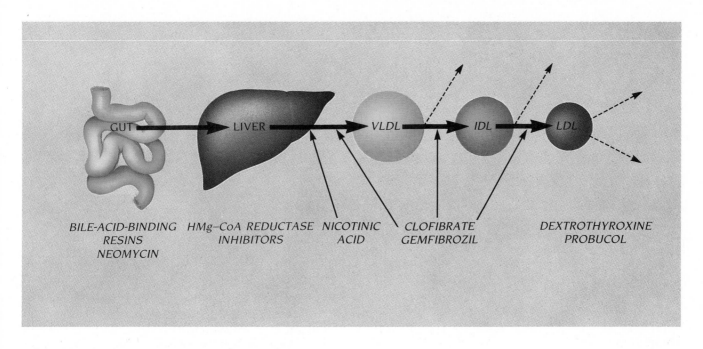

Figure 37–4 Sites of action of lipid-lowering drugs.

Drugs That Impair Intestinal Absorption

Bile-Acid-Binding Resins: Cholestyramine and Colestipol

The chemical structures of these agents are shown in Figure 37–5. The bile-acid-binding resins, which are insoluble in water, are unaffected by digestive enzymes and are not absorbed from the intestinal tract.

Mechanism of Action

Cholestyramine (Questran®) and colestipol (Colestid®) are cationic exchange resins that bind the bile acids and thus prevent their absorption from the intestine. The net result is increased fecal excretion of bile acids, and a compensatory increase of new production of bile acids from cholesterol in the liver. As a consequence, there is an increase in LDL receptors and in the activity of 3-hydroxy-3-methylglutaryl-CoA (HMg-CoA) reductase (the rate-controlling enzyme in cholesterol synthesis). The increased number of LDL receptors causes increased clearance of LDL from the plasma, and reduction in LDL cholesterol level. Patients who suffer from a genetic defect in the production of LDL receptors can not respond to therapy with the bile-acid-binding resins.

These agents lower the plasma LDL-cholesterol level gradually, over a period of 2–3 weeks. The effect is proportional to the dose and gradually disappears when treatment is stopped.

Generally, the level of VLDL increases during the first weeks of treatment and then decreases slowly to its original value. However, in patients whose VLDL and IDL levels are high before the start of treatment, the

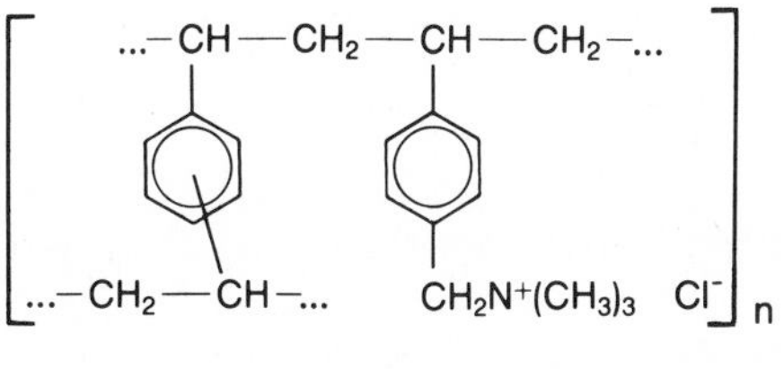

Cholestyramine (Questran®)

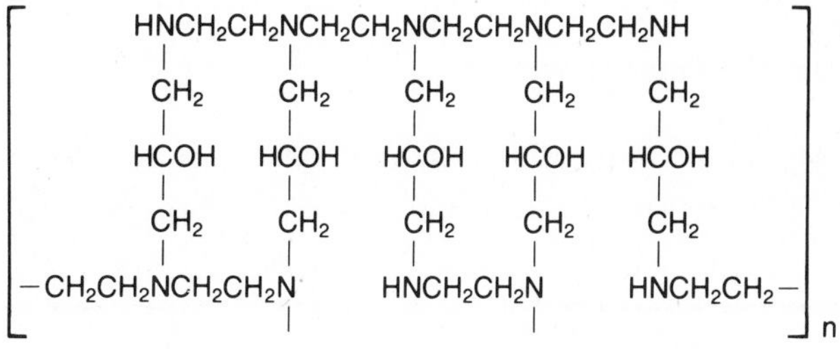

Colestipol (Colestid®)

Figure 37–5 Structural formulae of bile acid-binding resins.

GASTROINTESTINAL SYSTEM

increase in triglycerides that occurs when resin therapy is started may be greater and more prolonged. Therefore the resins are most effective when only the LDL level is elevated (Type IIa).

Side Effects

Nausea, abdominal bloating, indigestion, and constipation are common side effects. Since the resins bind the bile acids, they also impair the absorption of dietary fat; therefore, in high doses they may cause steatorrhea.

Since cationic resins have a high affinity for acid compounds of many kinds, they can also bind to, and impair the intestinal absorption of, such drugs as warfarin and similar anticoagulants, chlorothiazide, phenylbutazone, barbiturates, thyroxine, and digitalis glycosides. Therefore other orally administered drugs should be ingested either 1 hour or more before, or 4 hours after, these resins.

Neomycin

Neomycin sulfate is an aminoglycoside antibiotic (*see* Chapter 55) that is only poorly absorbed from the intestinal tract. Like the bile acid-binding resins, it interferes with the absorption of bile acids and cholesterol from the intestine. Therefore it can also reduce LDL levels by 20–25% without affecting HDL- or VLDL-cholesterol or triglyceride levels.

Associated **side effects** include nausea, ototoxicity, and renal toxicity. It is contraindicated in patients with intestinal disease, reduced renal function, hepatic disease, or congestive heart failure, because these disorders may impair the renal excretion of the small amount of neomycin that is absorbed, and thus increase its toxicity.

Drugs That Impair Synthesis of Cholesterol and VLDL

3-Hydroxy-3-Methylglutaryl-Coenzyme A (HMg-CoA) Reductase Inhibitors

Mechanism of Action

Mevinolin and **compactin** (Fig. 37–6) are potent competitive inhibitors of HMg-CoA reductase, the rate-limiting enzyme in cholesterol biosynthesis. The inhibitory effect is highly specific and reversible. By inhibit-

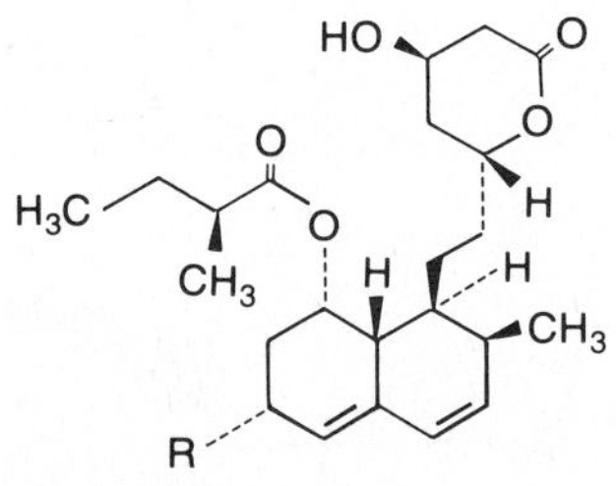

R=H: Compactin
R=CH₃: Mevinolin; Lovastatin (Mevacor®)

Figure 37–6 Structural formulae of HMg-CoA reductase inhibitors.

ing cholesterol synthesis in the liver, these drugs cause an increase in hepatic LDL receptors and therefore a reduction in plasma LDL.

Mevinolin decreases plasma LDL-cholesterol by 35–45% in normal humans without affecting plasma levels of VLDL and HDL. In patients with hypercholesterolemia, LDL levels decrease by 30% within 2 weeks of treatment. The extent of decrease can be even greater when HMg-CoA reductase inhibitors are combined with cholestyramine or colestipol. Mevinolin has recently been released for clinical use in Canada and the United States under the name **lovastatin** (Mevacor®). In early clinical trials in hypercholesterolemic patients it has been reported to lower plasma cholesterol levels by up to 40% or more.

Side Effects

Mevinolin (lovastatin) and compactin are generally well tolerated in short-term therapy. The long-term adverse effects include headache, gastrointestinal upset, and potentially severe myositis and renal failure. Because of the importance of HMg-CoA reductase in the developing fetus, these drugs should not be given to pregnant women.

Nicotinic Acid

Mechanism of Action

The antihyperlipidemic action of nicotinic acid (niacin), discovered in 1955, is unrelated to the role of nicotinic acid and nicotinamide as vitamins (*see* Chapter

49). Although the mechanism of action is not fully understood, there is some evidence that it involves inhibition of the release of free fatty acids from adipose tissue, and of their esterification to triglycerides in the liver. Nicotinic acid decreases production of VLDL in the liver, and this in turn decreases IDL and LDL levels in the plasma. Large doses can reduce VLDL levels by more than 50%, and lower plasma triglycerides correspondingly. LDL levels also fall, but much more slowly; the magnitude of the fall is related to the dose of the drug. Nicotinic acid alone can reduce LDL concentration by up to 15%; in combination with a bile-acid-binding resin, it can produce a reduction of 40–60%. In addition, nicotinic acid also tends to produce some elevation of HDL-cholesterol.

Side Effects

Pharmacologic doses of nicotinic acid produce significant side effects, all of which must be carefully considered by the physician. Peripheral vasodilatation occurs in most patients and results in a cutaneous flush that can be intense and accompanied by severe itching. This reaction is probably mediated by prostaglandins and can be reduced by acetylsalicylic acid. Symptomatic hypotension and transient vascular headaches have also been noted, and nicotinic acid can enhance postural hypotension caused by antihypertensive agents. Gastrointestinal disturbances, including peptic ulceration and bowel disease, are also common. Hepatic dysfunction, hyperglycemia, and abnormal glucose tolerance may occur even in nondiabetic patients taking this drug. Cardiac arrhythmias may occur in some patients during treatment with nicotinic acid.

Drugs That Impair Conversion of Plasma Lipoproteins

Clofibrate and gemfibrozil are the principal drugs in this category; their structural formulae are shown in Figure 37–7.

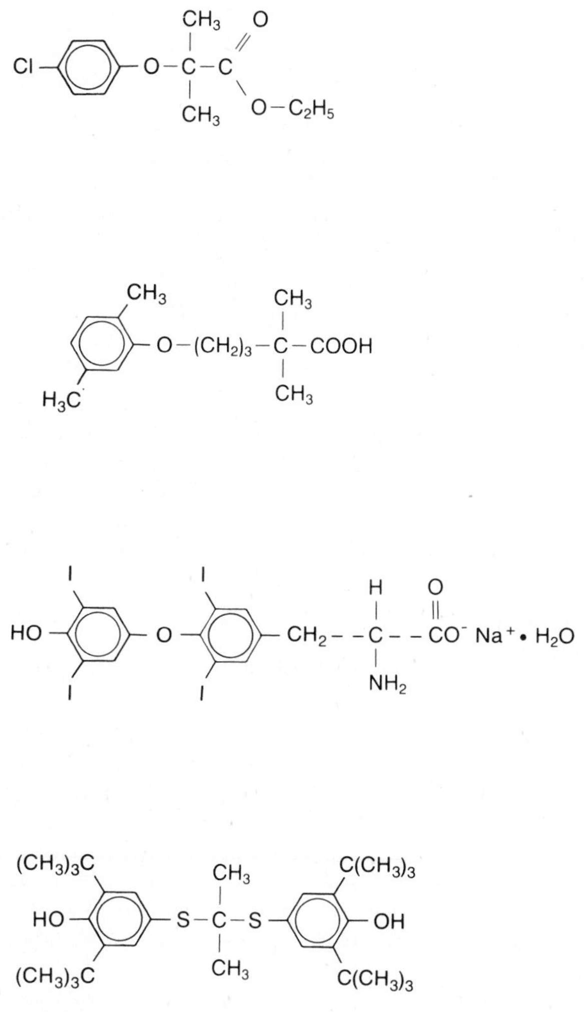

Clofibrate (Atromid®)

Gemfibrozil (Lopid®)

Dextrothyroxine sodium (Choloxin®)

Probucol (Lorelco®)

Figure 37–7 Structural formulae of drugs used to treat hyperlipoproteinemia.

Clofibrate

This drug (Atromid-S®) is an ethyl ester of *p*-chloro-phenoxyisobutyric acid (CPIB). After absorption, it is rapidly hydrolysed, releasing free CPIB. The pharmacologic effects are all due to the free CPIB.

Mechanism of Action

The mechanism of action of clofibrate is not fully known, but its primary action is to increase lipoprotein lipase activity. As a result, the rate of intravascular conversion of VLDL and IDL to LDL is increased, and the plasma VLDL and triglyceride levels fall rapidly. This action may initially increase LDL level, but in most cases the LDL also falls subsequently, as does the cholesterol.

In addition to its effect on plasma lipids, clofibrate inhibits platelet aggregation, decreases fibrinogen levels, and increases the fibrinolytic activity in the blood. It inhibits biotransformation of the active isomer of warfarin, so that the dose of warfarin may have to be reduced.

Therapeutic Uses

The effect of clofibrate on cholesterol level may be rather small in patients with asymptomatic hyper-cholesterolemia, but in familial dysbetalipoproteinemia the plasma triglyceride and cholesterol levels may decrease by as much as 80%. At present, this is its main therapeutic indication, though it also is occasionally useful in patients with severe hypertriglyceridemia who do not respond to nicotinic acid or gemfibrozil.

Clinical trials to date have not shown any significant effect of clofibrate in prevention of deaths from coronary artery disease. In one study it was actually found to increase mortality from noncardiac causes, including malignancies and other diseases.

Side Effects

Side effects of clofibrate include epigastric and abdominal pain, nausea, and diarrhea. The incidence of gallstones increases two- to fourfold. Alopecia, weight gain, myositis, and leukopenia may occur during long-term therapy with clofibrate. The drug is contraindicated in patients with impaired renal or hepatic function and in pregnant or nursing women.

Gemfibrozil

This drug (Lopid®) is a structural congener of clofibrate, and also lowers VLDL in hypertriglyceridemic patients. Its effect on plasma triglyceride levels is greater

than that of clofibrate, however, and it can increase HDL levels by up to 25%.

Mechanism of Action

The mechanism by which gemfibrozil lowers VLDL is not fully known. The drug appears to inhibit hepatic secretion of VLDL into the plasma, as well as increase the rate of its degradation by lipoprotein lipase. It has also been reported to inhibit lipolysis of triglyceride in adipose tissue and to impair fatty acid uptake by the liver. These actions might contribute to a reduction in the hepatic synthesis and secretion of VLDL.

Side Effects

The side effects, toxicity, and drug interactions of gemfibrozil are closely similar to those of clofibrate. All precautions relevant to clofibrate also apply to gemfibrozil.

Drugs That Increase the Clearance of LDL

Dextrothyroxine

Dextrothyroxine (D-thyroxine) is the synthetic dextro-isomer of thyroxine (*see* Chapter 44). It has relatively greater effects on plasma lipids than on other metabolic processes affected by thyroxine. Its structure is shown in Figure 37–7.

Mechanism of Action

D-Thyroxine increases the plasma clearance of LDL, possibly by increasing the number of functional LDL receptors. As a result, it lowers LDL-cholesterol levels by 5–25%, with no effect on HDL and only a slight reduction in VLDL. It also appears to increase the synthesis of bile acids from cholesterol, as a consequence of the increased hepatic uptake and degradation of LDL. The effects of D-thyroxine are synergistic with those of clofibrate.

Side Effects

These are related to the thyroid hormone-like properties of D-thyroxine, and include increased cardiac activity, which may precipitate anginal attacks and arrhythmias in some patients. Therefore the drug is contraindicated in those with a history of cardiac arrhythmias, and should be used with caution in patients with known coronary artery disease. It also potentiates the anticoagulant effects of warfarin and related drugs.

Probucol

This drug (Lorelco®) is chemically unrelated to any of those already described. Its structural formula is shown in Figure 37–7.

Mechanism of Action

The mechanism of action of probucol is poorly understood, and the results of its therapeutic use have been inconsistent. As a lipophilic agent, it is known to become incorporated into the LDL molecule and it has been shown to increase LDL clearance by non-receptor mechanisms. Therefore probucol can decrease LDL-cholesterol levels by 10–15%, especially when it is used together with appropriate dietary modification. The HDL-cholesterol concentrations are also lowered by probucol, often to a greater extent than those of LDL-cholesterol. Maximal effects on total cholesterol are apparent 1–3 months after the start of treatment. Plasma concentrations of VLDL and triglycerides are only slightly reduced.

Side Effects

Although probucol is fairly well tolerated by adults, it does tend to cause gastrointestinal upset (nausea, flatulence, diarrhea, and abdominal pain) in about 10% of patients. It has also been reported to produce electrocardiographic changes in some patients, and should probably not be given to those with evidence of recent myocardial damage or susceptibility to arrhythmias. Its ability to reduce plasma HDL levels may make it undesirable for use in patients with an already high LDL:HDL ratio. The hydrophobicity of probucol may also limit its clinical usefulness.

SUGGESTED READING

Blackburn GL, ed. A symposium: new approaches to cardiovascular therapy. Am J Cardiol 1987; 60:1G–93G.

Choice of cholesterol-lowering drugs. Med Lett Drugs Ther 1988; 30:85–88.

Goldstein JL, Kita T, Brown MS. Defective lipoprotein receptors and atherosclerosis: lessons from an animal counterpart of familial hypercholesterolemia. N Engl J Med 1983; 309:288–295.

Grundy SM. Recommendations for the treatment of hyperlipidemia in adults. A Joint Statement of the Nutrition Committee and the Council on Arteriosclerosis of the American Heart Association. Arteriosclerosis 1984; 4:445A–468A.

Lewis B, Pyörälä K, eds. Lipoproteins and atherosclerosis: current views, future trends. Eur Heart J 1987; 8 Suppl E:1–111.

Lipid Research Clinics Program. The Lipid Research Clinics coronary primary prevention trial results. I. Reduction in incidence of coronary heart disease. JAMA 1984; 251:351–364.

Lipid Research Clinics Program. The Lipid Research Clinics coronary primary prevention trial results. II. The relationship of reduction in incidence of coronary heart disease to cholesterol lowering. JAMA 1984; 251:365–374.

CARDIOVASCULAR SYSTEM

Chapter 38

PHARMACOTHERAPY OF HYPERTENSION

R.I. Ogilvie

Systemic arterial hypertension remains a major public health concern in spite of the availability of potent antihypertensive drugs. The overall prevalence of hypertension exceeds 10%, and rises in each decade of life. As it is an asymptomatic disease until some complication develops, detection is a major problem. Drug therapy may induce adverse effects resulting in poor compliance with instructions to take daily medications. Although drug therapy has resulted in less overall morbidity and mortality from cerebrovascular strokes, congestive heart failure, and renal failure, large-scale trials have failed to demonstrate a major reduction in deaths from myocardial infarction. Therapeutic trials are being used to define further the indications for starting drug treatment when the benefits of treatment (minus the risks and costs) exceed the risks and costs (minus the benefits) of no treatment. Greater attention is being paid to tailoring of therapeutic programs to individual patients to maximize efficacy and minimize toxicity.

A majority of hypertensive patients have primary or "essential" hypertension of unknown etiology, often associated with a family history of the disease and perhaps due to abnormal neurohumoral and renal regulation of peripheral vascular resistance and circulating volume homeostasis. The remaining patients have specific abnormalities such as renal artery stenosis or renal parenchymal disease producing excessive plasma renin concentrations, or diseases of the adrenal gland producing excess circulating steroids or catecholamines; they are classified as having secondary hypertension. Some of the secondary forms can be cured surgically. Antihypertensive drugs counter one or more of the pathophysiologic mechanisms maintaining a high total peripheral vascular resistance and arteriolar tone, which are a characteristic hallmark of persistent hypertension, but the precise mechanism for their antihypertensive effect may not be known.

ANTIHYPERTENSIVE DRUGS

Table 38–1 gives a classification of antihypertensive drugs based on their principal sites of action. These drugs are described in detail elsewhere. This chapter discusses some aspects of their use in systemic arterial hypertension.

Diuretics

The initial hypotensive effect of diuretics is associated with a reduction in extracellular fluid volume and circulating plasma volume due to natriuresis and diuresis, causing a decrease in venous return and cardiac output (Chapter 40). After 6 weeks of continuous therapy, intravascular volume and cardiac output return toward normal, and long-term pressure reduction is related to a reduction of total peripheral resistance by an unknown mechanism.

Diuretics as monotherapy are effective in a large proportion of patients with mild to moderate hypertension and are quite inexpensive compared to other groups of drugs. **Hydrochlorothiazide** and the related drug **chlorthalidone** have a flat dose-response curve for antihypertensive effect, but a steep dose-response curve for biochemical side effects. Low daily doses are used to limit increases in plasma renin activity, uric acid, blood sugar, creatinine, and cholesterol and to limit reductions in serum potassium. Hydrochlorothiazide can be combined with a potassium-sparing drug such as **amiloride, triamterene**, or **spironolactone** to prevent hypokalemia, muscle cramps, and fatigue. Of these three drugs, spironolactone is the only one with significant antihypertensive effects when used as monother-

TABLE 38–1 Classification of Antihypertensive Drugs Based on Their Principal Mode of Action

Diuretics

    Thiazides
    Indapamide
    Potassium-sparing diuretics
    Loop diuretics

Vasodilators

    Direct action on vascular smooth muscle:
      Hydralazine,* Minoxidil, Sodium nitroprusside,*
      Diazoxide,* Glyceryl trinitrate*

    Calcium antagonists:
      Verapamil, Diltiazem, Nifedipine

    Angiotensin converting enzyme inhibitors:
      Captopril, Enalapril

Drugs Acting on the Sympathetic Nervous System

    Centrally acting:
      α-Methyldopa, Clonidine, Guanfacine, Guanabenz

    Ganglionic blockers:
      Trimethaphan*

    Postganglionic blockers:
      Guanethidine, Reserpine

    Blockers of α_1 and α_2 adrenoceptors:
      Prazosin (α_1), Phenoxybenzamine (α_1, α_2),
      Phentolamine (α_1, α_2)

    Blockers of β_1 and β_2 adrenoceptors:
      Propranolol* (β_1, β_2), Nadolol (β_1, β_2),
      Metoprolol (β_1), Atenolol (β_1)

    Combined α- and β-blocker:
      Labetalol* (α_1, β_1, β_2)

* Parenteral form available for hypertensive emergencies.

apy. Another unrelated drug, **indapamide**, may have a direct vasodilator effect as well as being a diuretic. Loop diuretics such as **furosemide** are used to promote sodium and water loss in patients with markedly reduced renal function, but they are not as effective as the thiazides in consistently reducing blood pressure in patients with normal renal function. Diuretics can enhance the hypotensive effects of other drugs and prevent fluid retention associated with some vasodilators such as hydralazine and minoxidil.

Vasodilators

Vascular smooth muscle relaxation can be induced by interfering with contractile mechanisms (direct vasodilators, calcium antagonists, Chapter 36) or control mechanisms (sympathetic nervous system, renin-angiotension system, Chapters 17, 18, 31). Since mechanisms controlling the tone of large arteries, arterioles, and veins differ somewhat, vasodilator drugs can have differing effects on the circulation, and marked dose-response changes may occur. For example, small doses of glyceryl trinitrate and other nitrates have a prominent effect on large vessels, and much larger doses are required to reduce arteriolar resistance. Venodilatation can reduce venous return to the heart and cause a postural fall in blood pressure with orthostatic symptoms of poor cerebral perfusion. Intravenous sodium nitroprusside is used in hypertensive emergencies to reduce arteriolar resistance, but also in patients with severe congestive heart failure to reduce the cardiac afterload as well as preload by increasing venous capacitance.

In contrast, direct-acting vasodilators such as hydralazine and minoxidil have effects only on arteriolar resistance and therefore are not associated with postural hypotension. However, these two drugs can cause a reflex tachycardia due to baroreceptor activation, thus limiting their hypotensive effect and occasionally aggravating angina pectoris. Combination therapy with β-adrenergic blockers is required to control the reflex increase in sympathetic nerve activity. Stimulation of the renin-angiotensin-aldosterone system by these direct vasodilators can cause fluid retention and further attenuate the antihypertensive response unless concomitant diuretic therapy is instituted.

Direct-Acting Vasodilators

These drugs likely interfere with the smooth muscle contractile machinery by altering cGMP formation.

Hydralazine became a widely used oral therapy when it was shown that the addition of β-adrenoceptor blocking drugs reduced the baroreflex tachycardia associated with monotherapy. This combination permits lower hydralazine doses, reducing the development of tolerance resulting from fluid retention and the incidence of a lupus-like syndrome occasionally complicating its use. Headaches and flushing are common adverse effects.

Minoxidil is a potent orally active drug causing serious adverse effects (fluid retention, pericardial effusion, hirsutism); therefore its use is limited to patients refractory to other therapy.

Sodium nitroprusside is a most effective intravenous antihypertensive agent with a rapid onset and offset of effect in the order of minutes. It is used in hypertensive emergencies where careful titration of dose *vs.* hypotensive effect can be employed using continuously controlled pump administration.

Glyceryl trinitrate is commonly used to treat angina pectoris. Occasionally it is useful in patients with systolic hypertension by increasing large artery compliance. However, postural hypotension due to predominant venodilatation, tachycardia, headache, and rapid development of tolerance with continuous therapy limit its usefulness in chronic hypertension. In perioperative hypertensive emergencies it can be used as a continuous intravenous infusion.

Calcium Antagonists

These agents inhibit Ca^{2+} influx into cells by interfering with slow calcium channels in smooth muscle membranes. In addition, they may alter the availability of intracellular Ca^{2+} to the contractile machinery. The ratios of relative vasodilator to negative inotropic effects differ considerably, with **nifedipine** having the greatest vasodilator effect, and **verapamil** probably having the greatest negative inotropic effect. The greater arteriolar vasodilator effect of nifedipine is also associated with a baroreflex tachycardia, whereas **diltiazem** and verapamil have a frequency-dependent inhibitory effect on cardiac atrioventricular nodal transmission, reducing the heart rate response. A slow-release oral preparation of nifedipine is associated with less reflex tachycardia. Nifedipine also causes flushing and pedal edema, the latter presumably due to a greater precapillary than postcapillary arteriolar dilatation with capillary fluid transudation. None of these agents cause postural hypotension as venous tone is unaffected. Verapamil causes more constipation than diltiazem or nifedipine.

Angiotensin Converting Enzyme (ACE) Inhibitors

These agents prevent the conversion of angiotensin I to angiotensin II, thus decreasing a powerful influence on vascular smooth muscle tone. Angiotensin II not only directly constricts vascular smooth muscle but also increases sympathetic nerve activity and stimulates aldosterone secretion. In addition, ACE inhibitors also may enhance the vasodilator effects of prostaglandins and bradykinin, underlining the possibility of several different antihypertensive mechanisms acting cooperatively.

Captopril must be given in several doses per day whereas **enalapril**, a prodrug undergoing hepatic conversion to an active form with a longer half-life, can be administered once a day. Both drugs can cause hyperkalemia due to a reduction in aldosterone. The hypotensive effects of these drugs are enhanced in hyperreninemic states such as occur with circulating volume depletion and diuretic use. Combined therapy with diuretics can reduce dose requirements and prevent the hypokalemia commonly associated with diuretic use. Postural hypotension is uncommon because venodilatation is not a prominent effect and the cerebral autoregulatory curve is shifted to the left. In patients with bilateral renal artery stenosis, or with a single kidney with renal artery stenosis, these drugs may cause reversible renal failure associated with marked rises in serum creatinine. This is because glomerular filtration in these patients is highly dependent upon angiotensin-induced increases in postglomerular arteriolar tone. High doses of captopril have been associated with granulocytopenia and proteinuria. Commonly used lower doses rarely cause these abnormalities and may reduce proteinuria in patients with diabetic nephropathy. A dry, irritant cough occurs in some 5% of patients, and disturbances of taste somewhat less frequently.

Drugs Acting on the Sympathetic Nervous System

Centrally Acting Compounds

α-**Methyldopa** is a prodrug. After conversion to α-methylnoradrenaline by decarboxylation, the active form stimulates central α_2 adrenoceptors, resulting in a reduction of sympathetic outflow from the brain. **Clonidine**, an imidazoline derivative quite different from α-methyldopa in structure, also has a similar mechanism of action with central α_2-adrenoceptor stimulation. When given rapidly by intravenous infusion, or when larger plasma concentrations are achieved by oral dosing, clonidine can stimulate α_2 adrenoceptors peripherally and paradoxically increase blood pressure by arteriolar constriction.

In addition to α-methyldopa and clonidine, other drugs such as **guanfacine** and **guanabenz** also reduce blood pressure by decreasing central sympathetic outflow. All of these drugs rarely cause postural hypotension or tachycardia but are often associated with sedation, difficulty in concentrating, or fatigue. Occasionally, rapid withdrawal of clonidine leads to rebound hypertension with tachycardia.

Ganglionic Blockers

Trimethaphan is occasionally used intravenously for hypertensive emergencies in patients with a dissecting aortic aneurysm when effective hypotension must be attained without an increase in cardiac output or velocity of blood flow ejection. It inhibits transmission of impulses not only in the sympathetic but also in the parasympathetic system, because all autonomic ganglia are affected. The use of trimethaphan is limited by concomitant paralytic ileus, urinary retention, and rapid development of tolerance. Oral use of ganglionic blockers was abandoned decades ago because of these effects and severe orthostatic hypotension, impotence, impaired ocular accommodation, and xerostomia.

Postganglionic Blockers

Guanethidine and **reserpine** are examples of drugs that act on postganglionic neurons inhibiting noradrenaline* release. Both drugs also deplete neuronal noradrenaline stores. Orthostatic hypotension is a major adverse effect. This class of drugs is now considered obsolete.

α-Adrenoceptor Blockers

These drugs block the ability of endogenously released noradrenaline to cause vasoconstriction. **Phentolamine** (intravenously) or **phenoxybenzamine** (in-

---

* norepinephrine

travenously or orally) are useful in patients with hypertension induced by an excess of catecholamines such as is found with a pheochromocytoma. They block postsynaptic α_1 and α_2 adrenoceptors, but also block presynaptic α_2 adrenoceptors responsible for modulating noradrenaline release from the sympathetic nerve endings by feedback inhibition. As a consequence, α-adrenoceptor blockade with phenoxybenzamine or phentolamine may enhance local noradrenaline release and cause tachycardia. **Prazosin** is a much more useful drug for other hypertensive patients as it causes post-synaptic α_1 blockade but does not block presynaptic α_2 adrenoceptors. Thus tachycardia is less often induced unless the baroreflex is activated. In young patients, however, tachycardia may be prominent, and concomitant β-adrenoceptor blockade may be required. There is a significant venodilator effect of prazosin following the first dose, or with large dose increases, which can cause profound orthostatic hypotension. This "first-dose effect" can usually be prevented by initiating therapy and dose changes at bedtime. Tolerance to these venodilator effects usually develops rapidly, whereas there is no evidence for the development of tolerance to the antihypertensive effects.

β-Adrenoceptor Blockers

Soon after the introduction of these drugs for the treatment of angina pectoris, their antihypertensive properties were noted. In spite of decades of investigation, the responsible mechanism is still unknown. Administration of beta-blockers can initially increase peripheral vascular resistance by reducing cardiac output and blocking peripheral β_2 adrenoceptors, leaving unopposed α-adrenoceptor constrictor effects on arterioles. Continued therapy results in a reduction in blood pressure without a reduction in resting cardiac output. There does not appear to be any difference in the antihypertensive effects of beta-blockers that block both β_1 and β_2 adrenoceptors nonselectively, those that selectively block β_1 adrenoceptors, those with intrinsic sympathomimetic activity, and those with significant ability to reduce plasma renin activity. Blockade of presynaptic β adrenoceptors may reduce noradrenaline release from sympathetic nerve endings. Drugs that are poorly lipid-soluble, such as **nadolol** and **atenolol**, have less entry into the brain than **propranolol** or **metoprolol**, but they have equal hypotensive effects. The more water-soluble drugs generally have a longer plasma half-life, can be administered once a day, have fewer CNS adverse effects, but require dose adjustments in patients with renal failure. In larger doses, so-called β_1-selective blocking drugs such as atenolol and metoprolol produce increasing effects on β_2 adrenoceptors, and thus can also worsen asthma or peripheral vascular problems such as Raynaud's disease. Although resting heart rates may be higher during treatment with beta-blockers that have intrinsic sympathomimetic activity, such as

pindolol and **acebutolol**, the reduction in heart rate and in cardiac output responses to graded exercise is similar for all beta-blockers. Beta-blockers have additional advantages in patients with concomitant angina pectoris and provide secondary prophylaxis after myocardial infarction.

Combined α- and β-Adrenoceptor Blockade

Labetalol is a single molecule combining the properties of prazosin (α_1-blockade) with those of propranolol (β_1- and β_2-blockade). It is a weak α-adrenoceptor blocker and the β-blockade is approximately seven times more prominent; thus hypertension may be aggravated in patients with pheochromocytoma. It has all of the advantages and disadvantages of combined oral therapy with prazosin and propranolol. A parenteral form is available for use in hypertensive emergencies.

APPROACH TO THERAPY

Chronic Hypertension

Although drugs from every class can effectively lower blood pressure in a reasonable proportion of patients, the severity of the hypertension, the presence of complications, associated diseases or other diseases, and the likelihood of adverse effects greatly modify the choice for individual patients. Strategies to improve patient compliance, especially in the treatment of a disease such as hypertension, which is asymptomatic until some complication ensues, are of foremost concern. Monotherapy with a single agent taken once a day is ideal. It is essential to simplify dose schedules when more than one agent is required and to give careful attention to strategies to reduce adverse effects.

For over a decade, a "stepped-care" approach has been advocated in North America, with diuretics as the first step, and then adding in successive steps a beta-blocker and a vasodilator if the goal blood pressure is not achieved (below 140/90 mm Hg without adverse effects). More recently an individually tailored approach is being advocated, with closer attention to decreasing adverse effects and maximizing responsiveness. Some statements on this approach follow.

Monotherapy is desirable. In patients with mild hypertension, failure of one therapy should prompt substitution of another therapy, rather than the combined use of additional drugs, since the chance of a favorable response to the alternate drug remains high.

A favorable response without adverse effects may be found with different individual drugs for specific groups of patients. Younger patients may respond better to beta-blockers than older patients. Older patients may respond better to diuretics or calcium-channel blockers. Black patients often respond well to diuretics. Male patients may tolerate diuretics poorly because of the development of sexual impotence. Female patients often tolerate beta-blockers poorly because of the development of cold hands and feet and fatigue. Patients with lipid disorders can be treated with calcium-channel blockers, ACE inhibitors, prazosin, or centrally acting agents that do not alter plasma lipid profiles. These drugs have no effect on the blood sugar and thus may also be useful in diabetic hypertensive patients. Left ventricular hypertrophy, a complication of hypertension, may regress more rapidly when treated with agents interfering with the sympathetic nervous system, such as the centrally acting agents, α_1-adrenoceptor blockers and beta-blockers, or the calcium-channel blockers and ACE inhibitors, rather than with directly acting vasodilators such as hydralazine or minoxidil, which do not cause regression of ventricular hypertrophy even when adequate blood pressure control has been obtained. Other patient characteristics that may predict a beneficial outcome to specific drug treatment are being defined by clinical trials.

Hypertensive Emergencies

Hypertensive emergencies are best treated with parenteral agents that can be rapidly titrated to a goal blood pressure. Intravenous sodium nitroprusside is the most rapidly effective and titratable agent for pressure control in minutes. Intravenous labetalol is commonly employed in situations requiring pressure control in an hour or two. A loading dose of diazoxide, given by constant-rate infusion over 1–2 hours, may also be used. Trimethaphan is reserved for special situations, as discussed previously. Parenteral reserpine is not useful, because a dose-effect titration is not possible and adverse effects are common. Parenteral α-methyldopa is not very practical because the onset of hypotension is delayed, the response is not easily predicted, and profound sedation may ensue. Intravenous hydralazine combined with intravenous propranolol is not as effective as intravenous labetalol. Intravenous glyceryl trinitrate is rarely effective except in perioperative situations, particularly for patients undergoing cardiopulmonary bypass procedures.

Treatment of hypertensive emergencies requires careful dose titration of the hypotension to prevent inordinate reductions in perfusion of the brain, eyes, heart, and kidneys. Sublingual nifedipine is often useful to lower the blood pressure quickly, but occasionally an excessive response is obtained. Patients with acute pulmonary edema and severely elevated blood pressure may respond dramatically to sublingual glyceryl trinitrate. In all cases, other strategies must be considered to assure continued control and maintenance of the blood pressure with oral medications.

Long-Term Management

Education of the patient in the benefits of continued blood pressure control, surveillance for adverse effects, careful attention to associated conditions, and modification of risk factors that may alter morbidity and mortality are all important considerations in long-term management. Nonpharmacologic therapy is also essential and should always be considered as part of management. Pharmacologic regimens will likely be further refined by additional research efforts to develop a targeted approach to attain specific outcomes.

SUGGESTED READING

Genest J, Kuchel O, Hamet P, Cantin M, eds. Hypertension: pathophysiology and treatment. 2nd ed. New York: McGraw Hill, 1983.

Kaplan NM. Clinical hypertension. 4th ed. Baltimore: Williams & Wilkins, 1986.

Larochelle P, Bass MJ, Birkett NJ, et al. Recommendations from the consensus conference on hypertension in the elderly. Can Med Assoc J 1986; 135:741–745.

Logan AG. Report of the Canadian Hypertension Society's consensus conference on the management of mild hypertension. Can Med Assoc J 1984; 131:1053–1057.

Reviews of antihypertensive drugs. J Hypertens 1987; 5 Suppl 3:S1–S93.

Working Group on Hypertension in Diabetes: statement on hypertension in diabetes mellitus. Arch Intern Med 1987; 147:830–842.

RESPIRATORY, RENAL, AND BLOOD SYSTEMS

Chapter 39

DRUGS AND THE RESPIRATORY SYSTEM

W.A. Mahon

Drugs affect the respiratory system in a number of different ways, some by direct local action in the airways and some by remote actions in the central nervous system (CNS) with effects on the respiratory control mechanisms. The most important local drug effects on the airways are those that influence the volume and character of bronchial mucus secretion, and the degree of constriction or relaxation of bronchial smooth muscle. The most important CNS effects are those that diminish the sensitivity of the cough reflex, and those that alter the chemosensitivity of the respiratory control centres in the medulla and thus alter the rate and depth of respiration. These various categories of drug action are reviewed separately in the following sections.

DRUGS AFFECTING RESPIRATORY TRACT FLUID

The tracheobronchial tree is bathed in a mucus-containing fluid, a fibrous gel composed of mucoproteins, mucopolysaccharides, proteins, and fats. The fluid functions to protect the lung tissues by warming and moistening inspired air and by removing foreign airborne particles. Normal human respiratory secretion is 95% water, and adequate hydration and high relative humidity of inspired air are necessary for the production of normal mucus. The normal nasal humidification system maintains constancy of humidity and normal mucus movement as long as nasal breathing prevails. Oral breathing, in a dyspneic or unconscious patient, quickly leads to thickening of the bronchial fluid.

The rate of production of fluid averages about 100 mL/day, but varies with the rate of ventilation and the quantity of airborne material inspired. Calcium ions are believed to contribute to the viscosity of sputum, and the presence of excessive calcium is the one abnormality

linked to the very viscous secretions found in bronchiectasis and in cystic fibrosis. Infected or stagnant respiratory secretions contain DNA fibres from bacterial and phagocytic cells, which give purulent sputum its yellow or green color.

The respiratory tract fluid is produced from three sources: goblet cells of the epithelium, bronchial glands in the mucosa, and serous transudate from the mucosal vasculature. In bronchitis, goblet cells are greatly increased in number and produce extremely viscous sputum. Therefore, it has been traditional practice to administer drugs to stimulate secretion of an increased volume of more watery fluid. However, any agent that increases respiratory tract secretions or decreases their viscosity may act to the detriment of the patient unless the material is propelled upward by normal ciliary activity, and either expectorated by coughing or removed by mechanical suction. Otherwise, mobilized mucus will gravitate into the most dependent areas of the lungs, where it may impair respiratory function.

Antimucokinetic Agents

The reduction of respiratory tract fluid production may be accomplished by parasympatholytic drugs such as **atropine** (*see* Chapter 15).

Mucokinetic Agents (Expectorants)

Agents that increase the production of respiratory tract fluid are often used in order to prevent the drying out of secretions and the plugging of the airways with mucus, and to increase the productiveness of coughing. The most important of these agents are water or saline given as aerosols. The traditional expectorants, whether given by mouth (*e.g.*, **glyceryl guaiacolate**) or by vapor inhalation (*e.g.*, **menthol**, **camphor**, and lemon oils) are of dubious value. However, **potassium iodide** solution may be effective, and **ipecacuanha** (ipecac) apparently initiates a gastric reflex that results in vagal stimulation of the bronchial glands.

Mucolytic Agents

Mucolytic inhalants are mucokinetic substances that liquefy mucus and that are usually given by aerosol to aid the elimination of excess solidified mucus in patients with respiratory disease. Excess mucus may be liquefied by proteolytic agents and disulfide bond-cleaving agents. **Acetylcysteine** is the N-acetyl derivative of the amino acid L-cysteine. It possesses a reactive sulfhydryl group that splits the disulfide bonds of the mucin molecule and thereby reduces the viscosity of mucus. This drug is an extremely effective mucokinetic agent, but it is little used because it causes many side effects such as stomatitis, nausea, vomiting, rhinorrhea, and especially bronchospasm. **Pancreatic dornase** is a hydrolytic enzyme (deoxyribonuclease) that is of value in the treatment of purulent secretions whose viscosity is due to the presence of DNA. This drug is not available in Canada.

DRUGS AFFECTING CONTRACTION OF BRONCHIAL MUSCLE (ANTIASTHMATIC DRUGS)

Asthma

Bronchial asthma is a condition characterized by repeated attacks of paroxysmal dyspnea, due mainly to spasm of the bronchial smooth muscle and resultant narrowing of the bronchi. Initially the bronchospasm responds to bronchodilator drugs. In more severe cases, hypersecretion of viscous mucus and edema of the bronchial mucosa also occur and tend to impair the therapeutic effectiveness of bronchodilators.

The fundamental causes of asthma are still unknown. A number of trigger mechanisms are thought to act on an abnormally reactive bronchial tree. The trigger mechanisms are usually multifactorial in nature and are described in terms such as infective, allergic, exercise-induced, and psychogenic. In any individual these causes may vary in relative importance at different times. One way of classifying asthma is as "extrinsic," where causal allergens are demonstrable, or as "intrinsic" where they are not, but the distinctions are not clear. The allergic hypersensitivity response of extrinsic asthma conforms mainly to Type I and occasionally to Type III allergic reactions. Types II and IV possibly may be involved in intrinsic asthma.

The causes of bronchoconstriction in asthma may be

very complex. The variety of postulated mediators of bronchoconstriction is indicated in Table 39–1.

Bronchodilator Drugs

Many of the drugs that influence the calibre of the bronchi in asthmatic subjects act through the mediation of cyclic nucleotides and of calcium ions, which are considered to be important intracellular messengers, not only in bronchial smooth muscle cells but also in mast cells and the secretory cells of the tracheobronchial mucosa. β-Adrenoceptor agonists exert their effects by stimulating adenylate cyclase. Drugs that increase the intracellular concentration of cyclic AMP, such as β-adrenergic compounds, generally have a beneficial effect in asthma by relaxing bronchial smooth muscles and inhibiting mast cell disruption. Agents that increase cyclic GMP, such as cholinergic drugs, have an adverse effect on asthma; anticholinergics such as atropine or ipratropium have some therapeutic benefits as bronchodilators.

Sympathomimetic Agents

Although adrenoceptor agonists (*see* Chapter 16) may be administered by any route, delivery by inhalation results in the greatest local effect on bronchial smooth muscle with the least systemic toxicity. Aerosol deposition depends on the particle size, the pattern of breathing (tidal volume and rate of airflow), and the geometry of the airways. Even with particles in the optimal size range of 2–5 μm, 80–90% of the total dose of aerosol is deposited in the mouth or pharynx. Particles under 1–2 μm in size remain suspended and may be exhaled. Deposition can be increased by holding the breath in inspiration.

Use of sympathomimetic agents by inhalation at first raised fears about possible tachyphylaxis or tolerance to β agonists, cardiac arrhythmias from β_1-adrenoceptor stimulation and hypoxemia, and arrhythmias from fluorinated hydrocarbons in Freon propellants. However, the concept that β-agonist drugs cause worsening of clinical asthma by inducing tachyphylaxis to their own action has not been supported by sound clinical evidence.

Adrenaline* stimulates β_2 receptors and produces bronchodilatation in asthma. It also stimulates β_1 and α adrenoceptors and thus produces hypertension, tachycardia, and cardiac arrhythmias. It is used for treating the acute asthmatic attack and can be given subcutaneously in a dose of 0.5–1.0 mg. The drug has also been used by inhalation, but by this route it has been replaced by more selective β_2 agents.

Isoproterenol is a nonselective β-receptor agonist. Stimulation of β_2 adrenoceptors produces bronchodilatation, but because of β_1 stimulation, tachycardia also results.

---

* epinephrine

TABLE 39–1 Putative Chemical Mediators of Bronchoconstriction in Bronchial Asthma

Primary Stimulus	Mechanism	Chemical Mediator at Bronchial Muscle
Irritation of large airways	Vagal reflex	Acetylcholine
Type I immediate antigen–antibody interaction at		
• sensory nerve endings in large airways (?)	Vagal reflex	Acetylcholine
• mast cell	Release of histamine (which also may activate afferent vagal fibres)	Histamine
	Release of SRS-A by unknown mechanism	SRS-A
	Release of prostaglandins (?) by unknown mechanism	Prostaglandin $F_{2\alpha}$
Delayed Type I or Type III antigen–antibody interaction	Release of anaphyla-toxins, which cause histamine release	Histamine
	Activation of Hageman factor (XII), which promotes kinin production	Plasma kinins, e.g., bradykinin, kallidin
	Release of prostaglandins	Prostaglandin $F_{2\alpha}$

Ephedrine is a constituent of many older oral preparations for the control of asthma. It has some α as well as β_1 and β_2 effects, but its main advantage is its long duration of action.

Salbutamol* is a selective β_2 agonist. It is used as an aerosol, by intravenous infusion, and as an oral tablet. The aerosol administration minimizes side effects by delivering the drug directly to its site of action (thus permitting a lower dose), and is the method of choice for the use of this drug in the control of bronchoconstriction in chronic asthma or chronic obstructive pulmonary disease. The usual single dose delivered by an appropriate inhaler device (2 puffs) is 200 μg. The onset of action of the inhaled drug is almost immediate. When the drug is given by mouth as 5-mg tablets, the action begins within 30 minutes, rises to a peak between 2 and 4 hours, and gradually declines over a period of 6 hours. The drug causes an increase in

* albuterol

heart rate and skeletal muscle tremor when given by mouth. Other selective β_2-sympathomimetic agents with similar properties are **terbutaline, orciprenaline (metaproterenol), fenoterol,** and **isoetharine**.

These drugs are not inactivated by catechol-O-methyl transferase and so have a long duration of action compared to adrenaline. Table 39–2 shows the receptor activities and the durations of action of the sympathomimetic drugs. Figure 39–1 shows the structural relationship between salbutamol and isoproterenol. Specific β_2 stimulants are currently the drugs of first choice, and large doses in combination with methylxanthines and corticosteroids are used in the treatment of status asthmaticus.

TABLE 39–2 Receptor Binding Specificities and Duration of Action of Sympathomimetics

Agent	α	β_1	β_2	Duration
Adrenaline	+ + +	+ + + +	+ + +	±
Ephedrine	+	+ + +	+ +	+
Isoproterenol		+ +	+ + +	+ +
Orciprenaline		+	+ + +	+ + +
Salbutamol		+	+ + +	+ + + +
Terbutaline		+	+ + +	+ + + +

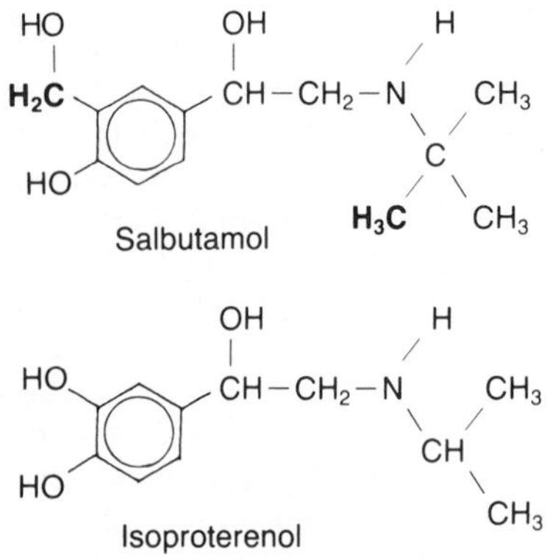

Figure 39–1 Structural similarity of salbutamol (albuterol) and isoproterenol.

Some studies have demonstrated that arterial oxygen tension (Pao_2) may decrease after administration of β agonists if ventilation:perfusion ratios in the lung worsen. This effect may occur, however, with any class of bronchodilator drug, and the significance of such an effect depends on the initial Pao_2 of the patient. Supplemental oxygen may be necessary if the initial Pao_2 is very low or if there is a large decrease in Pao_2 during treatment with bronchodilators.

Anticholinergic Drugs

Atropine competes with acetylcholine for muscarinic cholinergic receptors, and thus can cause a variety of effects including blurring of vision, increases in heart rate, and drying of secretions in the salivary glands and respiratory tract (see Chapter 15). This limits its usefulness as a bronchodilator. Atropine is best used by inhalation, which reduces, but does not eliminate entirely, these unwanted side effects.

Ipratropium bromide is a quaternary isopropyl-substituted derivative of atropine that has practically no central effect and shows some degree of bronchoselectivity. The actions of ipratropium bromide are otherwise similar to those of atropine, and its therapeutic use is confined to aerosol administration. The drug is administered by inhaler and each puff contains 20 μg. The exact place of ipratropium bromide in the treatment of asthma remains somewhat uncertain, and the drug appears to have little advantage over the selective β_2 agonists.

Methylxanthines

The three important methylxanthines are theophylline, theobromine, and caffeine. Their major source is, of course, beverages such as tea, cocoa, and coffee, respectively. Their effects on the various organ systems are as follows.

Central nervous system. In low to moderate doses, the methylxanthines, especially caffeine, cause mild cortical arousal with increased alertness and deferral of fatigue. In unusually sensitive individuals, the caffeine contained in beverages (e.g., 100 mg in a cup of coffee) is sufficient to cause nervousness and insomnia. Nervousness and tremor are primary side effects in patients taking large doses of aminophylline for asthma.

Cardiovascular system. The methylxanthines have direct positive chronotropic and inotropic effects on the heart. At low concentrations, these effects appear to result from increased calcium influx, probably mediated by increased cyclic AMP. At higher concentrations, sequestration of calcium by the sarcoplasmic reticulum is impaired, so that intracellular calcium concentration is increased, and myocardial contraction is strengthened (see Chapter 34). Methylxanthines have occasionally been used in the treatment of pulmonary edema associated with heart failure. These agents also relax vascular smooth muscle except in cerebral blood vessels, where they cause contraction.

Gastrointestinal tract. The methylxanthines stimulate secretion of both gastric acid and digestive enzymes.

Kidneys. The methylxanthines, especially theophylline, are weak diuretics. This effect may involve both increased glomerular filtration and reduced tubular sodium reabsorption. The diuresis is not of sufficient magnitude to be therapeutically useful.

Smooth muscle. The **bronchodilatation** produced by the methylxanthines is the major therapeutic action. Tolerance does not develop, but side effects, especially in the central nervous system, may limit the dose. In addition to this direct effect on the airway smooth muscle, these agents inhibit antigen-induced release of histamine from lung tissue; their effect on mucociliary transport is unknown.

Skeletal muscle. The therapeutic actions of the methylxanthines may not be confined to the airways, for they also strengthen the contractions of isolated skeletal muscle in vitro (see Chapter 19) and have potent effects in improving contractility and in reversing fatigue of the diaphragm in patients with chronic obstructive lung diseases. This **effect on diaphragmatic performance**, rather than an effect on the respiratory centre, may account for theophylline's ability to improve the ventilatory response to hypoxia and to relieve dyspnea even in patients with irreversible airflow obstruction.

Theophylline

This 1,3-dimethylxanthine is a plant alkaloid. It is poorly soluble and must be chemically complexed with other drugs to increase the solubility enough for clinical use (e.g., **aminophylline** = theophylline + diethylamine). It is the most selective of the methylxanthines in its effects on smooth muscle.

Mechanism of action. The major mechanism of action of theophylline as a bronchodilator is commonly believed to be its inhibition of phosphodiesterase and the consequent increase in cyclic AMP concentration in smooth muscle. However, inhibition of phosphodiesterase is not prominent at usual therapeutic doses of theophylline (10–20% inhibition occurs at blood concentrations regarded as therapeutic). It has been suggested that theophylline produces blockade of adenosine receptors, although this effect is probably not important for bronchodilatation. Alterations in smooth muscle Ca^{2+} concentration may also be influenced by theophylline, and this may explain the relaxing effect on bronchial smooth muscles. Theophylline has also been shown to inhibit the effects of prostaglandins on smooth muscle and to inhibit the release of histamine and leukotrienes from mast cells (see Chapters 30, 31, and 32). In normal subjects, intravenous administration of theophylline causes no bronchodilatation, whereas inhalation of a β_2-adrenoceptor agonist produces a definite response. In severe acute asthma, intravenous theophylline has been shown to have one-third of the bronchodilator potency of inhaled isoproterenol. There is, however, no doubt about the beneficial effects of theophylline, and this improvement of airway resistance may be due to a mechanism other than bronchodilatation. For example, it has been shown that theophylline increases contractility of the diaphragm, particularly of the fatigued diaphragm (*see* above).

Pharmacokinetics. There is marked interindividual variation in the hepatic transformation of theophylline. The clearance rate is influenced by so many different factors (Table 39–3) that it is essentially unpredictable in an individual. Therefore the dose necessary to maintain optimal serum concentrations (27–82 μmol/L, or 5–15 mg/L) varies widely, and must be controlled by actual measurement of the concentrations. The clearance of theophylline in males is 20–30% higher than that in females. There may also be a circadian variation in theophylline clearance. Cigarette smoking increases theophylline elimination by inducing the hepatic enzymes (*see* Chapter 4), and there is decreased biotransformation of theophylline in hepatic cirrhosis, congestive heart failure, and chronic pulmonary disease.

Theophylline toxicity is largely related to dose and plasma concentration. Serious toxic effects are uncommon at concentrations below 110 μmol/L (20 mg/L), although a significant percentage of patients have unacceptable side effects even when the plasma concentration does not exceed the usual therapeutic range. The most serious toxicities are cardiac arrhythmias, seizures, and respiratory or cardiac arrest. Minor adverse effects occur frequently; the commonest are anorexia, nausea, vomiting, and anxiety.

Calcium-Channel Blockers

Calcium-channel blockers have been shown to be effective in relaxing bronchial smooth muscle and are particularly useful for the treatment of exercise-induced asthma (*see* Chapter 36).

TABLE 39–3 Factors Influencing Theophylline Clearance

| Factor | Theophylline Clearance Is | |
	Decreased	Increased
Age	Prematurity >65 years	
Sex	Females	Males
Habits		Cigarette smoking
Drugs	Erythromycin	Phenobarbital
Diseases	Liver cirrhosis Congestive heart failure Chronic lung disease	

Asthma Prophylaxis

Anti-inflammatory Steroids

Glucocorticoid drugs such as **prednisone, prednisolone**, and **dexamethasone** (described in Chapter 47) are known empirically to relieve airway obstruction in bronchial asthma, but the mechanism of their action is complex and not fully understood. The possible actions include:

- anti-inflammatory activity;
- reduction of tissue sensitivity to antigens;
- inhibition of contraction of bronchial smooth muscle;
- mucolytic action;
- increased responsiveness of β_2 adrenoceptors.

In addition to their use for the relief of asthmatic attacks that are already in progress, glucocorticoids also find a prophylactic use for the prevention of attacks in patients who are subject to almost constant recurrence. However, the glucocorticoids can produce serious side effects such as Cushing's syndrome, peptic ulcer, osteoporosis, steroid myopathy, diabetes, sodium retention and hypertension, increased susceptibility to infection, and decreased responsiveness to stress (*see* Chapter 47). Therefore the chronic use of glucocorticoids must be avoided if at all possible. If it is necessary to use these drugs, minimum effective doses should be employed and therapy given on alternate days in order to minimize adrenal suppression. Short-term therapy is rarely harmful except in patients with concurrent diseases exacerbated by glucocorticoids, *e.g.*, diabetes.

Recently, glucocorticoid drugs such as **beclomethasone dipropionate** or **beclomethasone valerate** have been developed for administration by inhalation. Inhalation of these compounds is as effective as oral prednisone in patients starting on steroids. Only a small amount of the steroid administered in this manner is systemically absorbed. Therefore there is little or no effect on adrenal function, and the problem of growth suppression in children may be avoided. The major problem with this form of therapy to date has been the development of fungal infections in the oropharynx in about 10% of patients.

Because many patients taking oral steroids for asthma suffer some degree of adrenal suppression, reduction or discontinuation of their oral dose must be done very slowly. For a period of up to a year after discontinuation of chronic oral steroid therapy, oral or parenteral steroids must again be administered during episodes of severe infection or trauma to prevent additional crises.

Sodium Cromoglycate (Cromolyn Sodium)

Unlike the preceding drugs, this drug is used **exclusively** for the **prophylaxis**, rather than the treatment, of asthmatic attacks. It inhibits the release of mediators such as histamine and leukotrienes from the secretory granules of mast cells following the challenge of antigen interacting with specific IgE antibodies. The exact mechanism underlying the action of sodium cromoglycate (Fivent®, Intal®, and others) is not clear, but the drug is active only against Type I (immediate) allergic reactions, and not against delayed or immune reactions. Therefore it is used primarily for the prevention of allergic asthma, hay fever, and other acute allergic reactions.

However, sodium cromoglycate is also effective in asthma induced by exercise and by exposure to cold, dry air. Interaction of antibodies with mast cells is probably not involved in either of these types of asthma, but both are associated with rapid respiratory loss of heat, which may be a physical stimulus to mast cell degranulation. Therefore it is suggested that sodium cromoglycate acts as a nonspecific stabilizer of the mast cell membrane and/or granules.

Sodium cromoglycate is absorbed poorly from the gastrointestinal tract and therefore is effective only when deposited directly into the airways. Two methods of administration are currently used for asthma. In adults, the drug can be given by a "Spinhaler" apparatus that causes a capsule to be punctured so that its powdered contents are entrained into inspired air and deposited in the airways. The usual dose is 20 mg inhaled four times daily. In children, who may have difficulty in using this device, the drug may be given by aerosol. Other formulations, for topical use in the eye or nose, are intended for the prophylaxis of allergic rhinitis and conjunctivitis (hay fever).

There are very few toxic effects of sodium cromoglycate, because very little is absorbed systemically. Local side effects such as throat irritation and cough may follow inhalation of the dry powder. Rashes have been reported, as well as rare cases of anaphylactic reaction.

Anaphylaxis

Anaphylaxis is an acute Type I reaction to the administration of an antigen. It induces changes in the lungs that are similar to those of asthma, but while asthma is usually a localized reaction, anaphylaxis is widespread, involving the cardiovascular system. The signs of anaphylaxis include acute respiratory distress, asphyxia, angioneurotic edema, severe hypotension, and vascular collapse possibly leading to death.

The treatment of anaphylaxis is supportive. It is essential to support the vital functions before attempting to treat the cause of anaphylaxis. Cardiorespiratory resuscitation measures should be initiated promptly. The standard emergency drug, **adrenaline**, acts to support both the respiratory (bronchodilatation) and cardiovascular (increased cardiac output, vasoconstriction) systems.

Despite the possible contribution of histamine to anaphylaxis, the use of antihistamines is usually futile. Many mediators are responsible for the disorder, and antagonism of only one may have little noticeable effect. The histamine may already be present at receptor sites before antihistamine can be administered. Antihistamines are effective only when the lesions are not established or when the drugs are administered prior to the complete adsorption of the antigen. Even when antihistaminic drugs are given early, they offer only partial protection from the development of new lesions or the delayed complications of anaphylaxis.

Large doses of corticosteroids may be beneficial in reducing bronchospasm and inflammatory edema associated with anaphylaxis. Because their maximum biologic effect on bronchospasm does not occur until hours after administration, corticosteroids must be given as early as possible, *i.e.*, at the same time as the other therapy is started.

DRUGS AFFECTING THE COUGH REFLEX

Cough

The cough reflex is mediated by receptors located in the mucosa or deeper structures of the larynx, trachea, and major bronchi, and by mechanoreceptors that detect changes in bronchial intramural tension. Stimuli are transmitted *via* the vagus to the cough centre in the medulla. Efferent impulses originating from the cough centre are transmitted through cholinergic pathways to the abdominal and intercostal muscles and to the diaphragm, producing sudden explosive expiratory movements. The effect of coughing is to expel foreign particles that have entered the bronchial tree, and to expectorate sputum from the bronchial lumen. This may be beneficial to the patient, by protecting against damage by foreign bodies or bacteria, and by helping to clear the airways. However, repeated nonproductive coughing (*i.e.*, coughing that fails to clear mucus from the lower respiratory tract) exhausts the patient and disturbs sleep. Long-term coughing also may lead to the breakdown of elastic tissue in the lung, or damage to the tracheobronchial epithelium. It is therefore often helpful to give drugs to suppress the cough reflex.

Antitussive Drugs

Narcotic Antitussive Agents

Opiate narcotics (*see* Chapter 22) are most effective in depressing the cough centre. Although the precise mechanism whereby they exert their effects is uncertain, they appear to react with a variety of receptors identified at numerous sites in the central and peripheral nervous systems. There is some specificity found among various opiates with respect to their antitussive potency. For example, the ED_{50} for analgesia compared to the ED_{50} for cough suppression yields a ratio of 6.62 for codeine, 4.60 for hydrocodone, and 2.87 for morphine. **Codeine** thus appears to be a more effective cough suppressant relative to its analgesic activity. The antitussive dose of codeine is relatively low, and 10 mg may produce a 62% elevation of threshold to ammonia-induced cough for 60 minutes. The usual antitussive dose is 15–20 mg as required. Codeine also has significantly less respiratory depressant effect than morphine. The development of tolerance and physical dependence is a major drawback to morphine-like drugs, and for this reason, their long-term use as antitussive agents is discouraged. They can, however, be used for short-term cough suppression. Because of the low dose of codeine required, and its relatively low addiction liability, it may be more suitable than other narcotic drugs for long-term antitussive use.

Nonnarcotic Antitussive Agents

Dextromethorphan is a synthetic derivative of morphine that is an effective antitussive agent, suppressing the response of the cough centre but lacking analgesic or habituating properties. It is the d-isomer of levomethorphan, which is a potent opiate analgesic. This demonstrates that the analgesic activity, as well as the addictive properties, are exerted through receptors with stereospecificity, while the antitussive receptor sites lack the opiate stereospecificity (*see* Chapter 22). **Levopropoxyphene** is similarly an antitussive that lacks the analgesic activity of its isomer, dextropropoxyphene. Other nonnarcotic drugs that have some antitussive activity in addition to their other pharmacologic actions include **phenothiazines**, **antihistamines**, and **benzononatate**.

DRUGS AFFECTING CENTRAL RESPIRATORY CONTROL

Measurement of Respiratory Control Function

Normal functioning of the respiratory system keeps the hydrogen ion concentration at the central chemoreceptors constant, although in hypoxic emergencies the peripheral chemoreceptors can interrupt this $[H^+]$ regulation in favor of an increased supply of O_2. As a result of such regulation, the respiratory system matches the pulmonary exchange of O_2 and CO_2 to the cellular exchange that accompanies metabolism. The principal components of the system are shown schematically in Figure 39–2. The feedback nature of this system is important because changes in any one part

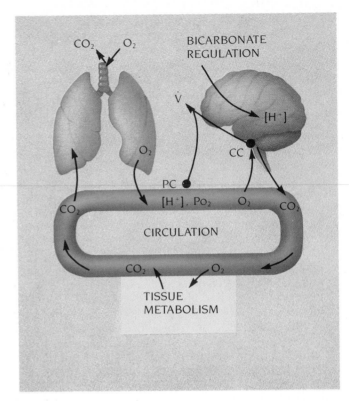

Figure 39–2 Schematic representation of the principal components of the respiratory control system. PC = peripheral chemoreceptors; CC = central chemoreceptors; $\dot{V}$ = airflow.

can affect other parts by altering the stimuli to central and peripheral chemoreceptors. The system, therefore, tends to keep ventilation at a level that matches metabolism despite changes in its components.

Unless CO_2 and O_2 levels are kept constant before and after drug administration, ventilation is a poor guide to the effect of a drug on respiration. Arteriolar P_{CO_2} is a better guide. Drug effects can often be assessed by examining the change in the system's ventilatory response to increasing P_{CO_2}. They can also be evaluated in relationship to decreasing P_{O_2}. Ventilation-P_{CO_2} response curves are usually measured at an inspired O_2 concentration of 30% so as to eliminate the variable contribution of the peripheral chemoreceptors. The slope of the ventilation-P_{CO_2} response curve is taken as an index of sensitivity of the central chemoreflex. An example of the use of the ventilation-P_{CO_2} response curve is shown in Figure 39–3, which illustrates the reduction of chemoreflex sensitivity with increasing levels of halothane anaesthesia. Note that at 2% halothane, sensitivity is almost zero but ventilation is still half its normal value. The P_{CO_2}, however, is markedly increased above normal. The system is on the brink of failure (sensitivity zero, CO_2 rising unchecked) but ventilation is only halved.

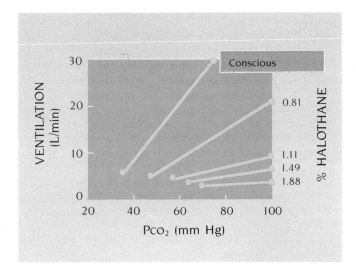

Figure 39–3 Ventilation-P_{CO_2} response curves at various levels of anaesthesia.

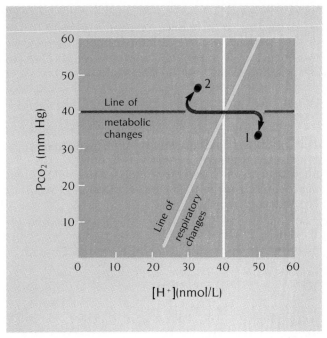

Figure 39–4 Respiratory changes in relation to arterial blood hydrogen ion concentration (*see* text for explanations).

Drugs Affecting Systemic Acid-Base Balance

These agents shift the ventilation-P_{CO_2} response curves to the left (increased arterial [H⁺]) or right (decreased arterial [H⁺]), but do not change the slope.

Acidifying Agents

Hydrochloric acid and **ammonium chloride** produce an increase in arterial blood [H⁺] (*i.e.*, decreased arterial blood pH), which stimulates ventilation slightly through peripheral chemoreceptor stimulation, but does not affect the central chemoreceptors because of the blood–brain barrier. An increase in ventilation quickly lowers P_{CO_2} at both central and peripheral chemoreceptors, and a decrease in P_{CO_2} at central chemoreceptors lowers [H⁺] there. The resultant withdrawal of central respiratory drive opposes the ventilatory increase driven by peripheral chemoreceptors. In the short term, the effect of the increase of arterial blood [H⁺] is to lower P_{CO_2} and increase ventilation only very slightly. Long-term changes (48 hours or more) are produced by regulation of central bicarbonate so as to restore central [H⁺] towards normal. These changes, therefore, produce an increase in ventilation and a reduction in P_{CO_2}. Significant variation exists among individuals with respect to their capacity for compensation by respiration (Fig. 39–4, point 1).

Carbonic Anhydrase Inhibitors

Acetazolamide slows the rate of CO_2 hydration in tissue and the rate of dehydration of carbonic acid in lungs, and prevents the renal absorption of bicarbonate.

All three factors thus lead to an increase in [H⁺] and the resulting increase in ventilation as described above.

Alkalinizing Drugs

Administration of **sodium bicarbonate** or **sodium lactate** produces a decrease in arterial blood [H⁺] (*i.e.*, increased arterial blood pH). This decrease withdraws the stimulatory effect of peripheral chemoreceptors on ventilation, but does not affect the central chemoreceptors because of the blood–brain barrier. A decrease in ventilation quickly results in an increase in P_{CO_2} at both central and peripheral receptors. The increase in P_{CO_2} at the central receptors results in an increase in [H⁺], and the resultant increase in central respiratory drive opposes the decrease in the peripheral respiratory drive. In the short term, the effect of the decreased [H⁺] in arterial blood is to raise P_{CO_2} and decrease ventilation, but only slightly. Long-term changes (greater than 48 hours) are produced by regulation of central bicarbonate so as to restore central [H⁺] towards normal, and thus to tend to normalize ventilation drive from the central chemoreceptors. These changes therefore produce a decrease in ventilation (the maximum decrease is equal to the ventilatory contribution of the peripheral chemoreceptors) with an increase in P_{CO_2} and normal central [H⁺], so that arterial [H⁺] increases towards normal. The amount of compensation by respiration varies widely among individuals (*see* Fig. 39–4, point 2).

Sodium bicarbonate is the agent most commonly used to correct metabolic acidosis. Because it can change respiration *via* these compensatory mechanisms, it is important to use it only for metabolic acidosis and not respiratory acidosis, which should be corrected by increasing ventilation. A hazard occurs with rapid intravenous injection of bicarbonate. As the bicarbonate-blood mixture passes through the lung, CO_2 "fizzes" off, transiently increasing alveolar and arterial P_{CO_2}. This CO_2 bolus reaches the cerebral circulation where it causes a transient increase in cerebral blood flow. Such an increase may be harmful, for example, during neurovascular surgery. Therefore, bicarbonate must be administered slowly.

Agents Affecting the Central Nervous System

Medullary Depressants

All anaesthetics, narcotic analgesics, sedative-hypnotics, alcohol, neuroleptics, and anxiolytics, and a variety of other drugs acting on the CNS depress the central chemoreceptor reflex control in a manner similar to that shown for halothane in Figure 39–3. Generally speaking, their effects on central chemoreceptor sensitivity are cumulative; the addition of an anxiolytic with little primary effect on ventilation may reduce chemoreceptor sensitivity so that an otherwise safe dose of anaesthetic may cause reduction of sensitivity to zero and produce failure of the system.

The peripheral chemoreceptor reflexes may not be depressed to the same degree and ventilation may then be supported through hypoxic drive. Administration of oxygen in such circumstances could stop ventilation altogether. Such an effect has been typically observed with barbiturate overdose. Few studies have tested the effects of depressants on the peripheral chemoreflex. Two agents, halothane and alcohol, have been shown to impair the peripheral reflex, probably through general vasodilatation.

Treatment for drug-induced respiratory depression is supportive, with artificial ventilation and maintenance of fluid, electrolyte, and acid-base balance. If respiratory depression results from overdosage with a narcotic analgesic or a related compound such as propoxyphene, a narcotic antagonist such as naloxone should be used to reverse the depression (*see* Chapter 22). The antagonistic effects of naloxone are short-lived relative to the respiratory depressant effects of opiate narcotics. Consequently the treatment with naloxone may have to be repeated several times at intervals of 30–60 minutes.

Medullary Stimulants

Analeptics. This class of drugs has been used as respiratory stimulants to reverse CNS depression and acute respiratory failure, but without great effectiveness. They are all CNS stimulants, and in large doses they can all produce convulsions. Agents such as **amphetamine, aminophylline, adrenaline, bemegride,** and **pentylenetetrazole** are of limited usefulness because of their short durations of action, narrow margins between therapeutic and toxic effects, and the possibilities of illegal use (amphetamine).

Nikethamide, ethamivan, and **doxapram** are most commonly used as respiratory stimulants. In common with all CNS stimulants, these agents increase the slope of the ventilation-P_{CO_2} curve (sensitivity). The action of an intravenous dose lasts for only 2–10 minutes and so these agents are administered by intravenous infusion.

Salicylates. Salicylate overdose induces a centrally mediated, powerful, and sustained stimulation of ventilation. Small doses shift the ventilation-P_{CO_2} response to the left while larger doses increase the slope. Very high doses cause respiratory paralysis.

The respiratory and metabolic disturbances from salicylate overdose require careful consideration for full understanding. Toxic doses can lead to respiratory alkalosis, metabolic acidosis, and respiratory acidosis depending upon the size of the initial toxic dose and the elapsed time without treatment (*see* Chapter 33).

The causal relationships leading to a renally compensated respiratory alkalosis are as follows. Central respiratory stimulation, which develops slowly due to slow diffusion of salicylates across the blood–brain barrier, leads to respiratory alkalosis (move down line of respiratory changes in Fig. 39–4). Renal compensation by bicarbonate excretion tends to restore [H^+] to normal (move horizontally to the right in Fig. 39–4), leaving the system with low P_{CO_2}, about normal [H^+], and impaired protection against metabolic acidosis (low bicarbonate).

Complicating this simple picture of a compensated respiratory alkalosis, and leading to metabolic acidosis, are the metabolic effects of salicylates, which include:

- uncoupling of oxidative phosphorylation and derangement of carbohydrate metabolism, leading to the accumulation of pyruvic, lactic, and acetoacetic acids;
- dissociation of salicylate in blood and the displacement of plasma bicarbonate;
- central vasomotor paralysis and impaired renal function.

In salicylate poisoning, as both dose and time since ingestion increase, the sequence tends to be from compensated respiratory alkalosis to a combined respiratory alkalosis and metabolic acidosis, to both metabolic and respiratory acidosis when respiratory depression occurs.

Except in extreme cases in which hemodialysis may have to be used, the treatment is supportive. Acid-base management depends upon careful evaluation of the patient's status and the factors involved (*see also* Chapter 33).

OXYGEN TOXICITY

Oxygen gas is used therapeutically in the treatment of many aspects of respiratory failure. While in most cases oxygen is benign, there are dangers associated with its overuse.

Ventilatory depression results when oxygen is administered to patients with central respiratory depression (elevated arterial Pco_2), because the oxygen decreases the sensitivity of the peripheral chemoreceptors to carbon dioxide.

CNS poisoning, causing **convulsions**, occurs when oxygen is breathed at pressures greater than one atmosphere (*e.g.*, hyperbaric chamber, diving). There is a wide variation both between and within individuals, but it appears that inspired O_2 at partial pressures below 1300 mm Hg is safe. It is believed that oxygen-induced seizures arise because oxygen at high partial pressure results in decreased GABA concentrations in nerve cells.

Prolonged breathing of oxygen concentrations above 60% produces an **inactivation of the alveolar surfactant**, which can lead to lethal lung damage. Retrosternal discomfort can occur after 6 hours of breathing 100% O_2 or 36 hours of 60% O_2. This type of damage is unlikely except in cases of long-term ventilatory support in respiratory care units.

Premature infants, who may require high concentrations of oxygen because of respiratory distress syndrome, risk blindness because of **retrolental fibroplasia**. High Po_2 leads to the obliteration of the developing blood vessels of the immature retina.

SUGGESTED READING

Cole RB. Drug treatment of respiratory disease. Monographs in clinical pharmacology. Vol 5. New York: Churchill-Livingstone, 1981.

Drazen JM, Austen KF. Leukotrienes and airway responses. Am Rev Respir Dis 1987; 136:985–998.

Hendeles L, Weinberger M, Johnson G. Monitoring serum theophylline levels. Clin Pharmacokinet 1978; 3:294–312.

Piafsky KM, Ogilvie RI. Dosage of theophylline in bronchial asthma. N Engl J Med 1975; 292:1218–1222.

Schwartz SL, Dluhy RG. Corticosteroids; clinical pharmacology and therapeutic use. Drugs 1978; 16:238–255.

RESPIRATORY
RENAL BLOOD

Chapter 40

DIURETICS

A. Marquez-Julio and C. Whiteside

The major function of diuretics is to inhibit renal tubular reabsorption of sodium. This natriuretic effect leads to reduction in extracellular fluid volume and to changes in electrolyte and acid-base balance. To understand fully the pharmacologic effects of diuretics, it is important to recall the mechanisms that control sodium homeostasis, and in particular the major role of the kidney in sodium regulation.

REVIEW OF RENAL PHYSIOLOGY

Sodium is the major extracellular cation and is the primary determinant of extracellular fluid (ECF) volume. The kidney regulates sodium and water excretion to maintain the ECF volume within narrow limits despite an irregular and often excessive dietary intake of sodium.

The filtered load of sodium first entering the renal tubules ($\approx 2.4 \times 10^4$ mEq/day) is equal to the product of glomerular filtration rate (GFR) and the plasma concentration of sodium. Sodium reabsorption then occurs at four major sites along the nephron: proximal tubule, loop of Henle, distal convoluted tubule, and collecting tubule and duct (Fig. 40–1 and Table 40–1). The bulk of sodium reabsorption necessary to maintain constancy of total body sodium occurs in the proximal tubule and loop of Henle. The fine-regulation of sodium reabsorption occurs at the distal sites, which may determine the rate of urinary sodium excretion. The control system regulating renal sodium excretion involves "sensor" and "effector" limbs. The sensor limb includes extrarenal volume receptors, located in the low-pressure capacitance areas (intrathoracic great veins or atria) and high-pressure resistance areas (arterial vasculature), that are capable of detecting changes in effective circulating blood volume. It also includes renal baroreceptors (juxtaglomerular apparatus, JGA), which sense the mean

arterial pressure entering the renal microcirculation. The effector limb is composed of multiple neural and hormonal factors that alter one or both of the two physiologic components involved in sodium excretion, namely renal blood flow and tubular transport of sodium.

The kidney is an autoregulatory organ. The intrarenal resistance vessels (afferent and efferent arterioles) maintain constant capillary blood flow and glomerular filtration rate over a wide range of mean arterial perfusion pressures. The filtered load of sodium, therefore, remains essentially unchanged during changes in arterial pressure. Thus, the control of tubular sodium reabsorption is the major determinant of ultimate sodium excretion.

In states of ECF volume contraction, both afferent and efferent renal arteriolar resistances increase (*via* sympathetic nerves and angiotensin II generation), maintaining the pressure gradient and thus maintaining GFR. The increase in efferent arteriolar resistance potentially leads to net changes in peritubular capillary hydrostatic forces in a direction that enhances movement of sodium and water into the capillary bed following reabsorption by the proximal tubule. In states of ECF volume expansion, when proximal sodium reabsorption is reduced, solute delivery *via* the lumen to the loop of Henle increases (Table 40–1).

The thick ascending limb of Henle's loop in the renal medulla is a major site of sodium reabsorption. Here, chloride ions are transported out of the lumen by a secondary active carrier mechanism. Sodium is passively cotransported by the same carrier. The rate of reabsorption is accelerated by increased delivery of sodium chloride to the carrier sites (Table 40–1). This, in turn, blunts the increased delivery of sodium to the distal nephron.

The medullary portion of the thick ascending limb of Henle's loop is also the major determinant of the countercurrent concentrating mechanism. Since this segment is water impermeable, the movement of sodium chloride out of the lumen in the absence of water creates hypertonicity of the medullary interstitial fluid. This

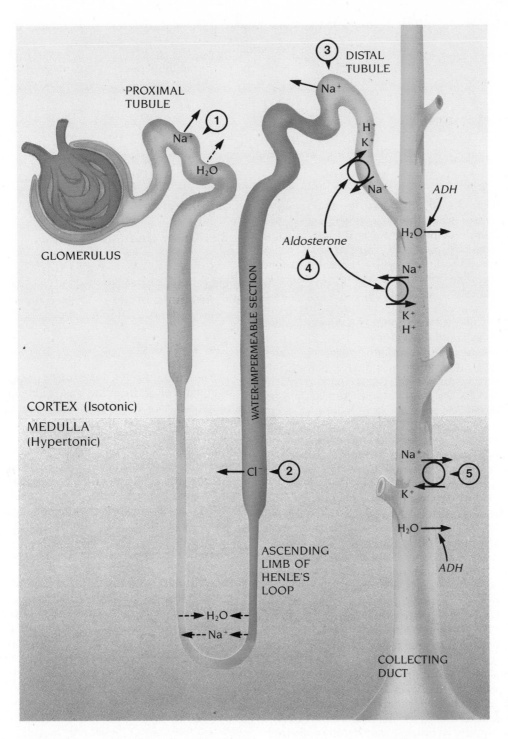

Figure 40–1 Sites of action of diuretic agents in the nephron: (1) carbonic anhydrase inhibitors, osmotic diuretics; (2) "loop" diuretics, organomercurials; (3) sulfonamide diuretics; (4) aldosterone antagonists; (5) other potassium-sparing diuretics; (———→) active transport mechanisms; (– – –→) passive transfer.

TABLE 40-1 Sodium Reabsorption in Major Nephron Segments (Derived from Studies in Rats)

	Percent Reabsorption of Filtered Load			
State of Hydration	Proximal Tubule	Loop of Henle	Distal Tubule and Collecting Duct	Percent Excretion of Filtered Load
Volume contraction	65	24	10	1
Volume expansion	45	40	10	5

(From Lassiter WE. Disorders of sodium metabolism. In: Earley LE. Gottschalk CW. eds. Strauss and Welt's Diseases of the kidney. 3rd ed. Boston: Little, Brown. 1979:1515.)

helps to establish the driving force for the osmotic movement of water from the collecting duct (in the presence of antidiuretic hormone, ADH) to produce a concentrated urine. As well, the transport of sodium and chloride out of the lumen of the cortical segment of the thick ascending limb of Henle's loop results in the formation of hypotonic tubular fluid or "solute-free water." Interference with sodium chloride transport in these segments will, therefore, alter the concentrating and diluting capacity of the kidney.

Mineralocorticoid-sensitive sodium transport occurs in the cortical collecting tubule and duct. It is associated with chloride reabsorption and potassium and hydrogen ion secretion. In states of volume contraction, an increase of sympathetic tone and a reduction of renal perfusion pressure (sensed by the JGA) cause release of renin. Angiotensin II is generated and, in turn, stimulates aldosterone secretion, which increases sodium reabsorption in the collecting duct.

The papillary collecting duct is capable of active sodium reabsorption. The primary effect of natriuretic hormone(s) may be inhibition of the sodium reabsorptive capacity of the collecting duct. This distal site may play an important role in determining the final urinary sodium concentration and, therefore, sodium excretion.

The fine-regulation of intrarenal blood flow and tubular reabsorption of sodium is controlled by humoral (e.g., prostaglandins, bradykinin, angiotensin II) and neural (sympathetic nervous system) factors. In states of normal sodium balance these influences are minor, but in disease states they can play a significant role. Local prostaglandin production, for example, maintains a degree of renal vasodilatation and directly stimulates tubular natriuresis. These effects are most pronounced in states of reduced effective renal perfusion (e.g., congestive heart failure, cirrhosis). In this setting, inhibition of prostaglandin synthesis may lead to further sodium and water retention and/or acute tubular necrosis (renal failure).

DIURETICS

Diuretic agents have been classified according to chemical structure and/or site of action (Fig. 40-1). A more clinically useful approach is to consider them also according to potency, as listed in Table 40-2.

Loop Diuretics ("High-Ceiling" Diuretics)

Mechanism and Site of Action

The loop diuretics (Fig. 40-2) directly inhibit the active chloride/passive sodium cotransport at the luminal membrane of the medullary segment of the thick ascending limb of Henle's loop.

Pharmacokinetics

Furosemide (Lasix®, Furoside®) is rapidly but incompletely absorbed from the gastrointestinal tract. In the circulation it is 91–99% protein-bound. Excretion is primarily via proximal renal tubular secretion, at the weak-acid secretory site. As with most diuretics, renal tubular secretion of furosemide is necessary for pharmacologic effect of the drug at the luminal membrane.

Ethacrynic acid (Edecrin®) is well absorbed from the gastrointestinal tract, and in the circulation it is 97% protein-bound. It undergoes partial hepatic metabolism. The major portion is secreted via the proximal renal tubular weak-acid transport sites and can then be reabsorbed at more distal nephron sites via pH-dependent nonionic diffusion (see Chapter 7).

Bumetanide (Bumex®), a sulfamoyl benzoic acid derivative like furosemide, is the third loop diuretic (approved for use in the United States but not in Canada). It is almost completely absorbed from the gastrointestinal tract, reaching peak blood concentrations within 30 minutes after an oral dose. In plasma, it is 90% protein-bound. The drug is partially metabolized by the liver, but more than 50% is excreted unchanged in the urine within 6 hours of administration.

The onset and duration of effect of these three drugs are summarized in Table 40-3.

Pharmacologic Effects

Loop diuretics are potent natriuretic agents that have the capacity to inhibit reabsorption of up to 20–25% of the filtered sodium load. This potency is related to the relatively large magnitude of sodium chloride transport occurring in this nephron segment and to efficiency of the chloride transport blockade.

The kaliuresis observed with loop diuretics is proportional to the increased rate of urine flow caused by these agents.

TABLE 40–2 Classification and Uses of Diuretic Agents

Class	Relative Natriuretic Potency	Chief Site(s) of Action	Major Indications	Major Complications
"Loop" diuretics Furosemide Ethacrynic acid Bumetanide Organomercurials	High (20–25%)*	Medullary ascending limb of Henle's loop	Pulmonary edema Resistant edema states	Vascular collapse, hypokalemia, hypochloremia, metabolic alkalosis
Sulfonamide diuretics Benzothiazides Non-thiazides	Moderate (5%)	Cortical ascending limb of Henle's loop Distal tubule	Edema states Hypertension	Hypokalemia, metabolic alkalosis, carbohydrate intolerance
Carbonic anhydrase inhibitors	Low (1–3%)	Proximal tubules	Urinary alkalinization Glaucoma	Hypokalemia, metabolic acidosis
Potassium-sparing diuretics	Low (1–3%)	Collecting tubules Collecting Duct	Ascites (spironolactone) Potassium-sparing effects	Hyperkalemia
Osmotic diuretics	Dose-dependent	Proximal tubules Loop of Henle	Cerebral edema	Acute volume overload Hypokalemia Hyponatremia

* Maximum % of filtered Na^+ load excreted (in parentheses).

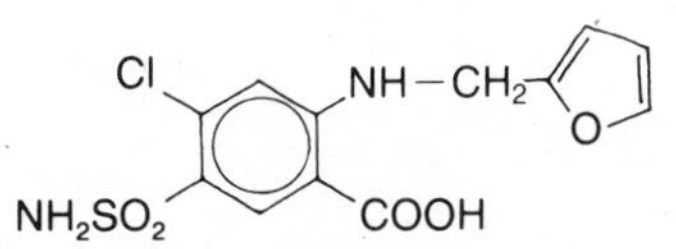

Figure 40–2 Structural formulae of loop diuretics.

TABLE 40–3 "Loop" Diuretics (Also Known as "High-Ceiling" Diuretics)

Drug and Route of Administration	Onset of Effect	Peak Effect	Duration of Action

Furosemide (Lasix®, Furoside®)
  p.o.
  i.v.
	
	15 min
	5 min
		
		1–2 hr
		30 min
			
			4–6 hr
			~2 hr

Ethacrynic acid (Edecrin®)
  p.o.
  i.v.
	
	20 min
	15 min
		
		2 hr
		45 min
			
			6–8 hr
			~3 hr

Bumetanide (Bumex®)
  p.o.
  i.v.
	
	30 min
	10 min
		
		1–2 hr
		45 min
			
			4½–6 hr
			~3 hr

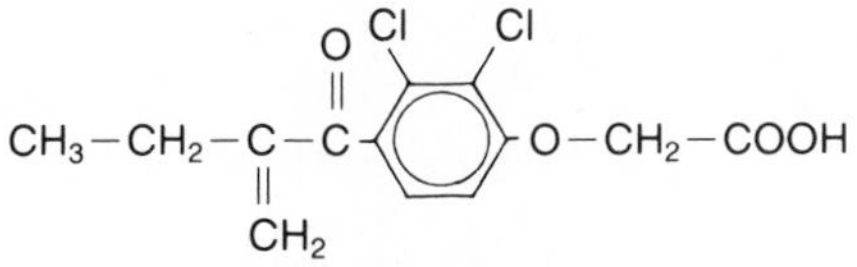

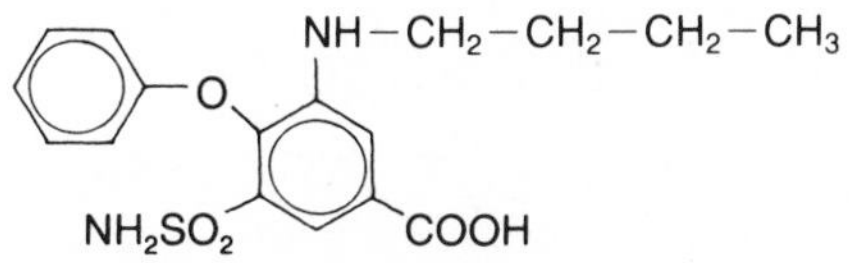

Since loop diuretics impair sodium chloride reabsorption in a water-impermeable segment of the nephron, they prevent the formation of medullary hypertonicity. Maximal urinary concentration is, therefore, impaired. Furthermore, in the presence of the diuretic, sodium chloride remains within the tubular lumen and "free water" cannot be formed. Thus, these agents also impair free-water clearance (*i.e.*, the renal capacity to form dilute urine).

All loop diuretics produce major calciuresis, which accompanies the increase in sodium excretion. There is evidence to suggest that this effect is due to inhibition of calcium reabsorption in the thick ascending limb of the loop of Henle.

Furosemide has a mild direct transient vasodilatory effect when administered intravenously. The exact mechanism of this effect is unknown, but may be related to induction of prostaglandin synthesis.

Adverse Effects and Toxicity

The most commonly encountered adverse effects of loop diuretics are intravascular volume depletion (which can lower blood pressure excessively) and hypokalemia (which may be associated with cardiac arrhythmias and muscle weakness). Chronic use usually leads to hypochloremic metabolic alkalosis. This is a result of large chloride losses in the urine coupled with distal sodium reabsorption in exchange for potassium and hydrogen ions (enhanced by aldosterone if intravascular volume depletion has occurred).

Frequently observed hyperuricemia is primarily a consequence of enhanced proximal tubular reabsorption of solute (including uric acid) when intravascular volume contraction occurs.

Carbohydrate intolerance can occasionally be observed, particularly in patients with prediabetic states. Hyponatremia is infrequent: the mechanisms involved in its genesis are similar to those that cause hyponatremia with sulfonamide diuretics (*see* below).

Acute administration of loop diuretics, usually when large doses are infused rapidly by the intravenous route, has produced deafness. The exact mechanism of this adverse effect is unknown, but there may be impairment of sodium extrusion from the endolymph to the perilymph in the inner ear. Although deafness is usually transient when caused by furosemide, there are reports of permanent hearing loss following ethacrynic acid administration.

Intravenous administration of ethacrynic acid has been associated with an increased frequency of gastrointestinal hemorrhage. This has been attributed to impairment of platelet aggregation.

Rare adverse effects of the loop diuretics include agranulocytosis, thrombocytopenia, and allergic phenomena (skin rashes, interstitial nephritis, *etc.*).

Drug Interactions

Three major groups of drug interactions are well recognized with loop diuretics. The most recently described, and likely the most common, is the blunting of the natriuretic effect of loop diuretics by most non-steroidal anti-inflammatory agents. Inhibition of intrarenal prostaglandin synthesis by the latter is

purported to be the mechanism of this interaction (as described in the review of renal function).

Less frequently seen is potentiation of the ototoxicity of aminoglycoside antibiotics and of the nephrotoxicity of first-generation cephalosporins (cephaloridine, cephalothin).

Drug interactions with other weak acids have been described and are due to competition between drugs for the secretory transport system. For example, probenecid, a uricosuric agent, delays the renal tubular secretion of the loop diuretics, thereby retarding their diuretic effect. High doses of furosemide have been reported to delay the excretion of tubocurarine and prolong its action.

Sulfonamide Diuretics

Currently available benzothiazide diuretics (Fig. 40–3) were developed during attempts to synthesize more effective carbonic anhydrase inhibitors (*see also* Fig. 10–4). The first member of this group to be studied extensively was chlorothiazide (Diuril®); the basic pharmacologic action of other analogs is similar to that of this agent. Somewhat different in structure, but with very similar pharmacologic profiles, are agents such as chlorthalidone (Hygroton®), quinethazone (Aquamox®),

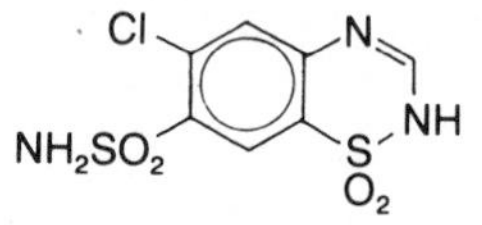

Chlorothiazide
(Diuril®)

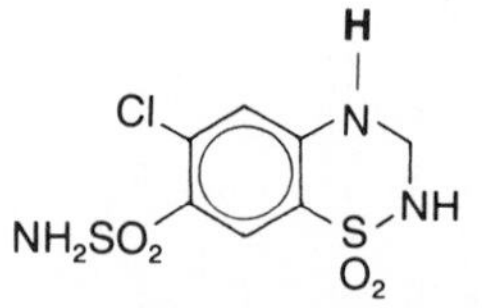

Hydrochlorothiazide
(HydroDiuril®,
Urozide®,
Esidrix®, *etc.*)

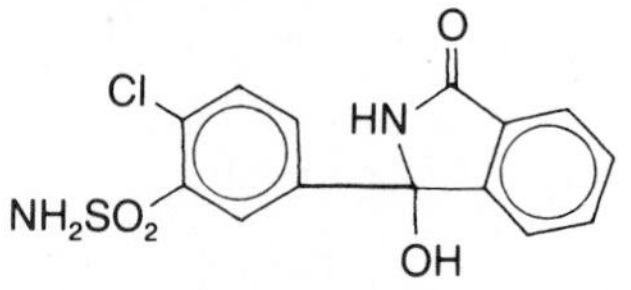

Chlorthalidone
(Hygroton®,
Uridon®,
Novothalidone®)

Figure 40–3 Structural formulae of sulfonamide diuretics.

TABLE 40–4 Sulfonamide Diuretics Available in Canada

Non-proprietary Name	Trade Name	Approximate Relative Potency	Usual Dose (mg/day)	Duration of Effect (hr)
Benzothiazides				
Hydrochlorothiazide*	HydroDiuril Esidrix and others	1	25–100	6–12
Bendroflumethiazide	Naturetin	10	2.5–15	6–12
Chlorothiazide	Diuril	0.1	500–2000	6–12
Methyclothiazide	Duretic	10	2.5–10	6–24
Polythiazide	Renese	10	2–15	24–48
Others				
Chlorthalidone*	Hygroton	0.8	25–200	48
Metolazone	Zaroxolyn	10	2.5–10	12–24
Quinethazone	Aquamox	1	50–100	18–24

* Agents most frequently used, least expensive.

and metolazone (Zaroxolyn®). Currently available sulfonamide diuretics are listed in Table 40–4.

Mechanism and Site of Action

Sulfonamide diuretics inhibit reabsorption of sodium from the lumen in the cortical ascending (diluting) limb of Henle's loop and the distal convoluted tubule. The exact cellular mechanism of action is uncertain. Inhibition of glycolysis and diminution of energy supplies (ATP) required for transport have been implicated.

Pharmacokinetics

Sulfonamide diuretics are rapidly absorbed from the gastrointestinal tract. The more substituted drugs (*i.e.*, with hydrophobic side chain) are more highly protein-bound. As well, they are more lipid-soluble and have a greater apparent volume of distribution. Sulfonamides are weak acids secreted into the proximal renal tubular lumen by an active (competitive) transport system for weak acids. Tighter protein binding parallels slower renal tubular secretion. Greater lipid solubility may result in increased reabsorption from the distal nephron. Most agents are excreted unchanged in the urine. The duration of action of the various sulfonamide diuretics in Table 40–4 relates to some of these pharmacokinetic properties.

Pharmacologic Effects

Sulfonamide diuretics are considered moderately potent natriuretic agents, capable of inhibiting reabsorption of up to 5% of the total filtered sodium load. The sites of action are proximal to the nephron segments responsible for potassium secretion. The increased sodium delivery to the collecting tubule results in increased sodium/potassium exchange and kaliuresis.

Since sulfonamide diuretics inhibit sodium chloride reabsorption in the water-impermeable cortical ascending limb of Henle's loop, they impair the ability of this nephron segment to generate solute-free water (*i.e.*, they impair free-water clearance).

Acutely administered benzothiazide diuretics decrease urine calcium excretion. Micropuncture and microperfusion studies suggest that this phenomenon is due to direct enhancement of calcium absorption in the distal convoluted tubule. Chronic thiazide administration significantly reduces urine calcium not only because of this distal reabsorption effect, but also because of enhanced fluid and solute reabsorption in the proximal nephron secondary to extracellular volume depletion.

Serum calcium (total as well as ionized calcium) becomes elevated following acute or chronic thiazide administration. This is partly due to the increased calcium reabsorption by the kidney. A parathormone-related action of thiazides on bone has also been implicated. Unless the recipient has a hypercalcemic tendency, this effect is not clinically important.

Adverse Effects and Toxicity

As with loop diuretics, sulfonamide diuretics frequently cause acute and chronic intravascular volume depletion and dose-related hypokalemia, metabolic alkalosis, and hyperuricemia.

Hyperglycemia and glucose intolerance have been observed with chronic use of sulfonamide diuretics. Controversy exists as to whether this occurs only in patients with prediabetic states. Recent studies suggest that this adverse effect may be common, but that it is slowly reversible in up to 60% of patients once the diuretic is discontinued. When sustained fasting hyperglycemia occurs in patients receiving sulfonamide diuretics, the benefits of continued diuretic use must be carefully weighed against long-term risks of diabetes mellitus. Many factors are postulated to contribute to glucose intolerance, including direct or hypokalemia-related inhibition of insulin release, as well as inhibition of insulin release and enhancement of glycogenolysis due to reflex sympathetic activity caused by intravascular volume depletion.

A recent randomized crossover trial in a hypertensive population has established that sulfonamide diuretics significantly increase plasma total cholesterol, VLDL-cholesterol, and plasma triglycerides. The magnitude of the lipid profile change is dose-related and can be prevented by weight reduction and a low-cholesterol diet. The cause of these changes in lipid levels is unknown.

Hyponatremia may arise as a complication of (thiazide) diuretic therapy, even when edema is still present. A combination of factors contributes to this untoward effect. In edema states with reduced effective circulating volume, intrarenal factors such as decreased GFR and increased proximal tubular sodium and fluid reabsorption diminish the delivery of tubular fluid to the diluting segments of the nephron. Inhibition of sodium chloride transport in the water-impermeable portions of the nephron (*i.e.*, diluting segments) impairs its capacity to generate free water (*i.e.*, dilute urine). If the nephron is unable to generate free water, excess extracellular-fluid water cannot be excreted efficiently. Intravascular volume contraction increases ADH secretion, overriding the effect of hyposmolarity. In the presence of ADH, water reabsorption in the collecting duct continues. Water accumulates in the ECF compartment and sodium concentration decreases (hyponatremia).

In an elderly population receiving thiazide diuretics for nonedematous pathologic states, profound hyponatremia has been reported recently. Although the same hormonal and intrarenal mechanisms might be operative, it is unclear why this side effect might be more prevalent in older patients.

Sustained hypercalcemia is very occasionally seen with sulfonamide diuretic use. Its presence should alert the physician to pathologic states that cause increased serum calcium (hyperparathyroidism, neoplastic disease, *see also* Chapter 48).

Sulfonamide diuretics occasionally produce gastrointestinal intolerance (nausea and vomiting), pancreatitis, and allergic manifestations (*e.g.*, skin rashes). Thrombocytopenia and agranulocytosis are rare toxic phenomena.

Drug Interactions

The major drug interaction currently recognized is the inhibition of the natriuretic and antihypertensive effects of the sulfonamide diuretics when nonsteroidal anti-inflammatory agents are used concomitantly. Inhibition of intrarenal prostaglandin synthesis is felt to be part of the mechanism involved in this untoward effect.

Carbonic Anhydrase Inhibitors (Acetazolamide)

Mechanism and Site of Action

Acetazolamide (Fig. 40–4) inhibits proximal renal tubular luminal brush-border carbonic anhydrase (CA). Normally CA catalyses the reaction:

$$H^+ + HCO_3^- \rightleftharpoons H_2CO_3 \rightleftharpoons CO_2 + H_2O$$

as shown in Figure 40–5.

Inhibition of CA results in delay in the conversion of intraluminal carbonic acid (H_2CO_3) to CO_2 and H_2O. The rise in luminal H^+ concentration provides a gradient against H^+ secretion from the tubular cell. The intracellular hydration of CO_2 to H_2CO_3 and subsequent production of H^+ and HCO_3^- is retarded. Therefore, intracellular H^+ available for secretion into the tubular lumen is also decreased. Since proximal tubular "reabsorption" of filtered bicarbonate (HCO_3^-) occurs indirectly by combining with secreted H^+ to ultimately form CO_2 and H_2O, which are immediately reabsorbed, CA inhibition causes HCO_3^- to remain in the tubular fluid. Furthermore, since sodium is the cation that accompanies the entry of HCO_3^- into the peritubular circulation, CA inhibition results in some natriuresis. This natriuresis is mild, partly because proximal sodium reabsorption will occur with a proportionately larger amount of chloride, and partly because more distal tubular sites reabsorb the sodium (partly by Na^+/K^+ exchange with resulting loss of potassium).

Pharmacokinetics

Carbonic anhydrase inhibitors, like thiazide diuretics, are well absorbed from the gastrointestinal tract, and excreted *via* proximal renal tubular secretion within 24 hours. Their natriuretic and urinary alkalinizing effects are of limited duration (2–3 days) because of factors unrelated to their pharmacokinetic properties.

Pharmacologic Effects

Acetazolamide is only a very mild natriuretic agent because of its proximal site of action, which does not alter sodium reabsorption in the more distal nephron.

Acutely, it will increase urinary bicarbonate excretion. Once sufficient bicarbonate losses accrue, a systemic metabolic acidosis occurs, and filtered tubular bicarbonate concentration also decreases. Distal tubu-

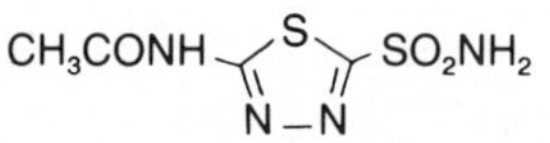

Figure 40–4 Structural formula of acetazolamide (Diamox®, Acetazolam®).

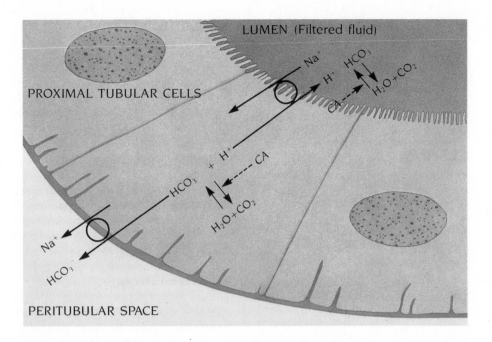

Figure 40–5   Site of action of carbonic anhydrase (CA) inhibitors.

lar secretion of H^+ is then sufficient to combine with luminal HCO_3^- to ultimately form H_2O and CO_2 and thus permit little HCO_3^- to appear in the urine.

When CA inhibitors acutely inhibit proximal sodium reabsorption, the sodium presented to distal sites (including collecting duct) is then reabsorbed in exchange for potassium, the net effect being some kaliuresis.

In the eye, CA inhibition is associated with decreased formation of aqueous humor.

Adverse Effects

The most frequent adverse effects seen with CA inhibitors are hypokalemia and systemic metabolic acidosis.

Allergic and toxic effects are similar to those of other thiazide diuretics. Acute renal failure caused by nephrolithiasis (acetazolamide may crystallize in acidic urine) has been described during chronic acetazolamide use in the treatment of glaucoma. A more recent congener, methazolamide (Neptazane®), has not caused this side effect.

Drug Interactions

No recognizable adverse drug interactions have been described. When CA inhibitors are combined with thiazide and loop diuretics, the natriuretic and kaliuretic effects of the drugs can be augmented.

Potassium-Sparing Diuretics

Aldosterone Antagonists (Spironolactone)

Mechanism and Site of Action

Normally, aldosterone acts on nephron segments beyond the distal convoluted tubule, stimulating sodium reabsorption in exchange for potassium and hydrogen ions. Spironolactone (Aldactone®; Fig. 40–6) and its major metabolite, canrenone, are inhibitors of aldosterone. Both bind competitively to cytosolic receptor sites for aldosterone prior to translocation into the nucleus.

Pharmacokinetics

Spironolactone is well absorbed from the gastrointestinal tract and rapidly undergoes hepatic biotransformation to canrenone, the major metabolite. Canrenone is highly protein-bound and has an elimination half-life of approximately 18 hours. Excretion occurs *via* the kidneys and the gastrointestinal tract.

Pharmacologic Effects

Aldosterone-stimulated sodium reabsorption in exchange for potassium and hydrogen ion, in the distal

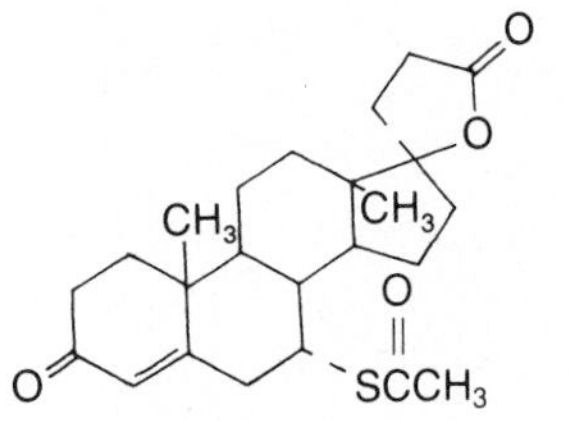

Figure 40-6 Structural formula of spironolactone (Aldactone®).

collecting tubules and ducts, accounts for 2–3% of total sodium reabsorption. Spironolactone therefore causes only a mild natriuresis.

Adverse Effects

The most potentially dangerous adverse effect of spironolactone is hyperkalemia. This occurs frequently because of inadvertent administration of spironolactone together with potassium supplementation, and/or to patients with moderate to severe renal insufficiency.

Other frequent side effects of spironolactone include an unpleasant peppermint aftertaste and nausea/vomiting. Its steroid molecular structure has been implicated in painful gynecomastia frequently noted in men. Other side effects related to the molecular structure include loss of libido, impotence, and menstrual irregularities.

Other Potassium-Sparing Diuretics (Triamterene and Amiloride)

Mechanism and Site of Action

Triamterene (Dyrenium®; Fig. 40–7) and amiloride (Midamor®) inhibit sodium/potassium countertransport in nephron segments beyond the distal convoluted tubule. However, they do not compete with aldosterone receptors. The specific mechanism of action of triamterene is still unknown. Amiloride directly inhibits the luminal sodium/potassium countertransport carrier.

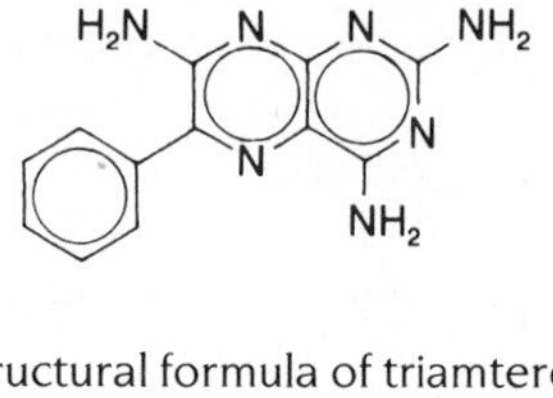

Figure 40-7 Structural formula of triamterene (Dyrenium®).

Pharmacokinetics

Triamterene undergoes prompt and essentially complete gastrointestinal absorption, whereas only 50% of amiloride is absorbed. Onset of diuretic effect is similar for the two drugs, occurring some 2 hours after ingestion. Duration of effect for triamterene is 7–9 hours, and up to 24 hours for amiloride.

Pharmacologic Effects

Since sodium/potassium countertransport in collecting tubules and ducts accounts for only 2–3% of total sodium reabsorption, only a mild natriuresis will occur with the potassium-sparing diuretics. The natriuresis is coupled with decreased potassium excretion.

Adverse Effects

The major adverse effect is hyperkalemia, which frequently occurs because of inadvertent concurrent potassium supplementation or because of moderate to severe renal insufficiency. Another frequent adverse effect is gastrointestinal intolerance.

Drug Interactions

Although not extensively studied, nonsteroidal anti-inflammatory agents oppose the natriuretic effect of triamterene. Furthermore, use of indomethacin together with triamterene has been reported to cause reversible renal insufficiency.

Osmotic Diuretics

Mannitol and **urea** have been utilized as osmotic diuretics. For this purpose these agents are administered intravenously; they are rapidly and freely filtered by the glomerulus. The hyperosmolarity caused by the high intratubular concentration of these solutes prevents sodium reabsorption by effectively diluting the intraluminal sodium concentration and by markedly increasing the tubular fluid flow rate. The overall effect is increased sodium and water excretion.

The adverse effects encountered with osmotic diuretics include hypokalemia and acute intravascular volume overload. The latter effect occurs because the osmotic agent increases the transfer of fluid to the intravascular compartment from interstitial sites.

Organomercurial Diuretics

Organomercurial diuretics were the first clinically useful group of diuretics. Like the modern loop diuretics, they inhibit chloride/sodium cotransport in the medullary thick ascending limb of the loop of Henle. Their exact molecular mechanism of action is not known.

These agents have fallen into disuse for various reasons. They require parenteral administration (i.m. or s.c.), and with protracted use they are potentially nephrotoxic. Development of safer and effective oral diuretic agents has rendered the organomercurial diuretics largely obsolete.

THERAPEUTIC APPLICATIONS

Edema

Diuretic agents are utilized primarily to enhance renal sodium excretion in abnormal clinical situations when the kidneys avidly reabsorb sodium and water despite the presence of an expanded ECF compartment (edema states).

Edema is the clinical manifestation of excess interstitial fluid. This is formed as an ultrafiltrate of plasma across capillary walls and has essentially the same sodium concentration as plasma. Increased accumulation of interstitial fluid occurs in disorders causing elevated hydrostatic pressure (e.g., congestive heart failure), reduced capillary oncotic pressure (hypoalbuminemia), or increased capillary permeability. Each of these conditions is associated with reduced mean arterial pressure due to either cardiac failure or reduced intravascular volume. This state of reduced "effective" circulating volume triggers the control systems regulating sodium balance, with the overall result of avid renal sodium reabsorption in an attempt to restore a normal circulating volume.

Another mechanism of edema formation is primary sodium retention due to kidney disease (e.g., acute glomerulonephritis). Inability of the kidney to respond appropriately to the increased effective circulating volume results in positive sodium and water balance. Reduction in GFR and increased activity of the renin-angiotensin system may also play a role in certain renal disease states. Expansion of both intravascular and interstitial compartments of the ECF rapidly becomes manifest as hypertension and edema.

The rational approach to the treatment of increased total body sodium and edema states includes dietary sodium and water restriction and the judicious use of diuretics. The underlying disorder and the physical state of the patient on examination will determine appropriate management and, when required, the appropriate choice of diuretic.

Pulmonary Edema

This is a life-threatening emergency that requires, among other therapeutic measures, a potent, rapidly acting diuretic agent. The diuretics of choice are the loop diuretics, and by convention furosemide is used most frequently. Its immediate vasodilatory action on venous capacitance vessels rapidly decreases cardiac preload while slightly decreasing total peripheral resistance and increasing renal blood flow. This transient effect, coupled with the prompt, large diuresis, has made furosemide a mainstay of therapy.

Congestive Heart Failure

Cardiac failure, from whatever causes, implies impairment of cardiac output. It is as a consequence of the attendant reduction of "effective" renal blood flow that renal retention of sodium and water occurs, through both reflex and hormonal effector pathways. Gradually, as sodium and water are retained, extracellular volume expands, ultimately leading to edema formation.

Therapy includes measures to enhance cardiac output (cardiotonic agents such as digoxin, arteriovenous dilators to decrease preload and afterload) and to minimize sodium and water retention (dietary sodium and fluid restriction, plus diuretics).

Diuretics in this setting have to be used with care and with close monitoring of the patient's clinical condition (orthostatic blood pressure changes, jugular venous pressure, etc.). The danger is that excessive use will cause contraction of intravascular volume with subsequent reflex vasoconstriction (mediated by catecholamines and angiotensin II). The attendant increase in preload and afterload will be detrimental to cardiac output. Furthermore, rapid contraction of intravascular volume may lead to symptoms of cerebral, coronary, and renal insufficiency, particularly in the elderly.

Diuretic "resistance" may be encountered with both loop and sulfonamide diuretics. A common reason is unsuspected excessive dietary intake of sodium and water. However, the other major cause of loss of natriuretic effectiveness relates to intravascular volume contraction. Once initial diuresis has occurred, time must be permitted for interstitial fluid to shift into the intravascular compartment before further diuretic intake is prescribed. For most diuretics this implies use on alternate days.

When diuretics are used in patients with cardiac disease, hypokalemia should be prevented, particularly if the patients are also receiving digitalis glycosides. They usually require 60–80 mEq potassium supplementation per day, through dietary manipulation and/or KCl replacement. Alternatively, potassium-sparing diuretics can be used concomitantly to maintain serum potassium above 3.5 mmol/L. Digitalis toxicity and inherent cardiac arrhythmias are more likely in the presence of hypokalemia.

Cirrhosis with Ascites

Hepatic cirrhosis frequently gives rise to portal hypertension, which impairs the venous return from the splanchnic bed. Hypoproteinemia may be present because of lymphatic exudation in the peritoneal cavity and/or diminished hepatic production of albumin. The net balance of hydrodynamic and osmotic forces then favors interstitial fluid formation in the peritoneal cavity, *i.e.*, the formation of ascites. The exact onset and mechanism of sodium and water retention by the kidney in cirrhosis are still controversial. ECF volume redistribution into the peritoneal cavity may reduce "effective" renal plasma flow, leading to sodium and water retention. Furthermore, hepatic insufficiency decreases aldosterone degradation, and secondary hyperaldosteronism is enhanced.

The control of ascites by means of diuretics makes life more tolerable for the patient. The diuretic of choice, in the absence of renal insufficiency, is spironolactone. Doses of up to 400 mg/day may be required. Thiazide diuretics may be added if spironolactone is insufficient to control the ascites. The loop diuretics should be reserved for resistant sodium retention.

Use of diuretics in cirrhotics can be associated with certain complications. Fluid shift from the peritoneal compartment is limited to about 700–900 mL/day. Danger of intravascular volume depletion exists if diuresis is too brisk. The resultant intravascular volume contraction will lead to renal hypoperfusion. If this is persistent, renal failure (hepatorenal syndrome) will occur.

Diuretic-induced hypokalemia and hypochloremic metabolic alkalosis are also undesirable. Systemic alkalosis favors the penetration of the blood–brain barrier by circulating toxic molecules that cause hepatic encephalopathy.

Renal Diseases

In those renal diseases associated with the nephrotic syndrome, peripheral edema may be severe and require diuretic use. Thiazide diuretics are usually quite adequate. As in all other edematous states, excessively brisk diuresis may only lead to acute intravascular volume contraction and, possibly, renal hypoperfusion.

Acute glomerulonephritis, with or without the nephrotic syndrome, is associated with avid renal sodium and water retention. Diuretic resistance is frequently encountered, and loop diuretics may be required to control the acute intravascular volume expansion (manifested as hypertension, plus pulmonary edema if severe) and the peripheral edema.

In progressive chronic renal failure the remaining functional nephrons reabsorb less sodium and water and thus maintain ECF balance. Nevertheless, if the primary renal injury has had associated nephrotic syndrome and/or abnormal renal sodium and water retention, the patients may have an excess of extracellular fluid volume requiring the use of diuretics. Thiazides are effective as long as GFR is above 20–30 mL/min. Below this level, only the more potent loop diuretics are effective.

Other Uses

Hypertension

Diuretic therapy is still one of the cornerstones of current antihypertensive therapy, and it is effective monotherapy in 60% of essential hypertensives (*see also* Chapter 38). In the absence of severe renal insufficiency (*i.e.*, if GFR > 30 mL/min), sulfonamide diuretics are the preferred drugs, being more effective than potassium-sparing diuretics or loop diuretics.

The antihypertensive action of diuretics is multifactorial. If the drugs are given in diuretic quantities (*e.g.*, hydrochlorothiazide or chlorthalidone 50–100 mg), the fall in blood pressure parallels the initial decrease in intravascular fluid volume. With continued use, despite the return of the intravascular volume to normal, blood pressure remains decreased. This sustained decrease has been ascribed to autoregulatory vasodilatation.

Recent studies have demonstrated that the antihypertensive effect of sulfonamide diuretics occurs with much smaller daily doses (*e.g.*, hydrochlorothiazide or chlorthalidone 12.5–25 mg), doses normally not associated with sufficient diuresis to decrease intravascular volume. The antihypertensive action in this circumstance may be through vasodilatation resulting from direct molecular or sodium effects on the vasculature.

In otherwise healthy hypertensive populations, diuretic-induced hypokalemia and serum lipid abnormalities may be detrimental. Serious ventricular arrhythmias have been recorded in prospectively studied hypertensives who became hypokalemic. Both the serum lipid abnormalities and the hypokalemia are dose-dependent. Therefore, smaller doses of sulfonamide diuretics should be used, and the agents chosen should have demonstrated peak antihypertensive effects at doses well below those needed for diuretic effects (*e.g.*, chlorthalidone: maximum antihypertensive dose 25 mg, diuretic dose 50–200 mg).

When diuretics must be used with other antihypertensive agents known to cause fluid retention, then the lower antihypertensive dosages may have to be increased to diuretic dosages.

Calcium Nephrolithiasis

In patients with idiopathic recurrent calcium nephrolithiasis, whether or not associated with abnormally elevated urine calcium (hypercalciuria), thiazide diuretics were demonstrated to be effective in preventing or significantly decreasing the frequency of stone formation. As reviewed earlier, this is due to both direct and reflex enhancement of urinary calcium reabsorption.

When thiazides are used for this purpose, moderate dietary sodium restriction is advised to maximize the hypocalciuric effect. States of hypercalcemia should be ruled out prior to onset of therapy, and serum calcium should be monitored during therapy.

Hyperparathyroidism

High serum calcium levels may be seen with hyperparathyroidism, either primary or secondary to malignancy (as well as with bone metastases). If serum calcium rises to the 15–16 mg/dL (3.75–4.00 mmol/L) range, profound neurologic disturbances and dehydration supervene, requiring emergency therapy. Together with adequate intravenous fluid replacement, loop diuretics are the treatment of choice because of their calciuric effects. Care must be taken to maintain electrolyte balance.

Diabetes Insipidus

Diabetes insipidus is a rare metabolic condition in which there is partial or complete lack of ADH secretion (*see also* Chapter 43). Renal collecting duct insensitivity to ADH is an equally rare condition called nephrogenic diabetes insipidus. In both states the kidneys are unable to reabsorb water from the collecting tubules and ducts. The consequence is the excretion of large volumes (usually > 10 L/day) of dilute urine, which requires replenishment through both oral and intravenous routes.

Sulfonamide diuretics have been used effectively to decrease urine volume in these conditions. When a sulfonamide diuretic is given, natriuresis occurs along with the water diuresis. Subsequent intravascular volume contraction then enhances isotonic proximal and distal tubular sodium chloride reabsorption (*i.e.*, accompanied by water). Less fluid reaches the collecting tubules and ducts, and urine volume decreases.

Special Uses of Carbonic Anhydrase Inhibitors

Carbonic anhydrase inhibitors are rarely used as diuretic agents because of their low efficacy.

They are used as urinary alkalinizing agents when it is desirable to maintain acidic substances in solution (*e.g.*, uric acid, cysteine, hemoglobin, myoglobin).

These diuretics have also been used to treat diuretic-induced metabolic alkalosis, and to enhance urinary excretion in patients with chronic obstructive disease of the airways and CO_2 retention (chronic respiratory acidosis).

Prior to the introduction of beta-blocker therapy for glaucoma, CA inhibitors, which decrease intraocular fluid production, were used regularly for this purpose.

CA inhibitors have been used rarely in the treatment of familial periodic paralysis and as anticonvulsant therapy.

SUGGESTED READING

Ansuini R, Pulito M, Pupita G, *et al*. Clinical pharmacology of loop diuretics: a comparative study. Int J Clin Pharmacol Res 1985; 5:113–121.

Brest AN. Clinical pharmacology of diuretic drugs. Cardiovasc Clin 1984; 14:31–38.

Corvol P, Claire M, Oblin ME, *et al*. Mechanism of antimineralocorticoid effects of spironolactone. Kidney Int 1981; 20:1–6.

Dikshit K, Uyden JK, Forrester JS, *et al*. Renal and extrarenal hemodynamic effects of furosemide in congestive heart failure after acute myocardial infarction. N Engl J Med 1973; 288:1087–1090.

Grimm RH, Leon AS, Hunninghake DB, *et al*. Effects of thiazide diuretics on plasma lipids and lipoproteins in mildly hypertensive patients. Ann Intern Med 1981; 94:7–11.

Murphy MB, Kohner E, Lewis PJ, *et al*. Glucose intolerance in hypertensive patients treated with diuretics: a fourteen-year follow-up. Lancet 1982; 2:1293–1295.

Reineck HJ, Stein JH. Mechanisms of action and clinical uses of diuretics. In: Brenner BM, Rector FC, eds. The kidney. 2nd ed. Philadelphia: WB Saunders, 1981:1097–1131.

Schrier RW, Anderson RJ. Renal sodium excretion, edematous disorders and diuretic use. In: Schrier RW, ed. Renal and electrolyte disorders. 2nd ed. Boston: Little, Brown, 1980:65–114.

Suki WN. Effects of diuretics on calcium metabolism (Editorial). Miner Electrolyte Metab 1979; 2:125–129.

Chapter 41

Drugs Affecting Hemostasis

W.H.E. Roschlau

The process of arresting the loss of blood from injured blood vessels (hemostasis) is of fundamental significance in health and disease. It involves vascular, platelet, and coagulation events, of which the response of blood platelets and the formation of fibrin are the major ones (Fig. 41–1). Usually the first or primary manifestation of hemostasis is the temporary closure of a vascular lesion by a "hemostatic plug" of aggregated platelets. Secondary or permanent hemostasis (referred to as blood coagulation and comprising the plasma phase of hemostasis) consists of the sequential interaction and activation of normally inactive plasma clotting factors that lead to the generation of prothrombin activator, the transformation of prothrombin into thrombin, and the formation of fibrin from fibrinogen. Permanent repair of a vascular lesion is achieved by endothelialization, organization of the platelet–fibrin seal, phagocytosis, and fibrinolysis (Fig. 41–6).

Disturbances of the hemostatic process may result in increased bleeding or increased clotting of blood.

Increased bleeding may be caused by clotting factor deficiencies or blood platelet abnormalities. Examples of inherited disorders are hemophilia A (classical hemophilia, factor VIII deficiency), hemophilia B (Christmas disease, factor IX deficiency), and von Willebrand's disease (factor VIII deficiency coupled with vascular and platelet defects). Acquired disorders of coagulation may be due to lack of vitamin K, or they may be associated with liver disease.

Thrombosis is the term applied to the excessive deposition of blood platelets and fibrin in the vascular system (in arteries, usually on the basis of atherosclerosis; in veins, as a consequence of diminished circulation, stasis, or inflammation). It is the misplaced response of the hemostatic process to hemodynamic alterations or lesions of the vessel walls. Depending on the underlying cause and location, thrombi may be platelet-rich or platelet-poor, multiple or solitary, microscopically small or filling whole vessel segments. (Clotting is the term normally applied to *ex vivo* blood coagulation, but also to *in vivo* conditions of thrombus formation where there is a relative absence of platelets and an abundance of fibrin.)

Embolism occurs when blood clots or thrombi become dislodged from their site of origin and are carried to remote parts of the circulatory system. Arterial emboli will travel towards the periphery, causing vascular occlusions and ischemia of the perfused organ or tissue. Venous emboli invariably reach the lungs *via* the pulmonary arterial circulation, with the predictable consequence of pulmonary embolism.

AGENTS AFFECTING PLATELET FUNCTION

A number of diverse compounds inhibit the aggregation of blood platelets both *in vitro* and *in vivo*, thereby reducing the likelihood of thrombus formation when administered to patients at risk. As shown in Table 41–1, these compounds comprise nonsteroidal anti-inflammatory agents, pyrimido-pyrimidine compounds, and a variety of unrelated agents that were found coincidentally to have effects on blood platelets.

The mechanisms of action vary between these groups of drugs, but they all in some way inhibit the release of platelet ADP following stimulation to aggregate. This "release reaction," shown schematically in Figure 41–2, can be elicited *in vitro* (and presumably also *in vivo*) by collagen, adenosine diphosphate, adrenaline, thrombin, and a variety of other substances. Platelet aggregation follows a set pattern (*see also* Chapter 30). Upon stimulation, platelets undergo membrane changes that lead to the intracellular synthesis of prostaglandin endoperoxides and thromboxane A_2 (from platelet phospholipids by the action of platelet cyclooxygenase). Thromboxane A_2 (TxA_2) is considered to be the specific stimulus for aggregation reactions. Also involved is

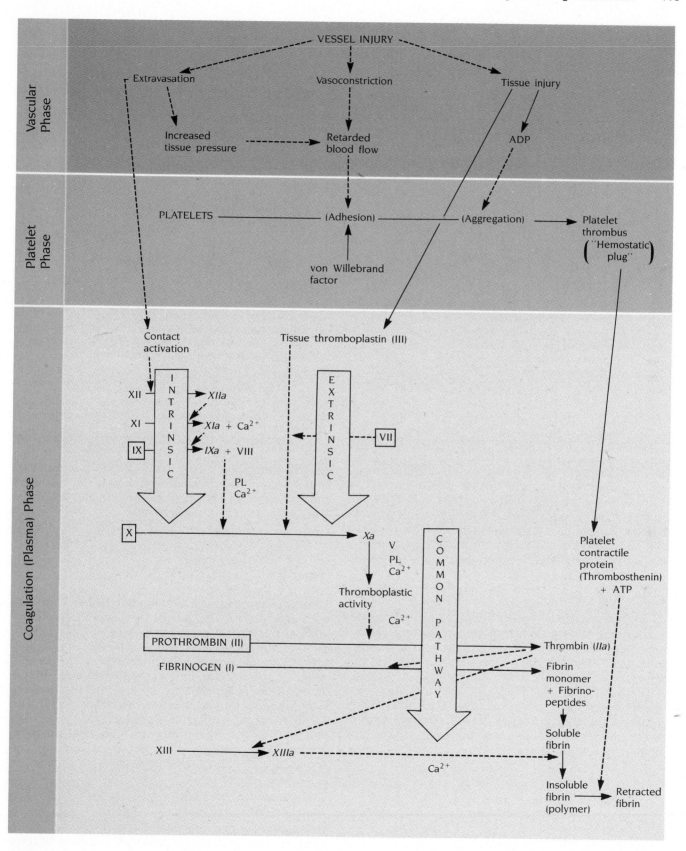

Figure 41-1 The hemostatic process. (Omitted for simplicity is the participation of prekallikrein and high-molecular-weight kininogen in the activation of factor XII.) Roman numerals designate clotting factors in the order of discovery. Italicized (active) clotting factors are subject to inactivation by heparin. Hepatic synthesis of boxed clotting factors is inhibited by coumarins. (PL = phospholipid; a = activated; – – → acts upon; —→ transforms into.)

TABLE 41-1 Inhibitors of Platelet Function

Compound	Mechanism of Action
Nonsteroidal Anti-inflammatory Agents (Acetylsalicylic acid, Indomethacin, Phenylbutazone, Sulfinpyrazone)	Inhibit ADP release reaction by inhibition of platelet cyclooxygenase, thus preventing synthesis of endoperoxides (PGG_2, PGH_2) and thromboxane (TxA_2). Variably inhibit platelet adhesion to collagen and subendothelium.
Pyrimido-pyrimidine Compounds (Dipyridamole)	Inhibit ADP release reaction by inhibition of platelet phosphodiesterase resulting in increased platelet cAMP. Inhibit platelet adhesion to collagen. Prolong platelet survival.
Prostaglandin I_2 (Prostacyclin)	Opposing system to thromboxane A_2. Prevents platelet adhesion to vessel wall components.
Hydroxychloroquine (antimalarial) Clofibrate (hypolipidemic) Propranolol (β-adrenoceptor blocker) Cyproheptadine (antihistamine) Penicillins (antibiotic) Hydrocortisone (steroid)	Various mechanisms proposed, including: inhibition of thromboxane synthesis; prolongation of platelet survival; inhibition of ADP release reaction; nonspecific platelet membrane actions.

a system of regulation of cyclic AMP content of platelets, which is thought to influence the transport of Ca^{2+} into platelets. Cyclic AMP acts to inhibit platelet adhesion, aggregation, and release of ADP.

Inhibition of platelet cyclooxygenase will prevent prostaglandin endoperoxide synthesis; inhibition of platelet phosphodiesterase will maintain high intracellular cAMP. Both mechanisms are recognized to interfere with normal platelet responses and are the basis for clinical use of platelet inhibition by "antithrombotic" drugs (Table 40-1). These are described in detail in Chapter 33.

Since antiaggregating agents are capable of profoundly disturbing the normal hemostatic mechanisms, their use may unmask unrecognized abnormalities in hemostasis resulting from hereditary absence of, or defects in, coagulation factors coexisting with normal bleeding time. Prolonged bleeding and possible spontaneous hemorrhage may result. Also, the combination of antiaggregating agents with anticoagulant drugs causes prolongation of bleeding time with occasional spontaneous hemorrhage.

ANTICOAGULANTS

There are many substances capable of preventing the coagulation of blood. Of clinical usefulness are those anticoagulants that can be administered *in vivo* without undue toxicity. Depending on their mechanism of ac-

tion, they are classified as (1) direct anticoagulants because they act on blood constituents and prevent their normal interaction directly in the streaming blood (*e.g.*, heparin), and (2) indirect anticoagulants because they interfere with the synthesis of clotting factors in the liver (*e.g.*, vitamin K antagonists).

Heparin

Heparin prolongs the clotting time of blood both *in vitro* and *in vivo*. The substance was discovered and originally extracted from dog liver in Howell's laboratory in Baltimore; it was named heparin in 1918. Subsequent development of the drug occurred in Toronto (Best, Charles, Scott) and Stockholm (Jorpes). Procedures for the commercial preparation of heparin were established by Charles and Scott (Toronto, 1933), and the first recorded use of this product was in 1935-36 by the Toronto surgeon Murray, who went on to introduce and evaluate heparin as a systemic anticoagulant of phenomenal versatility.

Origin and Chemistry

Heparin is a macromolecular, polymeric substance found in abundance in liver, lung, and intestinal mucosa. It is commercially extracted from bovine lung tissue and from hog and cattle intestinal mucosa. Heparin belongs to the class of mucopolysaccharides and is the strongest organic acid found in the body. Its chemical struc-

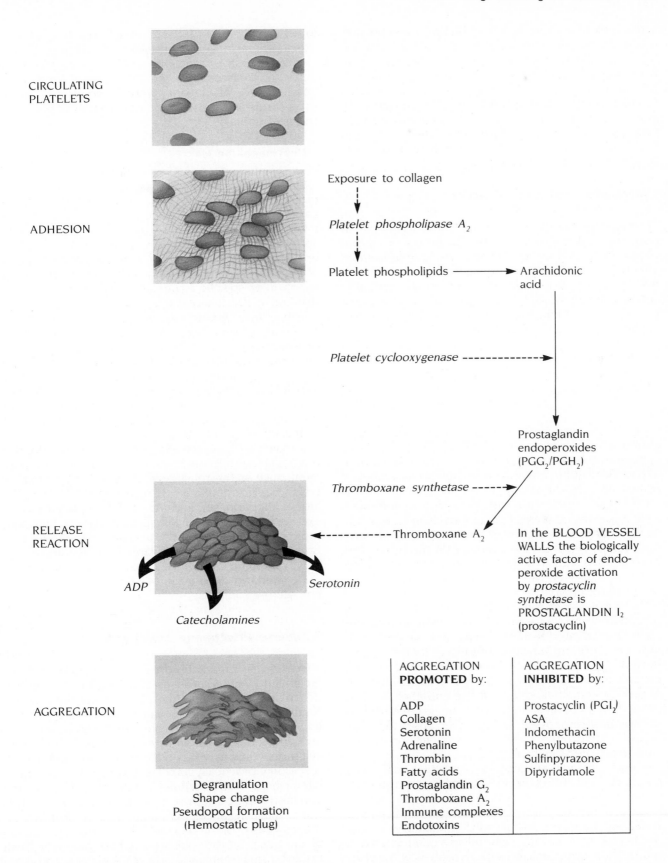

Figure 41–2 Schematic representation of platelet aggregation, the principal biochemical processes, and the agents at present known to promote or inhibit aggregation (*see also* Chapter 30). $--\rightarrow$ activates or acts upon; $\longrightarrow$ transforms into.

The following labels appear within the figure:

CIRCULATING PLATELETS

ADHESION

Exposure to collagen

Platelet phospholipase A₂

Platelet phospholipids → Arachidonic acid

Platelet cyclooxygenase ----→

Prostaglandin endoperoxides (PGG₂/PGH₂)

Thromboxane synthetase ----→

RELEASE REACTION

Thromboxane A₂

ADP

Serotonin

Catecholamines

In the BLOOD VESSEL WALLS the biologically active factor of endo-peroxide activation by *prostacyclin synthetase* is PROSTAGLANDIN I₂ (prostacyclin)

AGGREGATION

Degranulation
Shape change
Pseudopod formation
(Hemostatic plug)

AGGREGATION **PROMOTED** by:

ADP
Collagen
Serotonin
Adrenaline
Thrombin
Fatty acids
Prostaglandin G₂
Thromboxane A₂
Immune complexes
Endotoxins

AGGREGATION **INHIBITED** by:

Prostacyclin (PGI₂)
ASA
Indomethacin
Phenylbutazone
Sulfinpyrazone
Dipyridamole

RESPIRATORY RENAL BLOOD

ture is difficult to express, being a bundle of components of different chain length and molecular weight (average MW 15,000; low-molecular-weight heparins have been prepared experimentally and are being investigated for use as anticoagulants). The three principal monosaccharide building blocks are D-glucosamine, D-glucuronic acid, and L-iduronic acid, in addition to sulfuric acid. The drug is standardized in international and U.S.P. units, one unit having the activity of 0.01 mg of a sodium salt standard.

Mechanism and Sites of Action

Heparin interferes with clotting factor activations in both the intrinsic and extrinsic pathways of thromboplastin generation, and it has a strong antithrombin effect. The principal anticoagulant actions are due to the activation and acceleration of a plasma α_2-globulin, antithrombin III, which acts as heparin cofactor and protease (thrombin) inhibitor. The specific sites of action in the coagulation sequence are:

1. inactivation of factors IIa, IXa, Xa, XIa, XIIa, and XIIIa;
2. complexing of thrombin (factor IIa);
3. neutralization of tissue thromboplastin (factor III).

All of these anticoagulant effects of heparin take place exclusively in the streaming blood (and therefore also in isolated blood samples *in vitro*), which distinguishes heparin from other anticoagulants that act as inhibitors of clotting factor synthesis in the liver.

(At present under investigation are low-molecular-weight substances, oligosaccharide chains extracted from heparin, that bind more selectively to antithrombin III and accelerate the inhibition of thrombin. This property was shown to enhance the antithrombotic effects of smaller doses with less disturbance of other coagulation factors.)

There is evidence that heparin is taken up by vascular endothelium, where it reaches concentrations about 1000 times greater than those in plasma; the endothelium may therefore be considered the "target organ." Because of the strong electronegative charge of the heparin molecule, it serves to enhance or restore the negative electrostatic charge on the endothelium. This property of heparin is cited to explain its effectiveness in thrombosis prophylaxis when used in doses too small to cause detectable systemic anticoagulation during "low-dose" heparin therapy.

In addition to its anticoagulant activity, heparin has poorly defined effects on blood platelets, both stimulation and inhibition of aggregation having been reported. Heparin doses too small to cause anticoagulation have a clearing effect on postprandial (alimentary) hyperlipemia through activation and release of a lipoprotein lipase. This enzyme enhances the hydrolysis of triglycerides of chylomicrons and very-low-density lipoproteins, resulting in their rapid disappearance from the plasma into tissues (*see also* Chapter 37). Heparin also inter-

feres with numerous types of specific reactions and exerts a general influence on cellular permeability, allergic and inflammatory reactions, and on tissue growth. It must be stressed, however, that none of these additional actions of the drug were found to be adverse to its use as an anticoagulant, nor are they of particular therapeutic value.

Pharmacokinetics

Since heparin is very strongly ionized, and because of its molecular size, it is not readily absorbed by the gastrointestinal mucosa. Also, it is destroyed in the gastrointestinal tract and must therefore be given as an aqueous solution by intravenous injection or infusion, or by subcutaneous injection. Anticoagulant effects are obtained within minutes of a single intravenous application. (For specific routes and dosage regimens see the end of the chapter.)

In humans, heparin has an approximate half-life of 1.5 hours, which is inversely dose-dependent (*i.e.*, the rate of disappearance decreases with increasing dose). The drug is bound extensively to globulins and fibrinogen. It is therefore confined to the plasma volume. Due to this binding to inert carriers, but also to specific substrates, there is no correlation between the half-life determined by bioassay and the half-life of the anticoagulant effect of the drug.

A major pathway of elimination from the blood is the transfer of heparin to some extravascular compartment, such as the reticuloendothelial system. Heparin is also transformed to a varying extent by the liver (sulfatases, heparinase), and a partially degraded form is excreted in the urine. The large molecular size precludes rapid renal excretion of the unchanged form in significant amounts; after very large intravenous doses, however, some unchanged heparin may appear in the urine. Heparin does not cross the placenta, and it is not secreted in milk.

Adverse Effects and Toxicity

Heparin is remarkably free of undesirable side effects, and even large doses over long periods of time do not normally cause difficulties unless the blood is rendered temporarily incoagulable. A rare type of hypersensitivity has been observed, particularly with impure preparations, and prolonged use may in rare instances result in reversible osteoporosis or alopecia.

The only practically important danger lies in serious hemorrhage from **overdose**. If hemorrhage occurs, the administration of heparin must be discontinued. This will in most instances be sufficient to control hemorrhage because of the relatively short duration of action of the drug. Infusions of fresh whole blood or fresh frozen plasma (containing most of the elements required for coagulation) may sometimes be indicated to hasten restoration of coagulability.

The specific **antidote** for heparin is **protamine sul-**

fate. This strongly basic substance is used to neutralize excess heparin by formation of an inactive complex; this is its only use as a drug in medicine. Note, however, that protamine must be given with caution, since it is an anticoagulant in its own right.

Vitamin K Antagonists (Coumarin Compounds)

In the 1920s Schofield (Guelph) described a bleeding disease in cattle that were fed spoiled sweet clover silage (''sweet clover disease''). The hemorrhagic agent responsible for this condition was identified by Campbell and Link in 1939 as bishydroxycoumarin (dicumarol). Further developments yielded many congeners, such as warfarin sodium. All coumarin compounds are similar in structure and properties, but **racemic warfarin** has become the most widely used of the group following its initial marketing as a rodent poison.

Mechanism and Site of Action

The anticoagulant effect of all coumarin compounds depends on the depression of the vitamin K-dependent synthesis of clotting factors in the liver, thereby reducing their availability in the plasma. These are factors II (prothrombin), VII, IX, and X. Owing to a certain structural resemblance of coumarin compounds and vitamin K (Fig. 41–3), the drugs act as vitamin K antagonists or antimetabolites.

The only physiologic role of vitamin K is to promote the synthesis of these clotting factors (*see* Chapter 49), most likely by acting as an essential cofactor for microsomal enzyme systems that activate precursors by conversion of peptide-bound glutamic acid to γ-carboxyglutamic acid. This newly formed amino acid enables the protein to bind Ca^{2+} and to interact with phospholipids.

Warfarin and other coumarin-type anticoagulants interfere with the ability of the vitamin to catalyse the carboxylation and subsequent activation of clotting factor precursors. Thus, the administration of these drugs causes the appearance of biologically inactive precursors of the clotting factors in liver and plasma. The inactivity of the precursors is primarily due to an inability to bind Ca^{2+}, which prevents interaction with phospholipid-containing membranes, an important step in the activation of these clotting factors during coagulation.

Because the inhibition of vitamin K-dependent synthesis of clotting factors is competitive, vitamin K administration will result in displacement of coumarin compounds and resumption of normal clotting factor production. Vitamin K therefore is a specific antagonist used to reverse coumarin anticoagulant effects.

Pharmacokinetics

Coumarin compounds show varying rates of absorption from the gastrointestinal tract, that of bishydroxycoumarin being slow and erratic, while warfarin is rapidly and completely absorbed (Table 41–2). This absorption is a very important and clinically significant property, allowing oral administration of these drugs in routine anticoagulant therapy. (The drugs are therefore also referred to as oral anticoagulants.) Depending on the individual drugs, peak plasma levels are usually reached within 2–12 hours, the exact concentration varying from person to person. Peak anticoagulant effects (as measured with the prothrombin time), however, will not become apparent until about 24 hours after peak plasma levels were attained. This is because the inhibition of clotting factor synthesis is an indirect mechanism that requires time to be translated into a reduction of clotting factor activity in the circulating plasma. **Clinically significant anticoagulant effects can not be expected for about 30–60 hours**, depending on the dosage regimen (Fig. 41–4). Similarly, on cessation of treatment, it takes 2–5 days before normal clotting activity is restored.

Within the circulation, the drugs are almost entirely bound to plasma albumin so that exceedingly small amounts of free drug are present after therapeutic doses (Table 41–2). Of racemic warfarin, the most extensively investigated member of this group of drugs, the dextrorotatory form is converted to a secondary alcohol and the levorotatory form to 7-hydroxywarfarin. These inactive metabolites undergo some enterohepatic circulation and are excreted in the urine and stool.

Factors Affecting Activity; Drug Interactions

There are many factors that can affect the activity of these drugs (Fig. 41–5), and many drugs, when given concurrently, alter coumarin anticoagulant effects. This is of great clinical importance, since it involves a class of drugs with a narrow margin of safety and complex pharmacokinetic properties. Drug interactions can thus lead to serious hemorrhagic complications, or they may be the cause of therapeutic failure.

Pathophysiologic conditions that increase the anticoagulant response because of induced vitamin K deficiency are inadequate diet, intestinal disease, and inadequate bile flow. Hepatic disease may predispose to defective clotting factor synthesis. (Chronic alcoholics may experience bleeding episodes not from the metabolic effects of alcohol but from behavioral unreliability and noncompliance. On the other hand, induction of smooth endoplasmic reticulum in the livers of alcoholics can increase the rate of warfarin biotransformation, and thus reduce the anticoagulant effect.)

TABLE 41-2 Pharmacokinetics of Coumarins in Humans

Compound	Gastrointestinal Absorption	Plasma Protein Binding (%)	Plasma t½ (hrs)	Usual Daily Dose (mg)	Time to Peak Anticoagulant Effect* (hrs)	Duration of Effect After Stopping Drug (days)
Acenocoumarol	rapid, complete	?	~20	2–10	36–48	1½–2
Bishydroxycoumarin	slow, variable	99	10–30†	25–150	36–48	5–6
Phenprocoumon	complete	99	~160	1–4	48–72	7–14
Warfarin Na	rapid, complete	99.3	~45	2–15	36–72	4–5

* As measured with the prothrombin time.
† Plasma t½ increases with plasma concentration.

A **decrease in anticoagulant response** may be seen during pregnancy because of increased clotting factor activity in the mother (the fetus, however, remains highly susceptible to the drugs).

Some **drugs that enhance the response** to oral anticoagulants are acetylsalicylic acid and other compounds with platelet-inhibitory activity, as well as clofibrate (they cause an additive hemostatic defect by inhibiting platelet adhesion and aggregation); phenylbutazone has the added effect of inhibiting warfarin biotransformation, and to some extent also displacing warfarin from its albumin binding sites, and thus may cause severe hemorrhage during anticoagulant therapy. Disulfiram and trimethoprim-sulfonamide preparations inhibit the conversion and prolong the half-life of warfarin. Other drugs that prolong the prothrombin time by a variety of mechanisms are cimetidine, sulfinpyrazone, D-thyroxine, and anabolic steroids.

Drugs that diminish the response to oral anticoagulants by induction of hepatic microsomal enzymes are barbiturates and glutethimide. Their coadministration with anticoagulants requires significantly higher doses of the latter for therapeutic anticoagulation, predisposing these patients to serious hemorrhagic complications whenever the interacting drug dosage is changed without simultaneous adjustment of the anticoagulant as well. Rifampin reduces blood levels of oral anticoagulants. Cholestyramine increases the elimination of anticoagulants in the stool. Any drug or substance that interferes with the absorption of anticoagulants will also delay the attainment of therapeutic plasma levels or diminish the effects. (*See* Chapter 11 for further examples of drug interactions.)

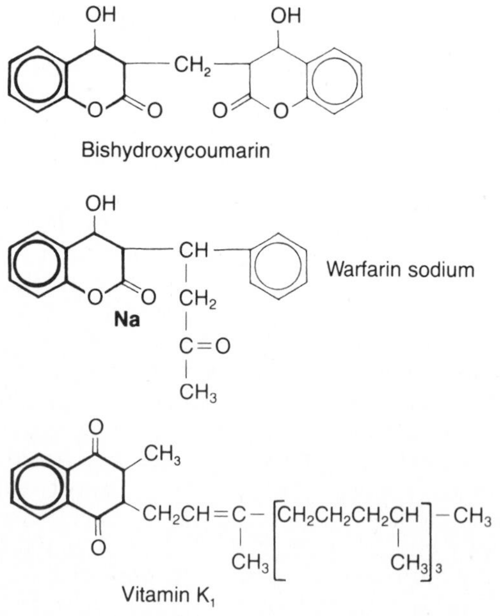

Adverse Effects, Contraindications, and Toxicity

Obvious contraindications for oral anticoagulant therapy are hemorrhagic diathesis, cerebrovascular hemorrhage, ulceration or bleeding from the gastrointestinal, genitourinary or respiratory tract, surgery on the central nervous system, and pregnancy. Bishydroxycoumarin and warfarin pass the placental barrier, leading on occasion to severe hypoprothrombinemia with cerebral injury in the newborn. These drugs are also secreted in the milk.

The most important complication of oral anticoagulant therapy is **hemorrhage**. Since **vitamin K** begins to reverse excessive coumarin activity within a few hours, with full correction of the coagulation defect within 24 hours, it is regarded as the **specific antidote**. Modest doses (5–10 mg vitamin K_1, also known as phytomenadione, phytonadione) are preferred because of long-lasting coumarin resistance after high doses of the vitamin. Plasma transfusions facilitate the reversal of excessive anticoagulation.

Figure 41-3 Coumarins and vitamin K_1.

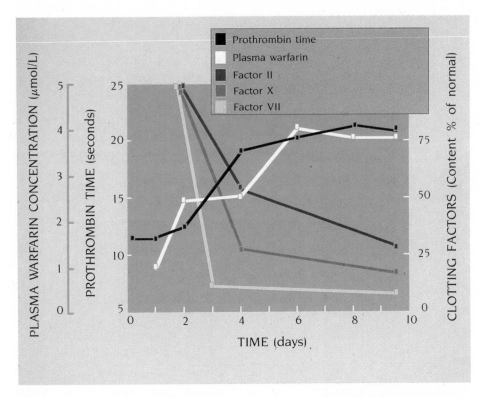

Figure 41–4 Schematic representation of the relationships between the administration of daily small doses of warfarin, fall in plasma clotting factor content, and prothrombin time response. Clotting factor t½: factor II = 60 hours, factor X = 40 hours, factor VII = 6 hours. Note the disappearance of clotting factors from the plasma in relation to their half-lives. Also note the initial lag between the measured plasma warfarin levels and prothrombin times, showing that the latter is a more meaningful indicator of the degree of induced clotting factor inhibition and coagulation impairment. Note also that a steady state is eventually obtained.

In Vitro Anticoagulants

Calcium ions (factor IV) are ubiquitous participants in almost all stages of the hemostatic process. They are required for the generation of prothrombin activator (thromboplastin) and in the conversion of prothrombin to thrombin. Removal of Ca^{2+}, therefore, will prevent coagulation of blood or plasma *in vitro* without interference with, or destruction of, the potential activities of other coagulation factors.

Calcium-removing agents such as sodium citrate, sodium oxalate, sodium fluoride, chelating agents, and ion-exchange resins are therefore used extensively for anticoagulation of transfusion blood, in the preparation of blood plasma, and in the performance of hematologic tests. Addition of molar equivalents of calcium (usually in the form of calcium chloride) to blood or plasma anticoagulated with these substances will restore the ability to clot, thereby providing, *in vitro*, some measure of control in the investigation of normally spontaneous and uncontrollable coagulation processes. (Con-

served anticoagulated transfusion blood will reacquire its coagulation characteristics when mixed with the calcium in the recipient's blood.)

FIBRINOLYTIC AGENTS

The removal of blood clots in the organism is normally accomplished by the physiologic process of fibrinolysis. This fibrinolysis is controlled *in vivo* by enzymatic processes involving the conversion of an enzyme precursor, **plasminogen**, into the proteolytic enzyme **plasmin**, a reaction that is mediated through activators or **kinases** (Fig. 41–6). Plasminogen activator is found in plasma as plasma activator, in urine as urokinase, in various tissues (including blood vessels) as tissue activator, and in body secretions. Therapeutic fibrinolysis (*i.e.*, thrombolysis, the dissolution of

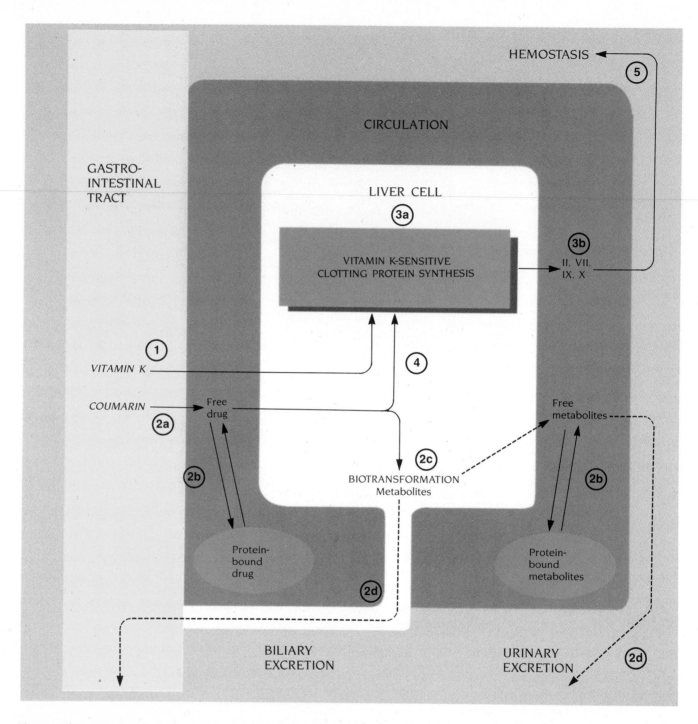

Figure 41–5   Sites at which drugs may modify the anticoagulant action of coumarins. (1) Vitamin K bioavailability; (2a) coumarin absorption; (2b) coumarin binding to albumin; (2c) coumarin biotransformation; (2d) coumarin excretion; (3a) prothrombin complex synthesis; (3b) prothrombin complex catabolism; (4) receptor affinity for coumarins; (5) hemostasis. (Modified from Koch-Weser J, Sellers EM, 1971.)

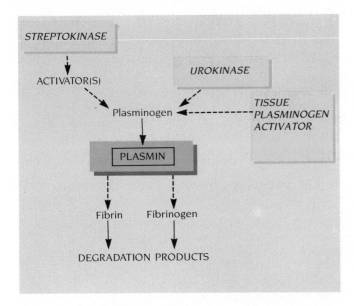

Figure 41-6 Fibrinolysis and sites of action of fibrinolytic agents. − − → activates or acts upon; ⟶ is transformed into.

blood clots) can be achieved by administration of activators of plasminogen, or with proteolytic enzymes. Because therapeutic fibrinolysis is complex and not without dangers to the patient, its use is at present reserved for limited indications in specialized treatment centres.

Streptokinase

This is a plasminogen activator derived from hemolytic streptococci. It has the longest history of clinical use, and the important concepts of thrombolytic therapy, indications, contraindications, and technique have been established with this agent in international collaborative trials. Streptokinase is antigenic because of its bacterial origin, with fever and allergic reactions being known risks and complications during therapy. Naturally occurring antistreptococcal antibodies cross-react with streptokinase and reduce its activity. Following its systemic administration, patients experience periods of increased hemorrhagic risk from generalized lysis of fibrin and fibrinogen.

Urokinase

This enzyme is derived from human urine, where it occurs in relative abundance, or from cultures of human kidney cells, or most recently by employing recombinant DNA technology (''genetic engineering'') in bacteria. It is used similarly to streptokinase to activate the patient's own plasminogen. The activator is nonantigenic, highly specific, but quite costly to

manufacture. It is recognized as a clinically acceptable and promising agent for systemic clinical thrombolytic therapy in the long term.

Tissue-Type Plasminogen Activator

This agent of human origin is manufactured by means of recombinant DNA technology. It has undergone extensive multi-centre trials and promotion as specific therapy for fresh thrombotic coronary artery occlusions. Tissue plasminogen activator is claimed to act preferentially on fibrin-bound plasminogen, with less systemic activity than streptokinase and urokinase on circulating fibrinogen. The drug is extremely expensive, and this fact, together with its currently narrow indication, might limit its use.

Plasmin

Plasmin is the naturally occurring species-specific fibrinolytic enzyme of mammals; it is prepared by *in vitro* activation of human plasminogen with streptokinase. It is inactivated by naturally occurring antiplasmins in plasma and serum, and it is unstable in solution. Its use in therapy, therefore, is limited.

THERAPEUTIC APPLICATIONS OF ANTITHROMBOTICS AND ANTICOAGULANTS

Abnormal tendencies of premature clotting and thrombus formation may be influenced therapeutically at various stages of the hemostatic process.

Antiaggregating Agents

Typically, arterial thrombi consist predominantly of platelet aggregates, platelets tend to be primarily responsible for thrombotic occlusions of cerebral vessels, and thromboembolic disorders in vessel grafts and heart-valve prostheses are usually caused by platelet deposits. It is therefore quite rational that antiaggregating agents are used with increasing frequency and extent in the prevention and treatment of arterial thrombosis and related cardiovascular and cerebrovascular disorders in which platelets play a predominant causative role. This therapeutic approach is relatively new, but several randomized trials have shown the usefulness of pharmacologic suppression of platelet activity to prevent strokes, transient ischemic attacks, and recurrent myocardial infarction. The drugs most extensively

TABLE 41–3 Characteristics of the Main Classes of Antithrombotic Drugs

Characteristic	Heparin	Coumarins	Platelet Inhibitors
Source	Natural	Synthetic	Synthetic
Principal Use	Short-term, intensive, controlled anticoagulation.	Long-term, sustained, controlled anticoagulation (thrombosis prophylaxis).	Long-term inhibition of platelet function (thrombosis prophylaxis).
Site of Action	Circulating blood (*in vivo* and *in vitro*)	Liver (*in vivo* only)	Circulating blood (*in vivo* and *in vitro*)
Mechanism of Action	Activates plasma antithrombin III. Inactivates factors IIa, IXa, Xa, XIa, XIIa, XIIIa. Complexes thrombin. Neutralizes tissue thromboplastin. Enhances negative charge on endothelium.	Inhibit hepatic synthesis of factor II factor VII factor IX factor X (all vitamin K-dependent).	Inhibit platelet cyclooxygenase and synthesis of TxA_2, causing failure to aggregate. Inhibit platelet phosphodiesterase, elevating platelet cAMP, causing failure to aggregate.
Tests for Evaluating the Degree of Clinical Effect	*In vitro*: Activated partial thromboplastin time; whole-blood clotting time.	*In vitro*: Prothrombin time.	*In vitro*: Platelet aggregation. *In vivo*: Bleeding time.
Route of Administration	Parenteral	Oral	Oral
Onset of Action	Immediate (10–20 minutes)	Delayed (after 12–24 hours)	Rapid (1–4 hours)
Duration of Action	2–4 hours i.v. 8–12 hours s.c.	2–5 days	5–7 days
Antidotes	Protamine sulfate (rapidly acting)	Vitamin K_1 (slowly acting)	No specific antidotes (fresh plasma)

investigated are **acetylsalicylic acid** (ASA, in low doses of 150–300 mg/day, or in high doses of 1 g/day or even higher, depending on conditions), **sulfinpyrazone** (800 mg/day), and **dipyridamole** (200–400 mg/day). Therapeutic inhibition of platelet aggregation can be estimated by measuring drug-induced prolongations of the **bleeding time**.

Heparin

The almost instantaneous and predictable anticoagulant effects of heparin through its direct interference with circulating procoagulants, as well as its relatively short duration of action and consequent safety, have made it the most attractive and useful agent in the prevention and treatment of the majority of thromboembolic disorders. The drug is particularly useful in short-term prophylaxis of thrombosis and in the acute treatment of a variety of life-threatening conditions of thromboembolic origin. (While the drug does not dis-

solve existing thrombi, it prevents the extension of thrombotic vascular obstructions and aids in the maintenance of blood circulation.)

In order to obtain therapeutic anticoagulation, the drug is preferably introduced directly into the blood stream, and the dose is titrated by repeated measurements of anticoagulant effects. The methods of measurement are the **activated partial thromboplastin time** or, now rarely, the **whole-blood clotting time**. The therapeutic objective is a prolongation of clotting times to approximately 2–3 times normal (pretreatment) values.

Several treatment schemes are used; typical examples and doses are:

- Intravenous injection—10,000-unit bolus, 5000–10,000 units q6h.
- Intravenous infusion—5000-10,000 units loading dose, 1000 units/hour (20,000 units/day) infusion rate.
- Subcutaneous injection (''low-dose heparin'')—5000 units q12h.

Intramuscular injections are painful, are frequently associated with hematoma formation, and should not be used.

Oral Anticoagulants

These agents are used primarily in the long-term (often life-long) prophylaxis of thrombosis in individuals at risk, and to prevent the recurrence of thrombophlebitis, venous thrombosis, or pulmonary embolism in patients with a respective history of thromboembolic disease. Because of the chronic nature of therapy, absolute compliance must be assured, and patients are usually thoroughly instructed in the type and use of their medication for reasons of safety and efficacy of anticoagulation.

The objective of oral anticoagulation is to obtain **maximal interference with coagulation with minimal hemostatic risk for long periods of time**. Dosages vary amongst individual drugs (Table 41–2). Therapy with warfarin, which is the drug of choice over all other coumarin-type agents, is usually initiated by administration of small doses and not a large loading dose. In this way the gradual development of hypoprothrombinemia may be observed, maintenance doses may be titrated, and the accidental occurrence of hemorrhage can be prevented (Fig. 41–4).

The commonly used method of control of therapy is the one-stage **prothrombin time** (Quick time) or variations thereof. It is essential that measurements be performed daily until a steady-state anticoagulation has been achieved and the patient has stabilized. Periodic measurements must then be performed for the duration of anticoagulant therapy. Results are expressed as a prolongation of the prothrombin time (normal =

approximately 12 seconds; therapeutic anticoagulation = approximately 25 seconds, or 1.5–2 times the control value).

SUGGESTED READING

Borden CW. The current status of therapy with anticoagulants. Med Clin North Am 1972;59:235–253.

deProst D. Heparin fractions and analogues: a new therapeutic possibility for thrombosis. TIPS 1986;4(12):496–500.

Genton E, Gent M, Hirsh J, Harker LA. Platelet inhibiting drugs in the prevention of clinical thrombotic disease. N Engl J Med 1975; 293:1174–1178(I); 1236–1240(II); 1296–1300 (III).

Jaques LB. The new understanding of the drug heparin. Chest 1985; 88:751–754.

Koch-Weser J, Sellers EM. Drug interactions with coumarin anticoagulants. N Engl J Med 1971; 285:487–494(I); 547–558(II).

Levine MN, Raskob G, Hirsh J. Risk of haemorrhage associated with long term anticoagulant therapy. Drugs 1985; 30:444–460.

Markwardt F, ed. Fibrinolytics and antifibrinolytics. Handbook of Experimental Pharmacology, Vol 46. Berlin/Heidelberg/New York: Springer-Verlag, 1978.

Ogston D. The physiology of hemostasis. Cambridge: Harvard University Press, 1983.

Packham MA, Mustard JF. Clinical pharmacology of platelets. Blood 1977; 50:555–573.

Roschlau WHE. Fungal proteases. In: Markwardt F, ed. Fibrinolytics and antifibrinolytics. Handbook of Experimental Pharmacology, Vol 46. Berlin/Heidelberg/New York: Springer-Verlag, 1978:337–450.

Symposium on Heparin. Meeting of the International Committee on Thrombosis and Haemostasis. Thrombos Diathes Haemorrh 1975; 33:17–123.

Weiss HJ. Platelet physiology and abnormalities of platelet function. N Engl J Med 1975; 293:531–541(I); 580–588(II).

RESPIRATORY RENAL BLOOD

Chapter 42

HEMATINIC DRUGS

W.H.E. Roschlau

"Anemia" is the term applied to conditions that manifest themselves in deficient numbers of circulating red blood cells or in abnormally low total hemoglobin content per unit of blood volume. Table 42–1 provides a classification of anemias; it indicates that the variety in etiology may require combinations of symptomatic and specific therapy for rational treatment and that lasting therapeutic benefits can usually not be expected unless the causative factors are identified and corrected.

A large number of drugs affect the blood and the blood-forming organs, either directly or indirectly, and many drugs exert known toxic effects on blood cells, hemoglobin, and hematopoietic organs. These are mentioned in the respective chapters in which these drugs are described. It is axiomatic that a drug with known hematotoxicity should not be administered unless the risks are recognized and weighed against the benefits, and proper hematologic surveillance is carried out.

NUTRITIONAL ANEMIAS

Many dietary factors are important for normal hematopoiesis, and a chronic lack or deficiency of one or more of these might eventually be reflected in deficient erythropoiesis and anemia. These "nutritional anemias" (*see* Table 42–1) form the largest group of treatable disorders and are most responsive to specific drug therapy.

Any nutrient deficiency arises from one or more of five basic causes: inadequate ingestion, absorption or utilization, or increased excretion or requirement. Nutritional anemias are all treatable by providing the deficient nutrient in appropriate form and dosage as a "drug." In addition, the therapeutic goal is to determine and, if possible, eliminate the cause of the deficiency.

Iron Deficiency

In states of constant blood volume and red blood cell values the amount of iron required daily depends on the average life span of erythrocytes and the total quantity of circulating hemoglobin. Iron balance is achieved by conservation of iron in the body. It is recycled from broken-down red blood cells into the bone marrow for hemoglobin production.

About 0.8% of circulating red blood cells are broken down daily. The quantity of hemoglobin thus removed and replaced daily is approximately 7.65 g, corresponding to 26 mg of iron. Total iron loss per day (intestine, urine, sweat) is probably not more than 1 mg, which is easily replaced from dietary sources (variously estimated at about 1.5–2 mg/day).

However, iron requirements are greatly increased during growth, menstruation, pregnancy, blood donations, and pathologic bleeding, *i.e.*, during periods of increased hematopoietic demands. Active growth and menstruation call for additional iron in excess of 1 mg/day. During pregnancy up to 6 mg may be required daily (Table 42–2), which cannot be met by diet alone.

Thus, iron deficiency anemia is essentially a symptom of negative iron balance rather than a primary disease. It begins with the gradual depletion of iron stores and leads, when untreated, to the development of **hypochromic microcytic anemia** (low plasma iron level, elevated plasma iron-binding capacity) (Fig. 42–1 and Table 42–3). The only effective therapy is supplementation of iron intake to correct the deficiency.

Iron Kinetics

Absorption of elemental iron and inorganic iron salts, whether dietary or medicinal, occurs from the gastrointestinal tract beyond the stomach. Iron must be ionized

TABLE 42–1 Etiologic Classification of Anemias

Excessive loss of blood
  Acute or chronic posthemorrhagic anemia

Deficient red blood cell production
  Deficient hemoglobin or DNA synthesis
    Iron deficiency ⎫
    Vitamin B$_{12}$ deficiency ⎬ So-called
    Folic acid deficiency ⎪ nutritional
    Other nutritional deficiencies ⎭ anemias
    Thalassemia
  Bone marrow abnormalities
    Hypoplastic and aplastic anemias
    Endocrine disorders
    Chronic renal failure
    Sideroblastic anemia

Excessive red blood cell destruction
  Due to intrinsic erythrocyte defects
    Hereditary enzyme deficiencies and/or
      membrane defects
    Hemoglobinopathies (*e.g.*, sickle-cell
      anemia)
  Due to extra-erythrocytic factors
    Reactions to incompatible blood, to
      chemicals and drugs, to infectious
      agents, to physical agents, antibody-
      mediated, hypersplenism, etc.

Note: Only the so-called nutritional anemias are discussed in this chapter.

and divalent (ferrous, Fe^{2+}) for easiest absorption. (Conversion of trivalent, *i.e.*, ferric, iron occurs readily in the gastrointestinal tract through gastric acid, ascorbic acid in food, and –SH or other reducing groups.) Iron may pass directly into and through the mucosal cells of the duodenum and upper small intestine into the blood stream, where it is attached to transferrin (a β_1-globulin binding two atoms of iron per molecule) for transport from sites of absorption or storage to sites of utilization, or it may be bound to and stored as ferritin in the intestinal mucosal cells for elimination by exfoliation. During situations of high iron demand, when iron stores become depleted, the absorption of iron is increased. Conversely, during iron overload, the absorption of iron can be blocked by increased ferritin storage in mucosal cells. Iron absorption is controlled by a combination of factors, such as serum iron levels, the amount of ferritin in duodenal mucosal cells, the degree of transferrin saturation, the state of iron stores, and the rate of erythropoiesis.

Iron turnover in the normal adult with about 4–5 g total body iron is approximately 35 mg/day. Of this, most enters the bone marrow for use in erythropoiesis, and about 1 mg goes into storage, extracellular fluid, and excretion. Iron entering the plasma under conditions of normal balance is that salvaged from aged red blood cells, return from storage, extracellular fluid, and intestinal absorption. Iron storage sites are the marrow, spleen, liver, and other reticuloendothelial structures, where iron is present as ferritin and hemosiderin. Excretion is by desquamation of iron-containing cells from bowel, skin, and genitourinary tract, and in bile, urine, and sweat. The normal loss is probably not more than 1 mg/day, but double that during menstruation. Iron provided to the fetus and placenta during pregnancy, together with losses during delivery and lactation, result in a net deficit of 200–500 mg for each pregnancy.

Pharmacologic Effects of Iron

Medicinal iron enters the total body pool and, in situations where there is an insufficient amount of the metal in the body to supply the demand for optimal hemoglobin production, it increases the rate of red cell production. The correction of hemoglobin iron deficiency is accomplished with ease and efficiency by administering the greatest amount that can be utilized. This amount is usually determined by the ability of the patient to tolerate the medication and by the absorptive capacity of the small intestine (which, as stated above, is controlled and regulated by various feedback mechanisms). The commonly accepted ceiling for iron absorption in a moderately severe anemia is about

TABLE 42–2 Estimated Iron Requirements to Balance Iron Losses

	Estimated Losses (mg/day)				Amount That Must be Absorbed to Maintain Optimal Hemoglobin Synthesis (mg/day)
	Normal Excretion	Menses	Pregnancy	Growth	
Men and postmenopausal women	1.0				1.0
Menstruating women	1.0	1.0			2.0
Pregnant women	1.0		3.0–5.0*		4.0–6.0
Children (average)	0.5			0.5	1.0
Girls (adolescent)	0.5	0.5		0.5	1.5

* Demand increases throughout pregnancy and fetal development.

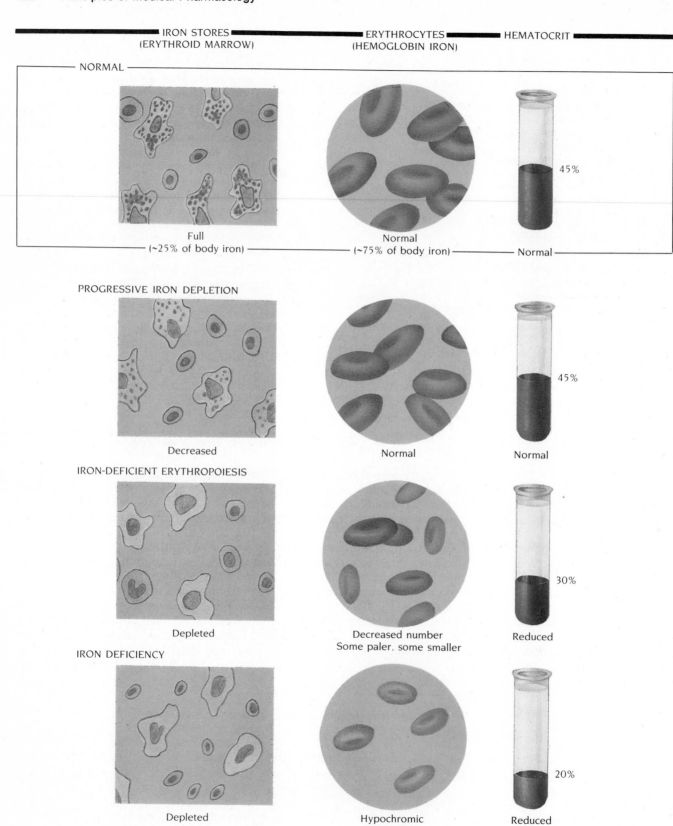

IRON STORES (ERYTHROID MARROW)   ERYTHROCYTES (HEMOGLOBIN IRON)   HEMATOCRIT

NORMAL

Full
(~25% of body iron)

Normal
(~75% of body iron)

45%

Normal

PROGRESSIVE IRON DEPLETION

Decreased

Normal

45%

Normal

IRON-DEFICIENT ERYTHROPOIESIS

Depleted

Decreased number
Some paler, some smaller

30%

Reduced

IRON DEFICIENCY

Depleted

Hypochromic
Microcytic

20%

Reduced

Figure 42–1   Development of iron deficiency anemia. Diagnosis of the anemia will become possible only after tissue iron stores are depleted, indicating that iron therapy is required beyond the time of symptomatic and hematologic improvement in order to replenish iron stores.

TABLE 42-3 Main Features of Nutritional Deficiency Anemias

Iron Deficiency Anemia (Hypochromic/Microcytic Anemia)		

Iron Requirements
 Greatest during growth, menstruation, pregnancy, blood donations, pathologic bleeding (likely
  conditions for iron supplementation).

Development of Anemia
 Decreased, and then depleted, tissue iron stores.
 Decreased hematocrit values (= fewer red blood cells; some paler, some smaller than normal).
 Decreased hemoglobin values (= hypochromic, microcytic RBCs).

Therapy
 Correction of iron deficiency:
  To restore hemoglobin synthesis and red blood cell production.
  To replenish depleted tissue iron stores.

Oral
 200–300 mg elemental iron per day for weeks or months.

Parenteral
 150 mg iron for each gram of hemoglobin deficit, plus 600 mg to replenish tissue stores, given
  over 1–3 weeks.

Megaloblastic/Macrocytic Anemia		
	Vitamin B$_{12}$	*Folic Acid*
Required for	Hematopoiesis; production of epithelial cells; and maintenance of myelin.	Purine and pyrimidine synthesis; amino acid interconversions.
Symptoms common to both types of deficiency	*Megaloblastosis*: Affects all proliferating tissues, specifically the hematopoietic system. *Macrocytosis*: Large stem cells in bone marrow; large cells with short life span in peripheral blood; "anemia."	
Additional symptoms	Damage to myelin with peripheral and other neurologic deficits.	
Development of anemia	Mainly due to impaired absorption of vitamin B$_{12}$ (pernicious anemia).	Mainly due to inadequate nutritional intake or utilization of folic acid.
Therapy	Cyanocobalamin (i.m.)	Folic acid (p.o./i.m.)

50–60 mg of elemental iron per day. If this amount enters the erythroid marrow, the rate of red cell production will increase to 2–3 times normal. To replenish depleted iron stores requires many more months of continued iron therapy after the anemia is corrected.

Adverse Effects of Oral Iron Preparations; Drug Interactions

These are localized mainly in the gastrointestinal system and are a result of physical intolerance. A dose-effect relationship has been shown for the incidence of nausea and upper abdominal pain, while the frequency of constipation and diarrhea is apparently unrelated to the size of dosage.

A potential drug interaction is the chelation of iron in the gastrointestinal tract. The absorption of tetracycline may be significantly impaired, which might require discontinuation of iron therapy during periods of oral medication with tetracycline antibiotics.

Toxicity

Acute effects from ingestion of toxic doses of iron (which may be any dose in excess of 1 g, usually about 5–10 g in fatal cases) appear in 30–60 minutes and consist of abdominal pain, nausea, vomiting, acidosis, and cardiovascular collapse, followed by coma and death if untreated. There is usually severe tissue damage to the gastrointestinal tract, the liver, and the kidneys (ulceration of the bowel, hepatic parenchymal cell necrosis, renal vascular congestion, and tubular degeneration). Treatment of this acute toxicity consists of gastric lavage and intravenous administration of iron-binding chelating agents (*e.g.*, deferoxamine, *see* Chapter 72); symptomatic therapy of peripheral vascular collapse; fluid and electrolyte replacement.

Chronic administration of iron to persons without iron deficiency may eventually lead to hemochromatosis, a condition characterized by excessive iron accumulation in all iron storage sites and in liver and pancreas.

Damage to these organs is in the form of cirrhosis, fibrosis, and diabetes; skin pigmentation may also occur.

Iron Compounds and Therapeutic Applications

Iron is usually administered orally as one of the iron salts. The oldest and most commonly prescribed form is **ferrous sulfate**, which also serves as the standard with which new iron preparations are compared. Other iron salts for oral administration, marketed under many trade names, are **ferrous ascorbate, ferrous fumarate, ferrous gluconate**, and **ferrous succinate**. Parenteral iron preparations are **iron dextran** (for deep intramuscular or intravenous administration) and **iron sorbitol** (to be used only intramuscularly).

Iron dosage must be calculated in terms of elemental iron rather than the iron salt. Approximate elemental iron equivalents per 100 mg of the orally administered salts are:

> ferrous fumarate = 32 mg,
> ferrous gluconate = 12 mg,
> ferrous succinate = 35 mg,
> ferrous sulfate = 20 mg.

Oral elemental iron requirements in deficient adults are, with great individual variations, about 60 mg/day (about 300 mg/day if allowance is made for incomplete absorption), which determines the size and frequency of dosage with the respective iron salts.

The dosage of parenterally administered iron must be calculated more precisely. For example, each gram of hemoglobin deficiency requires 150 mg of iron, and to this must be added 600 mg to replenish tissue stores. This total calculated dose is then divided into convenient daily doses and is given by injection over a period of 1–3 weeks.

Vitamin B$_{12}$ Deficiency

Defective gastrointestinal absorption of vitamin B$_{12}$ for very long periods of time (usually measured in years) will cause megaloblastosis. The condition is the result of blocked DNA synthesis in cells undergoing chromosomal replication, and occurs throughout the gastrointestinal tract, the cervix and vagina, and the hematopoietic tissues. The bone marrow of vitamin B$_{12}$-deficient patients shows a proliferation of erythrocyte precursors, and in the peripheral blood are found a combination of macroovalocytes, hypersegmented polymorphonuclear leukocytes, and giant platelets. These macrocytes have an abnormally short life span, and the condition is appropriately named **megaloblastic or macrocytic anemia**. In addition, vitamin B$_{12}$ deficiency may cause irreversible damage to myelin with resultant peripheral nerve and posterior or lateral column deficits. The basal metabolic rate is usually increased and hyperpigmentation of the skin may occur (see Table 42–3).

A familial, apparently immunologically based, abnormality of vitamin B$_{12}$ absorption, historically named "**pernicious anemia**" or "Addisonian anemia," may develop from lack of "gastric intrinsic factor of Castle," which binds ingested vitamin B$_{12}$ and protects it against destruction in the upper gastrointestinal tract, thus permitting its absorption from the ileum. However, even in the presence of intrinsic factor a number of intestinal diseases or defects can interfere with the absorption of the intrinsic factor-B$_{12}$ complex. Gastric atrophy and gastric surgery are common causes.

Vitamin B$_{12}$ is a cobalt-containing compound of rather complex structure; the term cyanocobalamin is accepted interchangeably with vitamin B$_{12}$ as the name of the active compound in humans. All requirements are usually met by a normal diet, and about 1 μg/day will maintain balance if gastric secretions are normal. Cyanocobalamin is stored in the liver (up to 90% of total). These stores become depleted very slowly, and it takes years for the development of megaloblastosis (see also Chapter 49).

Cyanocobalamin (vitamin B$_{12}$) is available for both oral and parenteral administration. The only established therapeutic use is in the treatment of vitamin B$_{12}$ deficiency. In pernicious anemia the preparation of choice is cyanocobalamin given by subcutaneous or intramuscular injection, since oral preparations cannot be depended upon because of the patient's inability to absorb the vitamin. Preparations of cyanocobalamin are nontoxic.

Folic Acid Deficiency

Folic acid (pteroylglutamic acid, Fig. 42–2) is required as a cofactor for purine synthesis, pyrimidine nucleotide synthesis, and amino acid interconversions. It is an essential vitamin for humans, but in bacteria it must be synthesized from para-aminobenzoic acid (see Chapter 56). The biologically active form is the tetrahydro derivative, folinic acid, produced by the action of dihydrofolate reductase on folic acid following its absorption (Fig. 42–2). (It is this step which makes folic acid vulnerable to the action of antibacterial and antineoplastic agents. See also Chapters 56 and 60.)

Folate deficiency results in **megaloblastic hematopoiesis** that is hematologically indistinguishable from that caused by vitamin B$_{12}$ deficiency. A striking clinical difference, however, is the absence of myelin damage (and its neurological consequences) in folic acid deficiency (see Table 42–3).

All physiologic requirements for folic acid (about 50 μg/day in adults) are usually met by a normal diet (see also Chapter 49). However, in situations of inadequate diet for long periods of time, chronic alcoholism (i.e., interference with the intermediary metabolism of folic acid), vitamin C deficiency (i.e., inability to reduce folic acid to its metabolically active form, tetrahydrofolic acid), chronic liver disease, and intestinal malab-

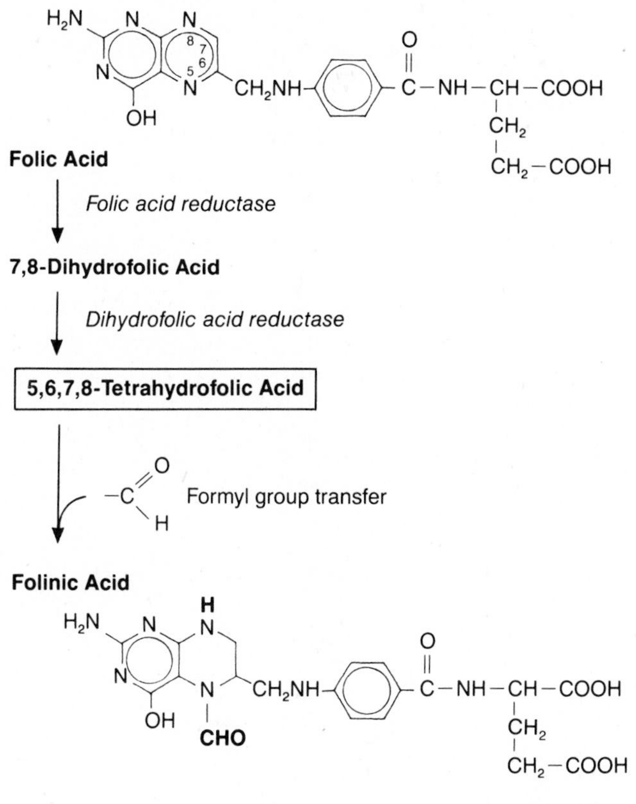

H₂N—[pteridine ring with positions 8,7,5,6]—CH₂NH—[benzene ring]—C(=O)—NH—CH—COOH
                                                                              |
                                                                             CH₂
                                                                              |
                                                                         CH₂—COOH

OH

Folic Acid

↓ *Folic acid reductase*

7,8-Dihydrofolic Acid

↓ *Dihydrofolic acid reductase*

┌─────────────────────────────┐
│ **5,6,7,8-Tetrahydrofolic Acid** │
└─────────────────────────────┘

↓   —C(=O)H   Formyl group transfer

Folinic Acid

H₂N—[pteridine/pteroyl ring with H, N, CHO]—CH₂NH—[benzene ring]—C(=O)—NH—CH—COOH
                                                                              |
                                                                             CH₂
                                                                              |
                                                                         CH₂—COOH

OH   CHO

Figure 42–2 Structural formulae of folic acid and folinic acid (N⁵-formyl-tetrahydrofolate, citrovorum factor, leucovorin).

sorption, a **macrocytic anemia** from folic acid deficiency may develop.

Total body stores of folic acid are about 5–10 mg, of which about half is found in the liver. The sole established therapeutic use of pteroylglutamic acid is in the treatment of folate deficiency. Folinic acid (citrovorum factor, leucovorin) is used as a specific antidote for the toxic effects of antineoplastic therapy with the antifol methotrexate (*see* Chapter 60). This antidotal action has been nicknamed "leucovorin rescue."

SOME OTHER DEFICIENCIES MANIFESTING AS ANEMIAS

Copper and Cobalt

Deficiencies in these metals are rare, but can be produced experimentally. Because copper and iron metabolism are interrelated, alleged copper deficiency anemias respond to iron therapy with or without copper.

Although primary cobalt deficiency has not been reported in humans, the metal may improve hematocrit, hemoglobin, and erythrocyte values in various types of refractory anemia not responding to conventional therapy.

Ascorbic Acid

Although quite rare, severe vitamin C deficiency may be associated with hypochromic anemia, which can be microcytic in conditions of chronic blood loss or macrocytic when associated with folic acid deficiency.

Pyridoxine

Pyridoxine, one of the three forms of vitamin B₆, produces a beneficial hemoglobin response in individuals suffering from a form of sideroblastic anemia that is characterized by abnormally large amounts of non-hemoglobin iron in erythrocyte precursors, hypochromic microcytic anemia, and other signs of severely disturbed blood regeneration. This pyridoxine-responsive anemia occurs sporadically in adult males as a possible familial condition; it is not due to nutritional pyridoxine deficiency. Pyridoxine therapy is thought to compensate for other unknown deficiencies in enzymes involved in normal hemoglobin synthesis (*see also* Chapter 49).

SUGGESTED READING

Beck WS. Metabolic aspects of vitamin B₁₂ and folic acid. In: Williams WJ, Beutler E, Erslev AJ, Lichtman MA, eds. Hematology, 3rd ed. New York: McGraw-Hill, 1983:311–331.

Beck WS. The megaloblastic anemias. In: idem, 434–465.

Bothwell TH, Charlton RW, Cook JD, Finch CA, eds. Iron metabolism in man, 3rd ed. Oxford: Blackwell, 1979.

Fairbanks VF, Beutler E. Iron metabolism. In: Williams WJ, Beutler E, Erslev AJ, Lichtman MA, eds. Hematology, 3rd ed. New York: McGraw-Hill, 1983:300–310.

Fairbanks VF, Beutler E. Iron deficiency. In: idem, 466–488.

ENDOCRINE SYSTEMS

Chapter 43

VASOPRESSIN, OXYTOCIN, AND OTHER OXYTOCIC DRUGS

S.R. George and B.P. Schimmer

Vasopressin and oxytocin are related nonapeptides that differ from each other by only two amino acids. Both hormones may have evolved from a single ancestral peptide, vasotocin, through molecular processing involving mutation and gene duplication. Du Vigneaud is credited with determining the structure of these peptide hormones and with their chemical synthesis. He was awarded the Nobel Prize in 1955.

Because of their structural similarities, the two peptides have similar pharmacologic activities, but these are expressed to different degrees. For example, vasopressin has greater antidiuretic and pressor activities and less uterotonic and milk-ejecting activities than oxytocin has.

Following the pioneering work of du Vigneaud, a large number of synthetic hormone analogs have been prepared and tested for separation of these various activities. Some of the analogs have markedly specific actions and have become clinically important drugs.

BIOSYNTHETIC AND ANATOMIC RELATIONSHIPS

The hypothalamus and the posterior lobe of the pituitary gland function together as a neurosecretory unit. The anatomic relationships of this unit are shown in Figure 43–1.

Site of Synthesis

Vasopressin and oxytocin are hormones associated with the posterior lobe (pars nervosa) of the pituitary gland. These two peptides, however, are not synthesized there; rather, they are made in specialized neurosecretory cells of the hypothalamus. **Vasopressin** is syn-

thesized in cell bodies that are localized predominantly in the **supraoptic nucleus**, while **oxytocin** is synthesized in cell bodies that are predominantly in the **paraventricular nucleus**.

Synthesis and Processing

Both peptides have molecular weights of approximately 1100 daltons, but are synthesized as larger precursor peptides (prohormones). The same precursor peptides are thought to give rise to the neurophysins (approximate MW 10,000 daltons), which are considered to serve as carrier proteins for vasopressin and oxytocin. The precursors are synthesized on membrane-bound ribosomes, packaged into secretory granules, and then enzymatically cleaved so that the hormones remain associated with the neurophysins only through electrostatic forces. The hormone-containing granules are transported to nerve terminals *via* unmyelinated axons. Most axons pass through the pituitary stalk and end in the posterior pituitary. Some axons only extend to the median eminence.

Secretion

Hormone secretion is triggered by electrical impulses that travel down the axons of the neurosecretory fibres to the nerve terminals. The secretory response is thought to involve: (1) influx of calcium to the cytosol, (2) fusion of secretory granules with the membranes of the nerve terminals, (3) emptying of the granule contents into surrounding capillaries, and (4) recapture of empty granules (as small vesicles) from the cell surface. Although it is believed that vasopressin and oxytocin are synthesized in separate neurons, most stimuli for secretion cause the release of both peptides. The type of stimulus, however, does determine the relative

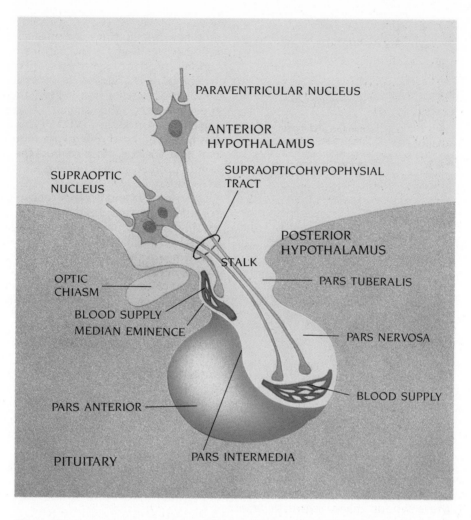

Figure 43–1 Anatomic structure and relationships of the hypothalamic-pituitary unit.

proportions of the secreted mixture. For example, thirst or hemorrhage causes preferential release of vasopressin; suckling stimulates the preferential release of oxytocin.

Role of the Posterior Pituitary Gland

From the above descriptions, it should be evident that the posterior pituitary is only a storage site for vasopressin and oxytocin. It is a physical, as well as functional, extension of the nervous system, organized into a specialized secretory apparatus. The posterior pituitary is composed of swollen, granule-filled, nerve terminals in juxtaposition to blood capillaries (*see* Fig. 43–1) and supported by pituicytes (glial cells). Lesions in the hypothalamic nuclei or in the supraoptico-hypophysial tract destroy the capacity for synthesis of vasopressin and oxytocin. Removal of the posterior pituitary, however, generally causes only a transient deficiency, because the nerve fibres terminating in the

median eminence remain functional and release sufficient amounts of these hormones.

CHEMISTRY

Structures

The structures of vasopressin and oxytocin are shown in Figure 43–2. In both hormones, six of the amino acids form ring structures by closure of the S–S bond between cysteines at positions 1 and 6; attached to the ring of each peptide is a tail of three amino acids. Opening the S–S bond results in a linear nonapeptide with no hormonal activity. For vasopressin activity, the tail must contain a basic amino acid—arginine in most mammals, lysine in the pig—at position 8, marked by the arrow in Figure 43–2.

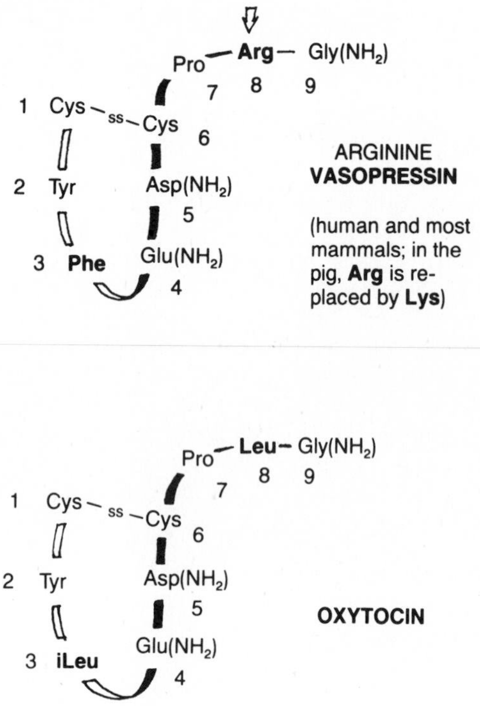

Figure 43–2 Amino acid sequences for vasopressin and oxytocin. The differences are at positions 3 and 8.

Hybrids of vasopressin and oxytocin, containing the ring structure of one and the tail of the other, have been synthesized. These hybrids, called oxypressin and vasotocin, have activities intermediate between those of the original hormones when tested in mammalian systems. Vasotocin is regarded as the "parent" hormone, since it is the natural form found in primitive species such as elasmobranchs and bony fish.

Rationales for Synthetic Analogs

Both vasopressin and oxytocin have a short half-life in the circulation (approximately 10 minutes), principally due to proteolytic degradation. An important site for proteolytic inactivation in both hormones is between the first two amino acids (cys–tyr). Cleavage of the peptide bonds in the tail also contributes to loss of activity. Over 300 synthetic analogs of vasopressin and oxytocin have been examined, in part for prolonged durations of hormone action. At present, synthetic analogs of vasopressin are the more important clinically.

At physiologic levels, vasopressin is important in water homeostasis (vasopressin also is known as antidiuretic hormone, ADH); however, as its name implies, vasopressin also has significant vasoconstrictor activity in pharmacologic doses. Therefore, another important rationale for the synthetic work has been to achieve greater separation of the antidiuretic and pressor actions of vasopressin. As shown in Table 43–1, there are four modifications that are important for enhanced antidiuretic action. Some combinations of these four modifications produce synergistic results. For example, 1-deamino-8-D-arginine-vasopressin (dDAVP) has an antidiuretic activity that is 2000 times greater than its pressor effect. The analog, 1-deamino-4-valine-8-D-arginine-vasopressin (dVDAVP), is even more potent but has been used only experimentally so far. Deamination at position 1 also renders the peptide more resistant to proteolysis, as does the substitution of D-arginine at position 8.

Other modifications can selectively increase the pressor effect of vasopressin and have clinical potential as local hemostatic agents during surgery. One such analog is 2-phenylalanine-3-isoleucine-8-ornithine vasopressin. It has a pressor:ADH ratio of 255; it is used for experimental purposes only.

Some of the smaller peptides produced by partial proteolytic cleavage of vasopressin have physiologic activities that differ from those of vasopressin. For example, removal of the terminal glycine (NH$_2$) from the side-chain yields desglycinamide arginine vasopressin (DGAVP), which retains the central actions of vasopressin (see below) but has greatly reduced peripheral activity. The side-chain of oxytocin, prolyl-leucyl-glycinamide, is a melanotropin release-inhibiting factor and has other central actions that are still under study.

VASOPRESSIN (ADH)

Physiology and Pharmacology

Antidiuretic Action

The major physiologic action of ADH in the human is on the reabsorption of water by the collecting ducts of the kidney. It probably acts to increase the permeability of the tubular epithelium to the passage of water.

TABLE 43–1 Modifications Affecting the Ratio of Antidiuretic to Pressor Activity of Vasopressin

Modification	ADH/Pressor Ratio*
Deamination at position 1	4
Substitution of Phe for Tyr	3
Substitution of Val or Thr for Glu (NH$_2$)	23
Substitution of D-Arg for L-Arg	28
1-Deamino plus 8-D-Arg	2000
1-Deamino-8-D-Arg plus 4-Val	>150,000

* Results are compared with arginine vasopressin, which is assigned a normalized value of 1.0.

Water, with some sodium and urea, moves from the tubular lumen into the interstitial fluid in response to an osmotic gradient, leaving solutes behind in more concentrated urine. The antidiuretic effect is extremely potent. Less than 0.1 μg per hour, administered by slow intravenous infusion, suppresses human urine flow completely.

The mechanism of action of ADH is shown in Figure 43–3. ADH, in sequential fashion, (1) interacts with a specific membrane receptor, (2) activates adenylate cyclase and causes cyclic AMP to accumulate, and (3) activates cyclic AMP-dependent protein kinase. The subsequent events are not well understood, though obviously protein phosphorylation is important. There is some evidence that one of the consequences of ADH-stimulated protein phosphorylation is stimulation of the formation of cellular microtubules, causing aggregation of membrane proteins and leading to the formation of molecular ''pores'' for water. As part of its action, ADH also stimulates the synthesis of prostaglandin E_1 (PGE$_1$), which serves in a negative feedback loop to inhibit ADH action. The adenylate cyclase system appears to be the target of the inhibitory influence of PGE$_1$.

Secretion of ADH can be stimulated or inhibited by osmotic, volemic, or nervous stimuli reaching cells in the supraoptic nucleus (Fig. 43–4).

ADH secretion is stimulated by:

- Hyperosmolality of plasma—e.g., by hypertonic saline injection. Secretion is responsive to as little as 1–2% change. The action is exerted through **osmoreceptors** located in the hypothalamus and other brain regions.
- Volume changes—e.g., hemorrhage or pooling of blood in the extremities on standing. As little as 6% change in blood volume affects ADH release by an action through stretch receptors and baroreceptors in thoracic vessels, atria, and carotid bodies.
- Drugs—e.g., ether, thiobarbiturates, cholinergic agonists (nicotine), clofibrate, tricyclic antidepressants.
- Noxious stimuli—pain, nausea, etc.

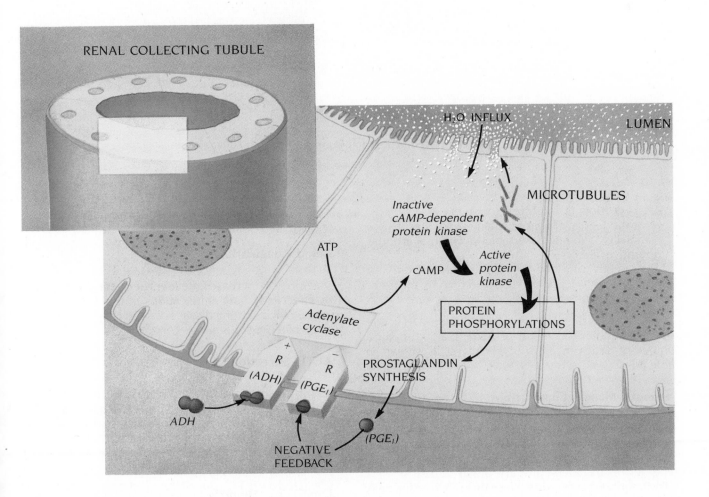

Figure 43–3 Mechanism of action of ADH on water reabsorption.

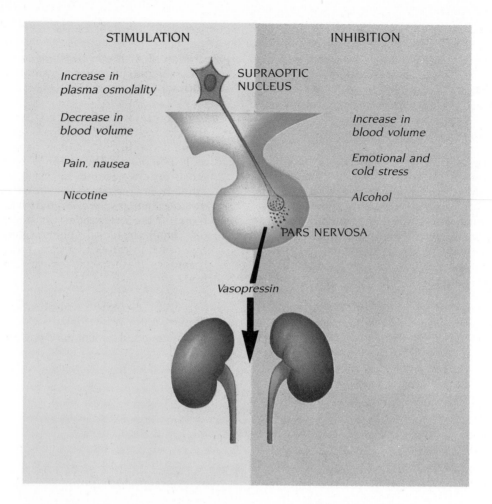

STIMULATION   **INHIBITION**

Increase in plasma osmolality

Decrease in blood volume

Pain, nausea

Nicotine

SUPRAOPTIC NUCLEUS

Increase in blood volume

Emotional and cold stress

Alcohol

PARS NERVOSA

Vasopressin

Figure 43–4 Factors involved in the stimulation and inhibition of vasopressin secretion. (Adapted from Ezrin C, 1979.)

ADH secretion is inhibited by:

- Hydration—drinking large volumes of water; hypo-osmolality and increased blood volume are the operative factors.
- Alcohol—by blocking nervous impulses from the midbrain; this action can be overcome by nicotine.
- Some nervous stimuli—*e.g.*, cold exposure.

In addition to stimulation and inhibition of ADH secretion, the antidiuretic action of ADH is affected by a number of drugs in a variety of ways, as shown in Table 43–2.

Smooth Muscle Contraction

At high dose, vasopressin causes the contraction of smooth muscle fibres in a number of tissues:

It causes pronounced vasoconstriction; the effect is general and includes coronary blood vessels.

The motility of intestinal smooth muscle, especially in the lower bowel, is increased.

Vasopressin stimulates uterine and cervical contractions, particularly circular smooth muscle. It causes short, frequent contractions without distinction between pregnant and nonpregnant uterus.

Blood Coagulation

Vasopressin increases the level of clotting factor VIII. This effect may have implications in the management of some blood clotting diseases and in prophylactic control of bleeding during surgery.

ACTH Secretion

Vasopressin stimulates ACTH release from the anterior pituitary. At one time, it was thought that ADH might be the corticotropin-releasing factor (CRF); now other peptides better fit the criteria for the physiologic CRF. Vasopressin, however, is synergistic with CRF in releasing ACTH.

Long-Term Memory

Vasopressin also is found in other parts of the brain; this fact suggests that vasopressin may have other physiologic roles in the CNS. When administered through normal routes, vasopressin improves the learning of new information and long-term memory. These effects are currently being tested in the treatment of amnesia and in the improvement of attention and memory in the elderly. Desglycinamide arginine vasopressin (*see* above) may be preferable for this, because it has negligible effects on the kidney and smooth muscle.

The mechanisms by which vasopressin causes its effects on smooth muscle, blood coagulation, ACTH secretion, and long-term memory are unknown, but they appear not to involve cyclic AMP-dependent pathways. They may be mediated by different subtypes of vasopressin receptors acting through the phosphatidyl inositol system.

Preparations

Desmopressin (DDAVP) is the 1-deamino-8-D-arginine synthetic analog of vasopressin. It has greater ADH potency, less pressor activity, and a longer half-life than vasopressin. Currently, it is the drug of choice in the treatment of diabetes insipidus. Preparations are supplied in isotonic saline as the acetate salt and are administered intranasally. DDAVP for injection (4 μg/mL) also is available.

Vasopressin injection (Pitressin®) is an aqueous solution for intravenous or intramuscular injection; the standard dosage form provides 10 IU/0.5 mL ampul. (The International Unit of vasopressin is defined by the pressor activity, in rats, of 0.5 mg of a U.S.P. standard posterior pituitary powder. One unit of activity cor-

responds to approximately 3 μg of purified arginine vasopressin.) The active principle may be purified from animal posterior pituitary (in which case it may have some contaminating oxytocic activity); more often, it is chemically synthesized. It acts for 3–4 hours.

Vasopressin tannate (Pitressin® tannate) is an insoluble suspension in oil for intramuscular injection. It is a long-acting (36–48 hours) preparation, supplied in ampuls of 5 IU/mL.

Available only in the U.S.A. and Britain are: **Posterior pituitary powder** ("Di-Sipidin")—used as a snuff, some is absorbed through the nasal mucosa; **crystalline lysine vasopressin** (Lypressin®; Syntropin®; Diapid®)—a synthetic preparation of lysine vasopressin, more stable than arginine vasopressin, and available as a nasal spray.

Therapeutic Uses

Relief of Diabetes Insipidus

This disease, caused by insufficient endogenous ADH, is characterized by excretion of large volumes of dilute urine (specific gravity about 1.002), extreme thirst, and copious intake of water. It can be congenital or can result from trauma to the supraopticohypophysial tract. Treatment consists of intranasal spray of synthetic vasopressin (DDAVP) or intramuscular injection of the long-acting form (vasopressin tannate in oil). The dose depends on the severity of the case, but typically is about 10 μg of desmopressin intranasally twice daily or about 2.5 IU of vasopressin in oil every 48 hours.

TABLE 43–2   Other Drugs Affecting Antidiuretic Action of ADH

Drugs	Mechanism of Action

Potentiators of ADH Action
  Acetylsalicylic acid (Aspirin)
  Chlorpropamide
  Indomethacin
	Inhibit renal prostaglandin synthesis. Chlorpropamide also stimulates ADH secretion.

Inhibitors of ADH Action
  Lithium carbonate
  Prostaglandin E$_1$
	Inhibit adenylate cyclase.

Colchicine Vinca alkaloids	Microtubular poisons.
Demeclocycline	Used clinically to treat SIADH.
Thiazide Diuretics Useful in treatment of nephrogenic or partial hypothalamic diabetes insipidus.	Unknown and paradoxical. Effects may result from systemic depletion of electrolytes, which in turn causes enhanced resorption of salt and water from the proximal tubule (*see also* Chapter 40, Diuretics).

Diagnosis of Diabetes Insipidus

The existence of polyuria and polydipsia is not synonymous with diabetes insipidus of hypothalamic origin. For example, similar symptoms are seen in diabetes insipidus of nephrogenic origin (failure of the kidney to respond to ADH). (*See also* Hays RM, 1985, for a brief description of other syndromes resembling diabetes insipidus.) Small doses of vasopressin (short-acting) are very effective in decreasing polyuria, thirst, and water intake in hypothalamic diabetes insipidus, but do not affect similar symptoms produced by other causes.

Stimulation of the Gastrointestinal Tract

Vasopressin is used specifically to expel gas postoperatively or before X-ray.

Local Hemostasis

This is achieved by intravenous infusion in the treatment of bleeding esophageal varices (the vasopressin causes strong splanchnic vasoconstriction, thus lowering pressure in the portal vein), or by specific arterial infusion to control active GI bleeding in the management of some cases of abdominal surgery.

Toxicity

Toxicity may result from overdosage or from pathologic conditions of hormone overproduction, such as ectopic tumors or CNS disorders. Secretion of too much ADH is known as syndrome of inappropriate antidiuretic hormone (SIADH). Symptoms include cerebral or coronary arterial spasm, water intoxication, pallor, nausea, and abdominal cramps.

OXYTOCIN

Physiology and Pharmacology

Milk Ejection

Milk ejection appears to be the major physiologic function of oxytocin. Oxytocin stimulates the contraction of myoepithelial cells of the breast during the postpartum period. These cells surround the channels of the glandular system and serve to squeeze milk out of the alveoli and ducts into larger sinuses. This is called "milk letdown" and is different from milk secretion. Suckling at the nipple of the breast is an important stimulus for the release of oxytocin.

Uterine Contraction

Sensitivity of the uterus to oxytocin increases rapidly during the **last trimester of pregnancy**, so that when labor is imminent, sensitivity to oxytocin greatly exceeds that to vasopressin. Oxytocin then stimulates slow, long-lasting peristaltic contractions of the upper uterine segment and relaxes the cervix. This is a useful type of contraction that results in delivery. Estrogen has a "priming action" on the uterus, increasing its sensitivity to oxytocin; progesterone renders uterine tissue more resistant. The effect of oxytocin on the **nonpregnant uterus** is slight.

The physiologic importance of oxytocin in the initiation of labor or in delivery is debatable. Arguments against the involvement of oxytocin include the observation that blood levels of oxytocin do not increase until labor is well advanced, and that parturition still proceeds in the absence of oxytocin (although prolonged labor has been reported).

Effects on the Corpus Luteum

Recent evidence suggests that oxytocin may also regulate the life span of the corpus luteum and thus play a role in the regulation of fertility. Included in this evidence are the observations that oxytocin administered to experimental animals shortens the life span of the corpus luteum and hastens the onset of estrus, while active immunization of animals against oxytocin has the opposite effect. These observations raise the possibility that oxytocin analogs may one day provide new pharmacologic approaches to contraception.

Vascular Effects

Oxytocin tends to relax circular fibres of smooth muscles and in large doses will lower blood pressure. Deep anaesthesia or concurrent use of ganglionic blocking drugs increases the likelihood of this potentially dangerous effect.

Mechanism of Action

The mechanism of action of oxytocin is not known. The hormone exerts its effects through specific cell-surface receptors. Cyclic AMP is not involved; induced changes in intracellular calcium may be important in muscle contraction.

Preparations

Oxytocin injection (Pitocin®; Syntocinon®) contains synthetic, pure oxytocin and is provided as an aqueous solution for intramuscular or intravenous injection, 10 IU/mL. (One unit is equivalent to about 2 μg of pure oxytocin. Oxytocic activity is bioassayed by measuring the drop in blood pressure in chickens; uterotonic activity parallels the decrease in blood pressure.)

Oxytocin citrate buccal tablets for sublingual administration contain 200 IU of synthetic oxytocin citrate per tablet.

Oxytocin nasal solution is a nasal spray containing 40 IU/mL of synthetic oxytocin.

Posterior pituitary injection (Pituitrin-S®) is made from posterior pituitary extract. This preparation contains both oxytocic and vasopressor activities in approximately equal amounts; the concentration is 10 IU/mL. When used in obstetrical doses, this preparation can cause coronary artery spasms. It is not available in Canada.

Therapeutic Uses

Stimulation of Labor at Term

Oxytocin is used primarily in the **induction of labor**. The aim is to determine the dose that just initiates labor without producing overly strong contractions, thereby avoiding damage to the fetus or uterus in the early stages of labor. Oxytocin is administered preferably by slow intravenous infusion of a diluted solution (initially 2 mU/min gradually increasing to 20 mU/min if necessary). The short half-life of oxytocin permits effective control through changing of infusion rates. The total dose required to initiate labor is on the average 4 IU (range = 0.6–12 IU). Oxytocin may be used in selected cases to **resume labor** if the uterus shows inertia during the first stage.

Contraindications for the use of oxytocin include situations that preclude normal vaginal delivery, predisposition to uterine rupture, or signs of fetal distress.

Control of Postpartum Bleeding

Bleeding may occur if the uterus relaxes too much during the interval of placental expulsion. Administration of oxytocin (approximately 5 IU) after the head is delivered will prevent excessive relaxation of the uterus during this stage. If oxytocin is administered again **after** the placenta is expelled, it will cause strong tetanic contraction and prevent postpartum bleeding.

Stimulation of Milk Ejection

Oxytocin is sometimes useful in relieving breast engorgement or in facilitating breast feeding when letdown is a problem. For these purposes, oxytocin is administered as a nasal spray a few minutes before feeding. Oxytocin is of no value in the case of inadequate milk production.

Toxicity

The toxicity of oxytocin is an extension of its physiologic effects. **Hypotension**, which may be enhanced by anaesthetics and ganglionic blockers, occurs on the basis of relaxation of vascular smooth muscle.

Symptoms of vasopressin activity may be elicited because of the structural similarity between oxytocin and vasopressin. They manifest primarily as water intoxication.

ERGOT ALKALOIDS AND OTHER OXYTOCIC DRUGS

A number of other agents, though chemically unrelated to oxytocin, are used clinically because of their ability to stimulate contraction of uterine muscle. Some of these agents are described briefly in this section.

Ergot Alkaloids

These compounds are derived from a fungus commonly known as ergot. For centuries, crude extracts of ergot were used by midwives as an obstetrical aid to hasten the onset and progress of labor. Their effects on uterine contraction, however, were vigorous and sustained. As a consequence, fetal anoxia and uterine rupture occurred with unacceptable frequency. In high concentrations, the extracts caused ergot poisoning characterized by marked vasoconstriction, giving rise to burning sensations in the extremities ("St. Anthony's Fire") and sometimes to gangrene, and CNS irritation (leading to convulsions).

With the isolation and purification of the various alkaloids of ergot, **ergonovine** and **methylergonovine** were identified and were found to have a highly selective action on the uterus, while causing minimal vasoconstriction. Structurally, they are simple amide derivatives of lysergic acid as shown in Figure 43–5.

In modern medicine, these ergot alkaloids are never used in the early stages of labor; however, because they are so effective in "clamping down" the uterus, they are used to control postpartum hemorrhage. The actions of the two ergot alkaloids are rapid and are exerted directly on the uterus. Effects are observed 8–10 minutes after an oral dose and almost immediately after intravenous or intramuscular injection. In very high doses, the toxic symptoms of ergot poisoning become evident.

Ergonovine differs from both vasopressin and oxytocin in its effects on the uterus (Table 43–3). Like

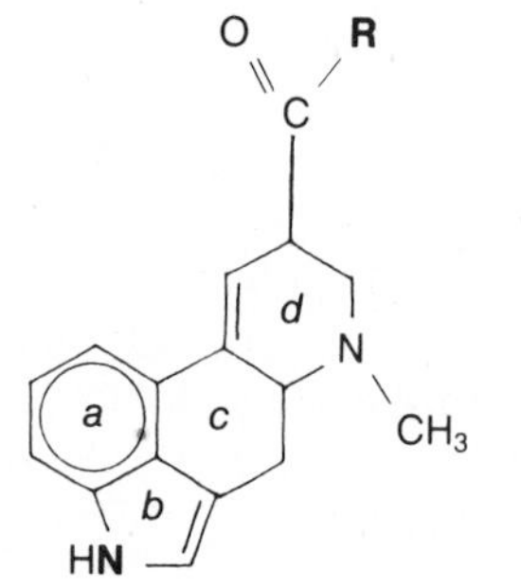

Lysergic acid	R = —OH
LSD	R = —N(CH₂CH₃)₂
Ergonovine (= Ergometrine)	R = —N—CHCH₂OH CH₃
Methylergonovine	R = —N—CHCH₂OH CH₂—CH₃
Methysergide	HN group on **b** ring replaced by CH₃N.

Figure 43–5 Ergot alkaloids.

vasopressin, it stimulates short, rapid contractions and contraction of the cervix in the **nonpregnant uterus**, causing pains akin to those of severe dysmenorrhea. Like oxytocin, it shows much more action on the **pregnant uterus**, particularly during labor and during the postpartum period, but has a longer duration of action.

Ergonovine maleate ("Ergometrine maleate"; Ergotrate maleate®) and **methylergonovine maleate** (Methylergobasine-Sandoz®) are available for injection (usual dose is about 0.2 mg i.m.) and as tablets (0.2 mg orally every 2–4 hours).

The **vasoconstrictor** activity of ergot alkaloids is most prominent in **ergotamine**, one of the amino acid-substituted alkaloids. Because of this property, ergotamine is used therapeutically in the treatment of **migraine headaches**. These headaches, which commonly affect one whole side of the head, are believed to be caused by dilatation of meningeal branches of the internal carotid artery.

Ergotamine tartrate is particularly effective in relieving this type of headache by causing prompt vasoconstriction. The drug is ineffective against other headaches because it is not an analgesic. It is used only for an incipient attack, not for routine maintenance therapy.

Bromocriptine (2-bromo-ergokryptine) is a semisynthetic ergot alkaloid that functions as a specific dopamine receptor agonist (cf. Chapter 9). It suppresses the production of prolactin and temporarily reverses effects of hyperprolactinemia including amenorrhea, galactorrhea, and infertility in women, as well as impotence and infertility in men. Therapeutic doses range from 2.5 to 7.5 mg of bromocriptine mesylate (Parlodel®).

Bromocriptine is also used in the treatment of acromegaly, suppressing growth hormone production in doses ranging from 7.5 to 40 mg/day, and as an adjunct in the treatment of Parkinson's disease with doses that may range up to 100 mg/day.

The use of bromocriptine is associated with a high incidence (68%) of mild side effects including nausea, headache, postural hypotension, and dizziness. At the higher doses cited above, additional side effects are seen, including abnormal involuntary movements, hallucinations, and mental confusion.

Prostaglandin E₂

Dinoprostone (Prostin® E₂, tablets of 0.5 mg) is used as an alternative to oxytocin, to induce labor when vaginal delivery is intended. As with oxytocin, the objective is to aim for the minimum effective concentration of prostaglandin by gradual administration of drug (0.5 mg/hour). Prostaglandin E₂ is equally effective on

TABLE 43–3 Comparison of Oxytocic Agents

| | ADH Activity | Smooth Muscle | | | | Onset | Duration |
| | | Blood Vessels | Gut | Uterus | | | |
				Nonpreg.	Preg.		
Oxytocin (injection)	+	–	o	± (cervix –)	+ + +	quick	short
Ergonovine (injection, oral)	o	+	o	+ +	+ + +	quick	long
Ergotamine (for migraine)	o	+ +	o	+	+ +	quick	variable
Prostaglandin E₂, F₂α							
(injection)	o	+ +	+ +	+ +	+ + +	slow	medium
(local)	o	o	o	+ +	+ + + (cervix –)		
Vasopressin (injection)	+ + + +	+ +	+ +	+ +	+ +	quick	short

Effects: + = positive; – = negative; o = none.

the pregnant and nonpregnant uterus; it generally has a slow onset of action and short half-life once absorbed. Other actions include stimulation of gastrointestinal smooth muscle leading to nausea, vomiting, and diarrhea (Table 43–3).

SUGGESTED READING

Ezrin C. The neurohypophysis. In: Ezrin C, Godden JO, Volpé R, eds. Systematic endocrinology. 2nd ed. Hagerstown: Harper and Row, 1979:45–53.

Gibbs DM. Vasopressin and oxytocin: hypothalamic modulators of the stress response: a review. Psychoneuroendocrinology 1986; 11(2):131–139.

Hays RM. Anti-diuretic hormone. N Engl J Med 1976; 295:659–665.

Hays RM. Agents affecting the renal conservation of water. In: Gilman AG, Goodman LS, Rall TW, Murad F, eds. Goodman and Gilman's the pharmacological basis of therapeutics. 7th ed. New York/Toronto/London: Macmillan, 1985:908–919.

Manning M, Lowbridge J, Haldar J, Sawyer WH. Design of neurohypophyseal peptides that exhibit agonistic and antagonistic properties of oxytocin and vasopressin. Fed Proc 1977; 36:1848–1852.

Robinson AG. DDAVP. N Engl J Med 1976; 294:507–511.

Tepperman J. Metabolic and endocrine physiology. 4th ed. Chicago: Year Book Medical Publishers, 1980.

Wilson JD, Foster DW. Williams' textbook of endocrinology. 7th ed. Philadelphia: WB Saunders, 1985.

ENDOCRINE SYSTEMS

Chapter 44

THYROID HORMONES AND ANTIHYPERTHYROID DRUGS

B.P. Schimmer and S.R. George

The thyroid gland synthesizes and secretes thyroid hormones required for the normal integrative functions of all body tissues. Thyroid dysfunction can lead to abnormalities in growth, development, metabolic regulation, and adaptive responses including acclimatization to heat and cold. This chapter deals with drugs used in the management of thyroid dysfunction, *i.e.*, thyroid hormone deficiency and thyroid hormone excess.

SYNTHESIS AND METABOLISM OF THYROID HORMONES

Figure 44–1 shows the principal features of the biosynthesis and metabolism of thyroid hormones. These steps are given in detail below.

Hypothalamic-Pituitary-Thyroid Unit

Thyrotropin-releasing hormone (TRH) is a hypothalamic peptide that functions to stimulate the release of thyrotropin (thyroid-stimulating hormone, TSH) from the anterior pituitary (Fig. 44–1). It is a tripeptide with the structure, L-pyroglutamyl-L-histidyl-L-proline amide (Fig. 44–2).

TRH also stimulates the release of prolactin and growth hormone, though the physiologic significance of these latter effects is uncertain. TRH has other effects within the CNS itself; for example, it counteracts the depressant effects of ethanol, barbiturates, and other hypnotic drugs. However, these effects are not yet well understood and have not found clinical applications at present. Factors that increase TRH levels include sleep, low ambient temperature, and noradrenaline.* Nonspecific stress (trauma, anaesthesia) reduces the level of TRH.

TSH is a pituitary glycoprotein (molecular weight about 28,000 daltons) made up of two chains—alpha and beta. The alpha chain is homologous and functionally interchangeable with the alpha chains of FSH and LH (*see* Chapter 45). TSH stimulates the production of thyroid hormones through interactions with specific receptors at the thyroid cell surface that are in close association with adenylate cyclase. Cyclic AMP appears to serve as the intracellular second messenger for the hormone. Stimulation of the synthesis and secretion of thyroid hormone occurs through actions of TSH on virtually each stage in the process (*see* Fig. 44–1). TSH also stimulates the growth of thyroid cells (excess TSH causes thyroid enlargement, *i.e.*, goitre) and maintains cellular structure. Circulating free thyroid hormone (*i.e.*, not protein-bound) exerts a negative feedback influence on TSH levels by rendering pituitary thyrotrophs insensitive to TRH (*see* Fig. 44–1).

Structure of Thyroid Hormones

The two active agents produced by the thyroid gland are **thyroxine** (tetraiodothyronine, T_4) and **triiodothyronine** (T_3). Their structures are shown in Figure 44–3.

The trisubstituted hormone T_3 has 4–10 times the activity of the tetrasubstituted compound T_4. The basic structural requirements for thyroid hormone activity seem to be two aromatic rings with an aliphatic side

---

*norepinephrine

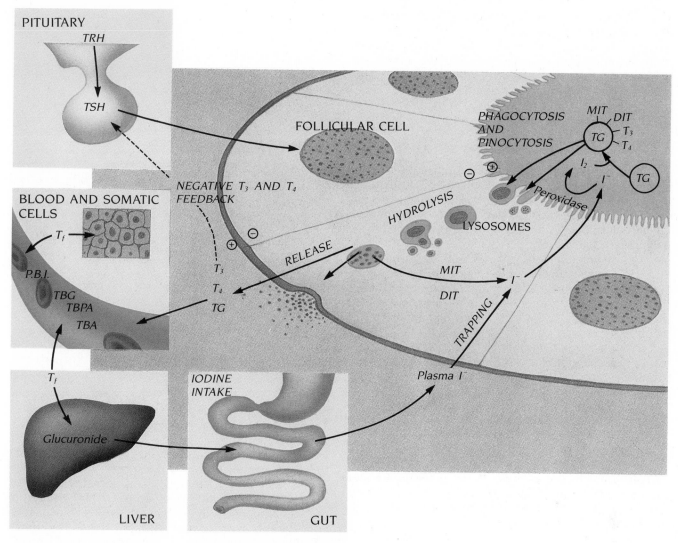

PITUITARY

TRH

TSH

FOLLICULAR CELL

PHAGOCYTOSIS
AND
PINOCYTOSIS

MIT DIT
TG T₃
T₄

I₂

TG

Peroxidase

I⁻

NEGATIVE T₃ AND T₄
FEEDBACK

⊖

⊕

HYDROLYSIS

LYSOSOMES

BLOOD AND SOMATIC
CELLS

Tᶠ

P.B.I.

TBG
TBPA

TBA

⊖

⊕

T₃

T₄

TG

RELEASE

MIT

DIT

I⁻

I⁻

TRAPPING

Tᶠ

IODINE
INTAKE

Plasma I⁻

Glucuronide

LIVER

GUT

Figure 44–1 Principal features of the biosynthesis and metabolism of thyroid hormone(s) (*see* text for abbreviations).

chain (an alanine side chain gives optimum activity). The iodine atoms and the ether bridge between the two rings maintain the two aromatic rings in a proper spatial alignment. Hormonal activity can be achieved with other bulky groups (methyl, isopropyl) in place of iodine. For example, DIMIT (*see* Fig. 44–3) has about 20% of the activity of T_4 and is of potential interest because it is more lipophilic than T_3 or T_4.

Biosynthesis of Thyroid Hormones

The points to be noted are shown in Figure 44–1:
1. Iodine (150 μg/day) is ingested in food and water and is absorbed into the blood as iodide.
2. Iodide is "trapped" by the thyroid gland by an active transport process leading to concentrations within the gland from 20 to several hundred times that in plasma.

Iodide is a non-threshold substance and is excreted readily *via* the kidney. In a sense the renal excretory mechanism competes with the thyroid I⁻-concentrating mechanism.

3. In the follicular lumen near the apex of the cells, iodide is oxidized to a more reactive form by a peroxidase.

4. In successive stages the iodine combines with tyrosine in glycoprotein molecules to form monoiodotyrosine (MIT) and diiodotyrosine (DIT).

In a subsequent oxidation reaction, probably involving the same peroxidase, the iodotyrosines are condensed to form T_3 and T_4. With a normal intake of iodine in the diet a lesser proportion of T_3 is produced. When the dietary intake is low, the proportion of T_3 becomes higher.

5. The iodinated thyroglobulin (TG) is a glycoprotein with a molecular weight of about 660,000 daltons and is stored in the acini of the gland. Its characteristic pink color after staining with eosin is well known.

6. The release of thyroid hormones from the gland is initiated by endocytosis of TG from the lumen into the cells of the follicle. Within the cell, TG is hydrolysed to amino acids by lysosomal enzymes; the iodine associated with MIT and DIT is reutilized; T_3 and T_4 are released into the circulating blood.

Transport and Metabolism

1. Most of the iodine in the circulation (about 90%) is in the form of T_4; 5% circulates as T_3. Both hormones are tightly bound to certain plasma proteins, with only a small fraction circulating as "free" hormone. The free hormone is considered to represent the physiologically active fraction. Unbound or "free" thyroxine (T_f) accounts for approximately 0.05% of the total T_4. T_3 is bound more loosely than T_4 (0.5% is free). Since the free hormone also is metabolized more rapidly than the bound, it follows that the half-life of T_4 in the circulation (about 7 days) is longer than that of T_3 (about 2 days).

2. Thyroxine-binding globulin (TBG) acts as a carrier for approximately 75% of the T_3 and T_4. The remainder is bound to thyroxine-binding prealbumin (TBPA) and to albumin.

3. Total T_4 is measured by isotope dilution techniques. Usual serum values are:

   hypothyroid <50 nmol/L (<3.5 μg/dL),
   euthyroid 60–155 nmol/L (4.7–12 μg/dL),
   hyperthyroid >160 nmol/L (>12.3 μg/dL).

Measurement of T_f provides a more sensitive indicator of thyroid function. The T_3-resin-uptake (T_3RU) test determines the extent of saturation of TBG and permits a rough calculation of the concentration of free hormone. Other assays for T_f, such as equilibrium dialysis, may be more accurate but are less readily available. Specific radioimmunoassays for T_3 and TSH also are helpful in diagnosis.

4. Thyroid hormones circulate to all tissues and are taken up in varying amounts. Metabolism either to the more potent T_3 or to "reverse T_3" (rT_3; monodeiodinated at the inner or α-benzene ring rather than the outer ring; metabolically inactive) accounts for 80% of T_4 degradation. Further metabolism results in the ap-

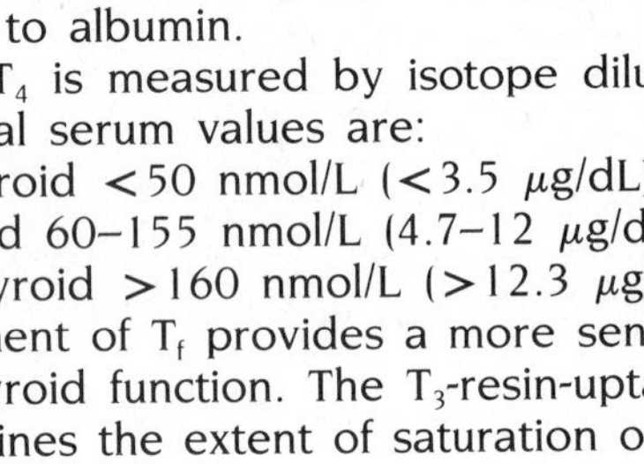

Figure 44–2 Thyrotropin-releasing hormone (TRH; L-pyroglutamyl-L-histidyl-L-proline amide).

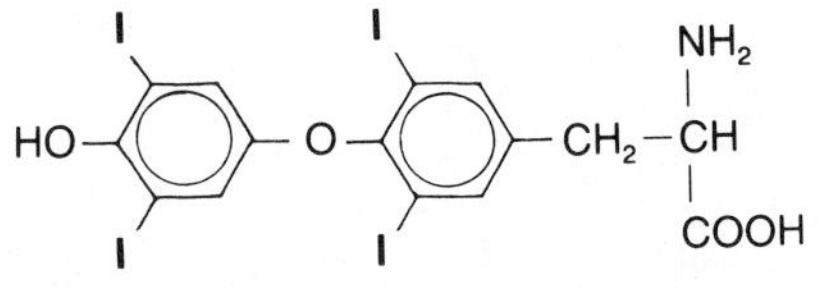

Figure 44–3 Agents with thyroid hormonal activity.

pearance of acetic and propionic acid derivatives of T_3 (metabolically active), various deiodinated derivatives, and iodotyrosines. The second major pathway for disposal of thyroid hormones is *via* conjugation in the liver and excretion in the feces.

5. Although the thyroid gland secretes some T_3, most of the active hormone (at least 70%) arises from deiodination of T_4 in peripheral tissues. Since T_3 is considerably more potent than T_4, it has been suggested that T_4 functions as a circulating "prohormone" for T_3.

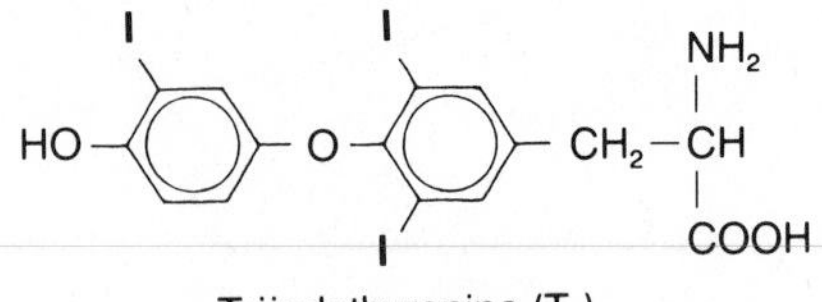

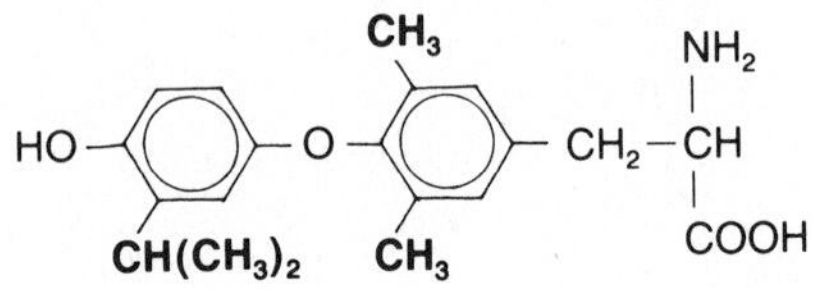

Autoimmunity and Thyroid Function

Graves' disease (diffuse toxic goitre; exophthalmic goitre) appears to be the major cause of thyroid hyperactivity (hyperthyroidism) in man. In Graves' disease, the circulating T_4 is high and TSH is found to be low. Thus excessive TSH production cannot be responsible for the growth and overactivity of the thyroid. The importance of immune phenomena in Graves' disease (and in chronic thyroiditis, or Hashimoto's disease) has been recognized for many years.

Circulating antibodies to thyroglobulin and to microsomal antigens, as well as cell-mediated autoimmunity, occur in both diseases. Circulating immunoglobulins that can stimulate the human thyroid can be demonstrated in most cases of Graves' disease. These thyroid-stimulating immunoglobulins (TSI), probably autoantibodies, are able to bind with and activate thyrotropin receptors and, like thyrotropin, produce an increase in the formation of cyclic AMP. As might be expected, administration of thyroid hormones does not suppress the action of TSI. A significant number of cases of Graves' disease undergo spontaneous remission, and may even progress to permanent hypothyroidism due to immune destruction of the thyroid.

A distinctive disorder often associated with Graves' disease is exophthalmos, a protrusion of the eyeballs and widening of the palpebral fissures. It is produced by an enlargement of external ocular muscles and associated connective tissue; however, there is no agreement as to its cause. Exophthalmos cannot be produced experimentally by administering thyroid hormone, nor does it occur in all hyperthyroid patients. Immune mechanisms, both cell-mediated and humoral, are currently regarded as likely pathogenic factors.

Thyroid Hormone in Pregnancy

Pregnancy, or estrogen treatment, increases the concentration of TBG, and this could lower the circulating level of free hormone. Feedback regulatory mechanisms compensate, however, and thyroid hormone synthesis increases enough to maintain a normal level of free (active) hormone.

Very little T_4 or T_3 can pass through the placenta. Thus, the fetus cannot depend on maternal hormone for its requirements. The amount of thyroid function necessary for normal development of the fetus is open to debate. While body growth is not affected in the athyreotic fetus, brain development may well be. There is agreement that, after birth, prompt and vigorous replacement treatment is essential in the management of neonatal hypothyroidism. Nevertheless, even prompt treatment after birth may not reverse all the effects of hypothyroidism on brain development. Consequently, current research is directed towards treating hypothyroidism *in utero*. Drugs such as DIMIT, which can cross the placenta, are of interest in this regard.

Hyperthyroidism also is of concern in pregnancy. While TSH and thyroid hormone cannot cross the placenta, thyroid-stimulating immunoglobulins will traverse the placenta and stimulate the fetal thyroid gland. In addition, labor and delivery may precipitate "thyroid storm," an extreme and life-threatening state of hyperthyroidism. The main concern usually is for the well-being of the mother.

ACTIONS

Thyroid hormones seem to be essential for normal function of all body tissues. They have profound influence on integrated processes such as differentiation and development, growth, and adaptation to environmental stress. There is a tendency to associate the specific actions of thyroid hormones with the signs and symptoms of glandular dysfunction.

With thyroid hormone deficiency (**hypothyroidism**) there is impairment of:

- growth of skeletal tissues;
- growth, development, and function of the central nervous system;
- synthesis of protein;
- absorption of carbohydrate;
- lipid metabolism (hypercholesterolemia);
- adrenal cortical and gonadal function;
- cardio-renal function (decreased pulse rate and GFR, *etc.*);
- over-all tissue metabolism (low BMR).

With excessive function (**hyperthyroidism**; thyrotoxicosis) the principal effect is an increase in metabolism of most (if not all) tissues, causing an increased basal consumption of oxygen (BMR) and an increase in the amount of energy expended as heat. Most other effects of hyperthyroidism follow from these: increased appetite, loss of weight, high pulse rate, high systolic pressure, increased water turnover by sweating, dyspnea, fine tremor of skeletal muscles, *etc*. Many of these changes resemble those of excessive activity of the sympathetic nervous system.

The mechanisms underlying the diverse actions of thyroid hormone are not known precisely. Direct actions of the hormone on mitochondrial and other cellular activities have been reported; however, these effects generally are seen with hormone concentrations above the physiologic range. In the current view, thyroid hormone binds to specific receptor proteins in the nuclei of many tissues. Thyroid hormone-receptor complexes stimulate transcription of specific genes, resulting in increased synthesis of important proteins such as:

- $(Na^+ + K^+)$-ATPase (may regulate BMR by rapidly hydrolysing the high-energy bond of ATP; the fall in ATP:ADP ratio stimulates mitochondrial oxidative reactions and results in excess production of heat—this factor likely contributes only modestly to the overall calorigenic effects of thyroid hormone);
- nerve growth hormone (CNS development?);
- β adrenoceptors (potentiation of cardiovascular and metabolic effects of catecholamines).

CLINICAL USE OF THYROID HORMONE

From the above, it can be seen that the administration of thyroid hormone is indicated as replacement therapy for treatment of hypothyroidism. The clear indication is frank thyroid deficiency (cretinism, myxedema). Cases of mild hypothyroidism also occur in which only one, or at most a few, of the symptoms are present. In such cases, laboratory tests help establish the diagnosis and treatment.

Preparations

Levothyroxine (sodium); *syn*. Sodium L-thyroxine, U.S.P., B.P. (Eltroxin®, Synthroid®):

This is a crystalline synthetic pure compound, prepared in oral tablets, in strengths ranging from 0.025 mg to 0.3 mg; it is also available in sterile lyophilized form for injection after reconstitution. Levothyroxine is measured chemically, and therefore there is no variability. Because of this uniformity it is preferred to thyroid powders or extracts.

Thyroid (U.S.P., B.P.), also called "desiccated thyroid":

This preparation consists of dried powdered gland in the form of tablets of 15–300 mg. It is standardized only in terms of I_2 content. Since some of the I-containing compounds in the glands are inactive, and their concentrations vary, there is a potential variability in potency of dried gland standardized in this way. Some preparations are standardized biologically, which is better.

Liothyronine (sodium); *syn*. L-triiodothyronine (Cytomel®):

This is a crystalline synthetic pure compound, in oral tablets of 5 and 25 μg.

Liotrix (Thyrolar®, available in U.S.A., but not currently available in Canada):

Liotrix is a combination of synthetic T_4 and T_3 in a ratio of 4:1; this ratio is thought to resemble closely the physiologic secretion ratio. The value of this combination is not clear, since T_3 is readily derived from circulating T_4. The mixture is supplied as tablets in several strengths.

Dextrothyroxine (Choloxin®):

This pure compound is used as a hypocholesterolemic agent (*see* Chapter 37). The rationale for this is based on the observation that it has approximately the same potency as L-thyroxine in lowering the concentration of cholesterol in blood, while having only one-quarter the potency to increase the general rate of metabolism. Thus, the objective is to produce a lowering of blood cholesterol with minimal effects (particularly cardiovascular) of hyperthyroidism. Nevertheless, because of its potential for metabolic and cardiovascular actions, other more conventional means of plasma lipid reduction are generally preferred. Serious adverse effects include angina in patients with a history of coronary artery disease, and cardiac arrhythmias.

Therapy of Hypothyroidism

In the treatment of hypothyroidism, it is usual to begin with a low dose of L-thyroxine (0.05 mg) daily, to avoid strain on the heart and adrenal cortex caused by a too rapid rise in metabolic rate before there has been some recovery from the effects of thyroid deficiency.

The full effect may take several weeks to develop, and therefore the dose should not be adjusted upward for at least 3 weeks. In the presence of cardiac disease, increments should be small and the intervals between them extended. By successive increments (0.05 mg L-thyroxine) the dose is eventually brought up to a maintenance level of approximately 0.15 mg thyroxine, depending on individual response. In the presence of concomitant adrenocortical dysfunction, glucocorticoid replacement therapy should be initiated before starting treatment with thyroid hormone.

Both dried thyroid and pure thyroxine have a prolonged action that takes up to 3 months to wear off completely after medication is stopped.

In infants and children the dosage is related to age and body weight and is adjusted to the level of circulating thyroid hormones. The dosage regimen is close to that of adults. Adequate dosage is extremely important for normal growth and mental development.

Triiodothyronine is much more rapid in action. Effects start to occur in 4–8 hours, reach a maximum in 24–48 hours, and wear off in a few days if medication is stopped. Therefore, the "evenness" of effect depends more closely on regularity of dosage, which makes it a difficult agent for routine use. It is also more expensive. The value of triiodothyronine lies in its relatively short duration of action; in certain cases repeated thyroid function tests may be desirable and these can be done a few weeks after stopping triiodothyronine medication. The dose of 25 μg is equivalent to 0.1 mg L-thyroxine.

THERAPY OF HYPERTHYROIDISM

When the thyroid gland is overactive, secreting excessive (thyrotoxic) amounts of thyroid hormones, the therapeutic objective is to interrupt synthesis and/or release. Several methods are available.

Ablation of Part or All of the Thyroid Gland

Two methods are in common use: surgical ablation and destruction by radioactive iodine (^{131}I-iodide). The choice depends upon such things as the experiences of the treatment centre and the age and physical status of the patient. Na[131]I is taken up and concentrated by the gland in the same way as ordinary I⁻. The uptake is especially great in the hyperactive gland, as in thyrotoxicosis. Where the normal gland takes up less than 40% of an administered dose, the hyperactive one may take up 80% or more. This concentration of ^{131}I causes intense local β irradiation, which destroys glandular epithelium, while the low concentration in the rest of the body causes no damage to other tissues. In some cases, more than one treatment may be required to achieve control. ^{131}I is also useful for treating thyroid carcinoma, including metastases, provided the cells still retain their I^--trapping mechanism (*i.e.*, they are not too undifferentiated).

Danger: If the thyroid gland has a large store of colloid, surgical manipulation or destruction by ^{131}I may release a flood of thyroxine into the circulation and cause "thyroid storm." Therefore one usually tries to block synthesis of hormone first, allowing the gland to become depleted before using definitive therapy. ^{131}I is not used in pregnant women because it crosses the placenta and can have potentially harmful effects on fetal tissues, especially thyroid. It also is not generally used in children.

Blocking I⁻ Uptake

ClO_4^- and SCN^- resemble halide ions in dimensions, distribution of charge, *etc.*, and probably act as competitive blockers of the I^--trapping mechanism. Theoretically this is a rational approach. Unfortunately, SCN^- has marked hypotensive effects and is too toxic for long-term therapy. $KClO_4$ is effective and for a time was used extensively. However, reports of aplastic anemia during continued treatment accumulated and enthusiasm for its use waned.

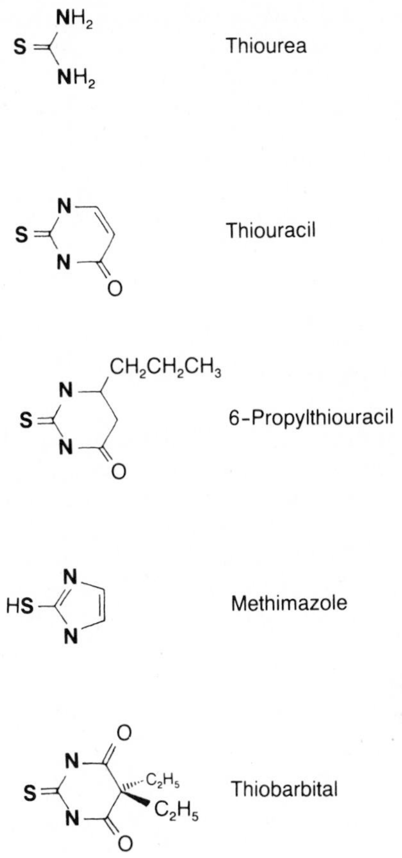

Inhibiting Synthesis of Thyroid Hormones

Synthesis of thyroid hormones can be inhibited by blocking the iodination of tyrosyl groups and the coupling of iodotyrosines to form T_3 and T_4.

Thiourea and **thionamides** derived from it (incorporating the thiourea grouping in some type of ring structure) (Fig. 44–4) act in this way. They do not interfere with the release of TH, and therefore (depending on the amount of stored hormone) the onset of clinical effect is slow. Several weeks may be required to produce a maximal effect.

Equivalent Dosage of Thionamides (initial daily dose):

- propylthiouracil   200–300 mg.
- methimazole and carbimazole   20–30   mg.

Actions and Properties of Thionamides

- They inhibit iodination of tyrosine and monoiodotyrosine.
- They inhibit coupling of iodotyrosines.
- Propylthiouracil inhibits deiodination of T_4 to T_3 in tissues; it also inhibits the deiodination of T_3.

Figure 44–4   Thiourea and derivatives.

- Half-lives are short (hours), so several doses are required per day.
- Propylthiouracil is being evaluated for use in the treatment of alcoholic liver disease. By lowering circulating levels of thyroid hormone, propylthiouracil may counteract the hypermetabolic effects of alcohol and thereby protect the liver from hypoxic necrosis (*see* Chapter 62).

Toxic Effects

All drugs of this group are capable of causing toxic effects (3% with propylthiouracil, 7% with methimazole). These are:

- agranulocytosis (most serious—reported in 0.5% of cases);
- drug rash, arthralgia, edema (in over 2% of cases), drug fever (very rare); and
- rare cases of hepatitis, lymph node swelling, loss of taste, *etc.*

In the physiologic scheme, the level of T_f is shown to control secretion of TSH by "feedback" to hypothalamus and anterior pituitary. With thiourea compounds, interruption of thyroxine synthesis may cause a gradual increase in output of TSH, making the gland larger, more friable, and harder to handle surgically.

Thionamides cross the placenta and are also secreted in milk. Infants born of mothers who are being treated with these drugs may show hyperplasia of the thyroid. If breast-fed, they may develop cretinism. Therefore, one uses the lowest possible dose and initiates bottle-feeding. If the dosage is low, the effect on the fetus is not serious because it is reversible.

Blocking Release of Thyroxine

Iodide is thought to inhibit the enzyme that splits thyroxine from thyroglobulin, as shown by accumulation of large amounts of colloid in the gland. There is some suggestion, also, that a large dose of I⁻ blocks the action of TSH on the gland because the epithelium becomes less hyperplastic. How both of these actions are achieved is not known. However, the gland becomes easier to handle surgically and symptoms are relieved rapidly, making iodide useful in the treatment of thyroid storm. Iodide in high concentrations may inhibit synthesis of thyroid hormone within the gland (Wolff-Chaikoff effect).

Iodide is not suitable for long-term therapy because the gland escapes from the effect of I⁻, the release of thyroxine is resumed, and the gland is so saturated with I⁻ that ¹³¹I will not be taken up. Therefore it is used only for a few weeks. The forms available are:
- Lugol's Iodine, B.P.;
- Strong Iodine Solution, U.S.P.;
- Saturated NaI or KI solution.

Of these, enough is used to give 60 mg of I⁻ per day.

Lithium (as the carbonate) is also effective in preventing release of thyroid hormones from the thyroid. It most likely acts by inhibiting the thyroid adenylate cyclase. Its place in the treatment of hyperthyroidism is unclear.

Symptomatic Relief

This may be produced by administration of β-adrenoceptor blockers such as propranolol (*see* Chapter 17). Propranolol acts quickly and is well tolerated. The usual contraindications for use of propranolol should be kept in mind, *e.g.*, bronchial asthma, chronic obstructive lung disease, and congestive heart failure. The similarity of many signs and symptoms of thyrotoxicosis to those of increased sympathetic activity has been mentioned, and the beneficial effect of a β-adrenoceptor blocker such as propranolol is consistent with the hypothesis that some of the effects of thyroid hormone are mediated by its action on β receptors. Reserpine, because of its ability to deplete catecholamine stores, has also been used for symptomatic relief. Its use is infrequent because of problems with depression and because of early reports, now questioned, indicating an increased incidence of breast cancer.

SUGGESTED READING

Chopra IJ. New insights into metabolism of thyroid hormones: physiological and clinical implications. Prog Clin Biol Res 1981; 74:67–80.

Cooper DS. Antithyroid drugs. N Engl J Med 1984; 311: 1353–1362.

Tepperman J. Metabolic and endocrine physiology. 4th ed. Chicago: Year Book Medical Publishers, 1980.

Van Herle AJ, Vassart G, Dumont J. Control of thyroglobulin synthesis and secretion. N Engl J Med 1979; 301:307–314.

Volpé R. The role of autoimmunity in hypoendocrine and hyperendocrine function. Ann Intern Med 1977; 87: 86–99.

Wilson JD, Foster DW. Williams' textbook of endocrinology. 7th ed. Philadelphia: WB Saunders, 1985.

Chapter 45

GONADOTROPIC AND GONADAL HORMONES

S.R. George and B.P. Schimmer

Gonadal hormones are important for conception, embryonic development, development at puberty (primary and secondary sex characteristics), and for the desire and ability to procreate. While not essential for life, they are essential for the individual's well-being. The economic and social significance of their use in control of fertility is a matter of worldwide concern.

For many decades it has been known that production and release of the gonadal hormones are controlled by the gonadotropic hormones of the anterior pituitary, and that in turn these are under the influence of factors (gonadotropin-releasing hormone) originating in the hypothalamus. Our current understanding of the subject has been facilitated by the determination of the chemical nature of hypothalamic and pituitary hormones and the development of specific radioimmunoassays that permit the measurement of low concentrations of hormones, or fragments of hormones, present in blood or tissues.

The principal features of these relationships are shown in Figures 45-1 and 45-2.

GONADOTROPIN-RELEASING HORMONE

Gonadotropin-releasing hormone is known by several names and abbreviations: GnRH, luteinizing hormone-releasing hormone, LHRH, LH-FSHRH. In 1971, LHRH was isolated from pig and sheep hypothalami, the amino acid sequence was determined, and the hormone then was synthesized chemically. It is a decapeptide with the structure:

PyroGlu-His-Trp-Ser-Tyr-Gly-Leu-Arg-Pro-GlyNH$_2$.

In the human, this peptide stimulates the release of luteinizing hormone (LH) and follicle-stimulating hormone (FSH) from the anterior pituitary. The quantal release of FSH is less than that of LH. It has been proposed that the decapeptide is the single hypothalamic hormone (GnRH) that controls the release of both LH and FSH from the pituitary gland. The quantitative discrepancy between release of LH and of FSH could be related to differential responses of gonadotrophs to the pulsatile secretion of GnRH or to feedback modulation by gonadal steroids altering the function of the hormone-producing pituitary cells. The existence of a separate specific FSHRH is still considered possible by some investigators.

There is evidence for central inhibitory opioid regulation of GnRH secretion, which may be relieved by adrenergic pathways. Higher dopaminergic pathways may also be involved, but their role is less well defined.

The secretion of GnRH is pulsatile, which is of major importance in the effects it produces on secretion of LH and FSH. Continuous administration initially stimulates but then inhibits the release of LH and FSH, apparently because of an altered response (a desensitization) of the gonadotropin-producing cells. Estrogens increase the sensitivity of LH-producing cells to GnRH.

The biologic half-life of GnRH is short, but analogs have been prepared that are less readily catabolized and are many times more potent as agonists, or act as antagonists of the natural hormone. The ability to stimulate or inhibit production of gonadotropins by appropriate use of GnRH or its analogs represents a new and powerful means of affecting fertility in males and females. Also, by controlling the production of gonadal hormones, GnRH analogs (Lupron®) may be useful in the treatment of hormone-dependent tumors (prostate, breast) and other rare conditions such as precocious puberty.

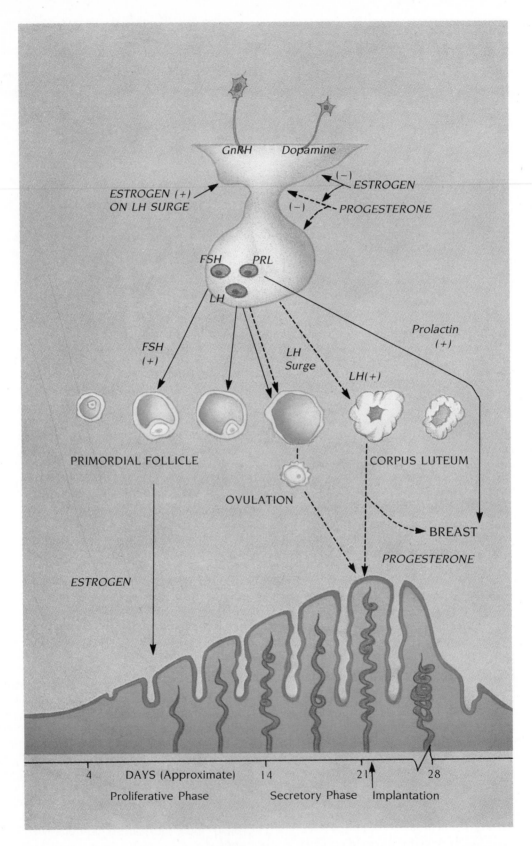

Figure 45–1 Physiologic relationships of gonadotropins and gonadal hormones and their influences on the ovary, uterus, and breast.

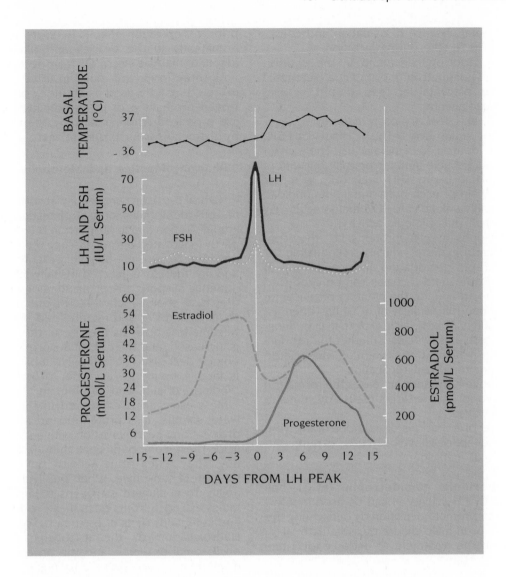

Figure 45–2 Approximate plasma concentrations of ovarian hormones and gonadotropins during a normal menstrual cycle. The change in body temperature through the cycle is shown on the top.

GONADOTROPINS

In the human there are two pituitary gonadotropins that act on the ovary or testis. Chemically they are complex glycoproteins that originate in the gonadotrophs of the anterior pituitary. FSH induces development of ovarian follicles and initiates and maintains spermatogenesis. In the female, LH (also called ICSH or interstitial cell-stimulating hormone) induces continued follicular development, followed by ovulation and corpus luteum formation. In the male, it stimulates androgen formation by the interstitial cells of the gonad.

Prolactin stimulates the function of the corpus luteum in the rat and mouse, but probably does not do so in the human. It is closely related chemically to growth hormone. Its release appears to be under inhibitory dopaminergic control from the tuberoinfundibular neurons, since pituitary stalk section may increase secretion of prolactin, with resulting galactorrhea. Some drugs (morphine, reserpine, metoclopramide, chlorpromazine) also produce this effect by inhibiting the release of dopamine or by blocking dopamine receptors. Dopamine, or dopamine agonists (bromocriptine), inhibit release of prolactin. Releasing factors for prolactin have also been described.

Prolactin, with other hormones (*e.g.*, ovarian and adrenal steroids, placental lactogen, thyroid hormone), plays a major part in the growth and development of the breasts during pregnancy and lactation. The increased blood levels of prolactin observed during this period may inhibit the secretion of gonadotropins or their action on the ovaries. This action probably ac-

ENDOCRINE SYSTEMS

counts for the usual absence of ovulation and consequent decrease in fertility during lactation.

An LH-like gonadotropin is found in the chorion (human chorionic gonadotropin, or hCG); a lactogenic hormone (human placental lactogen, or hPL) is also produced in the placenta.

FSH, LH, hCG, and TSH are each made up of an α and a β chain of amino acids. The α chains of FSH, LH, and TSH are identical (89 amino acids). The α chain of hCG is indistinguishable immunologically but differs from that of FSH, LH, and TSH chemically in minor degree. The β chain of each hormone is immunologically and chemically unique (112–115 amino acids). By itself, neither chain has biologic activity.

The four hormones are glycoproteins, *i.e.*, they contain abundant carbohydrate, which is responsible for preventing the rapid degradation and inactivation of the molecules. Both α and β chains can be produced in other tissues in addition to the pituitary or placenta, and this production (particularly of hCG) has been associated with malignant neoplastic growth in liver, lung, islet cells, and colon. It is not clear whether the production is specific for malignant replication or is associated with any (benign) rapid cell replication.

Each of the above hormones increases the formation of cyclic AMP in appropriate target tissues by stimulating adenylate cyclase.

Relatively pure preparations of gonadotropins from humans and other species have been used experimentally and in clinical medicine.

- **Human chorionic gonadotropin (hCG)** has predominantly LH activity. It can be used in infertile women to promote ovulation by duplicating the LH "surge," or in male children to stimulate interstitial cells in the treatment of undescended testicles.
- **Pregnant mare's serum gonadotropin** has both LH and FSH activity.
- **Menotropins for injection** (Pergonal®), gonadotropin prepared from urine of postmenopausal women, has FSH and LH activity. It is usually administered for 9–12 days, followed by an injection of hCG, in an attempt to simulate the LH surge and produce ovulation.
- **FSH and/or LH from human pituitaries.** There is no commercial source, but the preparation is effective in causing ovulation in selected cases.

ESTROGENS

Natural Products

The principal naturally occurring estrogen is 17-β-estradiol. It occurs in equilibrium with its oxidation product, estrone, but is largely hydroxylated to estriol

prior to excretion (Fig. 45–3). It is produced predominantly in the ovaries and placenta, but small amounts may be secreted from testes and adrenals.

All three forms are found in urine, and the amount excreted may be used as an index of endogenous estrogen production or of an administered dose. They are produced commercially by chemical synthesis or by extraction from pregnant mare's urine.

Pharmacokinetics and Metabolism

Natural estrogens are readily absorbed from the skin, mucous membranes, or gastrointestinal tract. After oral administration a high proportion is biotransformed and partly inactivated during passage through the liver. The natural estrogens are only very slightly soluble in water and are therefore injected (usually intramuscularly) as aqueous suspensions or as solutions in oil; however, they have enough polarity to be quickly absorbed from the injection site and metabolized. Esters of estradiol become less polar as the size of the ester substituent is increased, and the rate of absorption from oily solutions is decreased accordingly. In blood, the hormone is largely bound to a carrier protein, sex-hormone-binding globulin, and to albumin.

Most estrogen is converted in the liver into more water-soluble, less protein-bound substances by hydroxylation and conjugation with sulfuric or glucuronic acid. These compounds are then excreted by the kidney. They retain some activity, but less than that of the parent substance. When the liver is damaged, the ability to conjugate estrogens is impaired so that in males estrogen from testes may produce feminization, and in females signs of estrogen excess are observed. Hydroxylation of the estrogens is catalysed by microsomal enzymes, and the process is affected by drugs that induce these enzymes (*see* Chapter 4).

The synthetic analogs 17-α-ethinyl estradiol and mestranol (Fig. 45–4) are absorbed well after oral administration, but unlike the natural hormone they are inactivated very slowly in the liver and peripheral tissues. This slow inactivation is responsible for their potency and prolonged action.

Preparations

- **Esters of benzoic, propionic, or cyclopentylpropionic acid** are given by intramuscular injection for slow absorption from the site and for prolonged action.
- **Ethinyl estradiol**—an ethyne group at C-17 makes this compound stable in the GI tract, and it is absorbed well. The dose is 0.01–0.05 mg daily by mouth.
- **Mestranol** (3-H_3CO-17-α-ethinyl estradiol).
- **Conjugated estrogens**—pregnant mare's urine extract (Premarin®) contains natural conjugates, principally sodium estrone sulfate (60%) and sodium equilin sulfate (30%). They are effective orally or by injection.

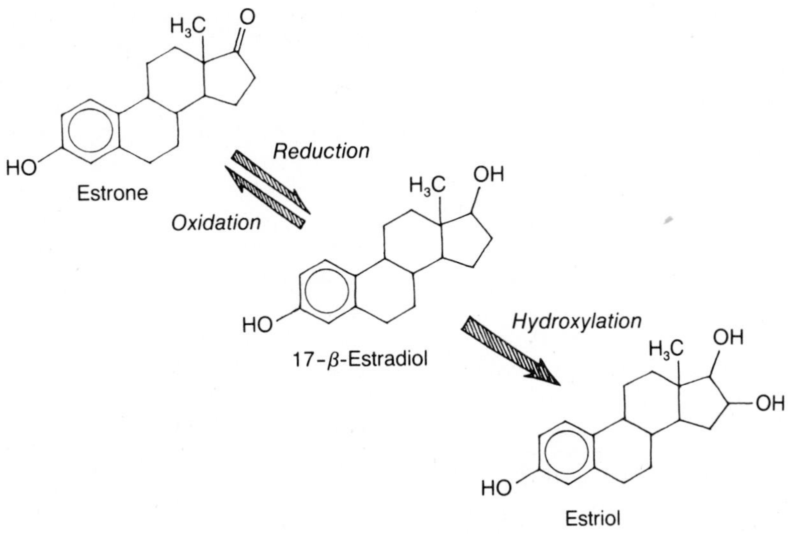

Figure 45-3   Natural estrogens.

- **Piperazine estrone sulfate** is a semisynthetic, water-soluble preparation; the usual dose is 1.5 mg daily by mouth.
- **17-β-Estradiol**—dermal patches are available for absorption through the intact skin (Estraderm®).

Synthetic Estrogens

Certain nonsteroidal substances are highly estrogenic. These compounds resemble natural estrogens in structure or spatial arrangement and thereby stimulate the same receptors in target tissues.

Diethylstilbestrol (DES). This is the simplest and most widely used of the synthetic estrogens. Despite its fairly simple chemical structure, it probably acts by assuming a conformation (Fig. 45–5) that enables it to bind to estrogen receptors.

Chlorotrianisene (TACE). Being very soluble in fat, this compound is stored in adipose tissue and is slowly released. Chlorotrianisene (Fig. 45–6) is converted in the liver to active estrogen.

The synthetics mentioned are equally effective by mouth or by injection, and they are cheaper than the natural estrogens.

Actions and Uses

The fundamental nature of action of estrogens at the cellular level is still unclear; however, estrogen is localized in the nuclei of cells of target tissues (uterine

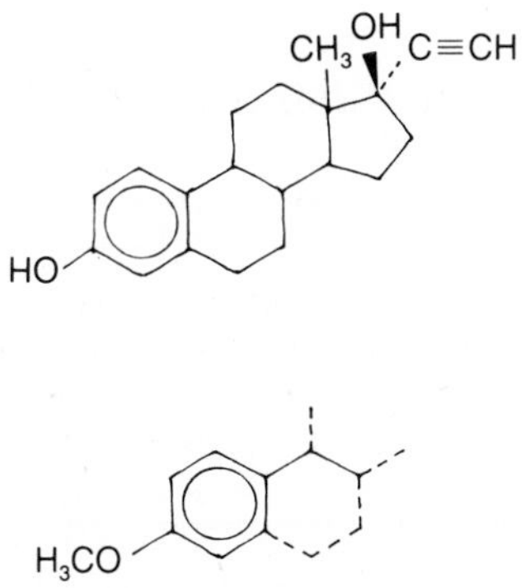

Figure 45-4   Structural formulae of (*upper*) ethinyl estradiol and (*lower*) mestranol, the C-3 methoxy derivative of ethinyl estradiol.

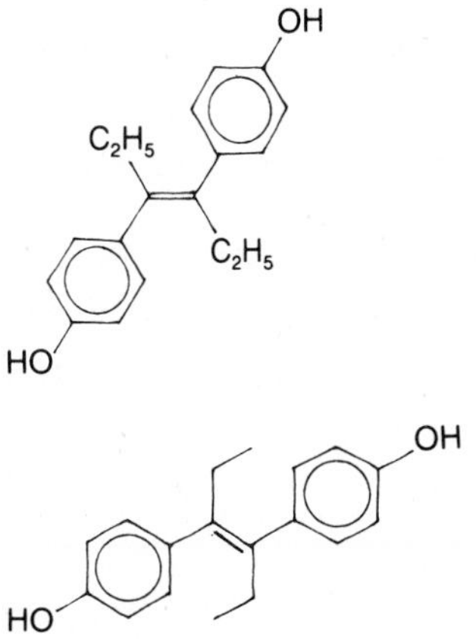

Figure 45-5   Formulae of diethylstilbestrol: (*upper*) structural formula; (*lower*) theoretical spatial arrangement (steroid form).

ENDOCRINE SYSTEMS

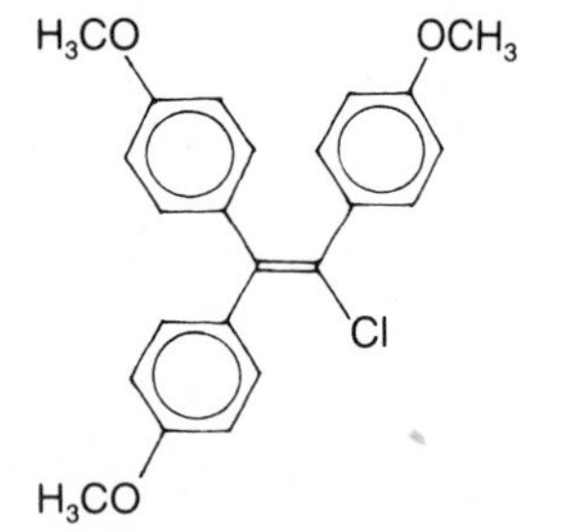

Figure 45–6 Structural formula of chlorotrianisene.

muscle, *etc.*) in association with specific receptor proteins. In such tissues a specific receptor (8S-protein) binds the steroid hormone, undergoes an activation process (conversion to a 5S-protein), and then interacts with nuclear chromatin. As a consequence, the production of messenger and ribosomal RNA is stimulated. This may not explain all the physiologic effects.

The **physiologic functions** of estrogens may be summarized as follows:

- Growth and development of reproductive organs.
- Development of secondary sex characteristics.
- Bone growth.
- Sexual behavior.
- "Priming" action for progesterone receptors.
- Feedback regulation of gonadotrophs, including stimulation of the preovulatory LH surge.

The **clinical uses** listed below are practically all consistent with some aspect of replacement therapy.

Menopausal symptoms. Following natural menopause or surgical castration, many patients show varying degrees of vasomotor instability, headache, emotional lability, *etc.* How much of this is physiologic, due to estrogen deficiency, and how much is due to other factors, is not clear. If severe symptoms require estrogens, the dose must be carefully and individually prescribed because overdosage can cause troublesome and serious toxic effects (*see below*). Cyclical administration, usually in combination with a progestin, is currently recommended.

Senile atrophic vaginitis. Local therapy, in the form of vaginal suppositories, may be used to avoid systemic effects.

Primary or secondary amenorrhea. Treatment may include simulation of natural cycles by substitution therapy with an oral contraceptive routine (*see* below). However, proper treatment depends on the underlying cause, and with the availability of accurate diagnostic techniques, an assessment of hormonal status and a rational approach to treatment is recommended.

Dysmenorrhea. In severe cases, continuous estrogen therapy in high doses from the beginning of the cycle suppresses ovulation and prevents the progesterone phase. Suspension of estrogen is followed by atyp-

ical but painless menstruation. This regimen has been supplanted in large part by using the combined estrogen-progestin oral contraceptive dosage schedule (*see* section on Fertility Control below).

Suppression of lactation. Postpartum administration of fairly large doses for 8–10 days stops lactation. This treatment is not used much currently, however. Bromocriptine is much better and avoids the dangers of high-dose estrogen.

Postmenopausal osteoporosis. Estrogens are often used, sometimes in conjunction with androgens. The anabolic effects of androgens and estrogens on the organic matrix of bone are complementary, even though effects on the primary and secondary sex organs are antagonistic. Thus, combined therapy may be more effective for osteoporosis, but the androgenic side effects, especially hirsutism, are often unacceptable for the patients.

Carcinoma of the prostate and breast. Estrogens are often used alone or in combination with surgical castration, especially when bony metastases are present. Like androgens, estrogens also promote Ca^{2+} retention by the kidney, so that there is a risk of hypercalcemia when unresponsive osteolytic lesions are present. In breast carcinoma in patients 5 or more years beyond menopause, estrogens often give better results than androgens; the explanation is unknown. In prostatic cancer, estrogen decreases androgens by shutting off LH and by increasing sex-hormone-binding globulin.

Contraception. Under normal circumstances, estrogens act with progesterone to inhibit the release of GnRH and gonadotropic hormones. This action is probably *via* the hypothalamus, although some direct action on the anterior pituitary occurs also. The axis is therefore turned off and ovulation does not occur. (*See* section on Fertility Control.)

"Morning after" contraceptive pill. Estrogen, given daily in high dosage for 5–6 days, is used for this purpose. Postulated effects include acceleration of passage of the fertilized ovum along the fallopian tube, as well as induction of withdrawal bleeding.

Hirsutism. Hirsutism resulting from excess androgens of ovarian origin may respond to estrogen therapy.

Adverse and Toxic Effects

- **Gastrointestinal upset** (nausea and vomiting) is the commonest disturbance; it is probably a local effect on the GI tract, because it usually occurs with fairly large doses of synthetic estrogens given by mouth.
- **Breast engorgement, endometrial hyperplasia, and bleeding** are the outcome of exaggerated normal actions of estrogens, and they may be quite uncomfortable and disturbing to the patient. Risk of endometrial carcinoma is increased if the estrogen is not combined with progestin.
- **Retention of Na^+ and water** occurs. As with androgens, resemblance to corticosteroids is shown by an effect on renal tubular reabsorption of elec-

trolytes. An increase in plasma renin substrate also occurs. Hypertension, weight gain, edema, or heart failure may occur. Caution is advisable in older patients.

- The use of estrogen predisposes in a dose-related fashion to **thromboembolic events**, such as thrombophlebitis, pulmonary embolism, myocardial infarction, stroke, and mesenteric and retinal thromboses. The risk is increased in smokers or in those over age 35.
- Stilbestrol has been implicated as the likely cause of the rare clear-cell **vaginal or cervical carcinoma** and more frequent benign abnormalities of the genital tract reported in a number of young women whose mothers received this drug during early pregnancy. In the male offspring, an increased incidence of genital abnormalities has been reported. Presumably the causal change was produced at a specific critical time of fetal development. The use of any estrogen in pregnancy is not recommended.
- Estrogen therapy may cause a lowering of LDL- and elevation of HDL-cholesterol.
- **Cholestatic jaundice** and an increased incidence of gallstones have been reported in patients taking estrogens. The formation of hepatic adenomas in long-term users is recognized.
- Carbohydrate tolerance may be impaired with estrogen therapy. Diabetics or those with positive family histories of diabetes should be followed closely.
- Onset of migraine **headaches** or exacerbation of migraine is experienced by some patients. Other nonspecific headaches may also occur.
- Many other **nonspecific effects** have been documented: appetite stimulation, depression, chloasma or hyperpigmentation, loss of scalp hair, rashes, pancreatitis, vaginal candidiasis, and post-pill amenorrhea.

Antiestrogens

Substances that modify or oppose the action of estrogens have been referred to as "antiestrogenic," and in this sense both progestins and androgens are antiestrogens. Other compounds, with a weak estrogenic effect, inhibit the action of potent estrogens by preventing their access to receptor sites. Clomiphene and tamoxifen belong to this group (Fig. 45–7). **Clomiphene** (Clomid®), an analog of chlorotrianisene, interferes with the "negative feedback" of estrogens on the hypothalamus and pituitary, resulting in an increase in the secretion of GnRH and gonadotropins. This stimulates ovarian function, and leads to maturation of multiple follicles, ovulation, and luteinization. It has been used successfully to treat infertility associated with anovulatory cycles. **Tamoxifen** (Nolvadex®) produces fewer toxic side effects and may have a greater blocking effect on peripheral target tissues than clomiphene. For this reason it is used in the palliative treatment of carcinoma of the breast, provided estrogen receptors are present in the tumor tissue.

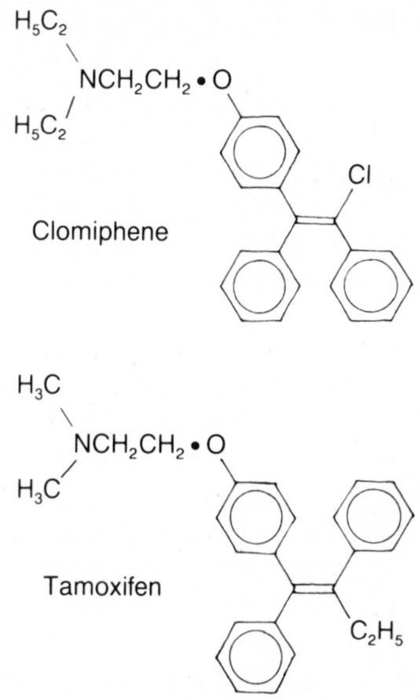

Figure 45–7 Structural formulae of clomiphene and tamoxifen.

PROGESTINS (Gestagens)

The chemical structure of **progesterone**, the natural hormone of the corpus luteum, is shown in Figure 45–8. It is also found in the placenta and adrenal cortex. For many years, it was the only progestin available, and because it is insoluble in water it had to be given in oily solution intramuscularly or as a microcrystalline suspension. This limited the clinical use, as did the scarcity of the substance. The development of orally active synthetic analogs has made wide use possible.

Metabolism and Excretion

Progesterone is biotransformed to pregnanolones and pregnanediol. The latter is conjugated with glucuronic acid in the liver and excreted *via* the kidney.

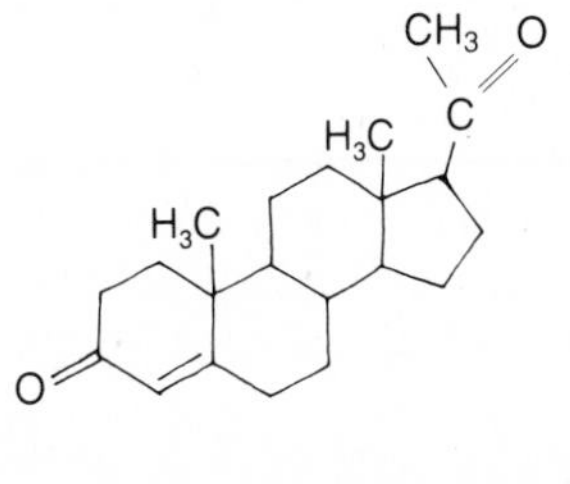

Figure 45–8 Structural formula of progesterone.

ENDOCRINE SYSTEMS

Actions and Uses

In the normal menstrual cycle, progesterone promotes secretory activity in an endometrium "primed" by estrogen in preparation for implantation of a fertilized ovum. In addition to its effect on the endometrium, it suppresses the production of gonadotropin and thus prevents further ovulation and further maturation of the follicles. Toward the end of the cycle the stimulation of the corpus luteum by LH decreases, and there is a consequent fall in the amount of progesterone produced (see Fig. 45–2). The abrupt fall in endogenous progesterone (or cessation of administration of exogenous progestin) produces local circulatory changes resulting in a shedding of the endometrium. If a fertilized ovum is implanted before this series of events takes place, hCG takes over the role of pituitary LH and supports the corpus luteum of pregnancy. The secretion of progesterone continues and the uterine endometrium is maintained as a favorable environment for pregnancy. Progesterone, with estrogen, prolactin, and other hormones, is important in breast development and lactation. It is also responsible for the rise in body temperature that occurs close to the midpoint of the menstrual cycle, corresponding with the time of ovulation.

The clinical use is based on these actions. By far the greatest use is as a component of oral contraceptive pills in combination with estrogen (discussed below in connection with fertility control). The availability of inexpensive oral progestins has also greatly extended the therapeutic uses, some of which are listed below:

- Dysfunctional uterine bleeding may be converted to regular cycles. A short period of twice-daily administration of a progestin, followed by sudden withdrawal, causes rapid shedding of endometrium and helps to control anovulatory bleeding.
- Endometriosis. When progestins are given for prolonged periods, the ectopic endometrial tissue undergoes some involution and develops areas of necrosis, thus presenting a decidua-like reaction.
- Progestins can be used to postpone menstruation, pre- or postoperatively, or for other reasons of convenience.
- They are used as adjunctive treatment of certain metastatic cancers, e.g., endometrial, breast, and renal.
- Progestins are the principal oral contraceptive agents (see section on Fertility Control).

Adverse Effects

- Thromboembolic events such as thrombophlebitis and pulmonary embolism have been reported.
- Edema and weight gain may result from fluid retention.
- Miscellaneous effects such as breakthrough bleeding, skin rashes, breast tenderness, and headache have been associated with progestins.

Many side effects relate to the androgenic action of 19-nor derivatives.

FERTILITY CONTROL

Decreasing Fertility

A decrease in fertility can be achieved in many ways:

- Interfering with fertilization by nonpharmacologic means, e.g., behavioral control, mechanical barriers.
- Impairing gametogenesis, e.g., by mitotic damage, due to alkylating agents, colchicine, nitrofurans.
- Interfering with maturation of gametes, e.g., by gossypol, a phenolic compound from cottonseed, which has been used in China as a male fertility inhibitor.
- Preventing ovulation: Suppression of gonadotropins by the use of 19-norprogestins, estrogens, or other agents. Prevention of gametogenesis by continuous dosage of long-acting analogs of GnRH, or possibly GnRH antagonists or antibodies.
- Interference before or at implantation by mechanical means (e.g., intrauterine device), or alteration of the endometrium by hormones (e.g., very low dosage of a progestin).
- Interference with gestation.

All these methods have been examined, but at present preventing ovulation is the most widely used.

Preparations

Some of the difficulties caused by newer synthetic compounds are related to their structural similarity to androgens, estrogens, progestins, and adrenal cortical steroids (Fig. 45–9). These newer compounds cross the lines between categories and have mixed properties. All are potent progestins, but norethynodrel has some estrogenic action; the others have some androgenic action, and all (as well as progesterone itself) have some corticosteroid-like activity.

The available commercial preparations (commonly known collectively as "the pill") include a small amount of estrogen, which acts with the progestin to inhibit both gonadotropins. Several manufacturers introduced a modification: sequential dosage starting with estrogen for 15–16 days followed by estrogen plus progestin for 5 days. This was withdrawn, but has been superseded by a "triphasic" regimen—a low dose of estrogen for 21 days combined with low but increasing doses of progestin for three successive periods of 7 days. When the oral contraceptive is discontinued, the endometrium is "shed."

The effectiveness of the combination oral contraceptives is beyond question—virtually 100%. The effectiveness of the sequential preparations appears to be

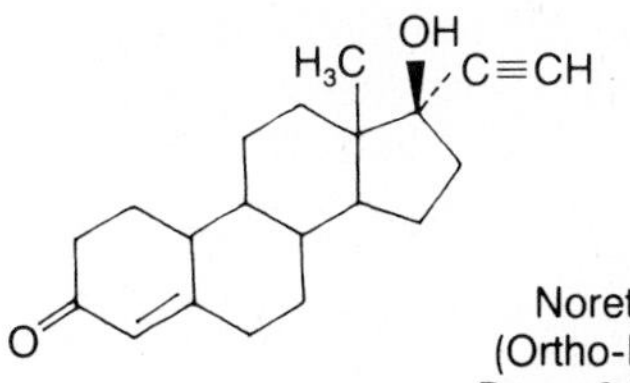

Figure 45–9 Synthetic progestogens used in oral contraceptive preparations.

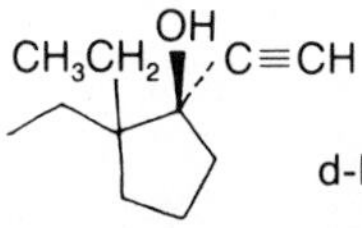

slightly less, and a low continuous dosage of progestin, the "mini-pill," is less effective again than the combinations. Generally, the incidence of side effects is low, and their nature depends to a large extent on the quantities of the two components in the combination pill.

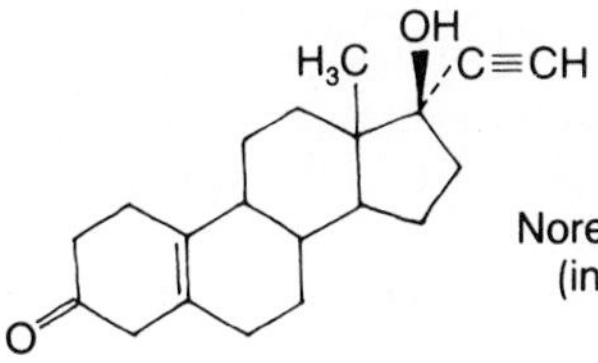

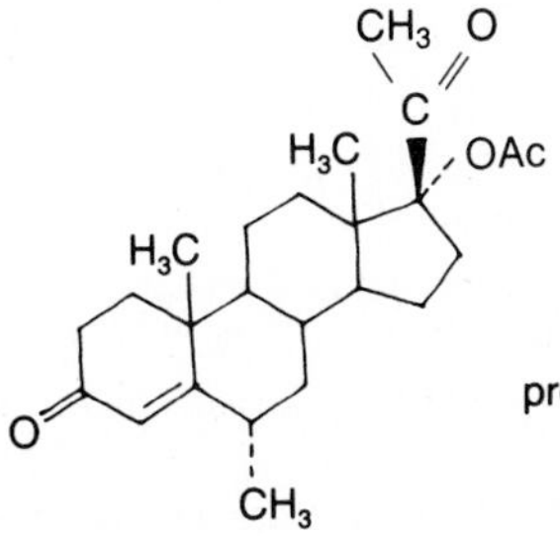

Side Effects

These were recognized soon after the use of the pill became widespread, and they include the separate side effects of estrogen and progesterone as described. Even the "low-dose" pills contain pharmacologic doses compared to the endogenous production of these hormones. The most common side effects are:

- Gain in body weight, mild edema, nausea, fullness

of breasts, headache, dizziness, depressed feeling.
- Changes in clotting factors (increase in factors VII, VIII, IX, X) and renin substrate; increase in concentration of thyroxine-binding globulin.
- Changes in carbohydrate metabolism, with a decrease in glucose tolerance.
- Occasional alteration in liver function tests, with elevation of SGOT, alkaline phosphatase, and serum bilirubin.
- Inhibition of lactation.
- In the adolescent, an acceleration in closure of epiphyses.

The "side effects" noted are adverse or potentially so. But there are also some very desirable features: peace of mind, fewer ovarian cysts, fewer benign breast lesions, fewer heavy and irregular periods, less dysmenorrhea. A decreased incidence of ovarian and endometrial carcinoma has been reported in users and previous users of the pill who are over the age of 40.

Gradually, evidence has accumulated that users of oral contraceptives have a higher incidence of most diseases of the cardiovascular system (thrombophlebitis, coronary disease, hypertension, cerebral vascular accidents). The incidence of gall bladder disease and of primary tumors of the liver is higher in users than in nonusers. Among young women, these hazards and the mortality associated with them are much less than the risks associated with pregnancy or abortion. In women over 40 years of age, mortality risks are still less than those associated with pregnancy; but in those over 40 who smoke, the risks are nearly three times those associated with childbirth.

Most of the early side effects, and probably the later ones related to intravascular blood clotting (acceleration of platelet aggregation, decrease in antithrombin III), are closely related to the dosage of estrogen. The lower dose of estrogen in most currently used preparations may be expected to lessen the incidence or severity of these effects. However, at least some progestins influence the clotting mechanism and have been shown to decrease the level of HDL-cholesterol. Thus, both components of the pill may contribute to the occurrence of fatal events such as myocardial infarction and hemorrhagic or thrombotic stroke. Genetic factors cannot be disregarded. For instance, increased risk of thromboembolic disease is about three times greater in women with blood groups A, B, or AB than in those with group O. This may be associated with the lower level of antithrombin III in persons of A, B, or AB groups. In summary, for myocardial infarction and stroke, oral contraceptives appear to multiply (rather than add to) the effects of age and other risk factors.

In terms of effectiveness and aesthetic acceptance, no method of contraception compares with the use of the combination pill. It seems clear that its benefits must be balanced against the costs involved. The costs are likely to be too high in the presence of the following

ENDOCRINE SYSTEMS

conditions, which are considered to be **absolute contra-indications:**

- Thromboembolic disease.
- Cerebrovascular disease.
- Impaired liver function.
- Carcinoma of the breast, or estrogen-dependent neoplasia.
- Undiagnosed bleeding.
- Pregnancy or suspected pregnancy.
- Classic migraine.

Combinations containing low doses of estrogen (less than 50 μg) are preferable, as they offer a low but effective dose with usually an acceptable level of side effects. Table 45–1 is a list of preparations available in Canada. With low-dose estrogen, "break-through" bleeding may occur, but other possible explanations of bleeding in patients using the pill are worth considering. For instance, the concurrent administration of substances that may induce microsomal enzymes of the liver may accelerate metabolism of estrogen, so reducing its effectiveness. This has been reported for tetracycline, rifampin, and ampicillin.

Usual Dosage

The dose is commonly 20–100 μg of ethinyl estradiol or mestranol with various amounts of a progestin, beginning on day 5 of the cycle and continuing for 21 days. Implants of a progestin (medroxyprogesterone) are effective for 3 months or more. The "mini-pill" (Micronor®) consisting of norethindrone 0.35 mg is taken continuously, but does not appear to be as effective as the combination.

Increasing Fertility

Stimulating ovulation and spermatogenesis might be expected to increase fertility. It had been suggested that after cessation of progestin administration fertility might be increased, but this has not proven to be the case. Indeed, a temporary decrease in fertility lasting several months is seen, except in patients with polycystic ovarian disease who may respond to the suppression of endogenous androgens by oral contraceptives with normalized ovulation and cycling for short periods after ovarian suppression.

Clomiphene citrate (*see* Fig. 45–7) is mildly estrogenic in the rat, but is antiestrogenic in the human. It stimulates ovulation (or spermatogenesis), presumably by blocking the negative feedback of endogenous estrogen on the hypothalamus, thus stimulating release of gonadotropins. Other means are effective, *e.g.*, FSH from a human source, followed by a large dose of hCG (to stimulate LH surge in the hope of causing ovulation). Judging from recent reports, multiple births may

occur more frequently than is usual. Lately, pulsed administration of GnRH (Factrel®) has been used successfully to increase fertility in males and females.

ANDROGENS

Physiology

The natural androgen produced in the Leydig or interstitial cells of the testis is testosterone (Fig. 45–10). In some tissues testosterone acts directly, while in others it is converted to more potent derivatives such as dihydrotestosterone. After binding to a specific receptor it becomes localized in the nuclei of target tissues (a similar mechanism to that of estrogens). Testosterone plays an essential role in spermatogenesis (initiated by FSH). Testosterone has a variety of physiologic effects, some of which are obviously related to male genital development (prostate, external genitalia), some to secondary sex characteristics (hair distribution, voice, *etc.*), and some of which are not obviously related to sexual development but to somatic development in general (development of skeletal muscle and organic matrix of bone). Most modifications of the testosterone molecule affect all these activities in equal proportions; for example, stanolone (androstan-17-ol-3-one), which resembles testosterone except that the 4–5 double bond is saturated, is a much weaker androgen and also a weaker anabolic hormone. All the modifications have a $-CH_3$ group at C-19 and are often referred to as C-19 steroids. Like estrogens, testosterone in blood is largely bound to a carrier protein, sex-hormone-binding globulin. Estrogen "competes" with androgen for the carrier protein and to some extent for receptors in target tissues. Examples of the actions of testosterone and its derivatives on various tissues are shown in Table 45–2.

Metabolism

In various tissues, but chiefly in the liver, testosterone is degraded in different ways, of which the most important are:

1. Reduction of the 3-keto group to $-OH$.
2. Oxidation of the 17-OH group to keto group.
3. Saturation of the 4–5 double bond.

These changes result in a large number of products, of which the most important quantitatively are shown in Figure 45–11.

These are all much less active as androgens. They are the main urinary excretion products of testicular origin, the so-called 17-ketosteroids. Others are found

TABLE 45–1 Representative Oral Contraceptives and Progestins

Estrogen	Progestogen	Product
Ethinyl Estradiol	Norethindrone	
35 µg	1.0 mg	Ortho-Novum 1/35
		Brevicon 1/35
35 µg	0.5 mg	Modacon
		Brevicon
35 µg	0.035, then 0.5 mg	Ortho 10/11
35 µg	0.5, then 0.75, then 1.0 mg	Ortho 7–7–7
Ethinyl Estradiol	Norethindrone Acetate	
50 µg	2.5 mg	Norlestrin 2.5/50
50 µg	1.0 mg	Norlestrin 1/50
30 µg	1.5 mg	Loestrin 1.5/30
20 µg	1.0 mg	Minestrin 1/20
Ethinyl Estradiol	d-Norgestrel	
50 µg	0.25 mg	Ovral
30 µg	0.15 mg	Min-Ovral
30–40–30 µg	0.05, 0.075, then 0.125 mg	Triphasil
Ethinyl Estradiol	Ethynodiol Diacetate	
50 µg	1.0 mg	Demulen 50
30 µg	2.0 mg	Demulen 30
Mestranol	Ethynodiol Diacetate	
100 µg	1.0 mg	Ovulen 1
100 µg	0.5 mg	Ovulen 0.5
Mestranol	Norethindrone	
100 µg	2.0 mg	Ortho-Novum 2
		Norinyl 2
100 µg	0.5 mg	Ortho-Novum 0.5
80 µg	1.0 mg	Norinyl 1/80
75 µg	5.0 mg	Ortho-Novum 5
50 µg	1.0 mg	Ortho-Novum 1/50
		Norinyl 1/50
Mestranol	Norethynodrel	
100 µg	2.5 mg	Enovid–E
	Norethindrone	
—	0.35 mg	Micronor
	Medroxyprogesterone Acetate	
—	5.0 mg	Provera
—	100.0 mg	Provera
	Medrogestone	
—	5.0 mg	Colpone

in smaller amounts, and most have a keto group. In the normal male, 70% of ketosteroids are derived from the adrenal cortex, the most important being dehydro-epiandrosterone. In the female almost all (98%) are from the adrenal cortex.

Since these natural modifications all result in loss of activity, synthetic changes for pharmacologic purposes are of two different types: those that modify solubility and susceptibility to enzymatic breakdown, and hence affect route and duration of action; and those intended to give some separation between androgenic and anabolic effects.

Modified Testosterones

Testosterone is readily absorbed from the GI tract, but it is altered and inactivated during passage through the liver before reaching the systemic circulation. If injected in oily solution, it is metabolized quickly (half-life generally 10–20 minutes). In order to modify its solubility in oil, so as to delay absorption and prolong its action, it has been converted to esters that are much less polar. The ester of propionic acid at the 17-OH position produces a steady effect when injected at 2-

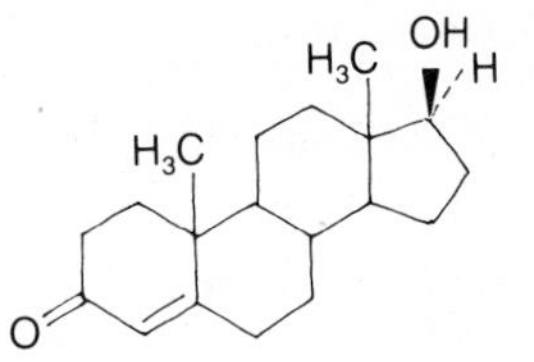

Figure 45-10 Structural formula of testosterone.

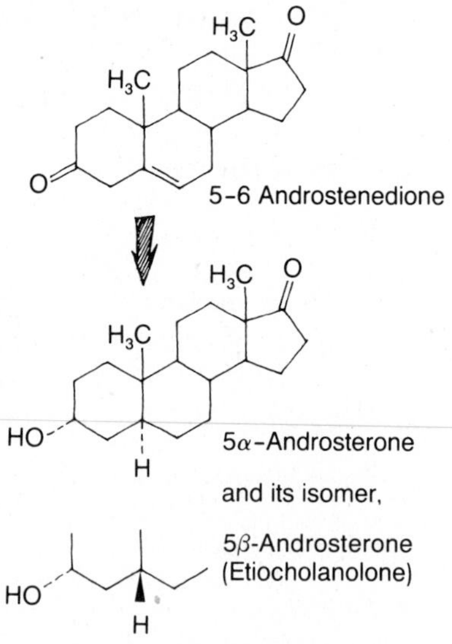

Figure 45-11 Metabolic products of testosterone.

to 3-day intervals. The cypionate (cyclopentylpropionate) and enanthate esters are effective for periods of up to 2 weeks. Crystals in aqueous suspension may also be injected intramuscularly. Compressed pellets of testosterone implanted in subcutaneous tissue afford slow release over periods of 4–8 months.

A different set of modifications consists of the addition of a methyl group at C-17 ("1" in Fig. 45-12) to yield methyltestosterone, or the insertion of an − F ("2") and − OH group ("3") in methyltestosterone to produce fluorohydroxymethyltestosterone (= fluoxymesterone, Halotestin®, see Fig. 45-12).

These changes facilitate absorption of the product through the oral mucosa, so that it can be administered as tablets placed under the tongue; this mode of administration bypasses the liver so that the same distribution through the body is achieved as by injection. In addition, these modifications result in slower metabolic inactivation of the compound, so that the effects are prolonged and the dose may be reduced.

Uses

1. Androgenic action suggests the first use, namely replacement therapy in cases of testicular hypofunction, whether primary, or secondary to pituitary failure.

TABLE 45-2   Examples of the Actions of Testosterone and its Derivatives

Intracellular Product	Examples of Actions
Testosterone	Development of structures derived from Wolffian duct Erythropoietin synthesis Pectoral muscle development Kidney hypertrophy
5α-DHT	Growth of genital tubercle, hair
Estradiol	Brain: behavioral effects Gonadotropin secretion Anabolic effects on some muscle
5β-DHT	Red cell production in bone marrow

Maintenance of secondary sexual characteristics, muscular development, and prevention of anemia are characteristic of androgenic action.

2. Normal growth depends on a combination of actions of growth hormone, insulin, thyroid hormones, and gonadal hormones. Dihydrotestosterone and testosterone bind to androgen receptors and initiate effects at the nucleus. The nuclear action results in increased production of specific RNAs and subsequently increased protein synthesis. Ultimately this results in the development and increased functional capacity of target tissues. As with other steroid hormones, the exact mechanisms are unknown. In any case, it leads to retention of nitrogen in the body, an increase in the mass of skeletal muscle, and an increase in the organic matrix of bone. Therefore, androgens are used with the other "growth" hormones in the treatment of pituitary dwarfism to promote skeletal growth. With higher doses there is a danger of earlier closure of epiphyses, limiting growth to an increase in thickness of bones.

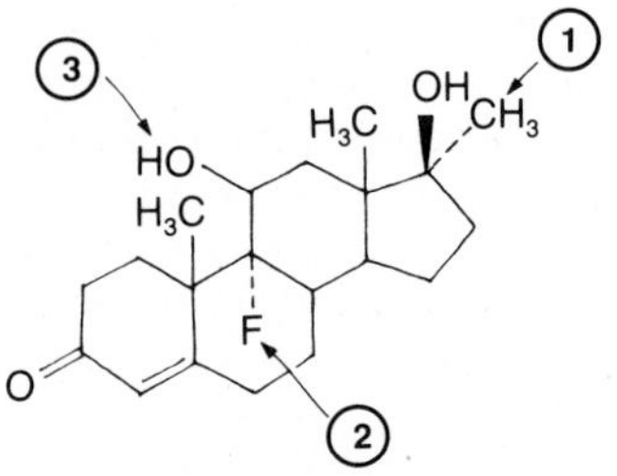

Figure 45-12 Structural formula of fluoxymesterone.

3. Carcinoma of the breast in the female is activated by estrogens and inhibited by androgens. Androgens are used therapeutically in such cases to reverse the normal endocrine balance. However, this means that other effects of androgens occur: changes in hair distribution, voice, external genitalia, *etc*. Therefore, they are used only in cases in which surgery, radiation, and other antitumor drugs cannot be used. Most often, these are cases with extensive metastases especially to the skeleton. Androgens cause regression of bony lesions in many cases, followed by reossification, for periods of a few months to 2 years or more. Patients with extensive bony metastases often show increased excretion of calcium, which may lead to calcium stone formation in the kidneys. Calcium excretion is sharply reduced by androgens, partly by recalcification of lesions and partly by renal action from increased tubular reabsorption. **Risk**: In some cases androgens do not stop growth of bony metastases and in a few cases may even make them worse; with continuing osteolysis and calcium release, the action of androgens causing calcium reabsorption in the kidney may cause hypercalcemia and muscular paralysis. Stopping androgens and giving EDTA may reverse this condition.

4. Anabolic effects of androgens are used in various situations: to offset catabolic effects of adrenal cortical hormones; in burn treatment; in senile osteoporosis; to speed recovery from chronic debilitating diseases or operations; in uremia to slow accumulation of nonprotein nitrogen; to increase muscle mass in athletes, *etc*. In athletes, only long-term use of anabolic steroids can be expected to improve competitive performance, and there are risks attendant on such use. National and international athletic federations disapprove strongly of the use of anabolic steroids for such purposes.

5. The mild anemia associated with hypogonadism is corrected by administration of androgens. Large doses have been observed to cause polycythemia. Androgens are used in the treatment of aplastic anemia, hemolytic anemia, and anemias associated with lymphomas, renal failure, and leukemia. The consensus is that in mild anemias androgenic steroids are beneficial, but in severe cases they are of little use. The action is on erythropoiesis, most likely by stimulating the secretion of erythropoietin from the kidney. As other cells of bone marrow are stimulated also, a direct effect also seems likely. For these purposes, androgenic effects *per se* are undesirable but unavoidable side effects. If anabolic effects could be separated from virilizing effects, the androgens would be much more useful for this purpose. This separation is claimed for newer synthetic modifications such as norethandrolone and nandrolone (Fig. 45–13). Analogous compounds, stanozolol (Winstrol®) and methandrostenolone (Dianabol®), are in use. Undoubtedly they are less androgenic than testosterone, but the extent to which they are less androgenic, and therefore better for this purpose, will have to be ascertained in long clinical trials.

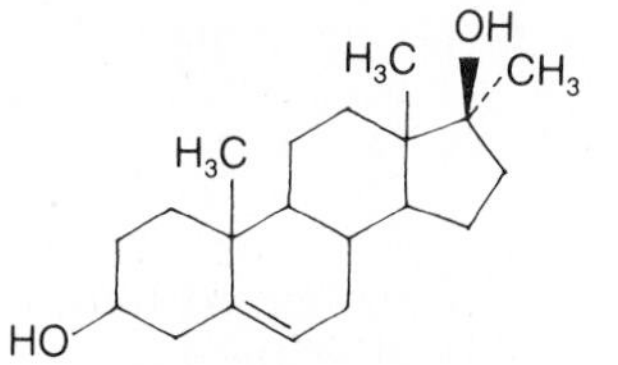

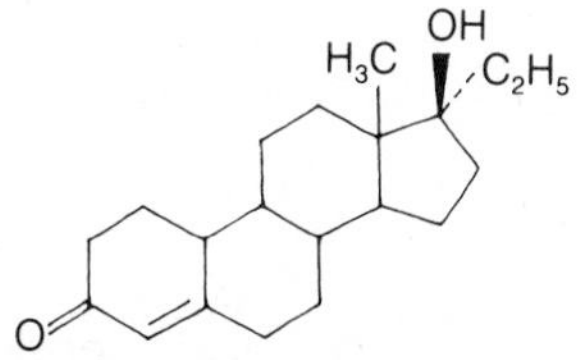

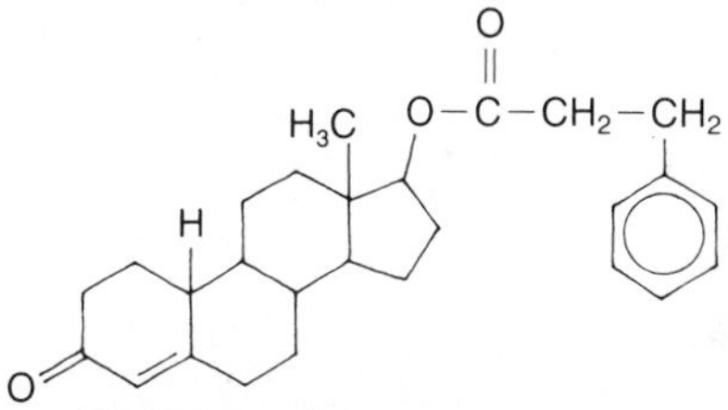

Figure 45–13 Some modified androgenic preparations.

Dangers

Virilization is the commonest side effect. All androgens can cause salt and water retention (compare their structures with those of corticosteroids) and should be used cautiously if heart failure is a threat.

Androgens with a methyl or ethyl group on C-17 cause abnormality of the bromsulphthalein excretion test and a rise in SGOT level. This appears to be a direct effect on the liver, related to dose, and not a sensitivity reaction (*see* Chapter 62). A high dose or prolonged use may cause dilatation of biliary ducts, cholestasis, obstructive jaundice, and even carcinoma. Anabolic-androgenic steroid administration also reduces output of testosterone and gonadotropins, thus causing a reduction in spermatogenesis.

SUGGESTED READING

Crowley WJ Jr. Development of a male contraceptive—a beginning. N Engl J Med 1981; 305:695–696.

Ferland L, Labrie F, Kelly PA, Raymond V. Interactions between hypothalamic and peripheral hormones in the control of prolactin secretion. Fed Proc 1980; 39(11): 2917–2922.

Kaufman DW, Shapiro S, Slone D, et al. Decreasing risk of endometrial cancer among oral contraceptive users. N Engl J Med 1980; 303:1045–1047.

Knobil E. Patterns of hormone signals and hormone action. N Engl J Med 1981; 305:1582–1583.

Pincus G. The control of fertility. New York: Academic Press, 1965.

Ryan AJ. Anabolic steroids are fool's gold. Fed Proc 1981; 40(12):2682–2688.

Shapiro S, Kaufman DW, Slone D, et al. Recent and past use of conjugated estrogens in relation to adenocarcinoma of the endometrium. N Engl J Med 1980; 303: 485–489.

Stadel BV. Oral contraceptives and cardiovascular disease. N Engl J Med 1981; 305:612–618 (part I); 672–677 (part II).

Szoka PR, Edgren RA. Drug interactions with oral contraceptives: compilation and analysis of an adverse experience report database. Fertil Steril 1988; 49(suppl 2):31S–38S.

Wilson JD, Foster DW. Williams' textbook of endocrinology. 7th ed. Philadelphia: WB Saunders, 1985.

Yen SSC, Jaffe RB. Reproductive endocrinology. Philadelphia: WB Saunders, 1986.

Chapter 46

INSULIN AND ORAL HYPOGLYCEMIC AGENTS

B.P. Schimmer and S.R. George

Diabetes has been recognized for centuries as a debilitating disease, characterized by excretion of large volumes of "sugar urine," excessive thirst, wasting of tissue (loss of nitrogen), and in severe cases the development of ketoacidosis, coma, and death.

An extract of pancreas, prepared by F.G. Banting and C.H. Best at the University of Toronto in 1921, contained an active principle (insulin) capable of controlling the hyperglycemia of diabetes. Since then, insulin has given life to millions of diabetics, but because diabetics may have children and live longer than before, the incidence and the absolute number of diabetics are increasing.

Two major classes of the disease are recognized: Type I, insulin-dependent diabetes mellitus (IDDM), and Type II, non-insulin-dependent diabetes mellitus (NIDDM). The first (Type I) often occurs in juveniles and is characterized by destruction of β cells of the pancreas, with resulting severe insulin deficiency and a tendency to ketoacidosis. The second (Type II) is often slow in onset, occurs in older age groups, and the hyperglycemia may not be due only to a lack of insulin.

The objectives of treatment are the same for both types—to maintain blood glucose within normal limits and to prevent the development of complications of diabetes mellitus.

INSULIN

Insulin is a protein with a molecular weight of about 6000 and is made up of two polypeptide chains (51 amino acids) linked by two disulfide bridges (Fig. 46–1). It is produced in the β cells of the islets of Langerhans initially as a precursor molecule, proinsulin (formed from a larger precursor, pre-proinsulin), which is cleaved by proteolytic enzymes to form insulin. Bovine insulin differs more from human insulin (three amino acids) than does that derived from the pig (one amino acid), which may explain the lesser antigenicity of pork insulin in therapeutic use. The differences are shown in Table 46–1.

Most of the insulin in the β cells of the pancreas (approximately 200 units) is packaged in secretory granules. Under appropriate stimulation the contents of the granules are released into the extracellular space by exocytosis. Some proinsulin and connecting "C" peptide are released into the circulation along with insulin, but do not contribute significantly to bioactivity. Plasma insulin measured by bioassay (insulin-like activity, ILA) differs qualitatively and quantitatively (higher) from insulin measured immunochemically (immunoreactive insulin, IRI). Therefore, some insulin-like activity must be ascribed to sources other than insulin from the β cells.

The molecule contains a high proportion of dicarboxylic acids (isoelectric point about pH 2), which enables it to combine readily with basic proteins without affecting its fundamental structure. This is an important fact utilized in the preparation of insulin for clinical use. In an acid medium it tends to polymerize into insoluble fibrils.

Physiology

The main physiologic stimulus for insulin secretion is a rise in blood sugar. Glucose produces a rapid release of insulin, as well as a secondary, slower release that raises blood levels of insulin for about an hour. This slow release is attributed to synthesis and release of new insulin, since it is inhibited by the protein synthesis inhibitor puromycin. Growth hormone also stimulates the synthesis of insulin, but probably does not have a direct effect on its release. Other factors that may enhance the release of insulin include secretin, pancreozymin, gastroinhibitory polypeptide (GIP), gastrin, glucagon, some amino acids (arginine, leucine), and

465

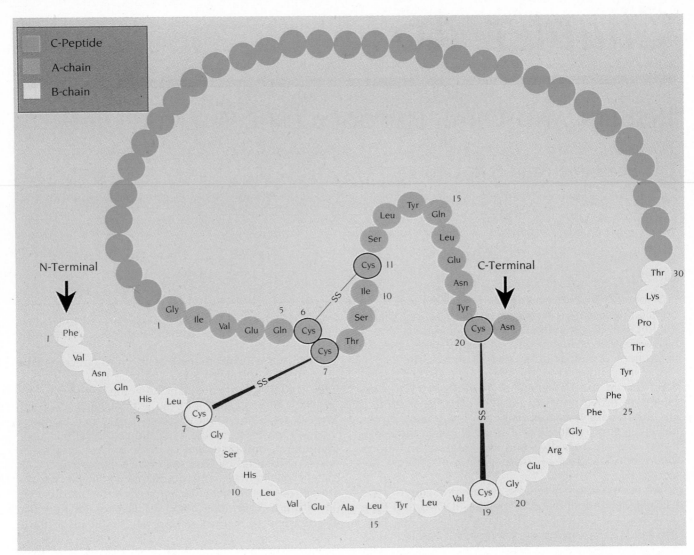

Figure 46-1 Structure of human insulin (A-chain = 21 amino acids, B-chain = 30 amino acids, connected by two of three disulfide bridges at positions A7–B7 and A20–B19). The proinsulin molecule contains a "C-peptide" of 31 amino acids, which is removed by proteolysis to form insulin.

free fatty acids (FFA). Drugs of the sulfonylurea group (tolbutamide, chlorpropamide) also stimulate release of insulin (Fig. 46–2).

TABLE 46-1 Species-Specific Structural Differences Between Human, Porcine, and Bovine Insulin (*cf.* Figure 46-1)

	A–8	A–10	B–30	C-Peptide Amino Acids
Man	Thr	Ile	Thr	31
Pig	Thr	Ile	Ala	33
Ox	Ala	Val	Ala	30

Autonomic mediators also influence secretion of insulin. Adrenaline and noradrenaline (through α receptors) inhibit the secretion induced by a rise in blood glucose. In contrast, substances that stimulate β_2 adrenoceptors increase insulin secretion, and beta-blockers inhibit it. Vagal stimulation and cholinomimetic drugs enhance the release of insulin.

Glucose taken orally has a greater effect on insulin secretion than glucose by injection, the likely explanation being that glucose taken orally concurrently stimulates the secretion of glucagon, "gut-glucagon," and digestive hormones. These in turn stimulate the release of insulin from the islet cells.

It has been shown that somatostatin, as well as inhibiting the secretion of growth hormone, inhibits the secretion of both insulin and glucagon by direct action

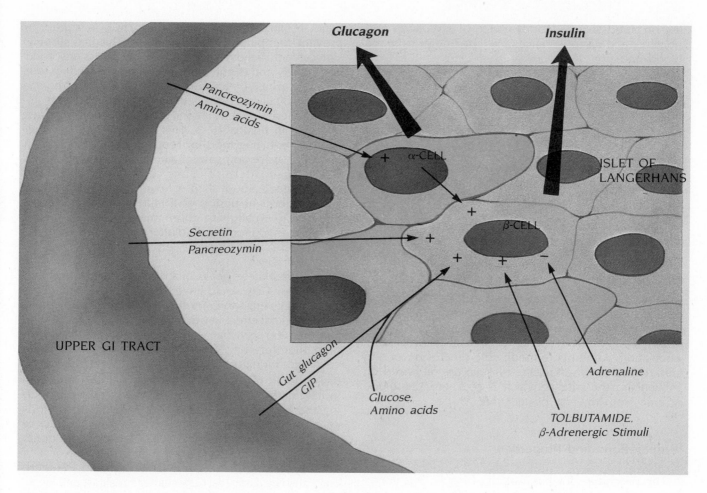

Figure 46–2 Factors involved in the stimulation (+) and inhibition (−) of insulin production and release.

on β and α cells of the pancreas. The presence of somatostatin has been demonstrated in the "D" cells of the islets of the pancreas, as well as in a large number of secretory cells throughout the gastrointestinal tract. Since it also inhibits the secretion of gastrin, secretin, cholecystokinin, pepsin, and HCl, its physiologic role seems complex.

The interaction of insulin with its receptors in cell membranes results in the activation of receptor-associated tyrosine kinase and possibly the generation of an intracellular second messenger. How these early signalling events are linked to the end-effects of insulin is not understood. End-responses to insulin include: (1) an alteration in the membrane that permits an increased rate of entry of glucose, amino acids, and ions such as potassium, magnesium, and phosphate into the cell, and (2) an increased utilization of glucose within the cell, which may be used to store energy (synthesis of glycogen, fat, protein), or be used as a fuel.

Insulin, perhaps by an intracellular mediator, may reduce the sensitivity of a protein kinase to cyclic AMP (thus decreasing the breakdown of glycogen) and at the same time produce an activation of glycogen synthetase. The facilitated diffusion mechanism stimulated by insulin, which transports glucose across the cell membranes of skeletal muscle and adipocytes, is not required in neurons, erythrocytes, or liver cells, and probably is not required in the intestine or kidney tubules.

Insulin is an anabolic and anticatabolic hormone. Glucose uptake and oxidative metabolism by muscle and other tissues are increased. This prevents breakdown of tissue protein and conversion of residual amino acids into glucose by the liver. It also prevents mobilization of fatty acids from fat depots, and breakdown of these by the liver with formation of ketone bodies. Indeed, fat synthesis from glucose is promoted by insulin. In the diabetic, these actions result in a lower-

ENDOCRINE SYSTEMS

ing of blood sugar, disappearance of glycosuria and polyuria, and disappearance of ketone bodies from the blood and urine.

Fate of Injected Insulin

Like any protein, insulin can be digested (and inactivated) in the gastrointestinal tract. Therefore, it must be administered by injection. When crystalline zinc insulin (or the noncrystalline amorphous insulin) at a neutral pH is injected subcutaneously, it is absorbed rapidly, and within minutes can be detected in the cells of liver, kidney, and muscle. These tissues (particularly liver and kidney) contain an enzyme, insulinase, that is of primary importance in degrading the hormone. After intravenous injection the plasma half-life of insulin is less than 9 minutes. Its volume of distribution approximates that of extracellular fluid. The fate of injected insulin is different from that of secreted insulin. About 50% of insulin secreted into the portal vein is destroyed in the liver and never reaches the general circulation. Attempts to modify the time of onset and duration of action of injected insulin are all based on influencing the rate at which it gets into the blood stream from the site of injection.

Preparations and Properties

The procedure for purification of insulin has undergone almost continuous refinement and modification, resulting in a great variety of preparations for specific therapeutic purposes (Table 46–2). In earlier days contamination with its precursors, with glucagon, and with other hormones produced in the pancreas was usual. This is no longer the case.

Insulin (Zinc Crystalline), Beef and Pork; Insulin Injection U.S.P.; Insulin Toronto

Crystalline zinc insulin (CZI) is a solution of purified insulin extracted from beef or pork pancreas, containing enough zinc to permit crystallization of insulin as a zinc salt, which is then redissolved. One mg of crystalline insulin = 22 units. It usually is given subcutaneously, although the intravenous route is used in emergencies. It lowers blood sugar within minutes and reaches a peak effect in about 4 hours. The blood sugar returns to its starting level after 8–12 hours. However, the duration and magnitude of effect depend on the dose and the individual patient.

Insulin (Protamine Zinc) Beef and Pork; Protamine Zinc Insulin Suspension U.S.P. (PZI)

PZI is formed by treating crystalline insulin with protamine at pH 7.2, causing a fine precipitate of prota-

mine insulin. A small amount of $ZnCl_2$ is added to prevent clumping of the precipitate. This fine suspension can only be given subcutaneously, and is absorbed very slowly and evenly. It has no short-term effect, but slowly reaches a maximum action by about 24 hours, then gradually wears off over the next 24 hours.

The different time relations of these preparations are idealized in Figure 46–3. This picture might be seen in subjects taking food in frequent small amounts, so that there were no peaks of alimentary hyperglycemia. The normal pattern of eating consists of taking three or four meals about 4 to 6 hours apart, followed by a long overnight period with little or no food. Therefore there usually are three main peaks of hyperglycemia—mid-morning, mid-afternoon, and early evening. Blood sugar is lower overnight and lowest in the early morning.

To control these peaks in a diabetic, Insulin Injection (Regular or CZI) would have to be given several times daily. PZI given in the morning would cover supper and have maximal effect in the early morning before breakfast the next day, but would be wearing off by lunchtime; therefore one would have the risk of inadequate coverage during the day and hypoglycemia during the night. Some of these shortcomings can be overcome in mild diabetics who are on small doses by distributing the bulk of food intake to coincide with periods of maximum insulin action or by altering the time of injection. In more severe cases, this cannot be done, and other modifications of insulin are useful.

Formerly, mixtures of regular insulin and PZI were used, the regular for fast effect after breakfast and lunch, PZI to cover after the supper period and overnight. To a considerable extent, such mixtures have been replaced by the following preparations.

Insulin (Isophane) Beef and Pork; NPH Insulin (Neutral Protamine Hagedorn)

This is a suspension of crystalline zinc insulin and protamine at neutral (7.2) pH. It contains less protamine than PZI, and is intermediate in duration of action between CZI and PZI. It is also available from beef *or* pork.

Lente Insulins

These are suspensions of insulin in acetate buffer at pH 7.2. The physical state and crystal size influence the rate of absorption from the site of injection.

1. **Insulin (Semilente); Prompt Insulin Zinc Suspension (U.S.P.)**—a suspension of amorphous insulin.
2. **Insulin (Ultralente); Extended Insulin Zinc Suspension (U.S.P.)**—large crystals, slow absorption, similar to PZI in duration of action.
3. **Insulin (Lente); Insulin Zinc Suspension U.S.P. (intermediate)** made up of 70% ultralente and 30% semilente—its effect is similar to that of NPH, but it has quicker onset.

TABLE 46–2 Summary of Available Insulin Preparations

"PARCOST" Name*	U.S.P. Official Name	Common Synonyms	Action (hours):		
			Onset	Peak	Duration
Rapid Action					
Insulin (Zinc Crystalline)‡ Beef, Pork, Beef and Pork†	Insulin injection U.S.P.	Regular‡; CZI‡; Toronto-Neutral‡	0.5	3–5	8–12
Insulin (Zinc Crystalline) Human Biosynthetic (rDNA Origin)‡			0.5	3–5	6–8
Insulin (Semilente) Beef and Pork	Prompt Insulin Zinc Suspension U.S.P.		0.5	5–10	14–16
Intermediate Action					
Insulin (Isophane) Beef, Pork, Beef and Pork†	Isophane Insulin Suspension U.S.P.	NPH; NPH–50	2.5	4–12	12–24
Insulin (Isophane) Human Biosynthetic (rDNA Origin)			1.5	4–12	12–24
Insulin (Lente) Beef, Beef and Pork†	Insulin Zinc Suspension U.S.P.	Lente; Insulin Zinc Suspension Intermediate	2.5	7–15	12–24
Prolonged Action					
Insulin (Protamine Zinc) Beef, Pork, Beef and Pork†	Protamine Zinc Insulin Suspension U.S.P.	PZI	4	10–30	36
Insulin (Ultralente) Beef and Pork	Extended Insulin Zinc Suspension U.S.P.	Ultralente; Insulin Zinc Suspension Prolonged	4	10–30	36

* Ontario Ministry of Health PARCOST Comparative Drug Index. February 1984.
† Available as single-species (beef *or* pork) and mixed-species (beef *and* pork) preparation; prescriber must specify.
‡ Only Regular (Crystalline Zinc) Insulin can be given intravenously.

Since 1975, all preparations in North America have been standardized at 100 U/mL. To avoid risk of incorrect dosage, the patient must use a syringe calibrated for this fairly recent standardization. Outside North America preparations of 20, 40, and 80 U/mL are encountered.

Sulfated Insulin (Beef and Pork)

Sulfated Insulin (Beef and Pork) is used in patients with insulin resistance. Insulin antibodies do not appear to bind to it.

Human Insulin

Human insulin is available as regular, lente, and isophane (NPH) Insulin. It is produced at present by two distinctly different techniques.

1. Recombinant DNA molecules introduced into bacteria direct the synthesis of the A chains and B chains of insulin. The two chains are purified and chemically combined to form the active hormone (Humulin®).

2. Substitution of threonine for alanine at position 30 of the B chain of pork insulin. This is a chemical conversion of porcine to human insulin (*cf.* Fig. 46–1 and Table 46–1).

Human insulin is absorbed more quickly from its site of injection than insulin from animal sources. Therefore, the duration of action of human insulin is shorter and doses must be adjusted to compensate.

Clinical Uses

Diabetes Mellitus

The most obvious use, as with any hormone, is for replacement therapy where the patient's own insulin is deficient. In milder cases (maturity onset) dietary control alone is often sufficient. If not, suitable therapy consists of giving a diet that is adequate for the patient's metabolic needs and adding insulin of a type and amount sufficient to keep the urine essentially free of sugar and ketones and the blood sugar within normal range.

ENDOCRINE SYSTEMS

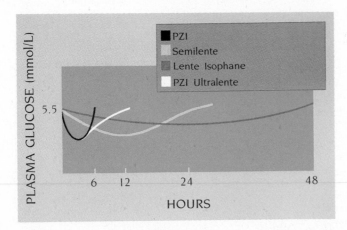

Figure 46-3 Usual patterns of blood sugar responses with different insulin preparations.

Diabetic Coma

This is an emergency situation because the patient may die of dehydration and acidosis. Intravenous fluid and crystalline zinc or regular insulin, intravenously and subcutaneously, are indicated. The soluble short-acting type of insulin is needed to achieve rapid and flexible therapy, since the condition of the patient can change rapidly with massive administration of intravenous fluid and electrolytes. A recent development is to administer 0.1 unit CZI per kg body weight per hour by infusion, which approximates the normal rate of insulin delivery to the periphery and produces a level of venous plasma insulin (about 100 μU/mL) close to that seen after a carbohydrate meal.

Diagnostic Test

Insulin is also used as a diagnostic test for growth hormone and ACTH secretion from the anterior pituitary.

Occasional or Historic Uses

A small dose of regular insulin before meals causes mild hypoglycemia, which stimulates appetite. This has been used in the past to increase food intake in patients with anorexia nervosa and other functional impairments of appetite.

Large doses of regular insulin were formerly used in serious depression or schizophrenia for the deliberate production of hypoglycemic shock, which is equivalent to electroshock or pentylenetetrazol (metrazol) convulsions in its effect on the patient's mental state.

Undesired Side Effects

The following side effects are usually encountered only in chronic use, *i.e.*, in diabetes.

Hypoglycemic Reactions

Mild reactions are common and are seen when a meal is missed, when an overdose of insulin has been taken, or when unusually heavy work has been done. The typical symptoms include sweating, weakness, hunger, "being ill at ease" (resulting from a compensating increase in the secretion of adrenaline), diplopia, and mental confusion; severe cases may go on to convulsions or coma. If the latter occurs, it is important to differentiate it from diabetic coma (Table 46-3).

Laboratory tests provide conclusive differentiation. Where rapid laboratory service is not available and diagnosis is uncertain, try intravenous glucose first. This will cure hypoglycemic coma in minutes, and will not do much harm to diabetic coma. The other way around, *i.e.*, giving insulin in hypoglycemic coma, may kill the patient.

Local Lipodystrophy

Irregular atrophy and lumpiness of subcutaneous fat may occur if repeated injections are given in the same place. To prevent this occurrence, the sites of injection may be rotated. This complication is less common with purified preparations of insulin.

Insulin Presbyopia

This visual disturbance is due to osmotic changes in ocular fluids; this occurs early in therapy, but is usually transitory.

Facial Edema

Edema of the face may occur (lasting for a few weeks), but it is not clinically important.

Insulin Allergy

Severe allergy, with urticaria, angioneurotic edema, *etc.*, occurs in 1-2% of patients. The allergic reaction is not usually due to insulin itself, but to traces of other proteins present. This can be overcome by use of highly purified recrystallized insulin or by switching to insulin from another species. Most insulins are beef-pork mixtures, but pure pork insulin is available, and most cases of allergy appear to be due to the beef component. As might be expected, human insulin is less aller-

TABLE 46–3 Differentiation Between "Hypoglycemic Shock" and Diabetic Coma

	Acute "Hypoglycemic Shock"	Diabetic Coma
Onset	Rapid	Gradual—over days
Acidosis, Dehydration	No	Severe
Preceding infection	No	Common, often with vomiting or diarrhea
Skin	Pale, sweating	Hot, dry
Respiration	Normal or shallow	Deep—"air hunger"
CNS	Tremor, mental confusion (even coma), occasionally convulsions; may have positive Babinski sign	General depression

genic than that from bovine-porcine sources; however, there is a potential risk of sensitivity to traces of *E. coli* protein in the recombinant form of the hormone.

Insulin Resistance

A total diabetic (*e.g.*, a pancreatectomized patient) usually requires from 30 to 50 units of insulin per day for control. A requirement of 200 units or more per day (clearly a high value) indicates that the patient is "resistant" to insulin. Occasionally 1000 or more units fail to control hyperglycemia and the frequent attendant ketoacidosis. In itself, ketoacidosis inhibits uptake of glucose by tissue cells. Infections, uremia, surgical trauma, and even anxiety tend to increase insulin requirements. In such cases the resistance may be due to increased secretion of adrenocortical hormones or to increased secretion of glucagon. With appropriate treatment of the underlying condition, resistance may disappear.

Less frequently, resistance is very severe, and other causes have been identified. Insulin-binding antibodies in large amounts have been demonstrated in plasma. As noted earlier, the antibodies may be selective for bovine rather than porcine insulin. Highly purified pork insulin and human insulin are available. A change in the number and nature of insulin receptors in cell membranes has also been implicated as a cause of variability in response to endogenous as well as exogenous insulin. Fewer receptors are present in the cells of obese Type II diabetics than of non-diabetics, and relatively high blood insulin levels are frequently observed in such individuals.

Problems and Prospects

As indicated earlier, insulin has dramatically increased life expectancy, but the complications of diabetes

mellitus—cardiovascular, renal, neural, and ocular—remain unpleasant prospects for the diabetic. It has been assumed that good control of blood sugar would prevent such complications, and there is indirect evidence supporting this assumption. Incontrovertible proof is hard to produce, but if obtained, would prove the need for rigid control and justify the attendant difficulties in achieving it.

It has been difficult or impossible in the past for ambulant patients to monitor blood glucose, so that most insulin-dependent and many non-insulin-dependent diabetics have had periods of hyperglycemia (and often hypoglycemia). Reliable methods for monitoring blood glucose at home, using a drop of fingertip blood, are now available. Also, it has been found that fractions of hemoglobin are slowly and irreversibly glycosylated during the life of the red cell. The concentration of the principal glycosylated fraction (HbA_1C) therefore reflects the time-averaged glucose level to which the hemoglobin has been exposed during the life of the red cell (about 120 days).

Along with these means of assessing the degree of control, attention has been paid to the continuous delivery of insulin from portable or implanted pumps in amounts determined by metabolic need. Two principal methods have been developed: the "closed loop," in which delivery is controlled by frequent automated measurements of blood glucose, and the "open loop" used in ambulant patients, in which delivery is controlled by a pre-set schedule based on times of food intake and physical activity.

ORAL HYPOGLYCEMICS

Sulfonylureas

Soon after the discovery of insulin, the search began for antidiabetic drugs that could be taken by mouth.

The substance known as synthalin (decamethylene diguanidine) was found to lower blood sugar, but produced damage to the liver.

In 1942, during investigation of antibacterial sulfonamides, French workers (Janbon, Loubatières, and colleagues) found that some of these compounds lowered blood sugar. The first compound used clinically (carbutamide) had a free para-amino group and therefore had antibacterial activity. Subsequent modifications of the sulfonamide molecule led to separation of these two pharmacologic actions, and currently used hypoglycemic compounds have no antibacterial effect (Fig. 46–4; see also Fig. 10–4).

These drugs appear to act essentially by causing release of insulin from the subject's own pancreas. Therefore they are useless in insulin-dependent diabetes, but are effective in mild cases with endogenous insulin production. Many of these can be controlled quite well with diet alone. Therefore, the main use of oral hypoglycemic drugs is with moderately severe cases that cannot be controlled by diet alone or in mild cases where the patient cannot or will not adhere to diet.

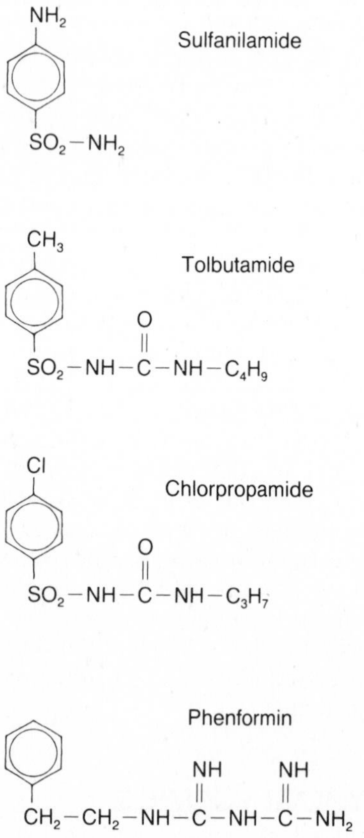

Figure 46–4   Sulfanilamide and selected oral hypoglycemics.

Preparations

Tolbutamide (Orinase®, Mobenol®, Novobutamide®) available in 0.5 g tablets; dose 1–6 tablets daily.

Chlorpropamide (Diabinese®, Novopropamide®) available in 0.25 g tablets; usual dose 1–2 tablets daily.

Acetohexamide (Dimelor®) available in 0.5 g tablets; dose 1–3 tablets daily.

Tolazamide (Tolinase®) available outside Canada in 0.1 and 0.25 g tablets.

Glyburide (glibenclamide, Diaβeta®, Euglucon®) available in 2.5 and 5.0 mg tablets; usual dose 5–10 mg daily.

Untoward Effects and Toxicity

Toxic reactions most commonly encountered are nausea and vomiting, which may be severe enough to prevent use; occasional flare-up of peptic ulcer is reported. Many patients report headaches, weakness, *etc.*, but these usually wear off after a short time. Rare cases of serious skin rash and leukopenia have occurred. An intolerance to alcohol (disulfiram-like) is common. In patients on chlorpropamide, obstructive jaundice due to plugging of fine intrahepatic biliary ducts has been reported. Also, since these drugs cause release of endogenous insulin, they can cause hypoglycemic reactions in patients with mild diabetes; these are usually insidious in onset and therefore may be hard to recognize.

Patients receiving chlorpropamide may occasionally develop hyponatremia and water retention, resembling the syndrome of inappropriate ADH secretion (SIADH). This is probably due to an effect on tubular cells, increasing their sensitivity to endogenous ADH. An increased formation and release of ADH has also been reported.

Secondary failure: About 75% of cases, chosen as described above, show good initial response to these drugs, but about 5–10% later stop getting any effect from them. Some will show a response if switched to another drug, but most do not. The reason is not known.

Biguanides

Phenformin or phenethylbiguanide (DBI) (*see* Fig. 46–4) is not a sulfonylurea, but a "throw-back" to synthalin. Because of the relative frequency of serious lactic acidosis in patients receiving phenformin it was taken off the market in Canada in 1978.

It does not release endogenous insulin, but appears to act directly on muscle to increase glycolysis. The sensitivity of tissues to insulin appears to be increased by biguanides. As would be expected, it is effective only in non-insulin-dependent diabetics.

Metformin, a closely related biguanide, is still in use.

As might be expected, its action is directly on tissue cells and its adverse effects resemble those of phenformin. Epigastric distress, nausea, vomiting, and diarrhea are most common, but lactic acidosis, particularly when renal or hepatic disease coexists, presents the real hazard.

Clinical Assessment

In 1970, a combined university group survey—University Group Diabetic Program (UGDP)—comparing insulin treatment with that by oral hypoglycemics found that after 4 years' observation the mortality rate (mainly cardiovascular) among those receiving tolbutamide was significantly higher than in those patients treated with insulin or with diet alone. Updated reports of the same group (1972) indicated that this was also the case with phenformin. The statistical basis of the original report was confirmed in late 1976, but questions were raised concerning the selection of subjects and the absence of a difference in nonfatal cardiovascular complications. Interpretation of the study is still unsettled. This puts the use of oral hypoglycemics in doubt once more. At the least, it seems clear that oral hypoglycemics do not reduce the incidence of cardiovascular complications of diabetes. There is no reason to believe that any one hypoglycemic drug currently available is much safer or much more effective than any other.

While reduction of hyperglycemia can be demonstrated, according to the UGDP (and other) studies, the long-term effectiveness of controlling blood glucose by oral hypoglycemic agents (tolbutamide or phenformin) is minimal. In spite of these observations, many specialists in diabetes administer oral hypoglycemics to non-insulin-dependent adult diabetics who have persistent fasting hyperglycemia of over 11 mmol/L (200 mg/dL) if this cannot be controlled by diet and exercise. Ideally, oral hypoglycemics should not be used as an alternative to dietary control.

ISLET–CELL TUMORS

Insulin-secreting tumors of the pancreatic islets are usually treated surgically. In adults and children, **diazoxide**, a non-diuretic thiazide with antihypertensive properties (*see* Chapter 36), has been used to control the hypoglycemic attacks that occur. It decreases the secretion of insulin (α-adrenergic action on β cells of islets) and causes release of catecholamines. Long-acting analogs of somatostatin (*e.g.*, Sandostatin®) also have proven effective as inhibitors of insulin secretion from islet-cell tumors, and Sandostatin currently is available as an investigational agent.

GLUCAGON

This is a polypeptide (29 amino acids, MW 3485) originating in α cells of the islets of Langerhans. Chemically it is similar to secretin and GIP. It activates the enzyme adenylate cyclase, resulting in an increase in cyclic AMP levels and subsequently in the activity of cyclic AMP-dependent protein kinase. The activated protein kinase in turn activates phosphorylase, causing glycogenolysis in the liver with release of glucose into the blood. Glucagon (1 mg) normally causes a 50–80 mg/dL increase in blood sugar, with gradual decline over 90 minutes or so.

The glucagon concentration in the blood of diabetics is higher than in non-diabetics and does not appear to be controlled by keeping glucose concentration within normal limits. It has been suggested that glucagon (and/or growth hormone) may be the cause of the microangiopathies and other long-term complications of diabetes. As noted earlier, somatostatin inhibits release of both glucagon and insulin.

Toxicity of glucagon is low: it sometimes causes nausea and vomiting. Its main use is as an alternative to glucose in treating hypoglycemia, especially in insulin shock therapy (easier to administer). It is also used experimentally in glycogen storage disease with results that are not too encouraging. Dosage varies between 0.5 and 2.0 mg subcutaneously or intramuscularly. It is inactive orally.

SUGGESTED READING

Albisser AM, Leibel BS. The artifical pancreas. J Clin Endocrinol Metab 1977; 6:457–479.

Brautigan DL, Kuplic JD. Proposal for a pathway to mediate the metabolic effects of insulin. Int J Biochem 1988; 20(4):349–356.

Bunn HF, Gabbay KH, Gallop PM. The glycosylation of hemoglobin: relevance to diabetes mellitus. Science 1978; 200:21–27.

Flier JS, Kahn CR, Roth J. Receptors, antireceptor antibodies and mechanisms of insulin resistance. N Engl J Med 1979; 300:413–419.

Freinkel M. Pregnant thoughts about metabolic control and diabetes (Editorial). N Engl J Med 1981; 304:1357–1359.

Kilo C, Williamson JR, Choi SC, et al. Insulin treatment and diabetic vascular complications. JAMA 1979; 241:26–27.

Steiner G. Diabetes and atherosclerosis, an overview. Diabetes (Supplement) 1981; 30:1–7.

Taylor SJ, Grunberger G, Marcus-Samuels B, et al. Hypoglycemia associated with antibodies to the insulin receptor. N Engl J Med 1982; 307:1422–1426.

University Group Diabetes Program. A study of the effects of hypoglycemic agents on vascular complications with adult-onset diabetes. Diabetes 1970; 19(2):747–830.

University Group Diabetes Program. Supplementary report on nonfatal events in patients treated with tolbutamide. Diabetes 1976; 25(6):1129–1153.

Wilson JD, Foster DW. Williams' textbook of endocrinology. 7th ed. Philadelphia: WB Saunders, 1985.

ENDOCRINE SYSTEMS

Chapter 47

ADRENOCORTICOTROPIC HORMONE AND ADRENAL STEROIDS

B.P. Schimmer and S.R. George

The normal physiologic relationships of the hypothalamic-pituitary-adrenal axis are summarized in Figure 47–1.

CORTICOTROPIN-RELEASING FACTOR

Corticotropin-releasing factor (CRF, corticoliberin) is a 41-amino-acid hypothalamic peptide, present in high concentrations in neurosecretory cells in the paraventricular nucleus. Its primary function is to stimulate the release of adrenocorticotropic hormone (ACTH) from the anterior pituitary gland. The neural factors that control CRF release are complex and not completely defined. Cholinergic pathways stimulate CRF release, whereas specific noradrenergic pathways are inhibitory. The input pathways to the system are multisynaptic, so all the transmitters probably have some effect. The release of CRF varies in a circadian pattern under basal conditions. Neural stimuli such as stress, trauma, infection, hypoglycemia, and anxiety override the basal controls and increase CRF release.

Vasopressin also stimulates the release of CRF from the hypothalamus and, at one time, was thought to be the authentic CRF. Vasopressin potentiates the action of CRF on ACTH release and may have physiologic as well as pharmacologic importance.

CORTICOTROPIN, MELANOCYTE-STIMULATING HORMONE, AND ENDORPHIN

Corticotropin (ACTH) (Fig. 47–2) is a protein with 39 amino acids, synthesized in the basophil cells of the anterior pituitary. The first 24 amino acids of ACTH are responsible for the hormonal activity of the peptide. Species variation occurs in the region from the 25th to the 33rd residue.

Like other peptide hormones, ACTH is derived from a larger precursor protein "pro-opiomelanocortin" (pro-opiocortin). Proteolytic cleavage of the precursor releases ACTH along with other important pituitary peptides as shown in Figure 47–3. Three melanocyte-stimulating hormones (MSH, melanotropin) with related structures, a lipid-mobilizing factor (β-lipotropin), and the opioid peptide β-endorphin (see Chapter 22) are all found as components of the same precursor, pro-opiomelanocortin.

Secretion of ACTH is regulated both by feedback from adrenal corticoid hormones and by neural mechanisms. Receptors for glucocorticoids are located within the hypothalamus and in other parts of the brain including the pituitary gland itself.

Neural control of ACTH is demonstrated by the wide variety of stimuli that increase ACTH secretion and therefore plasma corticoid levels. These stimuli include

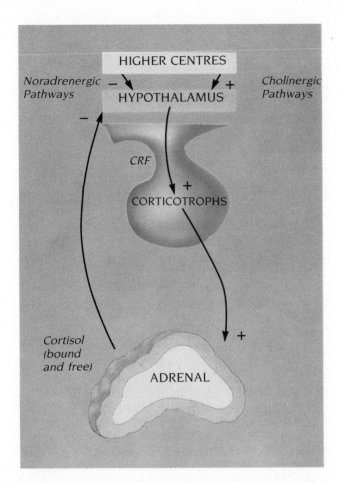

Figure 47-1 Functional relationships in the hypothalamic-pituitary-adrenal axis. (+) indicates stimulation of release, (−) indicates inhibition.

both physical and psychological stresses. Under these circumstances, feedback control does not appear to work in the same way. This might be analogous to rais-ing the thermostat setting—perhaps higher blood levels of cortical hormones are needed before ACTH output stops.

Those factors that regulate the secretion of ACTH similarly regulate the production of the other peptides associated with pro-opiomelanocortin. Notably, the opioid peptide β-endorphin is produced concomitantly with ACTH in response to stressful stimuli.

The most important physiologic effect of ACTH is the stimulation of the biosynthesis and output of adrenal cortical hormones. Administration of large doses to adrenalectomized animals produces lipolysis, ketosis, and hypoglycemia, but these probably do not have physiologic significance. Generally the effects of administration are similar to those observed after cortisol (also known as hydrocortisone), and therefore these can be considered together. However, it should be recalled that ACTH causes the release of other steroids from the adrenal cortex in addition to cortisol.

The basic action of ACTH is to stimulate the first step in the synthesis of adrenal steroid hormones, *i.e.*, the oxidative cleavage of cholesterol to pregnenolone in adrenal mitochondria. The further metabolism of pregnenolone occurs rapidly and is not under acute hormonal influence. The availability of cholesterol at the site of oxidative cleavage seems to be rate-limiting for steroidogenesis. ACTH exerts its effects by activating adenylate cyclase, increasing cyclic AMP, and stimulating the cyclic AMP-dependent protein kinase. The reactions intervening between the cAMP-dependent protein kinase and cholesterol metabolism are unknown.

ACTH also controls the cyclic diurnal secretion of adrenocorticosteroids (cortisol in humans) and maintains the structural integrity of the inner zones of the adrenal cortex. When ACTH levels are suppressed for prolonged periods (*e.g.*, following hypophysectomy or feedback inhibition by exogenous glucocorticoids), the inner zones of the cortex atrophy and secrete less steroid.

The actions of ACTH on the zona glomerulosa of the

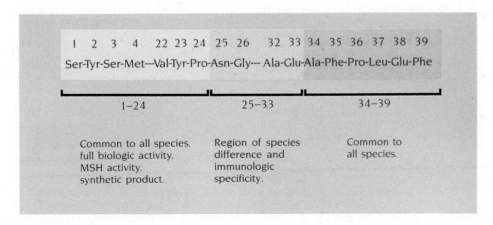

Figure 47-2 ACTH (corticotropin).

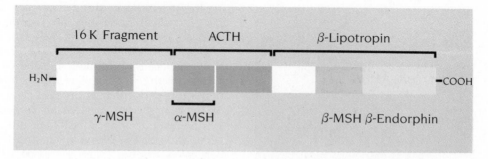

Figure 47-3 Biologically important peptides derived from pro-opiomelanocortin.

adrenal cortex do not appear to fit into this scheme. Angiotensin II and potassium are the major regulators of aldosterone production by the zona glomerulosa. Aldosterone secretion from the glomerulosa is stimulated by high levels of ACTH (equivalent to the levels encountered in response to stress), but secretion is not maintained despite continued administration. ACTH acts primarily to maintain the capability of the zona glomerulosa to respond to angiotensin II (a "permissive" effect possibly mediated by glucocorticoids).

ADRENAL INSUFFICIENCY AND TYPES OF ADRENOCORTICOID ACTION

After adrenalectomy or after complete elimination of adrenal cortical function by disease (Addison's disease), death occurs because of two types of disturbance:

1. Loss of Na^+ and water *via* the kidney, leading to dehydration and thus to shock.
2. Failure of glucose formation by the liver, leading to hypoglycemia, which causes muscular weakness and failure of CNS function.

The first of these can be corrected by aldosterone. Because of its action on water and mineral (electrolyte) metabolism, it is called a **mineralocorticoid**. The second set of effects is remedied by cortisol. Because of its action on intermediary metabolism of glucose and other substances, this steroid is called a **glucocorticoid**. Synthetic or semisynthetic substances with similar actions are also classified in the same way.

Mineralocorticoid Actions

Mineralocorticoids cause the renal tubule to retain Na^+, HCO_3^-, and water and excrete more K^+. As a result, serum Na^+ rises and K^+ falls. In the extreme,

alkalosis may occur. Retention of Na^+ and water leads to increases in blood volume and blood pressure.

Glucocorticoid Actions

Metabolic Effects

Liver metabolism is reset to a gluconeogenic mode. Protein in muscle, bone, and other tissues is broken down to amino acids. The amino acids are carried to the liver, deaminated, and converted to glucose. This results in **increases** in liver glycogen concentration, fasting blood sugar levels, and urinary N output. The proportions of carbohydrate and fat utilized by muscle are altered (increased mobilization and oxidation of depot fat; decreased utilization of glucose).

Effects on Blood and Lymphoid Systems

Erythrocyte and hemoglobin levels are increased. Circulating lymphocytes and eosinophils are decreased, due mainly to redistribution of these elements away from blood into other body compartments such as bone marrow, spleen, and lymph nodes and, to a lesser extent, to lymphocytolysis. The intensity of inflammatory responses is dampened by actions at multiple sites.

Renal and Cardiovascular Effects

The ability of the kidney to excrete a sudden load of water is maintained. Generally, a shift of water into cells is prevented, and extracellular volume is maintained. The excretion of uric acid is increased by decreasing renal tubular reabsorption of uric acid. Cardiac contractility and vascular tone are enhanced.

Effects on Other Endocrine Organs

The interaction of glucocorticoids with other components of the endocrine system is exemplified by the feedback inhibition of ACTH production. TSH production also is suppressed whereas growth hormone production is increased.

Other Effects

CNS effects include regulation of mood, increased sense of well-being, and increased motor activity. A direct action of glucocorticoids on the CNS is suggested by the presence of specific glucocorticoid receptors in the brain.

The ability of muscles to do prolonged work is maintained (independent of effects on carbohydrate and fat metabolism).

The production of gastric HCl and pepsin is increased.

Glucocorticoids regulate calcium uptake from the intestine, apparently by competitively inhibiting the action of vitamin D_3.

Effects on blood coagulation are unclear. Both thrombocytosis and thrombocytopenia have been reported following glucocorticoid administration. Nevertheless, caution is advised when glucocorticoids are used in conjunction with anticoagulants or ASA.

Many of these effects had been known for years; they were characteristically absent in Addison's disease and were restored upon replacement therapy with corticosteroids. **How** the effects were brought about, *i.e.*, the mechanism of action at the cellular level, was not known. It seems increasingly clear that most of the effects are produced by regulating the transcription of specific messenger RNA(s) and, as a consequence, the synthesis of the "controlling" enzyme proteins.

It came as a surprise when Hench and Kendall reported, in 1949, that one of the adrenal steroids, now known as cortisone (compound "E"), relieved pain, inflammation, and disability in rheumatoid arthritis. One great difficulty in studying the phenomenon or treating patients was that ACTH and the steroids could be obtained, at that time, only by extraction from pituitary or adrenal glands. The cost was high. This was changed drastically by chemical studies that led to the synthesis of steroids.

CHEMISTRY, KINETICS, AND SYNTHETIC ANALOGS

Structural Requirements

Adrenal cortical steroids are structurally related to progesterone (Fig. 47–4); however, to produce any activity as a corticosteroid, there must be an additional — OH group at C-21 (Fig. 47–5).

With these features, and no substitution at C-11, there is only mineralocorticoid activity (desoxycorticosterone).

With a β-hydroxyl group (— OH) at C-11 there is less mineralocorticoid activity, but glucocorticoid activity is observed (corticosterone, Fig. 47–6). A keto group (= O) at C-11 also confers glucocorticoid activity because of systemic metabolism to an 11 β — OH function. With — OH at position 17 as well, there is still less miner-

alocorticoid activity and much more glucocorticoid activity, though — OH at C-17 has no effect without oxygen at C-11. In the human, cortisol (hydrocortisone) is the predominantly secreted corticosteroid (Fig. 47–7).

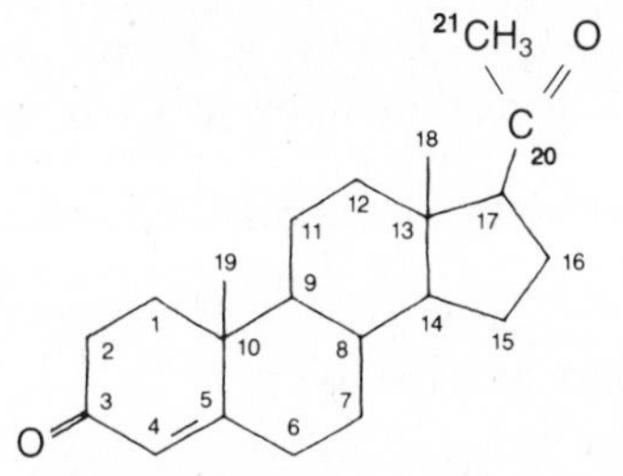

Figure 47–4 Structural formula of progesterone. The four rings that constitute the steroid nucleus are virtually coplanar. Chemical substitutions to the steroid molecule that reside *above* the plane of the rings are designated β and are conventionally represented by solid lines; substitutions made *below* the plane of the rings are designated α and are conventionally represented by broken lines, as shown in subsequent figures.

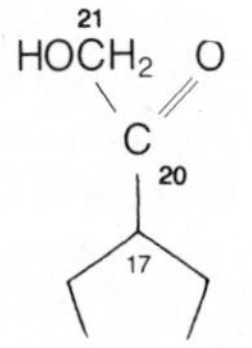

Figure 47–5 Characteristic side chain of the corticosteroids. The compound with a progesterone ring structure and this side chain is desoxycorticosterone.

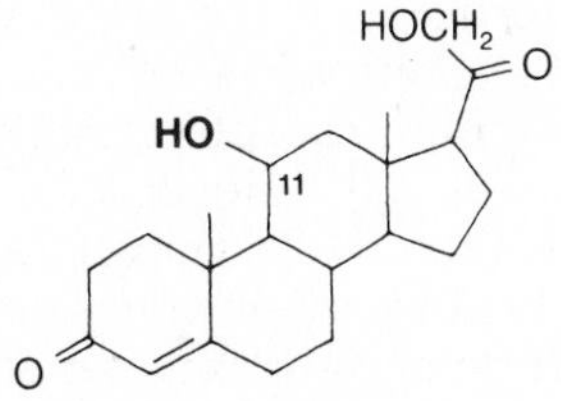

Figure 47–6 Structural formula of corticosterone.

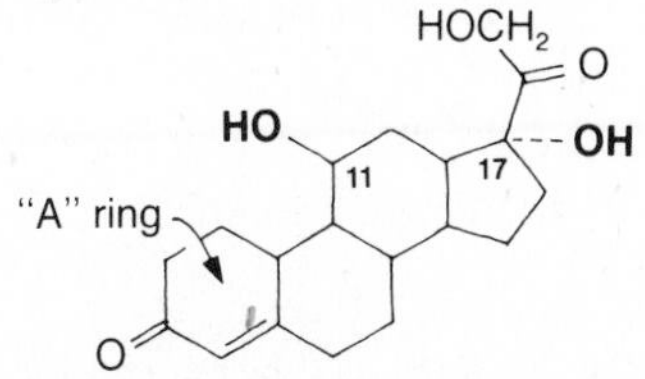

Figure 47–7 Structural formula of cortisol (hydrocortisone).

is the predominantly secreted corticosteroid (Fig. 47–7).

Aldosterone has an odd mixture of properties, because it has an aldehyde group at C-18 and – OH at C-11, which can form a cyclic hemiacetal (Fig. 47–8). The free form has – OH at C-11, and it is therefore a potent glucocorticoid. The acetal form has the – OH tied up, and therefore behaves like an 11-desoxy compound and is a potent mineralocorticoid. The latter predominates at physiologic concentrations so that glucocorticoid action is negligible.

Transport and Metabolism

The daily rates of secretion of adrenal steroids and their levels in plasma are given in Tables 47–1 and 47–2. Like most steroid hormones, cortisol in blood is predominantly (90–95%) bound to proteins (*see* Table 47–2). Most is bound to a specific globulin with high affinity, corticosteroid-binding globulin (CBG), and the remainder nonspecifically to albumin. Free cortisol is in equilibrium with the bound form.

Cortisol has a plasma half-life of about 90 minutes, and to a large extent is inactivated in the liver by reduction in the "A" ring and subsequent conjugation with sulfate or glucuronate. Analogs with a double bond between C-1 and C-2 or with a fluorine atom introduced into the molecule are biotransformed much more slowly, and the half-life is correspondingly increased.

Synthetic Analogs

A great impetus to the use of corticosteroids and to further developments was the discovery that the basic steroid could be obtained plentifully from a vegetable source, the Mexican yam. Selective modifications of the corticosteroid structure decrease the rate of metabolic inactivation of corticoids in the body. More importantly, these modifications enhance the affinity of corticosteroids for their receptors and increase their selective actions as mineralocorticoids or glucocorticoids. Taken together, these changes increase both the specificity and biologic effectiveness of a given dose. The relative effectiveness of several glucocorticoids is given in Table 47–3. Specific modifications include:

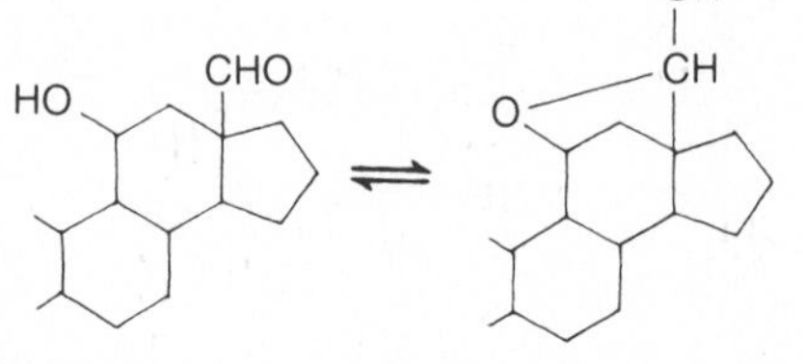

1. Insertion of a double bond between C-1 and C-2. This changes cortisol (hydrocortisone) to prednisolone, and cortisone to prednisone (Fig. 47–9). These are three to five times as potent glucocorticoids as the originals. Neither has appreciable mineralocorticoid activity.
2. Addition of a 6-methyl group to prednisolone gives methylprednisolone, which has a slightly greater anti-inflammatory potency than prednisolone.
3. Addition of fluorine to C-9 of cortisol gives fludrocortisone (Fig. 47–10). This addition markedly increases the affinities of the steroid for **both** the glucocorticoid and mineralocorticoid receptors. Fludrocortisone is ten times more potent than hydrocortisone as a glucocorticoid. Its activity as a mineralocorticoid, however, is far greater and approaches that of aldosterone. Pharmacologically, the mineralocorticoid activity of fludrocortisone predominates.
4. 9α-Fluoroprednisolone, analogous to the above, is not used medicinally, but is a starting point for other modifications. Addition of – OH at C-16 gives triamcinolone; addition of – CH₃ in the α position at C-16 gives dexamethasone; – CH₃ in the β position at C-16 gives betamethasone (Figs. 47–11 to 47–13). All are very potent glucocorticoids with minimal mineralocorticoid effect.
5. Addition of – F at C-6 of triamcinolone yields fluocinolone (Fig. 47–14) and increases the anti-inflammatory action still further. Fluocinolone is used topically.

TABLE 47–1   Steroid Secretion by the Human Adrenal Gland

Steroid	Daily Secretion Rate*
Cortisol (Hydrocortisone)	8–25 mg (14 mg)
Corticosterone	2–4 mg
Aldosterone	50–200 µg (100 µg)
Dehydroepiandrosterone	15–30 mg (20 mg)
Progesterone	0.4–0.8 mg
Androstenedione	1–10 mg
Testosterone	Trace
Estradiol	Trace

* Average values for the most significant steroids are given in parentheses. Values selected are somewhat arbitrary, and vary in different reports.

Figure 47–8   Aldehyde (*left*) and hemiacetal (*right*) forms of aldosterone.

TABLE 47–2   Usual Steroid Plasma Levels

Steroid	Plasma Level/100 mL	
	Total	Free
Cortisol (Hydrocortisone)	5–20 µg	1000 ng
Corticosterone	1 µg	100 ng
Aldosterone	3–15 ng	3 ng
Dehydroepiandrosterone	65 µg	65 µg

TABLE 47-3 Comparative Doses of Various Preparations to Achieve the Same Degree of Glucocorticoid Effect

Cortisone	25 mg
Cortisol (Hydrocortisone)	20 mg
Prednisone	5 mg
Prednisolone	5 mg
Methylprednisolone	4 mg
Triamcinolone	4 mg
Dexamethasone	0.75 mg
Betamethasone	0.6 mg

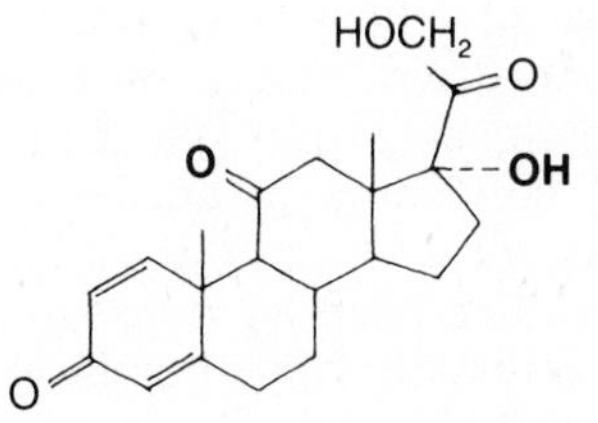

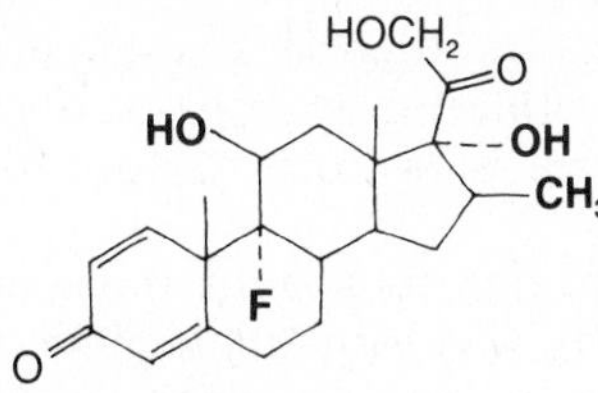

Figure 47-13 Structural formula of betamethasone.

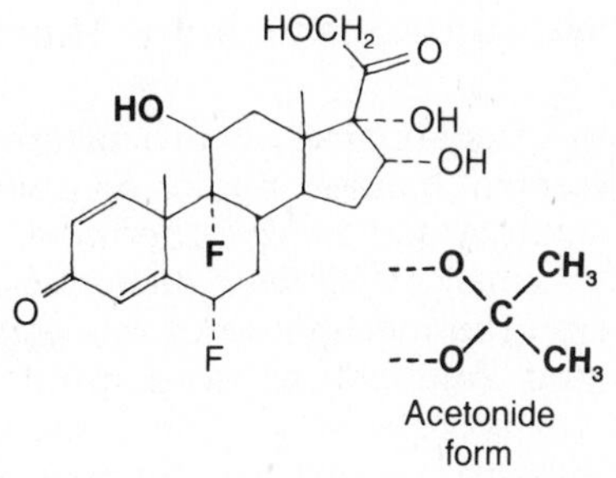

Figure 47-9 Structural formula of prednisone.

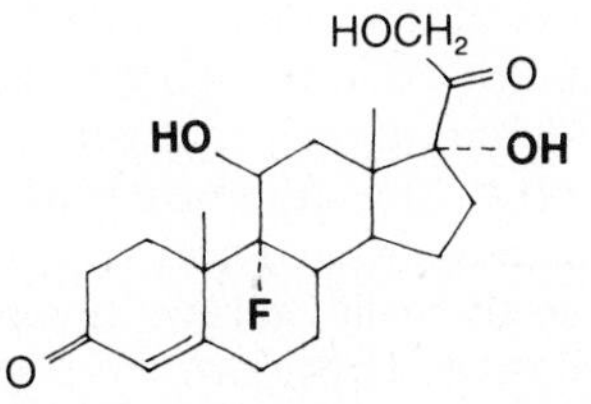

Figure 47-14 Structural formula of fluocinolone.

Figure 47-10 Structural formula of fludrocortisone.

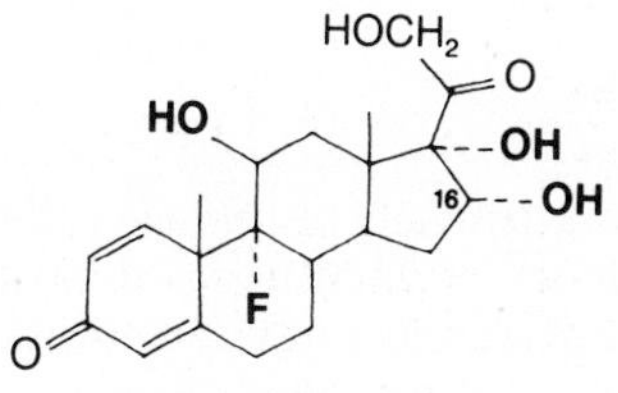

6. Beclomethasone (the 9α-chloro-analog of betamethasone) is used topically and as an aerosol for the treatment of asthma. Its effectiveness by the latter route makes it possible to reduce (or even eliminate) systemic therapy in severe chronic asthma.

CLINICAL USES

Replacement and Substitution Therapy

Primary or secondary adrenal cortical insufficiency as well as congenital adrenal hyperplasia are effectively treated with substitution of corticoids. These are the only uses for which the rationale is entirely clear. In cases with secondary insufficiency due to pituitary defects, the patient's own adrenal function can be maintained with injections of ACTH. However, therapy must be life-long, responses to ACTH are not always predictable, and resistance can gradually develop to ACTH as to any foreign protein. Therefore, the usual treatment for primary and secondary adrenocortical insufficiency is similar: providing exogenous corticosteroids.

Congenital adrenal hyperplasia is caused most often (in 95% of cases) by 21-hydroxylase insufficiency. As a consequence of this defect, circulating levels of cortisol fall and precursor steroids—including the adrenal androgens—rise, causing hypertension and virilization. Treatment with synthetic glucocorticoids suppresses

Figure 47-11 Structural formula of triamcinolone.

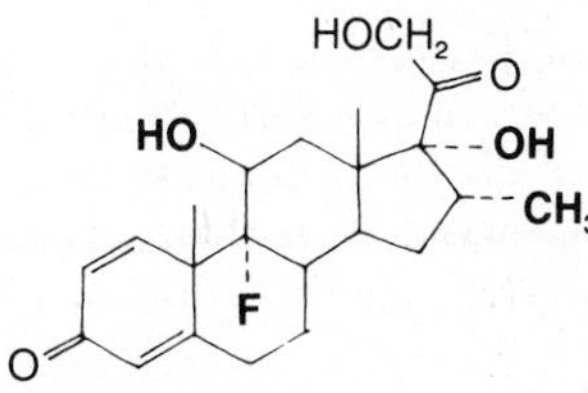

Figure 47-12 Structural formula of dexamethasone.

ENDOCRINE SYSTEMS

ACTH production by feedback regulation of the pituitary, shuts off abnormal steroid production by the adrenal gland, and substitutes a normal level of glucocorticoids.

Mineralocorticoid defects are the more acute threat to life, and therapy was formerly mainly with mineralocorticoids such as desoxycorticosterone acetate. However, best results are obtained with replacement of both types of corticoid, formerly as the natural extracts, now as the pure steroids.

Antiallergic and Anti–inflammatory Therapy

By far the most frequent use of corticosteroids today is not for replacement therapy, but for nonspecific treatment of inflammatory and allergic conditions, in doses that range from small physiologic ones to huge pharmacologic doses. The mechanism of this action is not really understood. Antibody titres seem not to be affected; instead, suppression of each stage of the inflammatory response seems to underlie both the anti-inflammatory and antiallergic actions of the glucocorticoids. Among the known components of the anti-inflammatory and antiallergic actions are decreases in capillary and leukocytic responses to local injury, inhibition of secretion of proteolytic and lipolytic enzymes (stabilization of lysosomes?), inhibition of fibroblast growth, and inhibition of scar formation. For these reasons, corticosteroids are used in many situations including:

- Rheumatoid arthritis—to reduce acute inflammation, and prevent scar deformity.
- Rheumatic fever—to prevent cardiac damage from scar formation.
- Collagen diseases, lupus erythematosus, *etc.*—to prevent fibrous proliferation.
- Severe asthma, serum sickness, *etc.*.
- Acute inflammation of the eye, where healing by scar would cause blindness.
- Topical application to skin for severe or chronic allergic or noninfectious inflammatory reactions.
- Nephrotic syndrome—to prevent or diminish proteinuria and increase serum albumin level.

Gout

In addition to the anti-inflammatory action, glucocorticoids block reabsorption of uric acid by the renal tubules, thus lowering blood uric acid levels. Their use for this purpose has been replaced to a considerable extent by that of phenylbutazone derivatives or allopurinol (*see* Chapter 33).

Malignancies

Lymphosarcoma, lymphatic leukemia, multiple myeloma, and **Hodgkin's disease** may show remission for varying lengths of time, from weeks to many months. This is not a specific antitumor action but is part of the normal glucocorticoid lytic effect on lymphatic and related tissues.

Synthetic glucocorticoids sometimes promote regression of **breast tumors**. This action is thought to be related to inhibition of the synthesis of adrenal androgens, which, in turn, can be metabolized to estrogens that promote breast tumor growth.

Glucocorticoids also have been used to treat hypercalcemia associated with tumor **metastases to bone** tissue. These metastases put out a prostaglandinlike substance that stimulates osteoclastic resorption of bone and releases calcium into the blood. Glucocorticoids lower blood calcium by decreasing calcium uptake from the intestine (anti-vitamin D_3 effect). (*See* Chapter 48.)

General Considerations About Therapeutic Uses

It must be stressed that the actions of corticosteroids against inflammation, allergy, gout, and malignancies are not curative but merely palliative and aimed at relieving symptoms. The common feature is suppression of inflammatory changes and scar formation while the drug is being given. If therapy is stopped, disease may recur in full force. Therefore, corticoids should not be used for minor conditions, but for (1) relief of acute allergic phenomena (short-term use), (2) relief of severe or potentially fatal symptoms, and (3) prevention of incapacitation by scar formation.

Diagnostic Uses

CRF is used diagnostically to release ACTH and thereby test the adequacy of pituitary corticotroph function. Synthetic CRF is available only for investigational purposes at present, not for general use.

ACTH is used to differentiate between primary and secondary/tertiary adrenal insufficiency. ACTH administration will stimulate cortisol production if there is no disease involving the adrenals directly, as in hypothalamic or pituitary disorders presenting with adrenal insufficiency.

Dexamethasone is used to test the suppressibility of the hypothalamic-pituitary-adrenal axis in patients with elevated levels of cortisol. Because dexamethasone is a potent glucocorticoid, low doses (1 mg) will inhibit the release of ACTH from the anterior pituitary in normal individuals. Some depressed or psychotic patients are resistant to small dexamethasone doses to which normal individuals are sensitive. In patients with elevated cortisol due to Cushing's syndrome, low doses of dexamethasone (2 mg) do not suppress ACTH or cortisol levels effectively. Higher doses of dexamethasone (8–16 mg) are used to distinguish pituitary-dependent Cushing's disease (suppressible) from adrenal tumors and ectopic ACTH-producing tumors (not suppressible).

PREPARATIONS

ACTH: This is available as a purified powder, or aqueous solution for injection subcutaneously, intramuscularly, or intravenously.

There are also depot forms, *i.e.*, ACTH to which carboxymethylcellulose, or zinc plus protamine, or gelatin is added, to slow the absorption and so give prolonged action over 24–72 hours after a single injection. These forms are used intramuscularly only.

Synthetic ACTH (cosyntropin, a peptide containing 24 amino acids, and marketed as Cortrosyn® or Synacthen®) is now available and is less likely to produce allergic reactions.

Corticoids: All glucocorticoids named in Table 47–3 are used. They are available in many forms, *e.g.*, oral tablets, ointments, lotions, ophthalmic drops, aqueous suspensions for intramuscular use, and solutions for intravenous use. The choice of one glucocorticoid over another is not clear-cut, except that 11-keto compounds are not effective topically. Absolute potency, in terms of dose (mg) required to produce a given effect, is not really important; the degree of separation of desired anti-inflammatory effects from undesired mineralocorticoid effects is important, and in this sense the newer glucocorticoids from prednisone onward are all better than cortisol or cortisone, but it is not really certain that the latest ones offer significant advantages over prednisolone or prednisone. Price is an important consideration in chronic treatment.

Desoxycorticosterone: The acetate (DOCA) was formerly the mainstay in chronic treatment of Addison's disease. It is available as an oily solution, a microcrystalline suspension, or as pellets for subcutaneous implantation.

Fludrocortisone has largely replaced DOCA because of its glucocorticoid activity as well as potent mineralocorticoid effect, and ease of administration by mouth. It gives full therapy when combined with small doses of cortisol.

Aldosterone is an extremely potent, but very expensive, mineralocorticoid and has less versatility than fludrocortisone; it is used only for research.

Hydrocortisone sodium succinate (Solu-Cortef®) is a water-soluble salt of cortisol for intravenous use. For instance, it is used before and after surgery in patients with relative adrenocortical insufficiency, or in Addisonian crisis.

TOXIC EFFECTS

Like other hormones, corticoids show toxic effects that are the logical outcome of exaggeration of their physiologic effects. Prolonged use with large doses causes some or all of the following:

- Salt and water retention, leading to edema, hypertension, and congestive heart failure. Excessive K^+ loss in urine at the same time may cause hypokalemia and muscular weakness. Excessive HCO_3^- retention may cause hypochloremic alkalosis. This is most likely to occur with mineralocorticoids, cortisone, or hydrocortisone (cortisol).
- Negative nitrogen balance and impaired glucose utilization may cause a diabetic state in prediabetic subjects. This problem is usually not too serious.
- Osteoporosis and impaired wound healing, including impaired synthesis of collagen, result from a catabolic effect on protein metabolism. The inhibition of growth in children receiving corticosteroids over long periods probably falls into this same category.

These first three groups of toxic effects make up most of the clinical picture of "iatrogenic Cushing's syndrome" (caused by the physician by overdosage with steroids or by patients taking more than was prescribed).

- Masking of infections by impairing the inflammatory defensive response. In the presence of infection, the use of corticosteroids presents a risk. Concurrent chemotherapy or antibiotic therapy may minimize the risk. Fibrosis is an important part of the defence reaction against tuberculosis, and corticosteroids may prevent this walling-off process and facilitate the spread of the disease. In herpetic keratitis, corticosteroids may allow the infection to spread and cause blindness unless effective antiviral chemotherapy is used concurrently (*see* Chapter 58).
- Perforation of viscera. Increased secretion of HCl and pepsin by the stomach, together with impaired healing, may cause peptic ulcers to perforate.
- Precipitation of mood disorders, ranging from euphoria to depression, and also psychoses in certain individuals. The mechanism here is not really known and is difficult to relate to the known physiologic effects.
- Exogenous glucocorticoids, through the negative feedback mechanism, suppress the secretion of ACTH, and thus secondarily reduce secretion from the patient's own adrenal cortex. If therapy is

stopped abruptly, the patient will be in adrenal cortical insufficiency. Therefore, dosage should be reduced gradually. Some clinicians have used ACTH during the period of glucocorticoid withdrawal to stimulate the patient's own cortex. While ACTH promotes the recovery of adrenal steroidogenic activity, its effect is only transient and does little to hasten recovery of adrenocortical function. After chronic treatment with glucocorticoids, the duration of suppression is not a matter of hours or days, but of months (perhaps permanent). Obviously, the dose, the duration, and the individual do influence the effects. There is some evidence that administration of glucocorticoids on alternate days in the treatment of chronic diseases may result in less negative feedback suppression.

- Avascular necrosis of bone, most notably of the femoral head, has been reported. This is more likely to occur with long-term use of higher doses of steroids, such as in the treatment of systemic lupus erythematosus, and in the immunosuppression protocol used after renal transplantation.

INHIBITORS OF ADRENOCORTICO-STEROID BIOSYNTHESIS

Metyrapone

Metyrapone (Metopirone®) is one of a group of chemicals (like amphenone) that interfere with the synthesis of cortisol and aldosterone in the adrenal cortex. It inhibits 11-β-hydroxylase, the enzyme responsible for the final step in the synthesis. Consequently the precursor substance (11-desoxycortisol, compound S), which is biologically inactive and does not inhibit ACTH secretion, is excreted in the urine. Because **less** cortisol is formed, the blood level falls, and in the normal person, this causes an increased release of ACTH. The increased levels of ACTH stimulate further steroid synthesis, so that with metyrapone the amount of 11-desoxycortisol synthesized (and excreted) increases.

This can be used as a test of pituitary function, because if a fall in blood level of cortisol does **not** produce a release of ACTH, synthesis of the cortisol precursor in the adrenal does **not** increase, and there is **no increase** in excretion. In hyperaldosteronism, metyrapone may be used to prevent aldosterone production, but in this case a glucocorticoid must be administered to replace that normally produced in the adrenal.

SUGGESTED READING

Corticosteroids and hypothalamic-pituitary-adrenocortical function (Editorial). Br Med J 1980; 280:813–814.
Imura H. Control of biosynthesis and secretion of ACTH: a review. Horm Metab Res (Suppl) 1987; 16:1–6.
McCann SM, Ono N, Khorram O, et al. The role of brain peptides in neuroimmunomodulation. Ann NY Acad Sci 1987; 496:173–181.
Taylor AL, Fishman M. Medical progress: corticotropin-releasing hormone. N Engl J Med 1988; 319:213–222.
Wilson JD, Foster DW. Williams' textbook of endocrinology. 7th ed. Philadelphia: WB Saunders, 1985.

Chapter 48

DRUGS ALTERING BONE METABOLISM

W.C. Sturtridge

Bone metabolism is a part of an integrated multi-organ system that also involves the gastrointestinal tract, the kidney, and control of extracellular concentration of calcium and phosphorus. Extracellular fluid calcium concentration is normally controlled within very close limits through the actions of parathyroid hormone (PTH), calcitonin (CT), and vitamin D. The major effects of parathyroid hormone on calcium control were first recognized in 1908 when MacCallum and Voegtlin showed that surgical removal of the parathyroids resulted in hypocalcemia and tetany. Calcitonin was not discovered as a hormone with actions on calcium and bone metabolism until after 1960, following the early research of Copp in Canada and Hirsch and Munson in the U.S.A. Although vitamin D has long been recognized as a fat-soluble vitamin important for prevention of rickets and osteomalacia, better understanding of its intermediary metabolism by the liver and kidney did not begin until about 1970.

A very large number of drugs and endogenous hormones may have pharmacologic or physiologic actions on bone metabolism. This chapter summarizes only those with major or primary effects on bone metabolism, and in particular those agents with therapeutic applications.

PHYSIOLOGY OF BONE

Structure and Mineral Metabolism of Bone

The histologic structure, metabolism, and density of bone are closely related to serum calcium concentration. Close physiologic control of serum calcium within a narrow range from 2.2 to 2.6 mmol/L is maintained by secretion of PTH and CT and production of 1,25-dihydroxy-vitamin D. These three hormonal substances act (1) on bone to control the transfer of calcium between extra- and intracellular fluid as well as bone resorption, formation, and mineralization; (2) on the gastrointestinal tract to regulate the absorption of calcium and phosphorus; and (3) on the renal tubule to regulate reabsorption of calcium and phosphate (Fig. 48–1). If intake of calcium is inadequate and increased percent absorption and renal reabsorption are not sufficient to maintain calcium balance, extracellular fluid calcium will be maintained at the expense of depletion of calcium from bone. It has been estimated that a calcium intake of about 1 g/day is required to maintain calcium balance in the normal adult. Net calcium absorption is normally about 15–45% of the oral intake when measured by isotopic calcium absorption methods. The duodenum has the greatest capacity for transport of calcium per unit length of intestine, but the major intestinal site of calcium absorption depends on the length of the bowel segment and intestinal transit time in addition to calcium concentration in the intestinal lumen. The largest fraction of the total calcium absorption occurs in the ileum.

Urinary excretion of calcium ranges up to 7.5 mmol/24 hours. Many factors affect total urinary calcium excretion including age, sex (males absorb and excrete more calcium than females), seasonal variations, exercise, and sodium and phosphorus intake. In adults, about 100 mL of plasma water is filtered by the kidneys every minute, but only about 1% of this filtered water and less than 2% of filtered calcium is excreted in the urine. The majority of the filtered load of calcium is reabsorbed by the renal tubules.

If input of calcium ion from absorption and reabsorption is not sufficient to maintain extracellular fluid calcium concentration in the normal range, calcium can be rapidly mobilized from bone under the influence of PTH. This transfer is mediated by osteocytes and osteoblasts, and only if the deficiency is prolonged is there an increase in osteoclast-mediated bone resorption secondary to sustained increase in PTH secretion.

483

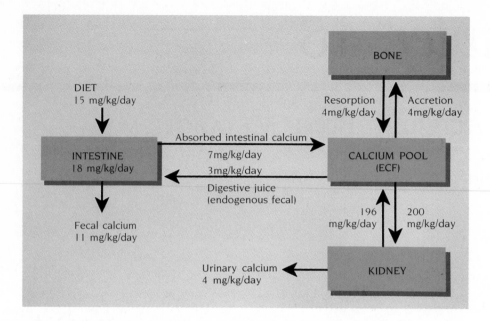

Figure 48–1 Calcium fluxes in the normal human adult who is in zero balance (on an average calcium intake).

Ninety-nine percent of total body calcium is in the skeleton. Radioisotopic studies with ^{45}Ca and ^{47}Ca indicate that 1% of skeletal calcium is freely exchangeable with extracellular fluid. Bone metabolic activity ensures that bone is not only continuously undergoing remodeling or turnover, but also that the readily exchangeable pool of calcium is maintained. The morphologic unit of compact bone is the osteon, which has been defined as "an irregular, branching and anastomosing cylinder composed of a more or less centrally placed cell-containing neurovascular canal surrounded by concentric, cell-permeated lamellae of bone matrix." At one level of an osteon, the predominant cells may be osteoclasts, and bone resorption the prevailing process, while at another level of the same osteon the predominant cell type may be osteoblasts, which are forming, depositing, and mineralizing the collagen matrix of bone (Fig. 48–2).

These two processes of bone resorption and formation are normally closely coupled. As matrix formation and mineralization continue, the active osteoblasts become encircled with mineralized matrix and become osteocytes lying within lacunae. Osteocytes are capable of active bone resorption (a process known as osteolysis) and transport of mineral ions to the osteoblasts *via* a cytoplasmic canalicular system. Osteolysis rather than osteoclast-mediated resorption is probably the primary metabolic activity of bone responsible for maintaining normal extracellular fluid concentration of calcium. The osteoclast is important for the resorption of bone in the remodeling process, but its contribution to the normal control of calcium homeostasis is minimal. Osteoclasts are derived from the

monocyte/macrophage system of cells of the hematopoietic system.

In predominantly trabecular bone the same cellular metabolic processes of bone prevail. However, osteoclast-mediated resorption and osteoblast synthesis of bone occur on the surface of trabeculae rather than within osteons.

Recent studies of osteoblasts have indicated that the term "osteoblast" describes heterogeneous cells of a common origin, but with differentiated functions. There is increasing evidence that cells of osteoblast lineage serve a central function in bone matrix turnover, stimulating not only synthesis of new matrix but controlling matrix resorption by osteoclasts as well.

Parathyroid Hormone (PTH)

A number of hormones play primary or secondary roles in controlling the metabolic activity of bone. Parathyroid hormone apparently has multiple effects on bone. It is a polypeptide composed of 84 amino acids and has a molecular weight of 9000. Within the parathyroid cell PTH is derived from larger polypeptide precursors. PTH promotes the release of calcium and phosphate into extracellular fluid, probably through stimulation of osteolysis by osteocytes. At the same time, PTH stimulates bone remodeling by increasing both resorption by osteoclasts and synthesis of bone matrix by osteoblasts. Other actions of PTH are: to enhance tubular reabsorption of calcium by an effect on the distal tubule; to increase the excretion of inorganic

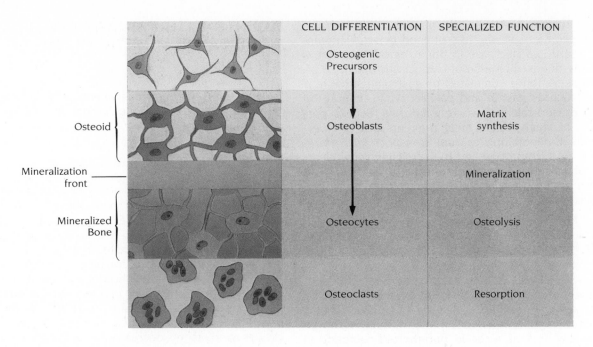

	CELL DIFFERENTIATION	SPECIALIZED FUNCTION
	Osteogenic Precursors	
Osteoid	Osteoblasts	Matrix synthesis
Mineralization front		Mineralization
Mineralized Bone	Osteocytes	Osteolysis
	Osteoclasts	Resorption

Figure 48-2   Cell differentiation and specialized functions of human bone cells.

phosphate by inhibiting tubular reabsorption of this ion; to increase HCO_3^- excretion and decrease H^+ excretion; and to stimulate production of 1,25-dihydroxy-vitamin D by the kidney through stimulation of 25-hydroxy-vitamin D-1-hydroxylase, thus contributing to increased intestinal absorption of calcium and phosphate. The actions of PTH on bone are normally synergistic with those of vitamin D metabolites, but the hypocalcemia of hypoparathyroidism can be corrected by adequate therapeutic doses of vitamin D and calcium.

While parathyroid hormone is of central importance in physiologic regulation of calcium and bone metabolism, to date it has not had pharmacologic significance. Recent development of synthesis of intact human PTH 1–84 by recombinant DNA techniques will likely lead to clinical testing in metabolic bone diseases such as osteoporosis. Bovine parathyroid extract and synthetic peptides of human sequence 1–34 and 1–38 are available for research purposes.

An interesting interaction occurs between PTH and thiazide diuretics (*see* Chapter 40). Some patients treated with thiazides show hypercalcemia as an undesired side effect. This is believed to be due to potentiation of the action of PTH, and may represent an unmasking of a subclinical hyperparathyroidism. The interaction of PTH with its receptor activates an adenylate cyclase, and raises the cAMP concentration within the target cells. Thiazides inhibit phosphodiesterase, thus increasing the cAMP concentration further.

Vitamin D

Vitamin D is obtained from dietary sources, or is derived from 7-dehydro-cholesterol in the skin by the action of light energy in the near-ultraviolet wavelength range. The precursor is converted to the biologically active metabolite 1,25-dihydroxy-vitamin D by enzymatic hydroxylations in the liver at the C-25 position, and in the kidney at the C-1 position (*see* Chapter 49). Vitamin D enhances gastrointestinal absorption of calcium and phosphate, augments the mobilization of mineral from bone, and increases the renal reabsorption of calcium and probably of phosphate. There are nuclear receptors for 1,25-dihydroxy-vitamin D, but there is no evidence that an adenylate cyclase system is involved in its actions. A direct action of vitamin D on mineralization of bone matrix has yet to be clearly demonstrated, but many authorities believe that such a physiologic role exists.

Calcitonin

The physiologic role of calcitonin in calcium and bone metabolism is unknown. Calcitonin is a 32-amino-acid peptide hormone with a molecular weight of 3500 that is produced and secreted by thyroid parafollicular cells. The acute administration of calcitonin lowers serum calcium and phosphate by inhibiting osteolysis and osteoclast activity and by decreasing renal tubular reabsorption of calcium. In sustained hypercalcitoninemia, there is a decrease in bone remodeling that is probably due to inhibition of osteoclastic activity. Calcitonin secretion is stimulated by gastrointestinal hormones such as gastrin and pancreozymin. It may be that increased calcitonin secretion during feeding, particularly of a high calcium meal, prevents excess hypercalcemia by inhibiting calcium transport into extracellular fluid from bone and by increasing renal clearance of calcium. Significant effects of calcitonin on calcium and phosphate absorption have not been demonstrated.

Other Hormones

Other hormones also play secondary roles in the control of bone metabolism. **Thyroid hormone** certainly has an effect on metabolic activity of bone cells and calcium metabolism. In hypothyroidism, bone turnover rate is low and, as a result, parathyroid secretion is increased to maintain normal serum calcium. Increased parathyroid hormone secretion rate results in increased production of 1,25-dihydroxy-vitamin D and increased calcium absorption. In hyperthyroidism, mobilization of mineral from bone is facilitated and PTH secretion is reduced. Although serum calcium concentration remains in the normal range, the decreased secretion of PTH results in elevated serum phosphate concentration.

Chronic administration of **adrenal steroids,** or adrenal cortical hypersecretion, leads to decreased gastrointestinal absorption of calcium, decreased synthesis of new bone matrix, and perhaps increased sensitivity of osteoclasts to PTH and decreased renal tubular reabsorption of calcium.

Sex hormones may affect the regulation of bone metabolism. When sex hormones are deficient, bone density tends to be diminished, probably due to an excessive degree of bone resorption. Although androgens may be aromatized to estrogens in peripheral tissues, no receptors for estrogen in bone cells can be identified. There is speculation that sex hormones may assist in the regulation of bone metabolism through calcitonin or a recently discovered glutamic acid-containing bone peptide of as yet uncertain functional significance.

Recent reports have suggested a correlation between high serum **prolactin** levels and decreased bone density. There does not appear to be a relationship between decreased bone density and plasma estrogen concentration in the presence of hyperprolactinemia. It has been reported that there is a positive correlation between elevated prolactin concentration and serum PTH. The significance of these observations so far remains unclear.

AGENTS WITH PRIMARY EFFECTS ON BONE/CALCIUM METABOLISM

Table 48–1 lists various agents with primary and secondary effects on bone/calcium metabolism.

Calcium

Various salts of calcium are available, such as calcium chloride ($CaCl_2 \cdot 2H_2O$); calcium gluconate ($[CH_2OH(CHOH)_4COO]_2Ca \cdot H_2O$); calcium lactate ($[CH_3CHOHCOO]_2Ca \cdot 5H_2O$); calcium carbonate ($CaCO_3$); and calcium citrate ($Ca_3[C_6H_5O_7]_2 \cdot 4H_2O$).

Many vital intra- and extracellular biologic processes, as well as membrane integrity and function, are dependent upon maintenance of adequate ionized calcium concentrations. Calcium salts are specific in the treatment of low calcium states. Long-term oral calcium dietary supplements decrease the rate of bone remodeling and maintain positive calcium balance.

Calcium chloride contains 27% calcium, calcium citrate 21%, calcium gluconate only 9%, calcium lactate 13%, and insoluble calcium carbonate, which is converted to soluble calcium salts in the body, contains 40% calcium.

If calcium chloride is administered intravenously, it is irritating to veins. Oral calcium supplements may cause gastric irritation, nausea, and constipation.

Calcium salts should not be taken orally at the same time as tetracycline because the absorption of tetracycline will be decreased by the formation of a calcium-tetracycline chelate. Similarly, the coadministration of fluoride or phosphates with calcium may be associated with decreased absorption due to formation of insoluble compounds in the gastrointestinal tract.

Administration of excessive calcium can lead to hyper-

TABLE 48–1   Agents and Drugs Affecting Bone Metabolism

Agents with primary effects on bone/calcium metabolism

Mineral salts: calcium, phosphate, fluoride
Hormones: vitamin D, calcitonin
Miscellaneous: diphosphonates, mithramycin

Agents with secondary effects on bone/calcium metabolism

Estrogens
Glucocorticoids
Thyroid hormone preparations
Thiazides

calcemic toxicity. Ingestion of large quantities of calcium salts, however, is unlikely to produce hypercalcemia unless there is also administration of large amounts of vitamin D.

Phosphate

Phosphate is an essential element of energy metabolism and in addition is essential for normal mineralization of bone matrix. It is absorbed from the gastrointestinal tract by active transport that is stimulated by vitamin D. About two-thirds of the ingested phosphate is absorbed and is balanced by an equal amount of phosphate excretion in the urine. In normal body fluids and tissues, phosphate ion has little pharmacologic effect, but phosphate supplements may be required to restore normal physiologic actions in phosphate depletion.

Effervescent tablets contain sodium acid phosphate together with potassium and sodium bicarbonate. Potassium phosphate solution for intravenous use is also available.

If large amounts of phosphate are administered, the unabsorbed phosphate has a marked cathartic action. Large quantities of divalent cations such as calcium or aluminum in the gastrointestinal tract will form insoluble salts and diminish phosphate absorption.

Fluoride

Fluoride is incorporated into bone as fluhydroxyapatite, which is resistant to resorption. More importantly, however, it appears to stimulate the synthesis of new bone matrix by osteoblasts. Precisely how or why this effect occurs is as yet unknown. At the same time, fluoride appears to retard the mineralization of the newly formed matrix.

Soluble fluoride compounds such as sodium fluoride (the official fluoride preparation currently in use to affect bone metabolism) are almost completely absorbed. Fluoride is probably concentrated only in calcified tissues or sites of extraskeletal calcification. The major route of fluoride excretion is the kidney.

The only known **pharmacologic effects** of fluoride other than on bone and teeth, where it inhibits dental caries, are toxic effects. (The fluoride dose to cause death in an adult is approximately 2.5–5 g of NaFl, taken in a single dose. It is estimated that the lowest acute toxic dose of water containing 1 ppm fluoride would be about 2000 L consumed at one time, if this were physically possible.) Fluoride inhibits some enzyme systems, including enzymes involved in anaerobic glycolysis and tissue respiration, and is an effective *in vitro* anticoagulant. It also inhibits glucose utilization by erythrocytes *in vitro*.

Adverse effects include gastric irritation in some patients and increased musculoskeletal pain and joint swelling of predominantly weight-bearing joints. Gastrointestinal distress is less with use of enteric-coated sodium fluoride tablets.

Dietary cations such as calcium or cations in nonabsorbable antacids retard fluoride absorption by forming poorly soluble compounds in the gastrointestinal tract.

Vitamin D

The mechanisms and sites of action of vitamin D are outlined above, and details of its metabolism may be found in Chapter 49. The pharmacologic effects of vitamin D have also been described above. In summary, vitamin D is a positive regulator of both calcium and phosphate through its actions on gut, kidney, and bone.

A large number of preparations containing vitamin D are marketed. Only four preparations need to be detailed structurally (Fig. 48–3), and the difference between them is largely in potency. However, there may be important differences in therapeutic application.

Gastrointestinal absorption of vitamin D is usually adequate when it is administered orally. Bile is essential for vitamin D absorption, so hepatobiliary disease may be associated with decreased absorption of vitamin D. Fat malabsorption may also impair vitamin D absorption.

The only adverse or toxic effects of vitamin D are those related to overtreatment and development of hypercalcemia and hyperphosphatemia. Impairment of renal function due to nephrolithiasis or nephrocalcinosis, localized or generalized decreases in bone density, and gastrointestinal complaints are the most common sequelae of vitamin D toxicity.

The important drug interactions involving vitamin D are with anticonvulsants and glucocorticoids. Phenobarbital and other anticonvulsants either interfere with the normal hydroxylations of cholecalciferol and ergocalciferol or interfere with target organ response. Glucocorticoids may also interfere with vitamin D metabolism and significantly inhibit the effect of 1,25-dihydroxyvitamin D on calcium absorption; effects on bone remodeling and calcium reabsorption are probably of secondary importance.

Calcitonin

The amino acid sequences of calcitonins from a number of different species have been determined, and the hormones have been characterized and synthesized. While the number of amino acids is 32 in all species, the amino acid sequence of calcitonin is quite different from one species to another, so that there is little immunologic cross-reactivity.

The primary effect of calcitonin is to inhibit osteoclastic and osteocytic bone resorption or mineral transfer through a direct effect on cellular activity. Other ef-

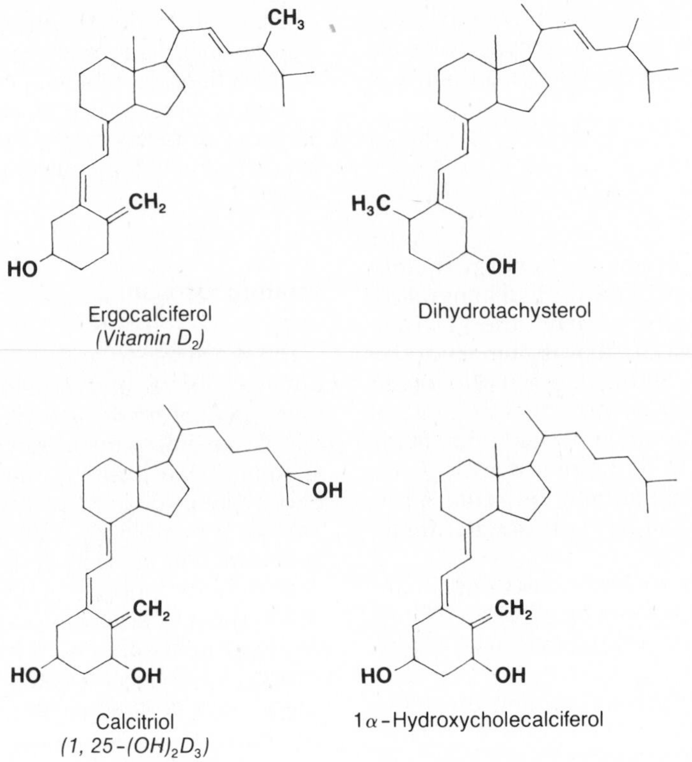

Ergocalciferol
(Vitamin D₂)

Dihydrotachysterol

Calcitriol
(1, 25-(OH)₂D₃)

1α-Hydroxycholecalciferol

Figure 48–3 Structural formulae of clinically important vitamin D preparations.

fects of calcitonin are more variable and are more species-dependent. In humans, synthetic salmon calcitonin inhibits tubular reabsorption of calcium, phosphate, sodium, potassium, and magnesium. Pharmacologic effects of calcitonin on intestinal absorption of calcium are still uncertain.

Calcitonin must be administered parenterally by subcutaneous or intramuscular injection. A preparation for intranasal administration has been tested in clinical trials but is not available for general use. Absorption of calcitonin from injection sites is rapid, although it is slowed by addition of gelatin to the vehicle. In the circulation the half-life of calcitonin is of the order of 20 minutes. It is weakly and insignificantly bound to protein and is catabolized in liver and kidney.

Calcitonin acutely lowers serum calcium and phosphate through inhibition of bone resorption. With chronic administration, the rate of bone remodeling is decreased and the urinary excretion of calcium and hydroxyproline is diminished in spite of decreased tubular reabsorption of calcium.

Calcitonin is relatively free of adverse effects, although a small minority of patients experience nausea and flushing following injection. Patients may become resistant to the actions of calcitonin because of antibody formation, since the preparation that is used pharmacologically is synthetic salmon calcitonin.

Drug interactions are uncommon, but the concomitant administration of calcitonin and thiazide diuretics may be associated with potassium depletion.

Diphosphonates

The diphosphonates are structurally similar to pyrophosphate and are adsorbed on the crystal surface of bone where they inhibit resorption and mineralization of bone. The only diphosphonate currently available clinically is disodium etidronate (Fig. 48–4).

The drug is effective orally but absorption is poor. Absorbed drug that is not taken up by bone is excreted unchanged by the kidney. There are no pharmacologic effects other than inhibition of bone remodeling.

With high doses or prolonged treatment there may be an increase in nonmineralized osteoid tissue and bone pain. No drug interactions or toxicity have been reported that are unrelated to bone.

A new agent, aminohydroxypropylidene disphosphonate (APD) has been tested in Europe and is an

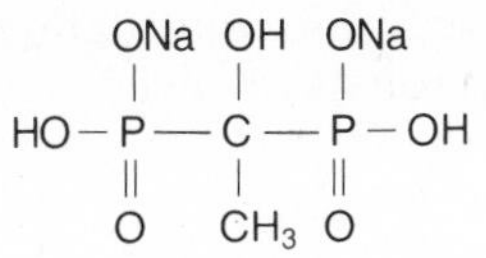

$$\begin{array}{ccccc} & \text{ONa} & \text{OH} & \text{ONa} & \\ & | & | & | & \\ \text{HO} - \text{P} & - & \text{C} & - & \text{P} - \text{OH} \\ & \| & & | & \| \\ & \text{O} & & \text{CH}_3 & \text{O} \end{array}$$

Figure 48–4 Structural formula of etidronate disodium (Didronel®).

investigational drug in North America. It is a potent inhibitor of bone resorption.

Mithramycin

Mithramycin is a cytotoxic antibiotic isolated from cultures of *Streptomyces tanashiensis*. It inhibits the synthesis of RNA without affecting protein synthesis. Osteoclasts appear to be particularly sensitive to its action.

Mithramycin has to be administered intravenously and little is known about its distribution, metabolism, or excretion. In hypercalcemic patients, low doses of mithramycin decrease bone resorption and plasma calcium concentration through a direct action on osteoclasts.

At antineoplastic doses, mithramycin is highly toxic to the liver, kidneys, and hematopoietic tissue. Severe hemorrhage may occur because of impaired synthesis of clotting factors and platelets.

THERAPEUTIC APPLICATIONS

Calcium

Calcium gluconate and calcium chloride, 10–20 mL in a concentration of 10%, are indicated for intravenous injection in the treatment of hypocalcemic tetany. A more dilute (0.3%) solution may be infused by slow drip to provide 1 g of elemental calcium a day in the management of hypocalcemia. Calcium gluconate is preferred because it is less irritating to veins than calcium chloride. For less severe hypocalcemia or to supplement dietary intake in osteoporosis or osteomalacia, calcium salts to provide 1–2 g elemental calcium a day are given orally.

Phosphate

Oral phosphate may be used in some circumstances as an adjunct in the management of hypercalcemia, where it probably decreases calcium absorption, or in

hypophosphatemia. Effervescent tablets of sodium acid phosphate provide 500 mg elemental phosphorus. Four to six tablets per day are prescribed in divided doses, but in many patients diarrhea limits the amount of drug that can be tolerated. In hypercalcemic patients, intravenous injection of phosphate may precipitate soft tissue calcification, but potassium phosphate may be given intravenously to correct severe hypophosphatemia ($\leq$ 0.3 mmol/L). The dose required to normalize serum phosphate in adult patients with normal renal function and normal serum potassium and calcium is 9 mmol of phosphorus as KH_2PO_4 in 0.5N saline as a continuous intravenous infusion over a 12-hour period (whereby the amount of potassium will be the limiting factor, because excess phosphate is excreted in the urine).

Fluoride

Enteric-coated tablets containing 20 mg of sodium fluoride may be given one to three times daily with meals in the treatment of osteoporosis, multiple myeloma, and otospongiosis. Serum fluoride concentration must be monitored frequently to ensure adequate but nontoxic levels. Sodium fluoride, stannous fluoride, and sodium monofluorophosphate are employed in dentifrices to reduce dental caries. Fluoridation of municipal water supplies has the same objective. Pharmacologic serum fluoride levels that stimulate bone matrix formation are of the order of 5–10 μmol/L; these may be attained with the daily ingestion of about 40 mg sodium fluoride (= 20 mg fluoride). Water fluoridation with the addition of 1 ppm fluoride produces lower serum fluoride levels of about 2 μmol/L.

Vitamin D

Vitamin D compounds are administered orally to increase calcium and phosphate absorption in diseases such as hypocalcemia, osteomalacia, osteoporosis, osteodystrophy, vitamin D deficiency, and hypophosphatemia. Doses vary considerably, depending on the indication for treatment and the preparation selected. Doses of 1.25 mg (50,000 IU) to 5 mg of ergocalciferol may be required in hypoparathyroidism, and up to 10 mg in vitamin D-dependent rickets, whereas this latter condition may respond to 0.25–0.5 μg of calcitriol. The usual dose of calcitriol or 1α-OH-cholecalciferol in hypoparathyroidism is 1 μg a day.

Calcitonin

It has been stated that the three consistently established indications for the use of calcitonin are Paget's disease of bone, hypercalcemia, and osteoporosis. However, calcitonin may be effective initially in treatment of hypercalcemia, but usually patients rapidly become refractory to it; this phenomenon most likely represents receptor down-regulation. Bone diseases with decreased bone density, such as involutional forms of osteoporosis with low bone turnover rates, are unlikely to benefit significantly from further decrease in bone turnover rate induced by calcitonin. Calcitonin is effective in diseases associated with increased skeletal remodeling, such as Paget's disease of bone. Synthetic salmon calcitonin administered subcutaneously or intramuscularly in doses of 50 MRC units, three times weekly, produces symptomatic relief from pain and reductions in bone remodeling and blood flow through affected areas. It has been suggested that calcitonin may decrease the spread of metastases of malignant disease in bone, with resultant decreases in bone pain and hypercalcemia. This indication for the clinical use of calcitonin needs further documentation in a well-controlled clinical study.

Diphosphonates

The only well-established clinical application of sodium etidronate is the treatment of Paget's disease of bone. The drug is available in 200 mg tablets for oral use at a dosage of 5–10 mg/kg/day. Heterotopic ossification following total hip replacement may occur in as many as 25–50% of high-risk patients. Preoperative treatment for 1 month and postoperative therapy for 3 months with sodium etidronate 20 mg/kg/day may decrease the risk and severity of heterotopic ossification. Therapeutic efficacy of sodium etidronate in treatment of hypercalcemia has not been established. Although other diphosphonates may be effective in this regard, none is commercially available at this time. To date, there is no conclusive evidence that the diphosphonates are effective in the treatment of osteopenic bone disease, although unsubstantiated claims have been made in this regard for alternating doses of phosphate and diphosphonate.

Mithramycin

Mithramycin is useful in treating patients with hypercalcemia associated with carcinoma and increased bone resorption. For treatment of hypercalcemia or hypercalciuria associated with malignant disease, the dose has been 25 μg/kg daily for 1–3 days, diluted in 5% dextrose and water and infused intravenously over 6 hours. The effect, however, is short-lived and treatment may have to be repeated at weekly intervals. At lower doses of 10–15 μg/kg/day for 7–10 days by intravenous infusion, mithramycin may provide substantial relief of pain in Paget's disease of bone.

SUGGESTED READING

Avioli LV. Calcitonin therapy for bone disease and hypercalcemia. Arch Intern Med 1982; 142:2076–2079.

Chambers TJ. Regulation of osteoclastic bone resorption. Bone Clin Biochem News and Rev 1988; 5:3–4.

Martin TJ, Raisz LG, Rodan GA. In: Martin TJ, Raisz LG, eds. Clinical endocrinology of calcium metabolism. New York: Marcel Dekker, 1987:1–61.

Nordin BEC, ed. Metabolic bone and stone disease. Edinburgh/London: Churchill Livingstone, 1973.

Nordin BEC, ed. Calcium, phosphate and magnesium metabolism. Edinburgh/New York: Churchill Livingstone, 1976.

Singer F, ed. Paget's disease of bone. New York: Plenum, 1977.

Sturtridge WC. Osteoporosis and Paget's disease. Medicine North America, May 1981:1171–1180.

Sturtridge WC, Wilson DR. Management of hypercalcemia. Drug Therapy, Jan 1982:108–112.

Vannatta JB, Whang R, Papper S. Efficacy of intravenous phosphorus therapy in the severely hypophosphatemic patient. Arch Intern Med 1981; 141:885–887.

Chapter 49

VITAMINS

L. Spero and M.J. Baigent

History

Scurvy was the first disease shown to be dependent on dietary factors. An early written account of scurvy and its treatment is found in the journals of Jacques Cartier who, in 1535, treated his crew with a decoction of the leaves of an "Anneda" tree as suggested by the Indians living at Hochelaga (now Québec). It was not until 1753, however, that James Linde described the treatment of scurvy with lime juice in his classical *Treatise on Scurvy*. In 1890, beriberi was shown by Eijkman to be due to a vitamin B_1 (thiamin) deficiency, likely precipitated by diets consisting mainly of polished rice. In the early part of this century, Hopkins and others demonstrated that humans could not survive on purified rations containing only carbohydrate, fat, protein, and minerals.

Since that time, 13 vitamins and many minerals and trace elements have been identified as essential to life. The term "Vitamine" was proposed by Funk in 1912 to designate a new food element vital for life. This term has been retained for historical reasons, although the final "e" was dropped to avoid the suggestion of chemical significance.

Vitamins are now recognized as a diverse group of organic chemicals that cannot be synthesized in the body, or not in sufficient amounts, to support normal tissue function. They must be supplied from exogenous sources (*i.e.*, foods or, in the case of vitamin D, by exposure to sunlight). They serve as coenzymes (*e.g.*, the group of B vitamins) or as regulators of specific cellular or tissue functions. More recently it has been recognized that vitamins A and D function as hormones, although the vitamin designation has been retained.

Recommended Intakes

Many countries, and scientific committees of international bodies such as the World Health Organization, have established recommended intakes for most of the essential nutrients (energy, protein, vitamins, minerals, and trace elements). These recommendations are revised periodically as new evidence of their physiologic relevance becomes available. In formulating these recommendations, it is assumed that diets will be based on a variety of foods so that even essential nutrients for which no specific recommendations have been established will be provided. Although a consistent daily intake of the essential nutrients is preferable, it is more practical and quite adequate to ensure that the daily intake averaged over a short period of time is at the recommended level.

Recommended intakes for the essential nutrients are based on the average physiologic requirements of normal healthy individuals, obtained experimentally from population studies. These requirements are the amounts that will prevent a nutrient deficiency and will allow for modest tissue stores. To these requirements is added a "safety factor," which allows for individual variability within a population. If the recommended intakes are set at two standard deviations above the average requirement, the physiologic needs of 97.5% of normal individuals are met. This means that the recommended intakes are well in excess of the requirements for most normal healthy people. They are not intended to be sufficient for therapeutic purposes, however, and they do not allow for losses of nutrients during commercial and shelf storage and food processing. Specific recommendations are given for the different age groups and sexes, and for pregnancy and lactation.

Where there are insufficient data to establish recommended intakes, "safe levels of intake" (expressed as averages) have been published to identify the minimal levels necessary to prevent deficiency, and upper levels beyond which toxicity is possible.

Recommended intakes for the vitamins as published by the governments of Canada and the United States, and by the World Health Organization, are presented in Tables 49–1, 49–2, and 49–3. Variations in recom-

TABLE 49-1 Recommended Nutrient Intakes (RNI) for Canadians (Vitamins per Day)

Age	Sex	Weight (kg)	Fat-Soluble Vitamins			Water-Soluble Vitamins		
			Vitamin A (RE)	Vitamin D (μg)	Vitamin E (mg α-TE)	Vitamin C (mg)	Folacin (μg)	Vitamin B_{12} (μg)
Months								
0–2	Both	4.5	400	10	3	20	50	0.3
3–5	Both	7.0	400	10	3	20	50	0.3
6–8	Both	8.5	400	10	3	20	50	0.3
9–11	Both	9.5	400	10	3	20	55	0.3
Years								
1	Both	11	400	10	3	20	65	0.3
2–3	Both	14	400	5	4	20	80	0.4
4–6	Both	18	500	5	5	25	90	0.5
7–9	M	25	700	2.5	7	35	125	0.8
	F	25	700	2.5	6	30	125	0.8
10–12	M	34	800	2.5	8	40	170	1.0
	F	36	800	2.5	7	40	180	1.0
13–15	M	50	900	2.5	9	50	150	1.5
	F	48	800	2.5	7	45	145	1.5
16–18	M	62	1000	2.5	10	55	185	1.9
	F	53	800	2.5	7	45	160	1.9
19–24	M	71	1000	2.5	10	60	210	2.0
	F	58	800	2.5	7	45	175	2.0
25–49	M	74	1000	2.5	9	60	220	2.0
	F	59	800	2.5	6	45	175	2.0
50–74	M	73	1000	2.5	7	60	220	2.0
	F	63	800	2.5	6	45	190	2.0
75+	M	69	1000	2.5	6	60	205	2.0
	F	64	800	2.5	5	45	190	2.0
Pregnancy (additional)								
1st Trimester			100	2.5	2	0	305	1.0
2nd Trimester			100	2.5	2	20	305	1.0
3rd Trimester			100	2.5	2	20	305	1.0
Lactation (additional)			400	2.5	3	30	120	0.5

Thiamin: 0.4 mg/1000 kcal. Minimum intake = 0.8 mg/day.

Riboflavin: 0.5 mg/1000 kcal. Minimum intake = 1.0 mg/day; add an extra 0.3 mg/day during pregnancy, and 0.4 mg/day during lactation.

Niacin: 7.2 NE/1000 kcal. Minimum intake = 14.4 NE/day.

Pyridoxine: 0.015 mg/g protein eaten; add an extra 0.3 mg/day during lactation.

Excerpted from Health and Welfare Canada, Ottawa, 1983.

mendations among these three dietary standards reflect differences in interpretation of the data used to establish the values, rather than differences in physiologic requirements between nationalities. For vitamins not listed, a specific recommended intake has not been set.

Vitamin Deficiencies

A vitamin deficiency may be classified as a primary deficiency, *i.e.*, an inadequate dietary intake; or as a secondary deficiency due to malabsorption, drug-

nutrient interactions, or increased vitamin needs due to physiologic stress or disease.

Inadequate Dietary Intake

In "westernized" cultures, deficiency may occur in individuals who are dieting vigorously to lose weight; among the poor who have insufficient incomes to purchase or prepare foods; in those who do not appreciate the need for, or who have life styles incompatible with, balanced diets (*e.g.*, "bachelor's scurvy"); in those who respond to gastrointestinal or other symptoms by

TABLE 49–2 Recommended Dietary Allowances (RDA) for Healthy People in the United States (Vitamins per Day)

	Age (years)	Weight (kg)	Fat-Soluble Vitamins			Water-Soluble Vitamins						
			Vitamin A (μg RE)	Vitamin D (μg)	Vitamin E (mg α-TE)	Vitamin C (mg)	Thiamin (mg)	Riboflavin (mg)	Niacin (mg NE)	Vitamin B₆ (mg)	Folacin (μg)	Vitamin B₁₂ (μg)
Infants	0.0–0.5	6	420	10	3	35	0.3	0.4	6	0.3	30	0.5
	0.5–1.0	9	400	10	4	35	0.5	0.6	8	0.6	45	1.5
Children	1–3	13	400	10	5	45	0.7	0.8	9	0.9	100	2.0
	4–6	20	500	10	6	45	0.9	1.0	11	1.3	200	2.5
	7–10	28	700	10	7	45	1.2	1.4	16	1.6	300	3.0
Males	11–14	45	1000	10	8	50	1.4	1.6	18	1.8	400	3.0
	15–18	66	1000	10	10	60	1.4	1.7	18	2.0	400	3.0
	19–22	70	1000	7.5	10	60	1.5	1.7	19	2.2	400	3.0
	23–50	70	1000	5	10	60	1.4	1.6	18	2.2	400	3.0
	51+	70	1000	5	10	60	1.2	1.4	16	2.2	400	3.0
Females	11–14	46	800	10	8	50	1.1	1.3	15	1.8	400	3.0
	15–18	55	800	10	8	60	1.1	1.3	14	2.0	400	3.0
	19–22	55	800	7.5	8	60	1.1	1.3	14	2.0	400	3.0
	23–50	55	800	5	8	60	1.0	1.2	13	2.0	400	3.0
	51+	55	800	5	8	60	1.0	1.2	13	2.0	400	3.0
Pregnant			+200	+5	+2	+20	+0.4	+0.3	+2	+0.6	+400	+1.0
Lactating			+400	+5	+3	+40	+0.5	+0.5	+5	+0.5	+100	+1.0

Excerpted from National Academy of Sciences, Washington DC, 1980.

TABLE 49–3 World Health Organization Recommended Intakes for Vitamins per Day

Age (years)	Weight (kg)	Vitamin A as Retinol (μg)	Vitamin D (μg)	Thiamin (mg)	Riboflavin (mg)	Niacin (mg)	Folic Acid (μg)	Vitamin B₁₂ (μg)	Ascorbic Acid (mg)
Children									
<1	7.3	300	10.0	0.3	0.5	5.4	60	0.3	20
1–3	13.4	250	10.0	0.5	0.8	9.0	100	0.9	20
4–6	20.2	300	10.0	0.7	1.1	12.1	100	1.5	20
7–9	28.1	400	2.5	0.9	1.3	14.5	100	1.5	20
Male adolescents									
10–12	36.9	575	2.5	1.0	1.6	17.2	100	2.0	20
13–15	51.3	725	2.5	1.2	1.7	19.1	200	2.0	30
16–19	62.9	750	2.5	1.2	1.8	20.3	200	2.0	30
Female adolescents									
10–12	38.0	575	2.5	0.9	1.4	15.5	100	2.0	20
13–15	49.9	725	2.5	1.0	1.5	16.4	200	2.0	30
16–19	54.4	750	2.5	0.9	1.4	15.2	200	2.0	30
Adult men (moderately active)	65.0	750	2.5	1.2	1.8	19.8	200	2.0	30
Adult women (moderately active)	55.0	750	2.5	0.9	1.3	14.5	200	2.0	30
Pregnancy (later half)		750	10.0	+0.1	+0.2	+2.3	400	3.0	50
Lactation (first 6 months)		1200	10.0	+0.2	+0.4	+3.7	300	2.5	50

Excerpted from Passmore R, Nicol BM, Rao MN. WHO Monograph Series No. 61, Geneva, 1974.

restricting their diet without medical advice; or in those who acquire restrictive or bizarre eating patterns from religious or philosophical convictions. Loss of appetite, poor dentition, and inadequate cooking facilities are common factors among the elderly. In poorly industrialized and economically depressed areas, extreme poverty and unsatisfactory food production are major factors.

Drug-Nutrient Interactions

A large number of therapeutic agents interfere with absorption and increase the rate of turnover of some vitamins. Common addiction chemicals such as alcohol, caffeine, and nicotine also interfere with vitamin metabolism. Little is known about the effects of illicit drugs.

Increased Vitamin Needs

Normal physiologic processes such as growth, pregnancy, and lactation impose higher requirements for vitamins. Increased needs for some vitamins may also occur in postsurgical, burn, or trauma patients and in a number of disease processes.

Megavitamin Therapy

The basis for advocating the consumption of very large doses of vitamins is the belief that the recommended intakes are inadequate for some individuals, and that greatly increasing the intake of certain vitamins will overcome symptoms purportedly due to a vitamin deficiency not previously recognized as such. In the case of the water-soluble vitamins used in some megavitamin therapies, it has been shown that intake greatly in excess of the recommended intake leads to excretion of the unchanged excess vitamin. Therefore, provided that vitamin stores are normal, increased intake does not result in increased tissue or plasma levels. In general, it would be fair to state that megavitamin therapy is difficult to rationalize on scientific grounds; its enthusiastic acceptance in some quarters is based largely on anecdotal evidence. It is probably fortunate that compliance with some of the recommended regimens is variable, and that on the whole the vitamins involved have low toxicity. Nevertheless, niacin and, more recently, pyridoxine have demonstrated toxicity. It is possible, however, that some of the observed megavitamin effects are pharmacologic in nature (rather than normal physiologic effects of the vitamin), and one must await the outcome of research in this area. At this time, megavitamin therapy is not a scientifically accepted medical practice.

FAT-SOLUBLE VITAMINS

Vitamin A

Structure, Dietary Sources, and Recommended Intake

Vitamin A, as the preformed vitamin, exists as all-trans retinol (the physiologically active form; Fig. 49–1), as long-chain fatty acyl esters of retinol (the main storage form in tissues), and as retinal (the active form in the retina). In the cells, retinol is converted to retinoic acid, also considered to be physiologically active. The cis-isomers have no significant vitamin activity. Vitamin A activity is also provided by β-carotene (provitamin A), which can be converted to retinol. Other members of the carotenoid group have marginal activity.

Preformed vitamin A, as retinyl esters, is found only in animal products, the major sources being liver, fish liver oils, milk and dairy products, egg yolk, and fortified margarine. β-Carotene occurs in plant foods such as green and yellow vegetables and yellow fruits.

Recommended intakes (*see* Tables 49–1, 49–2, and 49–3) are expressed as Retinol Equivalents (RE). In humans with a normal mixed diet, the activity of β-carotene is approximately one-sixth that of retinol because of incomplete absorption and inefficient conversion to retinol.

$$1 \text{ RE} = 1 \ \mu\text{g retinol,}$$
$$= 6 \ \mu\text{g } \beta\text{-carotene,}$$
$$= 12 \ \mu\text{g other carotenes.}$$

Older usage expressed the activity of vitamin A in U.S.P. units or International Units (IU). These were based upon biologic activity in the vitamin A-deficient rat, and 1 IU = 0.3 μg of retinol or 0.6 μg of β-carotene. Thus,

$$1 \text{ RE} = 3.33 \text{ IU retinol,}$$
$$= 10.0 \text{ IU } \beta\text{-carotene.}$$

One-third to one-half of the daily intake of vitamin A in mixed diets is β-carotene. In strict vegetarian diets containing no animal foods, β-carotene is virtually the sole source of vitamin A.

Pharmacokinetics

The preformed vitamin is well absorbed from the upper intestine by a carrier-mediated process at low intakes and by diffusion at higher doses. β-Carotene is cleaved to retinol mainly in the intestinal mucosal cells during absorption, and to a lesser extent by liver and other tissues. Bile salts enhance retinol absorption and are required for the absorption of β-carotene. Both vitamin A and β-carotene are transported from the intestine in the chylomicra *via* the lymph in a manner identical to that of fat absorption.

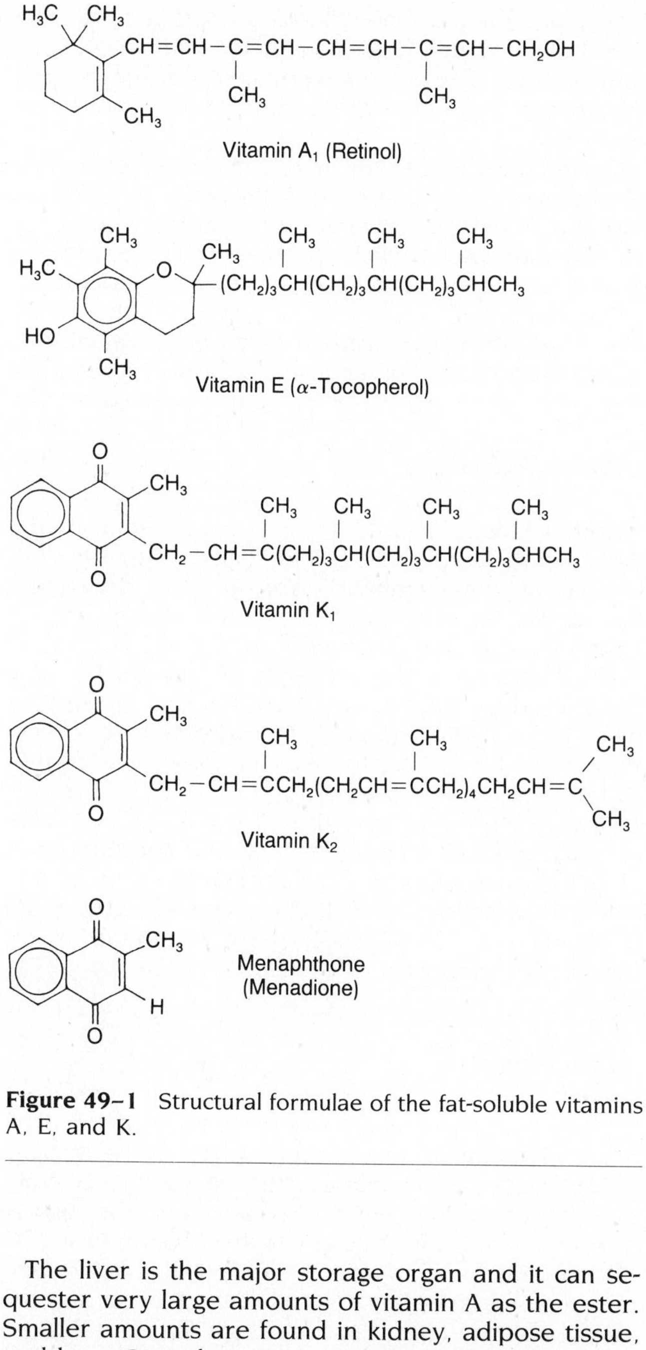

Figure 49–1 Structural formulae of the fat-soluble vitamins A, E, and K.

Physiology

In the retina of the eye, all-trans retinol is converted to the aldehyde and isomerized to 11-cis retinal, which then combines with the protein, opsin, in the rod cells of the retina to produce rhodopsin. This compound is responsible for vision in dim light. In the cone cells, iodopsin is similarly formed and is responsible for daylight vision.

Retinol (and likely retinoic acid) is required for normal cell differentiation, particularly of the mucus-secreting epithelial cells. In the absence of retinol, mucus-secreting cells are replaced by keratin-producing cells in many body tissues. This action may be exerted *via* the influence of retinol on gene expression in the nucleus. Retinol also serves as a carrier for mannose to effect its incorporation into cell surface glycoproteins, which appear to serve a number of functions including that of regulation of cell differentiation. The requirement for vitamin A in normal reproduction, bone development and growth, as well as its influence on the immune system, may be allied to the general function of cell differentiation.

Deficiency

Vitamin A deficiency is most prevalent in preschool children in Southeast Asia, parts of Africa, and South America because of poor intakes of both vitamin A and carotene. Also at risk are the newborn (especially the premature infant), since liver stores of vitamin A at birth are low. In the alcoholic individual, liver structure is affected (*see* Chapter 62) and storage of vitamin A is compromised. In the nonalcoholic adult, vitamin A deficiency occurs largely as a consequence of gastrointestinal abnormalities resulting in fat malabsorption. Deficiency symptoms include night blindness (nyctalopia), and keratinization of the epithelia of the cornea, conjunctiva, bronchorespiratory tract, genitourinary tract, gastrointestinal tract, and sweat glands. There is an increased frequency of infections of the respiratory tract, skin and mucous membranes, and the keratinization of the cornea (keratomalacia) may lead to blindness.

Therapeutic Use

Supplementation is necessary only to treat frank deficiency, or as a preventive measure in pregnancy, lactation, or infancy when dietary intakes are obviously inadequate. In the latter case, the supplement plus usual dietary intake should not exceed the recommended intake. In areas where intake of vitamin A is chronically inadequate, prophylactic intramuscular injections of 30–120 mg retinol given every 3–6 months to infants and small children have proved effective in reducing blindness induced by vitamin A deficiency.

Vitamin A palmitate, and more recently isomers of

The liver is the major storage organ and it can sequester very large amounts of vitamin A as the ester. Smaller amounts are found in kidney, adipose tissue, and lung. Stored vitamin A is released from the liver into the plasma as retinol, bound to a specific retinol-binding protein, by a tightly regulated process to maintain a constant supply of retinol to the target tissues. Normal plasma retinol levels are maintained at 30–70 μg/dL (1.05–2.45 μmol/L) and are not significantly reduced even in vitamin A deficiency until depletion of liver stores is well advanced. When large amounts of vitamin A, in excess of the normal requirement, are taken in chronically, they are not excreted but are stored in the liver and can ultimately exceed the hepatic storage capacity, resulting in toxicity.

retinoic acid, have proved effective in the treatment of various skin disorders, *e.g.*, acne vulgaris and psoriasis, albeit not without toxic side effects.

Toxicity

Vitamin A is highly toxic when taken in large amounts, either acutely or chronically. Hypervitaminosis A occurs most frequently as a result of overenthusiastic supplementation of children's diets or self-medication, but it may also result from the excessive consumption of retinol-rich foodstuffs (*e.g.*, a single serving of polar bear liver or chronic intakes of large portions of chicken or beef liver).

Acute toxicity may result from a single dose of about 200 mg (666,000 IU) of vitamin A in adults, or half of this amount in children. Toxicity signs include headache, nausea and vomiting, increased cerebrospinal pressure, blurred vision, and bulging of the fontanelle in infants. Larger doses cause extensive peeling of the skin.

Chronic toxicity may follow repeated intakes of vitamin A over long periods of time (3–6 months or more) in amounts greater than 10 times the recommended intake. There is an extensive array of symptoms that vary with the individual, the more serious including hepatotoxicity, hypercalcemia, hyperlipemia, spontaneous abortions, and fetal malformations. One fatality from apparent vitamin A toxicity has been reported in a newborn receiving 25 mg/day for 11 days.

In both acute and chronic toxicity, the symptoms are transient and disappear after withdrawal of the supplement. Toxic dose levels also vary considerably because of marked variation in individual sensitivity to large intakes.

Retinoic acid isomers, *e.g.*, etretinate and isotretinoin, used in the treatment of skin disorders, cause minor side effects including dryness of mucous membranes and conjunctivitis, but more importantly are teratogenic if taken in early pregnancy.

Large intakes of β-carotene produce an orange coloration of the skin. Hypercarotenemia is a benign condition that does not result in vitamin A toxicity because of the slow conversion of β-carotene to retinol.

Vitamin D

Structure, Dietary Sources, and Recommended Intake

The vitamin exists in two major precursor forms, 7-dehydrocholesterol and ergosterol, which are converted to their active forms cholecalciferol (vitamin D_3) and calciferol (vitamin D_2) upon exposure to ultraviolet radiation. Of major human importance is the photobiosynthesis of vitamin D_3 in the skin upon exposure to sunlight. The physiologically active form appears to be 1,25-dihydroxycholecalciferol or calcitriol (Fig. 49–2). Vitamin D levels are particularly high in fish liver oils.

Milk, margarine, and infant foods are fortified with vitamin D_3. Few natural foods contain the vitamin in significant amounts. The policy governing the choice of foods that may be fortified with vitamin D varies in different countries.

In climates where exposure to sun is year round, biosynthesis of vitamin D in the skin provides sufficient vitamin. In northern climates or in areas with heavy air pollution that occludes ultraviolet penetration, a dietary or supplemental source must be provided.

Recommended intakes are given in Tables 49–1, 49–2, and 49–3, and are expressed in μg vitamin D_3. As with vitamin A, older usage was in International Units, 1 IU of vitamin D_3 being equivalent to 0.025 μg.

Pharmacokinetics

Both vitamins D_2 and D_3 are absorbed from the intestine, the latter more completely. As with other fat-soluble vitamins, vitamin D absorption is dependent on normal fat absorption; it is thus dependent on hepatic and biliary function.

The first step in the activation of vitamin D_3 (now considered the prohormone form) occurs in the liver where it is hydroxylated to 25-hydroxy-D_3 (calcidiol). From there it circulates to the kidney where it is further hydroxylated to its active hormone form, 1,25-dihydroxy-D_3 (calcitriol). This latter hydroxylation is tightly regulated and responds to changes in serum concentrations of calcium and phosphorus. Parathyroid hormone and calcitonin are also involved. The major excretory route of vitamin D metabolites is the bile. (The details of this functional metabolism of vitamin D_3 are shown in Fig. 49–2.)

Physiology

Vitamin D has a primary role in the homeostatic regulation of serum calcium and phosphate levels through the promotion of intestinal absorption and renal reabsorption of calcium and phosphorus, and the resorption of calcium and phosphate from bone (*see also* Chapter 48). Maintenance of serum calcium levels permits mineralization and remodelling of bone and the maintenance of normal excitability in the central, autonomic, and somatic nervous systems. Because it is produced exclusively in the kidney in response to hypocalcemia and hypophosphatemia and exerts its function on specific target tissues, vitamin D is considered to be a hormone.

Deficiency

Vitamin D deficiency occurs mainly as a consequence of inadequate exposure to sunlight and/or as a consequence of dietary deficiency. It can also occur as a result of an increased requirement (*e.g.*, multiple pregnancies, lactation) or of a deficit in the 1-hydroxylation pathway of 25-hydroxy-D_3. Deficiency results in rickets in

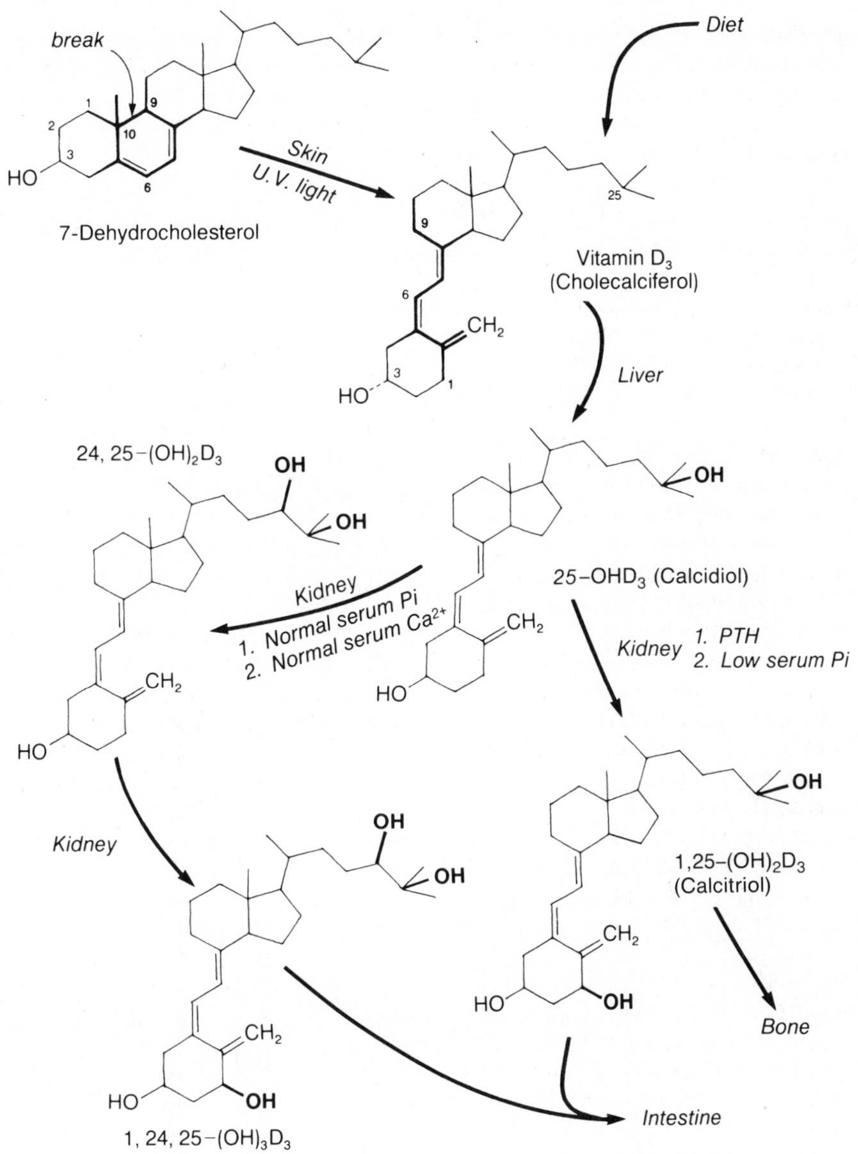

Figure 49–2 Current concepts of the functional metabolism of vitamin D_3.

children and osteomalacia in adults, as a consequence of decreased mineralization of bone and teeth. The matrix is decalcified, so that the bone is softened and may become grossly deformed. Rickets was formerly a major problem in Canada because of insufficient sunlight during the winter, but has been largely eliminated by vitamin D fortification of milk.

Therapeutic Use

Rickets due to inadequate exposure to sunlight can be reversed by 10 μg calciferol daily. Fully developed rickets and osteomalacia may require dosages of 0.1–1.0 mg calciferol daily, depending on the etiology of the disease. Since 45–50 μg calciferol daily can lead

to hypervitaminosis D, high-potency preparations are only available by prescription, and in most countries the addition of vitamin D to foods is restricted.

A form of vitamin D-dependent rickets that has a genetic rather than dietary etiology will respond to 1250–2500 μg (50,000–100,000 IU) of calciferol daily.

Toxicity

Hypervitaminosis D due to excessive intake is not uncommon. In Britain following World War II, school children were sometimes given ten times the recommended daily allowance in their supplemental orange drink. This led in extreme cases to hypercalcemia (1 in 10,000) and mental retardation (1 in 200,000). Symptoms of vitamin D toxicity include fatigue, headache, diarrhea, and hypercalcemia, which may lead to calcium deposition in kidney, heart, lungs, blood vessels, and skin. Hypercalcemia may also lead to an arrest of growth that cannot be fully reversed. This may be associated with irreversible effects on calcitonin production (*see* Chapter 48).

The amount of vitamin D that produces toxicity varies widely. Acute toxicity may occur after ingestion of 25–75 μg/kg (1000–3000 IU/kg). Chronic toxicity in adults occurs with doses as low as 250 μg (10,000 IU) per day over several months, or more commonly with doses approaching 1250 μg (50,000 IU) or more over several years. Infants and children may be sensitive to chronic intakes as low as 50 μg (2000 IU) per day.

Vitamin E

Structure, Dietary Sources, and Recommended Intake

Many tocopherols are known to have vitamin E activity. However, 90% of the vitamin E in animal tissues is d-α-tocopherol (RRR-α-tocopherol; *see* Fig. 49–1). Dietary sources are vegetable oils and wheat germ.

Recommended intakes of vitamin E (*see* Tables 49–1, 49–2, and 49–3) are given as mg d-α-Tocopherol Equivalents (TE). Older terminology used for vitamin E activity is the International Unit. 1 IU = 1 mg d,l-α-tocopheryl acetate (all-rac-α-tocopherol), the commercially synthesized form, or 0.9 mg d-α-tocopherol, the naturally occurring form.

Pharmacokinetics

Absorption of vitamin E, like that of other fat-soluble vitamins, depends on the integrity of fat-absorption processes in the intestine. Approximately 50% of dietary tocopherols are absorbed at normal intakes. Efficiency of absorption falls to less than 10% with pharmacologic doses, *e.g.*, 200 mg or more. Tocopherols are carried in the blood by plasma β-lipoproteins. The liver is the major storage site. Although large amounts are also deposited in adipose tissue, tocopherol in adipocytes is not readily available to other tissues.

Physiology

Vitamin E is an antioxidant and probably acts as a free radical scavenger in cell membranes to protect membrane polyunsaturated fatty acids from peroxidation. It appears to act in concert with other antioxidant systems in the cell, *e.g.*, selenium-dependent glutathione peroxidase and superoxide dismutase.

Vitamin E not located in the membranes likely serves as a protective antioxidant for other easily oxidized lipid-soluble compounds such as vitamin A.

It has also been suggested that vitamin E has a specific function as a repressor, regulating the synthesis of specific enzymes.

Deficiency

Vitamin E is accepted as an essential nutrient for humans, but while deficiency states have been clearly defined in animals, this is a subject of much debate in human health and nutrition.

Adults rarely develop a vitamin E deficiency due to poor dietary intake. However, individuals with chronic fat malabsorption or a genetic deficiency of β-lipoprotein, the plasma carrier for vitamin E, are at risk. In these individuals erythrocyte stability is diminished, resulting in decreased erythrocyte survival, although severe anemia does not usually ensue.

Premature newborns have limited tissue stores of vitamin E at birth and have intestinal malabsorption for the first few weeks of life. Decreased erythrocyte survival in these infants leads to a severe hemolytic anemia.

In many animal species vitamin E deficiency leads to male sterility and fetal reabsorption or abortion, muscular dystrophy, and pathologic changes in cardiac and vascular smooth muscle. In humans these syndromes are not observed in vitamin E deficiency, and evidence to support the efficacy of vitamin E in treating these disorders is anecdotal or based on small, poorly organized clinical trials.

Therapeutic Use

Correction of the deficiencies noted above may require up to 300 mg vitamin E. Vitamin E in high doses (about 300 mg) also appears to be effective in treating intermittent claudication in adults and to ameliorate oxygen-induced retrolental fibroplasia in premature infants. Claims for its efficacy in treating a myriad of other conditions (the effects of aging, cardiovascular disease, sexual dysfunction, *etc.*) are unfounded.

Toxicity

Vitamin E has extremely low toxicity, producing only mild gastrointestinal upsets or fatigue in some individuals.

Vitamin K

Structure, Dietary Sources, and Recommended Intake

Vitamin K exists in two forms, one of plant origin (phylloquinone, or K_1), and the other of bacterial origin (menaquinones, K_2) (*see* Fig. 49–1). A number of synthetic quinones have vitamin K-like activity, of which the most important is menadione (K_3). Sources in the diet are green leafy vegetables, cheese, egg yolk, and liver.

There is insufficient information to establish a recommended intake. One-half of the requirement may be met by intestinal bacterial synthesis. The requirement of vitamin K_1 may be between 0.03 and 1.5 $\mu g/kg$.

Pharmacokinetics

Vitamin K is readily absorbed by the usual pathways of fat absorption, and it is therefore dependent on the presence of bile salts. There is only limited tissue storage of vitamin K, and the stores can be depleted in 10–20 days.

Physiology

Vitamin K is required for the gamma-carboxylation (activation) of glutamic acid residues in a number of inactive precursors of biologically important proteins. The best known of these are prothrombin and at least seven other factors involved in the coagulation of blood (see Chapter 41).

Other vitamin K-dependent proteins have been identified, e.g., osteocalcin in bone and proteins in plasma and kidney cortex. The common feature of these proteins is their capacity to bind calcium, presumably at the gamma-carboxyglutamyl sites.

Oral anticoagulants of the coumarin class (including warfarin; see Chapter 41) are vitamin K antagonists and are useful in reducing thrombus formation in patients with ischemic heart disease. Paradoxically, vitamin K in megadose amounts has been reported to prolong the prothrombin time; a dose of 1200 IU may potentiate the anticoagulant effects of the coumarin drugs and cause bleeding.

Deficiency

Requirements are easily met in the diet and may also be met in part from synthesis by intestinal bacteria. In adults, deficiency is usually secondary to malabsorption or the administration of a vitamin K antagonist. In deficiency there is an increased prothrombin time and a tendency to hemorrhage.

Newborn infants, particularly premature ones, are susceptible to a vitamin K deficiency, "hemorrhagic disease of the newborn." Little vitamin crosses the placenta to the fetus, and the gut is sterile for the first few days of life. Human breast milk is sterile and contains little vitamin K, placing the breast-fed infant at further risk. Therefore, vitamin K is usually administered prophylactically to the newborn.

Therapeutic Use

The only rational uses of vitamin K are for the hepatic biosynthesis of clotting factors, especially as an anti-dotal agent in oral anticoagulant therapy (see Chapter 41), and in the prevention of hemorrhagic disease of the newborn.

Toxicity

Excessive doses of menadione (K_3) produce a hemolytic tendency and kernicterus in infants. It irritates mucous membranes and may depress liver function. Vitamin K_1 does not have these effects and, moreover, it is nontoxic in animals. In humans, flushing, dyspnea and death have occurred, but these may have been due to other constituents in the respective pharmaceutical dosage form of vitamin K_1.

WATER-SOLUBLE VITAMINS

B-Complex Vitamins

Thiamin (Vitamin B_1)

Structure, Dietary Sources, and Recommended Intake

Thiamin (Fig. 49–3) consists of a pyrimidine and a thiazole moiety. The major dietary sources are pork, beef, liver, whole or enriched grains, and legumes. Recommended intakes (see Tables 49–1, 49–2, and 49–3) are based on energy intake, but in instances of very low energy consumption the thiamin intake should not fall below the amount required for 2000 kcal (i.e., 0.8 mg/day).

Pharmacokinetics

Thiamin is absorbed from the upper small intestine by a carrier-mediated active transport process when intakes are less than 5 mg/day (well above the recommended intake). At higher intakes, passive diffusion contributes. Absorption is significantly impaired in alcoholics and in patients with folic acid deficiency.

The body pool is small, about 30 mg in the adult, half of which is in skeletal muscle and the remainder in heart, liver, kidney, and brain. Excess thiamin is not stored but is excreted in the urine. In addition to free thiamin, the urine also contains a number of catabolites of thiamin that arise as a consequence of the coenzyme action of thiamin.

Physiology

Thiamin pyrophosphate functions as a coenzyme in the oxidative decarboxylation of pyruvic and α-ketoglutaric acids, and in the "transketolase" reactions of the triose phosphate pathway.

ENDOCRINE SYSTEMS

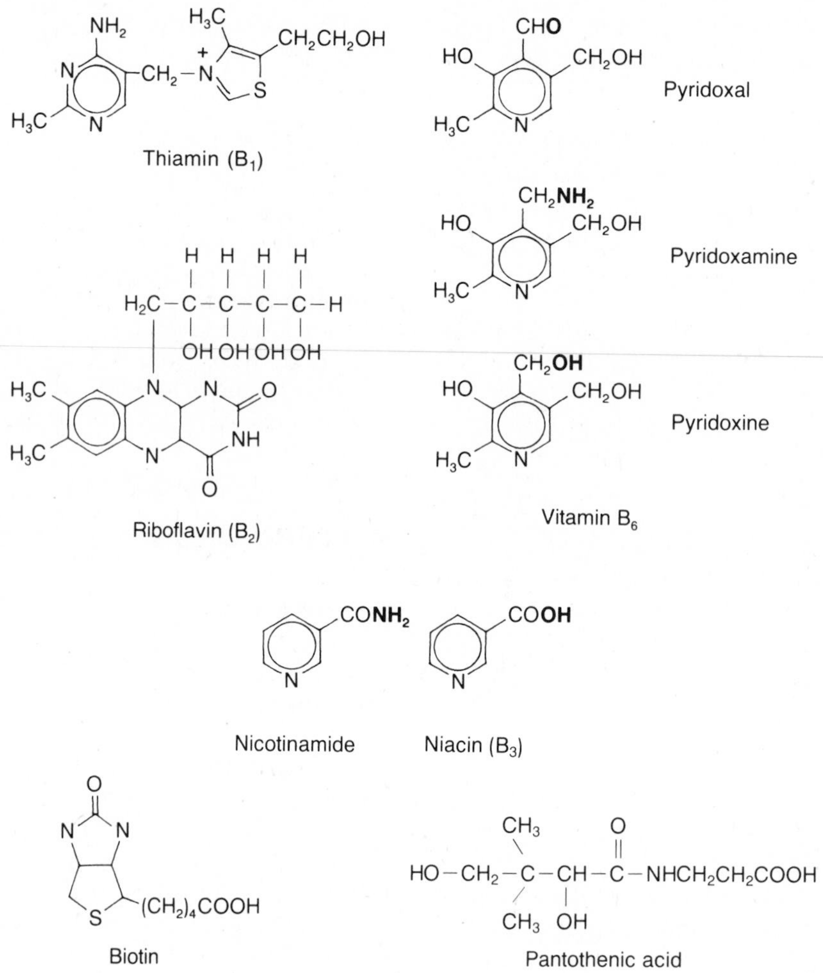

Figure 49-3 Structural formulae of the water-soluble vitamins of the B complex.

Thiamin is also required, likely as thiamin triphosphate, for nerve function in a reaction that is unrelated to its role as a coenzyme.

Deficiency

Beriberi is associated with the consumption of white polished rice diets as seen in Southeast Asia or of highly milled wheat diets. The deficiency has become much less common since the practice of fortifying foods with thiamin was adopted in most countries.

Acute deficiency (wet or cardiovascular beriberi) results from diets that are very low in thiamin and high in carbohydrates. Signs include edema, enlarged heart, ECG changes, and cardiac failure associated with increased cardiac output.

Slightly higher, but still inadequate, intakes produce a chronic deficiency (dry or neuritic beriberi), the essential feature of which is polyneuropathy with depressed peripheral nerve function, sensory distur-

bance, loss of reflexes and motor control, and muscle wasting.

Breast-fed infants whose mothers have a low thiamin intake are prone to infantile beriberi, which can be either acute or chronic. Cardiac failure and sudden death are seen with both forms.

In populations whose diet is not based on rice, thiamin deficiency is frequently seen in alcoholics because of a combination of poor diet and inhibition of the thiamin uptake mechanism by alcohol. It is the causal factor in three conditions often seen in alcoholics: alcoholic polyneuritis, indistinguishable from dry beriberi; a thiamin-responsive cardiomyopathy; and an encephalopathy known as the Wernicke-Korsakoff syndrome, that is characterized by impairment of memory, apathy, irritability, nystagmus, and oculomotor paralysis.

Therapeutic Use

Deficiency may be treated with 15-30 mg/day of thiamin hydrochloride. Pharmacologic doses of 50 mg/day are required for a few rare and poorly described thiamin-responsive inborn errors of metabolism.

Toxicity

No marked toxicity has been observed, and the very few isolated reports of alleged toxicity may have been due to individual hypersensitivity in patients receiving large amounts of thiamin intramuscularly.

Riboflavin (Vitamin B₂)

Structure, Dietary Sources, and Recommended Intake

Riboflavin (see Fig. 49–3) is a heterocyclic flavin linked to ribose, analogous to the nucleosides in RNA. It occurs predominantly in milk, liver, and enriched cereals. As with thiamin and niacin, the recommended intakes are related to energy intake but should not fall below the amount required for 2000 kcal (i.e., 1.0 mg/day; see Tables 49–1, 49–2, and 49–3).

Pharmacokinetics

Riboflavin is absorbed from the upper part of the ileum by a saturable active transport process. Bile salts facilitate absorption. The absorptive capacity is limited to 20–25 mg in a single dose. Riboflavin is distributed to all tissues; very little is stored.

Conversion of riboflavin to coenzymes occurs in most tissues. It is excreted in urine unchanged. Since there is little storage, urinary excretion reflects dietary intake. Excretion increases with conditions associated with tissue breakdown, such as weight loss, starvation, bed rest, and uncontrolled diabetes.

Physiology

Riboflavin phosphate (flavin mononucleotide, FMN) and flavin adenine dinucleotide (FAD) are involved in the metabolism of carbohydrates, fats, and proteins. In general, flavin dehydrogenases function as hydrogen carriers from specific substrates to the respiratory chain, resulting in the production of ATP (e.g., NADH dehydrogenase and succinate dehydrogenase). Other riboflavin enzymes not involved in energy metabolism include the d- and l-amino acid oxidases, pyridoxine-5-phosphate oxidase, and glutathione reductase.

Deficiency

Symptoms include cheilosis (vertical fissures in the lips), angular stomatitis (cracks in the corners of the mouth), glossitis, corneal vascularization, photophobia, seborrheic dermatitis, and a normochromic, normocytic anemia.

Therapeutic Use

For the treatment of deficiency, 5–10 mg orally (or intravenously) is administered along with other B complex vitamins, since ariboflavinosis is usually associated with other B vitamin deficiencies.

Toxicity

There is no known toxicity of riboflavin. Limited absorption, poor solubility, and urinary excretion of excess vitamin likely preclude the risk of toxicity even with megadoses.

Niacin (Nicotinic Acid, Vitamin B₃)

Structure, Dietary Sources, and Recommended Intake

Niacin (see Fig. 49–3) is a simple derivative of pyridine. The amide form, niacinamide (nicotinamide) is the physiologically active form. Tryptophan, an essential amino acid, can be converted to niacinamide adenine dinucleotide (NAD), one of the coenzyme forms, but less than 2% of tryptophan metabolism follows this pathway. Dietary sources are organ meats, peanuts, and enriched grains. In many cereal grains, especially corn, most of the niacin is bound in an unabsorbable form. Milk and eggs contain little niacin but are good sources of tryptophan.

Recommended intakes are expressed as Niacin Equivalents (NE) to take into account the presence of both preformed niacin and tryptophan in foods. As with thiamin and riboflavin, the niacin requirement is based on energy intake, but the intake should not fall below that required for 2000 kcal (i.e., 14.4 NE/day; see Table 49–1).

Pharmacokinetics

Niacin is readily absorbed from the intestine by a carrier-mediated facilitated diffusion at low intakes. It is distributed to all tissues. The vitamin forms are converted to the coenzyme forms in tissues. Niacin released from the breakdown of NAD can be reused within the cells. Little niacin is excreted as such in the urine; most is transformed to methylated derivatives prior to urinary excretion.

Physiology

Niacin in its amide form is part of nicotinamide adenine dinucleotide (NAD) and nicotinamide adenine dinucleotide phosphate (NADP). These function as coenzymes that serve as hydrogen carriers for many reactions catalysed by dehydrogenases. NAD is required in all of the major metabolic pathways involving the oxidative catabolism of carbohydrates, fats, and proteins to energy. NADP systems are common to biosynthetic reactions, and NADPH is required as a hydrogen donor for the cytochrome P-450 system (see Chapter 4).

Deficiency

In niacin deficiency (pellagra) the tissues most affected are the skin, the gastrointestinal tract, and the nervous system. Early signs are nonspecific and include lassitude, anorexia, weakness, mild gastrointestinal disturbances, and emotional changes such as anxiety, irritability, and depression.

As the deficiency progresses, a bilateral pigmented scaly dermatitis develops on areas exposed to the sun. In the gastrointestinal tract the mucosa becomes inflamed and atrophic, which may account for a profuse watery diarrhea. Glossitis, angular stomatitis, and cheilosis are frequent. Mental changes intensify to include confusion, hallucinations, memory loss, and frank psychosis (see also Chapter 25 for the significance of chronic niacin deficiency in alcoholics). Peripheral motor and sensory disturbances may also occur. Anemias are frequent, but they are likely due to associated deficiencies.

Therapeutic Use

In the treatment of pellagra the recommended oral dose is 50 mg given up to ten times a day, or 25 mg intravenously at least twice a day. Additional therapy with riboflavin and pyridoxine is usually carried out. The similarity between some mental signs of subclinical pellagra and those of schizophrenia has led to the "megavitamin" approach to the treatment of schizophrenia using large doses of niacin (3–6 g/day) together with ascorbic acid (3–6 g/day) and pyridoxine (600–1500 mg/day). In addition to the advocates of the megavitamin school, many psychiatrists use this regimen to satisfy patients' requests, in spite of the evidence (in the form of double-blind trials) of its ineffectiveness. Fortunately, neuroleptics are used in conjunction with megavitamin therapy. There is at present no valid reason for using megavitamin therapy alone for schizophrenia. Normal therapeutic doses can be used to treat both pellagra and subclinical pellagra.

Large doses of niacin (1–3 g/day) have been reported to lower serum cholesterol (see also Chapter 37). This appears to be a pharmacologic effect unrelated to its role as a vitamin.

Toxicity

One gram or more of niacin per day produces marked peripheral vasodilatation (flushing), an effect that is not shared by niacinamide. Doses over 3 g/day have been associated with activation of peptic ulcer, abnormal glucose tolerance, cardiac arrhythmias, and hepatotoxicity.

Pyridoxine (Vitamin B_6)

Structure, Dietary Sources, and Recommended Intake

The vitamin B_6 group consists of three naturally occurring pyridine derivatives: pyridoxal, pyridoxamine, and pyridoxine (see Fig. 49–3). They are present in low concentrations in virtually all plant and animal tissues. Recommended intakes (see Tables 49–1 and 49–2) are based on protein intake; thus, high protein intake increases the vitamin B_6 requirement.

Pharmacokinetics

It is well absorbed from the small intestine, likely by passive diffusion, although the vitamin in plant foods is in a glycosylated form of very low bioavailability.

The adult body pool of B_6 compounds is about 25 mg. The vitamin is excreted in the urine as both pyridoxal and its major metabolite 4-pyridoxic acid. Excretion reflects the dietary intake.

Physiology

All three forms of vitamin B_6 are physiologically active; they are interconvertible. The major coenzyme form is pyridoxal phosphate, which functions in amino acid metabolism in many pathways including decarboxylation, deamination, transamination, transsulfuration, heme synthesis, and the conversion of tryptophan to niacin.

Deficiency

A dietary deficiency of vitamin B_6 is uncommon because of the diversity of foods containing the vitamin, although epileptiform convulsions have been observed in infants fed a milk formula in which vitamin B_6 had been destroyed during processing. Deficiency symptoms include peripheral neuritis, seborrheic dermatitis and other skin lesions, and a B_6-dependent sideroblastic anemia resembling iron deficiency anemia. Inborn errors of metabolism that respond to high doses of vitamin B_6 have also been reported.

Vitamin B_6 deficiency can occur also as a result of interaction with certain drugs. Pregnant women and those taking oral contraceptives have shown abnormalities in tryptophan metabolism suggestive of B_6 depletion, which do respond to B_6 supplementation. Hydralazine, isoniazid, and penicillamine have similar effects, all of which appear to be due to inhibition of pyridoxal kinase, one of the enzymes that convert B_6 to its active form, pyridoxal phosphate.

Therapeutic Use

Pyridoxine is included in all B complex supplementation and is routinely used to prevent peripheral neuritis in patients receiving isoniazid. The efficacy of vitamin B_6 in amounts up to 200 mg/day in the treatment of sickle cell disease, asthma, premenstrual tension, and carpal tunnel syndrome has yet to be confirmed. Doses over 200 mg/day for prolonged periods may be toxic.

Toxicity

A transient physiologic dependence on vitamin B_6 has been reported in adults receiving 200 mg/day for a month. Therapeutic doses of 2–3 g/day for prolonged periods (from several months to 2–3 years) have caused incapacitating peripheral sensory neuropathy, which subsided slowly after withdrawal of the supplement.

Cyanocobalamin (Vitamin B₁₂) and Folic Acid

These two vitamins are discussed in Chapter 42, *Hematinic Drugs.* It is important to note that vitamin B_{12} is present only in foods of animal origin, and this fact has an obvious implication for life-time vegetarians.

Some of the folic acid in foods, particularly plant foods, is in a form conjugated with glutamic acid residues, which reduces its bioavailability. The increased requirement for folic acid in pregnancy makes the use of a supplement a necessity for many women.

Recommended intakes for vitamin B_{12} and folic acid (folacin) are given in Tables 49–1, 49–2, and 49–3. The recommendation for folic acid takes into account the variations in bioavailability.

Biotin and Pantothenic Acid

These two vitamins are usually included with the B complex vitamins. Other than the treatment of rarely occurring primary or induced deficiencies, they have no established therapeutic use. It is assumed that an adequate intake is provided in the diet. They are both virtually nontoxic. The structures are given in Figure 49–3.

Biotin

Biotin is widely distributed in the diet and may be synthesized by the bacterial flora. The usual intake is 100–300 µg/day, and this is considered adequate.

A naturally occurring deficiency is an extreme rarity. In two reported cases, large quantities of raw eggs (6–12 eggs/day) were consumed over periods of months or years. Raw egg white contains ovidin, which binds biotin and renders it biologically unavailable.

Experimental deficiencies are characterized by an-

orexia, nausea and vomiting, and a dry scaly dermatitis.

Biotin is involved in fatty acid synthesis as the coenzyme for acetyl-CoA carboxylase and other carboxylation pathways.

Pantothenic Acid

Pantothenic acid is converted to coenzyme A, which is involved in the intermediary metabolism of carbohydrates, fats, and proteins, as well as the many synthetic reactions involving acetylation. Intake is assumed to be above the 5–10 mg/day requirement, and no naturally occurring deficiency has been reported in humans.

Ascorbic Acid (Vitamin C)

Structure, Dietary Sources, and Recommended Intake

Ascorbic acid (Fig. 49–4) is structurally related to glucose. It is found in citrus fruits and vegetables, and as an additive in fortified tomato and fruit juices. This is the most labile vitamin, and it is easily destroyed by exposure to air and heat, and during prolonged storage.

The recommended intakes vary between 30 and 60 mg/day from country to country (*see* Tables 49–1, 49–2, and 49–3). A suitable intake has been hotly disputed among experts, and recommended intakes have undergone numerous revisions.

Pharmacokinetics

Vitamin C is well absorbed from the small intestine by a saturable active transport process. The efficiency of absorption decreases with increasing intake. The vitamin is distributed in most tissues throughout the body; the adult body pool is approximately 1500 mg. Excess vitamin C is not stored, and levels in leukocytes are used to estimate tissue levels. At plasma concentrations below 1.4 mg/dL (80 µmol/L), ascorbic acid is reabsorbed by the kidney; above that level ascorbic acid is actively secreted. A large number of metabolites also appear in the urine. Urinary excretion of ascorbic acid

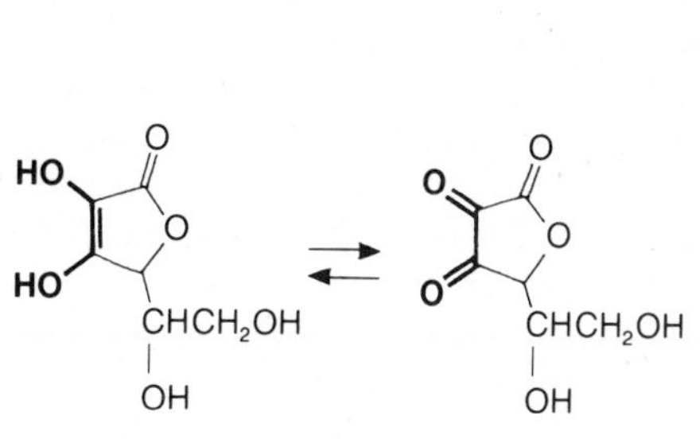

Figure 49–4 Structural formulae of ascorbic acid and its oxidation product, dehydroascorbic acid (both vitamin C).

ENDOCRINE SYSTEMS

closely reflects dietary intake. Tissue saturation occurs when the plasma level is between 1 and 2 mg/dL (56.8 and 113.6 μmol/L); women have higher levels than men, and cigarette smoking may drastically lower plasma ascorbate levels. All types of stress have a similar effect. If ascorbic acid ingestion is reduced following long-term supplementation with 250 mg/day or more, the kidney continues to secrete ascorbic acid. This results in a rebound phenomenon in which plasma ascorbate may fall to scorbutic levels (especially if prior ingestion was 2 g or more per day). There is a report that after daily ingestion of 10 g of vitamin C for a week, withdrawal resulted in frank symptoms of scurvy.

Physiology

Ascorbic acid appears to have a role in the maintenance of the cellular redox potential and is an important facilitator of the absorption of non-heme iron from the intestinal tract. It is involved in the synthesis of collagen and thus plays a role in wound healing and bone matrix formation. It is involved in tyrosine metabolism and is specifically required for the dopamine-β-hydroxylase step of catecholamine synthesis. Plasma ascorbate levels are decreased under stress, as are levels in the adrenal cortex where ascorbic acid plays a role in the synthesis of adrenal steroids.

Deficiency

Man, monkey, guinea pig, and fruit bat have lost the ability to synthesize ascorbic acid from glucose (the last enzyme in the series, L-gulonolactone oxidase, has been lost by these species). Dietary deficiency of ascorbic acid can therefore give rise, in these species, to the symptoms of scurvy, which include pathologic lesions of bones, teeth, gums, skin, and blood vessels. These all appear to be due to depolymerization of connective tissue and disappearance of collagen. Death ensues if the scorbutic state is not corrected. Infantile scurvy has been a problem, and Nutrition Canada reports that there may be clinical vitamin C deficiency among the Inuit (Eskimos) and the elderly.

Therapeutic Use

There is an increased requirement for ascorbic acid in pregnancy, lactation, tuberculosis, peptic ulcer, and other stress conditions, *e.g.*, surgery. This can be met by ingestion of 100–200 mg per day. Similar amounts are required by infants on high protein diets to prevent tyrosinemia. Scurvy is usually treated with 1–2 g/day until tissue saturation is attained.

Toxicity

Normal dietary levels are without toxicity. High dietary intake (in excess of 1 g/day) may cause diarrhea, and in some sensitive individuals it may promote the precipitation of cystine or oxalate stones in the urinary tract. At higher levels of ascorbate intake the possibility of rebound effects on withdrawal should be considered. There is a danger of scurvy in the newborns of mothers who ingested large amounts of ascorbate during pregnancy. There are also reports of false responses to some diagnostic tests.

Megavitamin C Therapy

Pauling, Stone, Szent-Györgi, and others have recommended taking 2–6 g of ascorbic acid daily for prophylaxis and therapy against the common cold, other virus infections, allergies, cancer, and aging. There have been a number of well controlled studies on the common cold, but no good studies on other aspects of megavitamin C therapy. Its use in the treatment of these states seems to have no foundation in fact. The studies on vitamin C and the common cold demonstrate no effect on the frequency of colds, but they do indicate that some respiratory symptoms are reduced and that there is a decrease in the number of days off work. Thus, there might not be an antiviral effect, but there may be an improved response to stress. On the basis of these trials and our knowledge of the pharmacodynamics of ascorbic acid, 250 mg/day would appear to be the maximum amount required to saturate the tissues; there would appear to be no justification for taking larger daily quantities.

SUGGESTED READING

Alpers DH, Clouse RE, Stenson WF. Manual of nutritional therapeutics. Boston/Toronto: Little, Brown and Company, 1983.

Machlin LJ. Handbook of vitamins: nutritional, biochemical and clinical aspects. New York/Basel: Marcel Dekker, 1984.

Passmore R, Nicol BM, Rao MN. Handbook of human nutritional requirements. World Health Organization Monograph Series No. 61, Geneva, 1974.

Recommended Dietary Allowances. 9th revised ed. Washington, DC: National Academy of Sciences, 1980.

Recommended Nutrient Intakes for Canadians. Ottawa: Health and Welfare Canada, 1983.

Shils ME, Young VR. Modern nutrition in health and disease. 7th ed. New York: Lea and Febiger, 1988.

GASTROINTESTINAL SYSTEM

—

Chapter 50

PHARMACOTHERAPY OF GASTROINTESTINAL ACID-PEPTIC DISORDERS

H. Orrego and L. Spero

Several pathologic processes affecting the upper gastrointestinal tract heal when gastric acid and pepsin activity are suppressed. Examples include gastroesophageal reflux and esophagitis, gastric and duodenal ulcers (including the ulcers associated with gastrin-producing tumors, the Zollinger-Ellison syndrome), stress ulcers, and several forms of gastritis. Duodenal ulcer is the most frequent and classic expression of these conditions and will be used as a prototype in this chapter.

Therapy in such situations can be directed to:

1. Decreasing the acidity and/or peptic activity of gastric juice by (a) neutralization of HCl or intraluminal inactivation of pepsin; (b) inhibition of the secretion of acid and/or pepsin.

2. Increasing the resistance of the mucosa or protecting the base of the ulcer from the action of acid and pepsin.

DECREASING GASTRIC ACIDITY

Control of gastric acidity is the basis for most methods of treating peptic ulcers. Gastric acidity can be reduced by neutralization of acid or by reduction of acid secretion. This can be achieved either by pharmacologic or by surgical means (Table 50–1).

NEUTRALIZATION OF ACID: ANTACIDS IN CLINICAL USE

The gastric antacids reduce the acidity of the stomach contents by neutralizing gastric HCl, but do not inhibit its secretion. Their duration of action depends upon (a) total acid-combining capacity and (b) duration of stay in the stomach.

Antacid effects in the fasting state rarely last longer than 15–30 minutes. On the other hand, when antacids are given in adequate dosage 1 hour after a meal, their effects can last for up to 4 hours. If the dose of the antacid is repeated 3–4 hours after the meal, a further prolongation is obtained.

The term "neutralization" in this context does not mean bringing the gastric pH to 7. The term is used to describe a decrease in acidity (or hydrogen ion concentration) to a pH above 4.5, at which pepsin activity is markedly decreased. Pepsin is completely inactivated above pH 6. Raising the pH from 1.0 to 3.5 eliminates 99% of the hydrogen ion in the stomach, and almost completely inhibits proteolytic activity.

Clinically desirable properties for a gastric antacid include: (a) prolonged effective neutralizing action when an acceptable amount is taken orally; (b) no induction of systemic disturbances of acid-base or electrolyte balance; (c) no interference with digestion or absorption; (d) no induction of constipation or laxative side effects. No one compound fulfills all these requirements.

The clinical efficacy of antacids in healing gastric and duodenal ulcers has been documented in a number of clinical trials. Gastric antacids in clinical use are classified as systemic or absorbable and nonsystemic or nonabsorbable agents (see Table 50–1).

Systemic Antacids

These agents (e.g., sodium bicarbonate, sodium citrate) are ingredients in many over-the-counter remedies, such as Eno's or Andrews salts. They are soluble and are absorbed from the digestive tract. One gram of bicarbonate will neutralize about 120 mL of 0.1 M HCl, and it is even possible to produce a slightly alkaline reaction in the stomach. It acts promptly but for

TABLE 50-1 Means of Reducing Gastric Acidity

Neutralization
    Systemic Antacids
        Sodium bicarbonate
        Sodium citrate
    Nonsystemic Antacids
        Aluminum hydroxide gels
        Magnesium trisilicate

Reduction of gastric secretion
    Pharmacologic
        Anticholinergics
        Histamine H_2-receptor antagonists
        Omeprazole
        Antigastrinics (proglumide, sulpiride)
        Prostaglandins
    Surgical
        Vagotomy
        Partial gastrectomy
        Total gastrectomy

an extremely short time. When absorbed, these agents can produce systemic electrolyte disturbances. Prolonged use of sodium citrate or bicarbonate carries a serious risk of inducing alkalosis.

Nonsystemic Antacids

These compounds are either not absorbed, or absorbed to only a very small extent. Thus, they do not produce systemic alkalosis.

Calcium Carbonate

$$CaCO_3 + 2HCl \rightarrow CaCl_2 + H_2O + CO_2$$

In the intestine, Ca^{2+} tends to be reprecipitated as $CaCO_3$, and NaCl is absorbed. Despite excellent acid-neutralizing action (1 g will neutralize 175 mL of 0.1 M HCl) it is now seldom used in clinical practice because it produces "rebound acid hypersecretion." This phenomenon is not related to its neutralizing capacity, but it is a consequence of a specific direct action of calcium both in the antrum, where it releases gastrin, and in the parietal cells (where H^+ is secreted). The net result of the administration of this compound is a very high nocturnal secretion of acid that offsets any beneficial effect of its high neutralizing capacity. Since some calcium will be absorbed by the proximal small bowel, hypercalcemia and its consequences may become a problem after chronic use of calcium carbonate.

Magnesium Hydroxide (Milk of Magnesia)

$$MgO + 2HCl \rightarrow MgCl_2 + H_2O$$

This is the most potent antacid in common use. In the bowel, most of the magnesium reacts with phosphate or bicarbonate to produce insoluble magnesium salts that are not absorbed. However, about 15–30% of the total amount of a dose of magnesium is absorbed and is rapidly excreted by the kidney. In patients with renal failure, dangerous toxicity can occur. The main limitation of treatment with magnesium preparations is the occurrence of diarrhea that can be severe and lead to fluid and electrolyte depletion. This has led to the use of mixtures with aluminum hydroxide. These mixtures have substantially less neutralizing capacity than plain magnesium hydroxide.

Aluminum Hydroxide Gel, Aluminum Phosphate Gel, Magnesium Trisilicate

$$Al(OH)_3 + 3HCl \rightarrow AlCl_3 + 3H_2O$$

$$2MgO \cdot 3SiO_2(xH_2O) + 4HCl \rightarrow$$
$$2MgCl_2 + 3SiO_2 + (x+2)H_2O$$

One gram of aluminum hydroxide will neutralize about 250 mL of 0.1 M HCl (or 25 mmol H^+). Aluminum hydroxide gel is a less potent buffer than the antacids described above. It has a pH of about 6. Fifteen millilitres of it will neutralize 15 mEq HCl to a pH of 4. It is effective in reducing the total load and concentration of acid but incapable of raising the pH of gastric juice to 6. Aluminum hydroxide gels also inactivate pepsin by adsorption and precipitation. This effect is especially marked at pH levels between 3 and 6. Aluminum hydroxide is amphoteric and relatively insoluble in water. Although aluminum ion is poorly absorbed by the small bowel, detectable plasma aluminum concentrations have been found after ingestion of aluminum-containing antacids.

The different salts contained in common antacid mixtures (aluminum hydroxide, magnesium hydroxide, magnesium trisilicate) vary widely in their potency. As shown in Table 50–2, there is a large number of different mixtures commercially available, which differ as much as 20-fold in acid-neutralizing capacity. However, in the choice of an antacid, potency is not the only factor that should be considered. Cost, taste, salt content, bowel habit, underlying diseases other than peptic ulcer, and side effects of the antacid are also important.

It has been reported that aluminum hydroxide tablets may sometimes fail to disintegrate properly in the

TABLE 50–2 *In Vivo* Neutralizing Capacity for Some Aluminum- and Magnesium-Containing Liquid Antacids

Antacid (Proprietary Name)	Capacity (mEq/mL)	Volume for 80 mEq (mL)	Na in 80 mEq (mg)
Delcid	7.1	11.3	26.0
Ducon	7.0	11.4	40.8
Mylanta II	4.1	19.3	30.9
Camalox	3.6	22.3	11.5
Aludrox	2.8	28.5	28.5
Maalox	2.6	31.0	34.7
Creamalin	2.6	31.1	18.7
Mylanta	2.4	33.6	26.2
Win Gel	2.2	35.6	8.8
Gelusil M	2.2	35.9	40.9
Riopan	2.2	36.2	5.1
Amphojel	1.9	41.4	49.7
A-M-T	1.8	44.7	53.6
Trisogel	1.6	43.5	155.2
Gelusil	1.3	60.1	85.6
Robalate	1.1	70.8	43.2
Phosphaljel	0.4	190.5	495.3

stomach, and thus be ineffective. For liquid preparations the dose usually recommended for duodenal ulcer (10–15 mL, one tablespoonful) is much too low. For hypersecretors, and for duodenal ulcer, a dose of 30–60 mL (Mylanta® or Maalox®) 1 hour and 3 hours after meals has been advised. In hyposecretors, and in patients with gastric ulcers, 15–30 mL of the antacids will generally suffice.

Complications of Antacid Use

No antacid is free of potential side effects and some of them, if these compounds are used to excess, can be severe. The more important complications are described below.

Milk-Alkali Syndrome

This syndrome is seen only in patients taking systemic antacids or calcium carbonate and large amounts of milk for prolonged periods. The symptoms are headache, irritability, weakness, nausea, and vomiting. The syndrome is characterized by hypercalcemia, mild alkalosis, calcification and stone formation in the kidney, and chronic renal failure. Experimental evidence suggests that some constituent of milk, possibly a protein, facilitates the intestinal absorption of calcium. The resulting hypercalcemia probably suppresses the secretion of parathyroid hormone and thus leads to increased

calcium excretion in the urine, where it precipitates to form calcium-based stones.

Renal Calculi, Osteomalacia, and Osteoporosis

Aluminum hydroxide combines with phosphate in the small intestine, forming insoluble salts that are excreted. While this loss is usually negligible, with very large doses substantial amounts of phosphate are rendered insoluble and are excreted in the stools. This leads to phosphate depletion and to a marked decrease in the urinary excretion of phosphate. This decrease is accompanied by hypercalciuria resulting from skeletal resorption and increased absorption of calcium from the intestine. The increase in urinary calcium excretion can produce urinary calculi, osteomalacia, and osteoporosis. Aluminum phosphate was introduced to eliminate this potential complication of the treatment with aluminum gels. However, aluminum phosphate is an extremely weak antacid.

Neurotoxicity

As aluminum is absorbed to a small degree from the gut, its deposition in brain has been implicated, but not proven, as an etiologic factor in the encephalopathy syndrome that occurs in patients with chronic renal failure and in patients with Alzheimer's disease.

Intestinal Effects

As mentioned above, magnesium-based antacids may induce diarrhea. Intestinal obstruction with aluminum gels has been reported, particularly in elderly patients with gastrointestinal bleeding or when there is barium in the gut. Although constipation has been reported to occur frequently in association with the use of $CaCO_3$, recently the accuracy of these reports has been questioned.

Sodium Ingestion

All commercial antacids contain sodium (*see* Table 50–2). Their use may therefore present problems where a low sodium intake is important (*e.g.*, in cardiovascular disease).

Interactions with Other Drugs

Aluminum hydroxide gel and other antacids can reduce the absorption of isoniazid, penicillin, tetracyclines, nitrofurantoin, nalidixic acid, sulfonamides, phenylbutazone, digoxin, and chlorpromazine. Systemic antacids, by raising the urinary pH, can decrease the excretion of amines (*e.g.*, quinine and amphetamine) and increase that of salicylates.

PHARMACOLOGIC INHIBITION OF GASTRIC SECRETION

Gastric acid secretion requires stimulation of H_2 histamine receptors, muscarinic acetylcholine receptors, and gastrin receptors on the parietal cell. Acetylcholine and gastrin act through an increase in cytosolic calcium. The pathways for this effect on intracellular Ca^{2+} appear to be different. Acetylcholine acts through muscarinic M_2 ("low-affinity") receptors to stimulate the membrane phosphatidylinositol cycle, and thus enhances the permeability for Ca^{2+} by activating calcium channels in the plasma membrane (see Chapters 13, 14, and 15). Both acetylcholine and gastrin may release Ca^{2+} from intracellular stores. The time course of the increase in Ca^{2+} differs for the two secretagogues, being shorter following gastrin stimulation. The responses to acetylcholine and to gastrin are additive (Table 50–3). Presumably, Ca^{2+} activates calcium-dependent protein kinases, as happens in other cells in which cholinergic stimulation occurs. Activation of the histamine H_2 receptors stimulates adenylate cyclase and the production of intracellular cAMP. This activates a cAMP-dependent protein kinase, which catalyses the transfer of high-energy phosphate from ATP to a protein that has not yet been identified, which activates the $(H^+ + K^+)$–ATPase, the proton pump of the parietal cell (see below). It has been postulated that the cAMP content of the cell determines the responsiveness to the secretagogues, gastrin and acetylcholine, that act through the Ca^{2+} messenger system. Therefore, histamine, by determining the content of cAMP of the parietal cell, modulates the responsiveness of the cell to both gastrin and acetylcholine.

Reduction in the level of any of these three agents (histamine, acetylcholine, or gastrin) will result in a marked decrease of the parietal cell response to the other two. The effects of acetylcholine can be blocked by specific muscarinic cholinergic antagonists, for which atropine is a prototype. The effects of histamine can be antagonized by histamine H_2-receptor antagonists. Gastrin secretion can be inhibited by hormones such as somatostatin or secretin, or by drugs such as proglumide, a specific gastrin receptor blocker.

The final step in the processes that lead to the gastric secretion of acid is the activation of the enzyme $(H^+ + K^+)$–ATPase, the proton pump. This enzyme is located in the membranes of vesicles of the resting parietal cells and of the microvilli of the secreting parietal cells. These membranes constitute the walls of the intracellular canaliculi into which acid is secreted. The proton pump is an ATP-splitting system that results in the transmural exchange of H^+ (from the cytosol into the lumen of the intracellular canaliculi) for K^+ (from the lumen of the intracellular canaliculi into the cytosol). The exchange is analogous to the Na^+–K^+ exchange by $(Na^+ + K^+)$–ATPase. The intracellular canaliculi drain into the lumen of the gastric glands and then into the lumen of the stomach. Therefore, an inhibition of the $(H^+ + K^+)$–ATPase will result in a decrease of the secretion of acid in response to every known secretagogue.

Muscarinic Anticholinergics

These drugs act by blocking cholinergic stimuli (vagal and intrinsic plexus reflexes). Their general pharmacology is discussed in Chapter 15. These drugs antagonize, competitively and nonselectively, all muscarinic actions of acetylcholine and other muscarinic agonists at effector cells innervated by postganglionic parasympathetic cholinergic nerves (Table 50–4). Because the conventional anticholinergics do not differentiate between muscarinic receptors in different organs, they have many side effects at effective doses.

Naturally Occurring Compounds

While atropine (Figure 50–1) has both central and peripheral actions, in the doses used for management of peptic ulcer its therapeutic action depends entirely upon (peripheral) postganglionic blockade. Atropine decreases gastric acid secretion during all phases in response to a meal, and during the interdigestive phase it may even induce anacidity. The effect on gastric secretion consists of a decrease in total volume and total acid production, without a change in the concentration of HCl in gastric secretion. While the usual doses of

TABLE 50–3 Major Physiologic Control of Acid Secretion and Specific Receptors

Pathway	Agent	Second Messenger System
Neurocrine	Acetylcholine	Ca^{2+} influx
Endocrine	Gastrin	Release of Ca^{2+}
Paracrine	Histamine	cAMP

The simultaneous binding of the 3 agents is necessary for maximal acid secretion.

TABLE 50–4 Muscarinic Cholinergic Antagonists

Naturally occurring compounds
  Atropine
  Belladonna alkaloids
  Scopolamine

Synthetic or semisynthetic analogs
  Quaternary ammonium compounds (methantheline, propantheline, glycopyrrolate)
  Tertiary amine compounds (oxyphencyclimine)

Pirenzepine, telenzepine

atropine have little or no effect upon intestinal motility, they do effectively suppress gastric and duodenal hypermotility in ulcer patients, with relief of pain. The dosages of atropine required in the treatment of ulcer patients usually produce side effects (see Chapter 15, *Autonomic Cholinergic Antagonists*).

Synthetic or Semisynthetic Analogs

The analogs are subdivided into quaternary ammonium compounds and tertiary amines. The former are poorly absorbed, have fewer central side effects, and show a more pronounced ganglionic blocking activity.

For equivalent doses, all these compounds are similar to atropine with respect to peripheral side effects and changes in gastric acid secretion.

Several synthetic cholinergic blocking agents are in use for reduction of gastric acid secretion, such as methantheline, propantheline (Pro-Banthine®), glycopyrrolate (Robinul®) and oxyphencyclimine.

Methantheline and **propantheline**, in usual doses, selectively block autonomic postganglionic cholinergic transmission. Much larger doses are required to block ganglionic and neuromuscular transmission. Propantheline is from two to five times as potent as methantheline.

Adverse Effects and Contraindications of the Conventional Anticholinergics

The main **adverse effects** are:

- increase in pulse rate (tachycardia);
- dryness of the mouth;
- blurring of vision, difficulty with near vision, photophobia;
- bowel discomfort;
- reduced esophageal transit, both primary (i.e., in swallowing) and secondary (i.e., in the clearance of reflux of gastric content from the esophagus), and decreased tone of the lower esophagus. Because of the latter effects, anticholinergics are contraindicated in patients with gastro-esophageal reflux symptoms.

The main **contraindications** of anticholinergics are:

- glaucoma;
- obstructive uropathy (abnormal emptying of bladder);
- obstructive disease of the gastrointestinal tract (pyloroduodenal stenosis);
- paralytic ileus;
- arrhythmias;
- acute hemorrhage (in order not to interfere with autonomic nervous system homeostatic mechanisms);
- severe ulcerative colitis;
- myasthenia gravis (see Chapter 19);
- gastroesophageal reflux.

Pirenzepine and Telenzepine

These new anticholinergic drugs are complex tricyclic compounds, related to the tricyclic antidepressants (Fig. 50-2). Although the mode of action is still controversial, pirenzepine and telenzepine, in contrast to the classic anticholinergics, seem to have a more selective antimuscarinic action, directed against the secretory function of the stomach rather than against the salivary glands and smooth muscle. Pirenzepine has been postulated to recognize both high- and low-affinity muscarinic receptors, while atropine recognizes only one type of high-affinity receptor. Pirenzepine is 200 times less potent than atropine at low-affinity receptors, but only about ten times less potent than atropine at high-affinity receptors (those involved in gastric secretion). Therefore, pirenzepine could block the high-affinity receptors with a dose as low as 10 mg (i.v.), without affecting the low-affinity receptors for which a dose of 100–200 mg would be necessary. If this selective action is confirmed, one would anticipate fewer side effects. The exact location of pirenzepine high-affinity receptors is not known, but the data suggest that they are not located in the parietal cell but at a neural site within the vagal pathway.

The effects of pirenzepine on gastric secretion are similar to those of the conventional anticholinergics, i.e., reduction of volume of acid secretion in response to vagal, histamine, and gastrin stimulation. It also

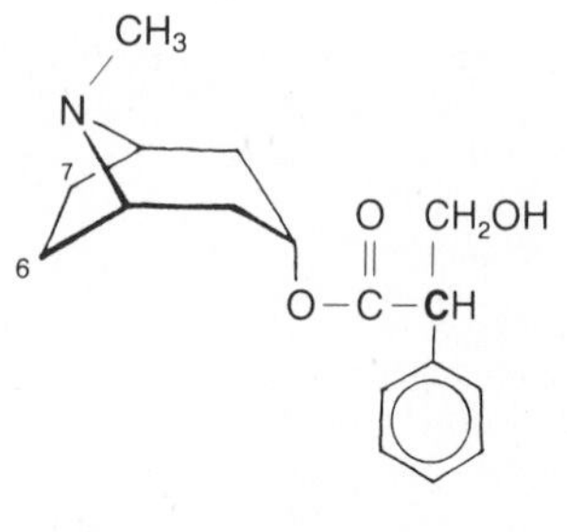

Figure 50-1 Structural formula of atropine.

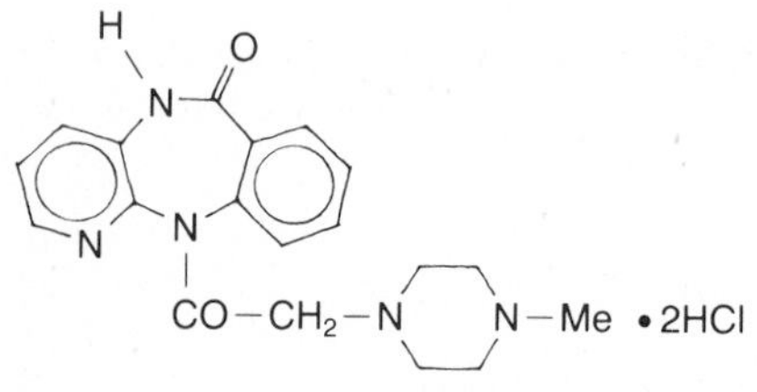

Figure 50-2 Structural formula of pirenzepine dihydrochloride, an anticholinergic agent related to the tricyclic antidepressants.

decreases pepsin secretion. The drug has the further advantage of being very hydrophilic, with a limited passage across the blood–brain barrier, and therefore it does not exhibit central nervous effects. Controlled studies have indicated that pirenzepine is superior to placebo and as effective as H_2-receptor antagonists in healing duodenal ulcers. With pirenzepine the incidence of dry mouth and blurred vision is approximately 14% and 2% respectively. Unlike previously available anticholinergic agents used in the treatment of peptic ulceration, pirenzepine is not contraindicated in patients with glaucoma or prostatic hypertrophy.

Telenzepine displays on the average a six-fold higher potency than pirenzepine for inhibition of the muscarinic receptors in the stomach, smooth muscle, and myocardium. When compared to atropine, the affinity of telenzepine for the muscarinic receptors involved in gastric acid secretion is five times as great.

Histamine H_2-Receptor Antagonists

Histamine stimulates gastric acid secretion through interaction with specific H_2 receptors, and its actions are blocked by specific H_2-receptor antagonists (Fig. 50–3). **Burimamide** was the first H_2-receptor blocker developed, but its use was limited by poor gastro-

intestinal absorption. **Metiamide**, a related compound, not only reduces stimulated gastric secretions but also suppresses nocturnal secretions after a single oral dose. However, it also was shown to produce agranulocytosis in a few cases. Metiamide cannot be used therapeutically in humans. This problem was solved with the synthesis of cimetidine, which has become one of the largest-selling drugs in the world.

It was believed that the imidazole ring was important for H_2-receptor recognition. This clearly is not the case, because ranitidine, a powerful H_2 antagonist, has a furan group instead of the imidazole, and famotidine, also more potent than cimetidine, contains a guanylthiazole ring. All of these drugs are described in detail in the following sections.

Cimetidine

Until 1982, cimetidine (Tagamet®) was the only H_2-receptor antagonist marketed in the United States and Canada. Cimetidine not only inhibits basal and stimulated acid secretion; it also decreases pepsin output and secretion, although to a lesser extent. If the cimetidine treatment is discontinued, episodes of ulcer formation can recur, but a maintenance dose of cimetidine may confer protection against recurrences. While use of the drug has resulted in a decrease in the num-

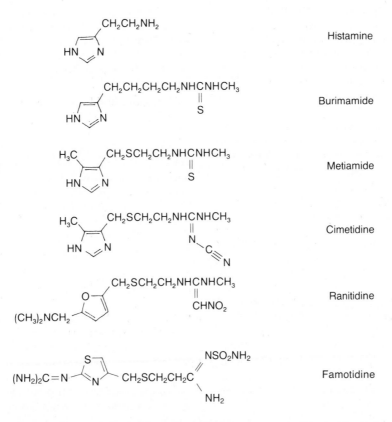

Figure 50–3 Structural formulae of histamine and of a number of H_2-receptor blockers (*see also* Chapter 32, H_1-receptor blockers).

ber of patients undergoing elective surgery for duodenal ulcer (surgical procedures to reduce acidity), it has not changed the number of operations for perforations and other complications of duodenal ulcer.

Pharmacokinetics

Cimetidine is readily absorbed after oral administration. About 30% of a dose of cimetidine is inactivated by the liver microsomal mixed-function oxygenase (MMFO) system (see Chapter 4) by conversion of the side-chain thioether moiety to the sulfoxide. The other 70% is excreted unchanged in the urine.

Adverse Effects

Side effects of cimetidine occur in only a small number of patients and, at least in short-term treatment, they are minor and in the majority of cases do not require discontinuation of the drug. The most commonly seen side effects consist of headache, dizziness, diarrhea, and muscular pain. Other side effects are:

Sexual dysfunction and gynecomastia. Cimetidine acts as a nonsteroidal antiandrogen and can induce a decrease in male sexual function and a reduction in sperm count. Gynecomastia (breast swelling and soreness of one or both nipples in males) has been reported in a small number of patients. This complication can result from either an increased level of serum prolactin (as a result of cimetidine blockade of dopamine receptors in the anterior pituitary) or from blockade of receptors mediating androgenic suppression of breast tissue responsiveness to normal male circulating levels of estrogens, gonadotropins, and prolactin. These effects are observed only when cimetidine is used in very high doses, such as those required for the treatment of Zollinger-Ellison syndrome.

Bone marrow dysfunction and granulocytopenia. Rare instances of reversible granulocytopenias of moderate degree, which may have been associated with cimetidine treatment, have been reported.

Liver changes. In a small proportion of patients, treatment with cimetidine has resulted in elevations of serum transaminases (SGOT and/or SGPT). Transaminase levels usually return to normal despite continuation of the drug therapy. Usually, there is no other evidence of liver dysfunction, although a few cases of cimetidine-induced cholestasis and hepatitis (see Chapter 62) have been reported.

Central nervous symptoms. Mental abnormalities have been observed, consisting of confusion, hallucinations, lethargy, agitation, restlessness, periods of apnea, and focal and general seizures. They are mainly seen in patients with severe liver disease, renal failure, or in the elderly or very young. The severity of symptoms increases with increasing serum concentrations of cimetidine.

Renal abnormalities. Small increases in serum creatinine and urea levels have been detected in patients treated with cimetidine. The mechanism for this increase has not been established.

Interactions with Other Drugs

Cimetidine binding to the hepatic MMFO inhibits the microsomal metabolism of a number of other drugs, resulting in higher blood levels and in enhancement of their effects. This has been shown to occur with diazepam, theophylline, warfarin, antipyrine, propranolol, meperidine, pentobarbital, chlormethiazole, chlordiazepoxide, lidocaine, phenytoin, and aminopyrine. The interaction of cimetidine with the metabolism of these drugs seems to depend more on the imidazole structure of cimetidine than on its H_2 receptor-blocking activity. On the other hand, cimetidine does not interact with the glucuronide conjugation of drugs (e.g., lorazepam or oxazepam).

Ranitidine

Ranitidine (Zantac®) is an H_2-receptor antagonist with a furan instead of an imidazole ring. The inhibitory effect of ranitidine on gastric acid secretion is, on a molar basis, up to eight times that of cimetidine. Ranitidine is also a more powerful inhibitor of pepsin secretion. One study has reported control of symptoms by ranitidine in a group of patients with the Zollinger-Ellison syndrome that had proven to be resistant to treatment with cimetidine. Ranitidine seems a most valuable alternative to cimetidine in the treatment of duodenal ulcer and the Zollinger-Ellison syndrome.

Pharmacokinetics

In contrast with cimetidine, which is predominantly excreted as the unchanged drug in the urine, approximately 50% of ranitidine is eliminated by hepatic biotransformation, and it undergoes significant presystemic conversion (first-pass effect; see Chapter 5). Consequently, patients with liver disease receiving the usual dose of ranitidine show increased blood levels of the drug due to both increased bioavailability and decreased elimination.

Adverse Effects

Ranitidine has minimal side effects. It has the advantage of not having the antiandrogenic or the prolactin-stimulating effects of cimetidine. Furthermore, it is less likely to inhibit the MMFO system in the liver (and therefore to induce clinically significant alterations in the biotransformation of other drugs) and does not increase serum creatinine or urea levels.

Famotidine

Famotidine (Pepcid®) may be unique because it is a slowly reversible, competitive H_2-receptor antagonist. Famotidine slowly dissociates from its active site on the parietal cell, and it is not displaced even by very high concentrations of H_2 agonists. It appears to be an effective and safe once-a-day therapy for the treatment of duodenal ulcer. Famotidine is 20–160 times as potent as cimetidine and 3–20 times as potent as ranitidine when compared on equimolar basis. The antisecretory activity has been demonstrated to last for 12 hours after a single 10-mg dose.

Pharmacokinetics

After oral administration, the onset of the antisecretory effect occurs within 1 hour, and it reaches its maximum within 1–3 hours. The bioavailability of oral doses is 40–45%. About 25–30% of an oral dose, and 65–70% of an intravenous dose, are recovered in the urine as unchanged compound. In patients with severe renal insufficiency, elimination half-life may exceed 20 hours and adjustment of dosing may be necessary.

Adverse Effects

Like ranitidine, famotidine has very low binding affinity for either cytochrome P-450 or for the androgen receptors. Therefore, it causes much less interference with the biotransformation of other drugs and also is less likely than cimetidine to have androgenic effects. A small number of patients receiving famotidine have suffered mild episodes of headache, dizziness, constipation, or diarrhea.

Substituted Benzimidazoles

At least three of these compounds, timoprazole, pricoprazole, and omeprazole, have proven to be powerful inhibitors of gastric acid secretion. **Omeprazole** (Fig. 50–4) is the only one that has been used clinically, and it is the most potent inhibitor of gastric acid secretion in existence. It has been shown to be efficient in promoting the healing of both gastric and duodenal ulcers. The suggested mechanism of action of omeprazole involves oxidation of key sulfhydryl groups in the gastric $(H^+ + K^+)$–ATPase enzyme, the final step in the process of acid secretion by the parietal cell (see above). Because the drug acts beyond the site of action of the two second messengers, Ca^{2+} and cAMP, omeprazole inhibits gastric acid secretion evoked by every stimulus.

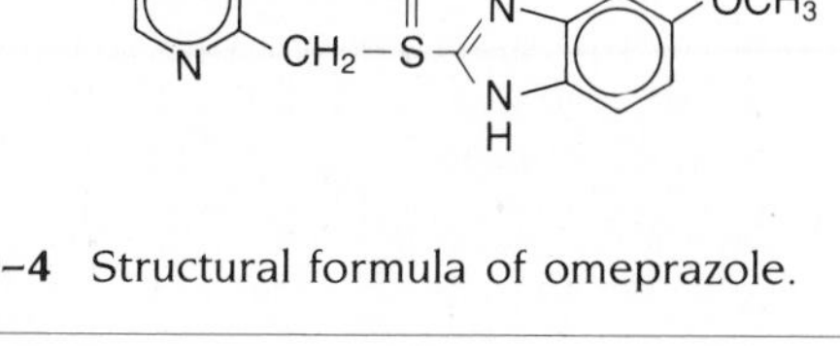

In the intact animal and in isolated gastric glands, the effect of omeprazole is related to the stimulation state of these cells. Omeprazole is a weak base and, therefore, it selectively accumulates in an acidic compartment of the parietal cells, probably the secretory vesicles or canaliculi. The binding to the $(H^+ + K^+)$–ATPase occurs only after a modification of the structure of the drug induced by acid. The accumulation in the gastric mucosa explains why, although the elimination half-life of omeprazole is short, the inhibition of gastric secretion persists for 22–24 hours, when omeprazole is no longer detectable in plasma. There is also an increasing inhibitory effect during the first days of repeated administration, which is in agreement with the long duration of action.

The requirement of an acid environment for the activation of omeprazole makes this drug specific for the parietal cell, as it will not inhibit other $(H^+ + K^+)$–ATPases that exist in a neutral milieu.

Pharmacokinetics

Omeprazole is rapidly absorbed in all species. Systemic availability is relatively high, provided the drug is protected from acid degradation in the stomach. The volume of distribution corresponds to the volume of extracellular water. The drug is about 95% bound to proteins in human plasma. It is eliminated almost completely by biotransformation, and no unchanged drug has been recovered from urine. The mean elimination half-life is about one hour.

Adverse Effects

Although omeprazole can interfere with the elimination of other drugs by inhibiting the MMFO system in the human liver, at the dose used for the treatment of duodenal ulcer (less than 30 mg/day) it is unlikely that this effect will be of significance in clinical practice.

Omeprazole administration triggers a pronounced increase in circulating gastrin in response to the almost complete inhibition of acid secretion that results from large doses of the drug. If the hypergastrinemia is maintained, fundal mucosal hyperplasia will ensue. In toxicologic experiments in rats maintained on very high doses of omeprazole for 24 months, carcinoid tumors, together with hyperplasia of parietal cells and of enterochromaffin cells, were observed. In humans treated with smaller doses for short periods of time, these abnormalities have not been seen.

Omeprazole is generally well tolerated, and the only

Figure 50–4 Structural formula of omeprazole.

other side effects reported have been rather nonspecific (tiredness, weakness, and headache).

Proglumide and Sulpiride

These drugs are now in use in several European countries. Proglumide [racemic-4-(benzoylamino)-5-(dipropylamino)-glutaric acid] is a derivative of glutaramic acid. The drug is a specific gastrin receptor blocker; it inhibits gastrin-stimulated acid secretion and the trophic effects of gastrin. Sulpiride is also being used in Europe. It is an antidopaminergic drug that inhibits gastrin secretion, probably acting at the level of the gastrin-producing cells in the gastric antrum.

PHARMACOLOGIC AGENTS THAT INCREASE THE RESISTANCE OF THE MUCOSA TO ACID-PEPTIC DIGESTION

Prostaglandins (Misoprostol, Enprostil, Rioprostil, Arbaprostil, and Trimoprostil)

These compounds (*see also* Chapter 30) belong to an intermediate category, in that they not only inhibit gastric secretion but also may increase the mucosal resistance to aggressive necrotizing factors. Exogenous prostaglandins (1) inhibit gastric acid secretion directly; (2) inhibit gastrin release by the antral gastrin cells; (3) inhibit pepsin secretion; (4) stimulate mucus secretion; (5) stimulate bicarbonate secretion; (6) increase mucosal blood flow.

Inhibition of acid secretion can be achieved with topical and systemic administration of prostaglandins, probably through an agonist action by E-type prostaglandins on high-affinity inhibitory receptors that exist on the parietal cells. Stimulation of these receptors decreases the histamine-stimulated accumulation of cyclic AMP, an effect that could account for the similar inhibitory properties of prostaglandins and H_2-receptor blockers. The inhibition of gastric secretion by prostaglandins is effective against stimulation of acid secretion by histamine, gastrin, and meals.

Certain methyl analogs of prostaglandin E_2 (enprostil) also inhibit gastrin release in response to a meal. Like the parietal cells, the gastrin-producing cells have high-affinity binding sites for the E_2 prostaglandins.

In animal studies, prostaglandins have been shown to protect the gastric mucosa against damage produced by several necrotizing agents. This property has been called "cytoprotection" and is independent of inhibition of acid secretion. The mechanism (and even the term cytoprotection) is still under discussion and has not been completely defined, but it probably depends on a prostaglandin-induced increase in the secretion of mucus and bicarbonate (the bicarbonate–mucus barrier), and also possibly on the increase in mucosal blood flow induced by these substances.

Prostaglandin analogs have been shown to be competent ulcer-healing drugs, but not better than other agents such as the H_2-receptor blockers. It has been claimed that they are not particularly effective for pain relief and that, in this regard, they have generally been inferior to cimetidine and ranitidine. It is not clear if the cytoprotective effects of prostaglandins play a role in the healing of gastric and duodenal ulcers. On the other hand, there is some evidence that prostaglandin analogs may reverse the deleterious effects of smoking on duodenal ulcer healing, and that they might be effective in preventing and treating the mucosal damage induced by nonsteroidal anti-inflammatory drugs and alcohol. It appears that the prostaglandin analogs may be particularly useful in patients in whom extended H_2-receptor blocker therapy has failed because of unknown factors that make these ulcers more resistant to the latter treatment.

Several prostaglandins are available for clinical use. **Misoprostol** (Cytotec®, marketed in Canada) is a synthetic methyl ester analog of prostaglandin E_1. It is a potent inhibitor of gastric acid secretion. **Enprostil** is a synthetic dehydroprostaglandin E_2 analog. This compound, which inhibits gastric acid secretion by acting directly in the parietal cells, also suppresses the increase in circulating gastrin that follows the administration of a meal or of cimetidine. **Arbaprostil** is the 15(R)-5-methyl analog of prostaglandin E_2. It is a stable compound that epimerizes in an acid environment from the [R] configuration at carbon 15 to the [S] configuration, the active form of the analog. It also suppresses acid secretion and reduces serum gastrin levels. **Timoprostil** and **Rioprostil** are still in the investigational stage and are derivatives of prostaglandins E_2 and E_1 respectively.

Side Effects

The most serious side effect of prostaglandins is diarrhea, which generally is mild, self-limited and of short duration. This side effect results from the prostaglandin-induced increase in cyclic AMP in the small intestinal mucosa. The reported frequency of diarrhea with misoprostol is 7–13%, with arbaprostil 34%, with enprostil 8–20%. Other side effects are nausea, vomiting, headache, abdominal pain, and cortical hyperostosis. Because prostaglandins are uterotonic, these agents have been shown to increase the incidence of uterine bleeding and of partial or complete expulsion of uterine contents in pregnant women. These actions limit their use in women of child-bearing age.

Carbenoxolone

Carbenoxolone (Bigastrone®) is a derivative of glycyrrhetinic acid (extract of licorice root). It has been claimed to increase the life span of gastric mucosal cells by 50%. It acts locally in the stomach, its site of maximum absorption. Carbenoxolone increases the production of mucus, altering the balance of its component sugars, and may slightly inhibit pepsin secretion, but it has no effect on acid secretion. Side effects, due to its mineralocorticoid-like activity, include sodium retention and hypokalemia. Carbenoxolone is thus contraindicated in hypertension, ischemic heart disease, and renal failure. In digitalized patients it increases digitalis toxicity. **Duogastrone** is a dosage form of carbenoxolone that releases the drug only in the duodenum. Its efficacy in the treatment of duodenal ulcers has not been demonstrated. Carbenoxolone preparations are no longer marketed in North America, but are still used in the United Kingdom and elsewhere.

Sucrose Octasulfate

Sucralfate® does not inhibit gastric secretion. Chemically, it is a complex aluminum salt of sucrose containing eight sulfate groups. In the presence of gastric acid (pH < 3–4) some $[Al_2(OH)_5]^+$ ions dissociate from the molecules and the residual compound becomes negatively charged. When the sucrose octasulfate molecules polymerize, they form a viscous paste-like substance, which is the active form of sucralfate. This substance adheres strongly to the gastric and duodenal mucosa. Furthermore, the negatively charged sucralfate polyanions bind selectively to the positively charged, partially denatured proteins at the base of the ulcer for at least 6 hours. Although sucralfate also binds to the normal mucosa, the affinity in this case is six times less than at the site of the ulcer crater. This barrier is thought to protect the ulcerated mucosa from further damage by acid, bile, and pepsin.

Because the mechanism of action of sucralfate requires conversion by acid into a highly charged polyanion, the antipeptic activity and the clinical efficacy of sucralfate are dependent on highly acidic pH values in the gastric lumen. Therefore, it should not be given in combination with antacids or with meals.

Sucralfate also directly binds pepsin and inhibits peptic activity. The drug also adsorbs bile acids and protects against bile-acid-induced gastric mucosal injury. Sucralfate appears to have additional protective actions, one of which is a significantly increased release of prostaglandin E_2 into the gastric lumen. This increase is completely abolished by indomethacin pretreatment, which markedly inhibits the protective action against ethanol-induced necrosis. Sucralfate also increases significantly the output of soluble mucus, even after inhibition of prostaglandin synthesis with acetylsalicylic acid.

The drug is only minimally absorbed from the gastrointestinal tract. The minute amounts of the sulfated disaccharide that are absorbed are primarily excreted in the urine. Several controlled clinical trials have shown that treatment with sucralfate results in duodenal ulcer healing more often than with placebos and as often as with cimetidine. Like the prostaglandins, sucralfate appears to overcome the adverse effect of smoking on ulcer healing.

Side effects are rare and mild (constipation or mild diarrhea, nausea, dry mouth, skin rash, dizziness).

Colloidal Bismuth

Colloidal bismuth subcitrate (De-Nol®) is a complex salt of citric acid. The trivalent $Bi(OH)_3$ and the trivalent citric acid can form a variety of different salts. The substance consists of molecules of different structure and size that, on the average, are so large that the aqueous solution becomes colloidal. In acid medium (pH < 5) colloidal bismuth precipitates. All these structures contain − COOH and Bi^+ groups that may bind to proteins.

Like sucralfate, the drug acts by increasing the mucosal resistance against endoluminal aggressive agents without inhibiting gastric secretion. In essence, colloidal bismuth subcitrate forms a protective film over the gastroduodenal mucosa. Other possible beneficial effects are (1) changes in mucus production and composition; (2) stimulation of intrinsic defence mechanisms (*i.e.*, increasing prostaglandin synthesis); (3) inhibition of pepsin activity; (4) bactericidal action against *Campylobacter pyloridis*, a bacterium that has been implicated in the pathogenesis of gastric ulcer. In *Campylobacter* gastritis, the microorganism is very sensitive to colloidal bismuth subcitrate, and its eradication results in histologic improvement.

The drug was not widely employed because of its unpleasant taste. Recently, chewing tablets have been introduced that have made this form of treatment much more acceptable to the patients. Several clinical trials have shown that colloidal bismuth subcitrate is a real alternative to the H_2-receptor antagonists in the treatment of gastric and duodenal ulcers.

Colloidal bismuth subcitrate has very few side effects. It can induce slight constipation and it also blackens the mouth and stool. The latter effect can lead to confusion with melena (blood in the stools).

GENERAL COMMENTS ON CHRONIC ANTACID THERAPY

Recent pharmacologic research has provided many alternatives for the treatment of gastric and duodenal ulcers. Despite the significant differences in potency, and mechanisms of action, none of the different new drugs offers a better healing rate for isolated episodes of ulcer activity than the treatment with antacids. In essence, all the agents that have been tried are approximately equal in efficacy. Therefore, the choice must be made in consideration of side effects, convenience of dosage, special intolerances, taste, cost, and particular circumstances of the patient, such as age or other diseases or treatments.

Clearly, for the treatment of ulcers it is not necessary to achieve a complete and prolonged suppression of gastric acid secretion. Furthermore, it has become apparent that a single nighttime dose of cimetidine or ranitidine (that does not affect the daytime acid secretion) is as effective as multiple daily doses in the treatment of duodenal ulcer. Actually, the lack of suppression of gastric acidity during the day may be beneficial as it could help in preventing the colonization of the stomach by bacteria and the marked increase in blood gastrin levels that follow a complete suppression of gastric acid secretion.

None of the anti-ulcer agents appears to prevent the ulcer from eventually recurring after termination of an acute course of therapy. Therefore, maintenance of the treatment with lower doses of these agents has been tried. The H_2 histamine-receptor blockers, sucralfate, and colloidal bismuth subcitrate have been shown to reduce the rate of ulcer recurrence and, apparently, to have decreased the incidence of ulcer complications. Trials with prostaglandins are now in progress and may provide new alternatives for the prevention of recurrences. Omeprazole, which causes a profound and long-lasting decrease in secretion of gastric acid, has the drawback of markedly increasing gastrin levels (not observed with sucralfate, colloidal bismuth subcitrate, or the prostaglandins). Omeprazole also has the potential for increasing the number of bacteria in gastric juice. Intragastric bacteria may reduce dietary nitrate to nitrite and thus facilitate the intragastric formation of N-nitroso compounds, which are carcinogenic in a variety of organs and animal species. Therefore, full-dose treatment with omeprazole is unlikely to be recommended for the long-term management of uncomplicated gastric or duodenal ulcers.

In the treatment of the Zollinger-Ellison syndrome, for which very large doses of H_2 antagonists are necessary for prolonged periods, ranitidine and famotidine are probably the H_2 antagonists of choice, because they are devoid of the antiandrogen effects associated with large doses of cimetidine. In these patients, omeprazole might provide a very important therapeutic alternative.

SUGGESTED READING

Bertaccini G, Coruzzi G. Pharmacology of the treatment of peptic ulcer disease. Dig Dis Sci 1985; 30:43–51.

Feldman M. Inhibition of gastric acid secretion by selective and nonselective anticholinergics. Gastroenterology 1984; 86:361–366.

Fordtran JS. Reduction of acidity by diet, antacids and anticholinergic agents. In: Sleissenger MS, Fordtran JS, eds. Gastrointestinal disease. Philadelphia: WB Saunders, 1973:718–742.

Heathcote BV, Parry M. Pirenzepine selectively inhibits gastric acid secretion: a comparative pharmacological study between pirenzepine and seven other cholinergic drugs. Scand J Gastroenterol 1980; 15(suppl 66):15–24.

Ippoliti AF, Maxwell V, Isenberg JI. The effect of various forms of milk on gastric acid secretion. Studies in patients with duodenal ulcer and normal subjects. Ann Intern Med 1976; 84:286–289.

Konturek SJ, Obtulowicz W, Kwiecien N, et al. Comparison of ranitidine and cimetidine in the inhibition of histamine, sham-feeding and meal-induced gastric secretion in duodenal ulcer patients. Gut 1980; 21:181–186.

Lam SK. Prostaglandins for duodenal ulcer. Clin Invest Med 1987; 10:232–237.

Salena BJ, Hunt RH. The limitations of current therapy in peptic ulcer disease. Clin Invest Med 1987; 10:171–177.

Strum WB. Prevention of duodenal ulcer recurrence. Ann Intern Med 1986; 105:757–761.

Chapter 51

LAXATIVES AND ANTIDIARRHEAL DRUGS

H. Orrego and L. Spero

Normal stools contain 60–80% water. The most satisfactory definition of constipation is the difficult passage of excessively dry, hard stools (*i.e.*, with less water than normal). Conversely, diarrhea can best be defined as the passage of voluminous stools containing an excessive amount of water (*i.e.*, more than 80%). There is no active transport of water; movement of water, therefore, follows the movement of electrolytes or of other osmotically active substances. Constipation can result from either an excessive absorption of solutes from the lumen, or from a decrease in their entrance into the lumen. Diarrhea results from either a decrease in absorption of solutes from the lumen, or their increased entrance into the lumen. While intestinal motility has been traditionally considered to be of major importance in the production of both diarrhea and constipation, most recent evidence is against this concept.

There is considerable circumstantial evidence that absorptive processes occur mainly in the villous epithelial cells, and that secretory processes take place especially in crypt epithelial cells. Secretion and absorption of solutes are linked to the activity of $(Na^+ + K^+)$–ATPase, to the nucleotides cyclic AMP and GMP, and to the concentration of calcium in these cells. In the ileum, the nucleotides have two actions: (1) inhibition of the neutral NaCl influx across the apical brush-border membrane of the epithelium, and (2) stimulation of either a coupled NaCl secretion or of the active secretion of Cl^-. In the colon, cyclic AMP stimulates only active Cl^- secretion. A number of substances, of which cholera enterotoxin is an example, increase cyclic AMP levels. The net effect throughout the small intestine of the increase in intracellular cyclic AMP is to cause a marked secretion of an isotonic fluid and a simultaneous decrease in the absorption of Na^+ and Cl^-. This results in severe diarrhea.

Calmodulin, a calcium-binding regulator protein, modulates several calcium-dependent cellular processes, including regulation of levels of cyclic AMP and GMP, activities of cyclic 3',5'-nucleotide phosphodiesterase and $(Ca^{2+} + Mg^{2+})$–ATPase, calcium-dependent phosphorylation in synaptic membranes, protein kinases, and microtubule assembly. Pharmacologic agents (*e.g.*, chlorpromazine, trifluoperazine, haloperidol, and calcium chelators) that inhibit calmodulin are also potent inhibitors of intestinal secretion, an observation that may suggest a role for calmodulin in the regulation of intestinal ion transport. Calcium influx into the cell is also necessary for intestinal secretion to occur, and it has been postulated that cyclic AMP may alter intracellular calcium pools. Cyclic nucleotides, calmodulin, and Ca^{2+} are major cellular messenger systems whose functions are closely interwoven. $(Na^+ + K^+)$–ATPase activity is essential for the active transport of sodium out of the cell at the lateral intercellular space and for the continuing high-luminal, low-intracellular gradient of Na^+ necessary for the active transport of many solutes.

Figure 51–1 depicts the possible interrelation of the two messenger systems (cAMP, calmodulin) with Ca^{2+} as a third messenger and the $(Na^+ + K^+)$–ATPase sodium pump. These interactions and the effects of the messenger are basic to the understanding of the mechanism of action of laxatives and antidiarrheal drugs.

LAXATIVES OR CATHARTICS

These agents have been traditionally divided into **mild** (aperients or laxatives) and **harsh** (drastics, cathartics, or purgatives). These terms imply potency and are subjective. A large dose of a "mild" agent will produce a "harsh" effect. Therefore, we will use only the term "laxative" throughout this chapter.

The most widely used classification of laxatives has no pathophysiologic basis and is especially directed to

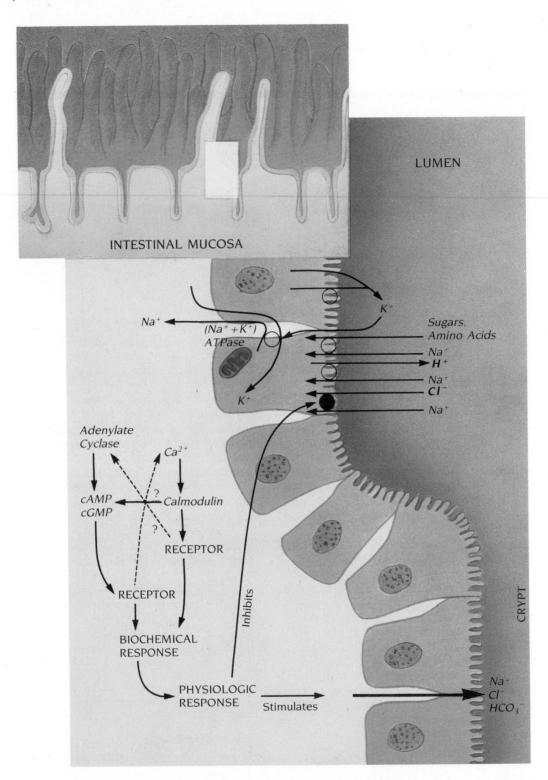

Figure 51-1 Mechanisms mediating and regulating the movement of solutes across the intestinal mucosa. The dashed arrows indicate relationships that are still not well established. The role of calmodulin is controversial. (Adapted from Cheung WY. Fed Proc 1982; 41:2253.)

the assumed effects of laxatives on intestinal motility. This is unfortunate since, as previously noted, the role of motility in the production of abnormally dry stools is, at best, doubtful. A conventional classification divides laxatives into irritant, bulk, emollient or lubricant, and wetting agents. However, since the action of laxatives is more clearly associated with an increase in fecal water excretion, a more appropriate classification should be based on this parameter.

The general mechanism of action of laxatives is the induction of a net accumulation of fluid in the intestinal lumen. This can be achieved by (1) an increase in secretion of electrolytes, (2) an increase in intraluminal osmolarity, or (3) a decrease in water (solute) absorption. According to these criteria, laxatives may be roughly classified as shown in Table 51–1.

This classification involves a degree of overlap because of the fact that most laxatives act through more than one mechanism, and also because our understanding of their mechanisms of action is still too fragmentary. Nevertheless, there is little doubt that this classification contains fewer assumptions and proven erroneous concepts than the more classical division, which still appears in many pharmacology textbooks.

Laxatives That Increase Secretion

Although some of these nonosmotic compounds may alter colonic motor function, such changes are not responsible for the increase in water excretion that these agents produce.

Anthraquinones

These are the most widely prescribed laxatives. They are found in the leaves, roots, or seed pods of various plants, such as aloe, cascara, rhubarb, and senna, and are present as glycosides as well as in the free forms. **Emodin** is the commonest of the anthraquinones and is present in amounts of 0.5% to 1.5% in all the plant preparations. The glycoside conjugates are absorbed only after hydrolysis, yielding the free anthraquinone and glucose. Hydrolysis occurs only in the large intestine by the action of the indigenous bacterial flora of the colon; this accounts, in part, for the delay in onset of action of these agents. The free anthraquinone is then reduced by the intestinal flora to the active anthral form. **Danthron** (1,8-dihydroxyanthraquinone) is a synthetic derivative that may be absorbed by the small intestine and/or alter the function of this portion of the bowel. **Cascara sagrada**, in usual doses, is the mildest of the anthraquinone laxatives. It is effective in about 8 hours and seldom causes colic. **Senna** is more active, is effective in about 6 hours, and usually causes some colic and griping. **Aloe** is the most irritant and can stimulate other visceral smooth muscles including the uterus. It acts in about 8–12 hours and usually causes considerable colic. **Rhubarb** is a relatively mild laxative that causes little discomfort.

It is widely believed that, once absorbed, the anthraquinones stimulate colonic myenteric nerve fibres and hence increase motility. However, this may occur only at toxic levels of these agents. There is substantial evidence that these substances inhibit $(Na^+ + K^+)$–ATPase and therefore the transport of Na^+ and of other actively transported solutes, leading to accumulation of water in the intestinal lumen. In addition to catharsis, these laxatives may induce spasmodic contractions and associated colic, which can be prevented by belladonna or atropine.

Castor Oil

Extracted from the **castor bean** (*Ricinus communis*), this preparation has been used as a laxative for hundreds of years. It may be absorbed to a limited extent. The active constituent of castor oil is ricinoleic acid, an 18-C aliphatic, mono-hydroxyl fatty acid. It is present as a triglyceride that is hydrolysed by pancreatic lipase to yield free ricinoleic acid. The laxative action takes place especially in the small bowel, the contents of which may be emptied into the colon within only 2 hours. A dose of castor oil is effective within 2–6 hours. Because the remaining unhydrolysed oil is also eliminated, the effects tend to be self-limiting.

The effect of ricinoleic acid results from an increase in luminal water content in the small and large intestines. This can occur as a consequence of several effects of this agent on the intestinal mucosa: (1) an inhibition of $(Na^+ + K^+)$–ATPase with the consequent decrease in the absorption of Na^+ and of the actively cotransported solutes (sugars, amino acids, *etc.*); (2) an increase in intracellular cyclic AMP, either as a response to an increased synthesis of prostaglandins (PGE_2) that stimulates adenylate cyclase activity, or

---

TABLE 51–1 Classification of Laxatives According to Their Effects on Intraluminal Fluid Accumulation

Laxatives That Increase Secretion
  Anthraquinone
  Castor oil (ricinoleic acid)
  Diphenylmethane laxatives
  Dioctyl sodium sulfosuccinate
  Bile acids
  Plant resins
  Saline
  Fibre

Laxatives That Decrease Absorption
  Liquid petrolatum
  Fibre
  Hydrophilic colloids

Laxatives That Increase Osmolarity
  Saline
  Lactulose
  Fibre

GASTROINTESTINAL SYSTEM

by a competitive inhibition of soluble cAMP-phosphodiesterase activity, or both; (3) by alterations of the mucosal surface structure. On electron microscopy, disintegration of microvilli and damaged villus tips have been observed.

Diphenylmethane Laxatives

Phenolphthalein. Before this agent causes laxation it must be absorbed, conjugated with glucuronide by the endoplasmic reticulum of the liver, and excreted in bile. Enterohepatic circulation also prolongs its duration of action. It loses the laxative effect in obstructive jaundice or after ligation of the bile duct.

Bisacodyl. This agent (Dulcolax®) is chemically similar to phenolphthalein. It is an effective laxative, acting 6–8 hours after oral administration. It can also be given in a rectal suppository and then it is effective in 20–60 minutes. When given orally it is active only after deacetylation, absorption from the small intestine, and excretion in bile. Like phenolphthalein, it has no laxative effect after bile duct ligation.

The effects of both phenolphthalein and bisacodyl are dependent on several actions of these agents that result in less absorption and more secretion of water by the intestine and are essentially similar to those described for ricinoleic acid: (1) Both drugs inhibit $(Na^+ + K^+)$–ATPase. (2) Bisacodyl increases adenylate cyclase activity and intracellular cyclic AMP. This direct effect is controversial in the case of phenolphthalein. (3) Both compounds increase the synthesis and release of PGE, resulting in an indirect increase in cyclic AMP. The role of PGE in the laxative effects of phenolphthalein and bisacodyl explains the reduction of their laxative effect after pretreatment with indomethacin. (4) There may be morphologic injury of the intestinal mucosa and increased permeability. These laxatives are cytotoxic to intestinal cells. (5) Bisacodyl has also been shown to raise the K^+ efflux across the colonic mucosa by 200–300%. It has been proposed that this effect depends on raised levels of intracellular Ca^{2+}, and it probably reflects an increase in mucosal K^+ permeability. There is evidence that both cyclic AMP and Ca^{2+} may have a role in modulation of mucosal border K^+ permeability.

Dioctyl Sodium Sulfosuccinate (DSS)

This compound (Colace®, Laxagel®, Regulex®) was developed as a synthetic wetting agent or a stool softener; this action is attributed to its ability to decrease surface tension and thus increase exposure of the stool surface to luminal water, resulting in fecal hydration. Actually, this theoretical action has never been proven. More recent studies have shown that DSS also acts through an increase in intraluminal water by mechanisms similar to those described for ricinoleic acid (inhibition of $(Na^+ + K^+)$–ATPase, increase in cyclic AMP, and cellular damage).

Bile Acids

Bile acids are often included in multi-ingredient laxatives. Dihydroxy (but not trihydroxy) bile acids produce fluid and electrolyte accumulation in the intestinal lumen by mechanisms similar to those described above. It is most likely that deoxycholate and other detergents stimulate and/or inhibit membrane-bound enzymes such as $(Na^+ + K^+)$–ATPase through nonspecific membrane perturbations.

Plant Resins, Colocynth, Jalap, and Podophyllum

Recently these substances have been shown to inhibit sodium transport by the intestine. The exact mechanism has been difficult to identify because these resins contain many different compounds, the precise functions of which have yet to be determined.

In summary, Table 51–2 shows the mechanisms that have been described for this group of laxatives.

Laxatives That Decrease Water Absorption (Emollient Cathartics)

Liquid Petrolatum

Some oils literally "lubricate" the fecal mass, prevent excessive dehydration of the material, and may inhibit water reabsorption by coating the gut wall. Almost the only oil preparation now in use is **liquid petrolatum**, a mixture of liquid hydrocarbons. It is indigestible but, nevertheless, in some people it is slightly absorbed. It interferes with the absorption of fat-soluble vitamins. It should always be taken at night on an empty stomach.

One problem with mineral oil is that it leaks past the anal sphincters. It has also been reported to interfere with healing of wounds in the ano-rectal area. It should not be used in very debilitated patients, the elderly, or patients with swallowing abnormalities because of the risk of aspiration and lipid pneumonia when mineral oil gains access to the lungs.

TABLE 51–2 Mechanisms of Action of Laxatives That Increase Secretion

Laxative	Increase in cAMP	Inhibition of ATPase	Mucosal Injury
Anthraquinones	o	+	o
Bile acids	+	+	+
Bisacodyl	+	+	+
Dioctyl sodium sulfosuccinate	+	+	+
Phenolphthalein	o	+	+
Ricinoleic acid	+	+	+

Fibre

Dietary fibre comprises a heterogeneous group of compounds that have in common the fact that they are not digested by the pancreatic or intestinal enzymes and therefore are not absorbed. This includes the carbohydrates cellulose and hemicellulose, and a non-carbohydrate substance, lignin. The main structural units of the carbohydrate components are a variety of monosaccharides. Lignin is made up of phenylpropane units. Cellulose is the best known constituent of fibre and is the most abundant organic compound found in nature. It is composed entirely of straight chains of 1-4-β-linked D-glucose molecules that form fibres that take up water and swell. Dietary fibre of different plant species can increase stool wet weight (Table 51–3) by several mechanisms: (1) by adsorption of water, particularly by cellulose; (2) by increasing stool bulk; (3) as a result of metabolism of fibre by the colonic flora, with production of volatile fatty acids (acetic, butyric, propionic) that have osmotic and secretory effects in the intestinal mucosa; (4) through sequestration of bile acids from the small intestine that, once released in the colon, have a secretory effect.

Hydrophilic Colloids, Bulk-Forming Laxatives

This group includes both natural and semisynthetic polysaccharides and cellulose derivatives that dissolve or swell in water, forming a viscous solution or emollient gel. These gelatinous masses, of greatly increased bulk when moistened with water, exert a mildly laxative action. In addition, bulk-forming agents may actually promote colonic fluid accumulation by delivering bile acids and fatty acids to the colon where they may interfere with water and electrolyte transport. Cases of esophageal obstruction, fecal impaction, and even intestinal perforation have occurred when these drugs are taken in the dry form. Fluids should always be administered concurrently. These agents have occasionally been used to provide relief in acute diarrhea because they form an emollient intestinal mass and absorb water. Because of their bulk, they have also been suggested as appetite suppressants in the management of obesity. **Agar**, **psyllium** (plantago), **methylcellulose**, and **sodium carboxymethylcellulose** are examples of hydrophilic cellulose derivatives.

TABLE 51–3 Colonic Response to 20 g/Day Dietary Fibre

Fibre Type	Increase in Fecal Weight
Bran	127%
Cabbage	69%
Carrot	59%
Apple	40%

Laxatives That Increase Osmolarity

Saline

The saline laxatives, of which **magnesium sulfate** (Epsom salts), **magnesium hydroxide** (Milk of Magnesia), and **sodium potassium tartrate** (Rochelle salt, Seidlitz powder) are examples, contain ions that are only slowly absorbed from the intestine, such as Mg^{2+}, SO_4^{2-}, and PO_4^{3-}. These ions retain fluid in the bowel lumen by virtue of their osmotic properties, and therefore they hasten the passage of the contents of the small intestine, causing a larger volume of fluid to enter the colon. This distends the colon, thereby stimulating it so that catharsis occurs quite quickly. Magnesium laxatives may stimulate the release of cholecystokinin (CCK), which in turn stimulates pancreatic and duodenal secretion and decreases water, sodium, and chloride reabsorption. CCK causes an increase in cyclic GMP without affecting cyclic AMP. As the kidneys normally handle whatever ions are absorbed, the saline laxatives act also, in some cases, as saline diuretics. When absorbed in sufficient quantity, Mg^{2+} can depress the central nervous system; however, this rarely occurs unless there is impaired renal function or prolonged retention of the saline solution in the intestine.

Lactulose (4-β-galactoside-(1,4)-D-fructose)

This disaccharide is resistant to hydrolysis by the small-intestinal disaccharidases. It has an osmotic effect in the small bowel, drawing water into the intestinal lumen. Thus, a large volume of fluid enters the colon. Once in the large intestine, lactulose is acted upon by the endogenous flora of the colon with the production of lactic acid and of short-chain, volatile fatty acids. As these acids have a low lipid solubility, their colonic absorption is very limited; therefore, they have an osmotic effect, retaining water in the lumen. They also have, like lactic acid, a secretory effect on the colonic mucosa. This mechanism applies also to other nondigestible disaccharides and to lactose in people with lactose intolerance (low intestinal lactase activity).

Side Effects of Laxatives

Cathartic colon syndrome. This is a frequent cause of diarrhea, abdominal pain, and cramps. In radiographs the colon appears dilated, hypomotile, and with few or absent haustral margins; sometimes areas of pseudostricture are observed. Morphologically, there is mucosal inflammation, hypertrophy of the muscularis mucosae, thinning or atrophy of outer muscle layers, and damage to submucosal and myenteric plexuses.

Dependence, almost **addiction**. This is a commonly seen side effect, especially in women, due to psychologic factors linked to the association of a regular bowel habit with physical and spiritual well-being. (The Greek

GASTROINTESTINAL SYSTEM

word *katharsis* means cleansing, and the Latin word *purgare* means to purify, to make clean.)

Hypokalemia. The loss of Na⁺ and water in stools results in a reduction of plasma volume, stimulation of the renin-angiotensin system, and increased serum levels of aldosterone. Aldosterone, in the colon and kidney, increases the reabsorption of Na^+ in exchange for K^+ that is then lost in stools and urine respectively.

Malabsorption. Chronic and continuous use of laxatives can lead to malabsorption of xylose and other carbohydrates, fat, fat-soluble vitamins, and calcium, and thus to the production of osteomalacia.

Disturbance of carbohydrate metabolism. Abnormal release of insulin and carbohydrate intolerance may occur as a consequence of hypokalemia.

Liver abnormalities. Therapeutic doses of **dioctyl sodium sulfosuccinate** (DSS) are taken up by the liver and excreted in the bile. Since the drug is toxic to hepatic cells *in vitro*, the possibility of similar toxicity *in vivo* has been studied. There is considerable evidence that DSS may facilitate gastrointestinal or hepatic-cell uptake of other drugs, potentiating their activity and possibly increasing their toxicity. Chronic hepatitis has been reported after use of the combination of dioctyl calcium sulfosuccinate (Surfak®) and the anthraquinone laxative danthron. DSS may have contributed to the liver damage caused by the laxative oxyphenisatin, which was withdrawn from the market because of hepatotoxicity. DSS and oxyphenisatin are more toxic to hepatic cells *in vitro* when added together in low concentrations than when either is added separately. Therefore, sulfosuccinate "stool softeners" may increase the risk of hepatotoxicity from other drugs, including some laxatives.

Increased loss of proteins by the intestine. With the sole exceptions of fibre and lactulose, all laxatives have been reported to cause an excessive loss of proteins by the intestine.

Unnecessary surgery. As a consequence of "cathartic colon," patients may undergo a variety of surgical explorations and operations (*e.g.*, laparotomy, adrenalectomy, partial pancreatectomy, bowel resection).

Indications for Laxatives

Most cases of constipation can be treated without the use of pharmacologic agents, simply by avoiding white flour and substituting whole wheat flour; by reducing the intake of food that contains no fibre; by eating plenty of fruit and vegetables; and by taking extra fibre in the form of unprocessed bran.

Laxatives should never be used on a regular basis simply to produce a daily bowel movement. Taking the above into consideration, about the only indications for the use of these potentially risky pharmacologic agents are to empty the bowel prior to elective colonic or rectal surgery; to empty the bowel before radiologic or endoscopic examinations; to minimize straining at stool in patients with cardiovascular disease or with hernia; and to prevent hard, abrasive bowel movements that elicit pain (the latter may best be achieved with emollient laxatives).

Comments on the Medical Use of Laxatives

The general practitioner rarely has a valid reason for prescribing these drugs. On the contrary, it is much more common for the physician to be faced with **chronic misuse** of these agents by patients who seem unable to break the laxative habit. The medical profession appears to have done little to counter frequent commercial claims that one "feels better" after a bowel movement; presumably one feels twice as well after two evacuations, and so on. The individual following this school of thought will ensure complete emptying of the large bowel with a suitable laxative. This is followed by 2 or 3 days' absence of bowel movements, leading to the assumption that constipation has occurred and must be treated with more laxatives, and the person thus acquires a "cathartic habit." Ninety percent of patients suffering from laxative abuse are women.

In North America, more than 200 laxative preparations are available over the counter. Laxative-induced diarrhea is a well-recognized clinical condition in which frequently the abuser conceals the fact that these agents are being consumed. Laxatives are generally prescribed for "constipation," but this is a very ill-defined abnormality. Contrary to popular belief, to be healthy does not imply a daily bowel movement. One healthy person can have two or three bowel movements daily, while another healthy person may have two or three bowel movements weekly. The most common form of self-diagnosed "constipation" seen by physicians is the "imaginary" or nonexistent variety. In imaginary constipation, the patient is persuaded by the social emphasis on "regularity" of bowel function, with at least one stool per day, that an abnormality exists that requires treatment.

Another problem is the use of a laxative for every illness or imagined pain. In cases of genuine intestinal disease, laxatives, because of their effects on the intestinal wall, may accelerate the disease process; in appendicitis, laxatives will increase the likelihood of rupture of the appendix, and it has been demonstrated that the mortality rate among subjects who have ingested laxatives is higher than among subjects not receiving these agents. **All laxatives must be avoided in persons with nausea, vomiting, cramps, colic, or other unexplained abdominal discomfort.**

DRUGS USED IN THE TREATMENT OF DIARRHEA

Diarrhea is the frequent passage of semifluid or fluid stools. Normally, more than 12 L of fluid containing electrolytes, proteins, nucleic acids, vitamins, *etc.*, from endogenous and exogenous sources, circulate through the intestine daily; of this volume only 100–200 mL are normally lost in the stool. Therefore, an interference with the reabsorption of this enormous volume of liquid can result in severe dehydration, and death, in a very short time (especially in children).

Abnormal bowel motility plays a secondary modulating role in the overall mechanism of diarrhea. It probably accounts for the production of the cramps and pain that commonly occur with this condition. The primary event responsible for the production of diarrhea is almost always an abnormality in the movement of fluid and electrolytes across the intestinal mucosa. Diarrhea can result from either malabsorption of solutes (and therefore of fluid), or hypersecretion of solutes, or a combination of both factors. Thus, treatment of diarrhea should be directed toward two essential objectives: (1) replacement of the fluid and electrolyte losses; (2) reduction of the water content of the stools by decreasing secretion and/or increasing absorption.

All antidiarrheal drugs act only by decreasing the water content of the stools. It is important, therefore, to emphasize that most of the antidiarrheal drugs provide only symptomatic relief from the condition that is causing diarrhea, that they can be potentially harmful, and that, without replacement of fluid and electrolyte losses, other treatments may be useless.

As in the case of laxatives, the traditional textbook classification of the antidiarrheal drugs has little pathophysiologic meaning. This classification divides the drugs into (1) adsorbents, including charcoal, kaolin, pectin, Sorboquel® (a polycarbophil resin plus an antimuscarinic agent), (2) astringents such as tannic acid, (3) protectives including bismuth salts, such as the subcarbonate, salicylate, subgallate and subnitrate, and chalk, (4) demulcents such as gums, pectin, and psyllium, and (5) opium derivatives.

Despite the fact that there are very few studies showing convincing evidence that the commonly used antidiarrheal compounds are useful in the symptomatic treatment of diarrhea, the sales of these products in the United States exceed 50 million dollars per year. (Comparable figures may be assumed for Canada, given the similarities in life style and drug promotion.) From the few rigorous studies it can be concluded that, of the agents listed above, only **bismuth salts**, the **opiate derivatives**, and to some extent **psyllium** are effective in decreasing diarrhea or in providing some solidification of the stool. No change in diarrhea has been observed with anticholinergics or with activated charcoal. Surprisingly, Sorboquel®, kaolin, pectin, and cal-

cium carbonate have been found to produce an actual worsening of the diarrhea.

Chronic treatment with opiate derivatives can lead to addiction; also, in patients with chronic ulcerative colitis, opioids may alter colonic motility, and, during active episodes of the disease, they can induce the serious complication called toxic dilatation of the colon. A decreased peristaltic activity may facilitate the penetration of the intestinal mucosa by bacteria and viruses. This also encourages the proliferation of pathogens and may result in a prolongation of the disease and possible symptomless carriage of bacteria. Reliance on antidiarrheal drugs may also delay the application of a more effective and specific treatment.

Bismuth Salts

One of the most widely used over-the-counter preparations is Pepto-Bismol®, which contains bismuth subsalicylate. This compound was previously available only as a liquid preparation, but now a solid, more convenient, tablet formulation is available. Bismuth subsalicylate has been shown to be a safe and effective means of reducing the occurrence of "traveller's diarrhea," a condition caused predominantly by a specific strain of enterotoxigenic *Escherichia coli*. The mechanism of the antidiarrheal effect is not clear. It could be attributed in part to an antimicrobial effect of the drug against *E. coli*. Also, bismuth subsalicylate can decrease diarrhea through an effect on cyclic AMP or on cyclic GMP, perhaps through the inhibition of prostaglandin metabolism. However, the drug has also been reported to be effective in the treatment of viral gastroenteritis, in which adenylate cyclase activation does not appear to occur, and in which prostaglandins do not appear to be an important pathogenic factor.

Bismuth subsalicylate is well tolerated; the most common side effects are blackening of the tongue and of the stools, and tinnitus caused by salicylate toxicity. People taking bismuth subsalicylate for the prophylaxis of diarrhea should be warned not to take other salicylate-containing medications at the same time.

Opium Derivatives

The use of opium (*see* Chapter 22) for relief of diarrhea and dysentery preceded by many centuries its employment for analgesia. Opium in various forms, such as **camphorated tincture (paregoric)** or, preferably, **codeine**, can effectively check diarrhea. Usually the opiate is administered together with one of the other agents such as bismuth, chalk, or kaolin. The central effects make the patient feel more comfortable and assure better rest. Because they are usually remarkably effective for the control of diarrhea, the opiates must be used with caution and full recognition that they are only providing **relief of symptoms** and not treating the cause.

The observed effects of morphine and related drugs on the bowel may vary widely, depending on the species, the dose, and the techniques of investigation. Therefore, the present discussion will concentrate on the effects observed in humans.

Morphine, Camphorated Tincture of Opium (Paregoric), Codeine

The antidiarrheal effect of opiates has been generally thought to be related to their effect on intestinal smooth muscle. Although this mechanism has been recently challenged in favor of the concept that the effect of the opiates on diarrhea is better explained by their action on the mucosa, increasing electrolyte transport from the lumen, the matter is still far from settled. Recent observations in humans given codeine have failed to show an increase in the rate of fluid absorption from the lumen. On the other hand, the drug did have an effect on motility, resulting in retention of luminal contents and therefore providing more time for the absorption of fluid and of electrolytes. This resulted in a slowing of the delivery of fluid from proximal to distal sites and in a reduction in stool volume. Therefore, at this time the possibility of these drugs acting through a slowing of intestinal transit cannot be ruled out. We will describe the effects of opiates both on motility and on the transport of fluid and electrolytes.

Effects of Opiates on Gastrointestinal Motility

Stomach. Morphine and related drugs cause a decrease in motility associated with an increase in the tone of the antral portion of the stomach. There is also an increase in the tone of the first part of the duodenum, which often makes therapeutic intubation exceedingly difficult and delays the passage of the gastric contents through the duodenum for as much as 12 hours.

Small intestine. Resting tone is increased and periodic spasms are observed. The amplitude of the nonpropulsive type of rhythmic contractions is usually enhanced, but propulsive contractions are markedly decreased. Water is more completely absorbed from the chyme because of the delayed passage of the bowel contents, and the viscosity of the chyme is thereby increased. Large doses of atropine, by inducing relaxation of the gastrointestinal sphincters, may counteract, in part, the gastrointestinal responses to morphine, but resection of the extrinsic nerves and administration of ganglionic blocking agents do not do so.

Large intestine. Propulsive peristaltic waves in the colon are diminished or abolished by morphine, and tone is increased to the point of spasm. The resulting delay in the passage of the contents causes considerable desiccation of the feces, which, in turn, retards their further advance through the colon. The amplitude

of the nonpropulsive type of rhythmic contractions of the colon is usually enhanced. The tone of the anal sphincter is greatly augmented and this, combined with inattention to the normal sensory stimuli for the defecation reflex due to the central actions of the drug, might further contribute to morphine-induced constipation.

Atropine partially antagonizes the spasmogenic action on the human colon, but it has little or no effect on the decreased propulsive activity produced by morphine.

Mechanism of action of opiates on bowel motility. Neither the administration of ganglionic blocking agents nor the removal of the extrinsic innervation of the bowel prevents the characteristic actions of morphine and its surrogates in the unanaesthetized animal. At present, it appears that morphine acts on nerve plexuses within the bowel wall, inhibiting the release of acetylcholine from axon terminals. The receptors on which morphine acts normally respond to the naturally occurring opiate-like peptide enkephalin, found specifically in the CNS and the gastrointestinal tract.

Biliary tract. Therapeutic doses of morphine, codeine, and other morphine surrogates can cause a marked increase in biliary tract pressure. The response begins within 5 minutes of injection, reaches its peak in 15 minutes, and persists for 2 hours or more. Symptoms often accompany the increased pressure and vary from epigastric distress to typical biliary colic. Indeed, some patients with biliary colic may experience exacerbation and not relief of pain when given these drugs. The spasm of the sphincter of Oddi prevents emptying and thus causes the intraductal pressure to rise; this effect is probably responsible for the elevations of plasma amylase and lipase that are sometimes found after patients have been given morphine. Such elevations may persist for 24 hours after therapeutic doses and may confuse the diagnosis of intra-abdominal pathology, especially when acute pancreatitis is one of the diseases under consideration. Biliary spasm is not, however, a consistent effect of therapeutic doses of morphine, and some patients show no changes in bile duct size or pressure. Atropine only partially prevents morphine-induced biliary spasm, but nalorphine prevents or relieves it.

Effect of Opiates on Intestinal Transport of Fluid and Electrolytes

Opiates have recently been shown to inhibit *in vivo* and *in vitro* the intestinal fluid accumulation induced by a variety of secretagogues such as prostaglandins, bisacodyl, vasoactive intestinal polypeptide, cholera toxin, and cholinergics. While the first four agents induce hypersecretion and diarrhea mainly through an increase in intracellular cAMP, the cholinergics act by increasing intracellular free calcium. Therefore it is likely that opiates inhibit secretion by more than one mechanism. The net effects of opiates on electrolyte transport are (1) an enhancement of absorption of Na⁺ and Cl⁻ and (2) inhibition of the secretion of these electrolytes. These effects might result from a blocking of the elaboration of cAMP by the opiates, or an inhibition of the actions of cAMP on the mucosa, or, more likely, from a combination of both mechanisms. Morphine inhibition of diarrhea induced by cholinergics could be related to the fact that morphine and calcium have antagonistic actions in several circumstances. Also, acute morphine administration decreases brain calmodulin activity. A similar action of opiates in the intestine could explain their effects on the absorption and secretion of fluid and electrolytes. Clearly, the mechanism of the antisecretory action of opiates is complex.

Diphenoxylate

Diphenoxylate (Lomotil®; Fig. 51–2) is an analog of meperidine (see Chapter 22), and its effects on GI motility and fluid and electrolyte transport are similar to those of morphine.

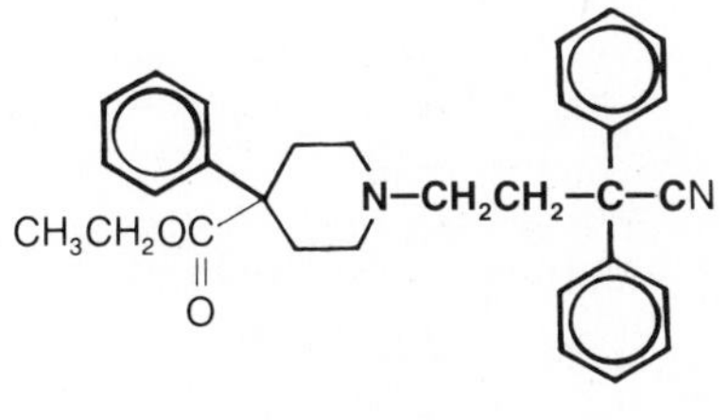

Diphenoxylate

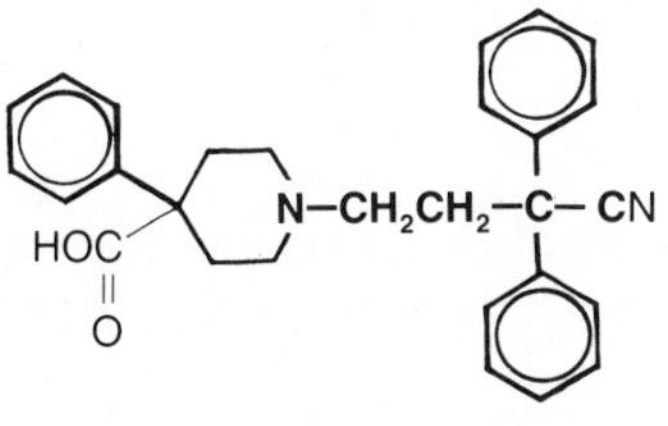

Difenoxin

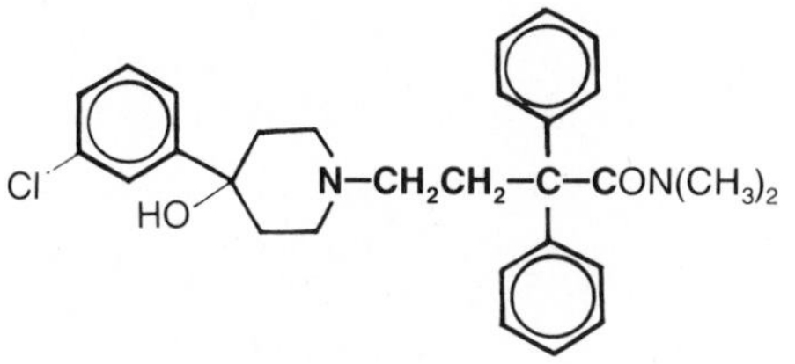

Loperamide

Figure 51–2 Structural formulae of diphenoxylate, difenoxin, and loperamide. (Common elements in bold face.)

Diphenoxylate has no analgesic activity in the therapeutic range, but at high doses the drug shows typical opioid activity. It is included in the Schedule of narcotic drugs. It has been used widely because of its efficacy, even though it has to be taken in four or more doses daily due to its short duration of action.

As diphenoxylate is a CNS depressant, it can potentiate the effects of barbiturates, neuroleptics, and alcohol. Because of its depressant action it should **not be used for more than 5 days** in the adult, and not at all in children. In the United States, atropine is included in Lomotil® (1/10 clinical dose) to "discourage" abuse.

The effects of overdose resemble those of morphine; both respiratory and cardiac arrest have been reported. With Lomotil®, atropine overdose effects have also been observed in the United States. Opiate-like **habituation** may occur, and the effects of overdose can be reversed by naloxone. Diphenoxylate sometimes increases cramping even while decreasing diarrhea; this also decreases patient acceptance of the drug.

Difenoxin

Difenoxin (Dioctin®, Lyspaten®; see Fig. 51–2) is the major metabolite of diphenoxylate. It has been synthesized, and in animal studies appears to be about five times as potent as diphenoxylate. Another advantage is that it also has a larger dissociation between antidiarrheal and opiate-like CNS effects. It is also marketed in combination with atropine sulfate. Like diphenoxylate, its principal side effects arise from its action on the CNS, an action that is responsible for the abuse potential of both agents.

Loperamide

This drug (Imodium®; see Fig. 51–2) is another opiate analog of the piperidine class with high affinity for both central and peripheral opiate receptors. It is related to both diphenoxylate and haloperidol. Its effects on gastrointestinal motility and on fluid and electrolyte transport by the intestine are similar to those of morphine. The fact that the effect of loperamide is blocked by naloxone lends weight to the hypothesis that it acts through specific opiate receptors. It is more effective than placebo in reducing acute or chronic diarrhea of varying etiology. Experimentally, it has been shown to prevent prostaglandin-induced diarrhea and to inhibit the secretion induced by cholera enterotoxin.

Loperamide is two to three times as potent as diphenoxylate, and its action is more rapid and prolonged. This drug has no analgesic activity, and even in high doses it is reported not to have CNS or cardiovascular effects. This may be due in part to the fact that the drug has a reduced passage through the blood–brain barrier. Disposition of orally administered loperamide is interesting in that the drug is biotrans-

GASTROINTESTINAL SYSTEM

formed by demethylation in the intestinal wall. The formed metabolites are then released back into the lumen. Only a small proportion of the administered dose is absorbed. This unique disposition reduces the amount of drug in the systemic circulation, and therefore the side effects are less frequent. About 7% of the administered drug is excreted in the urine. There is an efficient hepatic uptake followed by biotransformation and biliary excretion.

Loperamide has been used chronically (for more than 12 months) without any tolerance or dependence being demonstrated. A naloxone challenge in these chronically treated subjects did not precipitate withdrawal symptoms. Loperamide, in addition to its high antidiarrheal specificity, also has a wide safety margin. Nevertheless, despite the drug being certainly safer than other opiate analogs, there is still no consensus on whether the drug should be used in infants.

Adrenergic Compounds

Adrenergic agonists stimulate Na^+ and Cl^- absorption and also inhibit HCO_3^- and Cl^- secretion in the small and large intestines. They act on enterocyte receptors that inhibit adenylate cyclase, and thus decrease the stimulated rise in intracellular cyclic AMP. Also, the α_2-adrenoceptor agonists have a modest antimotility effect, which may increase the amount of time in which the luminal contents remain available for absorption.

Clonidine, a specific α_2-adrenoceptor agonist used primarily as an antihypertensive agent (see Chapter 18), has been shown to diminish castor oil-induced diarrhea and the diarrhea caused by naloxone-precipitated opiate withdrawal. Although the centrally mediated hypotensive and sedative effects of clonidine have so far limited its use as an antidiarrheal agent, it seems to be an effective treatment for diabetic diarrhea in patients with evidence of autonomic neuropathy. Diabetic patients treated with clonidine do not appear to develop hypotension, and preexisting postural hypotension is not aggravated.

Lidamidine is an amidinourea that is structurally dissimilar from clonidine and may cause less hypotension or sedation in its antidiarrheal dose range. It is an α_2-adrenoceptor agonist and appears useful in treating diarrhea in diabetics with autonomic neuropathy. Future development of α_2-adrenergic analogs that do not cross the blood–brain barrier, or with preferential gut action, would eliminate central side effects and make these ideal antidiarrheal agents.

Phenothiazine and Butyrophenone Neuroleptics in the Treatment of Secretory Diarrhea

The phenothiazine **chlorpromazine**, in well-tolerated doses, has recently been shown to be a potent antagonist of cholera toxin-induced cyclic AMP production. The drug has also been shown to reduce strikingly the fluid and electrolyte losses in patients with cholera. Also, a potent antisecretory effect of several neuroleptics has been reported in experimental diarrhea induced by PGE_1, theophylline, vasoactive intestinal peptide, heat-stable E. coli enterotoxin, and dibutyryl cyclic AMP. Chlorpromazine has been shown to act at two loci: (1) it inhibits adenylate cyclase, and (2) it blocks the mechanism through which the influx of Na^+ into the villus cell is inhibited by cAMP or dibutyryl cAMP. Recently, the antisecretory effect of the neuroleptics has been attributed to a direct inhibition of calmodulin, with which they form complexes and thus interfere with a variety of calcium-dependent biochemical events. The order of potency of the antisecretory activity of these drugs is: **trifluoperazine > chlorpromazine > haloperidol > chlorprothixene** (which is quite different from their order of potency of neuroleptic action; see Chapter 27).

The therapeutic potential of these drugs is high, as they seem to be very effective in reducing, or in turning off safely, the hypersecretory state that characterizes many diarrheas. Besides cholera, beneficial effects could be expected in diarrhea induced by bile acids, hormone-secreting tumors, salmonellosis, shigellosis, celiac sprue, diffuse regional enteritis, and certain E. coli strains. In all of these conditions, cyclic nucleotide-regulated intestinal hypersecretion has been considered to be at least partially responsible for the diarrhea.

Berberine

Berberine is an alkaloid from the plant Berberis aristata. It has been used for at least 3000 years in China and India for the treatment of diarrhea. The alkaloid has been shown to decrease the loss of fluid caused by both V. cholerae and the enterotoxin of E. coli. The effect appears to result from a specific inhibition of the action of enterotoxins on intestinal cells. Berberine has also a broad spectrum of activity against bacteria, fungi, and protozoa. Recent new trials with the substance have shown efficacy in the treatment of diarrhea in Indian children.

SUGGESTED READING

Beubler E, Juan H. Effect of ricinoleic acid and other laxatives on net water flux and prostaglandin E release by rat colon. J Pharm Pharmacol 1979; 31:681–685.

Donowitz M, Binder HJ. Effect of dioctyl sodium sulfosuccinate on colonic fluid and electrolyte movement. Gastroenterology 1975; 69:941–950.

Fedorak RN, Field M. Antidiarrheal therapy. Prospects for new agents. Dig Dis Sci 1987; 32:195–205.

Gaginella TS, Bass P. Laxatives: an update on mechanism of action. Life Sci 1978; 23:1001–1009.

Islam MR, Sack DA, Holmgreen J, et al. Use of chlorpromazine in the treatment of cholera and other severe acute watery diarrheal diseases. Gastroenterology 1982; 82:1335–1340.

Kramer D. Effect of antidiarrheal and antimotility drugs on ileal excreta. Am J Dig Dis 1977; 22:327–332.

McKay JS, Linaker BD, Higgs NB, Turnberg LA. Studies of the antisecretory activity of morphine in rabbit ileum in vitro. Gastroenterology 1982; 82:243–247.

Niemegeers CJE, Colpaert FC, Awouters FHL. Pharmacology and antidiarrheal effect of loperamide. Drug Dev Res 1981; 1:1–20.

Palmer KR, Corbett CL, Holdsworth CD. Double-blind, cross-over study comparing loperamide, codeine and diphenoxylate in the treatment of chronic diarrhea. Gastroenterology 1980; 79:1272–1275.

CHEMOTHERAPY

Chapter 52

PRINCIPLES OF ANTIMICROBIAL THERAPY

C. Prober

One of the greatest achievements of medical science has been the control and management of infectious diseases. The role of microbes in causing severe infections was not appreciated until **Louis Pasteur** formulated the germ theory in the years 1853 to 1867. During the years 1880 to 1910, pathogenic bacteria were discovered by the dozens. It was, however, not until the 20th century that therapy directed against these microbes was developed. This development of antimicrobial therapy can be divided into two historic periods—the era of synthetic compounds and the era of antibiotics.

The Era of Synthetic Compounds

Paul Ehrlich (1854–1915) was responsible for establishing a basic principle of chemotherapy. The importance of drug distribution as a determinant of drug action had been realized in the latter part of the 19th century. Struck by the observation that certain chemicals show a remarkable affinity for various materials (*e.g.*, the affinity of dyes for the proteins of wool), Ehrlich reasoned that if chemicals with antimicrobial activity could be targeted to be taken up in certain human tissues, they would exert there a chemical action against infecting microbes. Unfortunately Ehrlich's search for such "magic bullets" was initially rather nonspecific. He utilized chemicals designed to fix to proteins, carbohydrates, or fats, and therefore these chemicals interfered not only with the infecting microbes but also with host tissues. Ehrlich realized that a useful antimicrobial drug would have to be selectively toxic to the microbes, and he therefore began to investigate chemical modifications that would cause the toxic materials to be selectively taken up by the pathogens.

This led to the introduction in 1909 of an arsenic derivative, arsphenamine (**Salvarsan**), for the treatment of syphilis. Though this drug had considerable toxicity, it and its successor **Neosalvarsan** were the standard treatments for the disease throughout the world for over 40 years, until superseded by penicillin. With this discovery, Ehrlich not only developed an important chemotherapeutic agent, but also was responsible for beginning the systematic exploration of the molecular basis of antibacterial chemotherapy.

Within approximately three decades of Ehrlich's original work, a red tissue dye with antibacterial action was described. This substance, **Prontosil**, was the forerunner of the sulfonamides, substances that remain today some of the most important of the synthetic antibacterial compounds.

The Era of Antibiotics

The term "antibiosis" was coined in 1889 by Vuillemin and originally meant the antagonism between living creatures. This definition was refined by **Waksman** who, in 1942, defined antibiotics as substances produced by microorganisms and antagonistic to the growth or life of other microorganisms in high dilution. The first antibiotic was penicillin, a product of a *penicillium* mold. This was discovered by **Fleming** in 1928 and initiated the antibiotic era, which extends to the present and has been the subject of much historical, social, and biographical writing. Innumerable microbial products have been investigated since the discovery of penicillin, and a great variety of them have proven to be useful antibiotic substances. Pharmaceutical companies have been extremely active in the search for these products, and have made fundamental contributions to the development of antibiotic drugs.

Much work has been done in modifying the natural products (by removing some chemical groups and ad-

---

This chapter was revised by J. Uetrecht.

ding others) in attempts to enhance the beneficial effects while minimizing the toxic effects. The resultant modified end product is termed a semisynthetic antibiotic. Most antibiotics currently used in clinical practice are semisynthetic. Some desirable pharmacologic characteristics cultivated in these semisynthetic agents include: stability, solubility, diffusibility, activity in the complex environment of the body, and slow excretion. In addition, these agents are designed to possess as large a therapeutic index as possible (*i.e.*, the amount of drug causing toxicity far exceeds the amount of drug necessary for a therapeutic response).

The relationships between patient, infecting pathogen, and antimicrobial agent are illustrated in Figure 52–1. The therapeutic usefulness of a given chemotherapeutic agent is usually determined by its selective toxicity toward the pathogen.

MECHANISMS OF ACTION

The mechanisms of action of antimicrobial agents are based upon an attack on targets present in bacteria and other organisms but either absent or less vulnerable in human cells ("**selective toxicity**," a term formally introduced by Adrien Albert in 1951). These microbial targets include: the cell wall, the cytoplasmic membrane, cellular proteins, and cellular nucleic acids.

It is traditional to classify antimicrobial agents by their mechanism of action, a system that will be used throughout these chapters. In the following chapters the drugs to be described in relation to the sites of action mentioned above include:

- **Cell wall**—penicillins, cephalosporins, vancomycin, bacitracin, cycloserine.
- **Cell membrane**—polymyxins, colistin, nystatin, amphotericin B, imidazoles.
- **Cell proteins**—aminoglycosides, spectinomycin, tetracyclines, chloramphenicol, clindamycin, erythromycin.
- **Cellular nucleic acids**—griseofulvin, 5-fluorocytosine, rifampin, isoniazid, ethambutol, para-aminosalicylic acid, quinolones, sulfonamides, trimethoprim, pyrimethamine, sulfones.

The individual mechanisms of action are described in detail in the respective chapters.

BACTERIOSTATIC VERSUS BACTERICIDAL ANTIMICROBIALS

Bacteriostatic antimicrobial agents such as chloramphenicol, the tetracyclines, and erythromycin inhibit bacterial cell replication but do not kill the organisms;

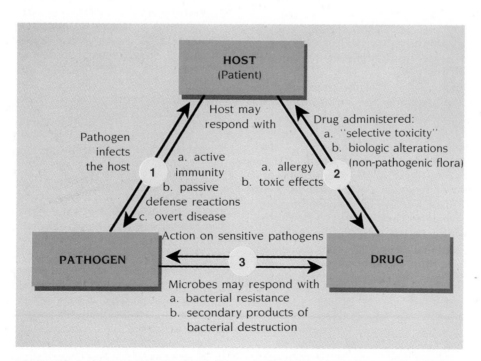

Figure 52–1 Host–pathogen–drug relationships in chemotherapy. (1) Pathogenesis of the infectious disease process. (2) Pharmacokinetics and -dynamics (*i.e.*, pharmacology) in the patient. (3) Microbiologic processes of drug–pathogen interaction.

that is, they stop bacterial growth and allow the host's immune factors to ultimately clear the infection. Theoretically, if host immunity is suppressed, or if the infection is in an area of poor immunologic surveillance (*e.g.*, cerebrospinal fluid or vegetations of subacute bacterial endocarditis), bacteriostatic drugs may not suffice as sole therapeutic agents.

Bactericidal antimicrobial agents such as the penicillins, cephalosporins, and most aminoglycosides cause microbial death by lysis. They therefore rely less on host immunity for clearing of bacterial infections.

Some antimicrobial agents, such as the sulfonamides and tetracyclines, are indeterminate in the extent of their action. They are bacteriostatic or bactericidal depending on the concentration of drug, the nature of the environment, and the specific microorganisms against which they are employed.

ANTIBIOTIC RESISTANCE

Most, if not all, microorganisms are capable of developing resistance to the action of antimicrobial agents.

Mutation

This is a rare, spontaneous, "normal" event that is not usually induced by antimicrobials. However, in relation to antimicrobials the mechanisms may include:

- Alterations of cell walls, or cell membrane components, that prevent the entry of drugs into cells.
- Alteration of the target or binding site for an antimicrobial inside the cell.
- Other indirect mechanisms by which previously susceptible cells may become nonresponsive to the action of drugs.

Mutation is not an important mechanism of resistance. Mutationally altered cells are often metabolically inferior to wild-type cells; they tend to be suppressed and diluted out in competitive growth of a bacterial population. Thus, they rarely give rise to a resistant strain. However, mutants may become a threat when selective antibiotic pressure on the wild-type organisms is maintained by suboptimal antibiotic exposure, extensive topical use of the drug, or other factors that allow resistant mutants to gain the competitive advantage.

Inheritance

This is the most common way for microbes to acquire resistance to antimicrobials. It is induced by exposure to antimicrobial agents, and it is transferable within a microbial population.

The genetic agents that confer antimicrobial resistance are the resistance plasmids (**R plasmids**), which may encode for resistance to as many as six or seven antimicrobial agents. Plasmids are extrachromosomal genetic elements in bacteria, ranging in size from less than one to more than a million daltons. Their main role is to allow bacterial evolution under greatly varying environmental conditions. They confer genetic properties that code for functions of particular advantage. Thus, plasmid-determined functions include replication, fertility, metabolism, virulence, resistance to toxic metals, *etc.*, in addition to resistance to antimicrobials.

Resistance plasmids are believed to arise from collections of foreign genes that are not normally part of a bacterium's chromosomes. These genes may have come from a variety of unrelated bacterial or fungal sources (such as antibiotic-producing microorganisms), and they must have experienced strong selective pressures to be assembled into resistance plasmids (such as may have been created by exposure to metals, halogens, and similar antibacterial agents of the preantibiotic era). Since their description by **Watanabe** in 1963, R plasmid activity and dissemination are recognized as the major threat to continued antibiotic effectiveness.

Examples of the products of R plasmid-coded activity are:

- Products produced in cell walls or cell membranes that interfere with transport systems or block pores (*i.e.*, antibiotics cannot enter the cell).
- Enzymes produced by microbes that modify the site of drug action (*i.e.*, the antibiotic will enter the cell, but the drug-binding site is lacking).
- Enzymes produced by microbes that destroy the antibiotic (*i.e.*, no active antibiotic remains).
- Substitute enzymes produced by microbes that are resistant to antibiotic action and replace antibiotic-sensitive essential enzymes. The substitute enzyme permits cell growth in the presence of antibiotic.

Dissemination of Resistance

Most R plasmids are transferable and conjugative, *i.e.*, they possess the sex-factor activity necessary to initiate **conjugation** between resistance-positive (R+) and resistance-negative (R−) bacteria. This conjugation leads to a direct transfer of complete R plasmids from one bacterial cell to another.

R plasmids can also spread among microorganisms *via* a bacteriophage vector. This process, called **transduction**, is limited to R plasmids that can be accommodated in a bacteriophage chromosome, *i.e.*, plasmids of smaller size.

R plasmids may be carried between microorganisms by direct DNA transfer, a process called **transformation.** This is the basis of recombinant DNA technology and "genetic engineering" with *Escherichia coli*. Although unproven in nature, it conceivably occurs through contact of plasmid DNA from lysed bacteria with recipient cells.

Resistance determinants can be transferred independently from the R plasmids by a process called **transposition** (*i.e.*, hopping from one plasmid to another, or to a chromosome, or to a bacteriophage). This is thought to be the "natural" construction of R plasmids from various genetic sources; the new resistance is then permanently transferred with its new vector. This process allows previously nontransferable forms to be joined to transferable R plasmids, which may be the most common basis of resistance in hospital environments.

Some known mechanisms of antibiotic resistance, relative to the mode of action of respective drugs, are shown in Table 52–1.

LABORATORY MONITORING

The rational use of antimicrobial agents requires careful laboratory monitoring. One important aspect of this monitoring includes determining the degree of activity of the selected antimicrobial agent against the infecting bacterial strain. This is termed **sensitivity testing**. Though most bacteria have a predictable sensitivity pattern (to be discussed in subsequent chapters for specific antimicrobial agents), there is sufficient variation to de-

mand that the degree of activity of a specific antibiotic against an organism causing a serious infection should always be assessed.

The principle of sensitivity testing is that the activity of the antibiotic against one or several specific bacteria can be determined *in vitro* under conditions that simulate the environment of the bacteria in the host. The two methods of performing sensitivity testing are the disc-diffusion method and the dilution method.

Disc-Diffusion Method

This was the earliest available method and is currently the most extensively used worldwide. Commercially available paper discs impregnated with specific amounts of antimicrobial agents are placed onto agar plates containing a standardized number (inoculum) of the bacteria to be tested. The antibiotic diffuses out of the disc into the agar, establishing a linear concentration gradient from the centre of the disc to some peripheral point in the agar. Bacteria on the agar are therefore presented with a continuous concentration gradient of antibiotic that inhibits or kills the bacteria for a variable distance around the disc. This resulting zone of antibacterial effect, the diameter of which is determined after an overnight incubation, is called the **zone of inhibition**.

The exact size of the zone (expressed in mm) reflects the degree of susceptibility or resistance, but the inter-

TABLE 52–1 Known Mechanisms of Antibiotic Resistance

Agent	Mode of Antibacterial Action	Microbial Resistance Mechanism
Sulfonamides	Block synthesis of tetrahydrofolic acid and cell-linked metabolic pathways.	R plasmid-coded, sulfonamide-resistant dihydrofolic acid synthetase.
Trimethoprim	Competitive inhibition of dihydrofolic acid reductase; blocks synthesis of tetrahydrofolic acid.	R plasmid-coded, trimethoprim-resistant dihydrofolic acid reductase.
Penicillins and Cephalosporins	Interfere with cell wall biosynthesis by interacting with penicillin-binding proteins.	Hydrolysis of the antibiotic's beta-lactam ring by beta-lactamase enzyme.
Tetracyclines	Inhibit protein synthesis by interaction with 30S and 50S ribosome subunits.	Interference with transport of drug into cell; cell unable to maintain drug.
Aminoglycosides	Bind to 30S (and 50S) ribosome subunit, cause translational misreading, inhibit peptide elongation.	Enzymatic modification of drug by R plasmid-coded enzyme; drug has reduced affinity for ribosome; reduced transport into cell.
Erythromycin and Lincomycin	Bind to 50S ribosome subunit; inhibit protein synthesis at chain elongation step.	Enzymatic modification of ribosomal DNA of sensitive cells renders ribosome drug-resistant.
Chloramphenicol	Inhibits protein synthesis by interacting with 50S ribosome subunit.	Drug inactivated by acetylation of –OH groups by chloramphenicol transacetylase. Interference with drug transport into cell.
Rifampin	Binds to bacterial RNA polymerase and blocks RNA synthesis (transcription).	Resistance arises by spontaneous mutation (no plasmid-coded mechanism known).

CHEMOTHERAPY

pretation of the results is based upon prior studies using dilution tests (see below), which have correlated zone sizes with the minimum amount of antibiotic required to inhibit the growth of the bacterium. Results are expressed in only three susceptibility categories: sensitive, intermediate, or resistant. These categories are based upon the approximated serum concentrations of the antimicrobial agent normally attained after a standard dose. Thus, sensitivity to a specific antibiotic, as determined by this system, is meaningful only if (1) the infection being treated is in the blood stream or in tissues having approximately the same antibiotic concentrations as that in the blood stream; (2) the patient is receiving a "standard dose" of the antibiotic; (3) the patient will attain the usual concentrations of the specific antibiotic in the circulation.

Although it is recognized that the disc-diffusion method of sensitivity testing is rather imprecise, in general it provides sufficient information to choose the appropriate antibiotic.

Dilution Method

This method of sensitivity testing can be carried out in agar or broth. A standardized inoculum of bacteria is exposed to varying concentrations (usually successive two-fold dilutions) of an antimicrobial agent. The minimum concentration of antibiotic required to inhibit the growth of the bacteria can then be determined. This **minimum inhibitory concentration (MIC)** can then be compared with the measured or predicted concentration of antibiotic at the site of infection, be that the blood, urine, cerebrospinal fluid, or other site.

In addition to the MIC, the **minimum bactericidal concentration (MBC)** can also be determined, especially if the original dilutions were done in broth. To measure the MBC, aliquots of broth from tubes showing no visible growth after overnight incubation are subcultured onto antibiotic-free agar. The MBC is represented by the lowest concentration of antibiotic that completely suppresses the growth of bacteria on the subculture. In general, the MIC and MBC of a bactericidal agent will be equal, whereas a bacteriostatic drug will have a large difference between the MIC and MBC. The clinical significance of the difference between MIC and MBC is unclear, and most reporting is in terms of the MIC.

Many laboratory variables may affect the results of a sensitivity test, such as size of the inoculum of bacteria used, the temperature of incubation, and the pH and cation content of the culture medium. These and other important variables are usually controlled in a consistent fashion by the laboratory providing this critically important information to clinicians; but clinicians must realize that, as with any test, external factors may influence observed results.

Another important aspect of sensitivity testing relates to assessing the *in vitro* effects of a **combination of antibiotics**. Two antimicrobial drugs acting together *in vitro* may be indifferent, antagonistic, or synergistic. When their combined action is no greater than that of the more active drug alone, they are said to be indifferent. When the activity of one is reduced by the presence of the other, they are said to be antagonistic. When their combined effect is significantly greater than that of either alone, they are said to be synergistic. Description of the precise mathematical definitions of these combined actions and of the methodologies available to test for these effects is beyond the scope of this chapter.

As early as 1952 it was suggested that the type of interaction of two drugs could be predicted on the basis of whether the component drugs were bactericidal or bacteriostatic. Two bacteriostatic drugs together would be additive, two bactericidal drugs together would be synergistic, and combination of one of each type would be antagonistic. It has become clear, however, that those generalizations do not apply to all combinations of antimicrobial agents. When a clinician deals with serious infections, especially those caused by relatively resistant microbes, the type of interaction can only be ascertained by direct synergy testing.

Determinations of Antimicrobial Concentrations

Another aspect of laboratory monitoring in the rational use of antimicrobial agents involves the determination of the concentrations of these agents. Though the approximate concentrations that will be attained in various body sites after standard therapeutic doses can be predicted from the literature, there is considerable interpatient variability. The only way of knowing what concentrations are attained after a given dose is to measure the plasma or serum levels. This is not so important for relatively nontoxic agents, which, at usual doses, generally attain concentrations several hundred-fold greater than the MIC of the bacteria being treated (e.g., penicillin in *Streptococcus pneumoniae* bacteremia). Here the margin for error is wide; however, for other agents that may attain concentrations only three- to four-fold higher than the MIC of the bacteria being treated (e.g., aminoglycosides in enteric aerobic infections), determining the attained concentrations is more important. In addition, the aminoglycosides have a low therapeutic index (i.e., narrow margin of safety) so that the determination of concentrations is also important for limiting concentration-related toxic reactions.

Serum Bactericidal Titres

The ultimate control of infection not only depends on the action of the antimicrobial agents but also reflects the resultant effect of many host factors, primarily immunologic. Therefore, a meaningful test of therapeutic activity should take into account all of these factors. Such a test is the measurement of serum bactericidal titre (SBT). Serum samples are obtained to coincide with anticipated maximum (peak) and minimum (trough) antimicrobial drug levels. The test is performed by adding a known inoculum of the bacterium isolated from the patient to serial two-fold dilutions of the serum. The minimum concentration (highest dilution) of the serum capable of inhibiting and ultimately killing the inoculated bacteria is determined. This test, which has been most widely used for the determination of therapeutic effectiveness in bacterial endocarditis and other serious infections, permits monitoring of therapeutic response and allows modification of the choice and dosage of various antimicrobial agents. Although controversial, for the highest probability of clinical improvement the peak SBT should represent a dilution of at least 1:8. Trough SBTs and other tests, such as the area under the concentration-time curve above the MIC, are being evaluated as methods of predicting outcome.

DETERMINANTS OF RESPONSE TO ANTIMICROBIAL THERAPY

Several factors must be considered when an antimicrobial agent is prescribed if therapy is to be successful. Antimicrobial agents are of no value in treating viral infections or in treating noninfectious ailments. Presuming that an established bacterial infection is being treated, the antibiotic must be active against the infecting bacteria. This implies a knowledge of the most likely pathogens and a knowledge of the spectrum of activity of the selected antimicrobial agent. If a bacterium has actually been isolated, then *in vitro* sensitivity testing is appropriate. The appropriate dose, route of administration, and duration of therapy must be selected for the specific patient, considering the specific site of infection. This is intended to maximize the chance of attaining adequate concentrations of the antimicrobial agent at the site of the infection. For certain antibiotics, especially those with a low therapeutic index, the actual measurement of the drug concentrations attained is indicated. Finally, successful therapy requires an assurance of compliance with the prescribed agents and dosage regimens, a factor that must be remembered in outpatient therapeutics.

Successful outcome may also require the employment of ancillary modes of therapy to assist antibiotic action. This might include surgical drainage of abscesses, removal of obstructions to urinary flow, or removal of foreign bodies such as intravascular catheters.

PHARMACOKINETIC FACTORS ESSENTIAL FOR OPTIMAL ANTIMICROBIAL THERAPY

The rational use of antibiotics requires some knowledge of their pharmacokinetics. Although it may

TABLE 52–2 Some Variables Influencing the Kinetics of Antimicrobial Agents

Variable	Mechanism of Effect	Example
Age	Decreased renal function early in life and late in life.	Need to decrease dose of aminoglycosides in neonates and elderly.
Renal function	Important for drugs dependent on renal excretion.	Need to decrease dose of aminoglycosides in patients with compromised renal function.
Liver function	Important for drugs biotransformed in the liver.	Need to decrease dose of chloramphenicol in patients with compromised liver function, *e.g.*, premature newborns.
Fever/Burns	Increased excretion or increased V_D of some drugs.	Need to increase dose of aminoglycosides.
Acetylation status	Important for drugs being acetylated.	Need to increase dose of isoniazid in rapid acetylators on regimen of once or twice weekly dosage.
Diabetes mellitus	Reduced absorption of certain drugs after intramuscular dosing.	Need to increase dose of intramuscular penicillins in diabetics.
Cystic fibrosis	Increased clearance and V_D of some drugs.	Need to increase dose of aminoglycosides in these patients.
	Altered absorption of some drugs.	Chloramphenicol palmitate malabsorbed because of lipase deficiency.
GI surgery	Altered absorption of drugs in patients with short bowel, *e.g.*, ileal bypass.	Ampicillin bioavailability is 15% of normal after small-bowel bypass.

not be necessary to know all kinetic details for each agent, the following are essential:

1. The **anticipated concentration** of the antibiotic **at the site of infection** to be attained after the selected dose. This implies knowledge of the serum concentration attained and the diffusion characteristics (distribution) of the antibiotic into the infected tissue. This concentration can then be related to the sensitivity of the infecting bacterium. It is generally desirable to attain antibiotic concentrations at the site of infection at least two- to four-fold in excess of the MIC of the infecting organism.
2. The **elimination half-life of the antibiotic.** This allows an approximation of the dosing interval that will result in maintenance of the desired concentration range.
3. The **sources of pharmacokinetic variation**. This implies some knowledge of biotransformation and elimination. If an agent is excreted primarily by the kidneys and the patient is in renal failure, it is necessary to recognize the need for dose adjustment. Similarly, if the agent is biotransformed in the liver and the patient is in hepatic failure, the dose may have to be adjusted. Some of the host variables influencing the kinetics of antibiotics, with examples from clinical practice, are outlined in Table 52-2.

In the chapters that follow, these variables will not be specifically considered for each antibiotic; rather, the discussion will refer to normal adult patients. It is important, however, to always consider sources of pharmacokinetic variation, for no patient will behave precisely in textbook fashion.

SUGGESTED READING

Albert A. Selective toxicity: the physicochemical basis of therapy, 6th ed. London: Chapman and Hall, 1979.

Conte JE Jr, Barriere SL. Manual of antibiotics and infectious diseases, 4th ed. Philadelphia: Lea and Febiger, 1981.

Gale EF, Cundliffe E, Reynolds PE, Richmond MH, Waring MJ. The molecular basis of antibiotic action, 2nd ed. London/New York/Sydney/Toronto: Wiley and Sons, 1981.

Garrod LP, Lambert HP, O'Grady F. Antibiotic and chemotherapy, 5th ed. Edinburgh/London/Melbourne/New York: Churchill Livingstone, 1981.

Koren G, Prober CG, Gold R, eds. Antimicrobial therapy in infants and children. New York/Basel: Marcel Dekker, 1988.

Kucers A, Bennett N McK. The use of antibiotics. A comprehensive review with clinical emphasis, 3rd ed. London: Heinemann, 1979.

Levy SB. Microbial resistance to antibiotics: an evolving and persistent problem. Lancet 1982; II:83–88.

Neu HC. General concepts on the chemotherapy of infectious diseases. Med Clin North Am 1987; 71:1051–1064.

Neu HC. Diagnostic laboratory procedures in infectious diseases. Ibid. 1987; 71:1065–1078.

Rosenblatt JE. Laboratory tests used to guide antimicrobial therapy. Mayo Clin Proc 1987; 62:799–805.

Timmins KN, Gonzales-Carrero MI, Sekizaki T, Rojo F. Biological activities specified by antibiotic resistance plasmids. J Antimicrob Chemother 1986; 18(Suppl C):1–10.

Whelton A. Antibiotic pharmacokinetics and clinical application in renal insufficiency. Med Clin North Am 1982; 66:267–281.

Wilkowske CJ, Hermans PE. General principles of antimicrobial therapy. Mayo Clin Proc 1987; 62:789–798.

Chapter 53

ANTIMICROBIAL AGENTS THAT ACT UPON BACTERIAL CELL WALL FORMATION

J. Uetrecht

All living cells, including bacteria as well as mammalian tissue cells, have **cell membranes** (plasma membranes) that are necessary for the functional integrity of the cells. These membranes have complex lipid structures that can be disrupted by surfactants (detergents). Surfactants can therefore have antibacterial action but will also damage mammalian cells.

Bacteria have much higher internal osmotic pressure than mammalian cells, and they require a **rigid outer cell wall**, external to the cell membrane, to prevent osmotic rupture in the isotonic medium of mammalian blood and tissues. These cell walls also maintain the shape of the bacteria. Mammalian cells do not have such cell walls.

During bacterial cell growth and division, the original cell wall must also enlarge and form a new septum between the two daughter cells so that, when they separate, each has a complete outer wall. This requires the synthesis of new wall material. Inhibitors of bacterial cell wall biosynthesis will therefore render growing bacteria vulnerable to osmotic rupture, without affecting mammalian cells. Since cell wall biosynthesis is complex, inhibitors can act at different points in the sequence.

MECHANISMS OF ACTION

The process of cell wall formation begins with conversion of L-alanine into D-alanine. Two D-alanine molecules are then linked together. **Cycloserine** competitively inhibits the conversion of L-alanine into its D-form and the linking of the two D-molecules. Since the D-ala-D-ala unit is needed for the synthesis of all bacterial cell walls, cycloserine is effective against Gram-positive and Gram-negative bacteria alike, as well as the tubercle bacillus. However, other antibiotics are superior in treating infections caused by most organisms, and cycloserine is used mainly against the tubercle bacillus.

The next step in cell wall synthesis is the linkage of the D-ala dipeptide to three other amino acids and an amino sugar, N-acetylmuramic acid, to form a sugar-pentapeptide. This in turn is coupled to a molecule of another amino sugar, N-acetylglucosamine (Fig. 53–1). The whole sugar-peptide structure, linked to a lipid carrier molecule, isoprenyl phosphate, is then transported from the cytoplasm to the exterior of the cell membrane, where the sugar-peptide unit is added on to the lengthening polymer chains (peptidoglycan strands) from which the new cell wall is being built. **Bacitracin** interferes with this process by binding to the isoprenyl phosphate to form an unusable complex inside the bacterial cell. **Vancomycin** prevents the transfer of the sugar-pentapeptide from the carrier molecule to the growing polymer chain on the outside of the cell membrane.

The terminal event in cell wall synthesis is a cross-linking of the peptidoglycan strands by connecting a D-ala of a sugar-peptide in one strand to a diaminopimelic acid unit in a sugar-peptide of an adjacent strand (Fig. 53–2). This is a transpeptidation reaction, which is catalysed by various enzymes that differ in different bacterial species. **Penicillins** and **cephalosporins** bind to the active site of the enzyme (in susceptible species) and prevent the formation of the cross-links.

This chapter contains portions of Chapter 52 in the 4th edition by C. Prober.

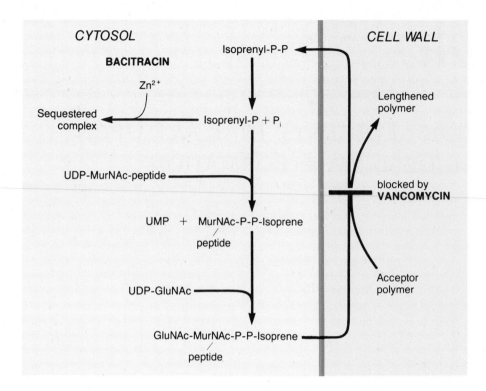

Figure 53-1 Sites of action of bacitracin and vancomycin as inhibitors of cell wall synthesis. UDP=uridine diphosphate; UMP=uridine monophosphate; MurNAc= N-acetylmuramic acid; GluNAc=N-acetylglucosamine.

These agents contain a **beta-lactam ring** that is chemically reactive because of ring strain (*i.e.*, the normal bond angle is 109°–120° but is forced by the ring to be 90°). The specificity of penicillins and cephalosporins for the transpeptidase involved in cell wall synthesis is due to the similarity of the antibiotic's three-dimensional structure to that of D-alanylalanine, which is the site on the peptidoglycan strand to which these enzymes bind. These transpeptidases are actually part of a group of proteins in bacterial cell walls called **penicillin-binding proteins** (PBPs), which have a high affinity for penicillins and cephalosporins. The degree to which the binding of beta-lactams to other penicillin-binding proteins contributes to their antibacterial activity is unknown, but is probably very important for the action against Gram-negative organisms. One such penicillin-binding protein cross-links lipoprotein to peptidoglycan in the wall of Gram-negative bacilli.

PENICILLINS

The penicillins are the most diverse of the antimicrobial agents. They are probably the most important group of antibiotics used for the treatment of infection. In 1928 Alexander Fleming fortuitously isolated penicillin from a sample of the mold *Penicillium notatum*, which was growing in his laboratory. However, it was not introduced into clinical medicine until 1941, when Florey, Chain, and associates devised suitable methods for large-scale culture of the mold and extraction of the penicillin. Since its original production, extensive chemical manipulation of the natural product has been carried out, resulting in a large number of natural and semisynthetic congeners with diverse pharmacokinetic characteristics and altered spectra of activity.

Chemistry

The basic structure of penicillin consists of a nucleus (6-aminopenicillanic acid, 6-APA) and side chains (acyl groups in amide linkage with 6-APA). The 6-APA nucleus has a thiazolidine ring connected to a beta-lactam ring (Fig. 53–3). In the natural penicillin, penicillin G, the R group is benzyl; the semisynthetic penicillins are synthesized by substituting other R groups for the benzyl group (Fig. 53–4).

The chemical reactivity of the beta-lactam ring, which confers antibacterial activity, is also responsible for **instability in an acid medium** (Fig. 53–5). The R group has a major effect on acid stability; an electron-withdrawing atom close to the beta-lactam, such as the oxygen in penicillin V or the nitrogen in ampicillin, con-

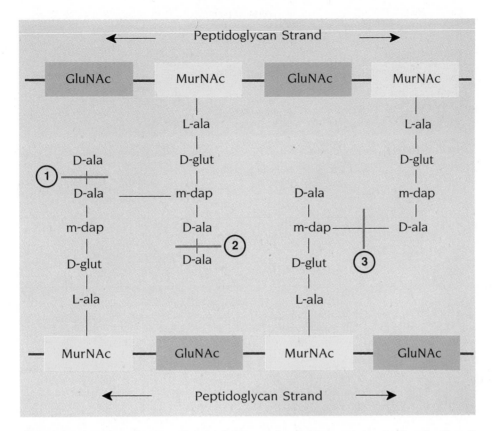

Figure 53–2 Sites of action of cross-linking and unlinking enzymes in *E. coli* cell wall synthesis. (1) Transpeptidase cleaves terminal D-ala and connects remaining D-ala to m-dap in peptide side chain on adjacent peptidoglycan strand. (2) Carboxypeptidase cleaves terminal D-ala from side chain of second strand, preventing further cross-linkage at that site. (3) Endopeptidase splits cross-link, providing site for transverse wall formation before divided bacteria separate. D-ala = D-alanine; L-ala = L-alanine; D-glut = D-glutamate; m-dap = m-diaminopimelate; GluNAc = N-acetylglucosamine; MurNAc = N-acetylmuramic acid.

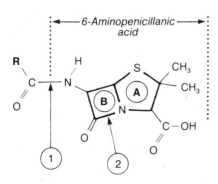

Figure 53–3 Structure of penicillin nucleus: *A* = thiazolidine ring; *B* = beta-lactam ring. Sites of penicillinase action: (1) = amidase; (2) = beta-lactamase.

fers relative acid stability. Cloxacillin and dicloxacillin are also relatively resistant to acid hydrolysis because of the electron-withdrawing effect of the heterocyclic ring.

The R group also controls the susceptibility to the **penicillinases**, produced by most *Staphylococcus aureus* and some other bacteria, which hydrolyse the beta-lactam ring and inactivate penicillins, causing the microorganisms to be resistant to the action of the antibiotics. Large bulky groups, such as those found in methicillin, prevent binding and, therefore, inactivation by these enzymes. Other penicillins that are resistant to penicillinase are oxacillin, cloxacillin, dicloxacillin, nafcillin, carbenicillin, and ticarcillin. Unfortunately, these bulky groups decrease binding to the transpeptidases and other penicillin-binding proteins that are responsible for the activity of penicillins; and, in general,

R SIDE CHAIN	CHEMICAL NAME	NONPROPRIETARY NAME
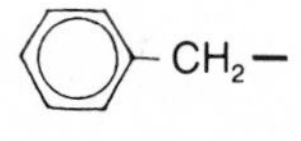 ⬡—CH₂—	Benzyl penicillin	Penicillin G
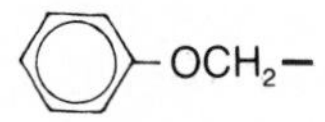 ⬡—OCH₂—	Phenoxymethyl penicillin	Penicillin V
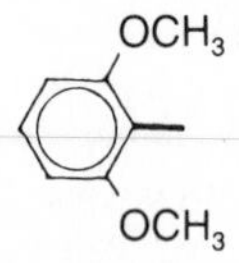 OCH₃ / OCH₃ phenyl	Dimethoxyphenyl penicillin	Methicillin
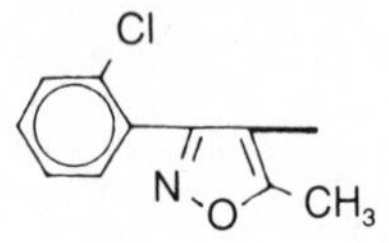 Cl isoxazolyl, CH₃	5-Methyl-3-*o*-chloro-phenyl-4-isoxazolyl penicillin	Cloxacillin
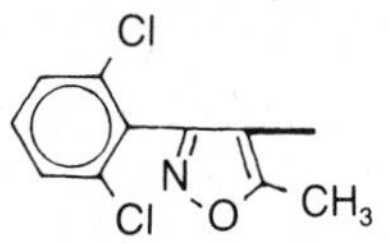 Cl / Cl isoxazolyl, CH₃	5-Methyl-3-(2,6-dichloro-phenyl)-4-isoxazolyl penicillin	Dicloxacillin
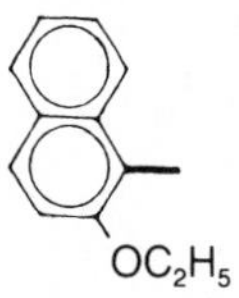 naphthyl OC₂H₅	2-Ethoxy-1-naphthyl penicillin	Nafcillin
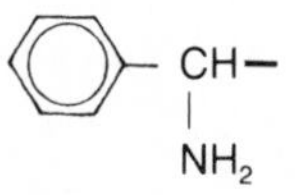 ⬡—CH—NH₂	α-Aminobenzyl penicillin	Ampicillin
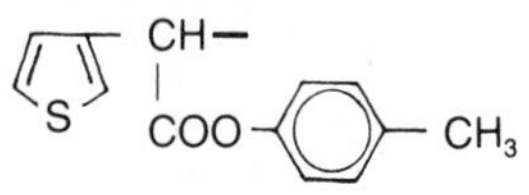 thienyl CH—COO—⬡—CH₃	α-*p*-Cresylcarbonyl-3-thienylmethyl penicillin	Ticarcillin
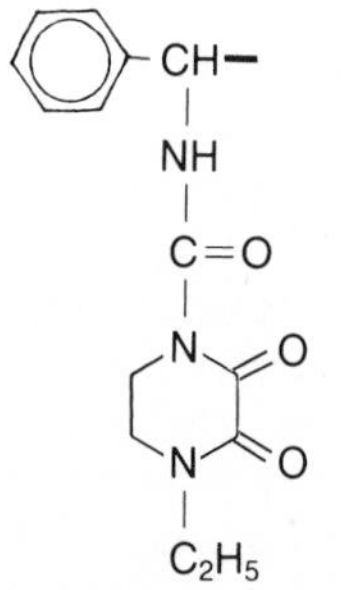 ⬡—CH—NH—C=O—piperazinedione—C₂H₅	α-[(4-Ethyl-2,3-dioxo-1-piperazinyl)-carbonyl-amino] benzyl penicillin	Piperacillin

Figure 53–4 Chemical structures of R side chains and names of various penicillins.

penicillinase-resistant penicillins are less active than penicillin G against organisms that do not produce penicillinase (see Fig. 53–4 and Table 53–1).

While most of the clinically significant microbial resistance to beta-lactam antibiotics is due to bacterial beta-lactamase activity, a new type of nonenzymatic penicillin resistance has been described in which one or more of the penicillin-binding proteins in the bacterial cell membrane are changed by mutation, rendering them less sensitive targets for penicillins. These resistant bacteria require several thousand-fold increases in MIC values for the beta-lactam antibiotics, and the newly resistant bacteria emerge as a significant fraction of the respective pathogenic flora.

Penicillin can also be reacted, via its free carboxyl group, with amines such as **procaine** and **benzathine** to form salts that have a low solubility. These salts are given by intramuscular injection and slowly release penicillin to provide a sustained level of antibiotic. Benzathine penicillin provides therapeutic levels for almost one month and measurable levels for about three months.

Bacterial Susceptibility

The penicillins can be divided into 3 groups based upon their antibacterial spectra. These groups are: narrow spectrum, beta-lactamase sensitive; broad spectrum, beta-lactamase sensitive; and beta-lactamase resistant.

The antibacterial activity of penicillins representative of each of these groups is outlined in Table 53–1. The attainable serum concentrations of these antibiotics that can be related to the MICs are discussed below.

Narrow-Spectrum, Beta-Lactamase Sensitive Penicillins

Penicillin G is the prototype of this group. The oral formulation representing this group is phenoxymethyl penicillin (**penicillin V**). As outlined in Table 53–1, penicillin G is very active against the majority of Gram-positive bacteria with the exception of penicillinase-producing S. aureus. Unfortunately the majority of S. aureus strains encountered in clinical practice are penicillinase producers. Penicillin G is also very active against Neisseria species and the Gram-negative anaerobes with the exception of Bacteroides fragilis. However, this antibiotic is not active against enteric Gram-negative organisms such as Escherichia coli, and hence the designation of narrow-spectrum.

The basis for the lack of activity of penicillin G against Gram-negative enteric organisms lies in the nature of the cell wall. Although Gram-negative organisms also have a cell wall composed of peptidoglycan and its synthetic enzymes, these organisms are surrounded by an additional membrane of lipopolysaccharide and a capsule, which are relatively impermeable to penicil-

lin. Furthermore, Gram-negative organisms have beta-lactamases in the membrane that contribute to the failure of penicillin to reach its site of action.

Broad-Spectrum, Beta-Lactamase Sensitive Penicillins

Modification of the R group (e.g., adding an amino group to make **ampicillin** and **amoxicillin**) leads to activity against some enteric Gram-negative organisms. As described earlier, this also increases stability to acid and does not significantly decrease activity against Gram-positive organisms, nor does it prevent hydrolysis by penicillinases. These agents also have increased activity against Group D streptococcus and Haemophilus species, although the emergence of penicillinase-producing Haemophilus species has made these agents inappropriate as the sole therapy for severe infections due to this organism.

Adding a carboxyl group (i.e., **carbenicillin** and **ticarcillin**) markedly increases activity against Pseudomonas but decreases activity against Gram-positive organisms. The newer ureidopenicillins (azlocillin, mezlocillin, and piperacillin) have even greater activity against Pseudomonas and other Gram-negative organisms and also have significant activity against Klebsiella.

Beta-Lactamase Resistant Penicillins

Cloxacillin is the representative of this group (Table 53–1). Other members include methicillin, oxacillin, nafcillin, and dicloxacillin. The principal bacteriologic advantage of this group of antibiotics is their high degree of activity against the penicillinase-producing staphylococci. They are, however, much less active than penicillin G against the other Gram-positive bacteria and are totally inactive against Gram-negative enteric organisms.

Pharmacokinetics

The degree of absorption of the various penicillin preparations from the gastrointestinal tract is variable and most dependent on their relative susceptibility to acid hydrolysis in the stomach (see Fig. 53–5). Penicillin V, ampicillin, cloxacillin, dicloxacillin, and oxacillin, which are quite acid-stable, are well absorbed. Penicillin G, methicillin, nafcillin, carbenicillin, ticarcillin, and piperacillin are more acid-labile and hence are poorly absorbed. These latter penicillins are, therefore, preferably administered parenterally. By this route these penicillins are rapidly and completely absorbed. Serum concentrations of the penicillins after representative doses are outlined in Table 53–2.

The volumes of distribution for the penicillins range from 0.1 to 0.3 L/kg. Their degree of protein binding is quite variable, as noted in Table 53–2. The penicillins spread widely throughout the body and enter all

TABLE 53-1   Median MICs (in μg/mL) of Some Penicillins

Bacteria	Penicillin G	Cloxacillin	Ampicillin	Ticarcillin	Piperacillin
Gram-positive					
Staphylococcus aureus, Penicillinase (−)	0.03	0.25	0.05	1.25	0.8
Staphylococcus aureus, Penicillinase (+)	25−>800	0.5	125.0	25.0	25.0
Streptococcus Group A	0.007	0.1	0.05	0.5	0.05
Streptococcus viridans	0.01	—	0.012	0.2	1.2
Streptococcus faecalis	2.0	25.0	0.38	34.0	4.0
Streptococcus pneumoniae	0.015	0.5	0.05	0.25	0.05
Listeria	0.1	—	0.1	2.5	1.25
Clostridium	0.06	—	0.05	0.5	—
Gram-negative					
Neisseria meningitidis	0.05	0.5	0.02	0.1	0.05
Neisseria gonorrhoeae	0.06	1.0	0.125	0.1	0.05
Haemophilus influenzae	0.16	—	0.05	0.5	0.25
Salmonella sp.	5.0	>250	2.0	4.0	4.0
Shigella	16.0	>250	6.0	—	—
Klebsiella	50.0	>250	50.0	50.0	4.0
Escherichia coli	64.0	>250	5.0	5.0	2.0
Pseudomonas aeruginosa	>400	>250	>400	25.0	10.0
Proteus mirabilis	32.0	>250	1.25	1.25	1.25
Bacteroides fragilis	32.0	—	25.0	37.5	—
Other Bacteroides	0.12	—	6.2	2.0	—

body fluids. Concentrations in brain and cerebrospinal fluid (CSF), however, vary depending upon the specific penicillin under consideration and on the degree of meningeal inflammation present at the time of dosing. The approximate concentrations attained in the CSF during treatment for meningitis are 25–30% of serum concentrations with penicillin G, ampicillin, carbenicillin, and ticarcillin. Methicillin, oxacillin, cloxacillin, and nafcillin, however, penetrate the CSF poorly.

The penicillins are not significantly biotransformed but are, rather, administered, distributed, and excreted in a biologically active form. Free penicillins are rapidly eliminated in the urine, with serum half-lives of less than 1 hour. They are mainly excreted by glomerular filtration and renal tubular secretion but also appear to lesser degrees in the bile. Renal tubular secretion takes place through the organic anion transport system and can be blocked, and the action of the penicillins prolonged, by probenecid. Probenecid may also increase serum concentrations by blocking distribution into tissues. In theory at least, therapeutic efficacy might be compromised by this action.

Adverse Reactions

Penicillins are of very low toxicity. Their specificity of action as antibiotics is such that they have little effect on mammalian cells. However, all penicillins have the potential to cause hypersensitivity reactions, neurotoxicity, nephrotoxicity, and hematologic toxicity.

Hypersensitivity reactions are the major type of toxicity seen with penicillin, and occur in about 5% of patients. The most serious of these occur immediately after exposure (in less than 30 minutes) and are mediated by IgE (anaphylaxis). The incidence of anaphylaxis is about 0.01% of treatment courses. The mechanism of these reactions also involves the chemical reactivity of the beta-lactam ring. Penicillins are the classic example of haptens (i.e., small molecules that are not immunogenic but bind to larger molecules, making them immunogenic) and react with the ε-amino group of lysine in proteins to make them immunogenic (see Fig. 53–5). This is the so-called major determinant because it is the major reaction that occurs, which can lead to a hypersensitivity reaction. There are also minor determinants composed mainly of penicilloic and penilloic acids. Although these determinants are quantitatively minor and are less commonly responsible for hypersensitivity reactions, a high percentage of the life-threatening immediate hypersensitivity reactions (i.e., anaphylaxis) are due to the minor determinants.

Accelerated reactions (occurring within 1–48 hours) are usually manifested by rash and sometimes fever. Delayed reactions (beginning more than 48 hours after exposure) can consist of skin reactions or other systemic reactions such as nephritis or serum sickness. In addition to these reactions, ampicillin and amoxicillin are commonly associated with a characteristic nonurticarial maculopapular rash. The mechanism of this rash is not understood, but it is not an "allergic reaction." It usually starts 3–4 days after the onset of therapy. For reasons not understood, this reaction is much more frequent in patients with viral infections, especially mononucleosis, or when penicillin is taken together with allopurinol.

In deciding on therapy for a patient with a history of "**penicillin allergy**" several facts should be kept in mind. The vast majority of patients who have been labelled as having a penicillin allergy will not have a reaction if given penicillin. This can be because that patient was never allergic to penicillin and the adverse event was due to some other factor. Examples of such factors include a viral infection for which antibiotic was inappropriately prescribed, causing a rash; some other drug or allergen to which the patient was exposed at the same time; or, in cases that had occurred many years before, it may have been due to impurities in earlier preparations of penicillin. Other patients may have had a nonallergic reaction such as an ampicillin rash. The other possibility is that the patient did have an allergic reaction to a penicillin but has lost the sensitivity to penicillin. Most patients who have had an allergic reaction to penicillin will lose their sensitivity after a period of about two years. Despite this fact, **the possible consequences make a past history of a severe reaction to a penicillin a contraindication to its use unless skin testing (which includes the minor determinant) indicates that the patient is not allergic to penicillin.** Alternatively, if the infection is life-threatening and can be adequately treated only with a penicillin (*e.g.*, bacterial endocarditis), a program of **desensitization** is indicated. Unfortunately, there is not a good correlation between the nature of the penicillin reaction history and the probability of a severe adverse reaction on re-exposure; therefore, most physicians would **elect to use an alternative antibiotic** irrespective of the nature of the past history of penicillin allergy. Although adequate skin testing would solve most of these problems, the minor determinant is unstable and is not commercially available; therefore, penicillin skin testing that includes the minor determinants is, at present, available in only a few centres.

Convulsions and other forms of **encephalopathy** may occur when extremely high doses of a penicillin have been prescribed. These reactions are more likely to occur in patients with renal insufficiency, a condition that predisposes to high serum concentrations of the penicillin. In addition, renal failure can lead to the accumulation of organic anions, which, like probenecid, inhibit the active anion transport system that pumps penicillin out of the CSF. These reactions are most closely related to the concentration of the penicillin in the CSF and have occurred more frequently in patients with meningeal inflammation or those who have received the drug by the intrathecal route.

Interstitial nephritis can occur during the course of therapy with any penicillin, although it is most frequently associated with the administration of methicillin. Hypokalemia may be a side effect of high-dose penicillin therapy because the penicillins act as nonreabsorbable anions.

Coombs test-positive **hemolytic anemia** may occur with excessive doses, or on an allergic basis, with any of the penicillins. **Neutropenia**, which is reversible upon discontinuing the drug, is also seen in some patients, especially those receiving methicillin, nafcillin, or cloxacillin. **Decreased platelet aggregation** has been noted at high concentrations of most penicillins, but has been most marked with carbenicillin and ticarcillin. This may predispose to bleeding diathesis.

Drug Interactions

High concentrations of penicillins bind to and inactivate aminoglycoside antibiotics (*see* Chapter 55) *in vitro* and *in vivo*. Therefore, penicillins and aminoglycosides should not be mixed in intravenous infusions, and when administered to the same patient their infusions should be separated in time.

TABLE 53–2 Serum Concentrations and Protein Binding of Different Penicillins

Agent	Dosage (mg and Route)		Serum Concentration (μg/mL)	Protein Bound (%)
Ampicillin	1000	i.v.	40	20
	500	p.o.	4–6	—
Cloxacillin	500	p.o.	8	95
Dicloxacillin	250	p.o.	8	95
Methicillin	1000	i.v.	20–40	35–40
Nafcillin	15/kg	i.v.	20–40	90–95
Oxacillin	1000	i.v.	40	90
	500	p.o.	4	—
Penicillin G	~670	i.v.	10	65
	500	p.o.	2	—
Penicillin G Procaine	800	i.m.	3	—
Penicillin G Benzathine	800	i.m.	0.1	—
Penicillin V	250	p.o.	2–3	80
Carbenicillin	5000	i.v.	200–300	50
Ticarcillin	3000	i.v.	150–200	50

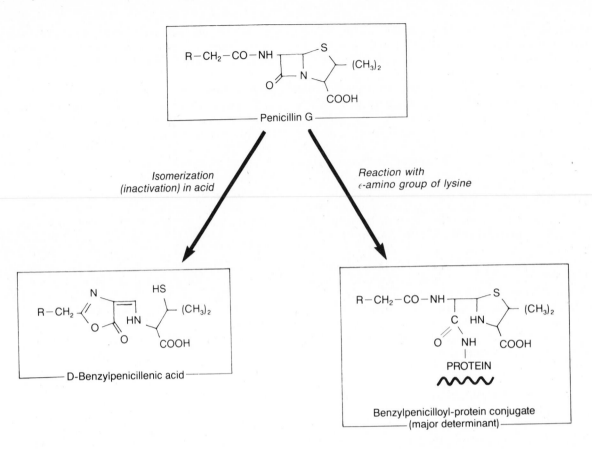

Figure 53–5 Inactivation of penicillin by acid, and reaction with protein to form the major determinant causing penicillin hypersensitivity reactions.

Penicillins and bacteriostatic drugs are often antagonistic *in vitro*, especially if the bacteria are exposed to the bacteriostatic agents first. The only *in vivo* example of this antagonism is the poorer outcome of *Streptococcus pneumoniae* meningitis treated with both penicillin and tetracycline than if treated with penicillin alone.

Probenecid, indomethacin, sulfinpyrazone, and high-dose aspirin (> 3 g/day) can block the tubular secretion of penicillins and may lead to prolonged high serum levels. Probenecid may also block the active transport of penicillin out of the CSF and thereby potentially lead to neurotoxicity.

Dosage Regimens and Routes of Administration

Penicillins may be administered by the oral, intramuscular, or intravenous route depending on the specific agent and the therapeutic indication. The dosages and regimens are dependent upon the specific agent, the infecting pathogen, and the seriousness and site of infection. The approximate daily dose of the penicillins that can be administered orally (penicillin V, ampicillin, cloxacillin, and oxacillin) ranges from 20 to 30 mg/kg. This amount is usually divided into four equal doses. The approximate daily dose of the penicillins that can be administered intravenously or intramuscularly (as in the treatment of serious infections requiring high blood levels of the antibiotic) is between 50 and 200 mg/kg for ampicillin, cloxacillin, methicillin, nafcillin, and oxacillin; 300 mg/kg for ticarcillin; 400–500 mg/kg for carbenicillin; and 100,000–200,000 IU/kg for aqueous benzyl penicillin G. (Penicillin G is prescribed in international units, 1 unit being equivalent to 0.6 μg). The parenteral penicillins are usually administered in 4–6 equal doses per day. The longer acting penicillin G preparations (procaine and benzathine) are administered as a single daily dose or as a single weekly to monthly dose respectively. The approximate unit dose for these penicillins is 1.2 million units.

It must be emphasized that those are only broad guidelines. Considerable variation is observed between clinicians and institutions, even for similar indications.

Therapeutic Applications

The penicillins belong to perhaps the most frequently prescribed class of antimicrobial agents.

Penicillins G and V are used for a variety of mild to severe infections proved or presumed to be caused by sensitive organisms. Examples of mild infections for which oral penicillin V would be indicated include pharyngitis, and skin and soft tissue infections, caused by Group A streptococcus. Moderate to severe infections treated with parenteral penicillin G include streptococcal pneumonia, meningitis caused by *S. pneumoniae* and *Neisseria meningitidis*, gonorrhea, and syphilis, to name a few.

Ampicillin is used to treat mild to severe Gram-negative urinary tract infections and meningitis caused by non-beta-lactamase-producing *Haemophilus influenzae*.

Carbenicillin and ticarcillin are used almost exclusively for *Pseudomonas* infections of the urinary tract, lung, and blood.

Cloxacillin, oxacillin, nafcillin, and methicillin are used almost exclusively for infections caused by staphylococci, including skin and soft tissue infections, pneumonia, osteomyelitis, endocarditis, and septicemia.

CEPHALOSPORINS

Cephalosporium acremonium, the first source of the cephalosporins, was isolated from the sea near a sewer outlet off the Sardinian coast. Crude filtrates from cultures of this fungus inhibited the growth of *S. aureus in vitro* and cured staphylococcal infections in man.

Since the original isolation of *Cephalosporium acremonium* and the identification of its active product, cephalosporin C, many semisynthetic derivatives and structurally related analogs have been developed. The newer derivatives possess an increasing spectrum of activity and diverse pharmacokinetic characteristics.

Chemistry

The nucleus of cephalosporin C (7-aminocephalosporanic acid, Fig. 53–6), which formed the basis for all early cephalosporins, is closely related but not identical to the penicillin nucleus, 6-aminopenicillanic acid. Analogous to that of penicillin, the chemical reactivity

of the beta-lactam ring is responsible for the antibacterial activity, acid instability, susceptibility to beta-lactamase hydrolysis, and the hypersensitivity reactions of the cephalosporins. The diversity of the cephalosporins is based on the R_1 and R_2 substituents placed on the parent structure (*see* Fig. 53–6). As with penicillin, the presence of electron-withdrawing substituents on R_1 near the ring leads to relative acid stability.

Bacterial Susceptibility

The evolution of cephalosporins and diversity of their properties has led to their division into three "generations." The original agents are referred to as first generation cephalosporins, and the most recently introduced are referred to as third generation cephalosporins. A list of representative cephalosporins from each generation is provided in Table 53–3. For the purpose of brevity the details of only one or two agents from each generation will be discussed, unless significant differences exist for other members. The antibacterial activity of cephalosporins representative of each of the three generations is outlined in Table 53–4. The attainable serum concentrations of these antibiotics that can be related to the MICs are discussed below.

In general, the spectrum of activity increases with each new generation of cephalosporins. This is primarily attributable to increasing stability to a wide range of bacterial beta-lactamases.

First Generation Cephalosporins

The prototype of this group of cephalosporins is **cephalothin**, which is not readily absorbed from the gastrointestinal tract. The acid-stable orally administered representative of this group is **cephalexin**. As outlined in Table 53–4, this antibiotic is very active against all staphylococci, pneumococci, and all streptococci except enterococci. Activity against aerobic and anaerobic Gram-negative organisms is limited, whereas it is ac-

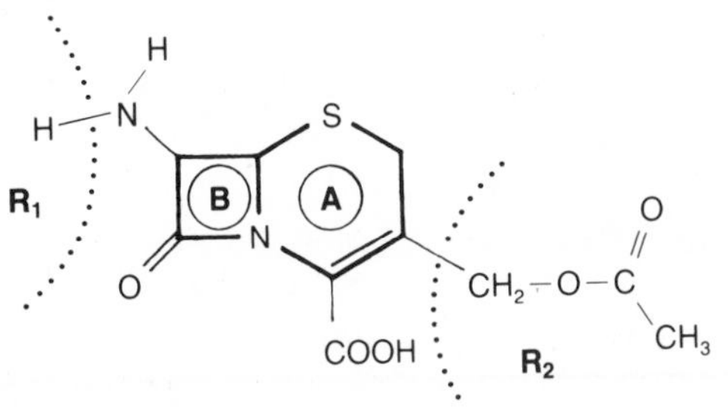

Figure 53–6 Structure of 7-aminocephalosporanic acid, the parent structure of cephalosporins, which are made by substitutions at R_1 and R_2. A = dihydrothiazine ring; B = beta-lactam ring.

CHEMOTHERAPY

TABLE 53–3 Generations of Cephalosporins

	First	Second	Third
Compounds for parenteral use	Cephalothin Cefazolin Cephaloridine Cephapirin Cephradine	Cefamandole Cefoxitin Cefuroxime	Cefotaxime Moxalactam Cefoperazone Ceftazidime Cefsulodin Ceftizoxime Ceftriaxone
Compounds for oral use	Cephalexin Cephaloglycin Cephradine Cefadroxil	Cefaclor Cefatrizine	

TABLE 53–4 Median MICs (in μg/mL) of Some Cephalosporins

Bacteria	Cephalothin	Cefamandole	Cefoxitin	Cefotaxime
Gram-positive				
Staphylococcus aureus, Penicillinase (−)	0.2	0.25	3.1	2.0
Staphylococcus aureus, Penicillinase (+)	0.4	0.5	3.1	2.0
Streptococcus Group A	0.1	0.06	0.4	0.01
Streptococcus viridans	—	0.5	1.6	0.125
Streptococcus faecalis	50.0	32.0	100.0	>128
Streptococcus pneumoniae	0.1	0.25	3.12	0.03
Listeria	4.0	6.0	25.0	25.0
Clostridium	0.4	0.12	1.0	0.25
Gram-negative				
Neisseria meningitidis	0.5	<0.125	0.12	0.004
Neisseria gonorrhoeae	3.1	<0.125	0.12	0.015
Haemophilus influenzae	6.3	0.5	8.0	0.03
Salmonella sp.	2.0	1.0	2.0	0.25
Shigella	125.0	2.0	25.0	0.25
Klebsiella	10.0	1.0	12.5	0.25
Escherichia coli	20.0	0.5	8.0	0.25
Pseudomonas aeruginosa	>200	>125	>400	16.0
Proteus mirabilis	10.0	1.0	6.3	0.1
Bacteroides fragilis	<25	64.0	16.0	8.0
Other Bacteroides	12.5	1.0	1.0	—

tive against *Clostridia* species and many of the other Gram-positive anaerobes. **Cefazolin**, another member of this generation, has somewhat more activity against aerobic Gram-negatives, especially against *E. coli* and *Klebsiella* species.

Second Generation Cephalosporins

Cefamandole and **cefoxitin** are two representative members of this group. Their Gram-positive spectrum is similar to that of the first generation cephalosporins, but they possess increased anti-Gram-negative activity. They are, however, inactive against *Pseudomonas* species. The principal advantage of cefamandole is its activity against *H. influenzae*, whereas that of cefoxitin is its broadened activity against anaerobic organisms.

It should be noted that, strictly speaking, cefoxitin is not a cephalosporin derivative but rather a cephamycin, a fermentation product of *Streptomyces*. **Cefaclor** is the prototype oral preparation of this group. Its activity mirrors that of cefamandole.

Third Generation Cephalosporins

Cefotaxime represents this rapidly increasing group of antibiotics. This generation retains most of the anti-Gram-positive activity of the first two generations but possesses in addition a remarkable amount of anti-Gram-negative activity including activity against many isolates of *Pseudomonas*. This latter attribute is especially prominent in such agents as cefsulodin, ceftazidime, and cefoperazone.

Pharmacokinetics

Parenterally administered cephalosporins must be given by that route because they are poorly absorbed from the gastrointestinal tract. Those for oral administration, on the other hand, are almost completely absorbed, and serum concentrations are similar to those obtained after equivalent doses of the parenteral preparations. Serum concentrations of some of the cephalosporins after representative doses are outlined in Table 53–5.

The volumes of distribution for the cephalosporins range from 0.1 to 0.4 L/kg and their degree of plasma protein binding ranges from 17% to 90% (see Table 53–5). The cephalosporins distribute widely throughout the body. The first and second generation derivatives, however, do not penetrate well into the CSF even in the presence of meningitis and, hence, must never be used to treat this infection. At least three of the third generation cephalosporins (cefotaxime, moxalactam, and ceftriaxone) do penetrate into the CSF to a sufficient degree (10–30%) to be potentially useful in the treatment of meningitis.

In general, the cephalosporins are not extensively biotransformed, but are distributed and excreted principally in a biologically active form. The primary route of excretion for most of the cephalosporins is renal (60–100%), although there are exceptions. For instance, cefoperazone, a third generation agent, is primarily excreted in the bile with only 20% appearing in the urine. Both glomerular filtration and tubular secretion are involved in the excretion of cephalosporins, although with some (e.g., cephaloridine, ceftriaxone, ceftazidime, and moxalactam) the amount of drug undergoing tubular secretion is negligible.

The elimination half-lives of the cephalosporins range from 0.5 to 8 hours depending on the specific agent, as noted in Table 53–5.

Adverse Reactions

As with most antibiotics, the full spectrum of **hypersensitivity reactions** including rash, hives, fever, eosinophilia, serum sickness, and anaphylaxis may occur. It is estimated that primary allergic reactions to the cephalosporins are seen in approximately 5% of cases. Reversible neutropenia and thrombocytopenia, both of which may have an allergic basis, have been observed occasionally.

The incidence of allergic reactions to the cephalosporins is increased in patients known to be allergic to penicillins. The precise frequency of such cross-reactions is, however, unclear; the estimated range has varied from 5% to 16%. Whether or not these reactions are due to cross-sensitivity is unknown because the sensitivity to penicillin was not confirmed by skin testing and, in addition, it may be that patients with a sensitivity to penicillin have a higher incidence of reactivity to immunologically unrelated drugs. It is generally held, however, that **all cephalosporins probably should be avoided in patients with a clear past history of anaphylaxis or immediate-type hypersensitivity to any of the penicillins**. It is reasonable, on the other hand, to consider their use in patients with a less severe type of reaction to the penicillins.

Adverse reactions related to the **route of administration** are also common with the cephalosporins. These reactions include pain with intramuscular injection, phlebitis with intravenous administration, and minor gastrointestinal complaints with oral preparations.

Therapy with the cephalosporins may lead to the development of a positive direct Coombs reaction, although it is not commonly associated with hemolytic anemia. The incidence of positive Coombs test is approximately 3%.

Some of the cephalosporins (e.g., cephaloridine) have been withdrawn from use because of **dose-related**

TABLE 53–5 Serum Concentrations, Half-Lives, and Protein Binding of Different Cephalosporins

Drug	Dosage (mg and Route)		Serum Concentration (μg/mL)	Protein Bound (%)	Half-Life (h)
Cephalothin	1000	i.v.	40–60	60–70	0.5
Cefazolin	1000	i.v.	90–120	85	1.5
Cephalexin	500	p.o.	15–20	low	0.5–1.0
Cefoxitin	1000	i.v.	60–80	70	1.0
Cefamandole	1000	i.v.	60–80	70	1.0
Cefaclor	200	p.o.	6	—	0.5
Cefotaxime	1000	i.v.	41	40	1.1
Cefriaxone	1000	i.v.	145	90	8.0
Cefoperazone	1000	i.v.	125	90	2.0
Moxalactam	1000	i.v.	70	43	2.3
Ceftazidime	1000	i.v.	83	17	1.8

CHEMOTHERAPY

nephrotoxicity, probably resulting from proximal tubular damage. Interstitial nephritis has been described with some of the other cephalosporins (*e.g.,* cephalothin), but this is rare. Although it has been suggested that some of the cephalosporins (*e.g.,* cephalothin) may enhance the nephrotoxicity of the aminoglycoside antibiotics, the evidence is not conclusive.

The third generation cephalosporins have also been associated with transient elevations of aspartate aminotransferase and alanine aminotransferase levels, reversible elevation of the blood urea nitrogen, and disturbances of vitamin K-dependent clotting function. This latter reaction is seen with cefamandole, moxalactam, and cefoperazone, which contain a methylthiotetrazole ring. This ring can be cleaved from the drug and inhibit vitamin K metabolism. This same structure also inhibits aldehyde dehydrogenase and can lead to a disulfiram-like reaction when the patient drinks alcohol (*see* Chapter 25).

Drug Interactions

As noted above, it is possible that some of the cephalosporins (*e.g.,* cephalothin) may enhance the nephrotoxicity of the aminoglycosides.

Cephalosporins may produce a "false-positive" glycosuric reaction with the Clinitest®.

Uricosurics such as probenecid may decrease the clearance of some cephalosporins by blocking renal tubular secretion.

Dosage Regimens and Routes of Administration

Cephalosporins may be administered by the oral, intramuscular, or intravenous route, depending on the specific agent and the therapeutic indications (*see* Table 53–3). In general, however, the intramuscular route is avoided, as these agents tend to cause pain upon injection. The approximate daily dose of the cephalosporins that can be administered orally ranges from 25 to 50 mg/kg. This amount is usually divided into four equal doses except for cefadroxil, which is divided into two doses. The approximate daily dose of the cephalosporins that are administered intravenously is 50–200 mg/kg. This amount is usually divided into 2–6 equal doses depending on the half-life of the individual agents (*see* Table 53–5). Agents with the longest half-lives (*e.g.,* ceftriaxone) may be administered every 24 hours whereas those with short half-lives (*e.g.,* cephalothin) must usually be administered every 4–6 hours.

As emphasized with the penicillins, these are only broad dosing guidelines, and considerable variation between clinicians is common.

Therapeutic Applications

The therapeutic applications of the cephalosporins are different for each of the three generations and, therefore, each will be considered separately.

First generation cephalosporins are rarely the antibiotics of first choice; however, they are useful for infections caused by penicillin-resistant staphylococci, *Klebsiella* species, and urinary tract infections resistant to penicillins and sulfonamides. This group of antibiotics is also useful for short-term perioperative prophylaxis for selected operations carrying a high risk of infections caused by Gram-positive organisms, but where Gram-negative organisms cannot be ruled out. They may also be useful in patients with a history of minor penicillin allergy but should not be administered to patients who have had immediate or accelerated penicillin reactions.

The broadened spectrum of activity of **second generation cephalosporins** increases their range of potential therapeutic applications, though they also are rarely the antibiotic of first choice. The activity of cefamandole against Gram-positive cocci as well as against beta-lactamase-producing *H. influenzae* makes it a theoretically attractive agent for infectious disease entities that might be caused by one or more of these organisms. Unfortunately, treatment failures, especially when *H. influenzae* is the pathogen, have limited the usefulness of this antibiotic, especially to pediatricians.

Cefoxitin, with its effectiveness against anaerobic and Gram-negative organisms, is a potentially useful single agent for the treatment of pelvic infections or peritonitis. Short-term perioperative prophylaxis for pelvic or abdominal operations is also a potential use of this antibiotic.

The group of ultra-broad spectrum **third generation cephalosporins** is relatively new to clinical medicine. Their most important indication is in the treatment of meningitis caused by Gram-negative aerobes. Although they have not replaced aminoglycosides, the third generation cephalosporins can sometimes be used instead of the more toxic combination of a penicillin and an aminoglycoside. Their indications also include the treatment of hospital-acquired Gram-negative aerobic infections or those otherwise rendered resistant to multiple antibiotics, and some intra-abdominal infections. Further indications await the completion of a multitude of clinical trials.

OTHER BETA–LACTAM ANTIBIOTICS

Several new beta-lactam antibiotics have been, or are being, developed that are neither penicillins nor cephalosporins (Fig. 53–7). One example is **imipenem**, a derivative of thienamycin, which is more stable than

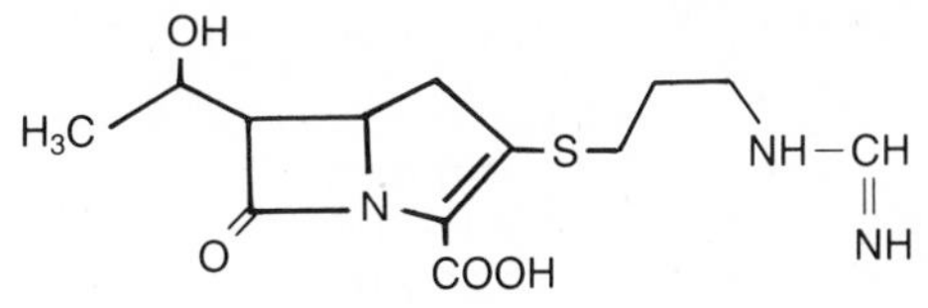

Figure 53–7 Structures of other beta-lactam antibiotics.

the parent drug. Imipenem has a very broad spectrum of activity including many strains of *Pseudomonas*, *Acinetobacter*, and anaerobic bacteria such as *B. fragilis*.

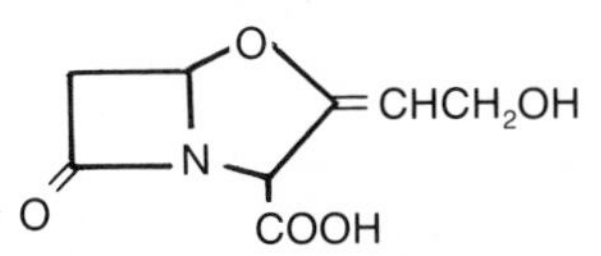

Another class of beta-lactams is the beta-lactamase inhibitors. They have poor antibacterial activity but are good "suicide" inhibitors of beta-lactamases. They are combined with penicillins to treat infections involving beta-lactamase-producing bacteria. Examples of such agents are **clavulanic acid** and **sulbactam.**

Clavulanic acid is a naturally occurring beta-lactam isolated from *Streptomyces clavuligerus*. Sulbactam is a semisynthetic penicillanic acid sulfone. Both compounds can be combined with beta-lactam antibiotics for the specific purpose of inhibiting many bacterial beta-lactamases and thereby extending the antibacterial spectrum of the respective antibiotics. Some current examples of combinations of a beta-lactam antibiotic with a beta-lactamase inhibitor are amoxicillin-clavulanic acid, ticarcillin-clavulanic acid, and ampicillin-sulbactam. In oral combination therapy, clavulanic acid and sulbactam have serum half-lives of about 1 hour, which is increased in neonates and the elderly. Excretion is primarily *via* the kidneys, but unlike that of the penicillins, it is unaffected by probenecid.

The combination of amoxicillin-clavulanic acid is useful in the oral treatment of otitis media, sinusitis, and infections of the lower respiratory tract and urinary tract caused by beta-lactamase-producing strains of pathogens. The combination of ticarcillin-clavulanic acid increases the activity of ticarcillin against beta-lactamase-producing strains of *S. aureus*, *H. influenzae*, *Neisseria gonorrhoeae*, *E. coli*, *Klebsiella*, and *B. fragilis*. The combination ampicillin-sulbactam has broad-spectrum activity in the treatment of infections caused by beta-lactamase-producing strains of *H. influenzae*, *Branhamella catarrhalis*, *Neisseria*, many anaerobes, *E. coli*, *Proteus*, *Klebsiella*, *S. aureus*, and *Staphylococcus epidermidis*.

VANCOMYCIN

Vancomycin was isolated from *Streptomyces orientalis*, an actinomycete found in soil samples from Indonesia and India. It was purified and characterized in 1956. The agent is not chemically related to any of the antimicrobial agents in present use. It is an unusual glycopeptide containing a chlorinated polyphenyl ether with a molecular weight of about 1500.

Bacterial Susceptibility

The primary activity of vancomycin is against Gram-positive bacteria. The vast majority of staphylococcal species including penicillinase-negative and -positive strains, and streptococcal species including enterococci, are killed by less than 1.6 μg/mL of this antibiotic. Gram-positive bacilli including *Clostridia* species are also very sensitive to vancomycin. Gram-negative bacteria are invariably resistant.

Pharmacokinetics

Vancomycin is not absorbed from the gastrointestinal tract. A single intravenous dose of 10 mg/kg in adults produces serum concentrations of 20–30 μg/mL at 1–2 hours after the infusion.

The volume of distribution of vancomycin is 0.5–0.9 L/kg. It is less than 10% protein-bound. It appears in various body fluids, and 20–30% is detectable in the cerebrospinal fluid when the meninges are inflamed.

Vancomycin is normally not biotransformed in the body. It is excreted by the kidneys, and about 80–90% of a dose can be recovered from the urine during the first 24 hours. Its serum half-life is 6–9 hours.

Adverse Reactions

Hearing loss has been associated with sustained high serum concentrations of vancomycin in excess of 60–80 μg/mL. Nephrotoxicity is rare at recommended doses. (The early reports of this complication may have been due to an impurity in the formulation.) A "red man" syndrome is manifested as flushing and a maculopapular rash on face, neck, trunk, and extremities during, or shortly after, intravenous administration. It is believed to be caused by histamine release and may lead to hypotension, tachycardia, shock, and cardiac arrest. This syndrome is most likely to occur if vancomycin is administered rapidly as an intravenous bolus; therefore, the dose should be infused over a period of 45–60 minutes.

CHEMOTHERAPY

Drug Interactions

Cholestyramine can bind vancomycin if the two drugs are administered together orally.

Dosage and Routes of Administration

Because vancomycin is not absorbed from the gastrointestinal tract, it should be administered orally only if high concentrations in the intestine are desired (*see below*). The recommended daily intravenous dose is 20–30 mg/kg divided into two or three doses.

Therapeutic Applications

The primary clinical use of vancomycin is in the treatment of severe staphylococcal and streptococcal (including enterococcal) infections in patients who are allergic to penicillin. In addition, some recently isolated multiply-resistant staphylococci and *S. pneumoniae* are sensitive only to this antibiotic.

Vancomycin is administered orally in the treatment of antibiotic-associated pseudomembranous colitis. This illness is caused by the toxin produced by *Clostridium difficile*.

BACITRACIN

This antibiotic, isolated from a strain of *Bacillus subtilis*, is a complex cyclic polypeptide composed of 11 amino acids, including one that contains a thiazole-type ring resembling that of penicillin, but no beta-lactam ring. As explained at the beginning of this chapter, it acts at a different point in the sequence of cell wall synthesis than do the beta-lactam antibiotics.

Bacitracin is poorly absorbed and its systemic use may damage mammalian cells. This is due to its property of complexing with lipids, including those that are essential constituents of mammalian plasma membranes. For these reasons its use is **restricted to topical application** in ointments and eye drops. It is active *in vitro* against staphylococci, streptococci, *H. influenzae*, *Corynebacterium*, *Neisseria*, and *Clostridium* species. All coliform bacilli, *Salmonella*, *Shigella*, *Proteus*, and *Pseudomonas* are resistant to this drug.

CYCLOSERINE

This antibiotic, D-4-amino-3-isoxazolidone, was derived from *Streptomyces orchidaeus* and *garyphalus* in 1955.

Bacterial Susceptibility

The most important activity of cycloserine is against strains of *Mycobacterium tuberculosis*, which are usually inhibited by 5–20 µg/mL. Strains of mycobacteria that become resistant to streptomycin, isoniazid, and para-aminosalicylic acid usually remain cycloserine-sensitive. *Mycobacterium kansasii* and *M. intracellulare* are often also sensitive to cycloserine.

Pharmacokinetics

When administered orally, cycloserine is rapidly absorbed from the stomach and small intestine. Peak serum concentrations are reached 3–4 hours after a single dose and are in the range of 20–25 µg/mL after a 500 mg dose.

The drug is highly diffusible and is distributed throughout body fluids and tissues. Cerebrospinal fluid concentrations approximate serum concentrations even in the absence of meningeal inflammation.

Approximately 35% of this antibiotic is biotransformed in the body, and about 50% of a dose is excreted unchanged in the urine in the first 12 hours. A total of 65% is recoverable over a period of 72 hours. Cycloserine has a serum half-life of 8–12 hours.

Adverse Reactions

The principal type of adverse reaction to cycloserine is neurologic. Psychoses, delirium, confusion, headache, convulsions, and tremor have all been reported. Neurotoxicity appears to be more frequent and severe at higher doses. While the antibacterial action of cycloserine depends upon its blockade of reactions involving L-alanine and D-alanine in cell wall synthesis, its neurotoxicity appears to result from competition with L-alanine for other enzymes, including transaminases required for synthesis of GABA in the brain. Pyridoxine, which functions as a cofactor in transamination reactions, may help to prevent these adverse effects. Drug interactions have not been reported.

Dosage and Route of Administration

Cycloserine is administered by the oral route at a daily dose of 10–15 mg/kg divided into two equal doses. The total dosage is limited by tolerance of the patient.

Therapeutic Applications

Cycloserine is a second-line agent used in the treatment of tuberculosis, and it may be used in the treatment of infections due to certain atypical mycobacteria. It may also be considered in the treatment of central nervous system *Nocardia* infections that are not responding to the standard sulfonamide treatment.

SUGGESTED READING

Allan JD, Eliopoulos GM, Moellering RC Jr. The expanding spectrum of beta-lactam antibiotics. In: Stollerman GH, ed. Advances in internal medicine. Chicago/London: Year Book Medical Publishers, 1986; 31:119–146.

Goldberg DM. The cephalosporins. Med Clin North Am 1987; 71:1113–1134.

Levine JF. Vancomycin: a review. Ibid. 1987; 71:1135–1146.

Neu HC. Beta-lactam antibiotics: structural relationships affecting *in vitro* activity and pharmacologic properties. Rev Infect Dis 1986; 8(Suppl 3):S237–S259.

Parry MF. The penicillins. Med Clin North Am 1987; 71:1093–1112.

Sykes RB, Bonner DP, Swabb EA. Modern beta-lactam antibiotics. Pharmacol Ther 1985; 29:321–352.

Thompson RL. Cephalosporin, carbapenem, and monobactam antibiotics. Mayo Clin Proc 1987; 62:821–834.

Tomasz A. Penicillin-binding proteins and the antibacterial effectiveness of beta-lactam antibiotics. Rev Infect Dis 1986; 8(Suppl 3):S260–S278.

CHEMOTHERAPY

Chapter 54

ANTIMICROBIAL AND ANTIFUNGAL AGENTS THAT ACT UPON CELL MEMBRANES

J. Uetrecht

MECHANISMS OF ACTION

Cytoplasmic membranes maintain the intracellular contents, both by controlling passive diffusion and by providing the mechanisms of active transport. Human and microbial cell membranes are similar in that they both possess lipid and protein structural elements. However, bacterial lipids are primarily phospholipids, and fungi contain sterols.

Polymyxins and **colistin** are large cyclic polypeptides with amino and carboxyl groups providing a polar face and hydrocarbon chains providing a non-polar face. Thus they act as cationic detergents, reacting with the phosphate group of cell envelope phospholipids. As a result there is disorganization of the cytoplasmic membrane, with leakage of the intracellular contents and cell death. Unfortunately, these agents can affect mammalian cell membranes in the same way, especially in the renal tubule where they are concentrated after excretion. Therefore they are used mainly topically, for superficial infections, but they can also be used for certain systemic infections if other, less toxic, antibiotics have failed.

Amphotericin B (Fig. 54-1) and **nystatin** have an analogous action on fungal cell membranes. Both of these antifungal agents have multiple conjugated double bonds (*i.e.*, they are "polyenes"; *see* Fig. 54-1), which cause them to interact preferentially with ergosterol, the main sterol in certain fungal cell membranes, rather than with the cholesterol of mammalian cell membranes. They produce hydrophilic channels through the fungal membrane, permitting leakage of essential cell contents.

The **imidazoles**, such as miconazole and clotrimazole, also exploit the requirement for ergosterol in the fungal cell membrane. These drugs inhibit the specific cytochrome P-450 that demethylates lanosterol, the precursor of ergosterol.

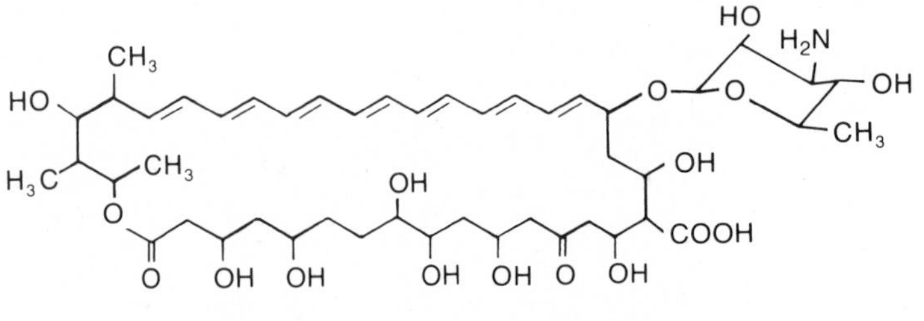

This chapter contains portions of Chapter 53 in the 4th edition by C. Prober.

Figure 54-1 Structural formula of amphotericin B.

POLYMYXINS AND COLISTIN

The polymyxins were discovered as antimicrobial agents in 1947. Polymyxin is a generic term for a group of closely related antibiotic substances (polymyxins A, B, C, D, and E, relatively simple basic polypeptides with molecular weights of about 1000) elaborated by various strains of an aerobic spore-forming rod, *Bacillus polymyxa*, which is found in soil. Polymyxin B, in the form of its sulfate, is the least toxic to humans. Colistin, which became available for clinical use in Japan in 1959, is also derived from a species of *B. polymyxa*. It is identical to polymyxin E but is supplied as the sulfomethyl derivative (methane sulfonate).

Bacterial Susceptibility

The activity of the polymyxins is related to a detergent action on the bacterial cell membrane, resulting in lysis of the organisms even in hypertonic media. This action is restricted to Gram-negative bacteria. *Enterobacter*, *Escherichia*, *Haemophilus*, *Klebsiella*, *Pasteurella*, *Salmonella*, *Shigella*, and *Vibrio* are sensitive to concentrations of 0.02–2 μg/mL. Most strains of *Pseudomonas aeruginosa* are inhibited by less than 4 μg/mL. Most strains of *Proteus* and some *Neisseria* are resistant to the drug. In general, the antibacterial activity of colistin is inferior to that of the sulfate derivatives.

Pharmacokinetics

The polymyxins, even in large doses, are not absorbed to a significant degree after topical or oral administration. The daily use of 2–4 mg/kg parenterally yields blood concentrations of 1–8 μg/mL, the peak occurring about 2 hours after intramuscular injection. Colistin blood concentrations tend to exceed polymyxin B concentrations after equivalent intramuscular doses. Intravenous doses of colistin result in peak serum concentrations approximately three times as high as those obtained after equivalent intramuscular doses.

The polymyxins are highly protein-bound; they do not diffuse well into body fluids, including the CSF, or into tissues or infective foci. Their main route of elimination is the kidney, but there is a lag in their excretion during the first 12 hours after an initial dose. Eventually, however, large amounts are excreted by this route and more than 60% of the administered dose can be recovered in the urine. Colistin, on the other hand, is more rapidly excreted *via* the kidney; about 40% is eliminated in the urine in the first 8 hours following injection. The serum elimination half-life of these agents is between 3 and 8 hours.

Adverse Reactions

The same detergent action that is responsible for the bactericidal effect can also be exerted on mammalian cell membranes, especially in the renal tubule where the drug is concentrated during excretion. Neurotoxicity and nephrotoxicity are the major severe adverse effects of these drugs. Lesser effects include drug fever, rashes, pain at the sites of intramuscular injection, and phlebitis after intravenous injections. Colistin tends to be less toxic than the sulfate derivatives.

Neurotoxicity is seen as transient paraesthesias and peripheral neuropathies. Severe reactions, such as ataxia or convulsions, may occur with large doses, especially in the presence of renal insufficiency. Neuromuscular blockade, which also appears to be dose-related, is of the noncompetitive type.

Nephrotoxicity (acute tubular necrosis with renal failure) is encountered with high doses of these agents. It will be rather common at doses greater than those recommended.

Drug Interactions

Neuromuscular blockade from muscle relaxants or general anaesthetics may be potentiated by the neurotoxic effects of these drugs.

Dosages and Routes of Administration

Polymyxin B is administered intramuscularly at a dose of 25,000–40,000 units/kg/day divided into two or three doses (10,000 units = 1 mg).

Colistin is administered intramuscularly or intravenously at a dose of 3–5 mg/kg/day divided into two or three doses.

The polymyxins are also available in numerous topical preparations such as creams, ointments, solutions, sprays, and eye drops. They are usually combined in these preparations with other antibiotics such as neomycin and bacitracin.

Therapeutic Applications

At the present time, the parenteral preparations of these agents have fallen into disuse clinically because of the availability of more efficacious, less toxic substances. The topical preparations of polymyxin B, however, are widely used because of its excellent activity against Gram-negative organisms, and its lack of absorption and hence of toxicity when applied superficially. Oral colistin has been used successfully as part of an oral decontamination regimen to prevent systemic infections in patients with acute leukemia and chemo-therapy-induced neutropenia.

NYSTATIN

Nystatin is an antifungal antibiotic that was isolated from *Streptomyces noursei* in 1950. It belongs to the group of polyene antibiotics. Its large, conjugated double-bond ring system is linked to an amino acid sugar, mycosamine.

Fungal Susceptibility

Nystatin is fungicidal against *Candida, Cryptococcus, Histoplasma, Blastomyces, Trichophyton, Epidermophyton,* and *Microsporum audouini in vitro* at concentrations ranging from 1.5 to 6.5 μg/mL.

Pharmacokinetics

Nystatin is too toxic for parenteral administration; it is therefore used only for the treatment of superficial mycotic infections. For these reasons the pharmacokinetics and toxic effects of parenteral nystatin need not be described. Very little, if any, nystatin is absorbed after topical or oral administration of pharmacologic doses.

Adverse Reactions

There are virtually no side effects related to the topical use of nystatin. The drug does not cause irritation or allergic reactions when applied to skin or mucous membranes. Nausea and diarrhea may occur following the administration of large doses orally.

Dosage Regimens and Routes of Administration

Many preparations of this drug (1 mg = 3500 units) are available, including oral tablets (500,000 units), oral suspension (100,000 units/mL), and vaginal tablets (100,000 units). Vaginal and skin creams are also available containing nystatin either alone or in combination with other antimicrobials (*e.g.,* bacitracin, neomycin, polymyxin B) or anti-inflammatory agents (principally steroids). Usually one tablet (orally or vaginally) or 5 mL of the suspension (swished in the mouth and swallowed) is administered 2–4 times per day. Topical application is usually made two or three times per day.

Therapeutic Applications

Nystatin is used almost exclusively for the treatment of mucosal or cutaneous candidal infections. However, some instances of oral candidiasis, especially those appearing as superinfections during the use of an antimicrobial agent, may fail to respond.

Nystatin has also been used prophylactically for the purpose of preventing yeast and fungal overgrowth in the bowels of patients receiving antibacterial agents or chemotherapy. There is no good clinical evidence to indicate that the incidence of systemic mycotic infections is reduced in such individuals.

AMPHOTERICIN B

Amphotericin is an antifungal compound that was isolated from *Streptomyces nodosus* in 1956. It exists in two forms, A and B: the latter, being more active, is used clinically. Amphotericin B is another polyene antibiotic; the basic moiety is aminodesoxyhexose, an aminomethyl pentose. It is closely related chemically to nystatin.

Fungal Susceptibility

Candida species, *Histoplasma capsulatum, Cryptococcus neoformans, Coccidioides immitis, Rhodotorula, Blastomyces dermatitidis, Paracoccidioides brasiliensis, Sporotrichum schenckii, Aspergillus, Cladosporium* species, *Phialophora* species, *Mucor,* and *Rhizopus* are usually killed by less than 1 μg/mL of amphotericin B. The drug is believed to act by binding to sterols in the fungal cell membrane, leading to formation of channels through which potassium is lost—a mechanism of action that is identical to that postulated for nystatin.

Pharmacokinetics

As would be expected from its structure (it is a large hydrophobic molecule; *see* Fig. 54–1), amphotericin B is poorly absorbed from the gastrointestinal tract. The intravenous injection of 0.5–1 mg/kg yields peak plasma concentrations of 1.5–2 μg/mL.

Data on the distribution of amphotericin B in both humans and animals are very limited. It is very lipophilic and it apparently distributes to cholesterol-containing membranes. This gives it a large volume of distribution of approximately 4 L/kg. Its degree of protein binding is greater than 90%. Only small quantities enter the CSF.

The primary route of elimination of amphotericin B is unclear. Only 2–5% of a given dose is excreted in biologically active form in the urine. The elimination of this agent is biphasic with an initial half-life of 24 hours, followed by a terminal half-life of 15 days, reflecting slow release from the large peripheral compartment.

Adverse Reactions

The main adverse reactions to amphotericin B are those that occur during intravenous infusions, or later as renal and hematologic toxicity.

Infusion reactions include fever, chills, headache, anorexia, nausea, vomiting, and thrombophlebitis. These reactions may be due to deoxycholate used to form a colloidal solution of the drug, or to the colloidal solution itself. They may be ameliorated by analgesics, antiemetics, antipyretics, heparin, or hydrocortisone.

Nephrotoxicity is a common and most important side effect of amphotericin B. Impairment of renal function and nephrotoxic reactions often limit the total amount of drug that can be administered. Early manifestations caused by the disruption of renal tubular cell membranes include hypokalemia, hypomagnesemia, and renal tubular acidosis. This drug also causes progressive impairment of renal function probably mediated by ischemia induced by renal artery spasm. This is manifested by rises in blood urea and serum creatinine, decrease in creatinine clearance, and the appearance of red and white blood cells, albumin, and casts in the urine. Such renal damage is usually reversible; however, permanent impairment and irreversible renal failure can occur and appear to be related to the total dose of drug used. Some degree of renal impairment has been demonstrated in 40% of adults who have received more than 4 g of amphotericin B. Recent evidence suggests that progression of amphotericin-induced nephrotoxicity may be limited by sodium loading to prevent proximal tubular uptake of the drug.

Hematologically, a normochromic, normocytic anemia may be associated with amphotericin B therapy. This is usually reversible and may be related to suppression of erythropoietin. Thrombocytopenia has also been noted occasionally.

Drug Interactions

Caution must be taken to monitor for hypokalemia in patients receiving digitalis preparations. Any drug that is renally excreted may accumulate as a consequence of the renal damage seen in most patients receiving amphotericin B. For example, the toxicity of 5-fluorocytosine (see Chapter 56), which is commonly administered with amphotericin B, is augmented.

Dosage Regimens and Routes of Administration

Amphotericin B is administered intravenously, though it is occasionally used topically, intraperitoneally, intra-

thecally, or by direct instillation into the bladder. There is no universal agreement on the method of intravenous administration. It is, however, common practice to treat fungal infections on the basis of a total dose of amphotericin B. That is, anywhere between 200 mg and 3–4 g of amphotericin B will be administered to treat a specific infection. The total amount of the dose will depend upon the specific infecting organism, the host, the site of infection, and the anticipated and observed responses to the treatment. In general, a daily dose of 0.5–1 mg/kg will be administered for as many days as it takes to attain the desired total dose. Some prefer to give this on alternate days, using a similar unit dose. Amphotericin B is the only antimicrobial agent that is administered on the basis of a total cumulative dose rather than on the basis of a daily dose administered for a specified period of time. The rationale for this method of administration is not entirely clear.

Therapeutic Applications

Parenteral amphotericin B is used for proven or highly suspected systemic fungal infections caused by susceptible organisms. Probably the most common infections treated with this drug in North America are disseminated candidiasis, aspergillosis, coccidioidomycosis, histoplasmosis, and mucormycosis. The topical formulations of amphotericin B are useful for the treatment of cutaneous or mucosal candidiasis. Intraperitoneal amphotericin B has been used successfully for the treatment of fungal peritonitis. Because of poor distribution to the CSF, it is either given intrathecally or combined with 5-fluorocytosine to treat fungal infections of the central nervous system (e.g., cryptococcal meningitis). Bladder instillation has been used to treat lower urinary tract infections (cystitis) caused by Candida.

TOPICAL IMIDAZOLE ANTIFUNGAL AGENTS

The topical imidazole antifungal agents are synthetic compounds that bind to the heme of cytochrome P-450s and inhibit ergosterol synthesis. Two major drugs in this class are **miconazole** and **clotrimazole**. They are lipophilic compounds with low water solubility at neutral pH, but the imidazole ring is ionized under acidic conditions and this greatly increases water solubility.

Fungal Susceptibility

These agents have a broad spectrum of activity including Epidermophyton, Microsporum, and Trichophyton species; Pityrosporon orbiculare and Candida albicans. They can be either fungistatic or fungicidal, depending on the concentration.

Adverse Reactions

Topical imidazoles seldom lead to adverse reactions although they can cause erythema, stinging, blistering, pruritus, and even urticaria.

Therapeutic Applications

The topical imidazoles are used to treat superficial fungal infections of the feet, perineum, nails, vagina, and mouth. In general, they are very effective and represent the treatment of choice for such infections. One consideration in the treatment of fungal infections of the nails is that penetration of topical agents into the nail is poor and systemic therapy with griseofulvin (see Chapter 56) is often required.

SYSTEMIC IMIDAZOLE ANTIFUNGAL AGENTS

Ketoconazole (Fig. 54–2) is the major imidazole used for systemic antifungal therapy, although miconazole can also be used systemically.

Fungal Susceptibility

Ketoconazole is usually active at levels of less than 0.5 μg/mL against *C. immitis*, *C. neoformans*, and *H. capsulatum*. Activity against *Candida*, *Aspergillus*, and *Sporothrix* usually requires levels from 6 to greater than 100 μg/mL.

Pharmacokinetics

Absorption of ketoconazole after oral administration is good; however, an acidic environment is necessary for dissolution of the drug and absorption is markedly decreased by antacids and histamine H_2-receptor blockers, or in patients with achlorhydria. The drug is highly protein-bound (90%). Distribution is limited and the level reached in the CNS is very low.

Elimination of ketoconazole is primarily due to hepatic biotransformation. The kinetics of ketoconazole appear to be dose-dependent; the half-life increases from 90 minutes after a 200 mg dose to almost 4 hours after an 800 mg dose.

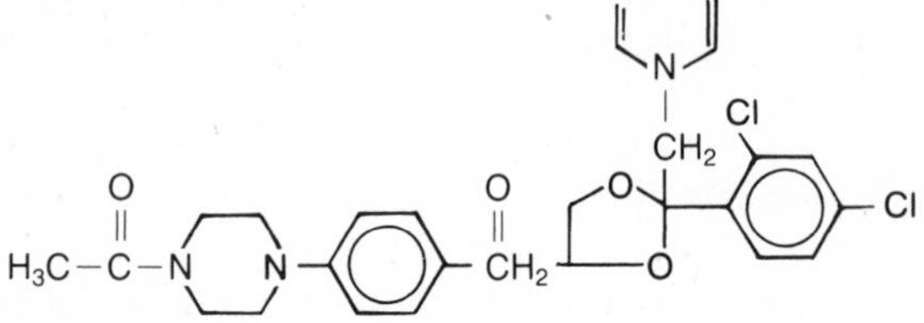

Adverse Reactions

The most common side effects of ketoconazole are nausea and vomiting. Mild, asymptomatic elevation of transaminases is observed in 5–10% of patients, and serious **hepatotoxicity** occurs with an incidence of approximately one in 15,000.

Although ketoconazole has some selectivity for the cytochrome P-450 that is involved in the synthesis of ergosterol, it also inhibits the metabolism of several other drugs in a manner similar to cimetidine (also an imidazole) and also inhibits the testicular synthesis of androgens. This is the probable mechanism for the observed association of ketoconazole with gynecomastia in some patients.

Dosage and Route of Administration

Ketoconazole is available in 200 mg tablets for oral administration. The usual dose is 200–400 mg per day. In cases of achlorhydria, the drug is dissolved in dilute hydrochloric acid and sipped through a straw to avoid contact with the teeth.

Therapeutic Applications

Ketoconazole is effective in the treatment of histoplasmosis involving the lungs, bones, skin or soft tissue, and disseminated disease. It is effective in nonmeningeal cryptococcal disease, but penetration of the CNS is not sufficient for the treatment of cryptococcal meningitis. It is also useful in the treatment of paracoccidioidomycosis, blastomycosis, and certain dermatomycoses. Its major limitation is its slow onset of action; therefore amphotericin B is usually the drug of choice in severe, acute fungal infections. There appears to be antagonism between ketoconazole and amphotericin B and so they are not combined.

SUGGESTED READING

Medoff G, Brajtburg J, Kobayashi GS, Bolard J. Antifungal agents useful in therapy of systemic fungal infections. Ann Rev Pharmacol Toxicol 1983; 23:303–330.
Terrell C, Hermans PE. Antifungal agents used for deep-seated mycotic infections. Mayo Clin Proc 1987; 62:1116–1128.

Figure 54–2   Structural formula of ketoconazole.

Chapter 55

ANTIMICROBIAL AGENTS THAT AFFECT SYNTHESIS OF CELLULAR PROTEINS

C. Prober

BACTERIAL PROTEIN SYNTHESIS

Protein synthesis occurs through translation of the genetic information coded in mRNA. This process takes place on the ribonucleoprotein particles, the ribosomes, and it consists of three stages: initiation, elongation, and termination (shown schematically in Fig. 55–1).

In general, the functional unit of bacterial protein synthesis is the 70S ribosome, which consists of two subunits: 30S and 50S. The mRNA attaches to the 30S subunit, and the anticodon of aminoacyl-tRNA is matched to the codon on the mRNA. The aminoacyl group attached to the tRNA is bound to the 50S subunit where peptide bond formation occurs. One of the proteins making up the 50S subunit is peptidyl transferase.

Initiation, *i.e.*, formation of the 70S ribosome, involves various initiation factors by which a 30S subunit combines with mRNA and tRNA, and then with a 50S subunit, to complete the 70S ribosome. The tRNA, initially bound to the "A" (aminoacyl) site of the ribosome, is translocated to the "P" (peptidyl) site, freeing the "A" site for additional tRNA.

The elongation stage is essentially a "request" by the codons of mRNA for additional aminoacyl-tRNA, which is first bound to the "A" site and then translocated to the "P" site. Various elongation factors are involved in this process, which is repeated until the message is read and the protein is completed.

Termination of the peptide chain occurs when a terminating codon is reached and the completed chain is discharged from the ribosome. Various termination factors are involved in the release of completed pro-

tein. The 50S and 30S subunits dissociate and join a pool of free subunits before recombining with a new messenger.

MECHANISMS OF INHIBITOR ACTION

Several antibiotics inhibit protein synthesis by interfering with translation. They bind to ribosomes and prevent normal peptide chain formation at one or more of several points, which include: peptide bond formation, translocation, and movement of the ribosomes along mRNA. The basis for selective toxicity to bacteria with relatively low toxicity to mammalian cells is that, with the exception of the tetracyclines, these agents do not bind to mammalian ribosomes. The structure of the mammalian ribosome is different from that of bacteria. The mammalian ribosomes are 80S and are not easily split into subunits.

Aminoglycosides bind tightly to the 30S subunit of the ribosome and inhibit protein synthesis at several points by blocking the normal activity of the initiation complex, interfering with tRNA attachment, and distorting the triplet codon of mRNA so that the message is misread and faulty proteins are formed. **Spectinomycin**, like the aminoglycosides, binds to the 30S ribosomal subunit, thereby inhibiting protein synthesis. It does not, however, cause misreading of the genetic code.

Tetracyclines also bind to the 30S subunit and act by blocking the binding of tRNA to mRNA. They also bind to mammalian ribosomes, but susceptible bacteria concentrate the tetracyclines and, therefore, the drugs can be used at a concentration that will kill bac-

---

This chapter was revised by J. Uetrecht.

557

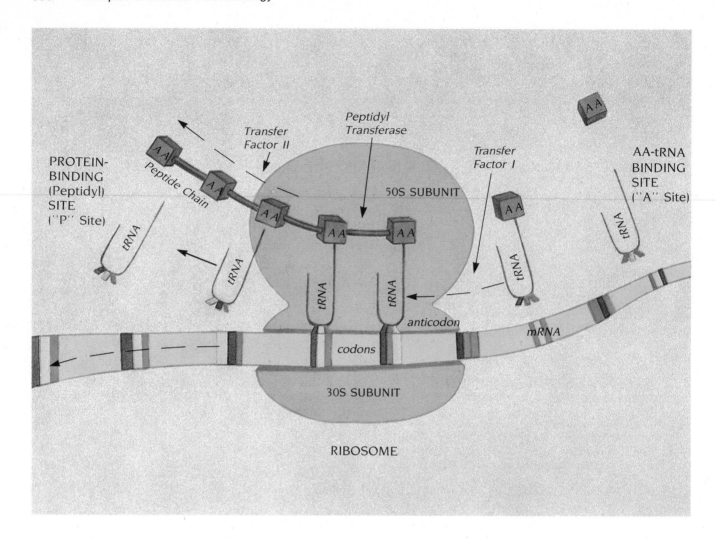

Figure 55–1   Schematic representation of basic elements and steps of bacterial protein synthesis (*see* text for explanations).

teria but have little toxicity to mammalian cells. In addition, these agents chelate essential cations, especially magnesium.

Chloramphenicol, clindamycin, and **erythromycin** bind to the 50S subunit. Chloramphenicol prevents peptide bond formation by inhibiting the responsible enzyme, peptidyl transferase, which is also located on the 50S subunit. Clindamycin inhibits the initiation of peptide chain synthesis, whereas erythromycin prevents chain extension of growing peptides on the ribosomes. The latter two drugs also block translocation or progression to the next codon on mRNA.

AMINOGLYCOSIDES

The aminoglycoside group of antibiotics includes a large number of structurally related compounds all derived from different species of *Streptomyces*. **Strep-**

tomycin was the first of this group to be discovered (1943) by means of a systematic examination of soil fungi. Subsequently, **neomycin** (1949), **kanamycin** (1957), **gentamicin** (1964), and **tobramycin** (1971) were discovered. Semisynthetic derivatives of these agents, including **amikacin** (1975) and **netilmicin** (1976), were then produced. The main impetus for the original search for these compounds was the lack of significant activity of the penicillins against Gram-negative organisms. The aminoglycoside class of antibiotics remains today our most important weapon against Gram-negative pathogens.

Chemistry

The members of this group of antibiotics are typified by the presence of amino sugars glycosidically linked (hence the name "aminoglycoside") to aminocyclitols (Fig. 55–2).

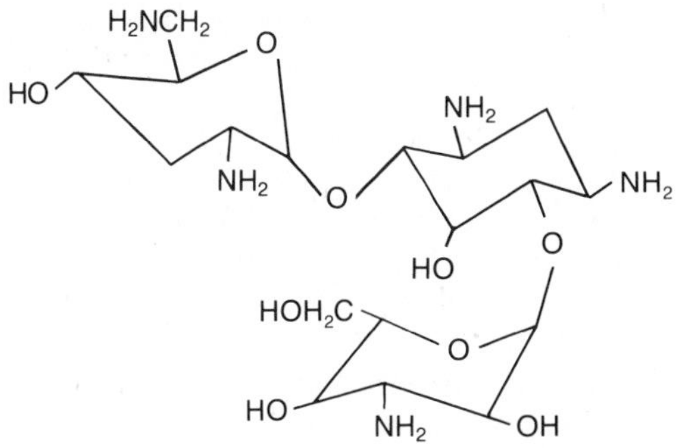

Figure 55-2 Structural formula of tobramycin, a representative aminoglycoside.

The bacterial susceptibilities, pharmacokinetics, adverse reactions, and drug interactions of all systemically used aminoglycosides are very similar, mainly because of their common physicochemical characteristics. The dosages, regimens, routes of administration, and therapeutic applications do differ somewhat, and these aspects must therefore be considered separately for each agent.

Bacterial Susceptibility

The aminoglycosides are active primarily against the Gram-negative aerobes and limited numbers of the Gram-positive aerobes (e.g., staphylococci). They are generally inactive against the Gram-negative anaerobes because an oxygen-dependent transport system is involved in their uptake by bacteria. Streptomycin is also quite active against bovine and human mycobacteria (MIC~0.5 μg/mL). Streptomycin, neomycin, and kanamycin are not active against Pseudomonas aeruginosa, but the other four agents in this group have varying degrees of activity against this organism (Table 55-1). Tobramycin is the most active against the majority of

P. aeruginosa isolates and netilmicin is the least active of the four. Other differences in the activity of the four most commonly used aminoglycosides against a variety of microorganisms can also be seen in Table 55-1. For instance, it should be noted that gentamicin is the most active against Serratia marcescens.

An important aspect of activity against Gram-negative aerobes is that increasing resistance has developed in hospitals and other enclosed environments after extensive use of aminoglycosides. This resistance results from either chromosomal mutations or plasmid-mediated R-factors that induce the bacteria to produce enzymes that can degrade some or all of the aminoglycosides. These enzymes cause aminoglycoside inactivation by acetylation, adenylation, or phosphorylation of specific amino or alcohol groups that are necessary for activity (see Fig. 55-2). Of the aminoglycosides represented in Table 55-1, gentamicin is susceptible to the largest number of these enzymes (nine of 12) and amikacin is susceptible to the smallest number (one of 12). It is thus not surprising that the development of resistance appears to be most common with gentamicin and least common with amikacin. When widespread resistance develops to one of the aminoglycosides being used in a particular hospital it is often beneficial to change to another aminoglycoside for some period of time.

Pharmacokinetics

Very little of the aminoglycosides is absorbed from the gastrointestinal tract even after oral administration of large doses. They are, however, rapidly absorbed after intramuscular injection and they can also be given intravenously. The concentrations of the various aminoglycosides obtained after specified doses are outlined in Table 55-2. Neomycin is not included in this table as it is too toxic to use systemically.

The volume of distribution of the aminoglycosides

TABLE 55-1   Median MICs (in μg/mL) of Aminoglycosides

Bacteria	Gentamicin	Tobramycin	Amikacin	Netilmicin
Gram-positive				
Staphylococcus aureus	0.39	0.5	1.8	0.5
Streptococcus Group A	6.3	>25.0	>200	4.0
Streptococcus viridans	4.0	—	>40	—
Streptococcus faecalis	25.0	25.0	>80	16.0
Gram-negative				
Haemophilus influenzae	1.0	0.8	5.0	1.0
Salmonella	0.78	0.4	0.8	0.4
Shigella	0.78	0.8	4.0	0.8
Klebsiella	1.0	1.5	3.0	1.0
Escherichia coli	3.2	2.0	2.0	0.7
Pseudomonas aeruginosa	4.0	1.6	6.0	8.0
Proteus mirabilis	1.0	1.0	2.0	1.0
Serratia marcescens	1.0	3.0	4.0	3.0

CHEMOTHERAPY

TABLE 55-2 Pharmacokinetics of Aminoglycosides

Agent	Unit Dose	Usual Serum Concentration ($\mu g/mL$)	Half-Life (h)
Streptomycin	500 mg	15–20	2.5
Kanamycin	7.5 mg/kg	25	2.0
Gentamicin	1.5 mg/kg	5–7	2.4
Tobramycin	2.0 mg/kg	6–8	2.0
Amikacin	7.5 mg/kg	15–30	1.5–2.0
Netilmicin	1.0 mg/kg	3.5–5.0	2.0–2.5

ranges from 0.25 to 0.7 L/kg. In general, it is lower in adults and higher in infants. The drugs are not highly protein-bound (less than 30%). They are distributed in all the extracellular fluids but do not generally attain sufficiently high concentrations in the CSF after parenteral administration to be of therapeutic benefit to patients with meningitis. The main site of uptake of the aminoglycosides is the kidney, which accounts for approximately 40% of the total antibiotic in the body. The cortex accumulates approximately 85% of this load, and the resulting concentrations are more than 100 times greater than serum concentrations.

The aminoglycosides are not significantly biotransformed by body tissues but rather are eliminated unchanged, primarily by the kidneys by glomerular filtration. The complete dose is usually not excreted during the first 1–2 days of therapy, but thereafter over a prolonged period nearly 100% elimination by this route occurs. The serum elimination half-life of these agents in normal adults ranges from 1.5 to 2.5 hours.

Adverse Reactions

The most important toxicities of the aminoglycosides are those affecting the inner ear and the kidneys.

Ototoxicity may be primarily vestibular or primarily cochlear (in both cases associated with ablation of hair cells). The agents most likely to cause **vestibular toxicity** are streptomycin and gentamicin. The most severe vestibular reactions were noted when streptomycin was used in high doses. Nearly 75% of patients who were given 2 g of streptomycin daily for 60–120 days manifested some vestibular disturbance, whereas reduction of the dose to 1 g daily decreased this incidence to approximately 25%. Inflammation of the meninges also appeared to predispose to ototoxicity, and repeated intrathecal injections of the drug caused earlier and more severe damage than did administration by other routes. The incidence of vestibular symptoms with gentamicin therapy is approximately 2%. This ranges from slight vertigo to an acute Ménière's syndrome. Damage is usually permanent, but patients may diminish their symptoms through adaptation.

The agents most likely to cause **cochlear toxicity** are

neomycin, kanamycin, amikacin, and tobramycin. The cochlear toxicity of neomycin is so severe that the systemic use of this agent is precluded. Irreversible deafness will occur from just 1–2 weeks of daily intramuscular therapy using 0.5–1 g. The frequency of hearing loss with tobramycin and amikacin is low, but it may occur without any warning and may be irreversible.

Risk factors that seem to predispose to ototoxicity include increased serum concentrations, prolonged use, advanced age, preexisting renal disease or hearing loss, and the concomitant administration of other ototoxic drugs (e.g., furosemide, ethacrynic acid; see Chapter 40).

The accumulation of the aminoglycosides in the proximal tubules of the renal cortex predisposes to the development of **nephrotoxicity.** This used to be common with parenteral neomycin therapy but appears to be rare with streptomycin therapy. The frequency with the other aminoglycosides is somewhere between these extremes, appearing to be reduced with amikacin, tobramycin, and perhaps netilmicin, though data on the latter agent are incomplete.

Early manifestations of nephrotoxicity include enzymuria, hypokalemia, glycosuria, alkalosis, hypomagnesemia, and hypocalcemia. The usual course is a nonoliguric renal failure of gradual progression. This nephrotoxicity is dose-related and generally reversible. Its incidence may increase with the concomitant administration of cisplatin, furosemide, ethacrynic acid, cephalothin, or cephaloridine, and is potentiated by volume depletion.

Another adverse reaction to the aminoglycosides is a competitive type of **neuromuscular blockade** (potency is less than 1% that of d-tubocurarine), which occurs most frequently after intraperitoneal administration. Hypersensitivity reactions to the aminoglycosides are infrequent, although a contact dermatitis is the most common side effect of topically applied neomycin. This usually occurs after prolonged use and is unlikely to be noted with short-term treatment.

Drug Interactions

Penicillins and cephalosporins react with the amino group of aminoglycosides and inactivate them; therefore, penicillins and cephalosporins should not be mixed in the same bottle with aminoglycosides. Inactivation can also occur in vivo, but this is of little clinical significance with the possible exception of patients with renal failure where the concentration of penicillin can be very high.

Another aminoglycoside interaction with the penicillins, which is of therapeutic advantage, is synergy against a variety of microbes. Penicillins synergistic with the aminoglycosides include penicillin G (vs. Streptococcus viridans), penicillin G or ampicillin (vs. enterococci or Listeria), cloxacillin (vs. staphylococci), and ticarcillin, piperacillin, or carbenicillin (vs. P. aeruginosa).

Some cephalosporins, specifically cephalothin and

cephaloridine, and also amphotericin B, may enhance the nephrotoxicity of the aminoglycosides. On the other hand, the cephalosporins often act synergistically with the aminoglycosides against *Klebsiella*.

Dosage Regimens, Routes of Administration, and Therapeutic Applications

Streptomycin

Adults are usually treated with 15 mg/kg/day intramuscularly, divided into one or two doses. The drug is often given only once or twice weekly in the initial treatment of tuberculosis. In the past, streptomycin was often administered intrathecally for the treatment of meningitis. This is an uncommon practice today because of its toxicity by this route and the availability of more acceptable therapeutic alternatives. It is primarily useful in the initial treatment of tuberculosis as a second or third drug. Streptomycin has also often been used in the management of *S. viridans* or enterococcal endocarditis, because of its synergistic activity with penicillin against many of these bacteria.

Neomycin

The drug is commonly used topically in combination with other antibiotics (to prevent the emergence of resistant bacteria) in the treatment of superficial staphylococcal or Gram-negative infections. Oral neomycin is also used to reduce the quantity of intestinal flora in patients with hepatic failure. Bladder irrigation with neomycin is used in the prevention or treatment of urinary tract sepsis in patients with indwelling urethral catheters or in those who have just undergone a urologic procedure (*e.g.*, cystoscopy).

Gentamicin, Tobramycin, Amikacin, and Netilmicin

The usual dosages and regimens of these four aminoglycosides are outlined in Table 55-3. They are administered by the intramuscular or intravenous route. Occasionally in the treatment of Gram-negative meningitis and other central nervous system infections these aminoglycosides are also administered by the intrathecal or intraventricular route in a single daily dose of 1–10 mg. Topical formulations (*e.g.*, ointments, ear drops, eye drops) are also on the market.

The most important indications for using one of these aminoglycosides are serious Gram-negative infections, including infections of blood, bones and joints, the respiratory tract, soft tissue and wounds, the urinary tract, and the central nervous system. These drugs are also invaluable in the empiric treatment of neutropenic febrile hosts who are at great risk of Gram-negative septicemia. They also act in synergy with the penicillins or cephalosporins against numerous bacteria (*see* Drug Interactions). The choice between the four aminoglycosides is influenced by several factors including the resistance pattern of organisms within the institution, the familiarity of the clinicians with the individual antibiotics, and the cost of each agent to the patient. If accumulating data confirm differences in toxicities between these aminoglycosides, this may also become a factor in choosing between drugs.

SPECTINOMYCIN

Spectinomycin is an antibiotic produced by *Streptomyces spectabilis*. The drug is an aminocyclitol. It is active against a number of Gram-negative bacterial species but is inferior to other drugs to which such microorganisms are susceptible. Its most important activity is that against gonococci, which it inhibits at concentrations of 7–20 μg/mL.

Absorption, distribution, and excretion of spectinomycin are similar to those of the aminoglycosides. A single dose of 2 g produces peak plasma concentrations of 100 μg/mL at 1 hour.

Local discomfort after intramuscular injection is the most common adverse reaction. The risk of oto- and nephrotoxicity is low because the drug is administered as a single injection in a dose of 35 mg/kg (up to 2 g). It is used exclusively for the treatment of gonorrhea suspected or proven to be due to a penicillin-resistant strain (or in a patient known to have penicillin hypersensitivity).

TETRACYCLINES

The development of tetracycline antibiotics was the result of systematic screening of soil samples from many parts of the world. The first tetracycline, chlortetracycline, was introduced in 1948. The most recent tetracycline congener is minocycline (introduced in 1972).

TABLE 55-3 Dosages and Regimens of Aminoglycosides

Agent	Usual Daily Total Dose (mg/kg)	Usual Number of Fractional Doses per Day
Gentamicin	4.5–5.0	3
Tobramycin	5.0–7.5	3
Amikacin	15–20	2–3
Netilmicin	4.5–6.0	3

Chemistry

The tetracyclines are all derivatives of the polycyclic substance naphthacenecarboxamide (Fig. 55–3). There are a number of these agents, including **tetracycline, chlortetracycline, oxytetracycline, demeclocycline, rolitetracycline, methacycline, doxycycline,** and **minocycline.** Of these, the three most commonly used are tetracycline, doxycycline, and minocycline.

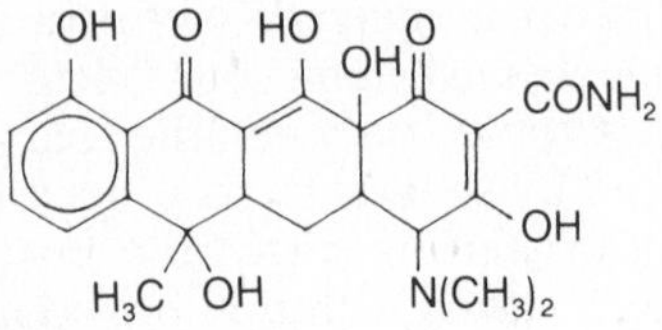

Tetracycline

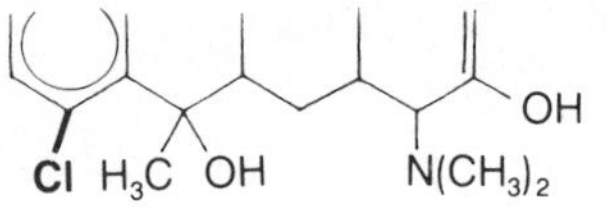

Chlortetracycline

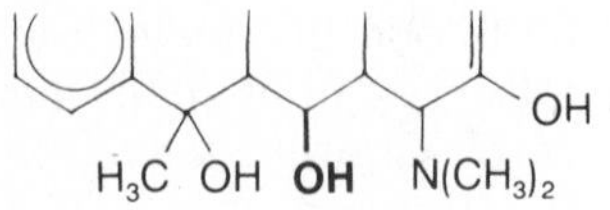

Oxytetracycline

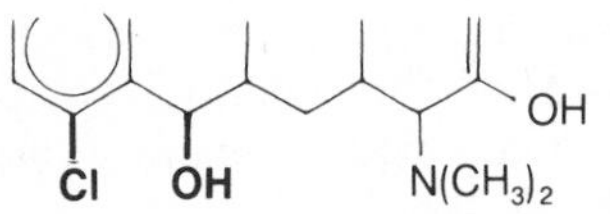

Demeclocycline

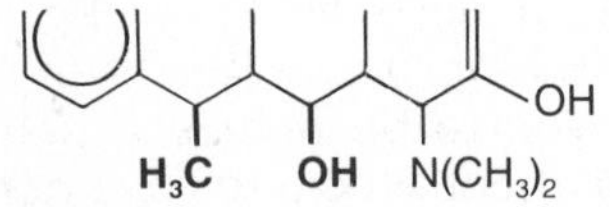

Doxycycline

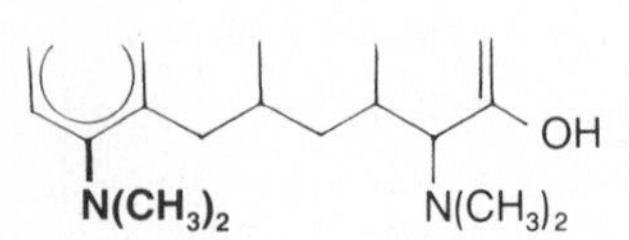

Minocycline

Figure 55–3 Structural formulae of tetracyclines.

Bacterial Susceptibility

The tetracyclines are active against a broad spectrum of bacteria. Susceptible strains include a wide range of Gram-positive and Gram-negative bacteria, *Mycoplasma, Rickettsia,* and *Chlamydia.* They are also very active against *Treponema pallidum.* The median MICs for three commonly used tetracyclines against representative organisms are shown in Table 55–4. Minocycline is generally the most active of the tetracyclines, especially against *Staphylococcus aureus.* Tetracyclines also have moderate activity against anaerobes, though only 40–60% of *Bacteroides fragilis* strains are now sensitive to clinically achievable concentrations.

Pharmacokinetics

All tetracyclines are absorbed adequately but incompletely after an oral dose. Absorption is most active in the stomach and upper small intestine and is greater in the fasting state. With the exception of minocycline, which does not have a hydroxyl group in the 6 position, the tetracyclines are unstable in the acid environment of the stomach.

Tetracyclines are effective chelating agents against various cations, with which they form poorly soluble complexes. Accordingly, absorption from the intestinal tract is impaired by milk and milk products and by the co-administration of aluminum hydroxide gels and calcium, magnesium, or iron salts. After a 250 mg oral dose of tetracycline to an average-sized adult, the serum concentrations are 2–3 μg/mL. After a 100 mg oral dose of doxycycline or minocycline, serum concentrations are 1–2 μg/mL. After parenteral administration, absorption is complete, serum concentrations being approximately twice those observed after an equal oral dose.

The volumes of distribution of the tetracyclines range from 0.4 L/kg for minocycline to 1–2 L/kg for doxycycline and tetracycline. Their protein binding ranges from 60% (tetracycline) to 80–95% (doxycycline). Tetracyclines are widely distributed, especially the highly lipid-soluble compounds minocycline and doxycycline. They enter the CSF quite freely, attaining concentrations 10–50% of those in the serum. Because of chelation of tissue calcium deposits, the drugs become markedly bound to bones, teeth, and neoplasms, in which they cause yellow fluorescence.

The main mode of elimination of most of the tetracyclines is renal glomerular filtration, but they are also eliminated to a greater or lesser extent *via* the biliary route. For most of the tetracyclines, 20–60% of the administered dose is found in the urine. Minocycline is recoverable in the urine and feces in significantly lower amounts than the other tetracyclines, and it

TABLE 55–4 Median MICs (in μg/mL) of Tetracyclines

Bacteria	Tetracycline	Doxycycline	Minocycline
Gram-positive			
Staphylococcus aureus	3.19	1.6	0.78
Streptococcus Group A	0.78	0.39	0.39
Streptococcus viridans	3.1	0.39	0.39
Streptococcus faecalis	>100	>100	>100
Streptococcus pneumoniae	0.8	0.2	0.2
Gram-negative			
Neisseria meningitidis	0.8	1.6	1.6
Neisseria gonorrhoeae	0.78	0.39	0.39
Haemophilus influenzae	1.6	1.6	1.6
Shigella	100.0	100.0	100.0
Klebsiella	50.0	50.0	25.0
Escherichia coli	12.5	12.5	6.3
Pseudomonas aeruginosa	200.0	100.0	200.0
Proteus mirabilis	>100	>100	>100
Serratia	200.0	50.0	25.0
Bacteroides fragilis	12.5	—	—
Other Bacteroides	0.25	—	—
Others			
Mycoplasma pneumoniae	1.6	1.6	1.6
Treponema pallidum	0.4	0.1	—
Chlamydia	2.0	2.0	2.0

appears to be biotransformed to a considerable degree. Doxycycline is excreted primarily in the feces (90%) as an inactive metabolite or perhaps as a chelate. The half-lives of these drugs range from 6 hours (tetracycline) to 24 hours (doxycycline).

Adverse Reactions

Hypersensitivity reactions to the tetracyclines are rare. **Gastrointestinal disturbances** (nausea, vomiting, and diarrhea) are common, and pseudomembranous colitis has been described.

Thrush and *Candida* vaginitis occur more frequently with the tetracyclines than with any other group of antimicrobial agents. These adverse reactions are related to the broad-spectrum nature of this type of antibiotic, which results in marked alterations of the normal flora.

Photosensitivity reactions may be caused by any of the tetracyclines, but are most frequent with doxycycline.

Tooth and bone deposition of these agents represents the most important side effect of the tetracyclines in pediatrics and is the reason these agents are **contraindicated in children** and, because they cross the placenta, during fetal development. The depositions are in the calcifying areas of teeth and bones, and they may discolor either deciduous or permanent tooth enamel. Bone deposition may result in temporary cessation of bone growth. This latter effect is reversible when the drug is discontinued.

Hepatotoxicity is an uncommon but serious adverse reaction, which has been described primarily after the intravenous administration of large doses of tetracycline to pregnant women. This reaction is usually fatal. The liver shows extensive fatty infiltration at autopsy.

Outdated tetracycline products have resulted in a "Fanconi-like" syndrome (renal tubular abnormalities), with acidosis, nephrosis, and aminoaciduria. Tetracyclines may also cause further increases in BUN and serum creatinine in patients with renal failure. These biochemical changes, as well as tetracycline-induced azotemia, have been attributed to an antianabolic effect of the drugs.

Benign increase of the intracranial pressure (pseudotumor cerebri) has been observed as a side effect of tetracycline therapy. It is reversible upon discontinuation of the medication.

Manifestations of neurotoxicity are observed frequently and almost exclusively with minocycline. Dizziness, weakness, ataxia, and vertigo appear within the first few days of therapy.

Drug Interactions

Antacids containing the divalent cations Ca^{2+}, Al^{2+}, or Mg^{2+}, and iron salts used in the treatment of anemia, can bind these antibiotics and may result in diminished absorption of the tetracyclines from the intestinal tract when administered concomitantly.

Diuretics, presumably acting by volume depletion, may aggravate the increases in BUN observed with the tetracyclines.

CHEMOTHERAPY

The combination of tetracycline and penicillin G represents one of the few *in vivo* examples of antibacterial antagonism. Patients with pneumococcal meningitis receiving this combined therapy were observed to have poorer clinical response than patients receiving penicillin G alone. This antagonism can be reproduced *in vitro*.

Dosage Regimens and Routes of Administration

Tetracycline is usually administered orally at a daily dose of 25–50 mg/kg divided into four equal doses. It may, however, also be administered intramuscularly (15–25 mg/kg/day) or intravenously (20–30 mg/kg/day). By these latter routes the dosing interval is 8–12 hours. Minocycline is usually administered orally in a daily dose of 4 mg/kg divided into two equal doses. When it is administered intravenously the dose and frequency of administration are the same. The daily dose of doxycycline by either the oral or the intravenous route is 5 mg/kg. It is usually administered in two doses orally, but in a single dose intravenously.

Therapeutic Applications

Possible clinical indications for the tetracyclines include acute exacerbations of chronic bronchitis, *Mycoplasma* pneumonia, gonorrhea and syphilis in penicillin-allergic patients, Q fever, psittacosis, brucellosis, rickettsial infections, and lymphogranuloma venereum. Minocycline, in general, has no therapeutic advantages over the other tetracyclines. However, because of significant salivary secretion, the drug is effective in eradication of meningococci from carriers. Doxycyline is unique among the tetracyclines in that it does not accumulate in renal insufficiency. It can therefore be used in the rare situation in which a tetracycline is the drug of choice in a patient with renal insufficiency. Doxycycline has also proven to be an effective chemoprophylactic agent against travellers' diarrhea induced by *Escherichia coli*. It may also be the drug of choice for genital tract infection with *Chlamydia* or *Mycoplasma*.

CHLORAMPHENICOL

Chloramphenicol was first isolated in 1947 from *Streptomyces venezuelae*, an organism found in a soil sample from Venezuela. After the structural formula of this antimicrobial agent was determined, it was prepared synthetically.

Chemistry

Chloramphenicol is a lipid-soluble compound lacking acidic and basic groups that could form salts. It is unique among natural compounds in that it contains a nitrobenzene moiety, which can be **reduced** by cytochrome P-450 (*see* Chapter 4). Antimicrobial activity requires the L(–) configuration of the dichloroacetamide side chain attached to one of the two asymmetric carbon atoms of the propanediol moiety (Fig. 55–4).

Bacterial Susceptibility

Most aerobic bacteria except *P. aeruginosa*, practically all anaerobes, and the majority of clinically important types of *Mycoplasma*, *Chlamydia*, and *Rickettsia* are susceptible to chloramphenicol at concentrations achievable in the serum. MICs of chloramphenicol against representative bacteria are outlined in Table 55–5.

Although chloramphenicol is bacteriostatic against most organisms, it is bactericidal *in vitro* against most

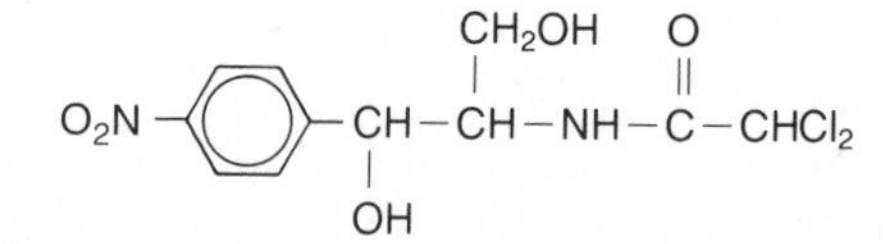

$$O_2N - \bigcirc - \underset{\underset{OH}{|}}{CH} - \underset{\underset{CH_2OH}{|}}{CH} - NH - \overset{\overset{O}{||}}{C} - CHCl_2$$

Figure 55–4   Structural formula of chloramphenicol.

TABLE 55–5   MIC Ranges (in μg/mL) of Chloramphenicol

Gram-positive bacteria	
Staphylococcus aureus	1.0–5.0
Streptococcus Group A	0.3–6.0
Streptococcus viridans	0.6–2.5
Streptococcus faecalis	6.3–>100
Streptococcus pneumoniae	0.06–12.5
Gram-negative bacteria	
Neisseria meningitidis	0.78–6.25
Neisseria gonorrhoeae	0.78–6.3
Haemophilus influenzae	0.2–3.5
Salmonella	0.75–5.0
Shigella	2.5–6.0
Klebsiella	0.5–25.0
Escherichia coli	3.0–50.0
Pseudomonas aeruginosa	8.0–1000
Proteus mirabilis	3.0–25.0
Serratia marcescens	2.5–5.0
Bacteroides fragilis	0.5–16.0
Other Bacteroides	0.1–16.0

strains of *Haemophilus influenzae, Streptococcus pneumoniae*, and *Neisseria meningitidis*. The mechanism of this bacterial killing action is not known.

Pharmacokinetics

Chloramphenicol is rapidly and completely absorbed from the intestinal tract. It is generally administered as the tasteless palmitate, which must be hydrolysed to free active base *in vivo* before absorption can occur. The peak serum concentration is approximately the same as that attained after a similar dose given intravenously, but the peak is not reached until 2 hours after an oral dose.

After an intravenous dose of 500 mg of the succinate form administered to an adult, rapid hydrolysis to the free drug results in serum concentrations of 6–10 μg/mL.

The volume of distribution of chloramphenicol is approximately 0.9 L/kg. It is 50–60% protein-bound. It diffuses into most body fluids and tissues, and unlike many other antibiotics, chloramphenicol penetrates well into the CSF even in the absence of meningitis. In the presence of meningitis, CSF concentrations often reach 70–80% of serum levels; brain tissue concentrations exceed those in the serum.

Chloramphenicol is converted in the liver to a highly water-soluble monoglucuronide, which has no biologic activity. Impaired liver function might reduce the rate of conjugation to glucuronic acid (*see* Chapter 4) and correspondingly increase serum concentrations of active drug. On the other hand, induction of liver microsomal enzymes by some drugs (*e.g.*, phenobarbital) may enhance the biotransformation of chloramphenicol, resulting in reduced serum concentrations.

About 90% of chloramphenicol is excreted in the urine, but only 5–10% of this is in the unchanged active form. Active chloramphenicol is excreted only by glomerular filtration, but the inactive derivatives (glucuronic acid conjugates) are also eliminated by tubular secretion. Only a small amount of chloramphenicol (2–3%) is excreted in bile, mostly in the inactive form, and less than 1% appears in the feces. The serum half-life of chloramphenicol is approximately 3 hours.

Adverse Reactions

The most feared complication of chloramphenicol therapy is **aplastic anemia**. It occurs in approximately one in 40,000 patients treated with this drug. The mechanism is unclear but appears to be due to the nitro group, because the analog in which the nitro group is replaced with a methylsulfone group has not been associated with aplastic anemia.

A second type of hematopoietic depression is dose-related. Serum concentrations in excess of 20–25 μg/mL

invariably result in reduced iron utilization by the bone marrow, and vacuolization of erythroblasts, megakaryocytes, and leukocyte precursors. Anemia, thrombocytopenia, and leukopenia result. This type of **marrow toxicity** is reversible and responds to discontinuance of the drug.

A toxic reaction to chloramphenicol observed almost exclusively in neonates is the **gray baby syndrome** (*see* Chapters 4 and 68). This is a form of circulatory collapse associated with excessive serum concentrations of unconjugated chloramphenicol maintained for several days due to immaturity of the glucuronyl transferase system in the liver of the neonate.

Drug Interactions

Chloramphenicol may inhibit the metabolism of phenytoin, oral hypoglycemic agents, and oral anticoagulants, with resultant phenytoin toxicity, hypoglycemia, or hemorrhage, respectively.

Some drugs such as phenobarbital can induce liver microsomal enzymes and, hence, increase the total body clearance of chloramphenicol. Acetaminophen, on the contrary, can prolong the half-life of chloramphenicol and lead to drug accumulation, perhaps because of reduction of its rate of biotransformation.

Dosage Regimens and Routes of Administration

The drug can be administered by the oral or intravenous route. The recommended dose by either route is the same, 50–100 mg/kg/day divided into four doses. Significant dose reductions are necessary in neonates (*see* above). Marked variations in individual patient kinetics necessitate the monitoring of serum concentrations and appropriate adjustments in dosage.

Therapeutic Applications

The most important indication for chloramphenicol therapy is in the pediatric patient with a probable or proven serious *Haemophilus* infection. Because ampicillin resistance is now common (10–40%) among *Haemophilus*, chloramphenicol must be used at the start of therapy, and continued until sensitivity testing indicates that ampicillin is effective against the organism involved.

Chloramphenicol is the drug of choice for the treatment of typhoid fever, and it is also effective in the treatment of rickettsial diseases, brain abscesses, and a variety of anaerobic infections. In the penicillin-allergic patient chloramphenicol is the drug of choice in treating infections caused by *H. influenzae, S. pneumoniae*, and *N. meningitidis*.

CLINDAMYCIN

Lincomycin, the parent compound of clindamycin, was isolated from the fermentation products of a soil streptomycete found in Lincoln, Nebraska, and called *Streptomyces lincolnensis*. Clindamycin is the 7-chloro-7-deoxy derivative of lincomycin. This family of agents is referred to as lincosamides.

Bacterial Susceptibility

The antibacterial activity of the lincosamides is very similar to that of erythromycin (*see* below). Clindamycin is generally more active than lincomycin. These agents show activity against Gram-positive organisms excepting the enterococci, and are inactive against Gram-negative aerobes with the exception of *H. influenzae*. They are also active against anaerobic bacteria, notably the cocci and Gram-negative rods. MICs against representative bacteria are given in Table 55–6.

Pharmacokinetics

Clindamycin hydrochloride is well absorbed from the gastrointestinal tract; a dose of 300 mg produces peak serum concentrations of 4–5 μg/mL, 1–2 hours after administration. The ester, clindamycin palmitate hydrochloride, is available as a suspension. This compound must be hydrolysed *in vivo* to the active base, but serum levels attained with it are nearly the same as those with clindamycin capsules.

The intramuscular and intravenous preparation is a 2-phosphate derivative. It, too, must be converted *in vivo* to its active form. Peak serum concentrations are higher after intravenous administration. After a 300 mg intramuscular dose the mean peak concentration is 4–5 μg/mL. After a similar intravenous dose the mean peak concentration is 14–15 μg/mL.

The volume of distribution of clindamycin is 0.6–0.75 L/kg. It is 90–95% protein-bound. It is widely distributed in the body and does not appear to be concentrated in any particular organ. Penetration into bone and across the inflamed meninges into the CSF is moderate, the concentrations reaching approximately 40% of those in serum.

After the administered compound is converted to active drug in the serum, biotransformation takes place primarily in the liver. Two metabolic derivatives are a demethyl and a sulfoxide form. The former is more active, and the latter is less active, than the base.

The main organ of clindamycin elimination is the liver, with only 8–28% of the drug being excreted in the urine. Thus, hepatic insufficiency has a more profound effect on clindamycin kinetics than does renal insufficiency. The half-life of clindamycin is normally 2–4 hours.

Adverse Reactions

Gastrointestinal disturbances represent the most important group of adverse reactions to clindamycin. Diarrhea, which is self-limited and subsides with discontinuance of therapy, occurs in up to 30% of cases. It may be associated with nausea, vomiting, and/or abdominal cramps. A more significant gastrointestinal side effect is pseudomembranous colitis. This relatively rare side effect, which occurs among clindamycin recipients at an estimated frequency variously reported as 1:10 to 1:10,000, was first described in association with this antibiotic. It is caused by overgrowth of toxin-producing *Clostridium difficile* in the feces. The varied incidence probably reflects the inconsistent presence of *C. difficile* in stools of patients in different locations and institutions. Almost every antibiotic has now been associated with this reaction.

Minor abnormalities of liver function tests occur with clindamycin use, and cardiovascular collapse has been described after rapid intravenous administration of lincomycin. No significant drug interactions have been reported with these agents.

Dosage Regimens and Routes of Administration

The usual recommended oral dose of clindamycin is 10–25 mg/kg/day, administered in four equal doses. The intravenous or intramuscular daily dose is 10–40 mg/kg, divided into two to four equal doses.

TABLE 55–6   Median MICs (in μg/mL) of Clindamycin and Erythromycin

Bacteria	Clindamycin	Erythromycin
Gram-positive		
Staphylococcus aureus	0.1	0.5
Streptococcus Group A	0.04	0.04
Streptococcus viridans	0.02	0.5
Streptococcus faecalis	100.0	1.5
Streptococcus pneumoniae	0.01	0.1
Gram-negative		
Neisseria meningitidis	12.5	0.78
Neisseria gonorrhoeae	3.1	0.94
Haemophilus influenzae	12.5	2.5
Salmonella	>100	>100
Shigella	>100	>100
Klebsiella	>100	>100
Escherichia coli	>100	>100
Pseudomonas aeruginosa	>100	>100
Proteus mirabilis	>100	>100
Serratia marcescens	>100	>100
Bacteroides fragilis	0.1	1.6
Other Bacteroides	0.1	1.0

Therapeutic Applications

Clindamycin is primarily useful in the treatment of a variety of anaerobic infections, including those caused by *B. fragilis*. Some examples of anaerobic infections that have been successfully treated with clindamycin, either alone or in combination with other antimicrobial agents, include intra-abdominal and pelvic infections, aspiration pneumonia, anaerobic pleuropulmonary infections, infected decubitus ulcers, and periodontal disease.

Clindamycin is a useful antibiotic in a variety of staphylococcal and streptococcal infections as an alternative to a penicillin, and the drug is also extensively used in the antibacterial treatment of acne vulgaris.

ERYTHROMYCIN

Erythromycin was discovered in 1952 in the metabolic products of a strain of *Streptomyces erythreus*, originally obtained from a soil sample collected in the Philippine Archipelago. It is a macrolide antibiotic, so named because it contains a many-membered lactone ring to which are attached deoxy sugars.

Bacterial Susceptibility

The antibacterial activity of erythromycin is very similar to that of clindamycin (*see* above). The agent is generally active against Gram-positive aerobes including most enterococci, and Gram-positive anaerobes. It is generally inactive against Gram-negative aerobes with the exceptions of *Neisseria* species, *Haemophilus*, *Bordetella*, *Campylobacter*, and *Legionella*. The Gram-negative anaerobes are not reliably sensitive. Erythromycin is also active against *Rickettsia*, *M. pneumoniae*, *Ureaplasma*, and *Chlamydia*. MICs against representative bacteria are shown in Table 55–6.

Pharmacokinetics

Erythromycin base is adequately absorbed from the gastrointestinal tract, although its activity is destroyed by gastric juice, and food in the stomach delays its absorption. These problems are overcome by enclosing the drug in acid-resistant capsules or by administering a stearate derivative. Another derivative, erythromycin estolate, is less susceptible to acid than the base, and food does not appreciably alter its absorption. Peak serum concentrations of erythromycin range from 0.5 to 1 µg/mL after a 500 mg oral dose of erythromycin base or stearate. Peak serum concentrations are two to four times higher when an equivalent dose of the estolate preparation is given. After intravenous administration of 500 mg of erythromycin, serum concentrations are approximately 5 µg/mL.

The volume of distribution of erythromycin is approximately 0.7 L/kg, and it is 70–75% protein-bound. It is distributed throughout the body water and tends to be retained longer in the liver and spleen than in the blood. Only very low levels are attained in the CSF even in the presence of inflamed meninges.

Only a small amount of erythromycin is excreted in its original form. It is presumed that the remainder is demethylated or otherwise degraded. Excretion occurs in both the urine and the bile, but only a fraction of the dose can be accounted for in this way. As noted above, a considerable amount is inactivated in the body. The half-life of erythromycin is approximately 1.5 hours.

Adverse Reactions

Gastrointestinal side effects, including nausea, vomiting, diarrhea, and abdominal cramps, are frequent after oral erythromycin.

Hepatotoxicity, which has been clearly documented with the estolate preparation only, is felt to be due to the propionyl ester linkage. Manifestations may include jaundice, fever, pruritus, rash, increased liver size, and eosinophilia. Liver histology reveals a hypersensitivity cholestasis with or without necrosis. This adverse reaction generally resolves when the antibiotic is discontinued.

Thrombophlebitis is a common side effect after intravenous administration. Ototoxicity, manifested as tinnitus and transient deafness, is a rare adverse reaction that has occurred more frequently after intravenous than after oral administration. No significant drug interactions of erythromycin have been reported.

Dosage Regimens and Routes of Administration

The usual recommended oral dose of erythromycin ranges from 20 to 50 mg/kg/day, divided into two to four equal doses. The daily intravenous dose is the same, usually administered in two doses.

Therapeutic Applications

Erythromycin is useful in the treatment of streptococcal and pneumococcal infections in patients who cannot tolerate penicillins. Additional indications for erythromycin therapy include the treatment of *Mycoplasma* infections (*M. pneumoniae* and *Urea-*

plasma), the eradication of *Bordetella pertussis* and *diphtheria* from the nasopharynx, *Chlamydia* infections, the treatment of Legionnaire's disease, the treatment of gonorrhea or syphilis during pregnancy, and in the eradication of *Campylobacter* from the stools of patients with *Campylobacter* gastroenteritis.

SUGGESTED READING

Brittain DC. Erythromycin. Med Clin North Am 1987; 71:1147–1154.

Edson RS, Terrell CL. The aminoglycosides: streptomycin, kanamycin, gentamicin, tobramycin, amikacin, netilmicin, and sisomicin. Mayo Clin Proc 1987; 62:916–920.

Feder HM Jr, Osier C, Maderaza EG. Chloramphenicol: a review of its use in clinical practice. Rev Infect Dis 1981; 3:479–491.

Francke EL, Neu HC. Chloramphenicol and tetracyclines. Med Clin North Am 1987; 71:1155–1168.

Klainer AS. Clindamycin. Ibid. 1987; 71:1169–1176.

Phillips I. Aminoglycosides. Lancet 1982; II:311–314.

Wilson WR, Cockerill FR III. Tetracyclines, chloramphenicol, erythromycin, and clindamycin. Mayo Clin Proc 1987; 62:906–915.

Chapter 56

Drugs Affecting Cellular Nucleic Acid Synthesis

C. Prober and J. Uetrecht

Direct Inhibitors of Nucleic Acid Replication

Rifampin, and perhaps griseofulvin, inhibit the replication of nucleic acids directly. **Rifampin** acts by inhibiting bacterial RNA polymerase, which is concerned with RNA replication. Human DNA-dependent RNA polymerase, on the other hand, is resistant to rifampin. **Nalidixic acid** and the newer **fluoroquinolones** inhibit DNA gyrase, which is responsible for introducing superhelical twists into double-stranded DNA. The superhelical twists facilitate unwinding of the strands, which is necessary for proper binding of certain proteins to DNA, for RNA transcription, and for DNA repair. It has been proposed that **griseofulvin** exerts its antifungal activity by inhibiting fungal DNA production. Griseofulvin also binds to microtubular protein and inhibits mitosis. It is also toxic to mammalian cells, and the basis for useful selective toxicity appears to involve the selective distribution of the drug to keratinized cells, especially those that are diseased.

5-Fluorocytosine (flucytosine) is also thought to inhibit the replication of nucleic acids directly. It appears that this drug enters susceptible yeast cells and is deaminated by cytosine deaminase to the antimetabolite 5-fluorouracil. 5-Fluorouracil is then incorporated instead of uracil into the fungal RNA. The genetic code is misinterpreted and growth stops. In addition, 5-fluorouracil is a close analog of thymine (the methyl group of thymine being replaced by a fluorine) and, after conversion to a deoxynucleotide, it inhibits thymidylate synthetase. 5-Fluorocytosine has a low intrinsic toxicity and the basis for its selective toxicity to yeast cells is its poor conversion to 5-fluorouracil in mammalian cells.

The precise modes of action of the two antituberculous drugs, **isoniazid** and **ethambutol**, are not known, but it is believed that they somehow interfere with the biosynthesis of nucleic acids in mycobacteria. One theory involves the observation that isoniazid is converted to isonicotinic acid by a peroxidase in mycobacteria. The isonicotinic acid appears to interfere with incorporation of nicotinic acid into NAD, which is necessary for the synthesis of mycolic acid, a molecule unique to the cell wall of mycobacteria. Exogenous isonicotinic acid is less effective because it does not penetrate the cell wall of the mycobacteria.

Indirect Inhibitors of Nucleic Acid Replication

Sulfonamides, sulfones, probably **para-aminosalicylic acid**, and the diaminopyrimidines (**trimethoprim** and **pyrimethamine**) inhibit the replication of nucleic acids more remotely by preventing the synthesis of folic acid by microbial cells. Folic acid functions as a coenzyme for the transfer of one-carbon units from one molecule to another, a step necessary for the synthesis of thymidine and the other nucleosides. Mammals require preformed folic acid (it is a vitamin for them; see Chapter 49). In contrast, bacteria can not use preformed folic acid, which can not enter the bacterial cell; instead, they must synthesize it intracellularly from para-aminobenzoic acid (PABA). Sulfonamides act by competitively inhibiting the incorporation of PABA into folic acid. The presence of an extraneous source of PABA (e.g., pus, blood, tissue exudates) can decrease the effectiveness of the sulfonamides as competitive binders. The diaminopyrimidines act as folic acid antagonists by depressing the enzyme dihydrofolic acid reductase, which is responsible for converting dihydrofolic acid to tetrahydrofolic acid (Fig. 56–1). The resulting depletion of folic or tetrahydrofolic acid within the bacterial cells inhibits the formation of coenzymes necessary for the synthesis of purines, pyrimidines, and other substances required for bacterial growth and reproduction. Although this does not usually result in

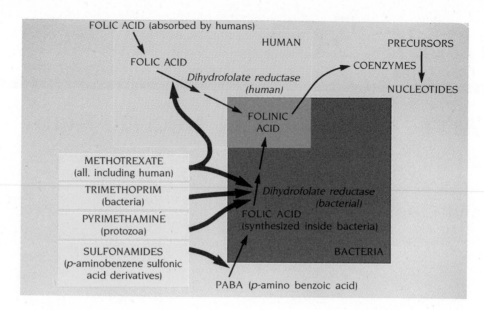

Figure 56–1 Sites of action of sulfonamides and inhibitors of dihydrofolic acid reductase (trimethoprim in bacteria, pyrimethamine in protozoa, methotrexate in all species including human). Because it binds to *human* dihydrofolate reductase, methotrexate is used as an antineoplastic drug of the antimetabolite class (*see* Chapter 60 for structure and mechanism of action).

cell death, the sulfonamides are selectively toxic to bacteria.

ANTIFUNGAL AGENTS

Griseofulvin

Griseofulvin was isolated from *Penicillium griseofulvium* in 1939, but was not used clinically as an antifungal agent until nearly 20 years later.

It inhibits the growth *in vitro* of various species of *Microsporum*, *Epidermophyton*, and *Trichophyton*. Minimum inhibitory concentrations against sensitive fungi range from 0.18 to 0.42 μg/mL.

Pharmacokinetics

Griseofulvin is reasonably well absorbed from the intestinal tract, although there is considerable variability and fluctuation in serum concentration in the same subject, or in different individuals receiving the same dose. A serum concentration of 1–2 μg/mL is attained about 4 hours after a 1 g dose. Concentrations are enhanced approximately two-fold if the drug is taken after a fatty meal rather than fasting.

The volume of distribution and degree of protein binding of this drug are unknown. Its half-life is 10–20 hours, and it reaches the skin, hair, and nails where it is concentrated in keratin.

Most of the absorbed drug is inactivated in the liver by dealkylation. This inactivation may be enhanced by barbiturates through induction of drug-biotransforming enzymes. The inactive metabolite of griseofulvin is excreted in the urine. A considerable proportion of an oral dose, which is unabsorbed, appears unchanged in the feces.

Adverse Reactions

Nausea, vomiting, diarrhea, headache, fatigue, and mental confusion may all occur with griseofulvin therapy but are uncommon.

Drug Interactions

The coadministration of barbiturates may increase the rate of biotransformation of griseofulvin, resulting in reduced serum concentrations.

Griseofulvin itself may induce liver microsomal enzymes and may increase the biotransformation of warfarin, thus diminishing its anticoagulant effect.

Therapeutic Applications

Griseofulvin is effective in the systemic treatment of dermatophyte infections caused by *Microsporum*, *Trichophyton*, and *Epidermophyton*. It is primarily useful in infections of the scalp, hands, feet, and nails, which are refractory to topical therapy.

5-Fluorocytosine (5-FC, Flucytosine)

5-Fluorocytosine was synthetized in 1957 as a cytosine antimetabolite for the treatment of leukemia. It was found to be ineffective for this purpose but was noted in 1964 to possess selective antifungal activity.

Fungal Susceptibility

The drug inhibits *Cryptococcus neoformans* and *Candida albicans* in concentrations of 0.46–3.9 μg/mL and kills them at concentrations of 3.9–15.6 μg/mL. Other fungi that are sensitive to this drug include the non-*albicans* species of *Candida* and *Torulopsis glabrata*. *Aspergillus* species are variably sensitive with MIC ranges of 0.48–500 μg/mL.

Pharmacokinetics

Flucytosine is well absorbed following oral administration. Peak serum concentrations of approximately 45 μg/mL are attained 2–6 hours after a 2 g dose.

The volume of distribution of 5-FC is 0.6–0.7 L/kg. It is approximately 10% protein-bound. It is well distributed in body fluids and tissues, and during the treatment of fungal meningitis it attains concentrations in the CSF that are 50–100% of those in the serum.

A small amount of 5-FC is converted to 5-fluorouracil, and approximately 90% of 5-FC is excreted unchanged *via* the kidney by glomerular filtration. It must be used cautiously in patients with impaired renal function. Unabsorbed 5-FC, usually less than 10%, is excreted unchanged in the feces. Its plasma half-life is 3–4 hours, which may increase to more than 100 hours in the presence of renal disease.

Adverse Reactions

Nausea and vomiting occur frequently. Dose-related hematologic toxicity with leukopenia may occur. Agranulocytosis and aplastic anemia have also been reported. There are no known drug interactions.

Dosage, Route of Administration, and Therapeutic Applications

Flucytosine is administered orally every 6 hours to provide a total daily dose of 50–150 mg/kg. It is most useful in the treatment of cutaneous and mucocutaneous candidiasis, *Candida* urinary tract infections, and in combination with amphotericin B in the treatment of cryptococcal meningitis. It may also play a therapeutic role as a synergistic agent in other systemic fungal infections caused by sensitive organisms.

ANTITUBERCULOUS DRUGS

Rifampin

Rifampin is a complex macrocyclic antibiotic produced by *Streptomyces mediterranei*, which was first isolated in 1959.

Bacterial Susceptibility

The drug is active against a wide range of Gram-positive and Gram-negative organisms (Table 56–1). However, resistance, which may emerge rapidly when it is used alone, limits its widespread use. Its strongest antibacterial attribute is its activity against the majority of *Mycobacterium tuberculosis* strains (MIC = 0.5 μg/mL or less).

Pharmacokinetics

Rifampin is well absorbed from the intestinal tract. A peak concentration of 8 μg/mL is reached approximately 2 hours after a 600 mg oral dose. Serum concentrations are lower if the drug is taken immediately after food.

The volume of distribution of rifampin is approximately 1.6 L/kg. It is 60–90% protein-bound. Rifampin penetrates well into most tissues and fluids including lungs, liver, pleural and ascitic fluid, bone, tears, saliva, and the CSF whether or not the meninges are inflamed. Concentrations in the CSF during therapy for tuber-

TABLE 56–1 Median MICs (in μg/mL) of Rifampin

Gram-positive bacteria	
Staphylococcus aureus	0.001
Streptococcus Group A	0.04
Streptococcus viridans	0.05
Streptococcus faecalis	4.0
Streptococcus pneumoniae	0.05
Gram-negative bacteria	
Neisseria meningitidis	0.016
Neisseria gonorrhoeae	0.2
Haemophilus influenzae	0.5
Klebsiella	10.0
Escherichia coli	5.3
Pseudomonas aeruginosa	20.0
Proteus mirabilis	3.9
Serratia	64.0
Bacteroides fragilis	0.26
Other *Bacteroides*	0.1
Mycobacterium tuberculosis	0.5

CHEMOTHERAPY

culous meningitis usually exceed 50% of serum concentrations.

Rifampin is deacetylated in the liver, and must also be inactivated elsewhere in the body to some extent, as a proportion of the dose remains undetected in excretion studies.

Rifampin is the antibiotic of choice for the chemoprophylaxis of contacts of patients with serious infections caused by *Haemophilus influenzae* and meningococci.

Isoniazid (INH)

Isoniazid was discovered in 1952. It is the hydrazide of isonicotinic acid and has proved to be the most useful antimicrobial agent for the treatment of tuberculosis (Fig. 56-2).

In vitro, INH is both tuberculostatic and tuberculocidal. The minimal tuberculostatic concentration is 0.025–0.05 μg/mL. The tuberculocidal effects of INH are exerted only against actively growing bacilli; resting organisms resume multiplication when drug contact is ended.

Pharmacokinetics

Isoniazid is readily absorbed after oral administration. Peak plasma levels of 1–5 μg/mL are attained 1–2 hours after an oral dose of 5 mg/kg.

The volume of distribution of INH is approximately 0.6 L/kg. It is poorly protein-bound, diffuses readily into all body fluids and cells, and is present, in varying concentrations, in all body organs. Cerebrospinal fluid penetration is variable, but CSF concentrations may be nearly equal to those in serum. Isoniazid penetrates well into the caseous material in the central parts of tubercles (from which the disease gets its name). Infected tissues retain the drug for long periods of time in quantities well above those required for tuberculostasis.

The main method of inactivation is acetylation in the liver by an enzyme, N-acetyltransferase, which converts INH to acetylisoniazid. This in turn is partly hydrolysed to isonicotinic acid and acetylhydrazine. Nonacetylated INH is excreted in the urine in its unchanged form or as its hydrazone conjugates. The rate of INH acetylation is genetically controlled. The amount of INH acetylation metabolites in the urine reflects the acetylator status of the patient. Over 90% of Orientals are rapid acetylators compared to about 45% of Caucasians and Negroes (*see* Chapter 12).

Approximately 70% of administered INH is excreted *via* the kidneys, but most of this is in an inactive form. Slow acetylators excrete about ten times more active INH in the urine than do rapid acetylators. The half-life of INH is 0.5–1.5 hours in rapid acetylators compared with 2–3 hours in slow acetylators.

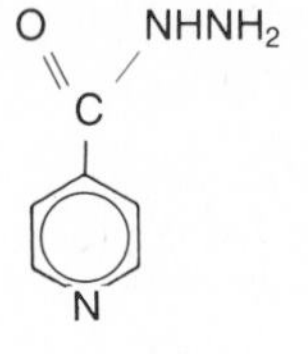

Adverse Reactions

Neurotoxicity and hepatotoxicity are the two most important side effects of INH. The incidence of neurotoxicity is higher in slow acetylators, but acetylator phenotype probably has no bearing on the incidence of hepatotoxicity. It was once thought that patients of the rapid acetylator phenotype had the highest risk of hepatotoxicity because the mechanism appears to involve an acetylhydrazine intermediate; however, although acetylhydrazine is formed more rapidly in rapid acetylators, it is also converted rapidly to nontoxic diacetylhydrazine.

Neurotoxic manifestations, including psychosis, confusion, convulsions, and coma, may occur with overdosage. Peripheral neuropathy may occur at therapeutic doses, but it is more common with larger doses than smaller ones, and in older or malnourished patients with pyridoxine deficiency. The administration of pyridoxine prevents this toxicity.

Hepatotoxicity is an age-related occurrence, being more prevalent in older patients. Hepatitis may progress to hepatocellular necrosis with jaundice if the drug is not discontinued. Alcoholics are more prone to this liver injury. An early transient rise in serum transaminases is noted in about 20% of INH recipients, but this does not, in itself, necessitate discontinuance of INH.

Drug Interactions

Aluminum hydroxide or other antacids may interfere with the absorption of INH. Also, isoniazid may inhibit the metabolism of phenytoin or anticoagulants, thereby causing excessively high serum concentrations and related toxicity.

Dosage Regimen, Route of Administration, and Therapeutic Applications

Isoniazid is usually administered orally in a daily dose of 5–10 mg/kg, divided into two equal doses. If pyridoxine is given concomitantly, its dose is 10 mg for every 100 mg of INH.

Isoniazid is a first-line tuberculocidal drug. It is used in combination with various other antituberculous drugs for the treatment of all types of tuberculosis. Also,

Figure 56-2 Structural formula of isoniazid.

it is the only agent known to be effective in chemoprophylaxis.

It is important to remember that approximately one in 10^6 tubercle bacilli is resistant to isoniazid and one cavitary lesion usually contains 10^7 to 10^9 bacilli; therefore, combination therapy (*e.g.*, isoniazid and rifampin) must be used to treat active disease to prevent the emergence of a resistant infection. This is in contrast to prophylactic therapy in patients with a positive TB skin test, where there are only a few dormant tubercle bacilli present and treatment with isoniazid as a single agent is appropriate.

Ethambutol

This drug was discovered in 1961 when randomly selected compounds were being tested for antituberculous activity. *In vitro* it is active against about 75% of strains of *M. tuberculosis* at a concentration of 1 μg/mL. It is a relatively simple molecule, consisting of two residues of aminobutanol connected by an ethylene bridge.

Pharmacokinetics

Ethambutol is well absorbed after oral administration. Peak serum concentrations of approximately 5 μg/mL are attained about 4 hours after a 15 mg/kg dose.

The volume of distribution of ethambutol approximates 1.5 L/kg. It is 20–30% protein-bound. There are no data available on its distribution to various body tissues. However, it is known that levels equal to 25–50% of the serum concentration are attained in the CSF when the meninges are inflamed.

Between 8% and 15% of absorbed ethambutol is converted to various inactive metabolites, which are excreted in the urine together with approximately 80% of absorbed drug in its active unchanged form. About 20% of an oral dose is unabsorbed and excreted unchanged in the feces.

Adverse Reactions

The most important adverse reaction to ethambutol is a **reversible retrobulbar neuropathy**, which results in defective red-green vision and eventual field constriction or blindness. The incidence of this reaction increases with increasing doses, reaching approximately 5% of patients at 25–50 mg/kg/day.

Dosage Regimen, Route of Administration, and Therapeutic Applications

Ethambutol is administered orally as a single daily dose of 15 mg/kg. Its main use is in combination with other antimicrobial agents to treat infections caused by *M. tuberculosis*. It is sometimes also used in the treatment of infections caused by atypical mycobacteria.

Para-Aminosalicylic Acid (PAS)

In 1940 and 1941 it was demonstrated that benzoic and salicylic acids increased the oxygen consumption of tubercle bacilli. It was speculated that similar compounds played a role in the normal metabolism of *M. tuberculosis*, and it was theorized that related substances might have an opposite effect. This led to the discovery of PAS, a drug that is chemically closely related to salicylic acid, and probably acts as a competitive antagonist of *p*-aminobenzoic acid.

Pharmacokinetics

PAS is well absorbed from the intestinal tract. Maximum serum concentrations of 50–150 μg/mL are attained 1–2 hours after a 2 g dose. The drug is 50–60% protein-bound. It is distributed throughout the total body water and reaches concentrations in the pleural fluid and in caseous tissues approximately equal to those in the circulation. It does not yield effective CSF concentrations, possibly because it is actively transported out of the CSF.

PAS is biotransformed in the liver mainly by acetylation. Over 80% of the drug is excreted in the urine by glomerular filtration and tubular secretion. Only 14–33% of the total dose is excreted in the urine as the active unchanged drug. The remainder is excreted as metabolites such as acetyl-*p*-aminosalicylic acid, *p*-aminosalicyluric acid, and other conjugated amines. The half-life of PAS is less than 1 hour.

Adverse Reactions

Nausea, vomiting, anorexia, abdominal cramps, and diarrhea occur to some extent in nearly all patients. These may be reduced by taking the drug with meals, or by the concomitant administration of antacids.

Drug Interactions

Para-aminosalicylic acid may enhance the effect of anticoagulants and inhibit the biotransformation of acetylsalicylic acid, thereby allowing toxic amounts to accumulate. Probenecid may inhibit tubular secretion of PAS, and PAS may impair the absorption of rifampin.

Dosage Regimen, Route of Administration, and Therapeutic Applications

The usual daily dose of PAS is 200–300 mg/kg administered orally, divided into two or three doses. This drug is useful as a second or third agent, in combination with other more effective agents, in the treatment of infections caused by *M. tuberculosis*. It may have a role in the initial treatment of such infections in young children who cannot be monitored effectively for the ocular toxicities of ethambutol.

QUINOLONE ANTIBACTERIAL AGENTS

The prototype drug is **nalidixic acid**, an old drug with limited use as a urinary antiseptic. The development of fluoroquinolones has greatly extended the antibacterial spectrum and usefulness of these agents. Two examples of the fluoroquinolones are **norfloxacin** and **ciprofloxacin**.

Bacterial Susceptibility

Nalidixic acid is active against most Gram-negative bacteria, excluding *Pseudomonas aeruginosa*, but it is inactive against all Gram-positive organisms. Nalidixic acid (Fig. 56–3) is bacteriostatic. Addition of a fluorine and removal of the ethyl side-group yields norfloxacin. The fluoroquinolones show activity against Gram-positive organisms and increased activity against Gram-negative organisms. The fluoroquinolones also are bactericidal. Their spectrum of activity includes *Staphylococcus aureus* (including methicillin-resistant strains), most streptococci, enterococci, and most other Gram-

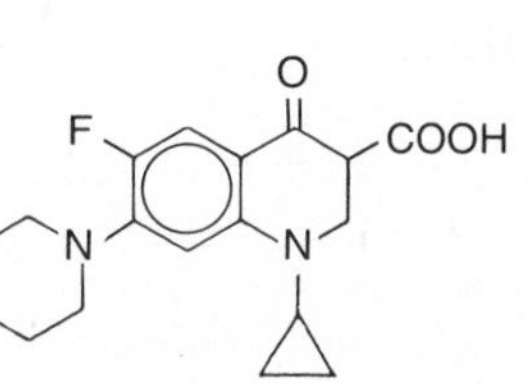

Nalidixic Acid

Ciprofloxacin

Figure 56–3 Structural formulae of nalidixic acid and ciprofloxacin.

negative enteric organisms, *H. influenzae*, and *Neisseria gonorrhoeae*. Addition of a piperazine ring, as in ciprofloxacin, increases fluoroquinolone activity against *Pseudomonas*.

Pharmacokinetics

The fluoroquinolones are well absorbed when given orally; they are available for both oral and parenteral administration. They penetrate well into most body fluids. The half-lives of norfloxacin and ciprofloxacin are about 4 hours, and these agents need be administered only every 8–12 hours. Elimination is about half by renal excretion and half by biotransformation, and the dose may need to be adjusted in renal and hepatic failure.

Adverse Reactions

Experience with the fluoroquinolones is still somewhat limited, but serious reactions appear to be uncommon. Seizure activity has occurred in patients treated with either norfloxacin or ciprofloxacin. Gastrointestinal disturbance (nausea and vomiting) is the most common side effect. Since the fluoroquinolones inhibit DNA gyrase, DNA damage is possible, but these agents do not appear to cause tumors in animals.

Therapeutic Applications

The major indication for the fluoroquinolones at the present time is for the treatment of urinary tract infections. Norfloxacin is very effective in the treatment of gonorrhea but does not eradicate concomitant *Chlamydia trachomatis*. However, newer agents have increased activity against *Chlamydia*. These appear to be very effective in treating pulmonary infections in patients with cystic fibrosis and in treating osteomyelitis. They decrease the need for hospitalization in these conditions since they can be given orally. The full potential of the fluoroquinolones is yet to be determined.

ANTIFOLS

Sulfonamides

Sulfonamides were the first group of synthetic antibacterial compounds for systemic use, based on Ehrlich's concepts of selective toxicity as outlined in Chapter 52. The original studies of the clinical effectiveness of sulfanilamide were reported by Domagk in 1935. At first, the claims pertained only to infections caused by hemolytic streptococci, but soon, with modifications of the molecule, activity against a wider range of bacteria was demonstrated.

Chemistry

All sulfonamides are amides of *p*-aminobenzenesulfonic acid (Fig. 56–4). Three basic features necessary for antibacterial action are: (1) a benzene ring with a sulfonic acid group, (2) an amide nitrogen on the sulfonic acid, and (3) a free amino group in the para position. The activity of the sulfonamides is also dependent on a negative charge on the amide nitrogen such that it mimics the carboxylate anion of *p*-aminobenzoic acid.

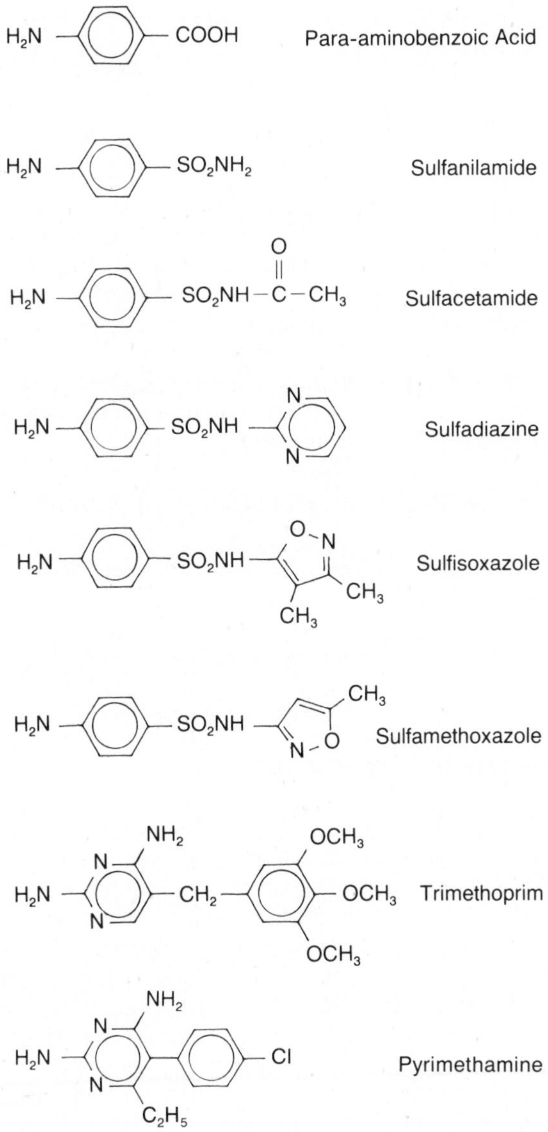

Figure 56–4 Structural formulae of para-aminobenzoic acid, some sulfonamides, trimethoprim, and pyrimethamine.

The free amino group in the para position represents the primary site of sulfonamide degradation.

Bacterial Susceptibility

The sulfonamides originally had a wide range of activity, but this range has been seriously compromised by acquired bacterial resistance. Gram-positive bacteria that are usually sensitive to sulfonamides include Group A streptococci, *Streptococcus viridans*, some *Streptococcus pneumoniae*, and *Nocardia*. Staphylococci are variably sensitive and *Streptococcus faecalis* is resistant. The most sensitive Gram-negative species are the *Neisseria*, many enterobacteria, *H. influenzae*, and *Bordetella pertussis*. Some representative bacteria and their median MICs are outlined in Table 56–2. Sulfonamides are also active against *Chlamydia*, *Toxoplasma*, and some *Plasmodium* species.

Pharmacokinetics

The sulfonamides are often classified on the basis of their pharmacokinetics, specifically on the basis of their half-lives. Hence, there are short-acting, medium-acting, long-acting, and ultra-long-acting forms. There are also those that are poorly absorbed from the intestinal tract. Some examples of the various forms of sulfonamides are listed in Table 56–3. These drugs are described below as a group, using sulfisoxazole (a widely used short-acting sulfonamide) as a representative. Where important differences exist between various agents, they are specifically noted below.

All sulfonamides (excepting sulfaguanidine and the other poorly absorbable derivatives) are well absorbed

TABLE 56–2 Median MICs (in μg/mL) of Sulfonamides and Trimethoprim

Bacteria	Sulfonamides*	Trimethoprim
Gram-positive		
Staphylococcus aureus	50.0	0.2
Streptococcus Group A	12.5	0.4
Streptococcus viridans	8.0	0.25
Streptococcus faecalis	100.0	1.0
Streptococcus pneumoniae	32.0	1.0
Gram-negative		
Neisseria meningitidis	5.0	8.0
Neisseria gonorrhoeae	4.0	12.0
Haemophilus influenzae	0.5	0.12
Salmonella	10.0	0.4
Shigella	4.0	0.4
Klebsiella	16.0	0.5
Escherichia coli	8.0	0.2
Pseudomonas aeruginosa	25.0	>100
Nocardia	12.5	>100

* Variations between individual sulfonamides occur.

TABLE 56–3 Forms of Sulfonamides*

Short-acting	Sulfanilamide
	Sulfacetamide
	Sulfadiazine
	Sulfisoxazole
Medium-acting	Sulfamethoxazole
Long-acting	Sulfamethoxypyridazine
	Sulfadimethoxine
Ultra-long-acting	Sulfadoxine
Poorly absorbable	Sulfaguanidine
	Sulfasalazine

* Not all of these drugs are official in all countries; currently preferred usage for the absorbable sulfonamides is in fixed-dose combination with trimethoprin.

after oral administration. Serum concentrations vary somewhat between the sulfonamides. The peak concentrations of sulfisoxazole after a 1 g dose range from 50 to 100 μg/mL. Intravenously injectable sulfonamides attain high plasma concentrations extremely well.

The sulfonamides are generally well distributed throughout the body, including the CSF. There is some variation in this distribution between individual agents. For instance, CSF concentrations of sulfisoxazole are approximately 30% of those in the serum, whereas the CSF concentrations of sulfadiazine are about 50% of serum concentrations. The volume of distribution of the sulfonamides is small, that of sulfisoxazole being 0.16–0.2 L/kg. Protein binding is very variable amongst these agents, ranging from 20% for some of the short-acting forms to over 90% for the long-acting drugs.

A percentage of the absorbed sulfonamide is acetylated in the liver to inactive conjugates. Individual acetylating capacity is variable in a manner analogous to that for INH. Some sulfonamides also undergo glucuronide conjugation to inactive metabolites in the liver.

Free and conjugated sulfonamides are excreted *via* the kidneys by both glomerular filtration and tubular secretion. The long-acting forms, which are more extensively protein-bound, undergo more complete tubular reabsorption and hence have prolonged half-lives. Since the sulfonamides and their metabolites are weak acids, their clearance is increased in alkaline urine. Minimal amounts of sulfonamides are excreted in the bile. Half-lives of the sulfonamides range from 2 hours to as much as 200 hours, depending on the individual agent. The half-life of sulfisoxazole is 5–6 hours.

Adverse Reactions

Hypersensitivity reactions ranging from a mild rash to severe Stevens-Johnson syndrome may occur. The latter reaction is an extreme form of erythema multiforme, characterized by bulla formation in the mouth, pharynx, anogenital region, and conjunctivae. Though rare, it produces serious morbidity when it does occur. It is more common in children, especially with long-acting sulfonamides.

Hematologic toxicity may also occur with sulfonamide use. Reactions include agranulocytosis, which is usually reversible on discontinuance of the drug, and hemolytic anemia in patients with G-6-PD deficiency. Aplastic anemia has also been described as a rare complication.

In the neonate, sulfonamides are contraindicated because they may displace bilirubin from protein binding sites and hence predispose these patients to the development of jaundice and even kernicterus (*see* Chapter 68).

Renal damage was common with older forms of sulfonamides that were poorly water-soluble. Patients developed crystalluria, which led to obstruction and hematuria. However, this reaction is rare with the more soluble congeners in use today. Nevertheless, renal damage on the basis of hypersensitivity may still be observed.

Drug Interactions

Sulfonamides may augment the action of oral hypoglycemic agents by displacing them from protein. Transient accentuation of hypoprothrombinemia may be observed when sulfonamides are given together with oral anticoagulants, because of displacement of the anticoagulant from protein binding sites and also perhaps because of inhibition of their biotransformation. Sulfonamides may also interfere with the biotransformation of phenytoin, with resultant increased serum concentrations of that drug.

Dosage Regimens and Routes of Administration

The usual daily dose of sulfisoxazole is 120–150 mg/kg orally, divided into four to six doses. Daily dosages, routes, and frequency of administration of some other commonly used sulfonamides are outlined in Table 56–4.

Therapeutic Applications

Common clinical uses of the sulfonamides include the treatment of acute, uncomplicated urinary tract infections; *Chlamydia* infections; *Nocardia* infections including those in the lung and central nervous system; *Toxoplasma* infections (in combination with pyrimethamine); and chloroquine-resistant *Plasmodium falciparum* malaria (in combination with pyrimethamine). The sulfonamides are also used prophylactically in patients with rheumatic fever who are allergic to penicillin; in contacts of patients with meningococcal infections, if the pathogen is known in advance to be sulfonamide-sensitive; and as a prophylactic agent for children with frequently recurring bouts of acute suppurative otitis media.

TABLE 56–4 Representative Sulfonamide Dosage Regimens

Agent*	Usual Daily Dose (mg/kg)	Route of Administration	Usual Number of Doses per Day
Sulfadiazine	120–150	oral	4–6
	100	intravenous	3–4
Sulfamethizole	30–45	oral	4
Sulfamethoxazole	50–60	oral	2

* Representative drugs; sulfamethizole is not official in Canada; sulfadiazine and sulfamethoxazole are available in fixed-dose combination with trimethoprim.

Trimethoprim

This drug, a 2,4-diaminopyrimidine, was first synthesized in 1956 as a result of a planned systematic study. It was designed at first as an antibacterial agent, but it was subsequently found to have valuable antiparasitic activity also.

Bacterial Susceptibility

Trimethoprim has an antibacterial spectrum similar to that of the sulfonamides, although it is more active than the sulfonamides against most bacterial species with the exception of *Neisseria*, *Brucella*, and *Nocardia*. The enterococci, which are resistant to the sulfonamides, are sensitive to trimethoprim, as are malaria parasites (*see* Chapter 57). The comparative activities of trimethoprim and the sulfonamides are shown in Table 56–2. As may be expected from its mechanism of action (*see* Fig. 56–1), trimethoprim is synergistic with sulfonamides against many bacterial species.

Pharmacokinetics

Trimethoprim is well absorbed from the gastrointestinal tract. A peak serum concentration of about 2 μg/mL is attained 1–2 hours after a 160 mg oral dose.

After absorption, trimethoprim is rapidly distributed in the body, and tissue concentrations often exceed serum concentrations except in the brain, skin, and fat. Its apparent volume of distribution is greater than total body water. Trimethoprim is 42–46% protein-bound.

A substantial proportion of trimethoprim is converted in the liver to at least five inactive metabolites, all of which are excreted in the urine. The amount of active (unchanged) drug excreted by this route during a 24-hour period ranges from 42% to 75% of an administered dose. A small amount of trimethoprim is excreted *via* the bile. The serum half-life is about 13 hours.

Adverse Reactions

Trimethoprim may cause nausea and diarrhea, especially at high doses. On rare occasions trimethoprim may also be associated with various blood dyscrasias, including agranulocytosis, thrombocytopenia, and anemia. Inhibition of folate synthesis leading to anemia is a problem only in patients who are already folate-deficient and who are receiving large doses of the drug. This anemia is reversible with the administration of folates, preferably folinic acid, and these measures do not interfere with the antibacterial/antiparasitic effects of the drug. Trimethoprim may inhibit creatinine secretion and thus increase the serum creatinine concentration. Adverse reactions are more common when trimethoprim is administered in combination with a sulfonamide (*e.g.*, sulfamethoxazole). The incidence of serious toxicity from this combination is especially high (about 50%) in patients with AIDS. The mechanism of this interaction is unknown.

Dosage Regimens and Routes of Administration

Trimethoprim is most commonly administered in a **fixed 1:5 ratio with sulfamethoxazole** (co-trimoxazole) or **sulfadiazine** (co-trimazine). The usual dose of the trimethoprim contained in these combinations ranges from 5 to 20 mg/kg/day, with the specific dose determined by the infecting organism and the severity of the infection. The combinations may be administered orally or intravenously, divided into two to four equal doses. An oral preparation of trimethoprim alone is also available. Its usual daily dose is 4 mg/kg, divided into two equal doses.

Therapeutic Applications

The combination of trimethoprim with a sulfonamide (*e.g.*, co-trimoxazole) is used extensively for the treatment of a variety of infections including urinary tract infections, prostatitis, exacerbations of chronic bronchitis, sinusitis, otitis media, shigellosis, salmonella bacteremias, traveller's diarrhea, nocardiasis, and *Pneumocystis carinii* pneumonitis (PCP). Septicemia and meningitis caused by multiply-resistant Gram-negative aerobes (*e.g.*, *Serratia marcescens* and *Pseudomonas cepacia*) have also been treated successfully with this combination. In addition, the combination of agents is often used prophylactically in patients with recurrent urinary tract infections, in immunocompromised patients at risk for PCP, and in neutropenic hosts to reduce the incidence of serious bacterial infections.

Trimethoprim alone appears to be as effective as the combination for many of the indications noted above including the treatment and prevention of urinary tract infections, for prophylaxis in neutropenic hosts, and for the treatment of lower respiratory tract infections excluding those caused by *Pneumocystis carinii*.

Pyrimethamine

This drug, which was first synthesized in 1951, is very similar to trimethoprim, also being a 2,4-diaminopyrimidine (*see* Fig. 56–4). It is more specific than trimethoprim in its activity against protozoal dihydrofolate reductases and is therefore useful in the treatment of protozoal infections. It is primarily active against *P. falciparum* and *Toxoplasma gondii* with lesser activity against other *Plasmodium* species.

Pharmacokinetics

Pyrimethamine is completely and regularly absorbed from the intestinal tract. Blood concentrations are prolonged and urinary excretion may persist for 30 days or more. Between 20% and 30% is excreted unchanged in the urine. The half-life is approximately 36 hours.

Adverse Reactions

Pyrimethamine binds to mammalian enzyme systems more strongly than trimethoprim; it is therefore more toxic. **Gastrointestinal** disturbances are common, and **hematologic** toxic effects such as megaloblastic anemia, leukopenia, and thrombocytopenia may occur if daily doses are administered without the concomitant administration of folinic acid.

Dosage Regimens, Route of Administration, and Therapeutic Applications

The drug is administered orally in one daily dose or divided into two equal doses. The total daily dose is 0.5–1 mg/kg, up to a maximum of 25 mg/day. The drug is given daily for the treatment of toxoplasmosis or malaria, and every second week for the prophylaxis of malaria. *See* Chapter 57 for its specific use (also in combination with a sulfonamide) in *P. falciparum* malaria.

Sulfones

The major sulfones used clinically are **dapsone (DDS)** and its water-soluble derivative **sulfoxone sodium**. Their mechanism of action is probably identical to that of the sulfonamides. Dapsone was first used against streptococcal infections, but is now used for the treatment of leprosy, dermatitis herpetiformis, malaria, and Brown Recluse spider bites rather than common bacterial infections.

Pharmacokinetics

Dapsone is slowly but almost completely absorbed from the gastrointestinal tract. Absorption of sulfoxone is less but it causes less gastric distress. Sulfoxone is hydrolysed to dapsone, which is the active agent. Distribution to most tissues is very good and the drug can accumulate in the skin, muscle, liver, and kidney. The major pathways of transformation involve N-acetylation and N-oxidation, which are reversible, and N-glucuronidation and N-sulfation, which lead to urinary excretion.

Adverse Reactions

The sulfones are aromatic amines, and their most common untoward effect, which occurs in most patients who are treated with 200–300 mg/day, is hemolysis of varying degree. Methemoglobinemia is also common. Anorexia, nausea, and vomiting can limit the use of dapsone, and sulfoxone is often better tolerated. An infectious mononucleosis-like syndrome occurs occasionally and can be fatal.

Therapeutic Applications

Dapsone is the primary drug used in the treatment of **leprosy**. The emergence of resistant strains has forced the search for alternate drugs. As mentioned earlier, dapsone can also be used in the treatment of chloroquine-resistant malaria, dermatitis herpetiformis, and Brown Recluse spider bites.

SUGGESTED READING

Cockerill FR III, Edson RS. Trimethoprim-sulfamethoxazole. Mayo Clin Proc 1987; 62:921–929.

Foltzer MA, Reese RE. Trimethoprim-sulfamethoxazole and other sulfonamides. Med Clin North Am 1987; 71:1177–1194.

Medoff G, Brajtburg J, Kobayashi GS, Bolard J. Antifungal agents useful in therapy of systemic fungal infections. Annu Rev Pharmacol Toxicol 1983; 23:303–330.

Reeves D. Sulphonamides and trimethoprim. Lancet 1982; II:370–373.

Sanders WE Jr. Rifampin. Annu Rev Intern Med 1976; 85:82–86.

Van Scoy RE, Wilkowske CJ. Antituberculosis agents. Mayo Clin Proc 1987; 62:1129–1136.

Chapter 57

Chemotherapy of Common Parasitic Infections

J.S. Keystone and J. Tetiuk

For organisms not covered in this section, students are referred to standard parasitology textbooks and the *Medical Letter Handbook*.

PROTOZOAN INFECTIONS

Amebiasis

Amebiasis is an intestinal infection by the protozoan *Entamoeba histolytica*. In the large bowel, the organisms are found in two forms: cyst and trophozoite. The motile trophozoite is the vegetative form, which maintains the infection by replication. Under an unknown stimulus, trophozoites, which normally live as commensals, will invade the intestinal mucosa and give rise to amebic colitis. Hematogenous spread to liver, lung, or brain may result in the formation of an amebic abscess. Under adverse conditions, trophozoites develop a protective covering and transform themselves into cysts. Cysts are transmitted by the fecal-oral route *via* flies, fingers, food, or fornication.

Amebicides can be divided clinically into two groups: those acting in the intestinal lumen, and those acting in the tissue.

Agents Acting in the Lumen

These agents act directly on organisms in the lumen of the bowel. They are often poorly absorbed from the intestine and are used primarily for eradicating the infection at that site. These drugs cannot eradicate trophozoites that have invaded the intestinal wall and beyond. Such drugs include halogenated quinolines, arsenical preparations, and diloxanide furoate.

Halogenated hydroxyquinoline derivatives. The only currently available agent is **diiodohydroxyquin**, a moderately effective and safe antiamebic compound. It functions by inactivating the enzymes or halogenating the proteins of the ameba. The drug is partially absorbed and can produce marked elevations of blood iodine levels. A previously available derivative, iodochlorhydroxyquin, was withdrawn from the Canadian market because of the problem of subacute myelo-optic neuropathy, which occurred after prolonged use of the drug.

Arsenical preparations. The administration of arsenicals involves the potential hazard of arsenic intoxication with resulting gastrointestinal symptoms, cutaneous disturbances, and drug-induced hepatitis. Arsenicals are contraindicated if renal or hepatic disease is present. In therapeutic doses, toxic symptoms are rarely observed. Arsenicals are excreted slowly, and hence prolonged use may lead to cumulative effects.

These drugs are very effective against the nonpathogenic amebae *Dientamoeba fragilis*, *Endolimax nana*, *Entamoeba coli*, *Entamoeba hartmanni* and *Iodamoeba bütschlii*, and also against whipworm (*Trichuris trichiura*).

The available arsenicals include **diphetarsone** and **carbarsone**. They are classified as emergency drugs in Canada, available with the authorization of the Health Protection Branch, Health and Welfare Canada.

Diloxanide furoate. This is a safe and highly effective agent for the eradication of *E. histolytica*. Toxicity is rare, but mild abdominal discomfort, increased flatulence, and occasional allergic reactions have been encountered.

Agents Acting in the Tissues

These substances act directly on organisms that have invaded tissues. Therefore, unlike those acting in the lumen, they must be well absorbed and reach high concentrations in tissue. Metronidazole has now replaced emetine, its less toxic analog dehydroemetine, and chloroquine as treatment for invasive amebiasis.

In asymptomatic persons passing cysts or trophozoites, in whom invasion has presumably not occurred, a lumen-active agent is all that is required. For symptomatic invasive amebiasis (intestinal or extra-intestinal) a drug acting in the tissues **plus** one acting in the lumen is needed.

Metronidazole (Flagyl®).   Metronidazole has been considered the drug of choice for the treatment of vaginitis caused by *Trichomonas vaginalis*, and it is also effective against the protozoan *Giardia lamblia* and some anaerobic bacteria such as *Bacteroides fragilis*. Although metronidazole has been promoted as being efficacious against all stages of amebiasis, it appears to be poorly effective in the lumen, but an excellent agent in the tissues. It is currently the drug of choice for invasive amebiasis, and should be used together with a lumen-active agent. A parenteral form of the drug is now available. Common adverse effects include nausea, vomiting, diarrhea, headache, and a metallic taste in the mouth. Alcohol should not be consumed during treatment with metronidazole because of a possible disulfiram-like reaction.

Recently, concern has been expressed about the ability of metronidazole to cause cancer and birth defects in experimental animals as well as gene mutations in bacteria. In high and prolonged dosage, it is carcinogenic in mice. It has been regarded by some clinicians as potentially dangerous in humans, although there are no data to support this claim. The drug should not be used for trivial indications.

Antibiotic amebicides.   These agents are transiently effective and act by altering the bowel flora, thereby depriving the amebae of nutrient. When they are used alone, relapses are frequent. Antibiotics such as **tetracyclines** and **paromomycin** are adjunct therapy, especially useful for symptomatic relief of severe amebic dysentery. Paromomycin also may be used as a lumen-active medication.

Giardiasis

This is an infection of the small bowel with the flagellate protozoan *Giardia lamblia*. The parasite resides in the upper part of the small intestine and exists in two forms: the trophozoite and the cyst. The latter is the infective stage of the parasite. The trophozoite, with its ventral sucking disc, is responsible for the damage to the upper small bowel. Water-borne epidemics have occurred as well as person-to-person transmission by the fecal-oral route. There is no invasion beyond the bowel lumen.

Metronidazole.   *See* above.

Quinacrine (Mepacrine) HCl (Atabrine®).   This drug is as effective as metronidazole in the treatment of giardiasis, but has potentially more adverse effects. These include gastrointestinal upset, psychosis, seizures (in predisposed patients), exfoliative dermatitis, and transient yellow discoloration of the skin. The drug is poorly tolerated in children, and like metronidazole it has a very bitter taste.

Furazolidone (Furoxone®).   This drug is the only liquid preparation available that is easy to administer and is well tolerated by children. It is no longer marketed in Canada, but is available as an emergency drug.

Malaria

Malarial parasites are protozoan organisms of the genus *Plasmodium*. Four species infect man: *Plasmodium falciparum* (malignant tertian malaria); *Plasmodium vivax* (benign tertian malaria); *Plasmodium malariae* (quartan malaria); and *Plasmodium ovale*.

Sporozoites are inoculated into humans from the salivary glands of a feeding female *Anopheles* mosquito. The organisms multiply in the liver and form tissue schizonts (**preerythrocytic stage**). The schizonts rupture and release merozoites into the blood stream. In *P. vivax* and *P. ovale* malaria only, some merozoites (hypnozoites) may lie dormant (**exoerythrocytic stage**) and later cause a relapse of malaria. This stage is not present in *P. falciparum* and *P. malariae*, which have a single passage through the liver. Merozoites released from the liver invade red cells and develop through a trophozoite into a schizont stage (**erythrocytic stage**). The red cell schizont ruptures and most of the released merozoites invade new red cells. Some merozoites develop into male and female gametocytes, which are ingested by mosquitoes that feed on the malaria patient. Mating of these gametocytes in the mosquito gut leads to sporozoite production and a completion of the malaria cycle (Fig. 57–1).

The modern classification of antimalarial drugs is based on the stage of the *Plasmodium* life cycle upon which the drugs act.

1.   **Tissue schizonticides:** Primaquine acts in the liver on the hypnozoite (exoerythrocytic phase) of *P. vivax* and *P. ovale*. Chlorguanide (proguanil) and pyrimethamine act in the liver on the preerythrocytic phase of *P. falciparum* only, whereas tetracycline acts on the preerythrocytic phase of all species.

2.   **Blood schizonticides:** Quinine, chloroquine, chlorguanide, pyrimethamine, sulfonamides, sulfones, clindamycin, and tetracycline act in the blood on the erythrocytic phase of all four species.

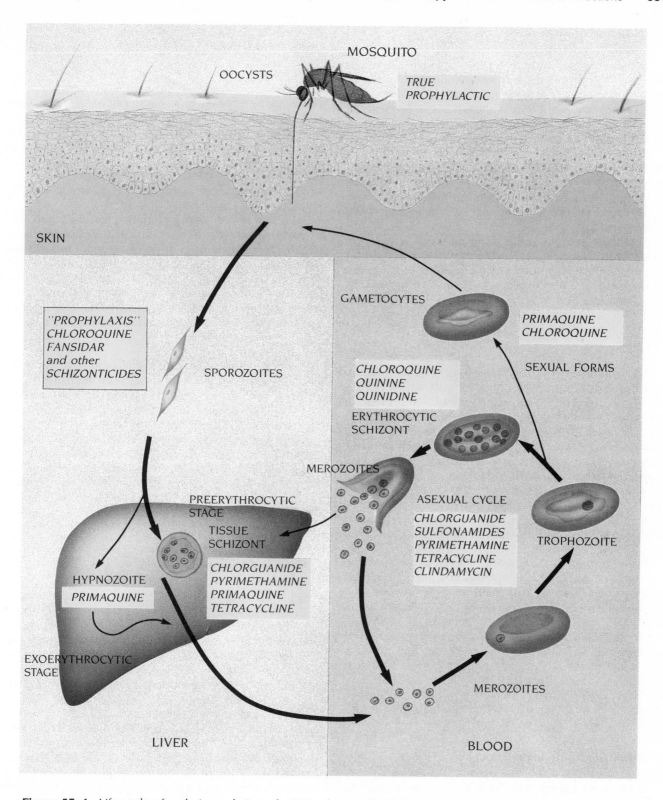

Figure 57–1 Life cycle of malaria, and sites of action of antimalarial drugs.

Tissue Schizonticides

Primaquine. Primaquine is at present the most effective member of a group of 8-aminoquinolines that destroy the exoerythrocytic (hepatic) forms of malaria. Its primary use is not in prophylaxis but in eradication of dormant hypnozoites of *P. vivax* and *P. ovale* after chloroquine has been used to clear the erythrocytic forms during a clinical attack of malaria. However, the drug can be used prophylactically to prevent late relapses of *P. vivax* in those who return from areas where *P. vivax* is highly endemic. *Plasmodium ovale* is so rare that prophylactic use of primaquine is unnecessary.

Hemolytic anemia is the principal adverse reaction associated with primaquine therapy. It is related to a genetic abnormality known as glucose-6-phosphate dehydrogenase (G-6-PD) deficiency, in which the red cells of susceptible persons (Mediterraneans, blacks, Asians, and Orientals) show a defect in the mechanisms that protect hemoglobin from denaturation (*see* also Chapter 12).

Chlorguanide (Proguanil; Paludrine®). Chlorguanide is a nontoxic antimalarial drug with a slow onset of action used for the suppression but not treatment of malaria. Its action is related to metabolic antagonism of folic acid. The greatest disadvantage of this drug is the development of resistance by plasmodia. Its major advantage is that it is a very safe drug. Chlorguanide must not be given with primaquine as it inhibits the degradation of the latter, and may lead to elevated primaquine levels with resultant toxicity. Chlorguanide is now being used in combination with chloroquine to prevent chloroquine-resistant *P. falciparum* malaria.

Pyrimethamine (Daraprim®). Alone, pyrimethamine is primarily used prophylactically. In combination with a long-acting sulfonamide such as sulfadoxine (sulfadimethoxine), it has been successfully employed in both the treatment and prevention of chloroquine-resistant *P. falciparum* malaria. Pyrimethamine is a slow-acting drug with antimalarial actions identical to those of chlorguanide. It blocks the enzyme dihydrofolic acid reductase, which is required for folinic acid synthesis. In large doses it has produced teratogenic effects in laboratory animals and should be administered with caution during pregnancy.

Blood Schizonticides

Quinine and quinidine. Quinine and quinidine are Cinchona alkaloids that are rarely employed alone as antimalarials because of frequent side effects. These include tinnitus, headache, nausea, and blurred vision (cinchonism). Quinidine is cardiotoxic (*see* Chapter 35), and electrocardiographic monitoring is required when the drug is used parenterally.

Because of their rapid schizonticidal action, they are currently used in combination with other slower-acting antimalarials for treatment of malaria due to chloroquine-resistant *P. falciparum*.

Chloroquine (Aralen®). Chloroquine is a 4-aminoquinoline that is highly effective against the erythrocytic phase of all species of malaria except *P. falciparum* strains in certain geographic areas. It is rapidly and almost completely absorbed from the gastrointestinal tract and is concentrated in the liver. The toxicity is quite low, but large doses may cause dizziness, headache, diarrhea and epigastric distress, and reversible disturbances of vision (blurring, corneal opacity, retinopathy).

Chloroquine is the **drug of choice for the treatment of malaria** except where chloroquine-resistant strains occur. Chloroquine-resistant *P. falciparum* malaria has been encountered with increasing frequency in South America, Asia, South East Asia, Oceania, and more recently in Africa. In such cases, combination therapy is required with quinine or quinidine and a slow-acting schizonticide such as pyrimethamine-sulfadoxine, tetracycline, or clindamycin.

Pyrimethamine–Sulfadoxine (Fansidar®). A combination of pyrimethamine and sulfadoxine can be used for the prevention and treatment of **chloroquine-resistant *P. falciparum* malaria**. However, recent reports have documented increasing *P. falciparum* resistance to this drug combination, particularly in South East Asia, Oceania, and the Amazon area of Brazil. Fatal cutaneous reactions to Fansidar (toxic epidermal necrolysis, Stevens-Johnson syndrome, and erythema multiforme) have been documented in approximately 1:20,000 persons using the drug for malaria chemoprophylaxis.

Malaria Chemoprophylaxis

Since no drug kills sporozoites, the term "malaria chemoprophylaxis" is a misnomer. With the exception of pyrimethamine, proguanil, and tetracycline prophylaxis of *P. falciparum* malaria only, most antimalarials act on the erythrocytic phase by suppressing the parasitemia and hence the symptoms of malaria. If chemoprophylaxis is continued beyond the preerythrocytic stage of *P. falciparum* and *P. malariae*, i.e., for 6–8 weeks after exposure to malaria, a "suppressive cure" of these species will result and no late recrudescence will occur. The additional weeks of prophylaxis will have no effect on curing *P. ovale* and *P. vivax* malaria, because these parasites may lie dormant in the liver to relapse at a later date. Only a tissue schizonticide, such as primaquine, will provide a "radical cure" of these latter infections.

Chloroquine is the drug of choice for suppression of all species of malaria except in areas where resistant *P. falciparum* strains occur, as noted above.

Malaria chemoprophylaxis for chloroquine-resistant areas of the world has become a very complex and controversial subject among those responsible for making recommendations. At present, there is no uniformity of opinion concerning optimal regimens for this purpose. To make matters worse, the **World Health Organization** recently declared that "**no available chemoprophylaxis regimen will guarantee protection against malaria.**"

In Africa, where chloroquine resistance occurs, weekly chloroquine and double-dose daily proguanil are recommended. In South East Asia and the Amazon area of Brazil, weekly chloroquine is added to daily doxycycline. In other areas of the world where chloroquine resistance is less well marked, chloroquine and Fansidar are recommended. In order to reduce the frequency of Fansidar reactions, travellers at low risk for malaria who enter chloroquine-resistant areas are given weekly chloroquine and are asked to carry a single treatment dose (3 tablets) of Fansidar. The latter is self-administered whenever fever develops in a situation where medical care is unavailable. Weekly chloroquine and Fansidar are recommended as an alternative regimen for high-risk travellers who are unable to use other, less toxic drugs. Mefloquine, a new quinoline methanol derivative, is effective for both prevention and treatment of chloroquine-resistant *P. falciparum* malaria but is not readily available.

Toxoplasmosis

This is a systemic infection by the intracellular coccidian protozoan *Toxoplasma gondii*. Although most mammals are susceptible to toxoplasmosis, the cat is the only definitive host in which the sexual cycle of the parasite occurs.

Pyrimethamine combined with **sulfadiazine** is the preferred treatment in humans. Since these drugs act synergistically on folinic acid synthesis, they should not be administered to pregnant women because of the teratogenic effects. Malaise, headache, and gastrointestinal side effects are common.

In order to minimize the marrow suppressant effects of these antifols, folinic acid is administered concurrently. Since the parasite cannot utilize exogenous folinic acid, but must synthesize its own, the addition of folinic acid (as Citrovorum Factor) does not reduce the efficacy of the pyrimethamine/sulfadiazine combination.

Spiramycin is an old antibiotic used for a new purpose—the treatment of toxoplasmosis. It is the drug of choice for toxoplasmosis during pregnancy because of the teratogenicity associated with the pyrimethamine/sulfadiazine combination. The drug has been shown to reduce the incidence but not the morbidity of congenital toxoplasmosis.

INTESTINAL HELMINTHIC INFECTIONS

Intestinal helminths are usually found inside the large and small bowel where they attach themselves to the intestinal mucosa. Unlike protozoa, helminths do not multiply in the human host. This means that the worm burden (*i.e.*, the total number of worms in the individual's gastrointestinal tract) may increase only when the patient is reexposed to infective eggs or larvae. Since human morbidity from helminthic infections is directly proportional to worm burden, it follows that reduction in worm burden, without a parasitologic cure, may produce an acceptable therapeutic result.

Extra-intestinal problems can occur from the systemic dissemination of eggs or larvae of certain worm species. **Hydatid disease** arises from the ingestion of hydatid tapeworms (*Echinococcus granulosus* and *Echinococcus multilocularis*) in the feces of dogs and related species. In the infected individual, larvae migrate from the intestine into the portal circulation and distribute to the liver, lungs, brain, and muscles, where they form hydatid cysts of increasing size that can rupture and become the source of multiple cyst infections with extensive tissue destruction. **Cysticercosis** arises from the ingestion of eggs of the pork tapeworm (*Taenia solium*). These eggs develop into cysticercus forms in muscles and other tissues, producing inflammation and granulomas.

Mebendazole (Vermox®). This drug acts by inhibiting glucose uptake into susceptible parasites, thereby leading to decreased ATP production and death of the organism. Mebendazole is very poorly absorbed from the gastrointestinal tract. It is an extremely safe drug with few side effects. However, patients with heavy *Ascaris lumbricoides* infections have manifested diarrhea, vomiting, and abdominal pain when treated with mebendazole. This parasite must always be eradicated first when multiple infections are being treated because of its potential to migrate within the bowel following irritation by an inappropriate drug.

Mebendazole has a broad spectrum of activity. It is the **drug of choice for trichiuriasis and hookworm infections** (especially *Necator americanus*). It is a second line drug for beef and pork tapeworm infections. The fact that mebendazole can be employed in the same dose for children over 2 years of age and for adults is an advantage in the treatment of large families for **enterobiasis** (pinworm). In addition to the uses shown in Table 57–1, mebendazole has been used successfully to eradicate hydatid cysts (*E. granulosus*), and to control the malignant hydatid (*E. multilocularis*).

However, because the drug is so poorly absorbed, its efficacy in the treatment of larval tapeworms (cestodes) is limited. A new derivative of mebendazole, albendazole, has much better intestinal absorption. Consequently, increased tissue levels of the latter drug lead to higher cure rates in the treatment of larval cestode infections, which include both forms of hydatid disease and cysticercosis.

Pyrantel pamoate (Combantrin®).   The anthelminthic activity of this drug is due to its neuromuscular blocking property. It induces spastic paralysis of the worm, which then "loses its grip" on the intestinal mucosa. Less than 50% of the drug is absorbed from the gut. It is well tolerated except for mild gastrointestinal upset, which has been reported infrequently. It is an excellent drug for **ascariasis, enterobiasis**, and **hookworm infections** with *Ancylostoma duodenale*. It is less effective for *N. americanus*.

Piperazine citrate (Entacyl®).   This drug exerts its action by inducing a flaccid paralysis of the worm, thereby causing it to detach from the intestinal mucosa. It is a relatively safe drug, which occasionally produces gastrointestinal upset, urticaria, and dizziness. It reduces the seizure threshold and is therefore contraindicated in patients with seizure disorders. It is very useful for the treatment of ascariasis, but less so for enterobiasis because of the required long duration of therapy compared with single dose alternatives.

Pyrvinium pamoate (Vanquin®).   This cyanine dye eliminates *Enterobius vermicularis* by inhibiting glucose uptake by the parasite. It is not absorbed by the intestine and hence is the only anthelminthic recommended for use in pregnancy. It is relatively nontoxic, occasionally producing mild gastrointestinal upset. Its chief disadvantage is that, as a dye, it colors the stool orange, staining underwear and bed sheets.

Thiabendazole (Mintezol®).   The mechanism of action of this drug is unknown. It is well absorbed, quickly biotransformed, and excreted in the urine. Of all the anthelminthics listed in Table 57–1, thiabendazole has the most frequent side effects. It often produces gastrointestinal upset, dizziness, and headache. Because of these adverse reactions and the availability of safer and more effective alternatives, thiabendazole, a broad spectrum anthelminthic, is now primarily used for the treatment of **strongyloidiasis**. Variable success has been shown in the treatment of toxocariasis (visceral larva migrans) and trichinosis. A safe topical preparation is extremely effective for **cutaneous larva migrans** (creeping eruption).

Niclosamide (Niclocide®).   On contact with **tapeworms**, niclosamide kills the scolex and proximal segments, causing the worm to release its hold from the gut wall. The worm is then evacuated (often in fragmented form) in the feces. The drug acts by inhibiting anaerobic metabolism of the tapeworm. Very little niclosamide is absorbed from the gastrointestinal tract and hence side effects are rare. Gastrointestinal upset is the most common side effect associated with the use of this drug. Niclosamide acts on adult intestinal cestodes only. It is without effect in cysticercosis.

Quinacrine (Mepacrine) HCl.   This drug is rapidly absorbed, strongly tissue-bound, and slowly excreted (*see also* under giardiasis). Its chief advantage in the **treatment of tapeworms** is its ability to kill the organism without causing the worm to disintegrate. Thus, the scolex can be recovered intact, the worm precisely identified, and eradication confirmed.

In addition, eradication of the "intact" worm is an advantage in the treatment of *T. solium* where worm rupture, with release of ova, might contribute to the spread of cysticercosis. On the other hand, the most frequent side effect of quinacrine HCl, nausea and

TABLE 57–1   Drugs Used in the Treatment of Common Helminthic Infections

Drug	Worm					
	Roundworm	Hookworm	Pinworm	Whipworm	Threadworm	Tapeworm
Mebendazole	+	+	+	+	+/−	+
Piperazine citrate	+		+			
Pyrantel pamoate	+	+	+			
Pyrvinium pamoate			+			
Thiabendazole		+/−		+/−	+	
Niclosamide						+

Roundworm: *Ascaris lumbricoides*.
Hookworm: *Ancylostoma duodenale; Necator americanus*.
Pinworm: *Enterobius (Oxyuris) vermicularis*.
Whipworm: *Trichuris trichiura*.
Threadworm: *Strongyloides stercoralis*.
Tapeworm: *Taenia saginata; Taenia solium; Diphyllobothrium latum; Hymenolepsis nana*.
The symbols indicate effective (+) or variably effective (+/−) use of these drugs in specific helminthic infections.

vomiting, may result in regurgitation of the worm and endogenous activation of ova in the small bowel with subsequent development of cysticercosis.

Praziquantel (Biltricide®). This is a broad-spectrum anthelminthic for the treatment of cestode and trematode infections. A heterocyclic prazine isoquinoline compound, praziquantel is readily absorbed, rapidly biotransformed in the liver, and largely excreted in the urine. No major side effects have been observed although abdominal pain and dizziness are not uncommon. Praziquantel increases the permeability of the worm's cell membrane to calcium ions, causing spastic paralysis of its musculature, followed by disintegration of its tegument.

Praziquantel is the safest and most effective drug against all three major species of schistosomiasis (*Schistosoma mansoni, S. hematobium,* and *S. japonicum*). With the exception of fascioliasis, it will become the drug of choice for the treatment of other trematode infections such as clonorchiasis, paragonimiasis, and fasciolopsiasis. In addition, it acts on adult tapeworms and is the therapy of choice for the larval cestode infection cysticercosis. In Canada, praziquantel is available as an emergency drug.

SUGGESTED READING

Drugs for parasitic infections. Med Lett Drugs Ther 1988; 30:15–24.

Goldsmith RS. Clinical pharmacology of the anthelmintic drugs. In: Katzung BG, ed. Basic and clinical pharmacology. 3rd ed. Norwalk: Appleton & Lange, 1987:641–664.

Hoffman SL. Treatment of malaria. Clinics in Tropical Medicine and Communicable Diseases 1986; 1:171–224.

Katzenstein DA. Drug treatment of amebiasis. In: Peterson PK, Verhoef J, eds. Antimicrobial agents annual 2. Amsterdam: Elsevier Science Pub BV, 1987.

Katzung BG, Goldsmith RS. Antiprotozoal drugs. In: Katzung BG, ed. Basic and clinical pharmacology. 3rd ed. Norwalk: Appleton & Lange, 1987:618–640.

Kumar V, Geerts S, Brandt JRA. Praziquantel. In: Peterson PK, Verhoef J, eds. Antimicrobial agents annual 2. Amsterdam: Elsevier Science Pub BV, 1987.

Lobel HO, Campbell CC. Malaria prophylaxis and distribution of drug resistance. Clinics in Tropical Medicine and Communicable Diseases 1986; 1:225–242.

Seidel JS. Treatment of parasitic infections. Pediatr Clin North Am 1985; 32:1077–1095.

Chapter 58

ANTIVIRAL AGENTS

S.L. Walmsley

The history of human antiviral chemotherapy is relatively short, with the first agent being licenced for clinical use in North America within the past two decades. Despite these new developments, the major approach to the control of viral infections is through prevention, including programs of vaccination.

A number of viral pathogens remain major therapeutic problems not only in the normal host but more significantly in the host whose immunity has been compromised by underlying disease or its therapy.

The development of antiviral agents has been slow because their effectiveness is closely related to cellular metabolism, and much had to be learned in this field before effective drugs could be devised. It was believed for a long time that viral replication was so closely coupled with normal cellular metabolism that antiviral therapy would not be possible without seriously compromising the host. However, extensive research has increased our understanding of viral metabolism, especially those aspects of viral genome replication that are different from host cell replication. This has led to the development of effective antivirals that are selective for the viruses.

Nonetheless, of the many antiviral drugs developed to date, few have had a sufficiently high ratio of therapeutic value to toxicity *in vitro* and in animal models to warrant proceeding to clinical trials in humans. Even fewer have shown sufficient clinical benefit to achieve licensure.

The current epidemic of human immunodeficiency virus (HIV) infections has had an enormous impact on the field of virology. Infections with this virus have become a major public health problem world-wide since their recognition in 1981. Investigation in this field has provided a serious challenge to those concerned with developing viral vaccines and antiviral drugs.

A great number of researchers have turned their efforts toward this problem, and although a solution to this epidemic is not yet in sight, remarkable advances have been made in our understanding of viruses, their replicative mechanisms, and potential targets for antiviral drugs and vaccines.

The mechanisms of action of antivirals currently available for clinical use include (1) the prevention of viral penetration and/or uncoating, (2) the selective inhibition of enzymes specific for viral metabolism, and (3) the shutting off of viral mRNA translation (*e.g.*, interferon). Immune modulating agents are also available for some viral infections. These drugs act to augment or modify the host response to infection.

There are many variables that may influence the outcome of antiviral chemotherapy. These include:

- type of underlying disease and immune competence of the host,
- age of the patient,
- stage of the illness at the time of initiation of treatment,
- dosage of antiviral agent utilized,
- ability of the virus to remain latent within its host,
- ability of the virus to penetrate the central nervous system,
- ability of the virus to change genetically over time, and
- development of resistance by the virus to the inhibitory action of the drug.

In clinical trials of antiviral agents, it is important that these variables be carefully considered during data analysis. It is also important to recognize that viral infections often follow an unpredictable course; some viral infections may improve even if the patient is treated with a placebo. For these reasons it is imperative that any trial of antiviral chemotherapy be double-blind and placebo-controlled until an agent with clinical efficacy is identified.

Antiviral drugs act at various points in the viral replication cycle, the key steps of which are shown in Figure

---

This chapter contains portions of Chapter 57 in the 4th edition by P.J. Middleton.

58–1. Given these various steps in viral replication it is possible to search for drugs that will cause a block at some point in the replication cycle. Thus, there are agents that

- interfere with virus attachment to host cell receptors, penetration, and uncoating,
- inhibit virion-associated enzymes such as reverse transcriptase,
- inhibit transcription of parental genome,
- inhibit translational processes of viral mRNA,
- interfere with viral regulatory genes,
- interfere with viral protein glycosylation,
- interfere with viral assembly, and
- interfere with release of virus from cell membranes.

The agents discussed in this chapter are limited to those that are currently, or will soon be, available for

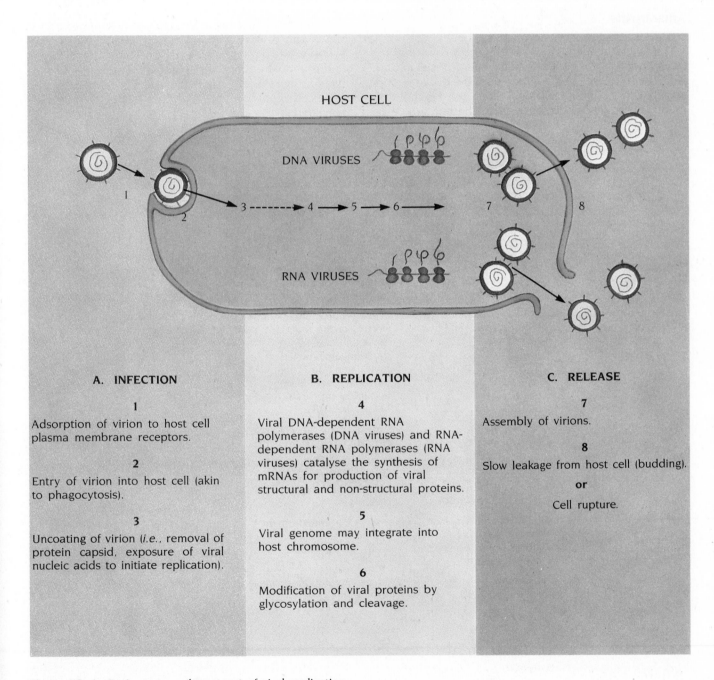

HOST CELL

DNA VIRUSES

RNA VIRUSES

A. INFECTION

1

Adsorption of virion to host cell plasma membrane receptors.

2

Entry of virion into host cell (akin to phagocytosis).

3

Uncoating of virion (*i.e.*, removal of protein capsid, exposure of viral nucleic acids to initiate replication).

B. REPLICATION

4

Viral DNA-dependent RNA polymerases (DNA viruses) and RNA-dependent RNA polymerases (RNA viruses) catalyse the synthesis of mRNAs for production of viral structural and non-structural proteins.

5

Viral genome may integrate into host chromosome.

6

Modification of viral proteins by glycosylation and cleavage.

C. RELEASE

7

Assembly of virions.

8

Slow leakage from host cell (budding).

or

Cell rupture.

Figure 58–1 Basic strategy (key steps) of viral replication.

clinical use (Table 58–1). One agent, methisazone, will not be discussed because its clinical utility was in the prophylaxis and treatment of smallpox infections, which no longer occur.

DRUGS

Amantadine

This antiviral agent is a stable hydrocarbon that has been chemically synthesized and has a peculiar cage-like structure (Fig. 58–2). It increases the dopaminergic activity in the striatum and was initially used in the treatment of Parkinson's Disease (see Chapter 20).

Antiviral Mode of Action

This is not fully known, but it is thought to interfere with the uncoating and nucleic acid release of certain RNA viruses. In vitro it is active against certain myxoviruses (type A influenza), a paramyxovirus (Sendai virus), and a toga virus (rubella).

Pharmacokinetics

Amantadine (as the hydrochloride, Symmetrel®) is slowly but probably completely absorbed by the oral route. It has a long half-life of approximately 15 hours and is almost entirely recoverable in the urine. Plasma half-life increases in the elderly and in patients with impaired renal function, and dosages are adjusted accordingly.

TABLE 58–1   Characteristics of Antiviral Agents

Drug	Mechanism of Action	Clinical Indications	Main Adverse Effects
Amantadine and rimantadine	Interference with uncoating of the virus	Prophylaxis and treatment of influenza A	Confusion, insomnia, anxiety
Idoxuridine	Inhibition of enzymes involved in viral DNA synthesis	Topical prophylaxis and treatment of herpetic keratitis	Local hypersensitivity reactions
Adenine arabinoside	Competitive inhibition of viral DNA polymerase	Herpes simplex encephalitis; herpes of the newborn; herpes infections in immunocompromised hosts; genital herpes; varicella-zoster in immunocompromised hosts; herpes keratitis	Gastrointestinal upset; CNS toxicity
Acyclovir	Inhibition of viral DNA polymerase	As for adenine arabinoside; Drug of choice	Transient increases in BUN and creatinine; thrombophlebitis
Ribavirin	Suppression of biosynthesis of guanosine-5'-monophosphate; blocks capping of viral mRNA	Influenza A and B; respiratory syncytial virus and paramyxovirus bronchiolitis and pneumonia	Macrocytic anemia; conjunctival injection; embryolethal in some animal species
DHPG	Inhibits DNA polymerase, thereby inhibiting DNA synthesis and terminating chain elongation	Serious CMV infections in compromised hosts	Bone marrow suppression; liver toxicity; hallucinations
Foscarnet	Inhibits DNA polymerase	CMV retinitis in compromised hosts	Transient increases in creatinine; anemia; nausea; tremor
AZT	Inhibits reverse transcriptase; chain terminator of DNA synthesis	Selected patients with AIDS and ARC	Anemia; leukopenia; neutropenia; ↓ vitamin B_{12}
Interferons	Activation of an endoribonuclease and phosphorylation of a peptide initiation factor	Herpes keratitis; rhinovirus prophylaxis and treatment; varicella-zoster infection in immunocompromised hosts	Headache; somnolence; gastrointestinal upset

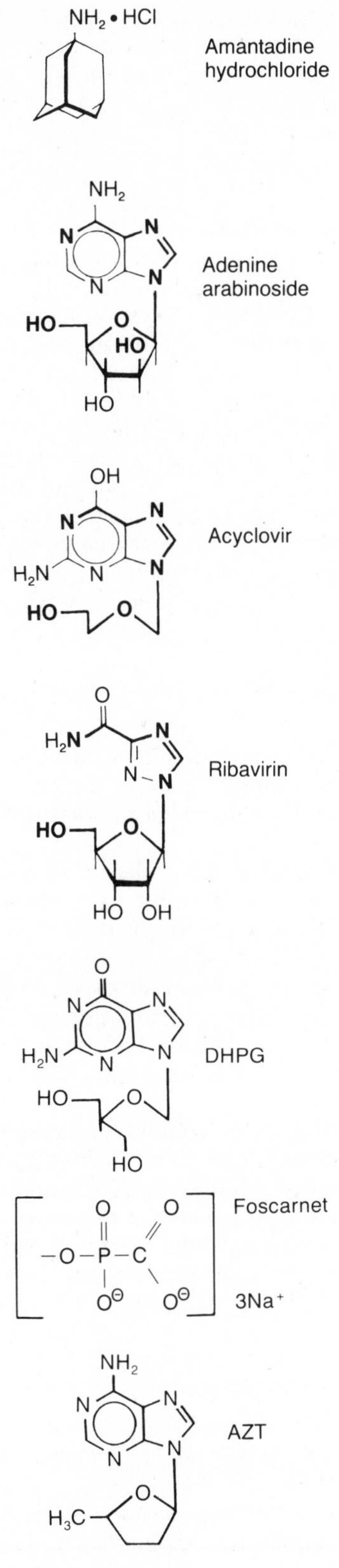

NH₂ • HCl

Amantadine
hydrochloride

NH₂

Adenine
arabinoside

HO—
HO
HO

OH

Acyclovir

H₂N

HO—O—

O

H₂N

Ribavirin

HO—O

HO OH

O

H₂N

DHPG

HO—O

HO

O   O

Foscarnet

—O—P—C—
O⊖   O⊖

3Na⁺

NH₂

AZT

H₃C—O

Figure 58–2 Structural formulae of some antiviral agents.

Adverse Reactions and Side Effects

These include difficulty in thinking, confusion, light-headedness, hallucinations, anxiety, insomnia, and a reduced seizure threshold. The approximate incidence of these primarily CNS manifestations is 3–7%. Very often they may occur within 48 hours of initiating therapy but are usually reversible despite continuation of therapy. Amantadine has also been found to be embryotoxic and teratogenic in animals.

Clinical Indications

Amantadine is currently used in chemoprophylaxis and chemotherapy of influenza A virus infections. It is compatible with influenza vaccine and may be used in combination therapy under epidemic conditions. As a chemoprophylactic agent, the drug has been found to reduce the incidence of clinical illness by 50–100% (as in persons at high risk, *e.g.*, patients with chronic respiratory or cardiovascular diseases). As a chemotherapeutic agent against influenza A virus infections, amantadine produces a diminution in fever in 50% of patients and a reduction in illness duration by 1–2 days if it is administered within the first 2–3 days of the onset of illness. It also results in reduced viral shedding.

Rimantadine

This antiviral agent is an analog of amantadine with identical mechanism of action. Its activity against influenza A viruses *in vitro* is four to eight times that of amantadine. It has also been found to be more efficacious against influenza A virus infections in animals. Until very recently, its use has been primarily in the Soviet Union. However, a clinical trial of its usefulness as a prophylactic agent against influenza A infections in humans, conducted recently in the United States, revealed that it is not more efficacious than amantadine but that it produces considerably fewer central nervous system side effects. This quality of rimantadine may soon make it the preferred agent.

Idoxuridine (IDU)

Mechanism of Action

Idoxuridine (Herplex®, Stoxil®) is an iodinated thymidine analog. The phosphorylated derivatives of this drug act by interfering with various enzyme systems involved in the synthesis of DNA, particularly DNA polymerase. It is also incorporated into DNA and may result in chain termination. IDU was originally synthesized in 1959, and was the first clinically effective antiviral nucleoside. It has demonstrable *in vitro* activity against herpes simplex virus, varicella-zoster virus, cytomegalovirus, vaccinia virus, and adenovirus.

Adverse Reactions

A number of serious adverse reactions, including bone marrow depression, hepatic injury, carcinogenicity, and teratogenicity, preclude its systemic use. Adverse reactions to topical use include pain, pruritus, inflammation, or edema.

Clinical Indications

Early clinical use of idoxuridine directed attention to the need for carefully controlled clinical trials. Initial uncontrolled trials suggested that this drug was effective in the treatment of herpes encephalitis. It was only after a carefully controlled double-blind study that the agent was shown actually to have a detrimental effect on the clinical course of that disease. The topical formulation of idoxuridine, on the other hand, has been employed with success in the therapy of herpetic keratitis since 1962. This remains its only clinical indication.

Adenine Arabinoside (Ara-A, Vidarabine)

This agent (*see* Fig. 58–2) was first introduced as an anticancer drug in 1960. Its antiviral activity was noted in 1964.

Mechanism of Action

Vidarabine is a nucleoside derivative that inhibits DNA synthesis by competitive inhibition of DNA polymerase. It may also be incorporated into viral DNA with resulting chain termination. It is primarily active against the DNA viruses including members of the herpes-group viruses, pox viruses, and adenoviruses.

Pharmacokinetics

When vidarabine (Vira-A®) is administered by intravenous infusion it is very rapidly deaminated to a hypoxanthine derivative. It may also be converted by phosphorylation to various phosphate nucleotides. The drug requires large administration volumes because of poor solubility. When it is given intravenously at a dose of 1 mg/kg, plasma levels of 1–2 μg/mL have been achieved, with a plasma half-life of approximately 1.5–3 hours. After an intramuscular injection of 1 mg/kg the peak serum concentration is only 0.2–0.3 μg/mL, but the half-life is prolonged to 10–16 hours. The differences in half-life are probably caused by protracted absorption from the intramuscular site. Most of the drug is excreted in the urine as an arahypoxanthine derivative. A dosage reduction of 25% has been recommended for patients with severe renal insufficiency.

Side Effects and Toxicity

The most important side effects are gastrointestinal upset consisting of nausea, vomiting, and diarrhea. Less commonly, but more importantly, central nervous system toxicities including tremors, ataxia, paraesthesias, dizziness, hallucinations, confusion, and even psychosis may occur. These CNS side effects are most common in patients with reduced renal function. Another problem with vidarabine therapy relates to its poor solubility, which necessitates a large fluid volume for administration of the drug. In patients being treated for encephalitis, this large fluid volume is relatively contraindicated. Other adverse reactions include skin rashes, weight loss, leukopenia, thrombocytopenia, anemia, megaloblastosis, and increased levels of aspartate transferase (AST, *syn.* SGOT).

Clinical Indications

Current clinical indications for vidarabine therapy include its topical administration to patients with herpetic keratitis, and its systemic administration to patients with herpes encephalitis or to neonates with disseminated herpes infections. Controlled clinical trials in these latter two groups of patients have demonstrated a reduction in mortality from approximately 70% to approximately 40%. Vidarabine has also been successfully employed for the treatment of varicella infections in hosts with compromised immunity, resulting in more rapid healing of the vesicular lesions and reduction in pain, as well as a reduced incidence of dissemination to internal organs.

Vidarabine has been largely replaced by acyclovir for serious herpes simplex and herpes varicella-zoster infections, because studies have shown increased efficacy and decreased toxicity of the latter. Vidarabine has been disappointing in the treatment of cytomegalovirus infections in compromised hosts.

Acycloguanosine (Acyclovir)

Mechanism of Action

This antiviral agent is a guanine derivative with an acyclic side chain (*see* Fig. 58–2). As a nucleoside derivative, it has a mechanism of action similar to that of vidarabine, but it displays a unique selectivity in action. It appears to be selectively taken up by virus-infected cells and converted to its monophosphate form by a virus-specific thymidine kinase. This monophosphate form is then converted to the active triphosphate form by cellular enzymes. The triphosphate form interferes with viral replication by inhibiting viral DNA polymerase. Acyclovir is much more active against the viral DNA polymerase than it is against cellular DNA polymerase. It may also be incorporated into the viral DNA and act as a chain terminator for viral DNA synthesis.

The spectrum of activity *in vitro* includes members of the herpes group of DNA viruses. It is most active against herpes simplex viruses and the varicella-zoster virus, and it is less active against cytomegalovirus and Epstein-Barr virus.

Pharmacokinetics

Acyclovir (Zovirax®) is slowly and poorly absorbed from the gastrointestinal tract. With multidose administration, steady-state concentrations are reached within 24–48 hours. Peak serum concentrations of 20 to more than 100 μmol/L are achieved following a 1-hour infusion of acyclovir at doses of 2.5–15 mg/kg.

The excretion of acyclovir is primarily *via* the kidneys, by both glomerular filtration and tubular secretion. There is minimal transformation of the drug *in vivo*. Dosage modification is required in the presence of renal insufficiency.

Adverse Effects

The topical and oral formulations of acyclovir are relatively free of side effects. The intravenous formulation results in transient increases in BUN and creatinine in approximately 5–10% of treatments, and local reactions consisting of thrombophlebitis or bullae formation have been noted in approximately 3% of patients.

Neurologic symptoms including lethargy, agitation, tremor, disorientation, and paraesthesia have been noted after intravenous infusion, especially in patients after bone marrow transplantation or with renal failure. Psychiatric symptoms including depersonalization, hallucinations, and hyperactivity have also been observed. Complicating illnesses and concomitant drug use may be contributing. These adverse reactions are reversible when acyclovir is discontinued.

Clinical Indications

The most important clinical use of **topical acyclovir** is for herpes genitalis infections. The drug has been found to be most effective in those patients suffering from their first episode of this infection. In such patients, topical application results in rapid decrease in viral shedding, reduced symptomatology, and prompt healing of lesions. The drug is less effective in patients suffering from recurrent episodes of genital herpes. Topical acyclovir also has been found to be of benefit in the treatment of mucocutaneous herpes infections in patients with compromised immunity. A liquid formulation of topical acyclovir is effective in the treatment of herpetic keratitis infections.

Oral acyclovir is effective in the treatment of first-episode genital herpes simplex infection. Effects include decreased duration of viral shedding, decreased time to crusting, and decreased duration of constitutional symptoms. Use of the drug does not alter the time to first recurrence. Oral acyclovir is associated with antiviral activity and, in some trials, with statistically significant but modest clinical effects in recurrent genital herpes simplex infection. Several placebo-controlled studies have shown that chronic suppressive treatment with oral acyclovir will reduce (but not completely prevent) recurrences of genital herpes.

Similarly, long-term suppressive oral acyclovir may decrease recurrences of mucocutaneous herpes simplex infections in compromised hosts such as transplant recipients and patients with AIDS.

Intravenous acyclovir (like the oral formulation) is effective in the treatment of first-episode genital herpes simplex infections in immunocompetent patients. Effects are less dramatic in recurrent episodes. It is also effective in the treatment of mucocutaneous herpes simplex infections in the compromised host.

Localized and disseminated infections due to varicella-zoster in immunocompetent as well as immunocompromised hosts respond to intravenous treatment. There is no effect on the incidence or the duration of post-herpetic neuralgia. In the compromised host, visceral dissemination of varicella-zoster herpes is decreased by treatment with acyclovir.

Two recent large randomized trials of acyclovir and vidarabine in the treatment of herpes simplex encephalitis demonstrated increased survival and decreased morbidity in patients treated with acyclovir. This is now considered the drug of choice in the treatment of herpes simplex encephalitis.

Early work comparing vidarabine and acyclovir in the treatment of neonatal herpes simplex infections showed the two drugs to be equally efficacious. Acyclovir is of no benefit in the treatment of severe cytomegalovirus infections in transplant recipients.

Ribavirin

This agent, 1-β-D-ribofuranosyl-1,2,4-triazole-3-carboxamide (Virazole®; *see* Fig. 58–2), was synthesized in 1972 as part of a major program to search for a compound with broad-spectrum antiviral activity. *In vitro* it inhibits a wide range of DNA and RNA viruses including myxoviruses, paramyxoviruses, arena, corona, bunya, RNA tumor, herpes, and pox viruses. In contrast, rotavirus, poliomyelitis, hepatitis B virus, and cytomegalovirus seem relatively insensitive to inhibition by the drug.

CHEMOTHERAPY

Mechanism of Action

The mechanism of antiviral effect is uncertain. Mechanisms proposed include (1) decrease in intracellular GTP, (2) inhibition of 5'-cap formation of mRNA, and (3) inhibition of the initiation and elongation of viral mRNAs through effects on RNA polymerase.

Pharmacokinetics

Biotransformation and tissue distribution have been extensively studied in rats, but this information is of limited value since the fate of the drug is significantly different in humans.

After oral administration in humans, the estimated serum half-life is 9 hours. Peak plasma levels of 1–2 μg/mL occur at 1–1.5 hours. Aerosol administration of the lyophilized agent by means of a small-particle aerosol generator delivering an estimated 0.8 mg/kg/hour achieves drug levels in respiratory secretions of 50–200 μg/mL, the actual concentration depending on ventilation and lung pathology. The half-life in tracheal secretions is 1–2 hours. The drug is biotransformed and secreted in the urine.

Adverse Effects

Aerosolized ribavirin is well tolerated except for mild conjunctival irritation in some patients. (The drug does precipitate in respiratory equipment, which may interfere with safe and effective ventilation.)

After oral administration, reversible increases in serum bilirubin, iron, and uric acid have been observed. The drug was found to be teratogenic and embryotoxic in small mammals during the first trimester. Prolonged use in animals has also caused a macrocytic anemia.

Clinical Indications

Ribavirin by aerosol is effective in the treatment of lower respiratory tract infections with the respiratory syncytial virus (RSV) in infants and young children with congenital heart disease, pulmonary disease, or immune deficiency. Infants treated with ribavirin showed a significantly faster improvement in their illness severity score. However, no differences were noted in viral shedding.

Other indications for ribavirin aerosols are respiratory infections secondary to influenza A and influenza B. Treated groups improve statistically more rapidly than controls; however, the clinical improvements are minimal. The drug cannot be used prophylactically for these infections.

In Sierra Leone, Lassa fever was treated with intravenous ribavirin. Mortality rates decreased significantly when treatment was initiated within the first 6 days of illness. Oral ribavirin was less effective.

Data on the use of ribavirin in HIV infection are conflicting and inconclusive.

9-(1,3-Dihydroxy-2-Propoxymethyl) Guanine (DHPG)

This drug is an acyclic nucleoside structurally related to acyclovir (see Fig. 58–2) but with increased potency against cytomegalovirus in vitro.

Mechanism of Action

In cytomegalovirus-infected cells, DHPG is phosphorylated by a cellular kinase, then further phosphorylated by other cellular enzymes to a triphosphate. DHPG-triphosphate competitively inhibits binding of guanosine to DNA polymerase, thereby inhibiting DNA synthesis and terminating DNA chain elongation.

Pharmacokinetics

Peak plasma levels of 20 and 50 μmol/L were obtained after intravenous infusions of 7.5 and 15 mg/kg/day respectively. Relationships between plasma levels, in vitro sensitivity, and therapeutic outcome have not been established. About 90% of an administered dose is excreted unchanged in the urine.

Side Effects and Toxicity

Bone marrow suppression with leukopenia is the major dose-limiting factor in therapy. Other observed adverse reactions include abnormal liver function tests, thrombocytopenia, nausea, myalgias, headaches, disorientation, and hallucinations.

Clinical Indications

DHPG has been used in the treatment of serious cytomegalovirus infections (retinitis, colitis, pneumonitis) in immunocompromised hosts, particularly those with AIDS or transplant recipients. Response rates are good (up to 80–90% for retinitis), but relapses are common (80–100%) shortly after treatment is discontinued. Intermittent-dose maintenance programs and intravitreal DHPG are currently being evaluated.

The drug is not licenced in any country (at the time of writing) but is available for compassionate use.

Foscarnet

This drug (trisodium phosphoformate hexahydrate) is a pyrophosphate analog (see Fig. 58–2) with potent in vitro virustatic effects against the herpes group of viruses through inhibition of DNA polymerases. Most of the drug is eliminated in urine. It is unstable at low pH and has a short half-life; it is therefore given by intravenous infusion.

Preliminary studies using foscarnet for cytomegalovirus retinitis in patients with AIDS have shown high response rates, but relapses occur in most patients within 1 month of drug discontinuation. The drug has also been used to treat serious cytomegalovirus infections in renal and bone marrow transplant recipients, and a topical preparation was used for mucocutaneous herpes simplex infections.

Adverse reactions include elevated serum creatinine, anemia, tremor, and nausea. Leukopenia has not been described. Toxicology studies in animals showed reversible dose-related changes in teeth, bone, and kidneys.

3'-Azido-3'-Dioxythymidine (AZT, Zidovudine)

This drug (see Fig. 58–2) was synthesized more than 20 years ago; however, no application of the agent was found until recently.

Mechanism of Action

AZT is a thymidine analog. It is converted by cellular enzymes to a triphosphate form, which is used by retroviral DNA polymerase (reverse transcriptase). Thus, AZT acts as a chain terminator of DNA synthesis. It has potent *in vitro* and *in vivo* activity against the human immunodeficiency virus.

Pharmacokinetics

The drug is well absorbed orally, and it penetrates the central nervous system. Peak plasma concentrations of 5 μmol/L are achieved with intravenous doses of 2.5 mg/kg or oral doses of 5 mg/kg. Average bioavailability of the oral drug is 60%; its half-life is approximately 1 hour. Little else is known to date.

Side Effects and Toxicity

Major reported toxicity includes nausea, myalgias, insomnia, headaches, and decreased levels of vitamin B_{12}. Anemia, leukopenia, and neutropenia are found in the majority of treated patients, being more marked with concurrent use of acetaminophen.

Clinical Indications

Zidovudine (Retrovir®) is under intensive clinical study in the United States and Canada to evaluate its efficacy in patients with AIDS and AIDS-related complex (ARC). In early studies, significant decreases in mortality and in the frequency of opportunistic infections were observed in patients treated with zidovudine compared to placebo. Although the drug is not a cure for AIDS, it has been licenced for use in selected patients with AIDS and ARC. The high frequency of adverse reactions requires that patients be carefully monitored while on the drug.

Interferon (IF)

The interferons are a family of **host range-specific** (*e.g.*, bovine IF is not crossprotective for humans) glycoproteins and are generated by a variety of stimuli. The human interferons are divided into three classes as follows:

1. **Leukocyte IF** (*syn.* αIF) is produced when null lymphocytes, B lymphocytes, and macrophages are stimulated by viruses, bacteria, foreign cells, and mitogens for B lymphocytes.
2. **Fibroblast IF** (*syn.* βIF) is produced in fibroblasts, epithelial cells, myeloblasts, lymphoblasts, and T lymphocytes when stimulated by viruses, polynucleotides, and inhibitors of RNA and protein synthesis.
3. **Immune IF** (*syn.* γIF) is produced in T lymphocytes when stimulated by foreign antigens, mitogens for T lymphocytes, galactose oxidase, and calcium ionophores.

More recently, interferons have been produced by means of recombinant DNA technology, thereby providing adequate quantities of pure interferon for clinical trials.

Interferons cause a range of biologic and biochemical effects. These include:

- antiviral action,
- immunoregulatory action,
- antitumor action,
- cell growth inhibition,
- macrophage activation,
- enhancement of cytotoxicity of lymphocytes,
- induction of new cellular proteins,
- alteration of initiation factor eIF-2, and
- induction of 2,5-oligoadenylic synthetase and activation of endonuclease activated by 2'-5'-oligoadenylic acid.

The interferon system is the earliest appearing host defense against viral infection, coming into operation within a few hours of infection. As the virus infection subsides and the titre of virus declines, there is a corresponding drop in the level of interferon. Several other lines of evidence strongly suggest a causal relationship between the interferon system and natural recovery from many viral infections of humans and animals. In addition there is increasing evidence that interferon may inhibit the growth of some tumors. Numerous trials are currently being carried out to determine the effects of the various interferons in the treatment of a variety of neoplasms, and as immunosuppressants (see also Chapter 61).

Mechanisms of Action

Interferons can be induced by active and inactive viruses, double-stranded RNA, and a number of other compounds. They tend to be species specific.

Interferon production appears to involve a depression of cellular genes induced by the presence of viral nucleic acid in the host cell cytoplasm. The interferon produced is released into the extracellular fluid and binds to specific cell receptors. This initiates a series of events leading to the production of two enzymes, protein kinase and 2,5-oligoadenylate synthetase. Protein kinase inhibits the formation of the initiation complex for protein synthesis, and 2,5-oligoadenylate synthetase activates a cellular endonuclease that degrades viral mRNA. Consequently viral protein synthesis is inhibited at two stages.

Pharmacokinetics

Doses of interferon given every 12 hours provide relatively steady serum levels. Maximum levels in blood following intramuscular injection are achieved in 5–8 hours. Interferon does not penetrate well into the CSF.

Adverse Effects

Interferons do produce undesirable side effects in their own right. When recrystallized recombinant interferon is administered in high dosage to humans (e.g., 100 million units i.m. per day) it can give rise to headache, somnolence, nausea and vomiting, fever, elevation of transaminase values, and neutropenia.

Clinical Indications

The **topical** application of interferon has been most extensively studied in the prophylaxis and treatment of rhinovirus infections. Recent clinical trials using this agent both prophylactically and therapeutically against these infections have been encouraging. The **intramuscular** injection of interferon has had demonstrable efficacy against varicella infections in the host with compromised immunity. Interferon, like other antiviral agents, has given disappointing results in the treatment of cytomegalovirus infections in bone marrow transplant recipients. There are no data on the use of interferon for either labial or genital virus infections. Gamma- and alpha-interferons have antiviral effects against HIV *in vitro*, but no immunologic improvements have been observed *in vivo*. Kaposi's sarcoma improves in approximately 40% of cases, but lesions eventually recur. Other uses are indicated in Chapter 61.

SUGGESTED READING

Balfour HH, Bean B, Laskin OL, *et al*. Acyclovir halts progression of herpes zoster in immunocompromised patients. N Engl J Med 1983; 308:1448–1453.

Collaborative DHPG Treatment Group. Treatment of serious cytomegalovirus infections with 9-(1,3-dihydroxy-2-propoxymethyl) guanine in patients with AIDS and other immunodeficiencies. Ibid. 1986; 314:801–805.

Dolin R, Reichman RC, Madore HP, *et al*. A controlled trial of amantadine and rimantadine in the prophylaxis of influenza A infection. Ibid. 1982; 307:580–584.

Fischl MA, Richman DD, Grieco MM, *et al*. The efficacy of azidothymidine (AZT) in the treatment of patients with AIDS and AIDS-related complex; a double-blinded placebo-controlled trial. Ibid. 1987; 317:185–191.

Hall C. Ribavirin: beginning the blitz on respiratory viruses? Pediatr Inf Dis 1985; 4:668–671.

Hayden FG, Albrecht JK, Kaiser, *et al*. Prevention of natural colds by contact prophylaxis with intranasal alpha-2 interferon. N Engl J Med 1986; 314:71–75.

McCormick JB, King IJ, Webb PA, *et al*. Lassa fever: effective therapy with ribavirin. Ibid. 1986; 314:20–26.

Pestka S, ed. Interferons part A. Methods in enzymology. New York: Academic Press, 1981.

Richman DD, Fischl MA, Grieco MM, *et al*. The toxicity of AZT in the treatment of patients with AIDS and AIDS-related complex. N Engl J Med 1987; 317:192–197.

Whitley RJ, Alford CA, Hirsch MS, *et al*. Vidarabine versus acyclovir therapy in herpes simplex encephalitis. Ibid. 1986; 314:144–149.

Chapter 59

ANTISEPTICS, DISINFECTION, AND STERILIZATION

E.L. Ford-Jones

Since foul odors were first associated with disease long before bacteria were discovered, people empirically attempted to minimize these odors and the suppuration of wounds by application of chemicals. As long ago as 450 B.C. a sort of chemical disinfection was practiced, as it was noted that water stored in copper or silver vessels was less likely to acquire a foul odor and taste than that stored in pottery vessels. At the time of Hippocrates, wine and vinegar were used in wound dressings. In 1847, the importance of hand decontamination was first appreciated when Semmelweis reduced the mortality rate of puerperal sepsis in an obstetrical unit from about 12% to less than 2% by requiring each student to wash his hands in chlorinated lime before performing examinations. Shortly after this, Pasteur introduced the concept of sterilization of surgical instruments by heat, and Lister began to use phenol to kill bacteria on instruments, dressings, and other operating materials and to spray carbolic acid over the wounds during an operation to kill bacteria before they could enter the wound. Such concepts, however, remained generally unpopular until the turn of the century.

Currently, 5–10% of adults entering hospital acquire an infection that was neither present nor incubating on admission to hospital and is therefore considered nosocomial (from the Latin *nosocomium* = hospital). Prevention of nosocomial infections depends in part on the effective use of antiseptics, disinfectants, and sterilization procedures combined with other measures to limit transmission of infection. In Canadian hospitals, Infection Control Committees composed of physicians, surgeons, pharmacists, nurses, and Central Sterile Supply staff among others are responsible for infection control activities. Each physician must understand the processes, their limitations, and methods of monitoring effectiveness. The major definitions follow.

Antiseptics are chemicals that are applied to living tissue to destroy bacteria or limit their growth.
Disinfectants are agents or processes applied to inanimate objects to destroy bacteria except spore forms.

Their main purpose is to eliminate the hazards of infection. Depending on the agent or process, mycobacteria, viruses, and fungi may also be eliminated.
Sterilization is the physical or chemical process of destroying all microorganisms including spore forms.
Germicides are agents that destroy pathogenic microorganisms, but not necessarily spore forms, mycobacteria, viruses, or fungi and are used on both living tissue and inanimate objects.
Fungicide is an agent that destroys fungi.
Sporidicide is an agent that destroys spores.
Virucide is an agent that destroys viruses.
Sanitizers are agents that reduce the number of bacterial contaminants to a safe level, to meet public health requirements.

PRINCIPLES OF INFECTION CONTROL

Antiseptics

There are few situations in which antiseptics are of proven therapeutic value. They are mainly used in prophylaxis, and they are applied locally because of toxicity that would make systemic administration unacceptable. Systemic absorption through broken skin, or permeable skin as in the infant of less than 32 weeks gestation, may result in toxicity. The following properties are desirable for antiseptics:

- potency and selectivity for the organism(s) concerned,
- low surface tension for ease of spread,
- retention of potency in the presence of inflammatory exudates,
- rapid and sustained action,
- absence of toxicity to skin or tissue, and noninterference with mechanisms of healing and tissue repair,

- nonallergenicity,
- lack of systemic absorption,
- pleasant aesthetic qualities (odor, color, lack of staining), and
- low cost.

Disinfectants

The properties listed above for antiseptics are equally desirable for disinfectants, and in addition, the disinfectants should be noncorrosive and otherwise nondamaging to instruments and materials. It is, however, of greatest importance to consider the purpose for which the disinfectant is used. Sterilization or thorough cleaning may be more appropriate, and disposable equipment may be more economical. Three categories of risk to the patient should be considered (high, intermediate or occasional, and low), which determine the stringency of asepsis required:

High risk: Equipment in contact with broken skin, mucous membranes, vascular system, or sterile body cavity where any form of microorganism could be harmful, *e.g.*, surgical instruments, urinary catheters, parenteral fluids.

Intermediate or occasional risk: Equipment in contact with mucous membranes and some nonintact skin where pathogenic organisms such as nonlipid-containing viruses, tubercle bacilli, and fungi could be harmful, *e.g.*, respiratory and ophthalmic equipment.

Low risk: Equipment not in close contact with the patient's mucous membranes, nonintact skin, sterile cavities, or vascular system, and where only significant numbers of bacterial pathogens would be harmful. Cleaning is usually adequate, *e.g.*, walls, ceilings, mattresses.

Sterilization

Once a decision is made that all forms of microbial life, including spore forms, must be killed, the method is selected on the basis of the ability of the material to withstand the process. Steam under pressure (autoclaving) is most widely used, and other gaseous or chemical methods are chosen only if equipment will not withstand autoclaving. Because ethylene oxide gas sterilization is more complex and expensive, it is restricted to objects that might be damaged by heat or excessive moisture. All objects processed in this way require special aeration to remove toxic residues of ethylene oxide.

Factors Influencing the Efficacy of Antimicrobial Agents or Processes

The Organism

The differences in response of microorganisms to chemical and physical agents are very great, bacterial endospores being most resistant, followed by tubercle bacilli, fungal spores, small or non-lipid viruses, vegetative fungi, medium-sized or lipid viruses, and vegetative bacterial cells. There is no evidence that the hepatitis viruses are unusually resistant. Among the vegetative bacteria, those with the highest lipid content, the Gram-negative organisms, are the most resistant. "Naturally occurring" organisms found in the hospital environment are often more resistant than those subcultured in the microbial laboratory, and this may reflect variations in temperature, pH, humidity, and growth factors present.

The Agent

Intrinsic or in-use **contamination** of many antiseptics and disinfectants, including benzalkonium chloride, chlorhexidine, hexachlorophene, iodophors, and phenolics, has been described following interaction with organic material or when they have been dispensed into unsterile containers.

Inactivation on contact with certain materials may occur, as in the case of benzalkonium chloride and cotton fibres.

Degree of dilution for use must be appropriate.

Duration of contact must be adequate. (Only incineration works immediately!)

Mechanical Cleaning

Good physical cleaning must precede any disinfection or sterilization process. Organic material will protect bacteria from penetration by the agent or directly inactivate certain agents. In a recent outbreak of *Serratia* species septicemia associated with a contaminated endoscope, the instrument had been gas-"sterilized" but not properly cleaned.

Evaluation of Antimicrobial Activity

Sterilization

This process is easy to monitor with well-recognized techniques, and this is the most reliable means of eliminating microbial life. Quantitative assurance of true sterilization is achieved through the challenge of a sterilizing process with 10^6 dried bacterial endospores, sterilization being defined as the state in which the probability of one spore surviving is $1:10^6$ or lower.

Disinfectants

Disinfectant tests have not been standardized. Many factors must be considered, such as choice of test organism, preparation of cell suspensions, neutralization of the disinfectant residues in subculture, and determination of the end point. There is some agreement over the need for three levels of testing, **in vitro**, **in vivo** (tests carried out in the laboratory under conditions simulating real life situations) and **in use**, but methodology and results vary widely. Evaluation of disinfection procedures is thus less reliable than that of sterilization processes.

Antiseptics

Although it might seem most reasonable to assess the value of antiseptics by measuring how effectively they reduce wound infections, as Semmelweis did, there are many variables in these situations, and antiseptics are therefore assessed on their ability to reduce numbers of resident and transient bacteria on the skin. Methods include culture of handwashing samples, bacterial counts in used gloves, contact plates, and skin biopsies. There is no satisfactory standard method for *in vitro* kinetic study of virucidal activity of antiseptics.

MECHANISMS AND SITES OF ACTION

Figure 59–1 and Table 59–1 show the main targets for antibacterial agents or processes.

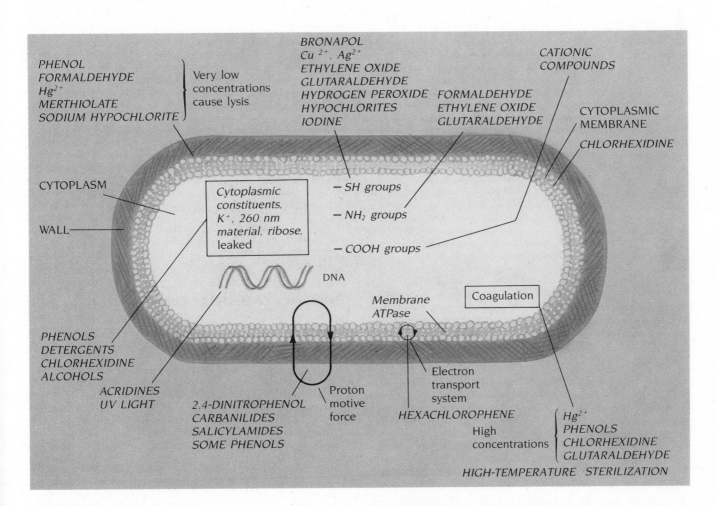

Figure 59–1 Diagram showing the main targets for nonantibiotic antibacterial agents. (Modified from Russell AD, Hugo WB, Ayliffe GAJ, 1982.)

TABLE 59–1 Cellular Targets for Nonantibiotic Antibacterial Agents

Nonantibiotic Antimicrobial Agent	Target or Reaction Attacked											
	CW	AMP	ETC	AT	ETG	AGMP	GC	R	NA	TG	AG	HRC
Acridine dyes									+			
Alcohols						+						
Anilides (TCS, TCC)		+				+						
Bronopol					+					+		
Chlorhexidine				+		+	+ + +					
Copper salts				+			+ + +			+		
Ethylene oxide				+	+					+	+	+
Formaldehyde	+										+ +	
Glutaraldehyde					+		+ +			+	+	+
Hexachlorophene		+	+				+ + +					
Hydrogen peroxide					+			+		+		
Hypochlorites, chlorine releasers	+				+					+	+	+
Iodine					+					+		
Mercury salts, organic mercurials	+				+		+ + +	+		+		
Phenols	+	+				+ +	+ + +					
β-Propiolactone					+					+	+	+
Quaternary ammonium compounds						+	+ + +					
Silver salts					+		+ + +			+		
Sulfur dioxide, sulfites					+						+	
Ultraviolet radiation									+			

Crosses, indicating activity, demonstrate the multiple actions of most compounds. Activity is nearly always concentration-dependent, and the number of crosses indicates the order of concentration at which the effect is elicited (*i.e.*, + = low concentration, + + + = high concentration). A cross in only one target column indicates the only known site of action of that agent. Note the range of reactions, varying specificity, and probable efficacy.

CW = Cell Wall; AMP = Action on Membrane Potentials; ETC = Electron Transport Chain; AT = Adenosine Triphosphatase; ETG = Enzymes With Thiol Groups; AGMP = Action on General Membrane Permeability; GC = General Coagulation; R = Ribosomes; NA = Nucleic Acids; TG = Thiol Groups; AG = Amino Groups; HRC = Highly Reactive Compounds.

RESISTANCE

Intrinsic Resistance

Gram-negative bacteria and mycobacteria are generally associated with a greater resistance to antiseptics and disinfectants, probably because of the unique character of the cell wall, which contains polysaccharide and lipid, leading to exclusion of agents that could otherwise act on intracellular targets.

Plasmid-Mediated Resistance

Bacteria occasionally contain small autonomously replicating cytoplasmic DNA strands called plasmids, which may contain genes for antibiotic resistance (*see also* Chapter 52). Such plasmids may determine resistance to mercury and organomercurials, cadmium, arsenic, and hexachlorophene, either by detoxification and removal of the agent from the bacterial cell, or by alteration of permeability of the cell surface. This resistance is often linked to plasmids that specify resistance to antibiotics.

Resistance of Bacterial Spores

The mechanism of resistance of spores to heat and chemicals is unknown, and a variety of different factors are probably important.

AGENTS

Table 59–1 summarizes the target structure or reaction of each antimicrobial agent.

Alcohols

Isopropyl and ethyl alcohol are effective in killing vegetative bacteria and mycobacteria but are not sporidicidal. The presence of water is essential for the activity of the alcohols, and the most effective alcohol concentrations are 60–70%. Concentrations less than 30% are ineffective. Coloring agents may be added to differentiate the alcohols from water or saline and prevent errors through inadvertent administration. They are corrosive and an antirust agent (0.1% sodium nitrite) must be added when they are used on metals. Killing requires between 1 and 30 minutes exposure to alcohol, depending on the organisms being attacked. A disadvantage is the failure of alcohol to exert any persistent effect.

Aldehydes

Glutaraldehyde is effective against bacteria, fungi and their respective spores, many viruses, and probably mycobacteria. It is supplied for disinfecting purposes as a 2% alkalinized solution. It is a popular high-level disinfectant and sterilizing agent because of its broad spectrum of activity, effectiveness in the presence of organic material, and noncorrosive qualities. It has, however, an irritating odor and the toxicity of the vapor to the user is largely unstudied. It must be removed with sterile water rinses before use of the disinfected object.

Formaldehyde has been a popular disinfectant in both liquid and gaseous states, but because inhalation of vapor may pose a carcinogenic risk to humans, its use is generally limited to the disinfection of dialysis equipment.

Antimicrobial Dyes

Triphenylmethane dyes are basic dyes that include crystal violet, brilliant green, and malachite green. They are used as local antiseptics because of their activity against Gram-positive bacteria and some fungi.

Biguanides

Chlorhexidine has a wide spectrum of antibacterial activity against Gram-positive and Gram-negative organisms, although it is not sporidicidal, virucidal, or fungicidal, or active against mycobacteria. It is an N^1,N^5-substituted biguanide that is available as a dihydrochloride, diacetate, and most commonly, gluconate. Its activity is reduced in the presence of organic matter, soap, and other anionic compounds, but at a 2–4% concentration it remains most popular because of its immediate and persistent effect in reducing bacterial counts. Administration directly into the middle ear may cause deafness, but the agent is otherwise nontoxic.

Chelating Agents

EDTA (ethylenediamine tetraacetic acid) may potentiate the activity of many antibacterial agents against many types of Gram-negative bacteria, but not Gram-positive bacteria. EDTA causes an increase in the permeability of the outer envelope of Gram-negative cells. It is used as a stabilizing agent in certain injections and eye-drop preparations.

Iodine

Iodine compounds are generally active against bacteria and other spores, yeasts, and viruses. Surface-active carrier agents such as polyvinyl pyrrolidone (povidone) solubilize iodine as micellar aggregates to form iodophors (iodine carriers); the concentration of free iodine is responsible for the antimicrobial activity. Below a certain critical micelle concentration, at which the free iodine is slowly liberated, the iodine is simply in aqueous solution, not free, and is therefore inactive.

Iodophors produce less pain, staining, and irritation than tincture of iodine and are also nonallergenic. Severe metabolic acidosis and iodism occur when the agent is applied to large surfaces such as burns or peritoneal cavities. Transient biochemical evidence of hypothyroidism occurs when it is routinely used in babies of less than 37 weeks gestational age.

Chlorine

Hypochlorites are effective against bacteria and many spore forms and viruses, although possibly not mycobacteria. The stability in solution is dependent on chlorine concentration, pH, presence of organic matter, and light. Chlorinated soda solution (Dakin's solution) contains 0.5–0.55% (5000–5500 ppm) available chlorine. Sodium hypochlorite solution (Javex) is a 6% solution that is used in a 1:20 dilution containing about 1000 ppm available chlorine.

Heavy Metal Derivatives (Silver, Mercury)

Silver nitrate has strong activity against staphylococcal and Gram-negative organisms. Silver sulfadiazine has excellent activity against Gram-negative organisms. Combination of silver oxide or nitrate with a high-molecular-weight polymer results in slow release of silver ions and reduces their protein precipitant effect.

Mercurochrome is only of historical interest and of no proven value as a skin antiseptic. Other organic mercury preparations, such as thimerosal (Merthiolate®) and nitromersol (Metaphen®), are also of very little value for disinfecting skin because they are only bacteriostatic.

CHEMOTHERAPY

Organic and Inorganic Acids

Both aromatic and aliphatic compounds are used. Salicylic, undecylenic, and benzoic acids are used in the topical treatment of fungal infections of the skin.

Phenols and Their Derivatives

Phenols have a wide spectrum of activity depending on para-substitutions of an alkyl chain up to six carbon atoms in length, halogenation, and nitration.

Cresols are ortho-, meta-, and paramethyl phenols, 3–10 times as active as phenol yet without increased toxicity.

Phenols with higher boiling points (up to 310°C) have decreased water solubility, cause less tissue trauma, have increased bactericidal activity, but are more readily inactivated by organic materials. As previously mentioned, thorough mechanical cleaning must precede any disinfection. These less toxic and more bactericidal derivatives of phenol are used today. Because of their association with hepatic disease in neonates, they are not used in the pediatric setting.

Hexachlorophene has good activity against Gram-positive organisms but is generally bacteriostatic rather than bactericidal. It is a chlorinated bisphenol compound. Repeated bathing of premature infants in hexachlorophene has been associated with vacuolar encephalopathy of the brain stem reticular formation. People who use the agent regularly, such as some operating room personnel, have detectable blood levels of it.

Surface-Active Agents

Depending on the predominance of the hydrophobic and hydrophilic group and, more specifically, ionization of the hydrophilic group, surface-active agents are classified as anionic, cationic, and nonionic. Cationic agents have strong bactericidal but weak detergent properties. Quaternary ammonium compounds are most commonly used and are active against Gram-positive organisms and, at higher concentrations, Gram-negative organisms. Because of the ease with which they may become contaminated, in the very rare instances in which they are still used as antiseptics, they should be dispensed in single-use containers. The practice of adding to a partially filled container (''topping up'') should be discouraged.

THERAPEUTIC USES

Disinfectants

Noninvasive devices, surfaces (walls, floors), and equipment such as beds and blood pressure cuffs con-stitute a lower source of infection than invasive devices and can probably be managed by good housekeeping techniques, separation of clean and dirty areas, and common sense in handling of equipment. In contrast, inadequately sterilized or disinfected invasive devices such as intravascular cannulae, urinary catheters, and respirator components present a major risk.

The therapeutic uses of disinfectants are best summarized in the chart produced by the Centers for Disease Control (CDC), Atlanta, U.S.A., and shown here as Table 59–2. Specific guidelines for certain disciplines such as dentistry and opthalmology are available (e.g., human immunodeficiency virus [HIV] is easily inactivated by simple and readily available physical and chemical agents including 1:10 dilution of bleach, alcohol, and heat [56°C for 10 minutes]).

Antiseptics

The distinction between pathogens and nonpathogens is becoming increasingly difficult as coagulase-negative staphylococci assume greater importance. Aerobic staphylococci, micrococci, and diphtheroids are distributed all over the body, with greater numbers in the axillae, groin, face, and under the nails; 20% are in the depths of the skin. Other organisms are thought not to survive in the skin because of the effects of drying, production of fatty acids by diphtheroids, and formation of bacteriocins by coagulase-negative cocci. Important pathogens such as *Salmonella* and *Pseudomonas* colonize the skin transiently, but also for longer periods of time where contamination is high, as in the intensive care unit. Regardless of the agent used, vigorous mechanical cleaning is essential.

Antiseptics and Operative Sites

As with surgical handwashing, chlorhexidine or povidone-iodine will satisfactorily reduce bacterial counts if applied for 2–5 minutes. The best results have been shown when the antiseptic is applied by vigorous mechanical activity by the gloved hand, as opposed to rubbing on with gauze or spraying.

Antiseptics in the Bath or Shower

A preoperative chlorhexidine or hexachlorophene bath or shower of the patient has been shown to reduce bacterial counts and infection rates.

Elimination of Bacterial Spores by Antiseptics

While the number of spores in a wound may be reduced by soaking with a compress of 10% aqueous povidone-iodine for 15–30 minutes, systemic penicillin prophylaxis is necessary in cases where gas gangrene and tetanus are potential hazards because of the presence of *Clostridium tetani* and *perfringens* spores.

TABLE 59–2 Methods of Sterilization and Disinfection

	Sterilization		Disinfection High-Level	Disinfection Low-Level
Object	Will enter tissue or vascular system, or blood will flow through the object		Will come in contact with mucous membranes but not enter tissue or vascular system	Will not come in contact with mucous membranes or skin that is not intact
Item Classification	Critical		Semicritical	Noncritical
	Procedure (See Key)	Exposure Time (hr)	Procedure (Exposure Time at least 30 min)*	Procedure (Exposure Time at least 10 min)
Smooth, hard surface	A B C D E	mr mr 10 18 6	C D E F G H I J	J L M N P
Rubber tubing and catheters†	A B E	mr mr 6	C E F H I	
Polyethylene tubing and catheters†‡	A B C D E	mr mr 10 18 6	C D E F H I J	
Lensed instruments	B C E	mr 10 6	C E	
Thermometers (oral and rectal)§	B C D E	mr 10 18 6	K	
Hinged instruments	A B C E	mr mr 10 6		

Key to Table 59–2

A Heat sterilization including steam or hot air, manufacturer's recommendations (mr).
B Ethylene oxide gas, manufacturer's recommendations (mr).
C Glutaraldehyde (2% aqueous solution—suitable data are not available to permit an adequate assessment of the comparative effectiveness of dilutions of 2% glutaraldehyde for high-level disinfection of in-use patient-care equipment).
D Formaldehyde (8%) - alcohol (70%) solution (corrosion inhibitor needed if formulated in hospital).
E 6% stabilized hydrogen peroxide (will corrode copper, zinc, and brass).
F Wet pasteurization at 75°C for 30 minutes after detergent cleaning.
G Sodium hypochlorite (1000 ppm available chlorine) (will corrode metal instruments).
H Phenolic solutions (3% aqueous solution of concentrate).
I Iodophor (500 ppm available iodine).
J Ethyl or isopropyl alcohol (70–90%).
K Ethyl alcohol (70–90%).
L Sodium hypochlorite (100 ppm available chlorine).
M Phenolic germicidal detergent solution (1% aqueous solution of concentrate).
N Iodophor germicidal detergent (100 ppm available iodine).
P Quaternary ammonium germicidal detergent solution (2% aqueous solution of concentrate).
mr Manufacturer's recommendations.

* The recommended exposure time for high-level disinfection, 30 minutes, is primarily based on an unpublished CDC study involving disinfection of used respiratory therapy equipment with 2% glutaraldehyde. This time and concentration may differ from those approved by the Environmental Protection Agency (U.S. agency that regulates disinfectant usage) for use on product labels. EPA-approved times are based on results from manufacturers' studies that are infrequently verified by EPA.
† Tubing must be completely filled for disinfection.
‡ Thermostability should be investigated when indicated.
§ Do not mix rectal and oral thermometers at any stage of handling or processing.
Modified from Centers for Disease Control. Isolation techniques for use in hospitals. 2nd ed. Washington, D.C.: U.S. Government Printing Office, 1975. (DHEW publication No. (CDC) 78-8314).

CHEMOTHERAPY

Antiseptics of the Nares

In personnel who are carrying an epidemic strain of *Staphylococcus aureus* that has been associated with disease in patients, creams containing neomycin in combination with chlorhexidine or other antimicrobial agents may reduce or remove the organism, provided that treatment is continued for 14 days or longer. Systemic (oral) antibiotics may also be required, because eradication of nasal colonization by staphylococci can be very difficult.

Antiseptics and the Mucous Membranes

Solutions of 1% or more chlorhexidine, as well as iodine, potassium iodide, or an iodophor, will all give a reduction in the number of potential pathogens.

Antiseptics at Vascular Catheter Sites

Although topical iodophors are widely used at catheter sites, there is insufficient evidence to suggest that it is necessary. Their use may be associated with a decrease in *Candida*, enterococcal, and Gram-negative infections, but the results are not statistically significant and staphylococcal infections may continue to occur. Use of strict aseptic technique during insertion of such intravenous catheters, followed by appropriate aseptic technique in maintaining the dressing, are the most important aspects of care of intravenous lines.

Urinary Antiseptics

In the noncatheterized patient, increasing numbers of adverse reactions to nitrofurantoin, particularly in older patients, have led to a need to reevaluate the role of this drug in the prevention and treatment of urinary tract infections.

In the catheterized patient, prophylactic continuous irrigations in closed catheter systems are unnecessary. Aseptic insertion and maintenance, specifically minimizing disconnections of the catheter, connecting tube, and bag, are most important.

Umbilical Cord Prophylaxis

Triple Dye (crystal violet, brilliant green, and malachite green) has long been used for the prevention of staphylococcal disease, although silver sulfadiazine has a greater effect against Group B streptococci. The need for anything other than application of 70% isopropyl alcohol to a moist cord has not been demonstrated.

Prevention of Gonococcal Conjunctivitis

One percent silver nitrate instilled in the eyes of the newborn at birth is considered adequate to prevent gonococcal conjunctivitis, although there are other topical antimicrobials such as erythromycin that may be more appropriate in view of the increasing recognition of chlamydial disease.

Antiseptics in Wounds

Most antiseptics have been used in the treatment of wounds at one time or another, but the removal of foreign or necrotic material and improvement of the blood supply is of greater importance than any direct antibacterial agents. Of the debriding agents, sodium hypochlorite (Dakin's solution) and hydrogen peroxide are most effective. The systemic absorption of other agents such as silver nitrate or hexachlorophene or an iodophor may result in undesirable side effects. In addition, hexachlorophene and other agents may be harmful to cartilage, synovia, and other soft tissues.

Antiseptics in Burn Patients

In contrast to wounds, burns benefit from the application of topical therapy. This is because of the large amount of nonviable tissue present. Serious subcutaneous infection subjacent to the burn wound is the single most important factor leading to burn death, and massive colonization of the wound is the source of potential invasion. The criteria for diagnosis of burn wound infection include a bacterial count of greater than 10^5 organisms per gram of tissue and histologic evidence of bacterial invasion of subjacent viable tissue. Topical therapy reduces the number of bacteria below the critical level necessary for invasion.

Mafenide (Sulfamylon®) was initially used in the therapy of burns but later abandoned when pain and respiratory alkalosis associated with carbonic anhydrase inhibition occurred.

The use of silver nitrate also has been abandoned. The silver, on contact with tissue, is precipitated as silver chloride, thereby limiting penetration beyond the surface tissue, and its successful use requires constant debridement. In addition, staining of clothing and linen, and electrolyte dilution from the absorption of large amounts of distilled water from the dressing, are problems.

Silver sulfadiazine combines the wide spectrum of activity of the silver ion and the antibacterial effect of the sulfonamide and is not inactivated by wound exudate or *p*-aminobenzoic acid. The release of sulfadiazine is slow enough to obviate toxicity.

Gauze impregnated with framycetin sulfate (Sofratulle®) is used in the management of burns in outpatients.

HANDWASHING

Handwashing is the most important single procedure in preventing the spread of nosocomial (hospital-acquired) infections.

Skin flora can be categorized as either resident or transient; resident flora survive and multiply on the skin and can be repeatedly cultured, while transient flora usually survive on the skin less than 24 hours, can be removed by detergents, and can be killed or inhibited by antiseptics. They are usually of low virulence and are implicated in infections only when surgery or other invasive procedures allow them to enter deep tissues. Transient flora, often found on the hands, can be acquired from colonized or infected patients and are frequently implicated in nosocomial infections.

The purpose of routine handwashing is simply to remove transient flora. In outbreaks of Gram-negative infections, a large percentage of hand cultures from physicians and nurses will yield the organism. Rhinovirus has been recovered from the hands of 40% of persons with rhinovirus infections and from as many as 90% with repeated sampling. The purpose of antiseptic handwashing is to reliably eliminate microorganisms when the hands are possibly contaminated with virulent microorganisms, and to reduce the number of permanent bacteria.

Routine Handwashing Indications and Techniques

Between patient contacts (other than those as brief as taking a blood pressure or shaking hands, which do not require hand washing), a vigorous washing with chlorhexidine 2% for 15 seconds is adequate. Hands should be rinsed, dried with a paper towel, and the towel used to turn off the faucet. A 2-minute "surgical wash" should antecede invasive procedures.

Because rings and cracked nail polish make microorganisms on the hand difficult to remove, personnel who take care of patients should be discouraged from wearing rings or nail polish while on duty; a single band is permissible. Wrist watches should not be placed in a way that prevents thorough washing, and should not be worn while giving direct patient care.

Because dermatitis may predispose to carriage of pathogenic organisms, efforts should be made to prevent it. Single-use packages of hand lotion are available. Multiple-use bottles should not be employed, because experience has shown that they have sometimes become contaminated.

Surgical Handwashing

Because perforations occur in approximately 25% of gloves worn by a surgical team, the hands must be scrubbed thoroughly before the gloves are put on. A 2-minute scrub with chlorhexidine or povidone-iodine is recommended and will reduce bacterial counts by 70–85% after one application and by 99% if used six times over a 2-day period.

Although chlorhexidine, hexachlorophene, and povidone-iodine all have a residual effect, chlorhexidine seems preferable because it is unaffected by the presence of blood on the skin. During a 3-hour operation, for example, there may even be a further fall in bacterial counts from that determined after the initial application.

SUGGESTED READING

Ayliffe GAJ. The effect of antibacterial agents on the flora of the skin. J Hosp Infect 1980; 1:111–124.

Buehler JW, Finton RJ, Goodman RA, et al. Epidemic keratoconjunctivitis. Report of an outbreak in ophthalmology practice and recommendations for prevention. Infect Control 1984; 5:390–394.

Dineen P. Local antiseptics. In: Drugs of choice 1980–1981. St. Louis: CV Mosby, 1980.

Ford-Jones EL. Antiseptics. In: Koren G, Prober CG, Gold R, eds. Antimicrobial therapy in infants and children. New York/Basel: Marcel Dekker, 1988:483–514.

Hospital Infections Branch: Atlanta, Georgia, USA: Centers for Disease Control Publications, 1981–1982, 1985.

Ibid.: Recommended infection-control practices for dentistry. Centers for Disease Control Publications, 1986; 35: 237–242.

Kaul AF, Jewett JF. Agents and techniques for disinfection of the skin. Surg Gynecol Obstet 1981; 152:677–685.

Russell AD, Hugo WB, Ayliffe GAJ. Principles and practice of disinfection, preservation and sterilization. Oxford/London/Edinburgh/Melbourne: Blackwell, 1982.

CHEMOTHERAPY

Chapter 60

ANTINEOPLASTIC DRUGS

C. Erlichman and I.G. Kerr

Neoplasia arises from transformed cells and is characterized by a cellular proliferation that is uncontrolled and occurs at the expense of the host. Cancers spread by invasion of the surrounding tissues and by metastasizing to distant sites. Tumors may possess great heterogeneity with respect to karyotype, morphology, immunogenicity, rate of growth, ability to metastasize, and responsiveness to antineoplastic drugs. Although surgery and radiation can often cure or control tumors locally, many patients eventually succumb to their diseases because of metastases to distant sites. Therefore, effective systemic treatment is needed if we are to cure most cancers. Most effective treatments for systemic disease presently employ either chemotherapy or hormonal agents, or a combination of the two. Immunotherapy has not proven to be very useful to date (*see* Chapter 61).

PRINCIPLES OF CANCER CHEMOTHERAPY

1. A "clonogenic" cell is one that has the potential for unlimited replication. Therefore, a single clonogenic malignant cell can give rise to sufficient progeny to kill the host. The effectiveness of chemotherapy will depend on its ability to eliminate **all** clonogenic cells.

2. The cell kill caused by antineoplastic drugs follows first-order kinetics, *i.e.*, a constant percentage or fraction rather than a constant number of cells is killed by a given therapeutic intervention. For example, a patient with cancer might harbor 10^{12} (or about 1 kg) malignant cells. A drug or drug combination that kills 99.99% of these cells (4-log kill) would reduce the tumor mass to about 100 mg (*i.e.*, a complete clinical remission). However, 10^8 malignant cells would remain viable, and

any clonogenic cells that remained would cause a recurrence of the disease.

3. Tissue culture and animal experiments have demonstrated the importance of a dose-response curve with cancer chemotherapeutic agents. However, the importance of such a dose-response effect in man is not clear. Therefore, one must consider factors such as drug concentration, drug exposure time, and frequency of drug administration, when defining an "adequate dose."

4. Tumor cells may grow in body compartments to which chemotherapeutic agents have limited access. These sanctuaries (*e.g.*, the central nervous system) protect malignant cells from systemically administered drugs. Local drug administration (*e.g.*, intrathecal chemotherapy) can be effective in eradicating malignant cells in such sites.

5. Most antineoplastic drugs have a low therapeutic index. As their mechanism of action is not specific for cancer cells, rapidly dividing normal body tissues may be damaged also (*e.g.*, bone marrow, gonads, oral mucosa, hair follicles).

6. High-dose intermittent schedules are believed to be more effective than schedules employing low-dose daily administration. These intermittent schedules allow time for recovery of normal host tissues between drug treatment cycles. Doses and schedules of drug administration are used to achieve maximum tumor cell kill and are limited by normal tissue tolerance.

7. Several drugs used together (combination chemotherapy) often are more effective than drugs used individually. In theory, drugs for combination chemotherapy are chosen because they have different mechanisms of action, are effective individually and have qualitatively different toxicities, so that each drug can be given at or near its individual maximum tolerated dose.

8. Theoretically, it would be best to start treatment early when there are small numbers of cancer cells (low tumor burden), when many of these cells may still be

in cycle (*see* below), and when there is a low probability of resistant cells. This principle has led to the development of adjuvant chemotherapy in recent years (*e.g.*, in the treatment of breast cancer and of osteogenic sarcoma). Adjuvant chemotherapy is the administration of drugs to patients who have no evidence of disease by currently available methods of investigation, but who are at high risk of developing recurrent cancer, according to current knowledge regarding the natural history of the disease. It is assumed that such patients have small numbers of cancer cells with a low probability of resistant cells.

9. Combined modality treatments are now being used more commonly. This involves treatment programs utilizing surgery, radiotherapy, and chemotherapy. Such an approach has been particularly successful in the treatment of childhood cancers.

CLASSIFICATION OF ANTINEOPLASTIC DRUGS

In order to classify antineoplastic drugs, a basic understanding of the cell cycle is necessary. This cycle can be characterized by five phases. G_0 is considered a resting phase when the cell is not dividing. G_1 is a phase associated with preparation of the cell for DNA synthesis. S phase is the phase of DNA synthesis followed by G_2, a resting phase prior to the cell under-

going mitosis. Finally, the cell enters M or mitosis, resulting in division into two cells.

Antineoplastic drugs may be classified by two schemes: according to where they act in the cell cycle, or according to their mechanism of action.

In the former case, antitumor drugs are characterized as **cell-cycle-independent** if they affect cells during any phase of the cycle including resting or G_0 cells, or **cell-cycle-dependent** if they affect only cells that are actively cycling at the time of exposure to drugs. If one specific phase of the cycle is the principal site of drug action, the agent is called **phase-dependent.** Examples of cell-cycle-independent drugs are chlorambucil and melphalan. Examples of cell-cycle-dependent drugs are 5-fluorouracil and methotrexate. Vincristine and vinblastine, which bind to microtubules during mitosis, are considered phase-dependent agents. Figure 60–1 illustrates where some of these drugs act in the cell cycle.

A more practical means of classifying these drugs is with respect to their mechanism of action. Six classes can be designated, as listed in Table 60–1. Figure 60–2 depicts the means by which these drugs interfere with cell replication.

In the following sections representative drugs from each class are discussed, and an overview of the more common clinically useful agents is given. Practical considerations for drug administration are outlined in Table 60–2. Some indications of the therapeutic uses of antineoplastic drugs are given in each section. In most cases, clinical uses were empiric in nature and the drug's mechanism of action was determined subsequently.

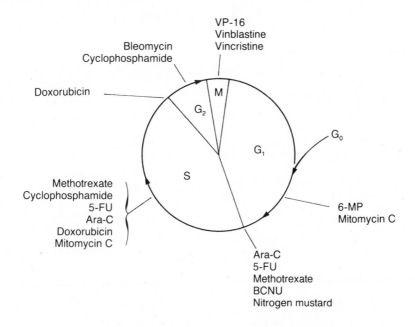

Figure 60–1 Sites of action of chemotherapeutic drugs in the cell cycle.

TABLE 60–1 Classification of Antineoplastic Agents According to Mechanisms of Action

Alkylating agents
 Nitrogen mustard (mechlorethamine)
 Melphalan
 Cyclophosphamide
 Chlorambucil
 Busulphan
 Bischloroethyl nitrosourea (BCNU)–carmustine
 Chloroethyl-cyclohexyl nitrosourea (CCNU)–
  lomustine
 Methyl-CCNU
 Cisplatin

Antimetabolites
 Methotrexate
 5-Fluorouracil
 Cytosine arabinoside (Ara-C)
 6-Mercaptopurine
 6-Thioguanine
 Hydroxyurea

Antibiotics
 Doxorubicin
 Bleomycin
 Mitomycin-C
 Actinomycin-D

Mitotic inhibitors
 Vincristine
 Vinblastine
 4-Dimethyl-epipodophyllotoxin ethylidene
  (VP-16)

Hormones
 Prednisone
 Diethylstilbestrol
 Medroxyprogesterone
 Tamoxifen

Miscellaneous
 Dimethyltriazenoimidazole carboxamide (DTIC)
 Procarbazine
 L-Asparaginase

ALKYLATING AGENTS

Alkylating agents are a chemically diverse group of drugs. The mustards, which include nitrogen mustard, melphalan, and cyclophosphamide, were among the first agents used to treat malignant disease. Their chemical structures (Fig. 60–3) demonstrate the presence of chloroalkyl groups (CH_2CH_2Cl), which are important in their mechanism of action.

These drugs are highly reactive substances that combine with a variety of biologically important molecules. The most important targets are pyrimidine and purine bases in DNA. Each chloroethyl group binds covalently to a N, C, or O atom in a target molecule. The mustard thus forms a bridge between two target sites, resulting in cross links within single DNA strands, between two strands of DNA, or between strands of DNA and nucleoproteins. These reactions either inhibit separation or result in abnormal separation of DNA during cell division, and this leads to subsequent cell death.

This group of drugs has many toxicities in common. The dose-limiting **toxicity** is bone marrow suppression, with neutropenia being predominant. The pattern and time to leukocyte nadir are demonstrated in Figure 60–4 for some of these agents. Nausea and vomiting are common but short-lived (usually less than 24 hours after administration). Alopecia of varying degrees is almost universal and occurs after two to four courses of treatment have been administered. Effects on the reproductive system and on the host's genetic material may cause serious side effects in long-term survivors. These drugs can induce amenorrhea in women and oligospermia in men. The degree and duration of these side effects depend on the duration of drug treatment and the patient's age at the time of treatment. Second malignancies in patients receiving long-term treatment with alkylating agents, and birth defects in infants of women inadvertently treated with these drugs during pregnancy, reflect the mutagenic effect of these agents on DNA.

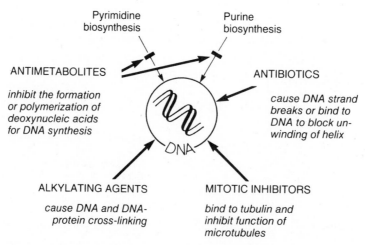

Figure 60–2 Mechanisms of action of major groups of antineoplastic drugs.

TABLE 60–2 Doses, Routes of Administration, Schedules, Elimination, and Toxicities of Antineoplastic Agents

Drug	Route of Administration	Dose* (mg/m^2)	Frequency[†]	Major Route of Elimination[‡]	Commonly Encountered Toxicities
Melphalan	Oral	9	daily × 4 q 4–6 wks	Renal	Leukopenia, thrombocytopenia, mild nausea, vomiting
Cyclophosphamide	Intravenous Oral	500–1000 100	q 3 wks daily × 14	Biotransformation	Leukopenia, thrombocytopenia, nausea, vomiting, cystitis, alopecia
BCNU (carmustine)	Intravenous	225	q 6 wks	Biotransformation	leukopenia, thrombocytopenia, nausea, vomiting, alopecia
CCNU (lomustine)	Oral	100–150	q 6 wks	Biotransformation	Leukopenia, thrombocytopenia
Me-CCNU	Oral	150–200	q 6 wks	Biotransformation	Nausea, vomiting, alopecia
Cisplatin	Intravenous	50–125	q 4 wks	Renal	Nausea, vomiting, mild myelosuppression, renal failure
Methotrexate	Oral Intravenous Intramuscular	25	2 days per week	Renal	Leukopenia, thrombocytopenia, mucositis, skin rash
5-Fluorouracil	Intravenous	500	daily × 5 or weekly	Biotransformation	Leukopenia, thrombocytopenia, diarrhea, mucositis
Ara-C	Intravenous infusion	100	5–10 days	Biotransformation	Myelosuppression, mucositis, neurotoxicity
6-Mercaptopurine	Oral	100	daily × 5	Biotransformation	Myelosuppression, cholestasis
Doxorubicin	Intravenous	75	q 3 wks	Biotransformation	Myelosuppression, nausea, vomiting, alopecia, cardiomyopathy
Bleomycin	Intravenous Intramuscular Subcutaneous	10–15	weekly	Renal	Skin and pulmonary fibrosis, fever, allergic reactions
Vincristine	Intravenous	1	weekly	Biotransformation	Neuropathy, SIADH
Vinblastine	Intravenous	6	q 1–2 wks	Biotransformation	Mucositis, myelosuppression
VP-16	Intravenous	90	daily × 2	Biotransformation	Myelosuppression, neuropathy

* Dose as a single agent.
[†] Frequency when given as a single agent.
[‡] "Renal" means renal excretion of unchanged drug. "Biotransformation" includes both hepatic and extrahepatic reactions; the metabolites may be excreted in the urine and bile.

Nitrogen Mustard

Nitrogen mustard (mechlorethamine), a highly reactive chemical, must be administered intravenously shortly after reconstitution. It was first used in 1942 in a patient with lymphoma and resulted in a marked diminution of lymph node masses. This agent requires great care during its intravenous administration. Extravasation of drug can result in severe local tissue necrosis, which may take months to heal. This drug has limited clinical utility today, but is still used routinely in the treatment of Hodgkin's disease. Although useful in the treatment of lung, ovarian, and breast malignancies,

it has been largely replaced by more stable alkylating agents.

Melphalan

Melphalan (L-phenylalanine mustard; Alkeran®) is an alkylating agent whose cellular uptake occurs *via* active transport systems for naturally occurring amino acids, located in cell membranes. It is administered primarily by the oral route. Bioavailability studies suggest that about 50% of an administered dose is ab-

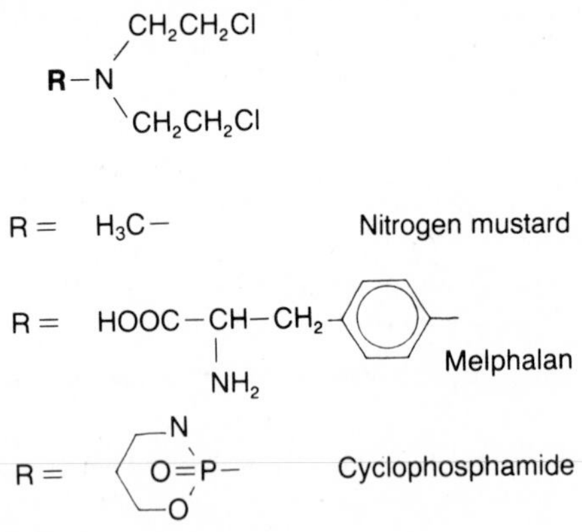

$$R-N\begin{cases} CH_2CH_2Cl \\ CH_2CH_2Cl \end{cases}$$

R = H₃C—   Nitrogen mustard

R = HOOC—CH—CH₂—⟨⟩—   Melphalan
         |
         NH₂

R = ⟨O=P—⟩   Cyclophosphamide
      |
      O

Figure 60–3 Structural formulae of mustard alkylating agents.

sorbed. The major clinical uses for this agent are in the treatment of multiple myeloma, ovarian cancer, and breast cancer. Common doses, frequency of administration, and route of elimination are summarized in Table 60–2.

Cyclophosphamide

Cyclophosphamide (Cytoxan®, Procytox®), which is inactive *in vitro*, is activated to alkylating metabolites by mixed-function oxidases found in hepatic microsomes. It can be administered orally or intravenously. Excretion of metabolites occurs primarily in the urine and may lead to a pattern of toxicity specific for this agent. The toxic metabolites may irritate the bladder mucosa, resulting in a chemical cystitis. The major method of treatment of this complication is prevention with adequate hydration, which decreases the concentration of metabolites in the urine and the duration of exposure of the bladder epithelium. This drug is probably the most commonly used alkylating agent clinically. It is ad-

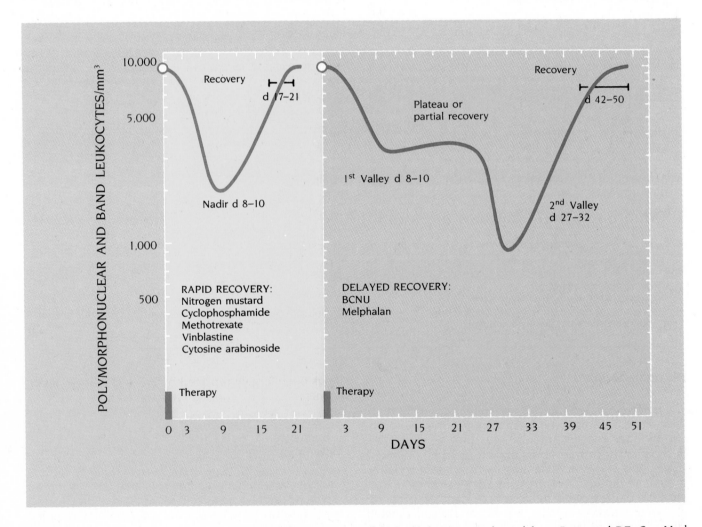

Figure 60–4 The effect of antineoplastic drugs on polymorphonuclear leukocytes. (Adapted from Bergsagel DE. Can Med Assoc J 1971; 104:31–36.

ministered in the treatment of leukemias, lymphomas, lung and breast cancers, and sarcomas. Cyclophosphamide dosages and schedule of administration are listed in Table 60–2.

Nitrosoureas

The drugs in this group, which includes BCNU (carmustine), CCNU (lomustine), and methyl-CCNU, are not mustards, because mustards have two chloroethyl substituents on the same N, whereas the nitrosoureas have only one. Nevertheless, it is believed that a major mechanism of action is alkylation. Their chemical structures are shown in Figure 60–5. The major difference between these drugs and other alkylating agents is their lipophilic character, which enables a significant fraction of these drugs to cross the blood–brain barrier and act against tumors in the CNS. Whereas most alkylating agents cause leukocyte nadirs about 10 days after administration, and recovery by day 21 to 28, the nitrosoureas cause two nadirs—one occurring at about day 10 and the other about day 28, with recovery by about day 42 (*see* Fig. 60–4). The mechanism underlying the two nadirs is unknown. Therefore, these agents are given every 6–8 weeks instead of the usual 3–4 weeks as for other alkylating agents. BCNU is administered only intravenously, while CCNU and meCCNU are administered orally. These drugs have been used in the treatment of lymphomas, lung cancer, and brain and gastrointestinal tumors.

Cisplatin

Cisplatin (*cis*-diamminedichloroplatinum) is a coordinated platinum complex with the two chlorine leaving groups in the *cis* position (Fig. 60–6). The drug's cytotoxic effects correlate with its DNA cross-linking activity, and therefore it may be considered as an alkylating agent. Cisplatin (Platinol®) is given intravenously, is highly protein-bound, and is slowly excreted by the kidneys. The major toxicities of this drug differ somewhat from those of the mustards. Nausea and vomiting tend to be severe and almost universal. Nephrotoxicity with progressively declining creatinine clearance is dose-limiting, but may be prevented in part by adequate hydration and mannitol-induced diuresis. Ototoxicity, manifested by high-frequency hearing loss, occurs not infrequently but usually is not dose-limiting. Renal tubular damage may result in magnesium wasting with associated hypomagnesemia. Whereas this problem is usually not clinically significant in adults, it can lead to seizures in children. Myelosuppression is much less of a problem with this drug than with the mustards. The major clinical utility of this drug is in the treatment of cancers of lung, head and neck, testis, ovary, and bladder. Table 60–2 lists common dosages and schedules for cisplatin administration.

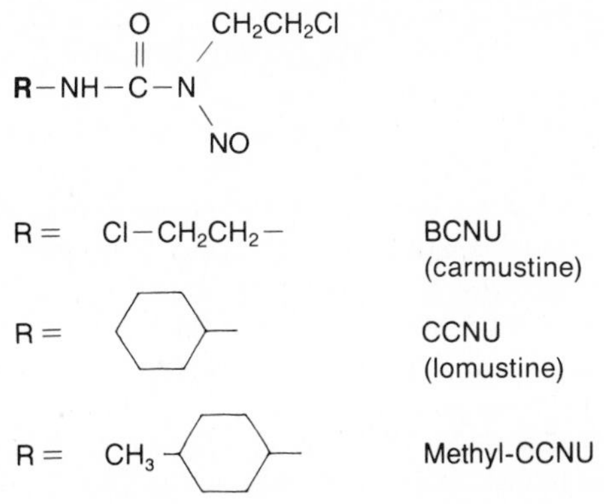

Figure 60–5 Structural formulae of nitrosoureas.

ANTIMETABOLITES

Antimetabolites are synthetic drugs that act as inhibitors of critical biochemical pathways in the formation of DNA, or as abnormal substitutes for naturally occurring nucleic acid bases, resulting in the formation of abnormal DNA. These agents tend to be cycle-dependent and affect both tumor cells and rapidly dividing normal cells. The most common toxicity of these drugs includes dermatological (skin rashes), gastrointestinal (stomatitis and diarrhea), and hematopoietic (neutropenia and thrombocytopenia) manifestations.

Methotrexate

Methotrexate (4-amino-N^{10}-methylpteroylglutamic acid), also called amethopterin, is a folic acid analog (Fig. 60–7) that competes with dihydrofolate (a naturally occurring folate) for binding to the enzyme dihydrofolate reductase (*see also* Chapter 56). This enzyme plays a central role in one-carbon transfer reactions that are necessary in DNA and purine biosynthesis. The competitive inhibition of this enzyme by methotrexate results in a cessation of DNA synthesis and decreased purine biosynthesis, with ultimate cell death. Leucovorin (folinic acid), the end-product of the

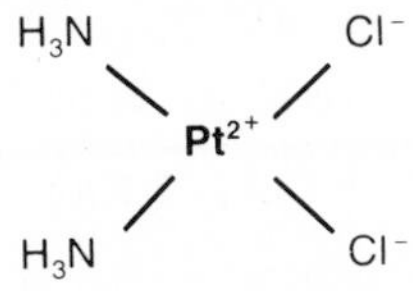

Figure 60–6 Structural formula of cisplatin.

dihydrofolate reductase reaction, may overcome the effect of inhibition of this pathway by methotrexate (*see also* Chapters 42 and 49).

Methotrexate can be given orally, intramuscularly, and intravenously. It crosses the blood–brain barrier readily and collects in body cavities and spaces such as pleural effusions. The parent compound and its hepatic metabolites are excreted by the kidney, but the excretion can be decreased by weak organic acids such as acetylsalicylic acid (ASA). ASA will also displace methotrexate from its binding sites on albumin. "High-dose" methotrexate, ranging from about 200 mg/m^2 to 20 g/m^2, has been administered to patients with cancer. With this treatment a high urine output must be maintained, and the urine must be kept alkaline in order to minimize the likelihood of drug precipitation in the renal tubules. Leucovorin must be administered shortly after such doses of methotrexate, to "rescue" normal tissues from drug toxicity. Otherwise, such high doses of methotrexate may be lethal.

The major clinical uses of this drug are in the treatment of leukemia, choriocarcinoma, sarcoma, breast cancer, and head and neck cancer. Methotrexate can be given intrathecally for meningeal leukemia or meningeal carcinomatosis. This will result in higher concentrations of methotrexate in the CSF than can be achieved by conventional doses given intravenously.

5-Fluorouracil (5-FU)

5-FU (Adrucil®, Efudex®) is a fluorinated pyrimidine analog of uracil (Fig. 60–8). To exert any cytotoxic effects, it must be converted intracellularly to the deoxynucleoside monophosphate (FdUMP) or the nucleoside triphosphate (FUTP). FdUMP binds to the enzyme thymidylate synthetase, which is necessary for the formation of thymidine phosphate, a critical precursor in DNA synthesis. The irreversible inhibition of this enzyme leads to the cessation of DNA synthesis. FUTP is incorporated into RNA, and the substituted RNA gives rise to the formation of abnormal proteins. These two actions are believed to be the cause of the cytotoxicity of 5-FU. The drug is usually given intravenously, since oral absorption is highly variable. Its elimination half-life is about 10 minutes. The major toxicities are leukopenia, skin rash, mucosal ulceration, and diarrhea. In addition, cerebellar ataxia is an uncommon toxic effect in patients receiving this drug.

Clinically, 5-FU is used in the treatment of breast and gastrointestinal cancers. Less frequently, it is used for the treatment of ovarian, lung, and bladder cancers.

Cytosine Arabinoside (Ara-C, Cytarabine)

Ara-C is an arabinoside nucleoside that differs from physiologic nucleosides by the presence of a β-OH group in the 2-position of the sugar (Fig. 60–9). It acts as an analog of a naturally occurring nucleoside, deoxycytidine, and is phosphorylated to Ara-cytosine triphosphate (Ara-CTP). Ara-CTP is a competitive inhibitor of DNA polymerase, an enzyme necessary in DNA synthesis and repair. By binding to this enzyme, it arrests DNA synthesis and replicating cells die. Therefore, this agent is more effective against cycling cells. (Note that an adenine arabinoside [Ara-A, vidarabine] is primarily active in blocking viral DNA synthesis, which makes it a useful drug to treat herpetic infections [*see* Chapter 58].)

The drug (Cytosar®) is given intravenously, either by frequent injections or by continuous infusion, since it is rapidly degraded (t½ = 7–20 min) by the enzyme cytidine deaminase found in blood. The parent compound and its inactive metabolite, uracil arabinoside, are excreted in the urine. Myelosuppression is the major dose-limiting toxicity, but gastrointestinal toxicity is also common. Central nervous system toxicity, with abnormal behavior and mentation, occurs uncommonly.

This agent is used primarily for the treatment of acute leukemias and may be given intrathecally for meningeal infiltration by leukemia.

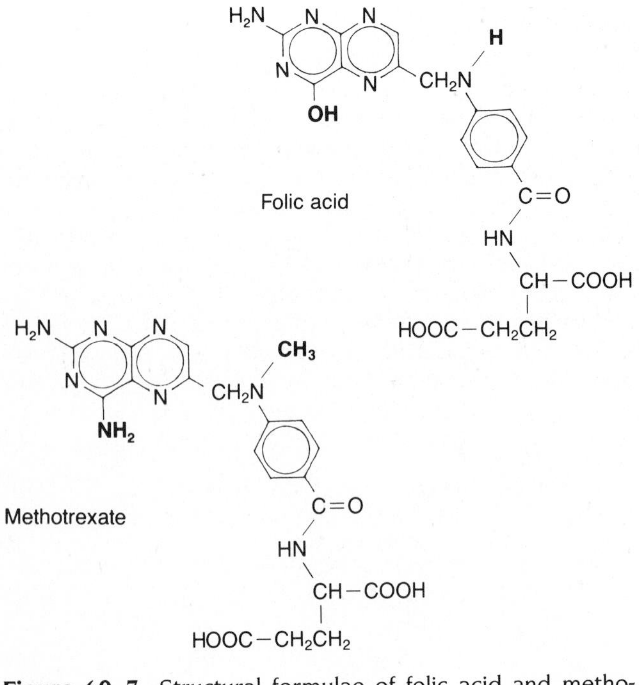

Figure 60–7 Structural formulae of folic acid and methotrexate.

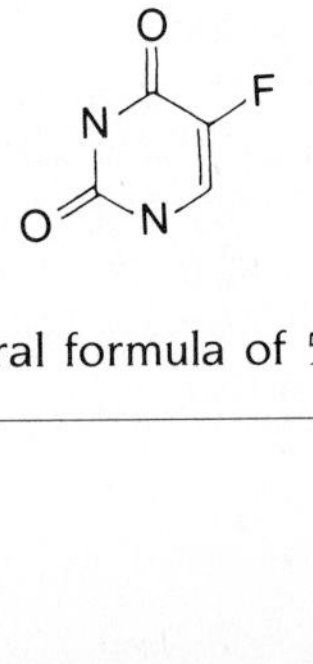

Figure 60–8 Structural formula of 5-fluorouracil.

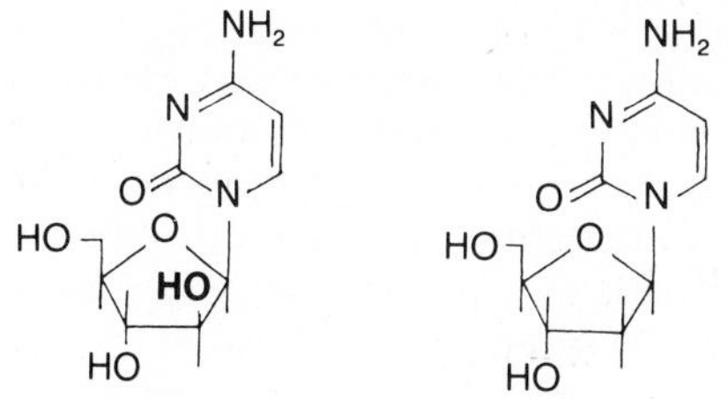

Figure 60–9 Structural formulae of cytosine arabinoside and deoxycytidine.

6-Mercaptopurine (6-MP)

6-MP (Fig. 60–10) is a thiopurine analog of hypoxanthine, a naturally occurring purine base. It is transformed intracellularly to ribonucleotide forms. These may be incorporated into RNA or DNA or act at several enzymatic steps of purine biosynthesis to inhibit purine formation.

6-MP (Purinethol®) is usually given orally and about 50% bioavailability has been reported. The drug is degraded by xanthine oxidase to 6-thiouric acid, which is devoid of antitumor activity. Allopurinol, used for the treatment of hyperuricemia, may inhibit the degradation of 6-MP and thereby increase its toxicity. The major toxicity of 6-MP is myelosuppression. Therefore, it is used clinically in the treatment of acute leukemia.

Azathioprine (Imuran®) was synthesized as a protected form of 6-MP and is believed to release 6-MP slowly at various sites in the body. It is used primarily as an immunosuppressive agent in patients receiving transplanted organs and in patients with severe rheumatoid arthritis resistant to other conventional treatments.

ANTITUMOR ANTIBIOTICS

In this section, two representative antibiotics used in cancer chemotherapy are described. These drugs are fermentation products derived from fungal cultures and subsequently isolated and characterized. Their mechanisms of action differ, and there are specific toxicities characteristic of each drug.

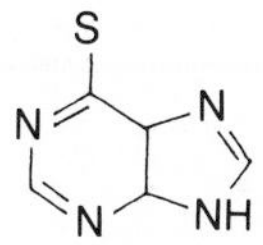

Figure 60–10 Structural formula of 6-mercaptopurine.

Doxorubicin

Doxorubicin (Adriamycin®; Fig. 60–11) is an anthracycline produced by *Streptomyces* species. Its mechanism of action is still speculative. At the cellular level it acts to chelate divalent cations, intercalates between strands of the DNA double helix, and undergoes oxidation-reduction of the quinone-hydroquinone group with free radical formation. It is potentially mutagenic, carcinogenic, and teratogenic.

The pharmacokinetics can be described by an initial plasma half-life of 10–15 minutes and a terminal half-life of 25–30 hours. It is widely distributed in body tissues and is approximately 75–80% protein-bound. The liver is the main site of biotransformation and elimination of the drug. Therefore, patients with hepatic dysfunction may need their doses adjusted.

Doxorubicin is one of the most useful antineoplastic drugs available, having activity against acute leukemia, lymphoma, breast cancer, lung cancer, and sarcomas.

Major acute side effects include myelosuppression, alopecia, local tissue necrosis (if extravasation occurs during intravenous administration), and ulceration of the oral mucosa. Its major chronic toxicity is cardiomyopathy.

Bleomycin

Bleomycin (Blenoxane®) consists of a mixture of antibiotic peptides with the predominant component being the A2 peptide (Fig. 60–12). Bleomycin produces DNA strand breaks through a complex sequence of reactions that involves the binding of a bleomycin-ferrous iron complex to DNA.

Its pharmacokinetics can be described by a biphasic plasma disappearance curve after intravenous administration, with half-lives of 24 minutes and 2–4 hours. It is effective only when given parenterally. The drug is eliminated primarily unchanged in the urine.

Bleomycin is useful in the treatment of head and neck,

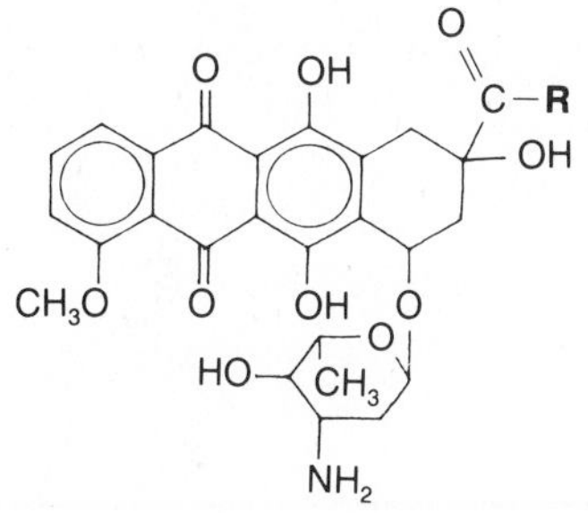

R = —CH₂OH   Doxorubicin
R = —CH₃   Daunorubicin

Figure 60–11 Structural formulae of anthracyclines.

testicular, and lung cancers as well as lymphomas. It has little myelosuppressive activity but may cause fevers, chills, rigors, hyperpigmentation, and skin thickening. Anaphylactoid reactions rarely have been reported with the administration of this agent. Its dose-limiting toxicity is the development of an interstitial pulmonary fibrosis.

MITOTIC INHIBITORS

This group of drugs is represented by the vinca alkaloids and the epipodophyllotoxins. They are extracted from plants and may be considered phase-dependent agents acting primarily during mitosis.

Vinca Alkaloids

The commonly used vinca alkaloids are vincristine (Oncovin®) and vinblastine (Velbe®) (Fig. 60–13). They are derived from the periwinkle plant, *Vinca rosea*.

The vinca alkaloids are able to bind to tubulin and thus inhibit spindle formation, resulting in metaphase arrest of cells undergoing mitosis. The pharmacokinetics of vincristine and vinblastine are somewhat different because of the side chain substitutions. Both drugs are given intravenously. Vincristine is cleared very rapidly with a terminal half-life of 2–3 hours, while vinblastine is eliminated more slowly with a terminal half-life of 20 hours. Both drugs are eliminated by hepatic biotransformation. They are useful in the treatment of lymphomas, breast cancer, testicular cancer, and sarcomas, usually as part of a combination chemotherapy protocol. Their major toxicities are slightly different, with neuropathy being the predominant dose-limiting toxicity for vincristine and myelosuppression for vinblastine. Vincristine can also cause a syndrome of inappropriate ADH secretion (SIADH).

4-Dimethyl-Epipodophyllotoxin Ethylidene (VP-16)

VP-16 (also called etoposide; Vepesid®; Fig. 60–14) is a glycoside derivative of podophyllotoxin with antimitotic properties. It causes metaphase arrest of dividing cells. It is usually given intravenously, although it can be given orally with approximately 50% absorption of the dose. After intravenous administration it is distributed rapidly, with extensive binding to plasma proteins, predominantly albumin. The terminal half-life ranges from 5.5 to 11.5 hours with a systemic clearance of 15–27.2 mL/m²/min. After 72 hours, 44% of the drug has been detected in urine, 29% as unchanged drug, and 15% as metabolites. In this same period, 16% was found in feces. It is a useful drug in the treatment of lymphomas and testicular and lung cancers. Its major toxicity is myelosuppression.

HORMONES

Some synthetic hormone analogs or antagonists are used in the treatment of hormone-dependent malig-

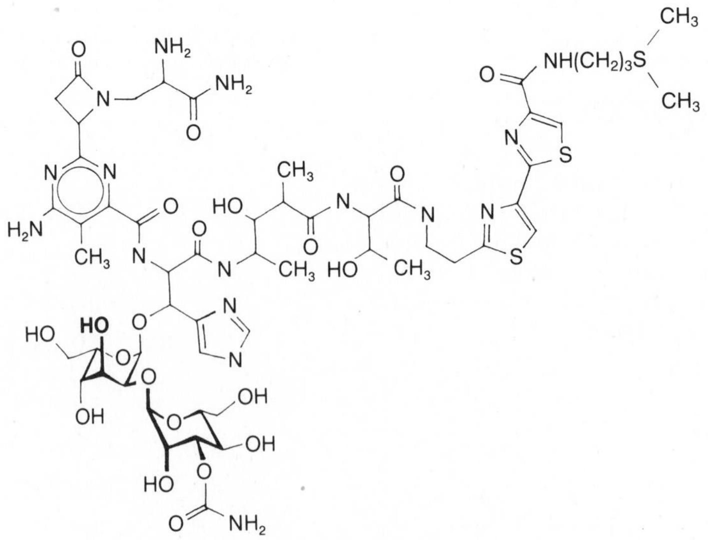

Figure 60–12 Structural formula of bleomycin A2.

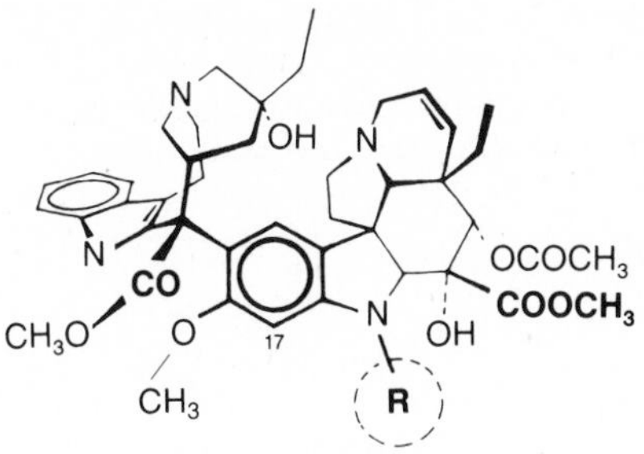

$$R = -CH_3 \qquad Vinblastine$$
$$R = -CHO \qquad Vincristine$$

Figure 60-13 Structural formulae of vinca alkaloids.

nancies. Details of their mechanism of action, pharmacokinetics, and toxicity are described in Chapters 45 and 47.

Prednisone, Estrogen Derivatives, and Medroxyprogesterone

These agents have useful roles in the treatment of cancer, either for their antitumor effect or for treatment of complications related to malignancy. Prednisone is often combined with other drugs in the treatment of leukemia, myeloma, lymphomas, and breast cancer. Glucocorticoids are also useful for treating patients with brain edema and hypercalcemia as a result of cancer. Estrogen derivatives (*e.g.*, diethylstilbestrol) and medroxyprogesterone are used for the treatment of breast, endometrial, and prostatic cancers.

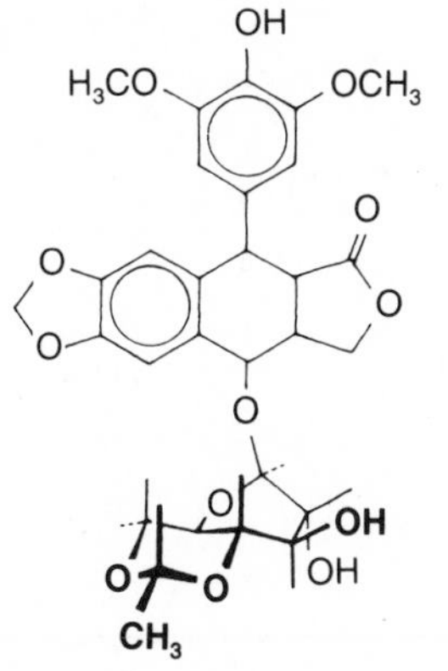

Figure 60-14 Structural formula of 4-dimethylepipodophyllotoxin ethylidene (VP-16).

Tamoxifen

Tamoxifen (Novaldex®, Tamofen®; Fig. 60-15) is a nonsteroidal antiestrogen analog of clomiphene. Although tamoxifen can bind to the cellular estrogen receptor, when this tamoxifen-receptor complex is translocated to the nucleus it inhibits DNA and RNA synthesis, instead of inducing synthesis, as estrogens usually do. This is probably due to successful competition of this complex for estrogen-receptor nuclear binding sites. Tamoxifen also alters prostaglandin production and decreases circulating levels of prolactin, LH, and FSH. The drug is given orally and undergoes extensive biotransformations. Some of the metabolites are long-lived and possibly contribute to the activity of the parent compound. It is very useful in the treatment of breast cancer. Toxicity is generally mild, although the drug can produce transient myelosuppression, menopausal symptoms, and a transient flare-up of breast cancer symptoms.

Aminoglutethimide

Aminoglutethimide (Cytadren®) is an inhibitor of aromatase, an important enzyme in the peripheral conversion of androgens to estrogens in extra-adrenal tissue. It also inhibits steroidogenesis by blocking conversion of cholesterol to pregnenolone. These two actions, together with administration of adequate hydrocortisone to prevent ACTH secretion, can depress plasma and urinary estradiol to levels observed in patients who have undergone surgical adrenalectomy. This antiestrogenic effect is useful in managing women with metastatic breast cancer. The drug undergoes extensive hepatic biotransformation. It also inhibits thyroxine synthesis, but in most cases this effect is associated with a compensatory increase in TSH leading to maintenance of a euthyroid state, so that thyroid replacement therapy for this problem is seldom necessary. Inhibition of steroidogenesis may require mineralocorticoid supplementation. The major side effects are skin rash, lethargy, drowsiness, and mild nausea.

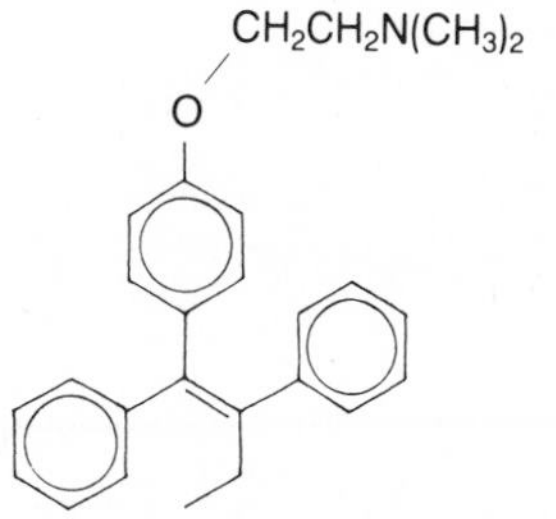

Figure 60-15 Structural formula of tamoxifen.

SUGGESTED READING

Chabner BA. Pharmacological principles of cancer treatment. Philadelphia: WB Saunders, 1982.

De Vita Jr VT, Hellman S, Rosenberg SA. Cancer, principles and practice of oncology. Toronto: JB Lippincott, 1982:156–197.

Erlichman C. The pharmacology of anticancer drugs. In: Tannock IF, Hill RP, eds. The basic science of oncology. Toronto: Pergamon Press, 1987; 292–307.

Chapter 61

Immunopharmacology

C. Erlichman

Immunopharmacology deals with the selective chemical control (enhancement, suppression) of the immune response in the treatment and prevention of disease. It is a new, fascinating, ill-defined, and complex area that holds great promise for the future. The goal is to identify agents that act on specific individual components of the immune system to enhance or block the action of those particular components while leaving everything else unaffected: the modern equivalent of Ehrlich's "magic bullet."

At present Rh Immune Globulin (IgG anti-D) is the only agent to approach this ideal. With few exceptions, therefore, present attempts to influence the immune response still rely on the exploitation of "side effects" of drugs that were originally introduced for other reasons. These immune system modulators are of two general types: (1) immunosuppressants, which suppress the immune response and are used to minimize rejection of organ transplants; (2) biologic response modifiers, which enhance or depress the immune response. These agents may be used in the treatment of conditions in which the immune response is depressed, such as cancer, and are often biologic substances derived from cells involved in the immune response, or are synthesized using recombinant DNA technology. Figure 61–1 is a simplified diagram showing components of the immune system and sites of action of some of these immune system modulators. This chapter serves to highlight the unique application of immune system modulators as immunopharmacologic agents.

IMMUNOSUPPRESSANTS

Prednisone

The corticosteroids were the first group of agents recognized as having lympholytic properties. Predni-

sone, the most commonly used immunosuppressant, reduces the size and lymphoid content of the lymph nodes and the spleen, although it has no toxic effect on proliferating myeloid or erythroid stem cells in the bone marrow.

Prednisone can suppress the inflammatory response of cell-mediated immunity and may suppress antibody synthesis. It is cytotoxic to certain subsets of T cells, and some of its diverse effects may be due to lysis of either suppressor or helper T cells. Plasma cells are less affected, but as the precursor lymphoid stem cells are sensitive to the drug, the primary response is diminished and, with continued use of the steroid, previously established antibody responses are decreased.

Continuous administration of prednisone increases the fractional catabolic rate of IgG, thus lowering the concentration of specific antibodies.

The corticosteroids also offset some effects of the immune response by reducing tissue injury from inflammation and edema. Prednisone is used in a wide variety of clinical conditions where the immunosuppressant properties of the drug account for its beneficial effects. These include autoimmune disorders (e.g., autoimmune hemolytic anemia, idiopathic thrombocytopenic purpura, systemic lupus erythematosus) and organ transplantation (e.g., kidney, bone marrow). Other uses and adverse effects are described in Chapter 47.

Azathioprine

At present azathioprine (Imuran®) is the drug most often used for immunosuppression in relation to organ transplantation. It is the precursor of mercaptopurine, which is the active molecule. Mercaptopurine, a structural analog or antimetabolite of hypoxanthine, interferes with nucleic acid metabolism (purine synthesis) during the wave of lymphoid cell proliferation that follows antigen stimulation, and is especially effective against T cells. Its toxic effects are primarily bone mar-

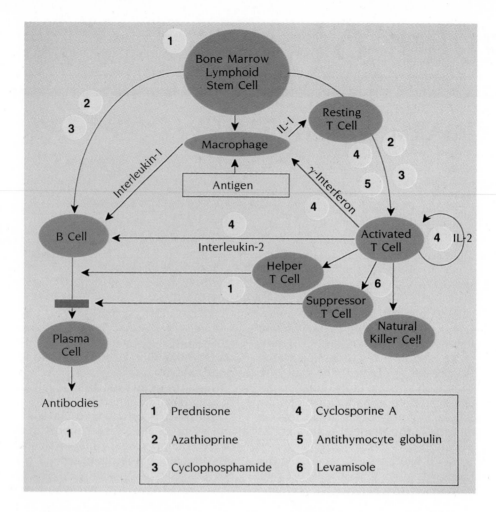

Figure 61–1 Sites of action of immune system modulators. (Natural killer cells are also known as cytotoxic cells.)

row depression and possible reactivation of viral hepatitis (*see* Chapter 60).

Cyclophosphamide

This alkylating agent is an antineoplastic drug that is also a potent immunosuppressor used chiefly in patients who do not tolerate azathioprine. It is a modified nitrogen mustard that destroys proliferating lymphoid cells, but that also alkylates some resting cells, rupturing the DNA double helix and inducing lethal mutations. Cyclophosphamide (Cytoxan®) was originally designed as an inactive nitrogen mustard precursor that would be converted to the active alkylating form at its site of action. Its adverse effects are those of the nitrogen mustards (*see* Chapter 60).

Cyclosporine A

This fungal antibiotic is one of many cyclosporins with a narrow spectrum of antibiotic activity, but with profound immunosuppressive effects on cell-mediated cytolysis in graft-host reactions and on delayed-type hypersensitivity. It has a remarkably specific affinity for lymphocytes, affecting both T cells and B cells in humans. Other cell types, including myeloid cells, are spared.

Cyclosporine A (Sandimmune®) interferes with early events during lymphocyte transformation and inhibits monocyte/macrophage function indirectly. In resting T cells this agent inhibits production of, and response to, interleukin-2 (IL-2), a lymphokine secreted by lymphocytes and macrophages that regulates the immune response. It can block IL-2 production by activated T lymphocytes but does not affect their IL-2 responsiveness. Cyclosporine A can suppress gamma-interferon and other macrophage growth factors, resulting in a decrease of interleukin-1. It appears that T cell suppressor function is not affected by cyclosporine A, thus shifting the balance in the immune system to promote natural immunosuppression.

The clinical use of cyclosporine A has been explored in organ transplantation and the treatment of autoimmune diseases. Studies of the clinical pharmacology of the drug indicate a large variation in bioavailability (5–90%), large amounts bound to erythrocytes and plasma proteins, and extensive biotransformation. The major route of elimination is biliary.

A major adverse effect of the agent is nephrotoxicity, which can be potentiated when the drug is administered together with amphotericin B, aminoglycosides, and co-trimoxazole. Other side effects include hirsutism; gingival hyperplasia; elevations of serum bilirubin, alkaline phosphatase, and transaminases; neurotoxicity; and a risk of lymphomas.

Antithymocyte Globulin

This product (Atgam®) is a concentrated gamma globulin, primarily monomeric IgG from hyperimmune plasma of horses immunized with human thymus lymphocytes. It reduces the number of T lymphocytes in thymus-dependent areas of the spleen and lymph nodes. Although it stimulates an antibody response in humans, this can be minimized by concomitant administration of other immunosuppressants such as azathioprine. The agent has been used to overcome graft rejections and to delay the onset of rejection. Other indications for its use have included aplastic anemia, T-cell malignancies, and graft-versus-host disease when reduction of T-cell function is considered important.

Common adverse reactions include fever, chills, leukopenia, thrombocytopenia, and skin reactions. Less frequently, arthralgia, chest and back pain, diarrhea, headache, and anaphylaxis may occur.

Immunosuppression Therapeutic Plan

Many immunosuppressive drugs are also antineoplastic agents, but the therapeutic plan differs for the two applications. For example, those cytotoxic agents that act primarily against proliferating cells act against both proliferating cancer cells and proliferating immune cells. But cancer cell proliferation is generally random while immune cell proliferation is "synchronized" in a burst of mitotic division after introduction of antigen, with a large proportion of the cells proliferating in one generation cycle. So, when drugs are used at the time of an implant, a large proportion of the initially small number of precursor cells can be destroyed by one high dose of the immunosuppressant, and long-term destruction is maintained with a low-dose daily schedule thereafter.

When the same drugs are used against cancer (see Chapter 60), they are given in high-dose pulses every 3–6 weeks in order to allow immune rebound between treatments.

IMMUNE MODULATORS

Levamisole

This drug is an anthelminthic agent that has been shown to potentiate immune responses in animals and humans. It is an imidazole derivative and it is thought to act by inhibiting the production of a substance by T suppressor cells that has immunosuppressive properties. A major side effect of this drug is arthralgia.

Interferons

These are a group of glycoproteins first identified as compounds that inhibit intracellular viral replication (see Chapter 58). Currently there are three major classes of interferons—α, β, and γ.

Interferons have been produced by stimulation of lymphocyte or fibroblast precursors, and now alpha-interferon is available through recombinant DNA technology. Alpha-interferon is derived from human lymphoblasts and beta-interferon from human fibroblasts. Gamma-interferon is also referred to as immune interferon.

Alpha-interferon can modulate antibody responses and enhance natural killer cell activity. It can be immunosuppressive because of antiproliferative effects. Gamma-interferon is a potent activator of macrophage function and may be antagonistic or synergistic in interactions with other lymphokines. Currently, alpha-interferon is approved for use in hairy cell leukemia, and it is being actively investigated in many other disease states.

Adverse effects have included fever, chills, hypotension, paraesthesias, and altered mental state. Neutropenia and elevated serum transaminases are commonplace.

SUGGESTED READING

Bennett WM, Norman DJ. Action and toxicity of cyclosporine. Annu Rev Med 1986; 37:215–224.

Patterson R, Norman P. Immunotherapy—immunomodulation. JAMA 1982; 248:2759–2772.

Pfeffer LM, ed. Mechanisms of interferon actions. Boca Raton: CRC Press, 1987.

Salvaggio JE, ed. Primer on allergic and immunologic diseases. JAMA 1982; 248(20).

CHEMOTHERAPY

SPECIAL TOPICS

Chapter 62

DRUGS, ALCOHOL, AND THE LIVER

H. Kalant and H. Orrego

Interactions between drugs and the liver are of pharmacologic interest in relation to two different questions: How do variations in liver function affect the fate of drugs and how do drugs (including ethanol) affect liver function? The first question is dealt with in several other chapters of this book and will therefore be mentioned only briefly in the present context. The second question will be covered in greater detail, in particular as it relates to alcoholic liver disease.

EFFECTS OF LIVER FUNCTION ON PHARMACOKINETICS

Basic Liver Functions Relevant to Drug Metabolism

Circulation

Normally the portal vein supplies about 70% of the liver blood flow and the hepatic artery about 30%, although the exact proportions vary from one species to another. Total liver blood flow amounts to about 25–30% of the cardiac output, but since the portal venous blood has already passed through the intestinal circulation, it is a low-pressure flow with low Po_2. The liver has low-resistance shunts that connect the junction of the portal venous and hepatic arterial flows directly to the terminal hepatic vein (central vein), bypassing the sinusoid. These shunts probably serve to permit portal venous blood to reach the systemic circulation when the perfusion pressure is too low to ensure flow through the sinusoids. The cost of this safeguard is that blood passing through the shunts is not exposed to the hepatocytes. Variations in blood flow and in intrahepatic shunting, therefore, markedly affect the delivery of drug to the liver. The importance of this factor in drug clearance is explained in Chapter 7.

Cellular Uptake Mechanisms

Free drug can enter the hepatocyte by passive diffusion or active transport; protein-bound drug can be taken up by pinocytosis. More than one mechanism may be involved in the uptake of the same drug. For example, free d-tubocurarine, which is actively transported across the cell membrane into the cytoplasm, is secreted into the bile, but protein-bound tubocurarine, which is taken up by pinocytosis, finds its way into lysosomes where it is stored and from which it can be displaced by quinacrine and other competing drugs. Mathematical analysis of hepatic uptake of drugs is considered in Chapter 7.

Storage

Storage can occur in lysosomes, as mentioned above, or by binding to intracellular proteins, as in the case of the antimalarial drugs. It seems likely that highly lipid-soluble drugs can also be stored within intracellular fat droplets.

Biotransformation

This is dealt with in detail in Chapter 4. As noted there, biotransformation can inactivate many drugs, but it can activate others and convert them into toxic compounds. The latter process will be of special interest in this chapter.

Biliary Secretion

Two separate phases contribute to the formation of the bile that is finally put out by the liver. The canalicular phase involves active secretion of Na^+, bile pigments, and drugs and their metabolites by the hepatocytes; this phase is induced by chronic treatment with phenobarbital. The bile-duct phase involves movement of electrolytes and water across the bile duct epithelium; it is under endocrine control and regulates the concentration and volume of the bile, and therefore its rate of movement down the biliary duct system. Biliary secretion may be an important factor in the fate of some drugs and of negligible significance to others.

Effects of Disturbed Liver Function on Pharmacokinetics

Circulation

Shock causes a fall in splanchnic blood flow, and within the liver the blood is diverted from the sinusoids to the low-pressure shunts. This reduces the delivery of drug to the liver cells and also decreases the supply of oxygen needed for most drug biotransformations. Both effects tend to prolong the half-life of the drug in the body. The same results can be produced by an extrahepatic portocaval shunt or by intrahepatic obstruction of blood flow due to swelling of the liver cells (inflammation, fat accumulation, hypertrophy of endoplasmic reticulum, osmotic swelling) or fibrosis (e.g., portal cirrhosis). Similar effects can be produced temporarily by vasoconstrictor drugs such as catecholamines and vasopressin, which can therefore alter the hepatic uptake of other drugs.

While the major effect of such circulatory disturbances is to reduce the rate of drug delivery to the liver, they can also decrease the rate of absorption of drug from the intestinal lumen. Increased intrahepatic pressure, with corresponding decrease in hepatic blood flow, also decreases the rate of flow through submucosal capillaries in the GI tract, and thus decreases the concentration gradient that maintains diffusion of drug from the lumen to the blood. For example, a recent study showed that in patients with portal hypertension the time to reach peak plasma concentration after an oral dose of the anti-inflammatory agent sulindac (*see* Chapter 33) was increased to 2.5 hours from a normal time of 1.2 hour.

The effect of such changes in drug delivery depends on the relative importance of hepatic biotransformation versus other routes of elimination for the individual drug in question. For example, the fate of digoxin will be unchanged because it is eliminated by renal excretion, while the half-life of digitoxin will be prolonged because it depends primarily on hepatic biotransformation. Similarly, the fate of ether will not be affected appreciably because it is primarily cleared by the lung, whereas halothane and methoxyflurane will have a longer sojourn in the body because they undergo a substantial degree of biotransformation in the liver. For most drugs, the effect of decreased hepatic circulation will be a decreased rate of elimination from the body.

On the other hand, this same effect can be protective if the drug is transformed into a toxic material in the liver. An interesting example is provided by the reduction of carcinogenicity of 3-methyl-4-dimethyl-amino-azobenzene (MDAB) in rats that have undergone a portocaval shunt operation. MDAB is biotransformed by three different reactions in liver microsomes (Fig. 62–1). Two reactions produce pharmacologically inert products, but the third forms an active compound that can bind covalently to DNA in the liver cell nucleus and act as a carcinogen. After a portocaval shunt, the liver is decreased in size, and microsomal drug-biotransforming activity is reduced. The pathway that leads to carcinogenesis is normally less active than the others, and therefore is selectively abolished by a reduction in hepatic oxygen supply. In one experiment, 73% of controls developed liver cancer after 11–20 weeks on MDAB, while only 5% of the animals with a shunt did so.

Hepatocellular Uptake

A reduction in functional liver cell mass can have two competing effects on the hepatic uptake of drugs:

1. Decreased plasma protein concentration, which often results from liver disease, can cause a significant increase in the free fraction of a drug that is normally extensively protein-bound, and this in turn can result in increased hepatic uptake. Many different types of drug are affected in this way. Some well-studied examples are amobarbital, cefoperazone, diazepam, morphine, phenytoin, propranolol, tolbutamide, and various nonsteroidal anti-inflammatory drugs. The increase in hepatic uptake of the drug is sometimes greater than the reduction in plasma albumin concentration, and it is possible that a qualitative change in the albumin may result in lower drug-binding affinity.

2. The decreased liver cell mass can mean a decreased uptake capacity. The actual result in any given case depends on the balance of these two factors. Usually, in severe liver disease, the effect of reduced cell mass predominates, and drug uptake is diminished. Several studies, for example, have shown a significant decrease in the clearance of antipyrine in patients with severe liver disease. There was an excellent correlation between the antipyrine clearance rate and the clearance of indocyanine green (Branch *et al.* Clin Pharmacol Ther 1976; 20:81–89) or the size of the liver estimated by ultrasonic scan (Halliwell *et al.* Br J Clin Pharmacol 1977; 4:393–394). Patients with severe cirrhosis also show greatly prolonged serum half-life times for phenobarbital, amobarbital, and hexobarbital.

Severe liver disease may also be accompanied by an increase in the apparent volume of distribution (*see* Chapter 5) for some drugs. This can be due to reduced plasma protein binding or to ascites, the ascitic fluid constituting an additional pool of extravascular fluid into which the drug can equilibrate.

Biotransformation

The effect of liver disease on the biotransformation of drugs after their uptake depends on the stage and

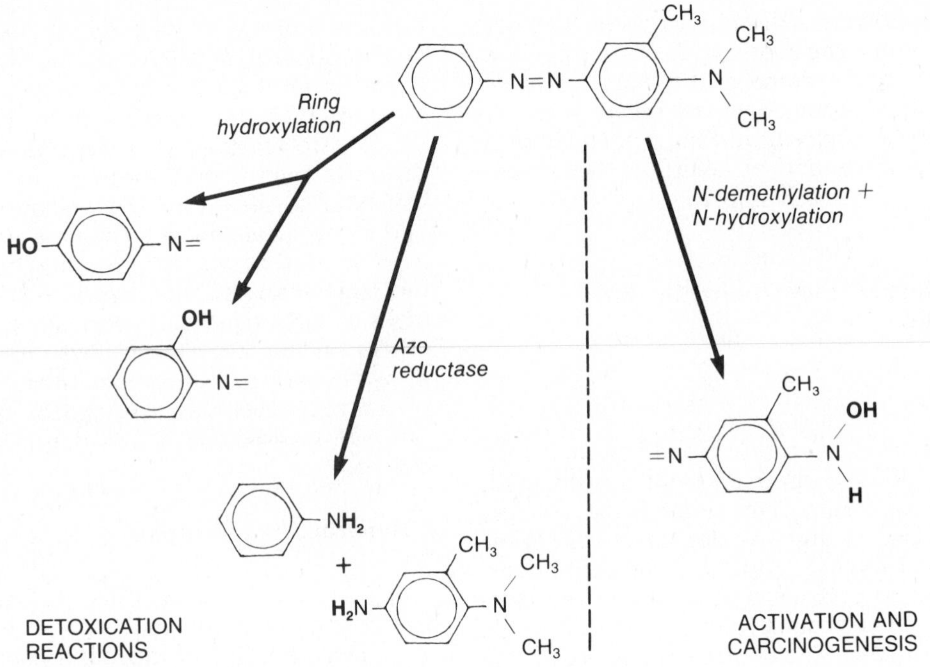

Figure 62-1 Pathways of biotransformation of 3-methyl-4-dimethylamino-azobenzene in the rat liver. The carcinogenic pathway, having the lowest activity, is the first to be depressed by a portocaval shunt.

severity of the disease. In mild disease, during the stage of recovery, there may be proliferation of liver cells to replace those previously damaged. During the phase of regeneration, all the constituents of the cytochrome P-450 pathway (*see* Chapter 4) may be increased, and the rate of biotransformation of barbiturates and many other drugs may actually be greater than normal.

However, in severe liver disease, punch biopsies have shown a 40–50% reduction in the cytochrome P-450 content and in the activities of N- and O-demethylases, pseudocholinesterase, and glucose-6-phosphate dehydrogenase (Schoene *et al.* Eur J Clin Pharmacol 1972; 4:65–73). There is a corresponding fall in the hydroxylation of phenobarbital, with an increase in the serum half-life of phenobarbital from 86 hours in healthy controls to 130 hours in cirrhotics (Alvin *et al.* J Pharmacol Exp Ther 1975; 192:224–235). Such changes are found in alcoholic hepatitis and active cirrhosis, but not in uncomplicated fatty liver or mild viral hepatitis.

These factors may require a decrease in dosage for some drugs. For example, patients with active liver disease may require from 15% to 65% reduction in dosage of various narcotic analgesics, nonsteroidal anti-inflammatory agents, long-acting benzodiazepines, digitoxin, beta-blockers, and verapamil.

Similar decreases in drug biotransformation by the liver may result from endocrine or other factors affecting the liver secondarily. For example, recent evidence in experimental animals indicates that progesterone and synthetic progestogens used in oral contraceptive pills prolong the sleeping time after a test dose of hexobarbital. Experimental kidney disease, in the stage of uremia, causes a fall in hepatic content of cytochrome P-450 and a decrease in drug-metabolizing activity. The mechanism of this effect is not clear; it may be due to endocrine disturbances or possibly to the accumulation of some hepatotoxic material that is normally excreted in the urine.

Bile Flow

The importance of reduction in rate of bile flow varies greatly from drug to drug. Some drugs (*e.g.*, d-tubocurarine) or drug metabolites (*e.g.*, hydroxybarbiturates) are secreted in high concentration in the bile and are significantly affected by changes in bile flow rate. For example, an infusion of saline or of sodium taurocholate, which increased the canalicular bile formation, resulted in increased biliary excretion of pentobarbital and its metabolites: 34% of a test dose appeared in the bile in control subjects and 46% after infusion of taurocholate. The ratio of pentobarbital to pentobarbital metabolites was not altered, so that the effect must have been exclusively on the flushing out of the biliary tree, rather than on the biotransformation reactions in the liver cell. Ligation of the bile duct caused the opposite change: sleeping time after thiopental, hexobarbital, or zoxazolamine was doubled 24 hours after bile duct obstruction.

In contrast, other drugs (e.g., digitoxin) are biotransformed in the liver, but the metabolites are passed back into the circulation and excreted by the kidney. Neither biliary obstruction nor bile flow stimulation affects their duration of action. Very closely related drugs may differ markedly with respect to their biliary excretion pattern. For example, after a test dose of the anticancer drug doxorubicin (see Chapter 60), only 20% of the drug appears in the bile in 24 hours, mainly as unaltered drug; with the more potent analog trifluoroacetyl-doxorubicin, over 80% appears in the bile, mainly as metabolites.

A general problem in such studies is that biliary excretion of a drug is normally investigated in animals or surgical patients with bile duct drainage *via* a catheter to the exterior. Therefore the results do not indicate what would happen in the intact subject when the bile reaches the intestine. If there is a significant degree of enterohepatic recirculation (see Chapter 1), the half-life for whole-body clearance might not be appreciably altered by a change in biliary secretion rate.

MECHANISMS OF DRUG-INDUCED LIVER DISEASE

Drugs can cause pathologic changes in liver histology and function by at least three different mechanisms. The type of damage differs according to the mechanism involved, and the speed of onset and the quantitative (dose-effect) relations also differ.

Indirect Extrahepatic Mechanisms

Drugs that produce major effects on circulation or respiration can cause liver damage by sharply decreasing the blood or oxygen supply to the liver, even temporarily. For example, massive release of noradrenaline* or adrenaline† causes a temporary **constriction of the splanchnic arterial bed**, including the hepatic artery. Drugs that produce shock (e.g., overdose of drugs such as quinidine that **impair myocardial contractility**) can produce an equivalent effect, not by constricting the visceral arteries but by decreasing the perfusion pressure that forces blood through them. **Respiratory depression**, by large doses of barbiturates or other hypnosedative drugs, causes poor oxygenation of the blood, so that oxygen supply to the liver is decreased even if the blood flow is not markedly affected.

All of these disturbances can lead to hypoxia of the liver, which, if severe enough, may result in degenerative changes or necrosis of liver cells. The damage tends to be periacinar, i.e., in the region of the terminal hepatic vein, formerly called the central vein. This is

---

* norepinephrine
† epinephrine

---

because the oxygen tension is normally highest at the confluence of the hepatic arterial and portal venous flows, at the proximal end of the sinusoid, and falls steadily as the blood moves along the sinusoid and oxygen is removed by the surrounding liver cells. Normally there is some oxygen reserve, and the Po_2 at the venous end, though lower than at the arterial end, is still high enough to meet the needs of the last liver cells along the sinusoid. However, if the arterial Po_2 falls, there may be insufficient oxygen left at the venous end and the cells suffer hypoxic damage. This is more likely to happen if the oxygen requirement of the cells is raised by high metabolic activity, such as increased urea formation due to a high-protein diet.

Drugs can also reduce hepatic blood flow by producing lesions of the intrahepatic blood vessels themselves. Oral contraceptives (see Chapter 45) and various anticancer chemotherapeutic agents (see Chapter 60) have been incriminated in the production of **thrombosis** of the large hepatic veins (Budd-Chiari syndrome) and of **veno-occlusive disease** of the small intrahepatic veins. The latter is a gradual constriction of the small veins by deposition of connective tissue around them. The same drugs, as well as a number of metallic poisons and vinyl chloride, have also been linked to perisinusoidal fibrosis and to gradual fibrous occlusion of the branches of the portal vein (hepatoportal sclerosis). Intravenous use of methamphetamine has been reported to cause **necrotizing angiitis**, a condition characterized by the formation of inflammatory nodules and microaneurysms in the walls of arterioles in the liver, brain, kidney, and other organs. These drug-induced vascular lesions are relatively rare, but they can be fatal when they do occur.

Some authors refer to the mechanisms of drug-induced liver damage described above as being due to "host idiosyncrasy," whereas those described below are considered "intrinsic toxicity."

Indirect Intrahepatic Mechanisms

Many drugs can cause liver injury by **interfering with an important metabolic pathway** and depriving the liver cell of an essential product. For example, tetracyclines and chloramphenicol (see Chapter 55) are antibiotics that can interfere with the synthesis of cell proteins, including the very-low-density lipoproteins that normally transport triglycerides out of the hepatocyte. Anticancer drugs (e.g., methotrexate, urethane, 6-mercaptopurine) can inhibit the synthesis of nucleic acids in normal cells as well as in malignant ones. Metabolism of ethanol by the alcohol dehydrogenase pathway inhibits the mitochondrial oxidation of fatty acids (see below) and the cytoplasmic oxidation of glycerophosphate, causing accumulation of triglycerides.

These metabolic disturbances typically lead to the production of fatty liver and other degenerative changes, and only occasionally (in severe cases) to liver cell necrosis. The effects are generally dose-dependent, but with a high degree of variability that possibly reflects differences in the degree of metabolic activity in the liver at the time the drug was given. The latency between the administration of the drug and the appearance of the damage ranges from several hours to several days. The percentage of exposed individuals who actually suffer liver damage is relatively low.

Another type of indirect cell damage is that due to **cholestasis** (obstruction of bile flow by precipitation of bile pigment within the bile canaliculi). Several steroids that are alkylated at position 17, such as the anabolic steroids and the synthetic estrogens and progestins used in oral contraceptives (Fig. 62–2), can inhibit the uptake of bile pigment from the plasma into the liver cell and its secretion into the bile. In addition, they decrease active secretion of Na$^+$ into the bile by the (Na$^+$+K$^+$)-ATPase of the liver cell and increase the permeability of the canalicular membrane to back-diffusion of water and some solutes from the bile canaliculi into the liver cell. Other compounds, such as

halogenated hydrocarbons, or chlorpromazine and a number of its derivatives, increase the permeability of the ductal epithelium, thus reducing the volume and the rate of bile flow along the canaliculi, and permitting the conjugated bile pigments to precipitate and form solid plugs blocking the canaliculi. The bile plugs lead to obstructive jaundice and mild degenerative changes in the liver cells that are secondary to the obstruction and are reversible when the drug is stopped.

Jaundice can also be caused by drugs that **interfere with the uptake of unconjugated bile pigments** from the circulating blood into the hepatic parenchymal cells. Examples include the antibiotics novobiocin and rifampin, and various radiopaque dyes used for X-ray visualization of the gall bladder. Since the bile pigments are prevented from being taken up into the liver and conjugated, they are poorly water-soluble, are not readily excreted by the kidney, and remain largely bound to serum proteins, where they can compete against the binding of other drugs.

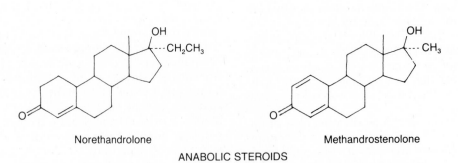

Ethinyl estradiol
SYNTHETIC ESTROGEN

Norethindrone   Norethynodrel

SYNTHETIC PROGESTINS

Norethandrolone   Methandrostenolone

ANABOLIC STEROIDS

Figure 62–2 Examples of C-17 alkylated steroids capable of causing cholestatic jaundice.

Direct Hepatic Toxicity

A number of agents including chloroform, carbon tetrachloride, furosemide, phenacetin, and acetaminophen are directly toxic to the liver cell. Unlike the indirect hepatotoxins, these direct-acting compounds show a **strict dose-dependence** with very **high reproducibility** experimentally and with a very **high incidence of damage** in exposed individuals. The **latency** between drug administration and onset of damage is very short, of the order of a few hours.

Some drugs appear to cause direct damage to the cell and mitochondrial membranes. An Oriental hornet venom was recently found to cause leakage of mitochondrial enzymes and electron-microscopic evidence of mitochondrial and plasma membrane damage in humans who had been stung repeatedly. Acetaminophen-induced hepatotoxicity in the rat was reported to cause a selective 52% drop in hepatocyte membrane $(Na^+ + K^+)$-ATPase 3 hours after the drug administration, whereas leakage of alanine aminotransferase and microscopic signs of necrosis were not found until 24 hours later. However, the typical lesion is **necrosis** (rather than fatty change, as caused by the indirect mechanisms). It tends to be widespread throughout the liver and indiscriminately located, though with a few of these drugs it may be zonal (periportal with some drugs and surrounding the terminal hepatic vein with others).

With a number of the direct hepatotoxins there is a **threshold dose** necessary to cause damage. For example, acetaminophen does not cause liver cell necrosis until the dose exceeds 300 mg/kg; beyond that, the damage is proportional to the dose. The reason for this appears to be that the damage is caused by a minor but highly reactive metabolite (Fig. 62–3) that can be inactivated by glutathione conjugation (*see* Chapter 4) to yield finally a mercapturic acid derivative that is excreted harmlessly in the urine. No damage occurs until the available glutathione is all used up and the toxic material is then free to react with essential constituents of the cell. Therefore, the damage by these drugs is increased by metabolic factors that reduce the cellular content of reduced glutathione and thus prolong the half-life of the toxic metabolite.

Since the damage is done by a **reactive metabolite** of the original drug, it can be prevented by blockers of drug biotransformation such as SKF 525A or increased by inducers of microsomal biotransformation reactions such as phenobarbital (*see* Chapter 4) or chronic ethanol ingestion. **Zonal distribution** of damage is seen with those drugs for which the biotransformation is localized to a specific zone (Fig. 62–4). The damage tends to occur at the point where the toxic metabolite is produced. For example, allyl alcohol is converted to acrolein in the periportal zone and produces necrosis there. In contrast, with acetaminophen the biotransformation and the damage are essentially

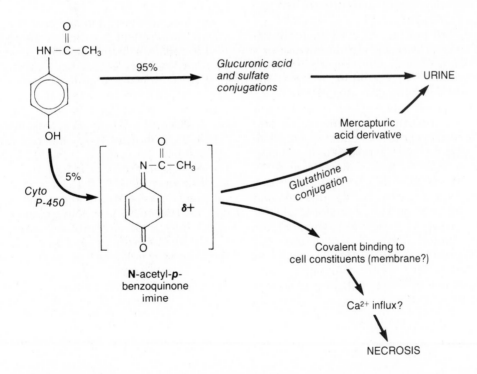

Figure 62–3 Probable mechanism of hepatotoxicity of acetaminophen. Covalent binding appears to occur only when the capacity for glutathione conjugation has been exceeded.

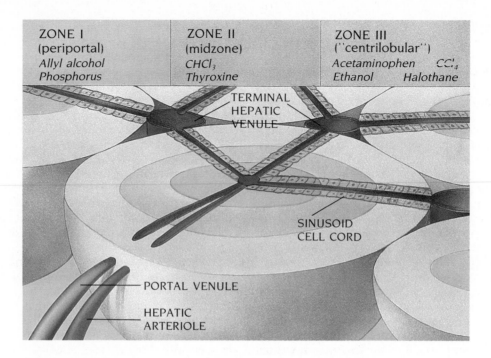

ZONE I (periportal)	ZONE II (midzone)	ZONE III ("centrilobular")
Allyl alcohol	$CHCl_3$	Acetaminophen CCl_4
Phosphorus	Thyroxine	Ethanol Halothane

TERMINAL HEPATIC VENULE

SINUSOID CELL CORD

PORTAL VENULE

HEPATIC ARTERIOLE

Figure 62–4   Zonal distribution of necrosis in the liver acinus, produced by various hepatotoxic agents.

centrilobular (Zone III). **Genetic variations** in drug biotransformation may also affect susceptibility to liver damage by the metabolites.

Numerous drugs can produce direct hepatocellular damage by mechanisms involving the production of a reactive intermediate. For example, liver cell necrosis after the administration of α-**methyldopa** is due to the formation of an epoxide intermediary metabolite, which acts as an arylating agent. This reaction is carried out by liver microsomes. **Halothane** is generally a safe anaesthetic, but a certain number of patients, especially those who undergo repeated exposure to it, develop fever, muscle and joint pains, nausea, anorexia, abdominal discomfort, and jaundice, which progresses to a Zone III hepatocellular necrosis. In rats, this damage is enhanced by pretreatment with phenobarbital. The explanation again appears to be the formation of a reactive metabolite. Under normoxic conditions the cytochrome P-450 system oxidizes the halothane to trifluoroacetate, but under hypoxic conditions it acts as a reducing system (see Chapter 4) and produces

a free radical that can bind covalently to the cell membrane (Fig. 62–5).

The mechanism of damage in all these cases appears to involve covalent bonding of the toxic metabolite to a vital cell constituent, possibly a membrane protein or a nucleic acid. Extent and severity of damage are proportional to the amount of covalent binding, which can be shown to occur about 1–2 hours before the appearance of cytologic damage. Glutathione can protect against such damage in at least three different ways: (1) detoxification of H_2O_2 and organoperoxides by a glutathione peroxidase reaction, (2) noncatalysed nucleophilic reaction of glutathione and drug to form stable adducts, and (3) the glutathione transferase reaction (see Chapter 4). The occurrence of cell destruction can be prevented if competing binding substances, such as cysteine or dimercaprol, are given early enough after the hepatotoxic drug. These substances can bind the toxic metabolite and prevent it from binding to the target constituents in the cell. In the case of CCl_4 poisoning, the toxic metabolite is the free radical,

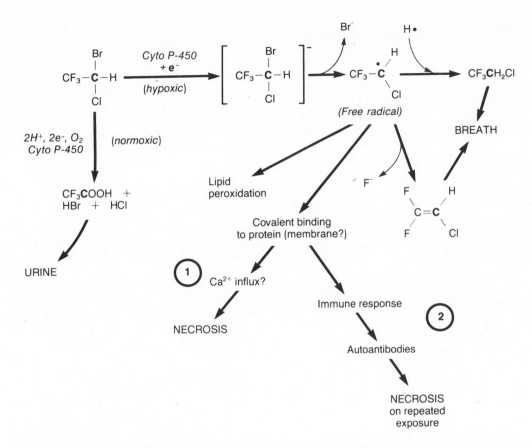

Figure 62–5 Postulated mechanism of hepatotoxicity by halothane. Pathway 1 would be the mechanism of necrosis produced by a single exposure to halothane, while pathway 2 is the suggested explanation of the increased risk on subsequent exposures. Both occur only under conditions of hypoxia in the liver, when the cytochrome P-450 functions as a reductase.

$CCl_3\cdot$, which can be "mopped up" by N-acetyl-cysteine or cystamine given up to 12 hours after the CCl_4. In contrast, drugs such as pyrazole or aminotriazole, which prevent the free radical formation, are protective only if given before or together with the CCl_4, but can do nothing against the $CCl_3\cdot$ if given after it has formed.

Recent evidence suggests that, after covalent binding has occurred, two different mechanisms are responsible for immediate versus delayed cell damage. **Immediate** damage, as in the case of halothane, appears to be due to altered ion permeability. Covalent binding of reactive intermediates to membrane proteins renders the membrane permeable to Ca^{2+}, which floods in along a concentration gradient and is the agent that finally kills the cell. In tissue culture, cell death can be prevented, even after covalent binding has occurred, by using a very low-calcium medium. Chlorpromazine, which hinders Ca^{2+} entry, also has a protective effect.

Delayed cell death, however, appears to be the result of an autoimmune reaction. The proteins that have been altered by covalent binding of the reactive drug metabolites can serve as antigens, giving rise to antibodies that may be able to attack the native proteins in previously undamaged cells. There is evidence that this may explain the increased risk of hepatotoxicity with repeated exposure to halothane, as well as the relatively long latent period. Similarly, tienilic acid (ticrynafen, a diuretic and uricosuric agent recently removed from the market because of hepatotoxicity) gives rise to a reactive intermediate that can alkylate a specific cytochrome P-450, converting it into an antigen. This gives rise to an antibody known as "anti-LKM$_2$" that reacts specifically with human cytochrome P-450$_8$ and decreases its ability to carry out hydroxylation of tienilic acid itself and of various other drugs. This antibody was found in the plasma of patients with ticrynafen hepatitis, but not in the plasma of patients who also received the drug but did not develop hepatitis. It is believed that the hepatitis was caused by the antibody attacking the native cytochrome P-450 in previously undamaged cells.

MECHANISMS OF ETHANOL-INDUCED LIVER PATHOLOGY

Alcoholic liver disease is the fourth commonest cause of death in white males in the United States. Worldwide, the annual mortality from alcoholic liver disease is no less than 310,000. The death rate due to this disease correlates quite well with alcohol consumption, which, during much of this century, increased steadily in every country except France.

Traditionally, alcoholic liver disease has been classified according to morphologic criteria into three categories: (1) fatty liver, (2) alcoholic hepatitis (liver cell necrosis and inflammation), and (3) cirrhosis, in which the normal lobular architecture of the liver is replaced by a nodular one. The nodules are surrounded by thick, fibrous septa. Some of these lesions appear to be of little consequence from the point of view of liver function. For example, fat accumulation (fatty liver) and, in certain circumstances, the presence of inactive cirrhosis (without associated alcoholic hepatitis) do not entail increased mortality risk.

Fatty Liver

This abnormality is thought to result mainly from the change of NAD to NADH during the metabolism of ethanol and acetaldehyde (see Chapter 25). The increase in hepatic NADH inhibits glycerophosphate dehydrogenase, leading to an elevated glycerophosphate level. The raised NADH also stimulates the synthesis and inhibits the oxidation of fatty acids by the liver. The decrease in oxidation of fatty acids is probably caused by the change in redox potential induced by alcohol, resulting in an increased transfer of H^+ into the mitochondria as malate, displacing the citric acid cycle as the normal donor of protons to the oxido-reduction chain, and resulting in an inhibition of the citric acid cycle and of fatty acid oxidation. The increase in both glycerophosphate and free fatty acids stimulates esterification of the fatty acids and the accumulation of neutral fat in the liver. Fatty liver, of itself, probably does not lead directly to hepatic fibrosis or cirrhosis.

For other examples of ethanol-induced disturbances of intermediary metabolism in the liver see Chapter 25.

Abnormalities Associated with Increased Severity of Liver Disease

The presence of necrosis, inflammation, Mallory bodies (accumulation of hyaline material in the hepatocytes), accumulation of collagen in the space of Disse, enlarged hepatocytes, and the presence of cirrhosis are all associated with increased severity of alcoholic liver disease. The abnormalities that are associated with a poor prognosis can be divided into two closely interdependent main groups, namely: (1) a reduction in the "functional" mass of the liver, and (2) the presence of portal hypertension and its consequences (ascites, encephalopathy, and renal abnormalities).

Three elements contribute to reduction of the "functional" mass of the liver: necrosis, compression of sinusoids by expanded hepatocytes, and interposition of exchange barriers of differing nature in the space of Disse.

Necrosis

The two most accepted general causes that have been postulated to lead to alcoholic hepatocellular necrosis are liver cell hypoxia and acetaldehyde-mediated liver cell damage.

Any theory postulating a mechanism for alcohol-induced liver cell necrosis has to account for the following facts: necrosis has a focal distribution; it occurs in Zone III of the liver acinus; and only a minority of those exposed to alcohol are affected.

The hypoxia theory. The liver has a high oxygen requirement, 60–70% of its blood supply is venous, and the perivenular zone of the acinus is normally in a state of hypoxia relative to the periportal zone. Therefore, this organ is highly susceptible to hypoxic cell damage. Preservation of normal liver function and hepatocellular integrity requires a fine balance between the consumption and the delivery of oxygen to the liver.

Oxygen tensions in the liver cells are lower in the perivenular areas (surrounding the "central vein"; Zone III) than in the periportal areas (Zone I), indicating that oxygen is removed during blood flow along the sinusoid, especially in Zone I. Oxygen tension in the portal vein is about 65–70 mm Hg, while in the hepatic veins it drops to about 30 mm Hg. The latter value constitutes an average oxygen tension resulting from a mixture of blood flowing through sinusoids of different lengths, and oxygen tensions as low as 2 mm Hg (approximately 0.1 mM) can be observed in some individual sinusoids. Moreover, there are diffusion barriers that might markedly reduce the availability of oxygen. Several studies of the redox potential of liver cells have shown that Zone III is normally in a partial state of relative hypoxia. If conditions of increased oxygen demand are not accompanied by a corresponding increase in oxygen delivery, the low oxygen tensions in Zone III could result in a critical **focal** hypoxic state and liver cell damage. Thus, situations that increase the requirements of the liver for oxygen, such as fever and hyperthyroidism, or that reduce oxygen delivery, such as anemia, congestive heart failure, and anaesthesia, can potentially result in hepatocellular necrosis.

Both acute and chronic administration of ethanol produce an increase in oxygen consumption by the liver (the hypermetabolic state) attributed, at least in part, to an increased utilization of ATP by the $(Na^+ + K^+)$-ATPase. The increase in ATP utilization leads to more availability of the phosphate acceptor ADP in the mitochondria, and therefore to an increase in the capacity of the mitochondria to oxidize NADH to NAD⁺. As a result, chronic alcohol ingestion leads also to an increase in the rate of ethanol metabolism (see Chapter 25).

The increase in oxygen uptake along the liver sinusoid results in a more pronounced oxygen gradient between Zone I and Zone III of the acinus, thus increasing the degree of hypoxia of Zone III. The degree of Zone III hypoxia induced by alcohol *per se* is not sufficient to produce liver damage, since most humans or animals chronically drinking large quantities of ethanol fail to develop hepatocellular necrosis, despite showing a marked increase in oxygen consumption by the liver. This probably reflects the protective effect of a compensatory increase in portal blood flow induced by ethanol, which can result in a normal mean oxygen tension in hepatic vein blood despite increased oxygen consumption by the liver. The alcohol-induced increase in portal blood flow has been attributed to the release of adenosine through interaction of two factors: acetate produced from the metabolism of ethanol, and the presence of hypoxia in the liver during the metabolism of ethanol. The bulk of the acetate generated in the metabolism of ethanol leaves the liver and is oxidized in extrahepatic tissues to acetyl-CoA, with the formation of 5'-AMP from ATP. 5'-AMP is metabolized to adenosine by the enzyme 5'-nucleotidase. It is also known that hypoxia *per se* releases adenosine, which lowers vascular resistance in the liver.

It has been postulated, therefore, that the production of cell necrosis requires the combination of two factors: the direct effect of ethanol on the liver that increases oxygen consumption and a precipitating factor that occurs at random and that decreases oxygen delivery to the liver. Among the random precipitating factors may be anemia, pulmonary insufficiency, excessive smoking, or sleep apnea.

The increase in oxygen consumption induced by both acute and chronic administration of ethanol requires thyroid hormone function as a **permissive** factor. Both thyroidectomy and the administration of the antithyroid drug propylthiouracil (PTU, see Chapter 44) markedly suppress or abolish both the acute and chronically induced hypermetabolic state. PTU administration markedly protected rats against liver necrosis induced by ethanol in the presence of low atmospheric oxygen tensions. Prolonged administration of PTU to patients with alcoholic liver disease resulted in an important decrease in mortality during a 2-year period of observation.

Acetaldehyde as a mediator of hepatocellular damage. Acetaldehyde, the initial product of alcohol metabolism, is a highly reactive metabolite that can bind to a number of molecules of biologic importance, including proteins such as hemoglobin, tubulin and albumin, DNA, phospholipids, and serotonin. Also, it can interact with dopamine and noradrenaline, yielding pharmacologically active and potentially cytotoxic compounds. It is not clear, however, whether these inter-

actions are related to cell necrosis, nor has an animal model been produced in which acetaldehyde has been involved as the direct cause of hepatotoxicity.

A number of investigators have proposed that acetaldehyde-mediated cell death might have an immunologic component. New findings have indicated that acetaldehyde *per se* can become a hapten when bound covalently to amino acid residues in macromolecules. The antibodies generated are directed against acetaldehyde-modified proteins independently of the nature of the carrier protein. If this happens on the surface of cells, it might be followed by cell lysis. Increased antibody titres against acetaldehyde-containing epitopes have been found predominantly in those alcoholics with alcoholic hepatitis characterized by cell necrosis and polymorphonuclear inflammation.

Acetaldehyde could account for the centrilobular localization of cell necrosis, since acetaldehyde, formed in the metabolism of ethanol along the sinusoid, is present in a higher concentration in blood leaving Zone III than in Zone I.

Hepatocyte Enlargement

Hepatomegaly is a nearly constant finding in alcoholic liver disease in humans and has also been observed in young rats fed alcohol chronically. This hepatomegaly is due to an increase in hepatocyte size rather than in the number of hepatocytes. In rats, 50–60% of the increase in liver weight induced by chronic ethanol administration can be accounted for by an increase in intracellular water, with a substantial reduction in the ratio of extracellular to intracellular water. An increase in intracellular K⁺ can osmotically account for 50% of the excess water retained in the hepatocytes. The nature of the intracellular anions accompanying the additional K⁺ is not clear.

The enlarged hepatocytes in the rat compress the sinusoids, resulting in an increased resistance to blood flow and, after a threshold in cell size is exceeded, in increased intrahepatic and portal pressure. In humans with alcoholic liver disease biopsies also reveal a marked reduction in the calibre of the sinusoids and in total sinusoidal area when compared to nonalcoholic patients with normal liver histology. Also, in such patients hepatocyte size correlates positively with portal pressure independently of the histologic diagnosis of fatty liver, alcoholic hepatitis, or cirrhosis. These findings are consistent with the concept that sinusoidal compression by the enlarged hepatocytes is one mechanism for portal hypertension in this condition. However, this postulate does not exclude the possible contribution of other factors such as compression by cirrhotic nodules, collagenization of the space of Disse, and fibrosis around the terminal hepatic vein. The compression of the sinusoids, by decreasing liver cell perfusion, can also interfere with the delivery of oxygen to the hepatocyte and thus potentiate the hypoxia in Zone III and increase the likelihood of liver necrosis in the presence of continued drinking.

Abnormalities in the Space of Disse

The following abnormalities have been described in chronic alcoholics: accumulation of collagen in the space of Disse, reduction of hepatocyte microvilli, capillarization of the sinusoids, and a marked decrease in the number of fenestrae in the sinusoidal endothelium. There is a very good correlation between the degree of accumulation of collagen in the space of Disse and both portal hypertension and severity of liver disease. These abnormalities not only decrease the calibre and elasticity of the sinusoids but can also restrict the exchange of substrates (and possibly of oxygen) from the sinusoids to the hepatocytes.

Cirrhosis

This is the end-stage of alcoholic liver disease and develops in about 10% of persons taking alcoholic beverages in excess. The condition is characterized by a loss of the normal architecture of the liver, formation of fibrous septa bridging the portal veins, and the formation of regenerative nodules. As a consequence of these abnormalities, hepatic vasculature is grossly distorted, with transformation of sinusoids into capillary-like structures and shunting of the blood from the portal venules to the hepatic vein. Much of the portal blood thus bypasses the hepatic parenchymal cells, and there is a progressive loss of the liver's important role as a filter for substances entering the circulation from the gastrointestinal tract.

The exact mechanism by which alcohol leads to cirrhosis has not been established. However, three mechanisms can contribute to fibrosis of the liver after prolonged alcohol abuse:
- There is evidence that alcohol itself can stimulate fibrogenesis and collagen synthesis.
- Necrosis of liver cells can result in fibrosis and scarring, especially in Zone III.
- Portal hypertension might induce collagen accumulation in the space of Disse.

The frequency of the development of cirrhosis is related to the degree and the duration of alcohol abuse. Most cirrhotics have consumed more than 80 g of absolute ethanol (equivalent to more than 250 mL of distilled spirits, i.e., over one-third of a bottle) daily for more than 10 years. Absolute alcohol intake seems to be the important factor, regardless of the type of beverage consumed.

Alcoholic cirrhosis is fatal within a few years, but the life span can often be prolonged substantially if the patient stops drinking alcohol, even though the fibrous scarring of the liver remains. The cause of death in alcoholic liver disease is either portal hypertension or metabolic failure of the liver cells. These can occur in the absence of histologic evidence of cirrhosis, and on the other hand a quiescent cirrhosis can be present without serious portal hypertension or hepatocellular failure.

The Production of Vicious Cycles

The severity of alcoholic liver disease depends upon the fact that the mechanisms described above can interact in such a way as to create a self-perpetuating "vicious cycle." Portal hypertension results in upper gastrointestinal bleeding, collateral circulation bypassing the liver, reduced functional blood perfusion of the liver, hypersplenism, and secondary anemia. All of these reduce oxygen availability to the liver and therefore, in the presence of continued alcohol intake, they increase the risk of hypoxic hepatocellular necrosis. Necrosis, on the other hand, triggers collagen deposition and leads to a reduction in hepatocyte microvilli and in the number of fenestrae as well as increased rigidity of the space of Disse. These effects interfere further with the optimum exchange of oxygen and nutrients between the blood and the hepatocyte. Also, cell expansion *per se*, which appears to be an important mechanism in the production of portal hypertension, can reduce sinusoidal perfusion through functional pathways. Furthermore, as a consequence of portal hypertension, the intra- and extrahepatic shunting of blood reduces the effectiveness of the compensatory mechanisms that normally increase portal blood flow in the presence of ethanol.

All of these cycles decrease oxygen availability to the liver cell. Other cycles may exist at lesser degrees of severity. Although in normal persons the blood levels of acetaldehyde following ethanol ingestion are extremely low, acetaldehyde levels increase in alcoholics, who metabolize alcohol at higher rates. The presence of liver disease in which acetaldehyde dehydrogenase is reduced will also diminish the removal of acetaldehyde. The latter may create an additional vicious cycle through the formation of adducts and immune complexes.

From the above, it is clear that in the presence of interactive systems the disease is self-fuelled, becoming less dependent on both external precipitating causes and amounts of alcohol consumed.

SUGGESTED READING

Davis M, Tredger JM, Williams R, eds. Drug reactions and the liver. London: Pitman Medical, 1981.

Israel Y, Kalant H, Orrego H, et al. Experimental alcohol-induced hepatic necrosis: suppression by propylthiouracil. Proc Natl Acad Sci USA 1975; 72:1137–1141.

Israel Y, Orrego H. Hypermetabolic state, hepatocyte expansion and liver blood flow: an interaction triad in alcoholic liver injury. Ann NY Acad Sci 1987; 492:303–323.

Klaassen CD, Watkins JB III. Mechanisms of bile formation, hepatic uptake, and biliary excretion. Pharmacol Rev 1984; 36:1–67.

Mitchell JR, Jollows DJ. Progress in hepatology. Metabolic activation of drugs to toxic substances. Gastroenterology 1975; 68:392–410.

Mitchell JB, Russo A. The role of glutathione in radiation and drug induced cytotoxicity. Br J Cancer [Suppl] 1987; 8:96–104.

Nies AS, Shand DG, Wilkinson GR. Altered hepatic blood flow and drug disposition. Clin Pharmacokinet 1976; 1:135–155.

Orrego H, Israel Y, Blendis L. Alcoholic liver disease: information in search of knowledge? Hepatology 1981; 1:267–283.

Szilagyi A, Lerman S, Resnick RH. Ethanol, thyroid hormones and acute liver injury: is there a relationship? Hepatology 1983; 3:593–600.

Timbrell JA. Drug hepatotoxicity. Br J Clin Pharmacol 1983; 15:3–14.

Zafrani ES, Pinaudeau Y, Dhumeaux D. Drug-induced vascular lesions of the liver. Arch Intern Med 1983; 143:495–502.

Zimmerman HJ. Hepatotoxicity: the adverse effects of drugs and other chemicals on the liver. New York: Appleton-Century-Crofts, 1978.

Zimmerman HJ, Maddrey WC. Toxic and drug-induced hepatitis. In: Schiff L, Schiff ER, eds. Disease of the liver, 5th ed. Philadelphia: JB Lippincott, 1987:591–667.

Chapter 63

Carcinogenesis and Mutagenesis by Xenobiotic Chemicals

A.B. Okey

In North America, more than one person in four will develop cancer; this can occur at any age, from infancy to senescence. Cancer is the cause of death for about one person in six. What are its causes? The epidemiologist John Higginson has been widely cited as stating (in 1979) that 60–90% of human cancers are primarily due to "environmental factors." By "environmental factors," Higginson meant not only environmental chemicals, but also other contributing elements such as diet and cultural and behavioral practices. These are collectively termed "lifestyle."

There is little doubt that exposure to xenobiotic (foreign) chemicals (in the form of drugs or environmental substances) is a major risk factor in the overall incidence of human cancer. Nearly one-third of cancer deaths in North America are related to the use of cigarettes and other tobacco products. Other medical, industrial, and environmental chemicals that are strongly implicated in the human cancer problem are summarized later in this chapter.

As illustrated in Figures 63–1 and 63–2, Canadian mortality rates from cancer at most anatomic sites have decreased, increased a little, or remained constant over the past 50 years. The important exception is lung cancer. In Canadian males, mortality from lung cancer has escalated rapidly since World War II. This rise is almost certainly the result of the increased frequency of cigarette smoking, a practice that became common in the male population around the time of World War I.

The lung cancer problem illustrates an important manner in which cancer differs from most other chemically induced toxic responses. That is, cancer usually appears only after a long **latent period**. Human cancers typically may not be clinically evident for as long as 10–20 years after exposure to the agent that caused the tumor. Obviously, this great time delay between exposure and cancer detection complicates identification of the responsible agent(s).

The concept of a latent period is further illustrated by cancer mortality data in Canadian females. Cigarette smoking did not become common in the Canadian fe-

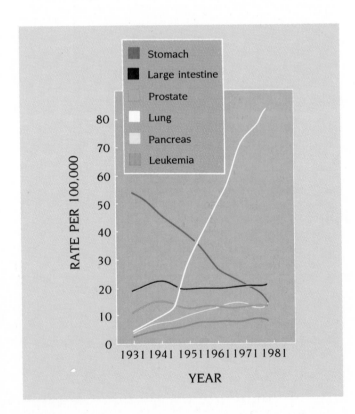

Figure 63–1 Age-standardized (25–74) Canadian mortality rates for six major cancer sites, 1931–1984 (male). (Courtesy of Ms. E. Mark, Bureau of Epidemiology, Health and Welfare Canada.)

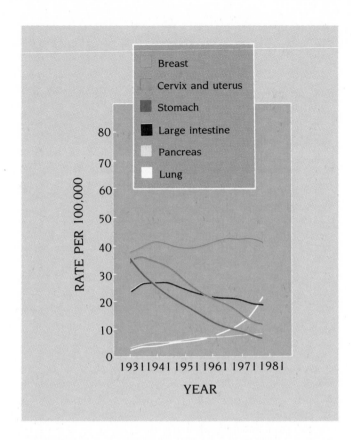

RATE PER 100,000

Breast
Cervix and uterus
Stomach
Large intestine
Pancreas
Lung

80
70
60
50
40
30
20
10
0

1931 1941 1951 1961 1971 1981
YEAR

Figure 63-2 Age-standardized (25–74) Canadian mortality rates for six major cancer sites, 1931–1984 (female). (Courtesy of Ms. E. Mark, Bureau of Epidemiology, Health and Welfare Canada.)

TABLE 63-1 Environmental Factors and Industrial Agents Implicated in Human Carcinogenesis

Ionizing radiation
Ultraviolet radiation

Aromatic amines
Arsenic
Asbestos
Aflatoxins
Benzene
Benzidine
Cadmium
Carbon tetrachloride
Chromium
Soots, tars, mineral oils
Tobacco smoke
Vinyl chloride

male population until World War II. As shown in Figure 63–2, mortality from lung cancer in Canadian females began to increase sharply around 1960. The rise in mortality from lung cancer in Canadian females is tragically reminiscent of the escalation that began in the male population two decades earlier. The most recent data indicate that in North America lung cancer has overtaken breast cancer as the leading cause of cancer-related deaths in females.

CHEMICAL CARCINOGENS: DIVERSITY OF ORIGINS AND CHEMICAL STRUCTURES

"Natural" Versus "Synthetic" Carcinogens

Tables 63–1 to 63–3 list several agents that have been reported to be carcinogenic. Notice that these lists include both "natural" and "synthetic" chemicals.

Although many of the carcinogens known are products of modern synthetic chemistry or are byproducts of industrial processes, the "natural world" contained carcinogens long before humans developed technological-industrial societies (Ames *et al.*, 1987).

For example, aflatoxin B_1, a potent liver carcinogen, is routinely formed by molds that contaminate improperly stored foodstuffs; polycyclic aromatic hydrocarbons such as benzo(a)pyrene are universally generated by partial combustion processes, including burning of wood and charcoal-cooking of food, as well as by internal combustion engines; safrole, a volatile oil from sassafras tea, is a carcinogen in mice and possibly in humans. Many other examples of naturally occurring carcinogens could be given. The point is that carcinogens are formed both by natural processes and by human activities.

Prevalence of Carcinogens in the Chemical World

It is important to understand that not all chemicals have carcinogenic properties, regardless of whether they are natural products or synthetic chemicals (Higginson, 1987). News reports in the popular media often give the incorrect impression that the majority of drugs and environmental chemicals cause cancer.

Table 63–4 gives some perspective on the prevalence of carcinogens in the overall spectrum of known chemicals. It can be seen that the number of **known** carcinogens is very small when compared to the number of existing chemical structures. In truth, however, the vast majority of chemicals, even those in common use, have not been adequately tested for carcinogenicity. Thus, it is impossible to state the magnitude of carcinogen exposure with any degree of accuracy. The methods

SPECIAL TOPICS

TABLE 63-2 Carcinogenic Anticancer Drugs

Drug	Species and Site or Type of Neoplasm Induced
Streptozotocin	Rat: kidney Chinese hamster: liver
Mechlorethamine	Mouse: lung
Chlorambucil	Mouse: papillomas
Melphalan (phenylalanine mustard)	Mouse: papillomas Human: hematopoietic system
Uracil mustard	Mouse: lung
Cyclophosphamide	Mouse: lung Human: bladder
Triethylene melamine (TEM)	Mouse: lung and thymus
Triethylenethio-phosphoramide	Mouse: lung Rat: lung
Dactinomycin (actinomycin-D)	Rat: mesothelioma
Doxorubicin	Mouse: fibroblasts *in vitro*

used to test chemicals for carcinogenicity are described later in this chapter.

Diversity of Chemical Types

It is immediately apparent, even from just the names of the agents listed in Tables 63-1 to 63-3, that carcinogens are found in a wide variety of chemical classes. There are no simple structure-activity rules by which a given compound can be designated as a carcinogen (or noncarcinogen) solely by virtue of its chemical structure.

This apparent lack of structure-activity relationships perplexed early workers in the field of experimental chemical carcinogenesis. Since carcinogens occurred in a wide variety of chemical classes, it was feared that there might be a very large number of mechanisms by which these diverse chemical structures caused cancer. Later evidence has shown that this is not so. The scheme diagrammed in Figure 63-3 provides a model that attempts to unify diverse chemical structures into a common pathway leading to cancer.

TABLE 63-3 Drugs Reported To Be Carcinogenic

Drug	Species and Site or Type of Neoplasm Induced
Nitrofurazone	Rat: breast
Nitrofurantoin	Rat: breast, lymphomas
Metronidazole	Mouse: lung, lymphomas
Phenacetin (acetophenetidin)	Human: kidney
Piperazine	Mouse: lung
Chloroform	Mouse: liver
Chloramphenicol	Human: hematopoietic system
Phenytoin	Human: lymphoreticular system
Penicillin G	Rat: sarcomas, fibromas, thyroid
Diethylstilbestrol (DES)	Mouse and rat: breast Human: vagina

CARCINOGENESIS AS A MULTISTAGE BIOCHEMICAL AND BIOLOGIC PROCESS

The purpose of the complicated diagram in Figure 63-3 is to provide a framework for examining the complex events in chemical carcinogenesis. The diagram emphasizes that cancer is the result of a progressive multistage process; this concept has been thoroughly described by Farber (1984). We will use the scheme in Figure 63-3 for reference as we examine particular stages in the carcinogenic process.

Direct-Acting Carcinogens

The common final target of most chemical carcinogens appears to be DNA. It is possible that specific RNA species or specific proteins might be the critical targets, but most present evidence and research focus

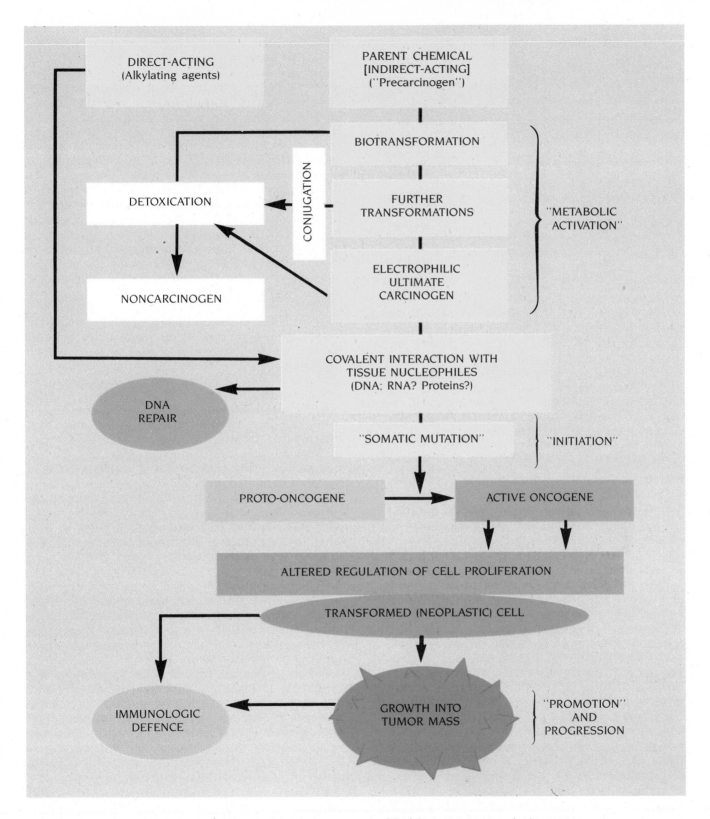

Figure 63–3 General mechanism of chemical carcinogenesis. (Modified from Gringauz and Okey, 1982.)

**TABLE 63–4 Cancer and Chemicals:
Numerical Considerations**

Total chemicals known (natural and synthetic)	>5,000,000
Chemicals in common widespread use	~50,000
Chemicals demonstrated to be carcinogenic in experimental animals	~1000
Chemicals for which there is strong evidence of carcinogenic activity in humans	~25–50

All numbers are estimates as of 1980.

on DNA as the critical target. Some drugs, such as alkylating agents used in chemotherapy of cancer, are chemically reactive in the form in which they are administered. These have the ability to bind directly to nucleophilic sites on DNA, RNA, and proteins. The ability of alkylating agents to bind covalently to DNA probably is responsible both for their ability to kill cancer cells (as therapeutic agents) and for their ability to induce new tumors.

Metabolic Activation into Ultimate Carcinogens

The term "ultimate carcinogen" refers to the chemical species that directly interacts with DNA. Most cancer-causing chemicals probably are not carcinogenic in the form in which they enter the body. Compounds such as polycyclic aromatic hydrocarbons (e.g., benzo(a)-pyrene) are chemically unreactive in their parent form and cannot form covalent bonds with DNA. Enzyme systems within the organism biotransform unreactive "pro- or precarcinogens" into chemically reactive (electron-deficient) products that can covalently interact with nucleophilic sites on cellular macromolecules. The general concept that most carcinogens are metabolically activated into their ultimate carcinogenic form arises from the work of several investigators, but especially James and Elizabeth Miller (1978).

As the scheme in Figure 63–3 suggests, metabolic activation requires more than one enzymatic step. Initial activation often is carried out by various species of cytochrome P-450 (see Chapter 4), but activation by reductases, peroxidases, and prostaglandin synthesis pathways also is well established. Regardless of the pathway(s), the final product (ultimate carcinogen) is a reactive electrophilic species.

Some specific examples of metabolic activation pathways are given in Figures 63–4 and 63–5. Figure 63–4 outlines the biotransformation processes that result in the conversion of the procarcinogen, benzo(a)pyrene (BP), into an ultimate carcinogenic form capable of cova-

lent binding to DNA. BP has been studied more than any other carcinogen. Although the activation scheme shown in Figure 63–4 is based on considerable experimental evidence, this is not the only pathway by which BP can be activated into an ultimate carcinogen.

The first step in activation of BP is its conversion into an arene oxide, BP 7,8-oxide. This first step is catalysed by a species of cytochrome P-450. BP 7,8-oxide then serves as a substrate for epoxide hydrolase, an enzyme that converts the oxide to a dihydrodiol by the addition of a molecule of water. The dihydrodiol is much more water-soluble than the parent compound, and it formerly was thought that the BP 7,8-oxide had been effectively "detoxified" by the action of epoxide hydrolase. Further investigation, however, revealed that the dihydrodiol undergoes a second conversion by P-450 to form BP 7,8-diol-9,10-epoxide. The diol epoxide is chemically reactive and capable of covalent binding to DNA; hence it is an ultimate carcinogenic form of BP.

Figure 63–5 indicates that species of cytochrome P-450 also are involved in the initial activation steps for structurally diverse carcinogens such as AAF (an aromatic amine), nitrosamines, vinyl chloride, and aflatoxins. Figure 63–5 also serves to reemphasize that metabolic activation commonly involves more than one enzymatic step before an ultimate carcinogen is formed. In the case of AAF, the initial step is formation of N-hydroxy-AAF catalysed by cytochrome P-450. The N-hydroxy intermediate then may follow one of several pathways leading to formation of a sulfate ester, an acetate ester, or a nitroxide radical. All these pathways are contenders for the generation of an ultimate carcinogen. The specific pathway depends upon the tissue. Sulfotransferase activity predominates in liver, whereas acyltransferase activity dominates in nonhepatic tissue such as the mammary gland. Both liver and mammary gland are susceptible to tumor induction by AAF, implying that different ultimate carcinogens can be formed from the same parent compound in different tissues by different metabolic pathways. Differences in metabolic capabilities among different tissues may in part explain why some carcinogens are tissue-selective in inducing tumors.

The discussion up to this point might imply that cytochrome(s) P-450 are undesirable and are harmful to the organism. There is no question that P-450 monooxygenases are capable of converting many types of compound into reactive intermediates that are toxic or carcinogenic. It should be recalled, however, that P-450-mediated reactions are the major pathways by which most hydrophobic drugs and environmental chemicals are converted to forms which can be conjugated and excreted (see Chapter 4).

Epoxide hydrolase also could be viewed both as a "beneficial" enzyme and as an enzyme deleterious to health. The determination of whether these enzymes are beneficial or harmful depends upon many complex factors such as dose and route of administration of their drug substrates, and the efficiency with which activation pathways are coupled with conjugating enzymes

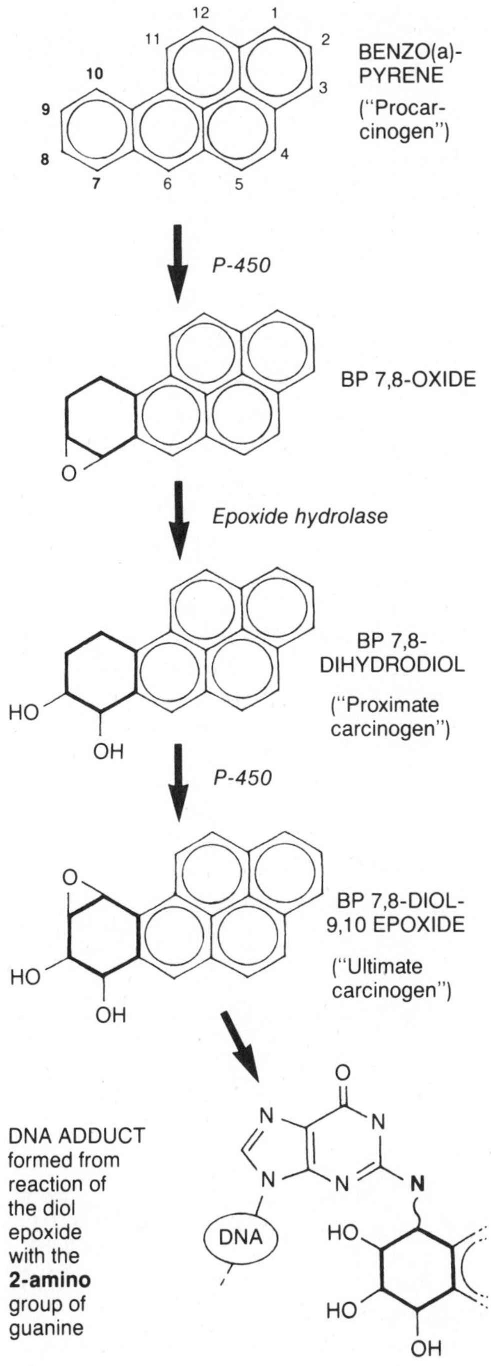

Figure 63–4 Metabolic activation of benzo(a)pyrene. Note: (1) Only the main activation pathway is shown. Many other metabolic products are formed from BP *via* several metabolic pathways involving P-450 species responsible for each step. (2) The enzymatic steps shown are stereospecific, but absolute and relative stereospecific products are not shown in this diagram.

(Okey *et al.*, 1986). The teleologic goal of P-450 and epoxide hydrolase is to facilitate the elimination of xenobiotic chemicals (*see* Chapter 4). Conversion of some xenobiotic agents into toxic or carcinogenic metabolites could be viewed as an accidental byproduct of the action of generally beneficial enzymes.

Detoxication

It should not be assumed that metabolic activation invariably leads to covalent attacks on critical macromolecules such as DNA. Most cells are well equipped with mechanisms that inactivate reactive metabolites before these metabolites strike critical targets. The predominant means of "detoxication" is *via* conjugation with glutathione (GSH), sulfate, or glucuronides (*see* Chapter 4). Cells that are deficient in GSH are known to be at high risk of cell death from reactive metabolites formed in the biotransformation of many drugs (*see* Chapter 62). GSH-deficient cells also may be at high risk for neoplastic transformation when exposed to carcinogens.

In normal cells, the majority of reactive metabolites probably are detoxified by conjugating enzymes or by reaction with noncritical protein targets. Cells at highest risk will be those that have an imbalance between the rate at which reactive metabolites are generated and the rate at which those metabolites can be conjugated and excreted.

Covalent Interaction with Tissue Nucleophiles

As stated previously, the primary target of ultimate carcinogens is believed to be DNA. Much of the progress in understanding chemical carcinogenesis has been made by tracing forward the route of parent compounds from their site of application through distribution to various tissues and through specific biotransformation pathways that convert procarcinogens into ultimate carcinogens.

In several instances the chemical identity of the ultimate carcinogenic form has been determined by chemical characterization of carcinogen adducts isolated from DNA. Carcinogen adducts (bound forms) have been detected on all four nitrogen bases in DNA and at several atomic sites within each base.

Initiation (Neoplastic Transformation)

Covalent binding of the ultimate carcinogen to DNA alters the genetic message. If the lesion in DNA is not

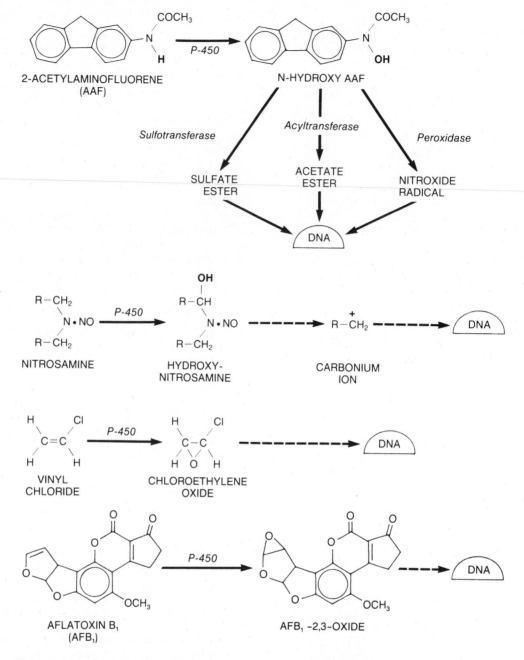

Figure 63–5 Examples of activation pathways for selected carcinogens.

recognized and repaired before cell division, the genetic lesion may be "fixed" as a mutation, which will be inherited by all progeny stemming from the altered cell. This permanent alteration is the initial cellular event in the cancer process.

Not all chemically induced mutations lead to cancer. Many DNA lesions probably are lethal to the cell bearing them. In addition, DNA-repair enzymes operate with high efficiency. Individuals who are genetically deficient in DNA-repair enzymes exhibit an increased risk for some, but not all, forms of cancer.

Over the past few years considerable excitement has been generated by the prospect that the primary targets of chemicals and other carcinogens might be a limited number of "cancer genes." As stated by Bishop (1987), "proto-oncogenes are the keyboard upon which carcinogens play." As a general model, it is proposed that the conversion of proto-oncogenes into oncogenes is a key event in the initiation of tumorigenesis (Fig. 63–3). Proto-oncogenes are normal cellular genes, most of which appear to code for cellular growth factors or growth factor receptors. When a proto-oncogene is damaged by a carcinogen (*i.e.*, undergoes mutation, chromosomal translocation, *etc.*) the resulting oncogene drives the abnormal cell division and abnormal cell differentiation that typify neoplastic growths.

Tumor Promotion and Promoters

In its simplest form, the multistage cancer process can be thought of as two major events: initiation (described above) and promotion.

Promotion refers to a poorly defined set of circumstances that permit initiated cells to proliferate into tumor masses. Several chemicals which are not in themselves "carcinogens" (*i.e.*, do not act as initiators) are able to promote development of tumors that have been initiated by other agents. Some tumor promoters are listed in Table 63–5.

Generally, initiators are thought to be agents that are capable of forming mutagenic electrophilic metabolites as previously described. Initiation can be accomplished by a single exposure to the initiating agent. The initiation process (mutationally-based) seems essentially irreversible.

In contrast, promoting agents do not appear to be mutagenic. In order to produce tumors experimentally, the promoting agent must be given after treatment with an initiator, and the promoter must be given repeatedly over a prolonged time period. The actions of promoters appear to be reversible, at least in early stages.

Very little is known about the mechanisms by which promoters act. Specific receptors have been identified that bind phorbol esters, but the means by which the phorbol receptor might be linked to tumor promotion and progression is unknown.

The diversity of chemical structure in agents classed as promoters is considerable. Present cancer research is giving great attention to the phenomenon of promotion, but no unifying hypotheses are yet available to explain the mechanisms of action of these structurally diverse agents.

DETECTION OF CARCINOGENS

Table 63–6 summarizes the major methods used at present to test chemicals for potential carcinogenic activity.

Long-Term Tests *In Vivo*

The ultimate "proof" that a given chemical is a human carcinogen can be obtained only by carefully designed epidemiologic studies and by rigorous evaluation of clinical observations. Given the multitude of drugs and environmental agents to which humans are

TABLE 63–5 Reported Tumor Promoters in Experimental Animals

Mouse skin tumors
 Phorbol esters from croton oil, *e.g.*,
  12-O-tetradecanoyl phorbol-13-acetate (TPA)
 Phenol
 Anthralin
 Hexadecane
 Iodoacetic acid
 Cigarette smoke condensate
 Extracts of unburned cigarettes
 Surfactants and detergents
 Benzoyl peroxide
 Abrasions or wounding

Rodent liver tumors
 Phenobarbital
 DDT
 Polychlorinated biphenyls (PCBs)
 2,3,7,8-Tetrachlorodibenzo-*p*-dioxin (TCDD, "dioxin")

exposed and the long latent period between exposure and tumor appearance, it is not surprising that confirmation of carcinogenicity in humans is a protracted and difficult process.

Bioassays in experimental animals (usually rodents) have until recently been the primary method of testing chemicals for carcinogenic potential. Rat tests often have been criticized as being irrelevant to the human cancer problem because such tests frequently employ doses that are greatly in excess of probable human exposure levels for the chemical in question. Although high doses are used in rodent bioassays, experience has shown that virtually all chemicals that induce a significant frequency of tumors at high doses also induce some tumors at lower doses (*see* below).

TABLE 63–6 Methods for Detection of Carcinogens

Long-term in vivo *tests*
 Clinical observations and epidemiology
 Bioassays in experimental animals

Short-term "screening" tests
 Mutational tests
  Bacteria (Ames' *Salmonella* test)
  Mammalian cells in culture
  Other prokaryotic or eukaryotic organisms
 Tests for chromosome damage
  Chromosomal abnormalities by cytogenetic
   assays
  Sister chromatid exchange
  Micronucleus formation
  Sperm abnormalities
 Neoplastic transformation of mammalian cells in
  culture
 Covalent binding of test compounds to DNA
  after "metabolic activation" *in vivo* or *in vitro*

High doses are employed in animal tests for a very practical reason—to increase the sensitivity of the assay. Thorough rodent bioassays for carcinogenicity of a **single chemical** typically cost in excess of $1 million and may require 2 to 5 years of research. High doses are used to reduce the number of experimental animals required. Usually a maximum of a few hundred animals can be studied, and it is necessary to test with doses that potentially can produce a high frequency of tumors. A chemical that caused cancer in 1 animal out of 1000 tested (for example, at low doses) would not be detected as a carcinogen, yet a similar increase in cancer frequency in the Canadian human population would afflict about 25,000 people.

Carcinogenic activity in rodents does not prove that a chemical will be a carcinogen in humans, but nearly all known human carcinogens are carcinogenic also in rodents. Any chemical that is a carcinogen in experimental animals must be considered a **potential** carcinogen in humans. Specific knowledge of the exact mechanism(s) by which cancers arise is required before any discrepancies in "animal testing" versus "human carcinogenesis" can be explained.

Short-Term "Screening" Tests

As stated in the previous section, *in vivo* animal tests are the definitive method for demonstrating carcinogenic activity. Because *in vivo* tests are expensive and time-consuming, less expensive short-term tests have been developed to cope with the thousands of chemicals that must be tested for potential carcinogenic activity.

Most of the screening tests devised are based on the premise that carcinogens act by damaging DNA. Bruce Ames (1979) has stated that "carcinogens are mutagens." Some cancer specialists believe that this oversimplifies the relationship between mutagenesis and carcinogenesis. Nevertheless, screening for potential carcinogens has been greatly facilitated by testing suspect chemicals for mutagenic properties.

Mutagenesis tests in bacterial systems are much quicker and cheaper than whole-animal tests for carcinogenesis. Bacterial mutational test systems are used in literally thousands of laboratories around the world and are especially valuable as an inexpensive screen in development of compounds that may have market potential.

Early attempts to correlate mutagenesis in bacterial systems with carcinogenesis in animals were compromised because the necessity for host-mediated metabolic activation of procarcinogens was not yet recognized. Present-day tests employ a combined system using mammalian liver enzymes (to activate procarcinogens) and *Salmonella* bacterial strains (to detect mutations). This system has shown that most carcinogens (approximately 90%) are mutagenic and that many mutagens are carcinogens.

The scientific study of carcinogenesis is not yet developed to the stage where any single test is considered adequate as an all-encompassing screen for carcinogenic chemicals. Rather, a battery of tests is required both *in vivo* and *in vitro*.

DOSE-RESPONSE CONSIDERATIONS IN CARCINOGENESIS

In general, the carcinogenic response, like other pharmacologic responses, is quantitatively related to dose (or to exposure). As illustrated in Figure 63–6, the frequency of tumors in a population increases linearly with the logarithm of the dose. This linear log–dose-response relationship has been shown experimentally to hold for several carcinogenic chemicals, provided that the carcinogen doses given yield a "medium" level of tumor response. At very high or very low doses linearity of the dose-response relationship is in question.

At very high doses, experimental animals may die from toxicity before tumors have an opportunity to develop to a detectable stage. It also is possible that high doses of some carcinogens might produce a higher tumor frequency than predicted by extrapolation of the linear middle portion of the dose-response curve.

The greatest difficulty, however, lies in **interpretation of the tumor response expected at very low doses.** Much of human exposure to potential carcinogens is of a chronic, low-dose nature. If the tumor dose-response curve is linear and originates at zero, there is no dose that will not produce a finite increase in tumor frequency. Only zero dose would yield zero response; *i.e.*, there is no "safe" dose for carcinogens.

The other possibility is that the dose-response relationship is not linear at very low doses. This includes the possibility that a "threshold" dose may exist, below which tumors are not induced.

To this date there has been **no satisfactory experimental definition** of the nature of the dose-response curve at very low carcinogen doses. A few large-scale experiments involving tens of thousands of rodents have been attempted, but these still have been inadequate to define response at very low doses. Partly this is inherent in the statistical uncertainty present when any rare event is measured. Only extremely large numbers of animals would reduce this uncertainty to a level where the nature of the response itself could be determined. It also is apparent that no experimental animal can be treated in an environment that is totally free from contamination by trace levels of other chemicals that are unwanted in the experiment. In addition, tumors that result from exposure to the test chemical are superimposed on a background of "spontaneous" tumors that are present in every experimental species. For these and other reasons, the tumor response at very low doses may never be adequately

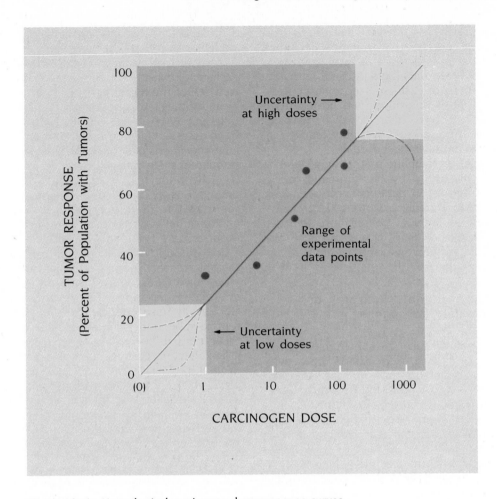

Figure 63–6 Hypothetical carcinogen dose-response curves.

defined by animal experiments.

Various mathematical models have been constructed to attempt to predict the magnitude of tumor response at very low doses. Each model requires certain assumptions that have not yet been experimentally validated. At the present time there is no conclusive answer as to whether there is a "safe" dose for any carcinogen. Regulatory agencies must make decisions about many potential carcinogens without having experimental evidence that might confirm risk at very low doses. As is true in other areas of toxicology, carcinogenic risk can be determined with greater assurance when the specific mechanism by which each agent acts is well understood.

VARIATION IN CANCER SUSCEPTIBILITY

The multistage model of carcinogenesis in Figure 63–3 suggests several levels at which individuals may vary in their response to carcinogens.

DNA-Repair and Immune Competence

Cells from individuals with genetically based deficiencies in DNA-repair are more sensitive than normal cells to the induction of mutations by chemicals, ultraviolet light, and ionizing radiation. Several DNA-repair deficiencies have been described in humans, including Bloom's syndrome, Fanconi's anemia, ataxia-telangiectasia, and xeroderma pigmentosum. Individuals with some of these diseases are more susceptible to certain cancers than are individuals with normal DNA-repair capacity. It is not yet clear, however, whether or not DNA-repair deficiencies invariably lead to increased risk of chemically-induced cancer.

The importance of the immune system as a defence against cancer is illustrated by the dramatic rise in cancer risk that occurred in patients receiving intensive immunosuppressive therapy following kidney transplantation. It is not yet known whether more selective immune suppression (such as with cyclosporine A) will reduce the cancer risk in transplant patients.

Imbalance in Enzymes that "Activate" or "Detoxify" Chemical Carcinogens

In experimental animals it can be shown that the risk of chemically induced cancer depends on the activity of various carcinogen-metabolizing enzymes. As noted previously, however, the relationship betwen enzyme activities and carcinogenesis is complex. Some enzymes (e.g., cytochromes P-450 and epoxide hydrolase) function both to "activate" certain carcinogens and to "detoxify" them.

In animals it generally appears that a high level of cytochrome P-450 in the **liver** protects peripheral tissues from chemical carcinogens, provided that the animal is exposed to the carcinogen by a route whereby the liver can clear the carcinogen from circulation before it is distributed throughout the body. Thus, if an animal ingests a carcinogen orally or is given an intraperitoneal injection, high hepatic P-450 activities enhance first-pass clearance of carcinogen by the liver and effectively reduce the carcinogen dose that is delivered to other tissues (Okey et al., 1986).

In contrast, if carcinogens are applied **directly** to tissues such as the skin or lung surface, tumor risk generally rises with increased P-450 activities in those tissues. In such cases metabolic activation occurs locally within the tissue (by P-450 and other enzymes), but this activation is not well coupled with conjugating systems or an excretory route.

Animal experiments such as these suggest that some variation in human susceptibility to chemical carcinogens might be due to variation in levels of carcinogen-metabolizing enzymes in different individuals. In 1973 Kellerman et al. reported that susceptibility to bronchogenic carcinoma (the most common form of lung cancer) was greatly increased in persons who had highly induced levels of aryl hydrocarbon hydroxylase (AHH; a cytochrome P_1-450-mediated enzyme activity that biotransforms benzo(a)pyrene and other aromatic compounds). Persons with highly inducible AHH were believed to be especially vulnerable to smoking-related

lung cancer, since smoking delivers carcinogenic substances directly to the lung.

Many further studies have attempted to confirm the Kellerman hypothesis, but there is no clear answer as to whether the hypothesis is correct. It has been technically difficult to phenotype humans for their levels of induced AHH. AHH activities in humans usually have been assessed in cultured lymphocytes, since liver and lung specimens cannot be obtained readily from large populations. Despite difficulties in assaying AHH activity in lymphocytes, recent improvements in the lymphocyte assay have been made and it has been reported that there is a positive correlation between an individual's AHH activity and the risk of lung cancer (Kouri et al., 1982).

Considerable effort has been expended on studying the role of "activating" enzymes such as AHH in human cancer. Less work has been done to determine the relative importance of "detoxication" mechanisms. Genetically based deficiencies in cell glutathione content have been identified in certain patients. Cells from these patients have an increased susceptibility to the killing effect of reactive metabolites formed from several drugs (Spielberg et al., 1981; see also Chapter 12). It is possible that patients with detoxication defects may also be at higher risk for chemically induced cancers. Overall, the highest risk would seem likely to occur in those tissues that exhibit a high level of activation enzymes coupled with a low capacity for conjugation or other detoxication pathways.

PREVENTION OF CARCINOGENESIS

The fact that cancer is a multiple-step process provides the opportunity for reduction in cancer frequency by intervention at several levels.

Selective Inhibition of Carcinogen Activation and Selective Enhancement of Carcinogen Detoxication

In experimental animals it is possible to use "chemoprophylaxis" to reduce cancer risk (Wattenberg, 1985). Chemical pretreatments can be given that inhibit activation pathways or stimulate detoxication pathways, thereby inhibiting tumor induction. For example, pretreatment of rats with phenobarbital partially protects them from induction of mammary tumors when they are later exposed to benzo(a)pyrene. Phenobarbital appears to protect by enhancing liver P-450 activities and increasing hepatic clearance of the carcinogen. Unfortunately, as previously described, phenobarbital also can promote development of liver cancer in rats treated with nitrosamines. At this time we do not have the ability to selectively switch on detoxication pathways and switch off activation pathways by chemical treatment.

Antioxidants

Several antioxidants have been demonstrated to inhibit chemical induction of tumors in experimental animals. Such chemicals include butylated hydroxytoluene (BHT), butylated hydroxyanisole (BHA), and vitamin E. Antioxidants may inhibit cancer by "scavenging" reactive metabolites before they can bind to DNA, but it is not at all clear what mechanism actually accounts for the anticarcinogenic action of antioxidants.

Retinoic Acid Analogs

Certain retinoic acid analogs (related to vitamin A; see Chapter 49) effectively inhibit chemically induced tumors in experimental animals. These substances now are entering clinical trials in persons exposed occupationally to "high-risk" potential carcinogens. The value of prophylactic treatment with retinoic acid analogs will not be known for several years. They must be administered continuously over a prolonged time to have effect. As with any chronic drug therapy, the possibility that the treatment itself might cause some toxic response must be weighed against the potential benefits (Bertram et al., 1987).

Avoidance

Considering the complexity of chemical carcinogenesis, it is obvious that no "all-purpose anticancer pill" yet exists, nor is any likely to be developed in the near future. The best method currently available for reducing cancer risk is avoidance of, or reduced exposure to, known causative agents.

We can never have a completely "clean" environment (that is, an environment totally free of carcinogens) since carcinogens arise from both "natural" and human processes. We can, however, avoid high-risk situations. Elimination of cigarette smoking would reduce human cancer mortality more than any other single public health measure. It is a continual source of frustration to scientists involved in cancer research that so little progress has been achieved toward a goal that would have such important benefits at so little cost.

SUGGESTED READING

Ames BN. Identifying environmental chemicals causing mutations and cancer. Science 1979; 204:587–593.

Ames BN, Magaw R, Gold LS. Ranking possible carcinogenic hazards. Science 1987; 236:271–280.

Bertram JS, Kolonel LN, Meyskens FL Jr. Rationale and strategies for chemoprevention of cancer in humans. Cancer Res 1987; 47: 3012–3031.

Bishop JM. The molecular genetics of cancer. Science 1987; 235:305–311.

Farber E. Cellular biochemistry of the stepwise development of cancer with chemicals: G.H.A. Clowes Memorial Lecture. Cancer Res 1984; 44:5463–5474.

Gringauz A, Okey AB. Carcinogens in foods and drugs. On Continuing Practice 1982; 9:17–26.

Higginson J [Interview]. Science 1979; 205:1363–1364.

Higginson J. Everything is a carcinogen? Regul Toxicol Pharmacol 1987; 7:89–95.

Kellerman G, Shaw CR, Luyten-Kellerman M. Aryl hydrocarbon hydroxylase inducibility and bronchogenic carcinoma. N Engl J Med 1973; 289:934–937.

Kouri RE, McKinney CE, Slomiany DJ, et al. Positive correlation between high aryl hydrocarbon hydroxylase activity and primary lung cancer as analyzed in cryopreserved lymphocytes. Cancer Res 1982; 42:5030–5037.

Miller EC. Some current perspectives on chemical carcinogenesis: presidential address. Cancer Res 1978; 38: 1479–1496.

Okey AB, Roberts EA, Harper PA, Denison MS. Induction of drug-metabolizing enzymes: mechanisms and consequences. Clin Biochem 1986; 19:132–141.

Spielberg SP, Gordon GB. Glutathione synthetase deficient lymphocytes and acetaminophen toxicity. Clin Pharmacol Ther 1981; 29:51–55.

Wattenberg L. Chemoprevention of cancer. Cancer Res 1985; 45:1–8.

SPECIAL TOPICS

Chapter 64

CHEMICAL TERATOGENESIS

P.G. Wells

Teratology, or the study of congenital defects, is derived from the Greek word *teras*, meaning monster. Interest in structural abnormalities in the newborn dates back to at least 5000 B.C. when Babylonian priests had a list of 62 malformations recognizable at birth. Since the 1960s teratology has expanded with the recognition of mutational and functional abnormalities or anomalies resulting from prenatal insult, sometimes in the absence of structural defects (Fig. 64–1). While the field is concerned with all causes of anomalies, this chapter is limited to teratogenesis associated with maternal exposure to drugs and environmental chemicals.

The study of chemical teratogenesis is relatively recent, dating from 1933, when Hale showed that maternal deprivation of vitamin A in pigs produced offspring without eyes (anophthalmia). Widespread scientific interest and public concern did not develop until 1960, with the first reports of teratogenicity associated with the sedative-hypnotic drug thalidomide, which was withdrawn from the market in 1961. While the thalidomide tragedy stimulated an enormous growth in basic and applied research in this field, we still know relatively little about how drugs and chemicals cause congenital anomalies, and even less about how genetic and environmental factors interact in individual unborn children.

Each year in the United States about 200,000 birth defects are reported (7% of all live births), while over 560,000 infant deaths, spontaneous abortions, stillbirths, and miscarriages are estimated to be due to defective prenatal development. These figures no doubt are underestimates of the problem since an unknown percentage of known defects are not reported and many defects, particularly functional and mutational anomalies, are not recognized. In other instances, there may be failure to recognize that the defect is associated with exposure to a drug or environmental chemical. About 20–30% of reported defects are thought to result from spontaneous genetic aberrations, while 6% are clearly related to drugs and chemicals, leaving the cause unknown in nearly 70%. Many cases of unknown causation probably result either from unrecognized exposure to drugs and chemicals, or from a complex interaction between a drug effect and genetic or environmental factors. One study found that the average woman takes 10 prescription or nonprescription drugs during her pregnancy, most of them without a physician's supervision. It has been estimated that over 125,000 women of childbearing age in the United States are exposed annually to potential chemical teratogens in their jobs, and presumably all women are exposed to some extent to the enormous array of environmental chemicals.

ASSESSMENT OF HUMAN RISK

There are a number of special problems in the detection of chemical teratogenicity and assessment of human risk that make this field of toxicology particularly difficult. Since the developmental process is complex and requires years for maturation, currently employed indices fail to detect many chemical effects. In the human population, fewer than 50% of abnormalities can be detected at birth. Over 30% of early embryos are estimated to die unrecognized, while 15% of recognized pregnancies abort spontaneously. In successful pregnancies, subtle biochemical or functional defects usually go unrecognized. In other cases, the defect may be detected, but the causal role of the drug may not be identified because it is expressed only under conditions of genetic predisposition, or of certain physiologic, pathologic, or environmental stresses that may go unrecognized. In this case, particularly susceptible individuals will not be distinguished from the general population by epidemiologic studies that cannot include sufficient detail about individual predisposing factors.

644

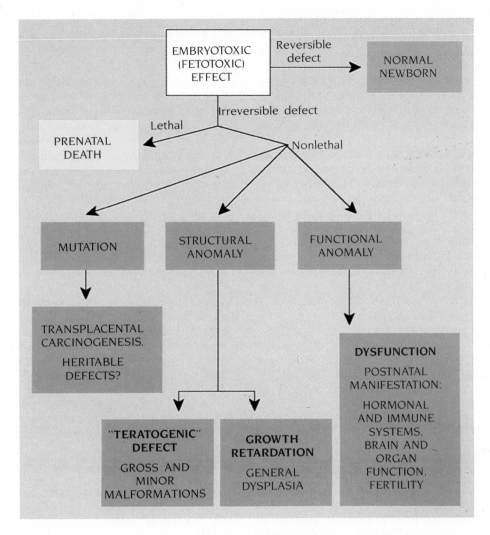

Figure 64–1 Consequences of chemical teratogenesis. (Modified from Neubert D *et al.* 1980.)

Most human teratologic studies are restricted to the perinatal period and fail to evaluate the maturational process. The frequency of defects detected at birth generally can be increased over six-fold by following the children for about 5 years. Some important structural defects (*e.g.*, cardiac anomalies), subtle behavioral deficits, or mutational anomalies may not be detected until even later. For example, infants exposed *in utero* to the transplacental carcinogen diethylstilbestrol did not develop vaginal adenocarcinomas until puberty. Unfortunately, long-term follow-up studies are too expensive and time-consuming to be employed for all drugs. Therefore teratologic evaluation often must depend upon retrospective epidemiologic studies and voluntary reporting of rare toxicities by astute physicians who have extensive records of their patients' histories.

During the clinical testing of new drugs, in studies on human volunteers and patients, pregnant women are rarely included. Therefore the fetal toxicity of most drugs can be assessed only after their use in the general population. Indeed, many drugs carry a warning that their safety during pregnancy and lactation has not been established. Once drugs are released for general use, epidemiologic studies can detect potent teratogens or drug-induced anomalies that are rare in the baseline population. However, such studies are less successful in identifying weaker teratogens or drugs that are teratogenic only in predisposed patients. Such potential predisposing conditions as physiologic differences, pathophysiologic influences, or concurrent drug use or chemical exposure seldom are discernible. Virtually never considered, especially in relation to environmental chemical teratogens, are such factors as the precise timing and magnitude of confounding influences, individual differences and gestational variations in drug disposition, and differences in specific, toxicologically critical pathways of drug bioactivation and detoxification.

To some extent, the teratologic risks can be reduced by preclinical studies employing *in vivo* animal models and *in vitro* tests, as discussed later. However, there are serious limitations of such methods. Thalidomide was found to be nonteratogenic in pregnant mice and rats, but unfortunately, in humans it proved to be an extraordinarily potent teratogen, causing embryolethality and a wide range of congenital anomalies in over 10,000 surviving children. Retrospective teratologic studies have shown the teratogenic dose in mouse and rat to be about 4000 mg/kg, compared with 0.5–1 mg/kg in humans.

Given the preceding discussion, one can begin to appreciate that relatively little can be stated as fact in the field of chemical teratogenesis. Teratologists disagree even about the identification of "known" human teratogens. However, Table 64–1 lists some drugs that are sufficiently potent teratogens for their effects to be recognized clearly above the spontaneous incidence of human congenital malformations. This list is not complete; if occupational and environmental chemicals, and additional categories of "probable" and "suspected" human and animal teratogens were included, this list would number over 800 (Shepard, 1983).

TERATOLOGIC PRINCIPLES

Direct Fetal Susceptibility: Critical Periods

The kinds and frequencies of anomalies caused by a teratogenic agent depend critically upon the developmental stage at the time of exposure. This so-called "critical period" is illustrated for several representative human organs in Figure 64–2. While the embryonic and fetal periods represent distinct developmental stages as illustrated, the term "fetal" will be used here to describe the entire prenatal period. The fetus is more susceptible to chemical insult than at any stage in its postnatal life because of the high rate of cellular prolifer-

TABLE 64–1 Proven or Seriously Suspected
Human Teratogens

Aminopterin*	Methylmercury
Androgens	Methotrexate*
Busulfan†	Phenytoin
Chlorambucil†	Procarbazine†
Colchicine	Progestins
Cyclophosphamide†	Radioiodine(^{131}I)
Diethylstilbestrol (Stilbestrol)	Thalidomide
Isotretinoin	Valproic acid
Mercaptopurine*	

* Antimetabolic anticancer drug.
† Alkylating anticancer drug.
This list is not complete, and refers primarily to drugs because of the lack of data in humans with respect to environmental chemicals.
Source: Primarily from Shepard TH. In: Shirkey HC, ed. Pediatric therapy. 6th ed. St. Louis: CV Mosby, 1980:94.

ation and differentiation, functional development and growth taking place over a relatively brief period of time. For example, the DNA content of the mouse fetus is increased about one million times within the first 11 days of gestation (21-day pregnancy), and 1000 times during the first 3 days of organogenesis.

The specificity of the critical period can be illustrated by considering the formation of the palate, which involves the horizontal convergence and fusion of the two palatal shelves. In the mouse, cleft palate (failure of the palatal shelves to close) can be induced by an appropriate teratogen only when this is administered between gestational days 8 and 13. However, even this "single" process is complex. Palatal closure involves initial cellular proliferation, synthesis of intercellular substances, elevation of the two palatal shelves from a vertical to a horizontal position, midline contact and fusion of the two shelves, and finally formation of a bony plate. Thus the critical period for any organ development actually is a continuum of discrete but interdependent processes that can be affected differentially by teratogens with different mechanisms, or by the same teratogen at different times. In the case of teratogens with different mechanisms, 6-aminonicotinamide induces cleft palates if administered at any time during palatal closure (days 8 to 13), while dexamethasone is effective only when given around day 13, 2,4,5-trichlorophenoxyacetic acid only around day 12, and tetrachlorodibenzodioxin (TCDD, dioxin) only between days 10 and 12 (Fig. 64–3). In the case of the same teratogen at different times, treatment of pregnant mice with 5-azacytidine on gestational day 15 produces an extreme reduction in brain size, particularly in the cerebral cortex, with abnormal layering of pyramidal cells in the hippocampus and a reduced corpus striatum. Later treatment, on day 19, produces damage in more restricted areas, with dead cells observed mainly within the subependymal and external granular layers of the cerebellum.

The one critical period that is not susceptible to the production of anomalies by teratogens is the initial development from fertilization to completion of the blastocyst. Since this stage involves little cellular differentiation, the cells have not achieved specific developmental roles, and damage at this stage either causes the death of the embryo or has no lasting effect. Established critical periods nevertheless are not absolute, since malformations occasionally have been demonstrated after chemical exposure during the preimplantation phase, while severe skeletal anomalies have been induced by teratogen exposure during the third trimester after the phase of organogenesis and limb formation.

Indirect Maternal Effects

In general, indirect insult to the fetus, mediated through effects on the mother, involves inadequate nutrient delivery, secondary either to maternal malnutrition or pathophysiology, or to reduced uterine blood supply to the fetus.

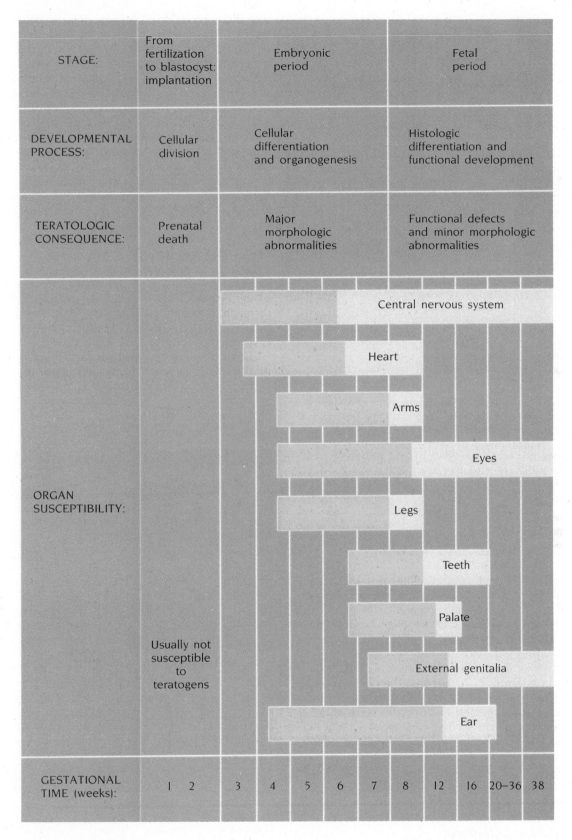

Figure 64–2 Human prenatal development and critical periods of susceptibility to teratogenic agents. Bars represent the organs, with their most susceptible period indicated in color.

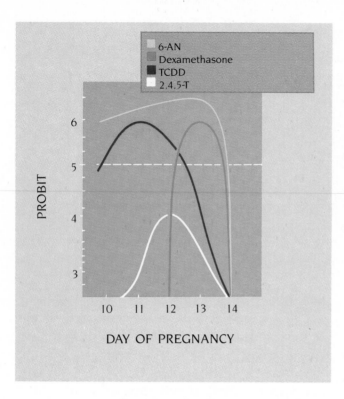

Figure 64–3 Time course of the susceptibility of NMRI mice to the induction of cleft palate by various agents. Doses given: 6-aminonicotinamide (6-AN) = 12 mg/kg; dexamethasone = 40 mg/kg; tetrachlorodibenzodioxin (TCDD) = 30 μg/kg; 2,4,5-trichlorophenoxyacetic acid (2,4,5-T) = 300 mg/kg. Differences in the period of maximum susceptibility suggest differences in the mode of action of the various compounds in inducing cleft palate. (From Neubert D et al. 1980.)

Maternal blood flow through the uterus to the placenta generally can be maintained at the expense of perfusion of other maternal organs; however, the homeostatic mechanisms can be overcome by high doses of drugs or endogenous substances that are vasoconstrictors (e.g., ergotamine, serotonin, bradykinin, angiotensin) or that reduce maternal cardiac function (e.g., propranolol). In humans, the consequences appear to be mainly a mild, reversible growth retardation rather than congenital malformations. In animals, treatment with vasoconstricting substances even at high doses produces resorptions without malformations. Thus, reduced uterine blood flow and its attendant deprivations generally do not produce measurable anomalies.

Teratologic Consequences

As indicated in Figure 64–1, teratogenesis can be viewed according to the major outcomes, namely, fetal death or structural, mutational, or functional abnormalities.

In the early stage of cellular division before differentiation, **fetal death** occurs in the absence of teratogenicity. During later developmental stages, often lower doses of a drug are teratogenic while higher doses cause fetal death. However, with some teratogens it is possible to induce a 100% incidence of anomalies such as cleft palate in the complete absence of fetal lethality (e.g., glucocorticoids in rodents), while other teratogens (possibly chloramphenicol in rodents) can induce fetal lethality without causing malformations. The latter case sometimes is difficult to establish, however, since malformed fetuses may die and be resorbed before detection. Teratogenicity cannot be estimated reliably if fetal lethality exceeds 50%. Since fetal death, teratogenicity, and growth retardation can be caused by different toxic mechanisms, the respective dose-response curves may be quite different, and their interrelation may vary at different times of gestation (Fig. 64–4). For example, dioxin induces about the same incidence of cleft palates (teratogenicity) in mice when given throughout gestational days 6 to 15, as throughout days 9 to 13, but fetal death is induced only when dioxin is given throughout days 6 to 15.

Chemically induced **mutations** can occur in fetal somatic cells, resulting in teratogenicity or transplacental

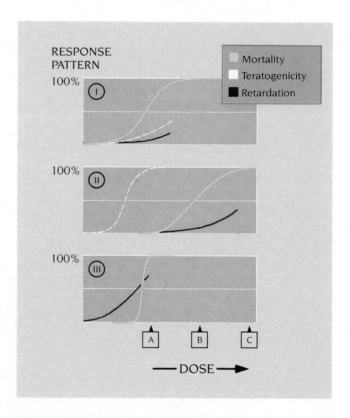

Figure 64–4 Hypothetical response pattern of an embryotoxic action. The three different effects have been evaluated separately; they may show quite different dose-response relationships. The outcome varies considerably, depending on the response pattern in early (I), mid (II), and late (III) gestation and the dose (A, B, C). (From Neubert D et al. 1980.)

carcinogenicity. There are no data concerning chemical mutations in fetal germ cells, and consequent hereditary disorders, in humans. Perhaps the best known human somatic mutation involved *in utero* exposure to the synthetic estrogen diethylstilbestrol, as a result of which female children developed a rare vaginal adenocarcinoma at puberty, and male children developed a spectrum of structural and functional reproductive anomalies. While the correlation between mutagenicity and carcinogenicity is estimated to be between 67 and 90%, their relationship to teratogenicity is less clear. Teratogenicity is more complex than mutagenesis, and not all teratogens would be expected to be mutagens and carcinogens.

Nevertheless, mutagens can initiate six of the nine teratogenic mechanisms listed in Table 64–2. Another point common to mutagens and teratogens is that many such chemicals are enzymatically bioactivated *in vivo* to a reactive intermediary metabolite, as discussed in subsequent sections (*see also* Chapter 4, *Drug Biotransformation*). These reactive intermediates or, in a few cases, the original reactive parent chemical generally are highly electrophilic and bind covalently or irreversibly to essential fetal cellular macromolecules such as DNA and proteins, thereby initiating either mutagenesis or teratogenesis. Retrospective surveys of experimental studies in animals suggest a high risk of teratogenicity (80–85%) from exposure to chemicals with *in vivo* and/or *in vitro* cytogenetic activity. The relationship for carcinogenic chemicals as a subgroup is more striking, with 92% also demonstrating teratogenicity. Aberrations of chromosome number can be caused by chemicals that affect microtubules and interfere with the role of spindle fibres in disjunction of chromosomes at anaphase of mitosis or meiosis; 64% of such chemicals were found to be teratogenic.

Functional anomalies are, for many teratogens, a more subtle indication of prenatal damage than overt structural malformations. The later fetal period is most susceptible to functional teratogenesis because of the high activities of histogenesis and functional maturation. The earlier embryonic period of organogenesis, which has little of these activities, is relatively insensitive to functional teratogenesis. Functional teratogenicity may include permanent "imprinting" of altered, discrete biochemical pathways; changes in organ function such as in the lungs or ears; and system deficits such as in the central nervous system (dysfunction and learning disabilities), the hormonal or immune systems, sexual function and fertility, and life expectancy. Since detection of such functional anomalies often requires decades of follow-up and is labor-intensive as well as costly, few human data are available in this field. Examples in humans include behavioral anomalies (low intelligence quotients and learning disabilities) in children exposed *in utero* to ethyl alcohol or to phenytoin, and possibly to acetylsalicylic acid (aspirin). Examples in experimental animals include a "permanently" induced cytochrome P-450 enzyme system in the offspring of pregnant mice treated with phenobarbital, and the

postnatal reduction in pulmonary oxygen consumption and respiratory rate in neonatal pups exposed *in utero* to excess vitamin A. Functional teratology can be produced over a wider gestational range than structural teratology, even up to the time of birth, as in the case of the developing central nervous system. Thus the traditional view of the first trimester of human pregnancy as the period of greatest teratologic susceptibility can no longer be considered accurate.

Cellular Mechanisms

The basic biologic mechanisms related to the early events in teratogenicity are listed in Table 64–2. Any given teratogen often initiates several mechanisms, and conversely, any given mechanism may be initiated by a variety of causes separate from, or complementary to, the effects of the potential chemical teratogen.

Pathogenesis is characterized by the appearance of

TABLE 64–2 Successive Stages in the Pathogenesis of a Developmental Defect

Mechanisms

Initial types of changes in developing cells or tissues after teratogenic insult:
  Mutation (gene)
  Chromosomal breaks, nondisjunction, *etc.*
  Mitotic interference
  Altered nucleic acid integrity or function
  Lack of normal precursors, substrates, *etc.*
  Altered energy sources
  Changed membrane characteristics
  Osmolar imbalance
  Enzyme inhibition

Pathogenesis

Ultimately manifested as one or more types of abnormal embryogenesis:
  Excessive or reduced cell death
  Failed cell interactions
  Reduced biosynthesis
  Impeded morphogenetic movement
  Mechanical disruption of tissues

Common pathways

Too few cells or cell products to effect local morphogenesis or functional maturation
Other imbalances in growth and differentiation

Final defect

Initiation of one or more mechanisms by the teratogenic cause from the environment leads to changes in the developmental system that become manifested as one or more types of abnormal embryogenesis. This in turn leads into pathways that seem often to be characterized by too few cells or cell products to effect morphogenesis or functional maturation, but the suggestion that this is a single common pathway for all developmental defects is conjecture. (Source: Wilson JG, 1977.)

demonstrable evidence of cellular and tissue damage. Increased cellular death is the most frequent sign of abnormal development, and the teratogenic process often, but not inevitably, involves some degree of focal cellular necrosis. Failure of either proper amount or sequence of cellular interaction and reduced biosynthesis of essential macromolecules such as DNA, RNA, proteins, and mucopolysaccharides can be important steps in teratogenesis. Impairment of morphogenetic movement, *i.e.*, of the migration or translocation of cells or groups of cells, is involved notably in neuronal maldevelopment. Finally, tissues can be traumatized mechanically by invasion of foreign materials or abnormal accumulation of tissue fluids or blood, resulting in anomalous development.

Genetic and Environmental Modulation

The genetic and environmental factors modulating teratologic susceptibility are poorly understood, and in many cases likely involve a complex interdependence. For most teratogens, it is not known whether the genetic predisposition or resistance is mediated *via* a pharmacologic mechanism, as discussed later, or *via* a biologic response mechanism. One example of the latter case may be the difference in susceptibility of various strains of mice to the induction of cleft palates. The inbred A/J mouse has a spontaneous incidence of cleft palates and is more susceptible than outbred mouse strains to induction of cleft palates by the anticonvulsant drug phenytoin. The palatal shelves of the relatively resistant outbred mice are oriented on a horizontal plane toward each other to start with, whereas the palatal shelves of the susceptible A/J mouse remain vertical and distant from each other until late in the closure period, thus being potentially more susceptible to developmental interferences. Other cases remain unexplained, such as resistance to thalidomide teratogenicity in rats and mice compared with an exquisite susceptibility in humans and to a lesser extent in rabbits. Conversely, the susceptibility of rodents and resistance of humans to salicylate teratogenicity also is unexplained, as are a multitude of other species and strain differences in teratologic susceptibility.

Environmental determinants of teratologic susceptibility are equally poorly recognized and understood. Stress and nutritional deficiency by themselves can increase the incidence of cleft palates in rodents and likely can potentiate the teratogenicity of many chemicals. Ambient temperature also can be important, as demonstrated in the case of 6-aminonicotinamide, a teratogenic chemical that also blocks temperature regulation in animals. In studies at room temperature, 6-aminonicotinamide produced a fall in maternal body temperature and the offspring were normal, while in studies conducted at 36°C with this chemical, normal maternal body temperature was maintained and there was a substantial increase in teratologic anomalies. In animals, a growing number of drugs and chemicals with or without their own intrinsic teratogenic activity have been shown to modulate the fetal damage produced by known teratogenic agents, but in most cases the underlying mechanisms are not known.

PHARMACOLOGIC PRINCIPLES

Placental Transfer and Fetal Chemical Disposition

Once believed to be a protective "barrier" isolating the fetus from harmful external influences, the placenta now is known to be more akin to a sieve, permitting ready access to the fetus of chemicals with a molecular weight under 600, while excluding only the largest (molecular weight above 1000) or most highly charged molecules such as heparin. Fetal blood concentrations of many chemicals are equivalent to maternal concentrations, and even some charged quaternary ammonium compounds can cross the placenta in limited quantities, possibly facilitated by a placental active transport process. (*See also* Chapter 68, *Perinatal Pharmacology*.)

While fetal factors such as a blood pH 0.1–0.15 unit below that of the mother and occasional differences in plasma protein binding of chemicals are theoretically important in determining chemical concentrations in fetal blood and tissues, such factors have not been shown to have a remarkable influence on chemical teratogenicity. For complete reviews of fetal drug disposition, *see* Mirkin (1978) and Waddell and Marlowe (In: Juchau, 1981).

Fetal Chemical Biotransformation

The principles of drug biotransformation are covered in Chapter 4 and are reviewed by Juchau and by Manson (In: Juchau, 1981) in specific reference to chemical teratogenesis. In general, most enzymatic pathways of drug biotransformation are at a much lower level of activity in the fetus than in adults. In animals, this activity for the most part is low or negligible until birth. In the human fetal liver, enzymatic activity is measurable as early as 6 weeks, but at midgestation it is only 20–40% of that in adults, with considerable interindividual variation. In nonhuman primates that have a midgestational mixed-function oxygenase activity similar to that in humans, activity increases four-fold from 10 days before to 10 days after birth. Enzymatic activity in fetal animals cannot be induced by chemicals such as phenobarbital and 3-methylcholanthrene until about 3 days before birth, although dioxin is an effective inducer of aryl hydrocarbon hydroxylase (AHH) activity earlier in gestation. In humans, enzymatic induction appears to occur much earlier, although still less than in adults.

The developmental activity for a number of important enzymes is shown in Figure 64–5. Within any one class of enzymes, the developmental activity for a specific isoenzyme and its substrates may vary considerably, as with the cytochromes P-450 (Fig. 64–5A). One of the glucuronyl transferases demonstrates high activity during the third trimester and perinatal period and declines rapidly thereafter, while the other transferase develops after birth (Fig. 64–5B). On the other hand, sulfotransferase activity in early fetal life can be equivalent to adult levels, although this pathway is capacity-limited for chemicals. The fetus also has significant prostaglandin synthetase activity, which may play a role in chemical teratogenesis. In general, however, the fetus is deficient in enzymatic activities for chemical biotransformation and thus often is unable to eliminate chemicals and detoxify reactive intermediates.

Teratogenic Specificity

The concept of "critical period" (previously discussed) can be restated here as **phase specificity**. Teratogens will cause markedly different anomalies depending on the phase of fetal development. For example, methylnitrosourea is a transplacental carcinogen in rats only if administered on gestational day 20, while earlier administration will cause a spectrum of structural and functional anomalies. This late susceptibility to carcinogenicity may be due to a requirement for a sufficiently developed fetal enzymatic system for bioactivation of the chemical to a carcinogenic reactive intermediate within the fetus, although other factors such as increased placental transport of a maternally produced reactive intermediate or processes involved in carcinogenic promotion cannot be excluded.

Drug specificity is closely linked to phase specificity. Many teratogens interfere with intermediary processes that occur only during discrete phases in development. These "specific" teratogens cause a limited number of anomalies or a characteristic syndrome of malformations. A partial exception to the principle of drug specificity is a limited group of "general" or "universal" teratogens that interfere with fundamental processes such as nucleic acid metabolism or protein synthesis occurring throughout the stages of cellular division and differentiation. Universal teratogens would include the cytotoxic anticancer drugs, such as cytosine arabinoside and 6-mercaptopurine. However, even the so-called universal teratogens may demonstrate a certain degree of specificity, as shown in Figure 64–6. Treatment of pregnant mice with 6-aminonicotinamide produces more limb defects when given on gestational

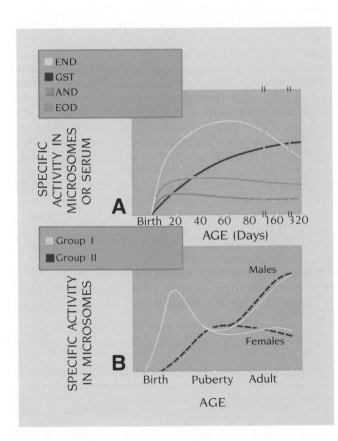

Figure 64–5 Developmental changes in activities of selected drug biotransformation enzymes in the rat. *A,* Hepatic monooxygenases and serum glutathione-S-transferase (AND = aminopyrine-N-demethylase, END = ethylmorphine-N-demethylase, EOD = ethoxycoumarin-O-demethylase, GST = serum glutathione-S-transferase). *B,* Glucuronidation of Group I and Group II substrates in males and females.

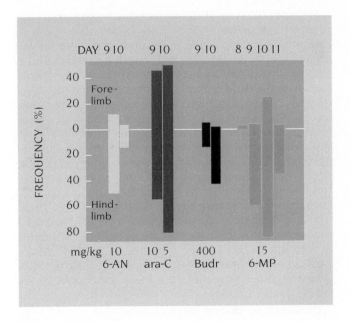

Figure 64–6 Frequency of limb abnormalities produced by various agents applied at different stages of pregnancy in NMRI mice, showing the great variability with different chemicals. 6-AN = 6-aminonicotinamide; ara-C = cytosine arabinoside; Budr = 5'-bromouracil deoxyriboside; 6-MP = 6-mercaptopurine. (From Neubert D *et al.* 1980).

day 9 than on day 10, while cytosine arabinoside is teratogenic on both days, if not more so on day 10. Furthermore, 6-aminonicotinamide preferentially affects the hindlimbs, while cytosine arabinoside affects both the forelimbs and hindlimbs.

Dose specificity also can affect both the type and the frequency of anomalies. For example, low doses of a number of teratogens given to pregnant mice on gestational day 10 cause polydactyly (*i.e.*, extra phalanges), while medium doses of the same teratogens reduce the length of phalanges and long bones without causing polydactyly, and high doses cause amelia (*i.e.*, the absence of entire limbs). In this case the malformation is more dependent upon the dose of the teratogen than on its mechanism of action. The lowest dose is thought to act by causing limited focal necrosis in the apical region of the developing limb bud, which responds with a compensatory overproduction of phalangeal cells, leading to polydactyly.

Chemical Mechanisms

Chemical mechanisms of teratogenesis can be classified into two general categories: (1) those related to the classical, reversible interaction of a chemical or its active metabolite(s) with a receptor and (2) those involving highly reactive chemicals or their respective reactive intermediary metabolites, which can bind irreversibly or covalently to essential cellular macromolecules, stimulate lipid peroxidation, and/or cause oxidant stress.

The specific, reversible interaction of drugs with their receptors is generally responsible for the intended therapeutic effects of the drugs and many of their side effects. Fetal toxicity caused by such an interaction is due to an exaggeration of the pharmacologic activity for which the drug is used therapeutically. On the other hand, fetal toxicity caused by the generally irreversible interaction of a reactive intermediate with fetal tissues is unrelated to the pharmacologic mechanism by which the drug exerts its therapeutic effect. In the case of environmental chemicals that have no therapeutic purpose, the discrimination is based only upon reversible binding to a receptor as opposed to the irreversible interaction of a reactive intermediate with tissues. These working definitions are not absolute, as illustrated by the exceptional case of the antineoplastic alkylating drugs, whose therapeutic effect of neoplastic cellular destruction is based on their covalent binding to DNA, which is also responsible for their teratogenicity.

Receptor-Mediated Mechanisms

Since fetal toxicity occurring *via* these mechanisms generally but not always represents an exaggerated therapeutic response, the toxicologic sequelae (including teratogenic effects) usually are predictable and proportional to fetal and maternal blood chemical con-

centrations, if not to the dose assimilated. The principles of such mechanisms are discussed in Chapter 65, *Adverse Drug Reactions*; the present discussion will be limited to teratogenesis.

The induction of cleft palates and limb anomalies in rodents by high doses of corticosteroids is an instructive example. While this does not constitute an exaggerated therapeutic response, it is an exaggeration of the physiologic role of endogenous corticosteroids in palatal development and is dependent upon reversible binding of the corticosteroid to its receptor. In general, the amount of glucocorticoid administered to pregnant mice and associated with the fetus correlates with the degree of inhibition of DNA and protein synthesis and with teratogenic susceptibility. The A/J strain of mice, which is highly susceptible to glucocorticoid teratogenicity, has the same endogenous maternal and fetal concentrations of corticosterone as the C57BL/6J strain, which is resistant. However, A/J mouse facial mesenchymal cells have two to three times more cytoplasmic glucocorticoid receptors than those from C57BL/6J mice, and this is reflected in an increased inhibition of growth and DNA synthesis in A/J compared with C57BL/6J mice.

Interestingly, receptor number in embryonic limb bud cells does not correlate with susceptibility to glucocorticoid-induced anomalies of the limbs. The positive correlation of receptor number with susceptibility to cleft palates is observed in a variety of mouse strains (Table 64–3). Conversely, in humans, cultured dermal fibroblasts from women, and children of women, with a history of cleft palates had fewer glucocorticoid receptors and were less responsive to glucocorticoid-induced inhibition of growth and DNA synthesis. Thus, while receptor numbers may play an important role in spontaneous and steroid-induced cleft palates, other processes must be contributive. Similarly, other substances such as cyclic AMP and various prostaglandins play a role in glucocorticoid modulation of palatal closure (*see* review by Greene, In: Johnson and Kochhar, 1983), but will not be discussed here.

The teratogenicity of narcotic analgesic drugs likely constitutes another example of a receptor-mediated mechanism, since the incidence of most anomalies in

TABLE 64–3 Maxillary Cytoplasmic Glucocorticoid Receptors and Cleft Palate Frequency (Mice)

Strain	Sites per Cell	Cleft Palate (%)
SWR/FR	83,960	100
SWR/NIH	61,500	100
DBA/1J	29,216	94
A/J	16,300	100
CBA/J	10,764	12
C57BL/6J	7,073	25

Source: Salomon DS. In: Johnson EM, Kochhar DM, eds. 1983:122.

animals can be reduced by pretreatment with narcotic antagonists (*see* review by Wells, 1988).

Reactive Intermediate-Mediated Mechanisms

A representative scheme for the enzymatic formation (bioactivation) of a potentially toxic, reactive intermediary metabolite (often an epoxide) and its various detoxification pathways is presented in Figure 64–7. This type of bioactivation is only one of several kinds reviewed in more detail by Juchau (1981). Glutathione S-transferases and epoxide hydrolases are critical enzymes for the direct detoxification of reactive intermediary metabolites. In a limited number of cases, however, these so-called detoxifying enzymes can be involved in the subsequent formation of an even more reactive and toxic intermediary metabolite. Glucuronyl trans-

ferases and similar transferase enzymes, while not directly involved in detoxifying reactive intermediates, can be quantitatively major pathways of drug elimination, thereby preventing much of a chemical from being metabolized *via* a bioactivating pathway.

Under normal conditions, a reactive intermediate is evanescent, being immediately detoxified and excreted. However, if bioactivation exceeds detoxification, the highly reactive electrophilic site on the chemical intermediate will bind covalently to nucleophilic sites on essential fetal cellular macromolecules such as DNA, RNA, protein, and phospholipids. If fetal repair mechanisms are inadequate, covalent binding of the chemical is thought to initiate a process, as yet poorly understood, that ends in cellular death or functional alterations. In a few cases, such as the antineoplastic alkylating drugs, the parent compound is sufficiently reactive to bind covalently without need for bioactivation. Chemi-

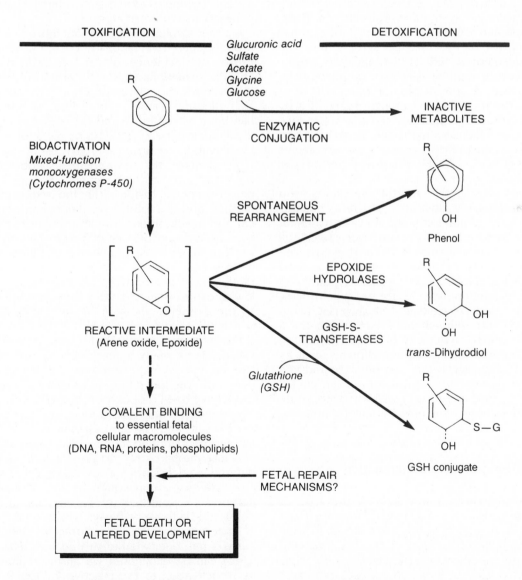

Figure 64–7 Role of bioactivation and detoxification in chemical teratogenesis.

cals believed to be bioactivated to a teratogenic reactive intermediate include thalidomide, phenytoin, and benzo(a)pyrene, although other mechanisms may be involved.

With some chemicals, bioactivation or certain detoxifying pathways may constitute a quantitatively minor route of metabolism and yet have major teratologic importance. For example, while only about 5–10% of the reactive arene oxide intermediate of phenytoin is hydrated and thereby detoxified by epoxide hydrolase, specific inhibition of this enzyme will dramatically increase the teratogenicity of phenytoin. It is not clear whether the reactive intermediate is formed in sufficient quantities by fetal tissues or is bioactivated in the mother and stable enough to cross the placenta. Given its early development of biotransforming enzymes, the human fetus may be capable of teratologically significant bioactivation.

Another enzyme system involved in the bioactivation of drugs, primarily to reactive free radical intermediates, is prostaglandin synthetase (Marnett and Eling, 1983; Halliwell and Gutteridge, 1985). The fetus has significant activity of this enzyme system, and the hydroperoxidase component of prostaglandin synthetase may cooxidize some drugs to a teratogenic reactive intermediate, as postulated for phenytoin (Fig. 64–8; Wells, 1988). Drug radicals may react directly with fetal tissues or may react with oxygen to produce toxic superoxide radicals, hydrogen peroxide, and hydroxyl radicals. In addition, by acting as the cofactor for reduction of PGG_2 to PGH_2, drugs may perturb the physiologic balance among the fetal syntheses of prostaglandins, prostacyclin, and thromboxanes, with potential teratologic consequences. The fetus has low concentrations of glutathione and low activities of glutathione reductase and glutathione peroxidase, all of which are critical for cellular protection against free radical damage. Thus, the fetus likely is at increased risk for free-radical-mediated cytotoxicity, although there is little information specific for chemical teratogenesis. A secondary principle illustrated by phenytoin is the potential contribution of more than one chemical mechanism to the teratogenicity of drugs; namely, a reversible, receptor-mediated interaction as well as irreversible interactions of reactive arene oxide and free radical intermediates. The relative teratologic contributions of these mechanisms may well vary with gestational age, strain, species, and environmental conditions.

Genetic and Environmental Modulation

Modulatory influences, particularly in the case of toxicologic mechanisms involving reactive intermediates, generally are complex and poorly understood. In addition to the complicating effects of the maternal and placental systems, modulating factors tend to affect multiple pathways of bioactivation and detoxification, with unpredictable teratologic consequences.

The **genetic determinants** of chemical teratogenesis have been evaluated for benzo(a)pyrene, which provides a useful model for discussion. Susceptibility of individual mouse fetuses from the same litter to benzo(a)pyrene teratogenicity has been correlated with their individual inducibility of aryl hydrocarbon hydroxylase (AHH). AHH, a cytochrome P-448 (P_1-450) isoenzyme controlled genetically by the Ah locus, is involved in the bioactivation of aryl hydrocarbons such as benzo(a)pyrene to teratogenic reactive intermediates. There is a remarkable variation in the induction of AHH activity among individual fetuses in the same litter following maternal administration of the inducer 3-methylcholanthrene. AHH activity in the responsive fetuses is from five to fifteen times as great as in the nonresponsive littermates. Littermates that are responsive to AHH induction are more susceptible to benzo(a)pyrene-induced malformations, and they have an increased amount of covalent binding of radiolabelled benzo(a)pyrene to **fetal** tissues compared with the AHH-nonresponsive littermates.

In other studies using pregnant inbred B6 mice which produce only AHH-responsive offspring, benzo(a)pyrene causes an incidence of fetal resorptions, stillbirths and malformations which is four-fold higher than that in inbred AK mice, which produce only AHH-nonresponsive offspring. Finally, metabolism of benzo(a)pyrene has been observed in mouse embryos induced with dioxin at as early as 3.5 days of gestation, with greater bioactivation occurring in AHH-responsive embryos.

In summary, the teratologic susceptibility to some chemicals appears to be genetically determined, the determinant can reside within the fetus rather than the mother, and this fetal determinant can be active very early in development. This also might explain why, in humans, it is possible that only one of fraternal (dizygotic) twins may be afflicted with a drug-induced anomaly or how only one of several children from the same mother may demonstrate a teratologic response following exposure *in utero* to a drug that had been taken by the mother in the same doses during all her pregnancies.

The observations above for the Ah locus likely are instructive for many other genetic systems which regulate other enzymatic pathways of bioactivation and detoxification for different chemicals. For example, there have been rare cases reported involving patients who are deficient in glutathione synthetase or epoxide hydrolases and have experienced life-threatening hepatotoxicity due to their inability to detoxify the reactive intermediates of certain drugs. Such genetically determined deficiencies would be expected to have serious teratologic consequences for pregnant women exposed to potential teratogens that are normally detoxified *via* these pathways. The potential importance of maternal glucuronyl transferase in chemical teratogenesis has been demonstrated for benzo(a)pyrene, which can be eliminated *via* glucuronidation prior to its bioactivation to the reactive 7,8-diol-9,10-epoxide intermediate. The embryotoxicity of benzo(a)pyrene is

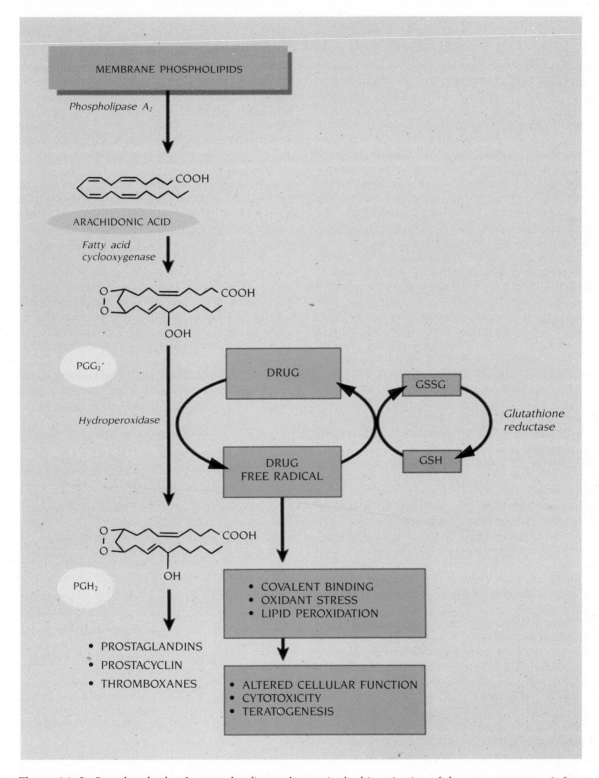

Figure 64–8   Postulated role of prostaglandin synthetase in the bioactivation of drugs to a teratogenic free radical intermediate. Fatty acid cyclooxygenase and hydroperoxidase are catalytic components of prostaglandin synthetase. (PGG$_2$ = prostaglandin G$_2$; PGH$_2$ = prostaglandin H$_2$; GSH = glutathione; GSSG = oxidized glutathione.)

significantly increased in Gunn rats, which have a genetic deficiency in glucuronyl transferase.

Relatively little is known about the **environmental determinants** that modulate chemical teratogenicity, particularly with teratogens that are bioactivated to a toxic reactive intermediate. Such determinants could include individual physiologic differences, concurrent pathophysiologic conditions, and exposure to other drugs or environmental chemicals. For example, in pregnant mice, the teratogenicity of phenytoin and similar drugs is potentiated by pretreatment with the epoxide hydrolase inhibitor trichloropropene oxide, the glutathione depletor diethyl maleate, the glutathione synthesis inhibitor buthionine sulfoximine, the glutathione reductase inhibitor bis-chloroethylnitroso-urea (BCNU), and the phospholipase A_2 activator tetradecanoylphorbol acetate (TPA). Conversely, phenytoin teratogenicity in mice is reduced by pretreatment with the prostaglandin cyclooxygenase inhibitor acetylsalicylic acid, the antioxidant caffeic acid, the free radical spin-trapping agent phenylbutylnitrone, and, under some conditions, the glutathione precursor N-acetylcysteine. Environmental factors with such effects on bioactivating and detoxifying pathways similarly would be expected to modulate the risk of teratogenesis in pregnant women exposed to certain potential teratogens. However, such possibilities have only recently been recognized in animal studies, and there are few data in humans on which to base any estimate of actual risk.

In addition, the complexities of developmental processes and maternal-placental-fetal interdependencies often preclude the straightforward predictions that are possible in other fields of toxicology. For example, in nonpregnant animals, induction of cytochromes P-450 generally will increase, while inhibition will decrease, the toxicity of chemicals that are bioactivated to a reactive intermediate. However, in pregnant mice, the teratogenicity of phenytoin and cyclophosphamide paradoxically is **decreased** by enzyme induction and **increased** by inhibition.

Thus it appears that enzyme induction and other environmental perturbations have complex effects *in vivo* relating both to simultaneous effects on multiple pathways of chemical bioactivation and detoxification and to confounding maternal effects. The underlying mechanisms for the most part are not understood and more studies will be necessary to identify and characterize the environmental determinants of teratogenesis, particularly with regard to human risk.

EXPERIMENTAL TERATOLOGY

The thalidomide tragedy clearly demonstrated the need for improved methods to detect potential chemical teratogens and elucidate their teratologic mechanisms. *In vivo* studies employing more nonrodent animal species are now combined with a battery of *in vitro* tests. *In vivo* studies of pregnancy are time-consuming and expensive, however, and are not practical for screening large numbers of drugs and chemicals. Furthermore, the chemical and biologic complexities of the maternal-placental-fetal interactions encountered *in vivo* generally preclude the elucidation of discrete teratologic mechanisms. Thus, *in vivo* studies are most useful for the ultimate teratologic testing of chemicals that have been prescreened *in vitro* and for applied aspects of teratologic research.

For the above reasons, a large number of *in vitro* teratologic methods have been devised, as shown in Table 64-4. This discussion will consider briefly four major categories: cells in culture, embryonic organs in culture, whole embryos in culture, and artificial embryos.

Differentiating embryonic **cells** in culture are used to study potential teratogens at various developmental stages, including cellular differentiation, cell-cell interactions, and cellular migration. This method is valuable particularly as a rapid prescreen for chemical teratogenicity and can provide mechanistic information as well.

Numerous types of **organs and tissues** in culture have been used in teratologic studies, including palate, limbs, kidney, sex organs, and skin. This method adds more

TABLE 64-4 *In Vitro* Tests for Screening Teratogenic Chemicals

Biologic Unit	Endpoints Measured
Virus	Plaque-forming units
Bacteria	Growth rate
Tumor cell	Number attached to surface
Prechondrocytes (chick, rodent)	Colonies formed and staining with Alcian blue
Neural crest cells (chick)	Morphogenesis of cell
Palate mesenchyme (human)	Morphogenesis of cell
Hydra attenuata	Regeneration of pellets to adult
Planaria	Regeneration of organ systems from fragments
Drosophila	Maturation of larvae or colonies formed from disrupted embryo
Xenopus laevis eggs	Malformations in embryos grown from eggs
Fish eggs	Malformations in free-swimming forms
Limb bud	Morphologic and chemical increment
Whole embryo (rodent)	Increase in somites, crown-length, protein, DNA, and malformations
Chick embryo	Malformation

Source: Shepard TH, *et al*. In: MacLeod SM, Okey AB, Spielberg SP, eds. Developmental pharmacology. New York: AR Liss, 1983:147.

dimensions to the developmental processes tested in cellular cultures. The explanted organ primordium consists of heterogeneous tissue components that progress through the organogenetic stages, thereby providing a measure of several developmental processes.

Whole embryos from mice or rats can be removed from the uterus at various developmental stages and cultured *in vitro*. This method permits the most comprehensive evaluation of the developmental process compared with the other *in vitro* systems. However, substantial facilities are required and the technique is labor-intensive and time-consuming. The embryo culture technique is suited ideally for mechanistic studies of chemical teratogenesis but is not readily applicable to general teratologic screening of large numbers of chemicals.

A number of nonmammalian life forms such as *Hydra attenuata* have been developed as "**artificial embryos.**" The adult Hydra are sheared into small pieces of tissue and compressed by centrifugation into an artificial "embryonic" pellet. This pellet "embryo" will develop into multiple adults within one week, undergoing a remarkable range of complex developmental processes somewhat analogous to mammalian prenatal development. Such model systems are useful in detecting teratogenic potential for large numbers of chemicals in a fairly quick and inexpensive manner.

SUGGESTED READING

Halliwell B, Gutteridge JMC. Free radicals in biology and medicine. New York: Oxford University Press, 1985.

Johnson EM, Kochhar DM, eds. Handbook of experimental pharmacology. Vol 65. Teratogenesis and reproductive toxicology. New York: Springer-Verlag, 1983.

Juchau MR, ed. The biochemical basis of chemical teratogenesis. New York: Elsevier/North-Holland, 1981.

Manson JM. Teratogens. In: Klaassen CD, Amdur MO, Doull J, eds. Toxicology: the basic science of poisons. 3rd ed. New York: Macmillan, 1986:195–220.

Manson JM, Zenick H, Costlow RD. Teratology test methods for laboratory animals. In: Hayes AW, ed. Principles and methods of toxicology. New York: Raven Press, 1982: 141–184.

Marnett LJ, Eling TE. Cooxidation during prostaglandin biosynthesis: a pathway for the metabolic bioactivation of xenobiotics. In: Hodgson E, Bend JR, Philpott RM, eds. Reviews of biochemical toxicology. Vol 5. New York: Elsevier Science Publishing Co., 1983:135–172.

Mirkin BL. Pharmacodynamics and drug disposition in pregnant women, in neonates and in children. In: Melmon KL, Morelli HF, eds. Clinical pharmacology: basic principles in therapeutics. 2nd ed. New York: Macmillan, 1978:127–152.

Neubert D, Barrach HJ, Merker HJ. Drug-induced damage to embryo or fetus. In: Grundmann E, ed. Drug-induced pathology. New York: Springer-Verlag, 1980:242–331.

Schardein JL. Chemically induced birth defects. New York: Marcel Dekker, 1985.

Shepard TH. Catalogue of teratogenic agents. 4th ed. Baltimore: Johns Hopkins University Press, 1983.

Wells PG. Analgesics: direct embryopathic effects, and indirect biochemical effects modulating the teratogenicity of other drugs and chemicals. In: Kacew S, Lock S, eds. Toxicologic and pharmacologic principles in pediatrics. New York: Hemisphere Publishing Corp., 1988:127–166.

Wilson JG. Current status of teratology. In: Wilson JG, Fraser FC, eds. Handbook of teratology. Vol 1. New York: Plenum Press, 1977:47–74.

Chapter 65

ADVERSE DRUG REACTIONS

C.A. Naranjo and U. Busto

All drugs have the potential to cause deleterious effects. While some adverse effects are detected in preclinical studies, some serious but relatively infrequent types of toxicity may become apparent only when the drug is used in a large population of patients over long periods of time. Consequently, the early detection and assessment of adverse drug reactions has become increasingly important.

From the time that humans first used different substances as medicines, toxic effects were observed. Reference to toxicity of drugs is found in the writings of several famous physicians of ancient times. For example, Hippocrates (460–377 B.C.) instructed his students and fellow physicians that they should "above all, do no harm"; this was obviously a reference to the potential hazards associated with remedies of that time. The balance between beneficial and toxic effects of drugs has been a continuing concern as medicine has progressed. Occasionally, wise laymen, such as Voltaire in "Le Médecin Malgré Lui," have expressed doubts about the proper use of drugs by physicians ("They poured drugs of which they knew little into bodies of which they knew less"). However, interest in the detection and prevention of serious drug toxicity reached a peak after the occurrence of the thalidomide disaster in 1961.

In that year there was a sudden outbreak of births of babies with the deformities known as phocomelia or micromelia. Astute physicians suspected that the development of these abnormalities was associated with the use of a new and presumably safe hypnotic, thalidomide, by the mothers of these babies during the first trimester of pregnancy, when the forelimb buds were forming and developing (*see also* Chapter 64). Case-control studies established that thalidomide was indeed the factor responsible for the malformation. All these events led to a reassessment of the methodology and regulations applied to the testing of the safety of drugs. As a consequence, more stringent legislation was implemented in several countries in order to improve the possibility of detecting serious toxicity before drugs were administered to humans. In recent years, new knowledge has been acquired concerning the diagnosis, assessment, mechanism, treatment, and prevention of adverse drug reactions. This chapter is a brief review of the most relevant knowledge.

DEFINITIONS, MECHANISMS, AND CLASSIFICATION

An adverse drug reaction (ADR) is any noxious, unintended, and undesired effect of a drug that is observed at doses usually administered therapeutically in humans. This definition excludes cases of drug overdose, drug abuse, or therapeutic errors.

The severity of ADRs is usually classified as mild, moderate, severe, or lethal. These terms are defined as follows.

Mild: No antidote, therapy, or prolongation of hospitalization is necessary.

Moderate: Requires a change in drug therapy although not necessarily discontinuation of the offending drug. It may prolong hospitalization and require specific treatment.

Severe: Potentially life-threatening, requires discontinuation of the drug and specific treatment of the adverse reaction.

Lethal: Directly or indirectly contributes to the death of the patient.

The adequate assessment and classification of ADRs requires a knowledge of the mechanisms by which they are produced. Adverse drug reactions are the result of an interaction between the characteristics of the administered drug, and some inherent or acquired characteristics of the patient that determine the individual pattern of response to drugs. Thus, there are some reactions that are determined principally by the drug (physicochemical and pharmacokinetic characteristics, formulation, dose, rate, and route of administration), others that are determined chiefly by the patient's characteristics (genetic, physiologic, or pathologic), and others in which both drug and patient variables are important.

ADRs can be dose-related (*e.g.*, CNS depression by sedative hypnotics). These reactions are the most common (about 95% of cases). In these cases the frequency and severity of the ADRs are directly proportional to the administered dose and therefore can be prevented and/or treated by adjusting the dosage to the patient's needs and tolerance. In some of these cases, impairment of drug elimination by renal disease (for drugs such as digoxin, predominantly excreted by the kidney) or liver dysfunction (for drugs eliminated after biotransformation in the liver) can contribute to the development of toxicity. The ADR can represent an extension of the usual pharmacologic effects of the drugs or an unusual toxicity caused by the drug and/or its metabolites. These reactions are usually predictable from animal toxicologic studies.

Other ADRs are not dose-related. These reactions are uncommon (less than 5% of cases) and are due to an increased susceptibility of the patient. The ADR is usually manifested as a qualitative change in the patient's response to drugs, and it may be caused by a pharmacogenetic variant (*see* Chapter 12) or an acquired drug allergy. Most reactions with a pharmacogenetic basis are detected only after the patient is exposed to the drug and therefore are difficult to prevent on first administration. An example of genetically determined toxicity is the polyneuropathy caused by isoniazid, a drug that is mainly biotransformed by acetylation. There is wide individual variation in the rate at which isoniazid and other drugs are acetylated. Within populations, there tends to be a clear separation of individuals into groups of slow or rapid acetylators, on the basis of differences in the activity of liver N-acetyltransferase. The neuropathic effects of isoniazid are more common in slow acetylators. Most such pharmacogenetic reactions can be prevented by avoiding readministration of the drug to the affected individuals.

The identification of a reaction as dose-related or not dose-related allows practical decisions concerning the treatment of an individual patient and/or the prevention of ADRs. The main features of these reactions are summarized in Table 65–1.

Allergic or hypersensitivity reactions have been classified into four main clinical types: type 1 (anaphylactic); type 2 (cytotoxic); type 3 (immune-complex-mediated); and type 4 (cell-mediated).

Type 1 or immediate hypersensitivity reactions involve interaction of the allergen (the drug) with IgE antibody on the surface of basophils and mast cells, resulting in the release of chemical mediators such as histamine, slow-reacting substances of anaphylaxis, kinins, and prostaglandins, which lead to capillary dila-

tation, constriction of smooth muscle, and edema. A type 1 reaction may be limited to cutaneous wheals and flares, but it can also result in life-threatening systemic anaphylaxis (characterized by shock and/or bronchoconstriction), asthma, or laryngeal angioneurotic edema. Anaphylactic reactions may occur after the injection of penicillin and other antimicrobials. Up to 25% of asthmatic patients may present intolerance to acetylsalicylic acid (ASA), which may cause severe bronchospasms. Drug-induced angioneurotic edema can occur with co-trimoxazole (trimethoprim + sulfamethoxazole).

Type 2 reactions consist of a complement-fixing reaction between antigen and antibody on a cell surface (*e.g.*, RBC, WBC, platelets), leading to lysis of the cell. Drugs are usually haptens, binding to a protein on the cell surface to constitute a complete antigen against which a specific antibody is formed. Subsequent antigen-antibody reactions with complement fixation may lead to hemolytic anemia (*e.g.*, after methyldopa, chlorpromazine), agranulocytosis (*e.g.*, after amidopyrine, cephalothin, sulfonamides), or thrombocytopenic purpura (*e.g.*, after ASA, quinidine, phenytoin).

Type 3 hypersensitivity reactions (toxic immune-complex reactions) occur when antigen-antibody complexes deposit on target tissue cells. Complement is then activated and causes tissue destruction by releasing lysosomal enzymes. This mechanism may cause glomerulonephritis, collagen diseases, and vasculitic skin eruptions. Drugs commonly implicated in these reactions are penicillins, sulfonamides, erythromycin, hydralazine, and nitrofurantoin.

Cell-mediated **type 4** allergic reactions arise from a direct interaction between an allergen (the drug) and sensitized lymphocytes, resulting in the release of lymphokines. Most cases of eczematous and contact dermatitis are cell-mediated allergic reactions. Common causes are topical antihistamines, para-aminobenzoic acid compounds, and mercury derivatives. Type 4 reactions are also responsible for serious drug reactions such as halothane-induced hepatitis.

EPIDEMIOLOGY OF ADVERSE DRUG REACTIONS

Drug Monitoring Methods

Drug monitoring is the systematic collection, recording, and assessment of information on adverse drug reactions. This information is collected to allow the early identification of severe ADRs, to determine the possible causal association of drugs and adverse events, to establish the frequency of ADRs, and to identify the factors predisposing to their development.

Estimation of the frequency of adverse reactions to a drug depends on the reliable identification of the num-

TABLE 65-1 Adverse Drug Reactions (ADRs)

	Dose-Related ADR	*Not Dose-Related ADR*
Nature of abnormality	Quantitative	Qualitative
Incidence	High	Low
Is ADR predictable?	Yes	No
In the presence of liver and/or kidney dysfunction	Increased toxicity, depending on the main route(s) of elimination of the drug in question	Not affected
Prevention	Adjustment of dose	Avoid drug administration
Treatment	Adjustment of dose	Discontinue drug administration
Mortality	Usually low	Usually high

ber of subjects presenting the adverse event (numerator) and the accurate estimate of the number of subjects exposed to the drug (denominator). The determination of these two numbers is generally difficult because the denominator is usually unavailable, and the numerator can be over- or underestimated. Information on adverse drug reactions is collected by using several methods that are briefly described below.

Spontaneous Communication to National Drug Monitoring Centres

Since the thalidomide disaster of the 1960s, several countries have established national drug monitoring centres to collect information on ADRs. These agencies encourage physicians and other health personnel to report any clinical event suspected of being an ADR. The system has met with varying success. The most active drug monitoring centres are located in the United Kingdom and Sweden, and they periodically report their findings. This system mostly collects information on the number of cases of ADRs, but is not designed to yield information on the number of prescriptions for various drugs. Another disadvantage is that the collection of information is highly dependent on the motivation of physicians to report the events. Therefore, under-reporting is common. However, these systems have obviously contributed to an early recognition of severe reactions, and thus they are still operative in various countries. In Canada, the Health Protection Branch, Health and Welfare Canada, has a Drug Monitoring Centre to which physicians can report information on suspected ADRs.

Cohort Studies

Another procedure frequently used has been the systematic collection of prospective information on drug therapy and adverse events in subjects with a particular characteristic (patient-oriented) or receiving a particular drug (drug-oriented). This system allows the collection of information on both the number of subjects with ADRs and the number of subjects receiving the drug. This procedure has been applied mostly to medical patients hospitalized in teaching hospitals. The best known example is the Boston Collaborative Drug Surveillance Program. In this and similar programs, information on the demographic and clinical characteristics of patients, the drugs administered to them, and the suspected ADRs is collected by trained nurse or pharmacist monitors. The data are subsequently analysed to establish the drugs most commonly inducing ADRs, the frequency of different types of ADR, and the factors predisposing to them. These procedures have provided information about the clinical use of and adverse reactions to the most commonly prescribed drugs. They have also been used to determine the clinical toxicity of drugs in subjects with special characteristics; for example, those suffering from renal or liver dysfunction. However, these data have obvious shortcomings, the most important being that the information has been collected in medical inpatients in university centres, making extrapolation of results to other populations difficult.

More recently, the postmarketing surveillance of a cohort of subjects receiving a new drug has gained popularity. These studies begin immediately after a new drug has been marketed, and the drug's performance is closely monitored during months or years when widespread use may result in the discovery of rare side effects or previously unknown drug interactions. Cohort studies are expensive and difficult to perform because large populations must be studied if the incidence of uncommon, but severe, ADRs is to be determined.

Case Control Studies

These studies are retrospective but useful for suggesting cause-effect relationships between drugs and adverse events. In the case of a suspected ADR, the relative use of the suspected drug is compared in subjects with the presumed drug-induced illness and in a matched control group without the illness. If the illness really is associated with the drug, those showing the adverse event will have had a greater exposure to the drug. This procedure was employed to discover the link between thalidomide and phocomelia. In his classic letter to Lancet, McBride reported that "...Congenital abnormalities are present in approximately 1.5% of babies. I have observed that the incidence of severe abnormalities in babies of women who were given the drug thalidomide...during pregnancy...(was) almost 20%." This method is very efficient when the undesirable event is clinically unique. However, when the adverse event is a common clinical occurrence such as jaundice, ulcer, or depression, it may be difficult to suspect that it is an ADR, and the event may be attributed to causes other than the drug. This is why so many adverse effects (e.g., ASA-induced bleeding) remained unrecognized for a long time. The most obvious limitation of this procedure is that it is retrospective; therefore, it is difficult to confirm the validity of the history of drug exposure. However, in spite of this problem it is a very useful method for generating hypotheses about possible drug-induced illness.

Frequency of ADRs

The reported incidence of ADRs varies widely from 1% or less to approximately 30%. This disparity is a reflection of the different methodologies used to detect and report the ADRs, the different populations surveyed, the different prescribing habits in various countries, and the inclusion or exclusion of mild reactions. However, most prospective studies show that the incidence of ADRs in hospitalized patients (excluding the mild ones) is between 10% and 20%. Admission to hospital due to an ADR is relatively common; several studies have shown that between 3% and 7% of patients are admitted to a hospital because of an ADR (e.g., digitalis intoxication). About 10–20% of ADRs occurring in hospitalized patients are severe. Drug-induced deaths occur in 0.5–0.9% of medical inpatients.

The drugs most commonly causing ADRs vary from one study to another. This reflects the differences in the populations surveyed and in the methods employed for collecting the data. Most studies have been conducted in hospitalized medical patients. In such patients, most reactions are caused by cardiac glycosides, diuretics, antimicrobials, anticoagulants, and nonsteroidal anti-inflammatory agents.

Factors Associated with ADRs

There are few well-conducted studies of factors that predispose to ADRs. However, epidemiologic studies in hospitalized patients have identified some of these factors.

Age

Most studies show that older subjects (over 60 years of age) are more susceptible to ADRs. For example, it has been consistently shown that, compared to younger subjects, the older ones are more likely to bleed during heparin treatment, are more sensitive to potent analgesics, are at a higher risk of developing digitalis toxicity, and are more likely to develop potassium depletion during diuretic therapy. Impaired drug elimination and/or increased receptor sensitivity to drugs have been proposed as likely mechanisms responsible for this increased susceptibility to ADRs. However, older patients usually have concomitant diseases and receive more drugs than younger patients; both of these factors are associated with a higher incidence of ADRs. The newborn, particularly when premature, is also more sensitive to some ADRs, probably as a consequence of incomplete development of enzymes involved in the biotransformation of drugs. The increased toxicity of chloramphenicol in the newborn may be explained by this mechanism (see also Chapters 4 and 68).

Sex

Several studies have shown that women are more likely than men to develop ADRs, especially drug-induced gastrointestinal symptoms. Women also appear to be more susceptible to the toxic effects of digoxin. In the over-60 age group, women are more likely than men to show bleeding induced by heparin.

Other Factors

It has been consistently found that patients on multiple-drug therapy have an increased probability of developing ADRs. This may be due merely to the additive risk of ADR when receiving several drugs or to drug–drug interactions.

A patient history of "allergic disorders" has been shown to be a predisposing factor to ADRs including those that are not allergic in nature. The predisposition to hypersensitivity reactions may be inherited, and close relatives may be at an increased risk (e.g., for idiosyncratic reactions to sulfonamides). It has also been shown that patients who have previously presented an ADR are more likely to develop a new adverse reaction. The disease state of the patient can also influence the susceptibility to ADRs. For example, impaired renal function predisposes patients to adverse reactions to those drugs that are mainly excreted by the kidneys. Hepatic dysfunction has a similar effect in relation to drugs that are inactivated in the liver. However, few drug monitoring studies have conclusively documented these relationships.

Important Adverse Reactions Detected Since the Thalidomide Reports

A recent study summarizing the most important ADRs identified since the occurrence of the thalidomide-induced congenital abnormalities, together with the drug monitoring method that contributed to their discovery, is shown in Table 65–2. It is of interest to note that a simple and relatively inexpensive procedure, the spontaneous reporting system (case reports), has allowed the identification of half of these reactions.

ASSESSMENT OF CAUSALITY IN INDIVIDUAL CASES OF ADRs

A major problem that a physician faces when evaluating an adverse event in a particular patient is to establish whether there is a causal association between the untoward clinical event and the suspected drug.

This can be particularly difficult because the manifestations of ADRs are not unique. The suspected drug is usually administered together with other drugs, and frequently the adverse clinical event cannot be distinguished from the symptoms of the underlying disease. Conventionally, the probability that an adverse event is associated with the administration of a particular drug has been classified as definite, probable, possible, or doubtful, as follows.

Definite: A reaction that (1) follows a reasonable temporal sequence after administration of the drug or in which the drug level has been established in body fluids or tissues; (2) follows a known pattern of response to the suspected drug; (3) is confirmed by improvement on removal of the drug and by reappearance on rechallenge; and (4) cannot be explained by the known characteristics of the patient's disease.

Probable: A reaction that (1) follows a reasonable temporal sequence after drug administration; (2) follows a known response pattern; (3) is confirmed on suspension of the drug ("dechallenge") but not on rechallenge; and (4) cannot be explained by the known characteristics of the patient's disease.

Possible: A reaction that (1) follows a reasonable temporal sequence; (2) may or may not follow a known response pattern; but (3) could be explained by the known characteristics of the patient's clinical state.

Doubtful: The event is more likely related to other factors than the suspected drug.

However, physicians often disagree on their assessment of the probability of ADRs. In an attempt to standardize the assessment of causality of ADRs, several algorithms of varying complexity have been developed. A simple method, the Adverse Drug Reaction Probability Scale (APS), is valid and reliable in a variety of clinical situations. The APS is a short questionnaire

---

TABLE 65–2   Ten Important Adverse Drug Reactions Detected Since the Occurrence of Thalidomide-Induced Reactions

Adverse Drug Reaction	Drug	Method of Discovery
Oculomucocutaneous syndrome	Practolol	Spontaneous communication (*i.e.*, Case reports)
Thromboembolism	Oral contraceptives	Case control
Nephropathy	Analgesics (especially phenacetin)	Case reports
Lactic acidosis	Phenformin	Cohort study
Deaths from asthma	Sympathomimetic aerosols	Case control
Subacute myelo-optic neuropathy	Clioquinol	Case reports
Vaginal cancer (in daughters)	Stilbestrol (maternal)	Case control
Aplastic anemia	Chloramphenicol	Case reports
Jaundice	Halothane	Case reports
Retroperitoneal fibrosis	Methysergide	Cohort study

Data from Venning GR, 1983.

(Table 65–3) that systematically analyses the various components that must be assessed to establish a causal association between drug(s) and adverse events (*i.e.*, pattern of response, temporal sequence, dechallenge, rechallenge, alternative causes, placebo response, drug levels in body fluids or tissues, dose-response relationship, previous patient experience with the drug, and confirmation by objective evidence). Each question can be answered positive (yes), negative (no), or unknown/ inapplicable (do not know) and is scored accordingly. The probability of the ADR is given by the total score, which can range from −4 (a drug-unrelated event) to +13 (a definitely drug-related event). The use of such procedures for assessing cases of ADRs observed in daily practice, as well as those reported in medical journals, should be encouraged.

Recently, a Bayesian Adverse Reaction Diagnostic Instrument (BARDI) has been developed. This method considers the assessment of the causality of ADRs as a special case of conditional probability. The application of this methodology to clinical practice has been simplified by the development of a microcomputer-based program.

DETERMINANTS OF THE DISCOVERY OF ADVERSE EVENTS INDUCED BY NEW DRUGS IN HUMANS

The toxicity of new drugs is assessed in Canada in animal and human studies as prescribed by Canadian law and described in Chapter 73. Nevertheless, the toxicologic studies in animals do not always predict the toxicity in humans. In addition, the discovery of ADRs in clinical trials assessing the efficacy and safety of new drugs depends on a variety of factors of which the most important are: (1) the relative frequency of drug-related and drug-unrelated events; (2) the mechanism of the drug toxicity (*i.e.*, dose-related or not dose-related reactions); (3) the number of subjects exposed to the drug; and (4) the methodology used for detecting ADRs. Since the contribution and limitations generated by these various factors are often ignored, it is appropriate to analyse briefly how they may influence the discovery of drug-induced illness.

TABLE 65–3 Adverse Drug Reactions Probability Scale

	Yes	No	Do Not Know	Score
Are there previous *conclusive* reports on this reaction?	+1	0	0	
Did the adverse event appear after the suspected drug was administered?	+2	−1	0	
Did the adverse reaction improve when the drug was discontinued, or a *specific* antagonist was administered?	+1	0	0	
Did the adverse reaction reappear when the drug was readministered?	+2	−1	0	
Are there alternative causes (other than the drug) that could on their own have caused the reaction?	−1	+2	0	
Did the reaction appear when a placebo was given?	−1	+1	0	
Was the drug detected in the blood (or other fluids) in concentrations known to be toxic?	+1	0	0	
Was the reaction more severe when the dose was increased, or less severe when the dose was decreased?	+1	0	0	
Did the patient have a similar reaction to the same or similar drugs in *any* previous exposure?	+1	0	0	
Was the adverse event confirmed by any objective evidence?	+1	0	0	
			Total Score:	

Note: To assess the adverse drug reaction, the questions are answered by inserting the pertinent score for each. The total score (which can range from −4 to +13) indicates the increasing probability of an observed event being drug-related. After Naranjo CA, *et al.* 1981.

Relative Frequency of Drug-Related and Drug-Unrelated Events

The manifestations of ADRs are usually nonspecific and the contribution of the drug must be distinguished from other possible etiologies. Accordingly, the discovery of an ADR depends on the relative magnitudes of two risks—the added risk of illness experienced by the users of a drug and the baseline risk in the absence of the drug. In the event that the drug-induced illness is frequent and severe, it is usually recognized very early during clinical use of the drug, and the identification is mostly based on well documented case reports in medical journals and/or from national drug monitoring centres. In contrast, when the drug-induced illness is less common, prospective investigation of cohorts of patients receiving the drug and/or retrospective case-control studies are indicated.

Mechanism of Drug-Induced Toxicity

The probability of discovery of an ADR may be determined by its mechanism. As described before, ADRs can be dose-related and dose-unrelated. Since dose-related ADRs are the most common, they are easier to detect in the early phases of human studies. In addition, animal studies are usually good predictors of the toxicity that must be ascertained in humans. In contrast, dose-unrelated ADRs (drug allergy and pharmacogenetically-based reactions) are peculiar to a group of subjects with very discrete genetic or immunologic characteristics. Therefore, these reactions are detected only when the new drug is administered to individuals with such a characteristic. These reactions are rarely detected in early clinical trials and generally are not predictable from toxicologic studies in animals.

Sample Size Required for Detecting Drug-Induced Disease

Clinical trials are usually short-term studies conducted in a few hundred patients before the drug is marketed. Therefore, only the most common acute dose-related ADRs are detected in the premarketing phase. A dramatic example of the limitation imposed by this factor is the case of the antipsychotic drug clozapine. Clozapine was introduced in Finland in 1975 when only about 200 subjects had been previously treated. Within the first 6 months of drug use, 17 cases of serious hematologic reactions (ten cases of agranulocytosis and seven of neutropenia) were reported to the Finnish national drug monitoring centre from among about 3,200 users, indicating that the risk of developing agranulocytosis or severe granulocytopenia during clozapine treatment was at least 0.6–0.7%. (For unexplained reasons, this frequency was 21 times higher

than in other countries.) Because of these reactions, the drug was withdrawn from the market. Recently, other drugs have been discontinued because of inadequate safety (e.g., benoxaprofen). These examples illustrate the importance of the close postmarketing monitoring of any new drug, irrespective of the safety shown in clinical trials. It also indicates the important role of physicians in evaluating the toxicity of newly introduced drugs by voluntarily reporting ADRs to national drug monitoring centres. No currently available method for detecting ADRs could have predicted such reactions; only the administration of the drug to a sufficient number of subjects resulted in the discovery.

Methods for Assessing ADRs

Methods for collecting information on ADRs in clinical trials are varied and consist of unstructured and structured interviews, physiologic and physical examinations, and laboratory tests. The procedures most commonly used are the unstructured interview, designed to eliminate suggestion of reactions to the patient, and a standardized list of symptoms (checklist). The frequency of symptoms elicited by these scales during treatment with the test drug is compared with the symptoms observed during treatment with a placebo. Those symptoms most commonly observed with the test drug are suspected of being ADRs. However, since the clinical manifestations of ADRs are usually nonspecific, the detected associations may be difficult to interpret. Therefore, despite the above-mentioned scales, a more definite assessment of individual cases of suspected ADRs is possible only by using the procedures for assessing causality mentioned above.

The discovery of ADRs also depends on the frequency of assessments and the validity, reliability, and sensitivity of the tests employed. Theoretically, if frequent assessments with a sensitive method are performed, all ADRs should be detected. In practice no such procedure exists. However, the systematic recording of all adverse events occurring during a drug trial greatly improves the chances of detecting ADRs.

CONCLUSIONS

The discovery and evaluation of ADRs depends on information collected in the preclinical and clinical studies. The most common dose-related acute ADRs are usually detected before a drug is marketed. However, uncommon ADRs or manifestations of chronic toxicity may become apparent only after the drug has been used in a large number of subjects for long periods of time. A more definite assessment of individual cases of ADRs should include the use of the APS or similar methods. Because knowledge about the clinical toxicity of a new drug will always be incomplete at the time of marketing, further investigation of the frequency and determinants of ADRs must be pursued in the post-marketing phase.

SUGGESTED READING

Bakke OM, Wardell WM, Lasagna L. Drug discontinuations in the United Kingdom and the United States, 1974 to 1983: issues of safety. Clin Pharmacol Ther 1984; 35:559–567.

Davies DM. Textbook of adverse drug reactions. 3rd ed. London: Oxford University Press, 1985.

Dukes MNG, ed. Meyler's side effects of drugs. Vol. 10. Amsterdam: Excerpta Medica, 1984.

Fletcher AP. Drug safety tests and subsequent clinical experience. J R Soc Med 1978; 71:693–696.

Jick H. The discovery of drug-induced illness. N Engl J Med 1977; 296:481–485.

Karch FE, Lasagna L. Adverse drug reactions: a critical review. JAMA 1975; 234:1236–1241.

Lane DA, Kramer MS, Hutchison TA, et al. The causality assessment of adverse drug reactions using the Bayesian approach. Pharm Med 1987; 2:265–283.

Naranjo CA. A clinical pharmacologic perspective on the detection and assessment of adverse drug reactions. Drug Info J 1986; 20:387–393.

Naranjo CA, Busto U, Sellers EM, et al. A method for estimating the probability of adverse drug reactions. Clin Pharmacol Ther 1981; 30:239–245.

Naranjo CA, Busto U, Sellers EM. Difficulties in assessing adverse drug reactions in clinical trials. Prog Neuropsychopharmacol Biol Psychiatry 1982; 6:651–657.

Naranjo CA, Busto U, Janecek E, et al. An intensive drug monitoring study suggesting possible clinical irrelevance of impaired drug disposition in liver disease. Br J Clin Pharmacol 1983; 15:451–458.

Shear NH, Spielberg SP, Grant DM, et al. Differences in metabolism of sulfonamides predisposing to idiosyncratic toxicity. Ann Intern Med 1986; 105:179–184.

Venning GR. Identification of adverse reactions to new drugs. I. What have been the important adverse reactions since thalidomide? Br Med J 1983; 286:199–202.

Chapter 66

BEHAVIORAL PHARMACOLOGY

L.A. Grupp and H. Kalant

Behavioral pharmacology refers to the study of how drugs affect behavior. This includes description of the changes in behavior produced by a drug, and exploration of the mechanisms by which the drug produces these changes. Such research draws on the knowledge and techniques of a number of different disciplines including anatomy, biochemistry, pharmacology, physiology, and psychology. Since human behavior differs in important ways from that of laboratory animals, new, behaviorally active drugs must ultimately be tested in humans. However, initial screening is done in various species, including rats, mice, cats, dogs, monkeys, and others. This chapter deals with the procedures used in animal studies.

The study of drug effects on learned behaviors and on certain instinctive or naturally occurring ones, such as locomotion, food and water intake, aggressive and sexual behavior, requires accurate and reliable methods for quantifying the rates and patterns of these behaviors, and sufficient control over the environment to diminish disturbing influences. All these measures are necessary because they provide a stable control or baseline level of performance against which drug effects can be observed and quantified. The following two sections identify some of the behaviors referred to later and describe the techniques used to measure them.

TYPES OF BEHAVIOR STUDIED

Instinctive Behavior

Locomotion

Locomotion refers to simple motor activity that forms part of exploratory behavior or other acts of general movement. It is measured by such means as counting the number of turns an animal makes in a running wheel, or the number of sectors traversed during a measured time period in a large open field that has been marked off in a grid pattern.

Sensory Function

Since the execution of behavior requires the use of one or more senses, drugs that affect sensory function can also affect behavior. For example, the sensation of pain has been extensively studied by means of the hot-plate or tail-flick tests. Typically, a rat or mouse is placed with its paws on a hot-plate (about 50°C = 120°F—**not** a stove element), or the tail is immersed in very warm water, and the latency to retract a paw or the tail, respectively, is measured. The test drug is given, and the procedure is repeated at various times after the dose. The drug effect is measured as the difference in latency between the predrug baseline and the postdrug tests.

Food and Water Intake

Food selection and total amount of food and water consumed, either per day or per meal, are measured. Again, the drug effect is measured as the change from predrug baseline.

Aggressive Behavior

This can be measured by placing two or more animals together in a cage and counting the number of spontaneous attacks, or the number of times an animal assumes a dominant or submissive posture. Alternatively, one can induce animals to fight by placing them on an electrified grid (the electrical current delivered by the grid is irritating rather than damaging). In this shock-induced aggression model, one can measure posturing and the number of attacks and bites.

Sexual Behavior

Receptive females are made available to their male counterparts and the frequency of sexually-related behaviors of both the female (the lordosis posture) and the male (mounting, intromission, ejaculation) is measured. Drug-treated animals can be compared with placebo-treated animals, with respect to the frequencies of these behaviors.

Learned Behavior

Many types of learning tasks have been used to test the effects of drugs. For example, the effect of cannabis has been tested in rats learning to find their way through a series of mazes of increasing complexity to earn a food reward at the exit from each maze. However, two special types of learning that have been very extensively used in drug studies are classical conditioning and operant conditioning.

Classical Conditioning

This kind of training or learning procedure is best illustrated by reference to a well-known experiment with dogs by the Russian physiologist I.P. Pavlov. A tuning fork was sounded, followed in 10 seconds by the presentation of some powdered food. Dogs salivate when food is presented to them. Initially the sound did not elicit any salivation; however, after a number of pairings of the sound and the food, the sound came to elicit salivation. The dog had learned that the sound of the tuning fork predicted the presentation of food and had learned to salivate at the sound in preparation for the food. In the language of learning theory, the sound was the **conditioned stimulus** whose presentation initially did not elicit an **unconditioned response** (salivation), but which through repeated association with the food (**unconditioned stimulus**) came itself to elicit the salivation as a **conditioned response**. The effect of drugs on the acquisition and maintenance of this conditioned response can be studied.

Operant Conditioning

This second type of learning involves a procedure whereby the probability of occurrence of some particular behavior can be either increased or decreased, depending upon the consequences of the behavior. For example, if a food pellet is presented to a hungry animal every time it presses a lever, it is highly likely that the animal will repeat its lever-pressing behavior until its hunger is satisfied. The lever press is termed an **operant** response because the animal operates on its environment to change it in some biologically significant way; the food pellet is termed a **positive reinforcer** because it reinforces or strengthens the behavior that resulted in its presentation (*i.e.*, the lever-press

response). The whole process is termed **positive reinforcement**. Similarly, if a lever-press avoids the presentation of an unpleasant stimulus (*e.g.*, an air blast), the lever-press is again termed an **operant**; the air blast is termed a **negative reinforcer** because it strengthens the response that avoids the negative or unpleasant event. The whole process is termed **negative reinforcement**. Finally, if the lever-press results in the delivery of a painful stimulus (*e.g.*, a foot-shock), the animal is reluctant to perform the response again. The process is called **punishment**, and the foot-shock is the **punisher**.

The animal may be required to learn to make the response according to a specific "schedule." For example, reinforcers can be presented or avoided either after a specified number of lever-press responses (fixed ratio, variable ratio), or after a specified period of time has elapsed (fixed interval, variable interval) since the last presentation of the reinforcer. For example, a fixed-interval (FI) 60-second schedule of food reinforcement indicates that a food pellet will be delivered as a result of the first response that occurs at least 60 seconds following the last food delivery. A fixed-ratio (FR) 10 schedule indicates that one food pellet will be delivered for every 10 presses of the response lever. These formulae, which specify the relationship between responding and the delivery of the reinforcer, are termed **schedules of reinforcement** and generate very stable and reliable patterns of responding. Drug effects are easily and effectively measured against such artificially generated but stable control levels of behavior.

In the following sections we will examine (1) the behavioral effects of drugs that alter neurotransmitter function, (2) some of the behavioral factors that determine drug action, (3) the effects of drugs on the processes of learning and memory, and finally (4) the stimulus properties and (5) reinforcing properties of drugs.

DRUGS, NEUROTRANSMITTERS, AND BEHAVIOR

When a drug enters the central nervous system, it alters the ongoing activity of the neurochemical systems in different ways and produces behavioral effects. The drug action may take various forms, such as a direct effect on ionic permeability; a change in the release, synthesis, or re-uptake of a neurotransmitter; or a blockade of receptor sites. Since different neurotransmitter systems coexist in many brain areas, drug-induced changes in the activity of one system may, by shifting the balance of activity, affect behavior as much by altering activity in the other systems as by acting directly on its own target system. Thus, in order to establish a causal relationship between behavior and a particular neurotransmitter system, a number of complementary experimental approaches must be taken. For example, if a change in behavior follows upon a reduction in the level of a neurotransmitter, then (1) blocking the receptor sites for that transmitter should have a similar effect on behavior and (2) replacing that neurotransmitter should cause behavior to return to normal. In the remainder of this section we will examine the relationships between some neurotransmitter systems and behavior, examine how drugs that modify neurotransmitter function also modify behavior, and see how similar behaviors can sometimes be related to the activity of a number of different neurotransmitters.

Serotonin (5-HT)

Serotonergic activity is decreased by a number of agents, including synthesis inhibitors (e.g., parachlorophenylalanine, or PCPA), receptor blockers (e.g., methysergide), agents that interfere with storage (e.g., reserpine), and neurotoxins that selectively destroy serotonin-containing cell bodies (e.g., 5,7- or 5,6-dihydroxytryptamine). **When serotonergic activity is decreased**, a number of behavioral changes occur. The following list provides some examples of these changes:

1. There is an increase in the sensitivity to a number of different painful stimuli, as shown by a decrease in the threshold stimulus required to make a rat or mouse escape a hot-plate or jump in response to an electric shock.
2. The increased sensitivity to painful shock leads to faster acquisition of an avoidance response by animals after depletion of brain serotonin by PCPA.
3. Decreasing 5-HT levels by the administration of reserpine or PCPA, or damaging the serotonin-containing cell bodies of the entire raphe nucleus, leads to a suppression of the electroencephalographic (EEG) signs of both slow-wave and paradoxical sleep and produces insomnia. This state may last as long as 2 weeks before compensatory mechanisms restore a more balanced sleep function.
4. When two rats are placed on an electrified grid, they tend to approach, attack, and bite each other (shock-induced aggression). When a mouse is introduced into a rat's cage, the rat may suddenly attack the mouse and kill it by breaking the neck (muricide). These are both considered to be experimental models of aggression. Serotonin depletion, produced by PCPA or by raphe lesions, often leads to an increase in these aggressive behaviors.
5. In male rats, serotonin depletion leads to an increase in sex-related behaviors such as mutual grooming, scratching, and sniffing of the genitalia. Castrated males will show a temporary increase in sexual behavior after injection of PCPA. After serotonin depletion, males will increase the frequency with which they engage in heterosexual activities if a female rat is present, or mount other males if no female is present.

In general, agents that **increase serotonergic activity** (such as the monoamine oxidase inhibitors or the precursor 5-hydroxytryptamine) antagonize the effects described above.

In addition, **5-HT agonists** have a very marked effect on eating and drinking. They reduce food intake, especially in the form of non-protein calories, and increase water intake. Serotonin re-uptake inhibitors, which increase 5-HT concentration at the receptor, have been used clinically to help obese patients lose weight by inhibiting appetite.

Acetylcholine

Modification of central cholinergic function by agonists (e.g., nicotine, arecoline, carbamylcholine; see Chapter 14), cholinesterase inhibitors (e.g., physostigmine), and antagonists (e.g., mecamylamine, atropine, scopolamine; see Chapter 15) produces a number of characteristic effects on behavior:

1. Both atropine and physostigmine produce a dissociation between behavior and the apparent state of consciousness indicated by the EEG pattern. Atropine produces an animal that is behaviorally awake but whose EEG is that of a sleeping animal. Physostigmine, on the other hand, produces an animal that appears to be sleeping but whose EEG is that of an awake animal.
2. Anticholinergic agents usually increase spontaneous locomotor activity, unless this is already elevated prior to drug administration. In that case, either no change or a decrease in activity results. Conversely, agents such as physostigmine, which increase cholinergic activity by inhibiting cholinesterase, lead to a decrease in general motor activity.
3. Stimulation of cholinergic synapses in the hypothalamus and limbic system has profound effects on feeding and drinking. Direct application of tiny crystals of a cholinergic agonist to these areas produces rapid and copious drinking in water-satiated animals, or increases drinking by thirsty animals. These effects can be blocked by the administration of atropine.
4. Physostigmine can disrupt the performance of a previously acquired shock avoidance response, and this disruption can be prevented by pretreatment with the receptor blocker atropine.

Catecholamines (Dopamine and Noradrenaline)

Catecholamine levels can be altered by drugs that inhibit synthesis (e.g., α-methyl-p-tyrosine, AMPT) or degradation (e.g., MAO inhibitors) of dopamine (DA) and noradrenaline (NA), block their re-uptake (e.g., cocaine), interfere with their storage (e.g., reserpine), or destroy catecholamine-containing cell bodies (e.g., 6-hydroxydopamine, 6-OHDA). Additionally, a large variety of selective DA and NA antagonists (e.g., pimozide and phenoxybenzamine, respectively) and agonists (e.g., apomorphine and clonidine, respectively) are also available. (*See* Chapters 13, 16–18, and 27.) The behavioral effects of alteration of catecholamine systems in the brain include the following:

1. Both DA and NA play a role in locomotor activity. A decrease in catecholamine levels, by the administration of reserpine or AMPT, leads to a profound decrease in spontaneous locomotor activity, which can be reversed by the administration of their common precursor, L-dopa. L-Dopa given alone produces an increase in locomotor activity. The relative contribution of DA and NA systems to this behavior is the subject of much investigation. Locomotor activity following catecholamine depletion can be restored by the DA agonist apomorphine, but not by the NA agonist clonidine; this suggests a primary role for DA. On the other hand, the combination of apomorphine and clonidine produces an even greater effect than apomorphine alone. It thus appears that both DA and NA play a role in spontaneous locomotor activity, with NA exerting a modulatory effect.

2. Reduction of catecholamine levels by the administration of 6-OHDA produces increased levels of aggression in animals tested with the shock-induced fighting paradigm. The increase can be antagonized by the DA agonist apomorphine. The functional relation between catecholamines and 5-HT in the control of aggressive behavior is not yet known.

3. The application of NA directly to certain areas of the hypothalamus elicits feeding in a totally satiated animal. Other α-adrenergic agonists also increase feeding, while β-adrenergic agonists decrease it, and each effect can be blocked by the corresponding receptor blocker. Current theory states that the alpha system inhibits satiety and thereby turns feeding on, while the beta system turns feeding off. DA also plays a primary role in feeding: the selective destruction of DA-containing cell bodies in the striatum can result in both aphagia and adipsia, to the point that the animals must actually be force-fed to insure their survival. The relationship among these two neurotransmitter systems and cholinergic and serotonergic systems in the control of food and water intake is as yet not fully understood.

4. A variety of drugs that decrease catecholaminergic activity, including inhibitors of synthesis and those that interfere with storage, attenuate the performance of a previously acquired shock-avoidance response. This attenuation effect can itself be reduced by the administration of the precursor L-dopa.

The foregoing lists of behavioral changes produced by modification of neurotransmitter activity merely scratch the surface. They are only intended to illustrate the huge range of behavioral alterations that have been studied, and to indicate the complexity of behavioral interactions among the neurotransmitter systems.

EFFECTS OF DRUGS ON BEHAVIOR CONTROLLED BY SCHEDULES OF REINFORCEMENT

One way to examine the effects of drugs on behavior is to administer a test drug to an animal that is performing a task, and observe the ensuing change in its performance. The procedures of operant conditioning afford stable behavioral baselines against which drug effects can be meaningfully assessed. Figure 66–1 illustrates this point. Hungry pigeons were trained to peck a key in order to receive brief access to a hopper of grain. Some birds were required to make 50 pecks to earn each reward (FR 50), while others obtained the grain for the first peck that occurred at least 15 minutes following the last grain delivery (FI 15'). When responding had stabilized, the pigeons were tested after the injection of the inactive drug vehicle (saline) and then after a number of doses of pentobarbital. This drug had similar effects on responding maintained by the two different schedules: lower doses tended to increase response rate while the higher doses decreased it. However, one major difference was also apparent, namely, that at the 1-mg and 2-mg doses the response

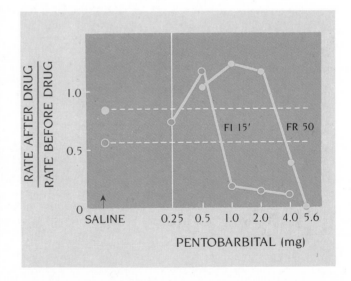

Figure 66–1 Change in response rate as a function of pentobarbital dose on two different schedules of reinforcement. (*See* text for experimental conditions.) Solid circles represent animals responding on an FR 50 schedule of reinforcement, open circles represent a different group of animals responding on an FI 15' schedule of reinforcement.

rate was increased under the FR schedule but decreased under the FI schedule. Thus, the same dose of pentobarbital produced opposite effects on responding on the two schedules of reinforcement.

The interpretation of such findings depends upon the type of hypothesis from which one starts. The "behavioral mechanisms" approach is based on the hypothesis that drugs act on behavior by influencing processes involved in either the learning of a new behavior (such as motivation or memory) or the ability to perform it once it has been learned (e.g., stimulus perception or response output capability). In contrast, the rate-dependency hypothesis states that the **direction** of effect of a drug on the rate of responding (i.e., either increase or decrease) depends on the predrug (i.e., saline-tested) rate of occurrence of the behavior. Specifically, if the rate of responding is low before drug, a postdrug increase in the rate is likely to ensue at the low and intermediate drug doses, while a decrease usually occurs at the highest doses. If the predrug response rate is high, a postdrug decrease in rate will be found even at low and intermediate doses. Rate-dependent effects on performance under schedules of

positive reinforcement have been seen with barbiturates, benzodiazepines, antipsychotics, and stimulants. The rate-dependency hypothesis predicts that, if predrug rates of responding are similar, drug effects will be similar regardless of the nature of the reinforcer controlling the behavior. Figure 66–2 illustrates this by showing that different doses of the stimulant d-amphetamine produce remarkably similar changes in response rate regardless of whether the behavior is controlled by positive reinforcement (food presentation) or negative reinforcement (shock termination), independently of the type of schedule. Similar results are seen for the antipsychotic drug chlorpromazine.

Although rate of responding is an important determinant of drug action, it is not the only operative factor and therefore should be considered to modulate rather than totally determine the effects of drug action. This is highlighted best by a number of studies of the role of antianxiety agents in punished responding. Specifically, if rate of responding were the sole determinant of the effect of a benzodiazepine such as diazepam, then at equivalent predrug response rates

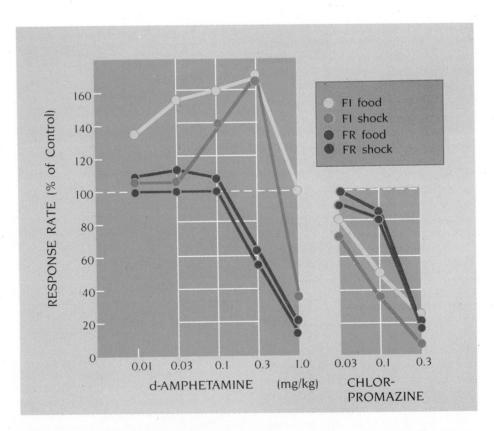

Figure 66–2 Effect of different doses of d-amphetamine or chlorpromazine on lever pressing by rats, maintained by schedules of food presentation or shock termination. The 0.3 mg/kg dose of amphetamine increased the rate of responding on FI performance (which has low baseline rates) but decreased the rate on FR performance (high baseline). Note that the change in response rate for each of the two schedules as a function of dose is similar, regardless of whether responding is maintained by positive (food) or negative (shock) reinforcement.

this agent should increase responding to the same extent, regardless of whether the responding is being punished or not. However, it has been shown unequivocally that low rates of punished responding are increased more than equivalently low rates of unpunished responding. Presumably other factors, such as the emotional and motivational state of the animal, are operating to produce this result.

Two other paradigms, in which drug effects are often tested, are assumed to be models of conflict, anxiety, and negative affect in humans. In the **escape-avoidance model**, a rat must learn to make a certain response in order to escape from a painful shock, or to avoid the shock when a warning signal is given. In the **approach-avoidance conflict model**, the animal learns to make a certain response to win a food reward, but when it has learned to do so, the experimenter then causes the same response to produce a punishing shock as well as the reward, and the animal begins to show behavioral disturbances reflecting the conflict between the drives to make the response and to avoid it. Drugs such as anxiolytics (Chapter 26), neuroleptics (Chapter 27), and antidepressants (Chapter 28) can reduce the avoidance, escape, and conflict behaviors seen in these models, which are therefore used as predictors of similar effects of new drugs on conflict and anxiety in humans.

Part of the difficulty in assessing these effects is that, although the test drug could be acting by reducing anxiety, it might also be acting by reducing the intensity of pain sensation and thus diminishing the effectiveness of the stimulus that generates the anxiety or conflict. One way to distinguish between these possibilities is to measure the effects on both the escape and the avoidance behaviors. For example, chlorpromazine alters avoidance responding at doses that do not alter escape responding, but secobarbital decreases both escape and avoidance behavior at all doses. Chlorpromazine is therefore likely operating through its effect on mood or motivation, secobarbital at least in part through its effect on the sensory stimulus produced by the shock.

DRUG EFFECTS ON LEARNING AND MEMORY

The ability of the brain to modify its output as the result of some previous experience is one of the most important yet least understood of its functions. This process of modification actually involves two separate but related processes: learning and memory. Learning refers to a semipermanent change in behavior as a result of the occurrence of some prior event. Memory refers to the registration of information in some manner that permits its later recall into consciousness. It involves three separate steps: registration of the information in a transitory short-term memory, followed by its consolidation into a more durable long-term trace, and the eventual retrieval from long-term storage when necessary. In what follows, we will consider those agents that influence the processes of learning and memory.

Pituitary Peptides

Hypophysectomized animals, which lack ACTH, show deficits in learning a shock-avoidance response, and in inhibiting the response once the shock is discontinued (extinction). The administration of ACTH to these animals normalizes both their learning and extinction of the avoidance response. It appears that this effect is not necessarily related to the endocrine action of ACTH, since the effect is obtained with fragments of ACTH (α-MSH and β-LPH, see Figs. 22–3 and 47–3), which do not act on the adrenal glands. Current thinking suggests that this peptide works by modulating neurotransmitter activity in the brain in such a way as to increase arousal and heighten attention to motivationally relevant stimuli.

Vasopressin acts to **delay** extinction of a learned shock-avoidance response. Its behaviorally relevant activity can also be dissociated from its vasopressor and antidiuretic effects (see Chapter 43).

Drug Effects

Strychnine, which at high doses produces convulsions, acts by blocking postsynaptic inhibition (see Chapter 21), thereby enhancing neuronal transmission. Both pretrial and posttrial injections of low doses of this drug facilitate the acquisition of a visual discrimination task as well as a maze-learning task. Other strychnine-like drugs, such as picrotoxin, bemegride, and pentylenetetrazol, have similar effects.

Amphetamine acts by promoting the release and blocking the re-uptake of both DA and NA from nerve endings. Injections of this drug have been reported to improve learning, perhaps through its effects on attentional mechanisms. Yet its ability to reduce fatigue and increase arousal raise the possibility that the improvement is related more to the ability to perform the task rather than to a real effect on the central processes related to learning.

The turnover of acetylcholine in the rat hippocampus has been shown to be increased while the animal is learning a new task to obtain a food reward. In keeping with this finding, anticholinergic drugs such as scopolamine or atropine impair learning, while drugs that increase cholinergic activity, such as physostigmine, have been reported to facilitate learning. These effects are of central origin, since the quaternary derivatives that do not pass the blood–brain barrier (e.g., atropine methylbromide) are ineffective. As with amphetamine, the facilitation is presumed to be related to improved attention.

Protein Synthesis Inhibitors

A vast amount of research has been devoted to exploring the possibility that all memories are encoded in terms of a change in the composition, quantity, or concentration of RNA in nerve cells. In turn, this change in RNA would direct the synthesis of a slightly different amount or type of protein molecule. The changes in both the RNA and the protein may be important for memory processes. Indeed, RNA synthesis and metabolism are both increased in trained animals compared to untrained ones. Furthermore, the administration of protein synthesis inhibitors (*e.g.*, puromycin, anisomycin, and cycloheximide) can produce amnesia and impaired retention of a previously learned task. Further research is needed to elaborate fully the role of RNA in memory.

STIMULUS PROPERTIES OF DRUGS

Meaning of "Stimulus Properties"

Discriminative stimuli are stimuli that enable an organism to discriminate or distinguish between two or more alternative situations in which a particular response will have different outcomes. For example, a rat may be trained in an operant chamber to press one or other of two levers to obtain a small food pellet as a reward. A signal light can then be added as a discriminative stimulus: *e.g.*, when the light is on, the rat will be rewarded only for pressing on the left-hand lever, while only presses on the right-hand lever will be rewarded when the light is off. The rat soon learns to discriminate correctly according to the presence or absence of the signal light.

Discriminative stimuli are said to set the occasion for a response because they signal that a reinforcer is available if the correct response is made. Responding tends to occur in the presence of a discriminative stimulus and to cease when the stimulus is removed or when a different stimulus appears. It is in this sense that responding is deemed to be under stimulus control. A mundane example is the traffic signal. A green light is the discriminative stimulus for the motorist to remove his foot from the brake and place it on the accelerator because this response allows him to proceed through the intersection in relative safety.

Drugs may also be thought of as stimuli. In this context, drugs do not **produce** stimuli, rather they **are** stimuli. This is best illustrated by comparing the action of a visual stimulus with that of a drug such as morphine. Each acts on specialized receptors that are selective only for that particular stimulus and not for any other. The impingement of the stimuli on the receptors causes biochemical reactions to take place that eventually initiate or modify a neuroelectrical response registered in the central nervous system. Both an ex-

teroceptive stimulus such as a light and an interoceptive stimulus such as a drug can act as (1) unconditioned stimuli that can elicit an unconditioned reflex response; (2) conditioned stimuli (*see* section Classical Conditioning); (3) reinforcing stimuli (*see* section Operant Conditioning); (4) discriminative stimuli—those that set the occasion for a response. In the present section we will examine drugs in their role as discriminative stimuli.

Methods of Study

Two procedures are typically used to study the discriminative stimulus properties of drugs.

State-Dependent Learning

In the State-Dependent Learning procedure, one group of animals is trained to perform a response in the non-drugged condition, while a second group is trained to make this response while under the influence of a certain drug. Once training is complete, the groups are subdivided, and half of the animals in each group are tested in the drugged condition, and the other half in the non-drugged condition. Figure 66–3 illustrates the design of such a procedure and the four groups obtained. If state-dependent learning has occurred, the animals will perform the task correctly only when tested under the same conditions (either drugged or non-drugged) as were present during training. If the drug simply impaired the animal's ability to perform the response, animals of both groups would do worse when tested under drug than when tested without drug.

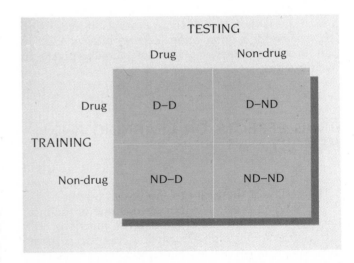

Figure 66–3 Experimental design used in studying State-Dependent Learning. D-D: group trained and tested with drug; D-ND: group trained with drug and tested without drug; ND-D: group trained without drug and tested with drug; ND-ND: group trained and tested without drug.

In a typical experiment, one group of animals is trained to escape a shock by making a right turn in a T maze while under the influence of pentobarbital, while a second group is trained to turn left when the saline vehicle is given. Upon testing, the first group is observed to make the correct response under pentobarbital but to respond randomly under saline, while the second group responds randomly under pentobarbital and correctly under saline. State-dependent learning has been demonstrated for a variety of drug classes whose representatives include ethanol, pentobarbital, scopolamine, morphine, amphetamine, cannabis (THC), and mescaline.

Drug-Discrimination Procedure

In the Drug-Discrimination Procedure animals are trained to make one response after a drug injection and a different response after an injection of either the drug vehicle or a different drug. In effect, the subjective state produced by the effects of the injection gains stimulus control over behavior.

In an experiment typical of this procedure, an animal pressing a lever while under the influence of a given drug obtains food, but if it presses the lever after getting the saline vehicle it receives electric shock. Animals given such differential training eventually learn to press under drug and to withhold pressing under saline. Drug-discrimination has been shown with the same drugs as state-dependent learning. The difference between drug-discrimination and state-dependent procedures lies in the objectives and the training techniques. In drug-discrimination studies, the purpose is to see whether the subjective effects produced by one drug are similar to, or different from, those produced by another drug. Therefore animals are trained to associate different responses with the different effects of two drugs (or a drug and its vehicle). In state-dependent learning, the purpose is primarily to see how a specific drug interacts with the learning process; therefore the animals are trained under the influence of only one drug, and then tested either with the same drug or its vehicle. However, drug-discrimination information can also be obtained by testing in addition with a drug other than that used in training; if it also elicits the state-dependent response, it must have produced a state similar to that caused by the training drug.

Generalization Gradients

One way to examine the control exerted by drug stimuli is to determine the drug-generalization gradient associated with that drug. Typically a discrimination based on a certain drug and dose is established, and testing is then carried out with a number of different doses of the same drug or with a number of different doses of a different drug. In the former case, the purpose is to find out how strong the drug test stimulus

has to be for the animal to react to it in the same way as to the training stimulus; in the latter case, the purpose is to see whether the test drug stimulus is perceived as qualitatively similar to, or different from, the training drug stimulus. What results is a drug-generalization gradient, which refers to the strength of responding to different values of a drug stimulus.

Figure 66–4 illustrates a typical generalization gradient for groups of rats trained to press one lever under the influence of a 1 mg/kg dose of d-amphetamine and to press a second lever under saline. Typically, drug-generalization gradients, like those for sensory modalities, show a progressive decrease in responding the more the test stimulus or dose decreases in strength from the training stimulus or training dose. However, the sensory generalization gradients show a peak when the intensity of the test stimulus equals that of the training stimulus, with responding dropping off at values greater or lower than the training stimulus, whereas drug gradients do not drop off at higher drug doses but tend to plateau. Figure 66–5 gives drug generalization gradients for animals trained to discriminate alcohol from saline and then given generalization testing with alcohol, a barbiturate, and a benzodiazepine. These gradients illustrate that even drugs of different classes share certain stimulus properties when care is taken to use equivalent doses.

Discriminability

Operationally defined, this refers to those properties of a drug that render it an effective discriminative stimulus. Discriminability can be measured in terms of (1) speed of acquisition of discrimination, and (2) maximum degree of control of behavior attained by a drug as the dose is increased (i.e., if drug A at any dose does not exert as great a degree of stimulus control as a second drug B even after similar training histories, then drug B is a more effective discriminative stimulus). Drugs may differ in their discriminability in terms of both potency and efficacy. Thus, if one drug is more potent in its stimulus effects than another and therefore can exert comparable stimulus control at a lower dose, it is said to possess greater discriminative potency. Similarly, if one drug is better able to produce a set of stimulus conditions than another drug regardless of dose, it possesses greater discriminative efficacy even though the two drugs may share certain other stimulus properties.

In this regard drugs are sometimes more effective than exteroceptive sensory stimuli in controlling behavior, and can retain this control even after a lengthy period in which the animal receives no drug. One reason for this might be that, since drug stimuli are interoceptive, it is harder to shut them out by shifting attention away from them, and the animal can attend to them without having to perform any orienting response such as is required with light, sound, touch, or other sensory stimuli.

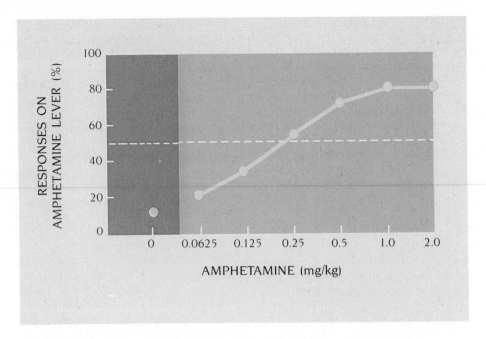

Figure 66–4   Example of drug-generalization gradient obtained in rats for responses on the amphetamine lever as a function of the size of test dose of amphetamine. The animals were trained with a dose of 1.0 mg/kg.

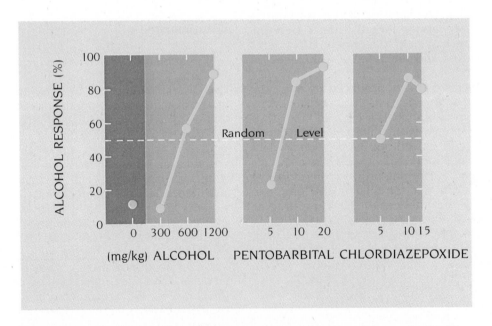

Figure 66–5   Examples of drug- and cross-drug-generalization gradients obtained in rats for responding on the lever appropriate for the alcohol-state, as a function of various test doses of alcohol, pentobarbital, and chlordiazepoxide. The animals were trained with an alcohol dose of 1200 mg/kg.

Mechanisms of Stimulus Control Exerted by Drug Stimuli

It appears that a drug must act centrally in order to be readily discriminable. Thus, amphetamine and atropine become effective discriminative stimuli, but their peripherally acting counterparts hydroxyamphetamine and atropine methylbromide do not.

Drug-induced changes in the functioning of a sensory system may produce alterations in perception that differ dramatically from those when no drug or different drugs are administered. These changes may form the basis of a discrimination.

In order to determine the pharmacologic systems involved, animals well-trained on a drug discrimination may be pretreated with a given antagonist and the resultant effect on the discrimination noted. In a typical experiment, morphine may be established as a discriminative stimulus, and the performance of the animal is noted after it has been pretreated with an opiate antagonist such as naloxone. An alternative method is to prevent the acquisition of a drug discrimination by interfering with the presumed neuropharmacologic substrate. For example, pretreatment with the catecholamine-depleting drug α-methyl-p-tyrosine (AMPT) can effectively impair the acquisition of stimulus control by amphetamine, which acts by releasing the catecholamines DA and NA from nerve endings.

DRUGS AS REINFORCERS

In the previous sections we have seen that psychoactive drugs have stimulus properties of their own, can alter ongoing behavior maintained by positive and negative reinforcement, and can influence basic biologic functions such as eating, drinking, sleeping, and learning. However, drugs can also modify behavior by acting as reinforcers or punishers in their own right. If a certain behavior (e.g., pressing a lever) results in self-administration of a psychoactive drug, the consequences of that drug exposure may positively reinforce the preceding behavior (i.e., increase the probability that the animal will go back and press the lever again), or may punish it (i.e., decrease the probability of pressing the lever again or stop it altogether). Psychomotor stimulants (e.g., cocaine, amphetamine), opiate narcotics (e.g., heroin, morphine), and some CNS depressants and anxiolytics (e.g., pentobarbital, diazepam) are positive reinforcers and can generate avid self-administration by animals and humans. The reinforcing properties of these drugs are believed to contribute

to their risk of generating drug dependence or abuse (see Chapter 67). On the other hand, neuroleptics (e.g., chlorpromazine, haloperidol), antidepressants (e.g., amitriptyline), narcotic antagonists (e.g., nalorphine), and hallucinogens (e.g., LSD, mescaline, and THC) are not self-administered by animals and can act as punishers (i.e., cause avoidance of the behavior that results in self-administration) or negative reinforcers (i.e., strengthen behavior that results in removal of the drug). Caffeine, nicotine, and ethanol under certain circumstances also act as punishers, especially in nonhuman subjects.

These latter examples illustrate an important limitation of the assessment of drug abuse potential in animals: all drugs that are readily self-administered by animals also show dependence or abuse potential in humans, but not all drugs that generate such problems in humans are readily self-administered by animals. Ideally, therefore, one would wish to study dependence liability directly in humans, but this is difficult for various reasons, including moral and ethical concerns about the administration of potentially dangerous or addicting drugs to humans, and the presence of confounding variables such as uncontrolled differences in nutritional status, cultural and psychological background, and previous drug experience. For these reasons, studies of drug self-administration in experimental animals are still important in the investigation of abuse or dependence liability of a drug. Various methods have been developed for this purpose (see Chapter 67).

SUGGESTED READING

Carlton PL. A primer of behavioral pharmacology. New York, San Francisco: WH Freeman, 1983.

Dews PB. Studies on behavior. I. Differential sensitivity to pentobarbital of pecking performance in pigeons depending on the schedule of reward. J Pharmacol Exp Ther 1955; 113:393–401.

Iversen SD, Iversen LL. Behavioral pharmacology. 2nd ed. New York: Oxford University Press, 1981.

Kelleher RT, Morse WH. Escape behavior and punished behavior. Fed Proc 1964; 23:808–817.

Kubena RK, Barry H. Generalization by rats of alcohol and atropine stimulus characteristics to other drugs. Psychopharmacologia 1969; 15:196–206.

Kuhn DM, Appel JB, Greenberg I. An analysis of some discriminative properties of d-amphetamine. Psychopharmacologia 1974; 39:57–66.

Seiden LS, Dykstra LA. Psychopharmacology. A biochemical and behavioral approach. New York: Van Nostrand Rheinhold, 1977.

Thompson T, Dews PB. Advances in behavioral pharmacology. Vols 1–3. New York: Academic Press, 1977.

Chapter 67

DRUG ABUSE AND DRUG DEPENDENCE

H. Kalant and L.A. Grupp

ADDICTION, DEPENDENCE, AND ABUSE

Since the beginning of this century the term "addiction" has been applied to the compulsive use of opiates, alcohol, and certain other potent CNS drugs. Despite numerous attempts, no fully satisfactory definition of drug addiction has ever been made that differentiated it clearly from what most people would consider "habit." By 1964, the best attempts of the World Health Organization Expert Committee had produced the following definition:

"Drug **addiction** is a state of periodic or chronic intoxication, detrimental to the individual and to society, produced by the repeated consumption of a drug (natural or synthetic). Its characteristics include:

1. an overpowering desire or need (compulsion) to continue taking the drug and to obtain it by any means;

2. a tendency to increase the dose;

3. a psychic (psychological) and sometimes a physical dependence on the effect of the drug."

In contrast, **habituation** was supposed to produce detrimental effects (if any) on the individual only and not on society as a whole; there was supposed to be little or no tendency to increase the dose; the desire to take the drug was not supposed to be so intense; and no physical dependence was supposed to occur.

It became obvious that these distinctions were quite arbitrary. The above definitions appeared to attribute all the importance to the drug, rather than to the interaction of drug, individual, and society. Value judgments were heavily involved. For example, if a drug was illegal and someone craved it to the point that he would commit a crime to obtain it, then this was interpreted as damage to society and to the individual, filling the requirements for addiction. If a different person craved a different drug equally strongly, but it was obtainable on prescription and he had a negligent physician who gave him as much as he wanted, then no crime was

committed and the case might be classed as habituation.

For this and other reasons, it became clear that both terms were unsatisfactory, and the W.H.O. committee recommended that they be replaced by the single term **drug dependence**, which would include all degrees of intensity of desire for the drug, all degrees of damage to both the individual and society, and all degrees of both physical and psychological need to continue using the drug.

Despite this recommendation, the term "addiction" continues to be widely used, and unfortunately there has been a change in its meaning since the W.H.O. Expert Committee gave the definition above. Because of excessive preoccupation with heroin and other morphine-like drugs, and with the dramatic (but relatively harmless) withdrawal reaction to which they can give rise, there has been a growing tendency to equate addiction with physical dependence, and even with physical dependence of the opiate type.

In an effort to avoid the confusion caused by these changing definitions, the new term "**hazardous use**" was introduced. This is an operational term based purely on empirical epidemiologic considerations, with no implications about dependence. It means use of a drug in such amounts and frequency as to carry a significantly greater risk of physical, mental, or social harm than would be expected in the normal population of the same age, sex, and socioeconomic status. This is a useful term for public health considerations, but there is still a need for mechanistic terms to describe the processes leading to such levels of consumption.

In contrast to the terms "dependence" and "hazardous use," both of which can be defined operationally, "**drug abuse**" is essentially a value judgmental term, with different uses and meanings for different people. Some consider it to be synonymous with "**nonmedical use**," any use of drugs for other than recognized therapeutic purposes being considered abuse. Yet alcohol is rarely employed therapeutically in modern medicine, but most use of alcohol is not considered abuse. Others equate the term with **heavy or excessive use**, but there is no generally accepted definition of "heavy" or "excessive," and in any case it is not clear how these terms differ from "hazardous use." Still others apply the term "drug abuse" to illicit use, including **any** use of an illicit drug (such as cannabis or LSD) or **nonapproved use** of a licit but restricted drug (such as amphetamine or cocaine). In reality, the term "drug abuse" means any drug use that the speaker, or society at large, does not approve of. Because of the subjectivity and vagueness of this concept, many experts in this field believe that the term is useless and should be abandoned. However, like "addiction," "drug abuse" continues to be widely employed even in scientific and clinical publications, and the reader must usually guess what the writer meant by it.

The term "abuse potential" is used to describe the degree of risk that a drug will be used for nonmedical purposes. Its operational measurement and significance are described later in this chapter under behavioral dependence.

The essential feature of addiction, as defined by the W.H.O. in 1964, is not tolerance or physical dependence, but compulsive drug-taking, i.e., a behavior rather than a postulated metabolic alteration. This is what is generally referred to as psychological dependence. A somewhat more descriptive term, which will be used in this chapter, is **behavioral dependence**, or "stimulus-controlled self-administration of drugs," as explained in the section on behavioral dependence. Many people consider this unimportant, because one can be "psychologically" dependent on chewing gum, work, television, and so forth. This is totally wrong. It can not be emphasized enough: **Behavioral dependence is the central problem in drug addiction, while tolerance and physical dependence are merely consequences of the drug-taking.**

If we accept this concept, the terminology becomes a matter of relatively little importance, and classification of drugs as "addictive" or "nonaddictive" is an oversimplification. It is the interaction among the drug, the user, and the environmental context that determines whether or not dependence arises. (The drugs to which this chapter refers are psychoactive drugs, i.e., those that primarily affect consciousness, perception, mood, and behavioral responses to the internal and external environment. One rarely, if ever, hears of "addiction" to digitalis, sulfonamides, or warfarin.) The questions of real concern to the patient and the physician, as well as to society at large, are the following:

1. Why does the user experience a "desire" or a "need" to use the drug? In other words, what initiates use, how does dependence arise, and what keeps it going?
2. How intense is the dependence, and to what extent does it control the user's life style? (Remember that the original meaning of the word "addicted" was "sentenced or given over to" something, in this case to the use of a drug.)

3. What are the consequences of this behavior, to the user, to the user's family and immediate associates, and to society at large?

In order to understand "abuse" and "dependence," it is necessary to examine normal or socially accepted patterns of use of psychoactive substances, and then see what differentiates these normal patterns from unacceptable or harmful ones.

SOCIALLY APPROVED USE OF PSYCHOACTIVE DRUGS

History of Drug Use

Virtually every society in human history has had at least one psychoactive drug that was used in a way that was approved by that society and incorporated into its customs and traditions. The type of drug used was originally a matter of chance, depending on what natural products with suitable pharmacologic properties were available in the region. The drugs used in preindustrial societies covered the whole spectrum of psychoactive drugs. A few examples are given in Table 67–1.

With the development of travel and trade between regions and nations, drugs native to one part of the world have become accepted and highly appreciated in other areas. Common examples are coffee, tea, and tobacco. The development of chemistry and industrial technology led to the isolation of pure active ingredients from natural products and the synthesis of highly potent derivatives, analogs, and substitutes. These are generally much less bulky and more stable than the natural products, and their use has spread around the world as a function of travel, commerce, education, communication, and availability of money for nonessentials.

Usually the first members of a society to adopt new drugs from another society are the wealthy and well-informed who come into contact with other cultures. Business people, diplomats, performing artists, and university students on foreign fellowships are frequently involved. Since they are prestigious figures in their own societies, their new patterns of drug use tend to be imitated by others.

Social Functions of Psychoactive Drug Use

The universality of drug use and the ease with which one society adopts the drugs of another suggest that drug use must have important social functions. The earliest known role was a **religious** or magical one. The red color of wine has made it a symbolic substitute for blood in the religious sacraments of many socie-

TABLE 67–1   Examples of Psychoactive Substances with Socially Accepted Uses in Various Parts of the World

Society	Preparation	Pharmacologic Agent or Category
Arabia, East Africa	Khat (q̂at)	Cathinone—central stimulant
Bolivian Indians	Coca	Cocaine—central stimulant
North American Indians	Tobacco	Nicotine—ganglionic cholinergic agonist
Indonesia	Betel	Arecoline—like nicotine
Southeast Asia	Opium	Morphine and other opioids
India, North Africa	Cannabis	Tetrahydrocannabinol—sedative
Amazon Indians	Kaapi, epena	Indole derivatives—hallucinogens
Southwest Amerinds	Mescal	Mescaline—hallucinogen
Universal	Beer, wine, etc.	Ethanol—sedative

ties, both ancient and modern, including our own. The feeling of warmth, due to alcohol-induced vasodilatation, has made it symbolic of the spirit of life itself, as indicated by such names as "spirits," eau de vie, akvavit, and even whisky (from the Gaelic for "water of life"). The hallucinogenic effects of peyote, epena, kaapi, and ololiuqui are used in the religious rites of various South and Central American populations to attain an other-worldly state in which contact with the gods is sought.

At a later stage, drugs were incorporated into **secular ceremonies**, such as passing around the kava bowl at the start of a Polynesian council meeting, smoking the pipe of peace among North American Indians, passing the "joint" at early marijuana parties before its use became widespread, and drinking toasts with alcohol at weddings or other special events.

From such uses, drugs gradually came to be used for **conviviality** in social gatherings, to increase pleasure and facilitate social interaction. In general, the drugs favored for this type of use have been either stimulants (khat, coffee, coca) or low doses of sedatives that produce disinhibition of behavior and emotional expression (alcohol, cannabis).

With increasing secularization of a society and progressive loosening of social controls over individual behavior, drug use for individual **private pleasure** became steadily more common. The use of wine with meals, smoking a cigarette at coffee break, and drinking caffeine-containing soft drinks as refreshments are among the many examples of such use.

The last stage of evolution of socially accepted drug use is **utilitarian**, at both individual and corporate levels. Individual utilitarian use is illustrated by the use of alcohol by salesmen who entertain clients during business negotiations, or by tense, nervous, depressed, or angry people who drink to feel better or to be able to release sentiments that they are unable to express when sober. Corporate utilitarian use is illustrated by commercial enterprises that create employment and profits from the manufacture, advertising, and sale of alcohol, tobacco, and other drugs and by the governments that gain large revenues from sale, customs duties, and taxes on these items.

Factors Governing the Extent of Use

The most important factor is the **degree of social acceptance or rejection** of a drug. For example, orthodox Moslems and Mormons do not use alcohol on religious grounds, even though societies around them use large amounts. At the same time, Moslem society accepted the use of cannabis when European and North American societies still rejected it as an alien practice that was in some way disreputable.

Social upheaval or rapid reorganization may suddenly weaken the conventional attitudes that control alcohol and drug use in stable times. If these substances are readily available, major epidemics of excessive use may occur at such times of crisis, and disappear when stability returns. Examples include the "gin epidemic" during the Industrial Revolution in England, the methamphetamine epidemic in Japan after its defeat in 1945, and the heroin epidemic among American troops in Viet Nam in the 1960s and 1970s.

Legal controls work best when they are in harmony with the prevailing social values and attitudes. For example, the move to enact Prohibition (of alcohol) in the U.S.A. was in keeping with popular sentiment before and during World War I, because the female suffrage movement and the temperance movement both saw alcohol-related problems as a major factor working against the well-being of women and children. The result was that Prohibition was at first highly effective in reducing both alcohol consumption and the death rate from alcoholic cirrhosis and other alcohol-related illnesses.

The law also works as an effective deterrent of drug use if it provides severe penalties and is seen to be strictly enforced and with a high degree of probability that offenders will be caught and punished. Alcohol rationing was enforced strictly by the German occupation forces in France during World War II, and this brought about a sharp fall in the death rate from cirrhosis, which rose rapidly again after the liberation of Paris in 1944.

In contrast, the law is not an effective deterrent when it is not in keeping with prevailing attitudes and also when it is seen to have a low probability of being applied successfully against the majority of offenders. The eventual failure of Prohibition was due largely to public disillusionment with the apparent lack of uniformity and effectiveness of enforcement. In the past two decades, American and Canadian laws prohibiting the use of cannabis appeared to be at odds with a large segment of public opinion; there is some evidence that public opinion has become less accepting of cannabis in the last few years, and the law may now be more in harmony with public attitudes.

Price is a very important factor; this is not the price in currency units of the day, but in "real" or "constant" units, *i.e.*, corrected for inflation and expressed in relation to average income and cost of living. In Ontario, Trinidad, and other jurisdictions in which studies have been done, there is almost a mirror-image relationship between the cost of alcohol expressed in these terms and the per capita consumption (Fig. 67-1) and the frequency of various alcohol-related problems, such as cirrhosis death rate or frequency of alcohol-related driving accidents. The relatively slow increase in alcohol consumption and in cirrhosis death rate in the U.S.A. after the repeal of Prohibition in 1933 probably reflects the influence of the severe economic depression at that time.

A closely related factor is **ease of availability**. When liquor stores in Ontario were changed to the self-service type, with all the goods available in open racks rather than held in a stockroom and brought to the counter by the clerk, the volume of sales rose quite substantially.

Occupational factors often relate to ease of access. For example, employees of breweries, distilleries, wineries, and drinking establishments are at higher risk of alcoholism, and physicians, nurses, and pharmacists are at increased risk of dependence on licit opioids, anxiolytics, and other psychoactive drugs.

Travel and mass communication facilitate the spread of drug use by giving large numbers of people the chance to learn about new drug practices. The methamphetamine ("speed") epidemic in Japan was brought to North America by American occupation troops stationed in Japan in 1945. The popularization of cocaine in North America and western Europe in the past two decades has probably been greatly assisted by the enormous publicity and initial glamorization that the drug received in the mass media.

Relation to Individual Use

It is very important to know how the extent of use of a drug by a whole population is related to the level of use by individual members of that population. Theoretically, for example, the average per capita consumption could increase even if the number of heavy users decreased; this would occur if large numbers of former nonusers all began to use small amounts while the smaller numbers of heavy users all used less. In that case, an increase in per capita consumption might not

be a cause for worry. Alternatively, increased per capita consumption might mean that all users, including the heavy users, were consuming more, and this would probably mean a major increase in drug-related problems.

This question is studied by examining the **distribution-of-consumption curve**. If the user population is surveyed and the percentage of users is determined for each interval in a scale of average daily consumption, the results can be plotted in a histogram or on a continuous curve. Conceivably one might find a bimodal curve, with the large majority of moderate users grouped around one mode near the low end of the consumption scale and a small number of heavy users clustered around a second mode near the high end. This would be the case if heavy users were qualitatively different from moderate users and responded to different controlling factors. In reality, however, the distribution-of-consumption curves for different drugs and populations all prove to be unimodal, with a large majority of users in the lower range of the scale, and smaller and smaller numbers at progressively higher levels of intake (Fig. 67-2).

Even more important, when there is a change in the mean per capita consumption of the whole population, it comes about through a corresponding displacement of the whole curve. Thus, an increased mean consumption reflects an upward shift of the modal level of use, a decrease in the numbers of users below the mode, and an increase in the numbers above the modal level. This is accompanied by an increased incidence and prevalence of drug-related problems of health, behavior, and economic function. The opposite happens when the mean per capita consumption falls.

This means that heavy users respond to the same controlling factors as light users do. Genetic or individual psychological factors may be responsible for their average daily consumption being high rather than low, but they respond in the same direction as light users do to changes in price, legal status, availability, and social attitudes. This has been demonstrated experimentally in a study employing alcoholic and nonalcoholic volunteers. Half of each group were allowed to buy alcoholic drinks at half price during a "happy hour"; the other half were not. The alcoholics drank much more than the nonalcoholics, but within each group the "happy hour" subgroup drank at least twice as much as the regular-price group (Table 67-2).

The conclusion is that **"drug abuse" is inseparable from drug use**, and that no method is yet available for selectively reducing "drug abuse" without reducing drug use by the whole population. In other words, the social functions that make psychoactive drug use so universally prevalent carry with them an inevitable price in the form of problems resulting from higher levels of use. Social policy on drugs must take this into account in deciding what level of such price is acceptable in return for what level of social pleasure or functional benefit. At the same time, the goal of research and education is to find ways of reducing the width

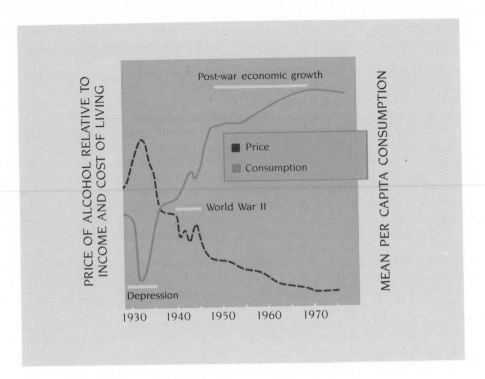

Figure 67–1 Inverse relation between the real price of alcohol and mean per capita consumption in Ontario over a 50-year period. The vertical scales are logarithmic. (From data provided by R.E. Popham and W. Schmidt, Addiction Research Foundation of Ontario.)

of the distribution-of-consumption curve, so that a given modal value will be accompanied by fewer individuals in the upper part of the range.

BEHAVIORAL DEPENDENCE

Since social, legal, economic, and other factors mentioned above appear to have comparable effects on the levels of alcohol and other drug use by light users and heavy users, it seems likely the same mechanisms control use at all levels, differing only quantitatively and not qualitatively in dependent and nondependent users. This section deals with a conceptual framework for these mechanisms and controlling factors.

Drug-Taking as Reinforced Behavior

People use psychoactive drugs for many different reasons. Some may use alcohol, barbiturates, or opiates for relief of boredom, tension, anxiety, or pain. Others may use them for a more positive type of pleasure associated with feelings of relaxation, joviality, "euphoria," or even physical visceral sensations that they find

intensely gratifying. Still others use amphetamines or other stimulants to achieve feelings of heightened alertness, endurance, and power (also referred to as "euphoria," a rather inadequate word). Others use drugs because their social group does, and there is pressure on them to conform. The only thing common to all these motives is the feature that the use of drugs is somehow **rewarding** to the user, whether by producing positive pleasure, by relieving displeasure, or by winning approval of the user's peers.

In the experimental analysis of drug-taking behavior, drug-taking is viewed as an operant response that is

TABLE 67–2 Effect of Purchase Price on Consumption of Alcohol by Volunteer Subjects in a Long-Term "Model Economy" Experiment

Subjects	Mean Number of Drinks Consumed	
	"Happy Hour" in Effect*	No "Happy Hour" in Effect
Moderate drinkers	20.9	10.1
Alcoholics	117.6	49.6

* In the "happy hour" condition, drinks were available at half price for 3 hours each day. From Babor TF, *et al.* 1978.

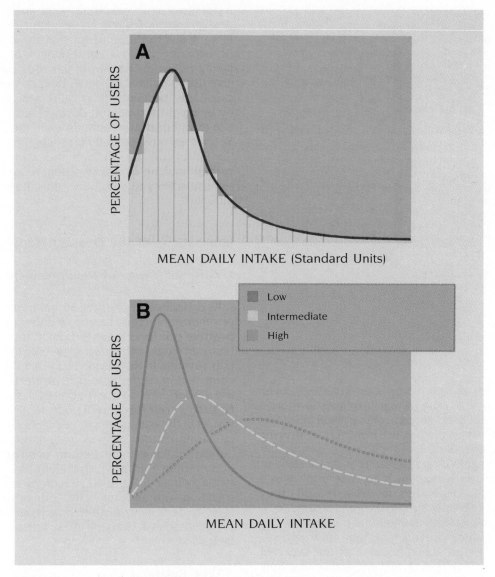

Figure 67–2 Schematic representation of distribution of consumption of alcohol or other psychoactive drugs in a population. *A*, Distribution shown as a histogram and as a smoothed unimodal skewed curve. *B*, Relation between shape of the curve and mean per capita consumption by three different populations with low, intermediate, and high per capita consumption.

reinforced by the effects it produces (*see* Chapter 66). The basic concept is shown schematically in Figure 67–3. If a stimulus of some kind disturbs the previously satisfied, quiescent state of an individual, it gives rise to a need to respond (*i.e.*, a "drive state") in such a way as to restore the satisfied state. Some stimuli (*e.g.*, hunger, thirst) and drive states (sex drive or self-preservation) have instinctual response patterns. Others, particularly those involved in interpersonal relations, have a wide range of possible responses that are markedly affected by personal experience and social rules and norms. Drug-taking is one such possible response, which may or may not be available to a given individual, depending on the society to which the person belongs, the time, the circle in which that

person moves, the economic situation, and so forth.

That form of response that gives rise to the most prompt and effective satisfaction of the drive is **reinforced**, *i.e.*, the next time that this stimulus gives rise to the same drive state, there is a greater probability that the same response will be repeated. For example, if a hungry animal learns to press a lever to obtain a food pellet that relieves its hunger, the lever-pressing response is said to be reinforced, and the food pellet is the reinforcer (*see* Chapter 66). Similarly, drugs may function as reinforcers, and the drug-taking response is reinforced by their effects. The reinforcing effects of the drug may then come to motivate further drug-taking behavior by themselves, in the absence of any other identifiable drive state. However, most drugs also

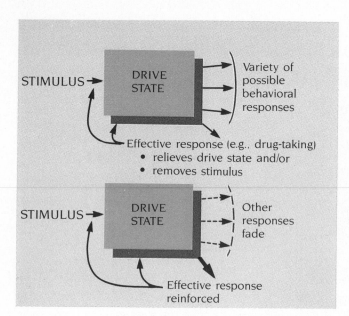

Figure 67-3 Schematic illustration of reinforcement, as applied to drug-taking.

have some unpleasant, punishing (aversive) effects, even in the same range of dosage that produces reinforcement. The strength of reinforcement in a given individual therefore depends on the balance between reinforcing and punishing effects.

The role of the individual's personality, temperament, background, and environment is to determine which drugs are likely to be chosen, for what reasons they are rewarding, and how strong the reinforcement is. For example, an aggressive ambitious person, striving to master everything around him, may find amphetamines or cocaine attractive because of the sense of increased energy, confidence, and endurance that they often produce. Others, who would like to be active and assertive, but actually find themselves tired and depressed much of the time, may like these drugs for the same reasons. A passive inadequate person associated with deviant groups in a large city is likely to use alcohol and opiates. A teenager motivated mainly by the desire to conform to his group will use whatever is the "in" thing, whether this is alcohol, or marijuana, or LSD, or solvent-sniffing. Obviously these various drives do not give rise specifically to drug-taking responses, but if drugs alleviate the drives, the drug-taking response will be reinforced. However, other responses may also be effective. The same drive stimulus (e.g., anxiety) may give rise to alcoholism in one person, overeating in another, and psychoneurotic symptoms in another, depending on which form of behavior provides the most acceptable, effective, and rapid satisfaction of the drive in any given person.

In behaviorist terms, drug dependence is simply the consequence of such frequently and strongly reinforced drug-taking behavior, so that this behavior becomes a dominant response that increasingly replaces other possible responses that are less effective (see Fig. 67-3). It is implicit in this concept that the drug effects must be experienced as a consequence of an active drug-taking behavior. Receiving the drug passively will not give rise to behavioral dependence. Animals or humans can easily be made physically dependent on a drug by being given repeated doses of sufficient size to give rise to withdrawal symptoms when the drug is stopped. Yet, if they have played no role in the drug administration, they will go through the withdrawal reactions without making efforts to obtain more drug. For drug-seeking activity to occur, they must be behaviorally conditioned.

Implications of the Operant Model

Different Types of Reinforcement

As described in Chapter 66, reinforcement (by drugs or other reinforcers) can be of different kinds. **Primary positive reinforcement** is thought to result from direct pharmacologic activation of a "reward" or reinforcement system in the brain. The exact location, neuronal composition, and physiologic properties of this system are under intensive experimental study at present. **Negative reinforcement** occurs if the drug-taking results in the elimination or prevention of an unpleasant or harmful state, such as frustration, boredom, pain, hunger, or anxiety. **Secondary positive** reinforcement occurs when a drug, which initially has no primary reinforcing effect of its own, becomes reinforcing by association with another active primary reinforcer. This topic is dealt with further in a later section in which the methods of studying drug self-administration are described.

Time Relations

For the effects of a behavioral response to be reinforcing, those effects must be experienced quite soon after the response is made. Therefore a drug that produces its reinforcing effects rapidly is more likely to give rise to repeated drug-taking than one that has a slow onset of action. Thus, heroin is much more addictive than, for example, methadone (see Chapter 22).

Route of Administration

It follows from the preceding point that the route of administration will have an important effect on the speed of reinforcement, and therefore on the probability of producing dependence. For example, heroin is more likely to cause dependence if taken intravenously than if taken by mouth. The same is true of cannabis when it is smoked, compared to when it is swallowed.

Genetic Predisposing or Protective Factors

Genetic factors may influence the sensitivity of an individual to either the reinforcing or the punishing effects of a drug. The sons of alcoholic fathers, even when adopted in very early infancy by nonalcoholic families, are three to four times more likely to become alcoholics themselves than the similarly adopted sons of nonalcoholic fathers. What is inherited is probably not a biologic need for alcohol, but either a greater sensitivity to its reinforcing effects or a greater resistance to its punishing effects.

Conversely, a high proportion of Oriental people have genetic variants of alcohol dehydrogenase and acetaldehyde dehydrogenase that result in faster oxidation of ethanol to acetaldehyde and slower oxidation of acetaldehyde to acetate (see Chapter 25). Therefore the ingestion of ethanol produces in them a high steady-state level of acetaldehyde that causes very unpleasant effects (flushing, tachycardia, nausea, and dizziness), which greatly decreases the likelihood of further drinking, or at least of heavy drinking.

In rats and other experimental animals, selective breeding over a number of generations can yield strains that will voluntarily consume high or low amounts of a drug or that will show greater or lesser sensitivity to drug-induced changes in behavior. Many groups of clinical investigators are currently looking for genetic markers that might help to identify, during childhood, those individuals at greatest risk of becoming dependent on alcohol or other drugs in adult life. It must be emphasized, however, that genetic factors simply affect the degree of risk; they are not the sole cause, and the majority of drug-dependent individuals do not have any identifiable genetic predisposition.

Motivational Factors

In experimental animals, the existence of an aversive motivational state (e.g., fear or approach-avoidance conflict; see Chapter 66) can increase the intake of ethanol and other sedative or anxiolytic drugs (see Chapter 26). Food restriction, leading to chronic weight reduction, can increase the intake of a wide range of drugs of different pharmacologic classes, even those that do not provide calories or directly reduce appetite. In humans, periods of heavy drinking or drug use are often triggered by situational changes that produce worry, fear, disappointment, anger, or frustration.

Stimulus Control

Environmental stimuli that are regularly associated with the availability and use of a drug can become discriminative stimuli, in the presence of which the drug-seeking behavior occurs. The drug-taking is then said to be under stimulus control, rather than being a "voluntary" act. Such stimuli, by their repeated association with the reinforcing effects of the drug, can also be-come conditioned reinforcers that produce brief drug-like reinforcing effects. For example, if a light is used regularly to indicate to a rat that it can obtain a drug injection by pressing a lever, it will eventually start to press the lever just to obtain the signal light. Humans who repeatedly experience the "rush" on self-injecting heroin or amphetamine into a vein often come to feel a brief "rush" on simply inserting a needle into the vein, even if the syringe is empty.

These conditioned responses are eventually extinguished if the conditioned stimuli do not continue to be paired with the drug from time to time. However, while they are present they may contribute to the phenomenon of drug-craving and the risk of relapse into drug use. Addicts who have been in hospital or prison for months or years, without any craving for drugs, have been known to feel a compulsion to take drugs within hours of returning to the environment in which they had regularly done so.

Role of Physical Dependence

Physically dependent subjects whose drug use is interrupted for any reason may, on feeling withdrawal symptoms (which constitute a new type of drive stimulus), learn that by making an appropriate drug-taking response they produce rapid satisfaction of the drive, with corresponding reinforcement of that response. In the case of humans, the response may consist of either self-administration of the drug or demanding and promptly receiving it.

The conditioning of behavior, i.e., to take more drug in response to certain stimuli arising during the withdrawal syndrome, may well explain the high relapse rate among drug-dependent people. Since these stimuli are not really specific (e.g., intestinal hypermotility, muscle tension and tremor, or hyperirritability), they can also occur as a result of physical illness or emotional disturbance. When they do, even though the person has not been using drugs for some time, these stimuli can evoke the conditioned drug-taking response just as if they were part of a withdrawal reaction.

Intensity and Significance of Behavioral Dependence

Since many different factors, as noted above, can enter into the creation of conditioned drug-taking behavior, and each can vary widely in degree, it is not surprising that the resulting behavioral dependence can also vary greatly in degree from trivial to an overwhelming compulsion that dominates all other behavior. It may be directed toward a drug or substance that is intrinsically rather harmless, or to one that is toxic and gives rise to serious physical consequences. The drug selected may be cheap and legally available, so that no social harm may result, or it may be expensive or illegal, so that the user or his family are deprived of other necessities, or he obtains more money by theft or other illegal means and he risks arrest and prison. In other words, behavioral dependence is neither harmful nor harmless in itself; the degree of harm depends on what consequences it brings in the individual case.

Methods of Studying Drug Self-Administration

The ultimate aim of studying drug self-administration is to understand the causes and controlling factors of drug use and drug dependence in humans, so that these factors can be manipulated for preventive or therapeutic purposes. However, a number of ethical and practical problems make it difficult to conduct experimental studies of drug self-administration in human subjects. Therefore much effort has been expended in developing suitable models in experimental animals. The underlying assumption is that fundamental behavioral and pharmacologic processes giving rise to drug self-administration are common to all higher species. Within certain limits, this assumption appears to be correct.

Oral self-administration can be produced quite simply by putting the drug in the food or the drinking water, so that the animal is forced to consume the drug while satisfying its physiologic need for food or water. However, such obligatory consumption tells us nothing about the reinforcing properties of the drug and is not relevant to the human situation, in which a choice is almost always available. Therefore the appropriate animal models always include a choice between drug solution and water, and consumption is measured in terms of both absolute amount of drug ingested and relative volumes of drug solution and water consumed.

Intravenous self-administration involves the implantation of an indwelling venous catheter, connected *via* a motor-driven infusion pump to a reservoir of drug solution. When the animal presses a lever that closes the pump circuit, the pump is activated and delivers a preset dose from the reservoir. Automatic programming equipment controls the number and spacing of lever-presses required to activate the pump. This set-up is illustrated in Figure 67–4. One advantage of the intravenous route is that the taste of the drug, which is often aversive to animals, is no longer a problem. A second advantage is that the drug effect is usually very rapid in onset, so that, if the drug has primary reinforcing properties, they can be demonstrated more easily. A third is that it is not necessary to have a second catheter and pump for water, since the animal can drink water normally.

Both oral and intravenous methods can be used to study the influence of the factors that control drug self-administration, including those described in the preceding sections. The intravenous studies are particularly useful for investigating primary reinforcing properties of drugs, *i.e.*, their ability to generate repeated self-administration without the need for other external inducements. This is often referred to as their "abuse potential." Central stimulants, such as cocaine and amphetamine, are the most potent in this regard. Mor-

phine and heroin are quite effective, but the newer agonist-antagonist opioids (*see* Chapter 22) are not. Some barbiturates, benzodiazepines, and methaqualone are moderately effective, but alcohol is only weakly and unreliably reinforcing in this type of experiment. Cannabinoids and hallucinogens such as LSD and mescaline are aversive; after experiencing their effects, the animal will not press the lever again.

It is common practice to "train" the animals to self-administer cocaine, then to substitute the drug under study. If the animal continues to self-administer this drug with a response rate greater than for saline, the drug is considered to be reinforcing. The "relative abuse potential" of different drugs, *i.e.*, their relative strengths of reinforcement, can be assessed by use of the **progressive ratio method**. After a stable response rate has been established on a fixed-ratio schedule (*see* Chapter 66), the number of responses required to obtain one drug injection is systematically increased in logarithmic steps. This makes the subject work progressively harder for the same amount of drug. The ratio value at which drug self-administration ceases or falls below some defined criterion is a measure of the relative reinforcing strength.

In general, drugs that animals will self-administer are also self-administered by humans. But humans will take some drugs that animals will not. This probably reflects the importance of non-drug factors in self-administration by humans.

TOLERANCE AND PHYSICAL DEPENDENCE

Many drugs give rise to the phenomenon of increase in tolerance when they are taken repeatedly or chronically. In other words, it becomes necessary to take progressively larger doses to achieve the same degree of drug effect. This may be illustrated graphically as a shift in the dose-response curve (Fig. 67–5). It may be produced in two quite different ways:

Metabolic Tolerance

The reactions by which the drug is detoxified, in the liver in most instances, may become more active. As a result, it is necessary to take a larger dose in order to maintain effective concentrations of the drug in blood and brain for the same length of time. This form of tolerance is not likely related to physical dependence, because it is really equivalent to taking smaller doses of drug.

Common examples include tolerance to long-acting barbiturates and, to some extent, alcohol. Metabolic cross-tolerance is also important for drugs that are biotransformed by hepatic microsomal enzymes. Induc-

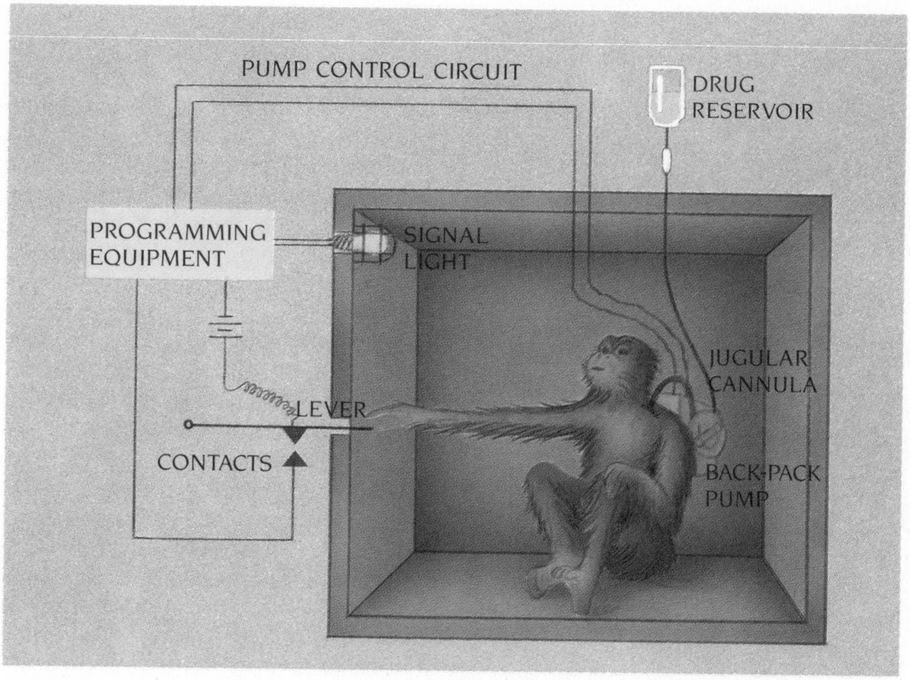

Figure 67-4 Schematic representation of apparatus for investigating reinforcing properties of drugs by the self-administration model in experimental animals (monkeys). Similar set-ups have been used with rats and other species.

tion of the cytochrome P-450 system by barbiturates or by phenytoin, for example, can cause increased rates of biotransformation of many other drugs (*see* Chapter 4).

Target Tissue Tolerance and Physical Dependence

Tolerance as Adaptation

The brain or other tissues on which the drug acts may undergo some adaptive change that tends to off-set the effect of the drug. For example, if ethanol or barbiturates or benzodiazepines cause depression of neuronal excitability, changes in ion fluxes, and impairment of neurotransmitter release, the adaptation might consist of changes in the cell membrane that facilitate both passive and active ion fluxes and neurotransmitter release and increase the excitability of the neuron. These changes would tend to compensate for the effect of the drug and produce an apparently normal functional state while the drug is present (tolerance).

Relation to Physical Dependence

When the drug is withdrawn, the same changes give rise to hyperexcitability because they are no longer balanced by the drug effect. The hyperexcitability therefore constitutes a **withdrawal syndrome**, which may range from sleeplessness, tremor, and irritability to hallucinations and tonic-clonic seizures. The severity depends upon the degree of adaptive change in the nervous system, which in turn depends on the degree and duration of exposure to the drug. Since the withdrawal reaction is abolished by a fresh dose of the drug, it constitutes evidence of **physical dependence** on the drug.

Drug-Specific Withdrawal Patterns

The particular characteristics of the withdrawal syndrome depend on the adaptive changes induced by the drug, which in turn depend in part on the pharmacologic actions of the drug. Thus, morphine suppresses gastrointestinal motility and constricts the pupil; the morphine withdrawal syndrome includes intestinal hypermotility and diarrhea, and pupillary dilatation. Amphetamine causes hyperactivity and euphoria, and the withdrawal reaction is characterized by profound fatigue and depression. It is a common error to think that a drug does not cause physical dependence if it does not cause a morphine-type withdrawal reaction: this is obviously quite illogical. There is no reason why a central stimulant such as cocaine should produce a withdrawal reaction similar to that of morphine. Because of the differences in pattern of physical and behavioral dependence commonly seen with different types of drugs, the W.H.O. Expert Committee recom-

SPECIAL TOPICS

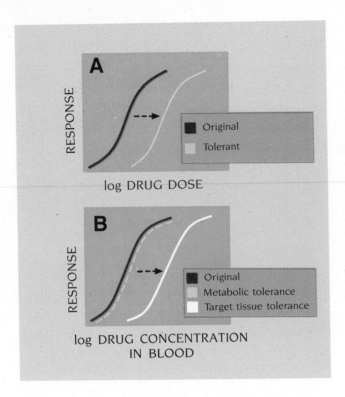

Figure 67–5 *A*, Shift in *dose*-response curve illustrates tolerance, but gives no indication of the mechanism. *B*, Metabolic tolerance does not alter the *concentration*-response curve, but target tissue tolerance shows a shift in the concentration-response curve similar to that in the dose-response curve.

mended that one should refer to drug dependence of the morphine type, of the barbiturate type, of the amphetamine type, of the cannabis type, and so forth.

Intensity

The intensity of withdrawal reaction is also related to the time course of action of a drug. For example, a drug that acts relatively slowly and for a relatively long time, because of slow distribution, high plasma protein binding, and slow biotransformation or excretion, frequently gives rise to less intense withdrawal symptoms than a drug that acts quickly, intensely, and briefly. Presumably the slow elimination of the drug permits some measure of physiologic readaptation to occur while the drug concentration is falling. This probably explains the less intense withdrawal reaction after methadone than after heroin or morphine.

Non-Drug Factors in Tolerance

Tolerance is not simply a physiologic adaptive response to the physical presence of the drug. Rather, it is a response to the functional disturbance produced by the drug. This depends not only on the kind and amount of drug, but on the sensitivity of the individual, on the type and level of ongoing activity at the time the drug is taken, on the environment in which it is taken, and on the individual's previous drug history.

Individuals, strains, and species with greater **initial sensitivity** to a drug will experience greater functional disturbance on their first use of the drug than more resistant subjects do, and therefore they will have a greater stimulus to the development of tolerance.

The same dose of a drug produces tolerance more rapidly if the subject is alert and **performing** some task under the influence of the drug than if the drug is taken at rest. This is particularly true if the drug effect causes the **loss of some reinforcer** for which the subject is working.

Tolerance, especially to relatively low doses of a drug, may be **environment-specific.** For example, an animal that receives a dose of morphine every day in the same environment, and has its body temperature taken each time to monitor the hypothermic effect of the drug, shows much greater tolerance in that environment than it does if the drug administration and temperature measurement are then carried out in a different environment. The environmental stimuli become conditioned stimuli; they bring on tolerance more rapidly as a conditioned response.

A subject who has a **history of having been tolerant** to a drug previously and who has then reverted to normal sensitivity after stopping the drug reacquires tolerance and physical dependence more rapidly on resuming drug use than on the first time around.

These observations show that tolerance is not a unitary process, but a complex phenomenon with many components. The same dosage of the same drug can therefore give rise to wide interindividual variations in the degree and rate of development of tolerance and physical dependence, and even within the same individual at different times and with respect to different effects of the drug. Many different biochemical mechanisms have been proposed to explain tolerance; so far, none can account for all the behavioral complexities of the process.

CROSS-TOLERANCE AND TRANSFER OF DEPENDENCE

If two drugs cause essentially similar pharmacologic effects *via* essentially the same mechanisms, one might anticipate that adaptive changes that arise from the use of one drug will also confer tolerance to the other, *i.e.*, there will be **cross-tolerance**. In fact, it has been noted clinically for many years that alcoholics are unusually resistant to general anaesthetics, barbiturates, and other hypnosedatives. Recent measurements have shown that the minimum alveolar concentration of halothane required for anaesthesia (*see* Chapter 23) rose from 0.76% in normal subjects to 1.31% in a group of alcoholics. The same transfer of tolerance is seen from one narcotic analgesic to another, and from alcohol and barbiturates to other hypnosedatives and anxiolytics. There is also transfer of tolerance from LSD to mescaline and other related hallucinogens, but this is a different type of tolerance (*see* Chapter 29).

Conversely, when one drug in a cross-tolerance group is withdrawn, another in the same group can be used to decrease or abolish the withdrawal symptoms, *i.e.*, there is a **transfer of physical dependence** (*i.e.*, cross-dependence). In fact, new synthetic narcotic analgesics are tested for dependence liability by testing their ability to prevent withdrawal symptoms in heroin addicts or in heroin-dependent monkeys. When one treats delirium tremens or other alcohol withdrawal symptoms by giving a barbiturate or a benzodiazepine, one is really using this transfer of dependence therapeutically. It is still necessary to gradually reduce the dosage of the substitute drug, or nothing will have been accomplished except to replace one drug problem by another.

TREATMENT OF DRUG DEPENDENCE

From the nature of dependence, it is obvious that the goal of treatment is to stop the undesired drug-taking response from continuing to be self-reinforcing. Psychological and social therapy, in the form of counselling and individual and group psychotherapy, are aimed at building up other behavioral responses for problem-solving (*i.e.*, for removing the drive stimuli) that are, at the same time, reinforced by social approval and that increase the patient's self-esteem. In other words, long-term treatment of drug dependence requires more than just getting the patient through a withdrawal period with the aid of a tranquilizer—it requires a process of behavioral retraining to enable the patient to make different and more helpful responses to the stimuli that have habitually elicited drug-taking behavior.

Pharmacologic agents can help in various ways:

1. Substituting a less reinforcing and legally available drug for a more reinforcing and illicit one, *e.g.*, methadone maintenance for heroin addicts. Note that the **methadone is not a treatment of the dependence.** It simply permits the patient to satisfy his drug need legally and under medical supervision and control. The treatment is the social and psychological rehabilitation that should be going on while the patient comes to the clinic regularly to receive the methadone.

2. Substituting a less reinforcing drug, which can then be gradually reduced in dosage to avoid a major withdrawal reaction, *e.g.*, methadone withdrawal therapy in heroin dependence, benzodiazepines for withdrawal from alcohol.

3. Use of specific blockers to prevent the drug from producing its usual reinforcing effect, *e.g.*, naltrexone to block heroin action, or α-methyl-*p*-tyrosine to block amphetamine ''high.'' The failure of the drug-taking behavior to provide the anticipated reward should lead to **extinction** of this conditioned behavior. Remember that narcotic blockers are not used in this way until withdrawal from the narcotic is complete; if used too soon, the blockers will precipitate a severe withdrawal reaction.

4. Aversive agents that interact with the drug to produce an unpleasant instead of a rewarding effect, *e.g.*, disulfiram in the treatment of alcoholics.

While reinforcement blockers and aversive agents are sound in theory, they have had rather limited success. This is because many patients are unwilling to take them and thus to cut themselves off from the possibility of deriving a pleasurable experience from their drug of dependence. Others may agree to take the blocker or aversive agent, but can simply stop taking it if they change their mind. Therefore, the effectiveness of these drugs depends very heavily on the patient's motivation.

Counter-conditioning is a behavioral counterpart of this approach aimed at eliminating stimulus control of drug self-administration. Stimuli that are associated with drug-taking are repeatedly paired with a very aversive stimulus such as electric shock or apomorphine-induced nausea. Unfortunately this technique is also not very successful. It reduces drug self-administration while the aversive conditioning is in progress, but the benefit seldom lasts after the course of conditioning is finished.

5. Chemotherapy of emotional disturbances that may be contributing to the problem drug use, *e.g.*, lithium or tricyclic antidepressants in many individual cases of alcoholism or barbiturate dependence, in which there may be an underlying depression playing an important causal role.

6. The most recent approach has been to test drugs that are thought by some researchers to act directly on the reinforcement mechanism(s) in the brain in such a way as to reduce the reinforcing effects of alcohol and other self-administered drugs. A number of serotonin re-uptake blockers (*e.g.*, citalopram and fluoxetine—*see also* Chapters 31 and 66) have been tested, but it is too early to assess their value.

SUGGESTED READING

Babor TF, Mendelson JH, Greenberg I, Kuehnle J. Experimental analysis of the "Happy Hour": effects of purchase price on alcohol consumption. Psychopharmacology 1978; 58:35–41.

Brady JV, Lukas SE, eds. Testing drugs for physical dependence potential and abuse liability. NIDA Research Monograph Series No 52. Rockville, MD: Nat Inst Drug Abuse, 1984.

Efron DH, Holmstedt B, Kline NS, eds. Ethnopharmacologic search for psychoactive drugs. Washington D.C.: US Dept HEW, 1967.

Fishman J, ed. The bases of addiction. Berlin-Dahlem Konferenzen: Life Sci Res Rep 8, 1978.

Kalant H, Kalant OJ. Drugs, society and personal choice. Toronto: Addiction Research Foundation, 1971.

Kalant H, LeBlanc AE, Gibbins RJ. Tolerance to, and dependence on, some non-opiate psychotropic drugs. Pharmacol Rev 1971; 23:135–191.

Kissin B, Begleiter H, eds. Social aspects of alcoholism. The biology of alcoholism, Vol 4. New York: Plenum Press, 1976. [See especially articles by Schmidt W, deLint J, 275–305 and Popham RE, Schmidt W, deLint J, 579–625.]

Lindros KO, Ylikahri R, Kiianmaa K, eds. Advances in biomedical alcohol research. Alcohol Alcohol, 1987; Suppl 1.

Popham RE, Schmidt W, deLint JE. The prevention of alcoholism: epidemiological study of the effects of government control measures. Br J Addict 1975; 70:125–144.

Chapter 68

PERINATAL PHARMACOLOGY

P. Rajchgot and S.M. MacLeod

Whenever a drug is administered, the pharmacologic outcome is the result of a complex interplay between a number of factors determining drug concentration in biologic fluids (and ultimately in target tissues or at specific receptor sites) and the constitution of the individual receiving the drug (including both genetic and environmental factors). It is generally understood that the relationship between drug and recipient will be defined by such factors as absorption, distribution, binding to tissue and serum proteins or receptors, biotransformation in the liver or elsewhere, and renal or nonrenal excretion (Fig. 68–1). During pregnancy such a simplified scheme is complicated in that all variables exist in duplicate, affecting both maternal and fetal drug disposition. In the newborn our knowledge of pharmacokinetics is incomplete, and this complicates the formulation of general principles that can be extended to all drug therapy in the neonatal period.

CHARACTERISTICS AND PHARMACOLOGIC UNIQUENESS OF THE FETO-PLACENTAL UNIT

Teratology

A major concern of obstetrician and pediatrician alike is the risk to the fetus arising from maternal drug ingestion. A drug or foreign compound that produces permanent structural or functional changes in the offspring is a teratogen (see Chapter 64). The most infamous teratogen was thalidomide, which, when finally identified as the cause of major limb deformities (phocomelia) in the newborn, led to more stringent drug controls. However, despite requirements for drug manufacturers to carry out teratogenicity testing in experimental animals, one cannot be certain that human teratogenicity will be detected prior to marketing of new drugs. One of the major problems lies in species susceptibility. For example, unlike the human, the rat fetus exposed to thalidomide is virtually not susceptible to its teratogenic effect. Furthermore, the background risk for development of spontaneous malformations in the general population is 2–3%. Thus, in order to be certain that a two-fold increase in risk for a relatively common malformation such as anencephaly was due to a given agent, 20,000 exposures to the agent would need to be studied. It is this need for such large numbers that makes drug dysmorphogenesis studies difficult to design and evaluate.

During human gestation three critical periods of development take place. The first occurs during embryonic development prior to implantation of the conceptus in the maternal endometrium. Because of the totipotent nature of embryonic cells during this period, cell damage leads either to death of the conceptus or to replacement of the damaged cells by healthy ones. Teratogenesis is less likely to occur during this time. After implantation there is rapid cell differentiation into various organ structures, and it is during this phase of organogenesis in the embryo that risk of teratogenesis is greatest. After the embryonic period (about 8 weeks) developmental changes continue in some organ systems, and this period of special development in certain systems constitutes the third critical period. At any time prior to birth, both the fetal central nervous system and palate, for example, may still be susceptible to damage.

It appears that, if the dose is high enough, most agents are teratogens. At therapeutic doses, however, genetic susceptibility may be the major determinant of damage. For example, certain strains of mice are susceptible to the development of cleft palate on exposure to cortisone in doses that do not affect other strains in this way. Investigations suggest that the teratogenic poten-

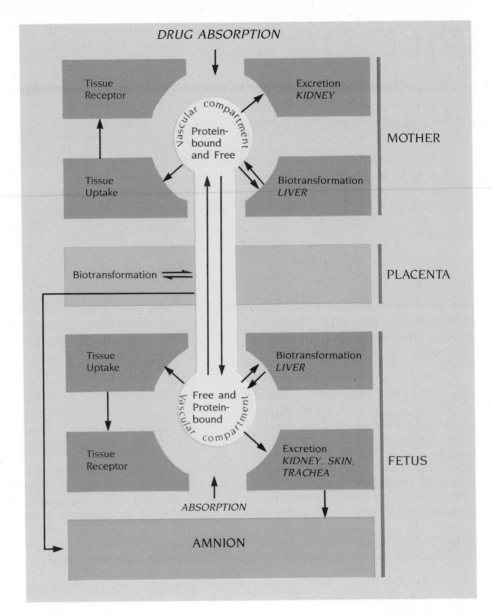

Figure 68–1   Drug distribution and disposition in mother and fetus *in utero*.

tial of drugs may be related to intermediate metabolites, produced by maternal or fetal tissues during gestation, which might bind with fetal cell DNA or other macromolecules. Thalidomide-induced phocomelia may be explained pharmacologically by the finding that liver tissue preparations from 18- to 20-week-old human fetuses could produce a metabolite of thalidomide (likely an arene oxide) that was toxic as determined *in vitro* by human lymphocyte killing. Tissue from species such as monkey and rabbit, which are sensitive to the teratogenicity of thalidomide, also produced a toxic

metabolite. However, rat liver preparations did not form a toxic metabolite and, as noted earlier, thalidomide is not teratogenic in the rat. The ability of a drug to stimulate its own biotransformation to reactive intermediates in certain genetically predisposed fetuses might be responsible for production of some malformations. Furthermore, a teratogenic event may ultimately be responsible for malignant potential of some cells; for example, exposure *in utero* of female fetuses to diethylstilbestrol predisposes to vaginal carcinoma in adult life.

Feto-Placental Transfer

In pharmacologic terms, disposition of drugs is qualified by designating compartments as hypothetical sites of drug accumulation and elimination. A simple example is the representation of plasma and cerebrospinal fluid as two distinct compartments. The feto-placental unit, because of its complexity, is not just another compartment but has its own particular properties of drug absorption, distribution, and elimination (see Fig. 68-1, and Table 68-1).

The bulk of any drug entering the fetus must do so via the placenta. Drugs reach the placenta almost totally from the maternal circulation, and their ultimate rate of transfer depends not only on their ability to diffuse across membranes, but also on the amount of drug reaching the site of exchange. This in turn is dependent on vessel distribution and blood flow. Placental blood flow increases throughout pregnancy, and although the placenta is not innervated, hormonal mediators or autacoids may influence blood flow (for example, autoregulation by prostaglandins).

The permeability of the placental barrier to drugs is limited to a quite narrow range of molecular sizes. In general, the placenta is impermeable to drugs with molecular weights greater than 1000 (e.g., heparin) and quite permeable to drugs with molecular weights less than 600 (e.g., penicillins and aminoglycosides). Intermediate-sized compounds such as thyroxine or erythromycin will have limited or variable access to the fetal circulation.

In general, drugs that are highly lipid-soluble traverse placental membranes rapidly. Ionized hydrophilic compounds such as salicylates may find entry across membranes only via pores. Most drugs are weak acids or bases and their degree of ionization is pH-dependent. An acidic drug tends to become charged when the pH

is alkaline, and a basic drug is charged when the pH is acidic. Since the pH of the fetal blood is slightly less than that of maternal blood, basic compounds will tend to be trapped on the fetal side of the placenta. An example of a weak acid is salicylic acid with pK_a 3.0 (the pH at which ionized and nonionized fractions are equal). Mepivacaine, pK_a 7.8, is a weak base. In pathologic states such as maternal alkalosis or fetal acidosis, there will be increased trapping of basic drugs such as mepivacaine on the fetal side.

Protein Binding

Protein binding also affects drug transfer. The amount of binding depends on the quantity of serum proteins (both albumin and globulins) present. The fetus at the time of delivery has lower total serum proteins than the mother, but the proportion of albumin is higher. Salicylate, which is largely bound to albumin, reaches higher fetal than maternal concentrations at delivery. On the other hand, deficiency of α_1-acid glycoprotein, a globulin, in the fetus leads to decreased binding of basic drugs such as propranolol and lidocaine.

Endogenous small molecules, e.g., bilirubin and fatty acids, may compete for binding to proteins and thus alter drug binding.

Distribution

Once a drug enters the fetus it distributes to various tissues. A variable proportion of umbilical venous blood (between 10% and 90%) will bypass the liver in the 10- to 20-week-old human fetus via the ductus venosus. The reason for this variability is not clear, but drugs that are eliminated by the liver will remain active in the fetus when a significant part of umbilical and fetal systemic blood bypasses the liver.

Some drugs accumulate in the amniotic fluid compartment by urine excretion as well as via exchange across nonkeratinized fetal skin. Keratinization takes place at 24–26 weeks gestation, after which time the skin is an unlikely transfer site. Some drugs exchange across respiratory epithelium. As term gestation approaches, net tracheal fluid flow is outward, with amounts of up to 100 mL/kg possibly exiting from the fetal lung each day.

TABLE 68-1 Factors Determining Placental Drug Transfer

Factor	Effect on Transfer
Placental blood flow	Increased drug delivery to placental membranes as blood flow increases.
Molecular size of drug	Decreased transfer of drug across placental membrane as molecular size increases.
Lipid solubility of drug	Increased transfer of drug across placental membrane as lipid solubility increases.
pK_a of drug – basic drugs:	Increased ion trapping on fetal side.
– acidic drugs:	Decreased ion trapping on fetal side.
Fetal pH (which is slightly less than maternal pH)	Increased ion trapping of basic drugs on fetal side.

Implications for Drug Transfer During Delivery

Because of certain characteristics of the feto-placental unit described above, the fetus is at some risk at the time of delivery. Inhalational anaesthetic agents are lipid-soluble and will cross the placenta rapidly. Transfer of these compounds from mother to fetus would be determined generally by placental blood flow. Nitrous oxide attains 80% of the maternal concentration in the fetus 3 minutes after induction, and 95% in another half-hour. The nonvolatile anaesthetic thiopental is largely nonionized at the pH of blood and reaches feto-maternal equilibrium within 12 minutes after injection.

Protein binding of drugs also has important implications for drug distribution at delivery. Bupivacaine, for example, is 90% protein-bound in the mother. At equilibrium the fetal drug concentration is only 24% of maternal because of considerably lower protein binding in the fetus (50%). However, in a situation such as severe maternal preeclampsia with hypoproteinemia secondary to protein loss in the urine, the free unbound maternal bupivacaine would rise and lead to more of the drug reaching the·fetus.

Drug Biotransformation

The pregnant mother and, in turn, the fetus are exposed to many foreign chemicals or xenobiotics during the gestational period. Some estimates suggest exposure rates of three to ten drugs per pregnancy, in addition to a myriad of environmental toxins. Early work showed that nonprimate fetuses had a very low capacity to biotransform foreign compounds because of inadequate enzymatic systems in liver and other tissues. After birth, metabolic capacity accelerated rapidly. More recent studies have shown that primates, including man, behave quite differently. Smooth endoplasmic reticulum, with which xenobiotic-biotransforming enzymes are associated, develops before mid-pregnancy in human and other primate species, and enzymatic systems necessary for drug transformations are present and functional early in gestation. In rodent fetuses, this enzyme system develops very late in gestation, or after birth.

There are several ways in which the body deals with drugs and other foreign compounds (*see* Chapter 4). Generally, chemicals are converted from hydrophobic to more hydrophilic forms that can be excreted by the kidney. The mechanisms of biotransformation include oxidation, reduction, hydrolysis, and conjugation. The first three of these mechanisms constitute phase I reactions during which intermediate metabolites are often formed. These intermediate metabolites are further converted to more polar substances by conjugation with various compounds, especially glucuronide, during phase 2 of biotransformation. It is the accumulation of intermediate metabolites that has potential toxicity for the fetus.

Monooxygenation, an oxidation reaction, takes place in the smooth endoplasmic reticulum and is dependent on cytochrome P-450 (or related hemoproteins). During prenatal life, the liver and adrenal glands are the major sites of P-450-dependent monooxygenation. Agents metabolized by this system include diazepam, acetaminophen, and phenytoin. However, during much of fetal life the enzyme activity is only basal and cannot

be stimulated by inducers such as methylcholanthrene and phenobarbital until the last few days of gestation.

These enzymatic systems are also present in the placenta. Maternal cigarette smoking, which is a potent inducer of maternal hepatic drug-metabolizing enzymes (*see* Chapter 4), does not stimulate fetal hepatic enzyme activities, but it does affect placental activity of a cytochrome-associated monooxygenase system specific for hydroxylation of aryl hydrocarbons.

Of the phase 2 reactions (glucuronidation, methylation, acetylation, sulfation, glutathione conjugation, and others), glucuronidation is the most important. During fetal life, glucuronyl transferase activity is low but present, especially in liver and kidney. Phenobarbital can accelerate development of glucuronyl transferase activity during late prenatal or early postnatal life in humans. The maternal capacity for drug biotransformation is the major determinant of drug concentration in steady-state conditions. On the other hand, if only single doses of drugs are given, *i.e.*, a non-steady-state situation, fetal metabolic potential may have an important role in clearing some drugs from the fetus, since the fetus will not be exposed to a "steady" maternal drug concentration.

Although fetal drug-metabolizing capacity may not be important as a determinant of drug clearance, this activity is nonetheless significant. As mentioned previously, drug biotransformation involves intermediate metabolite production. Clearance of these metabolites by phase 2 reactions, particularly conjugation with glucuronides, may not be as well developed in the fetus and premature infant as their production by phase I cytochrome P-450-dependent reactions. Therefore, there may be a relatively greater accumulation of intermediate metabolites than is observed in older children. Such metabolites may be more or less active than the parent drug, and fetal tissues may be more or less sensitive than adult tissues to the **harmful** effects of the intermediates. Despite their small quantity, these active intermediates could lead to teratogenesis, mutagenesis, and carcinogenesis, presumably by covalent binding to cellular macromolecules such as DNA (*see* the section Teratology). For example, it has been suggested that epoxide formation from phenytoin in fetal tissue leads to teratogenesis. In nonprimate experiments, fetal tissues were shown to convert benzo(a)pyrene, a common product of hydrocarbon combustion, to mutagenic metabolites.

Another interesting characteristic of the xenobiotic metabolizing system is its apparent hormonal regulation. Progesterone and somatotropin may suppress drug biotransformation during fetal and neonatal life. In the rat fetus glucocorticoids may trigger hepatic glucuronyl transferase activity towards some substrates. Exposure of the newborn rat to hormones, in particular androgens, during a critical neonatal period can establish or imprint permanent sex-dependent differences on metabolism involving hepatic microsomal monooxygenases.

Receptors

Drugs usually exert their effects through interactions with particular cellular receptor sites. Receptor sites must be present in the fetus for such drugs to be pharmacologically effective. Autonomic control has been demonstrated in animal fetuses during gestation. In the human fetus isoproterenol exerts positive inotropic effects on the heart, and propranolol has a negative effect, just as in postnatal life. Noradrenaline in the human fetus causes contraction of the ductus arteriosus and the ductus venosus. Examination of human fetal ileum suggests that β-adrenergic function begins to develop before α-adrenergic function.

It has been suggested that pharmacologic responses to bronchodilator drugs seen during maturational development may be related to receptor differences. Interest has focused on the incomplete development of β-adrenergic receptors as a possible explanation for the relatively low activity of β-adrenergic agonist drugs in infancy. Pulmonary β_2 functions, including surfactant release, mucus secretion, ion transport, and fluid secretion in tracheal epithelium; airway and vascular smooth muscle tone; mediator release from mast cells; and transvascular and transalveolar fluid and protein exchange, may differ from the norm of adults or older children. Maturation of β adrenoceptors may include a change in the number or affinity of receptors, or an alteration in postreceptor events. The receptors may be influenced by both local and remote factors; the former mechanisms involve regulation by catecholamines and the latter involve a number of noncatecholamine hormones, such as corticosteroids, thyroid hormones, and sex hormones. The development of receptors is thus a complex process, influenced by maturational changes occurring in the rest of the lung and the body.

Cholinergic receptor function is also present in the human fetus. Ileum and esophagus both respond to acetylcholine, and fetal heart rate increases when atropine is given to the mother. Vasomotor tone in the fetus probably does not reach full maturity until sometime after birth. Anaesthetic agents given to the mother

at the time of delivery may impair reflex autonomic function in the newborn and complicate the prediction of some drug action.

Interactions of other types of receptors with agents other than autonomic drugs have also been investigated in the fetus and newborn, in particular receptor interaction with digoxin and insulin. In the case of digoxin it is generally believed that infants, in contrast to adults, tolerate relatively large doses. Binding experiments using cord red blood cells indicate that the number of digoxin receptor sites per tissue unit is twice as great in the neonate as in the adult. However, receptor affinity for digoxin is less in the neonate. Consequently, doses for the neonate should be relatively greater than for the adult. Studies of fetuses of diabetic mothers show that insulin receptors on monocytes in the fetus increase when maternal diabetes is poorly controlled, resulting in an increased sensitivity of the neonate to insulin. With good maternal control, the number of fetal insulin receptor sites has been shown to remain normal.

Perinatal Renal Function

Renal function in the neonate is underdeveloped, and mature anatomic glomerulo-tubular balance is not reached until 1 year of age. Functionally, both glomerular filtration rate and renal plasma flow are lower at birth than in the older child and adult, and the ability to secrete organic compounds is restricted.

Some aspects of renal maturation remain to be clarified, and caution must be exercised when it is necessary to use drugs that depend on glomerular filtration for their elimination, such as aminoglycosides, which display prolonged half-lives of elimination in the premature and full-term newborn (Table 68–2).

Some drugs such as penicillin, an organic anion, are eliminated by tubular secretion, a function that is also relatively underdeveloped in the newborn. However, after birth, exposure to organic anion substrates such as those resulting from milk ingestion may augment the secretory capacity of the kidney. Drugs themselves may

TABLE 68–2 Selected Aminoglycoside Pharmacokinetics in Relation to Age and Weight of the Newborn

Drug	Age/Weight	Elimination $t\frac{1}{2}$ (hours)*	V_d (mL/kg)	Renal Cl_p (mL/min/1.73 m^2)
Amikacin	<4 days and <2000 g	7.1	563	21.3
	>7 days and >2000 g	4.9	594	36.4
Gentamicin	<1500 g	13.9	782	12.2
	>2500 g	4.5	519	34.0
Netilmicin	<1500 g	5.6		
	>2500 g	4.4		
Tobramycin	<1 week and <1500 g	8.5	431	11.0
	>1 week and >2500 g	4.0	435	35.9

* Note that the elimination half-life of these aminoglycosides is between 2 and 2$\frac{1}{2}$ hours in the adult with competent renal function.

also stimulate tubular transport of other closely related compounds; for example, oxacillin has been shown to enhance dicloxacillin secretion.

Prostaglandins may have a regulatory influence on renal blood flow. The prostaglandin synthetase inhibitor, indomethacin, reduces glomerular filtration rate in premature infants, an effect that may be secondary to altered hemodynamics and that is of particular importance in drug therapy. For example, toxic digoxin levels have occurred in neonates treated with both indomethacin and digoxin for patent ductus arteriosus.

PERINATAL DRUG DISPOSITION

Maternal Analgesia and Newborn Sedation

Narcotics, particularly meperidine, are frequently used for analgesia during delivery. Meperidine reaches equilibrium between maternal and umbilical venous blood fairly rapidly (2–3 hours), thus exposing the fetus to some risk of toxicity. Excessive exposure of the fetus to meperidine can lead to severe ventilatory depression and hypotonia in the neonate at delivery. The elimination half-life of meperidine in the neonate is 7–32 hours (i.e., two to seven times as long as in the adult). Furthermore, the neonate metabolizes meperidine to the potentially more toxic normeperidine. Thus, the risk of toxicity is prolonged because normeperidine levels do not peak until 24–36 hours after birth. Risk is further enhanced in the newborn because there is relatively little protection against penetration of drugs into the CNS. The blood–brain barrier matures during the first month of life, but prior to its full development the neonate is highly sensitive to many drugs acting on the central nervous system, including narcotic analgesics and sedatives.

Drug-related toxicity is also seen in the fetus exposed to narcotics taken by an addicted mother. There is an increase in both morbidity (low birth weight) and mortality of the fetus. In the immediate neonatal period, withdrawal symptoms may include tremors, hypertonicity, and seizures. Withdrawal of the mother from the drug during gestation might also harm the fetus. Studies in the rat indicate that maternal withdrawal during gestation is associated with fetal deaths; this finding suggests that methadone maintenance treatment throughout pregnancy is advisable in addicted humans.

Human newborns produce enkephalins and endorphins. Enkephalins are found both in the brain and in the gastrointestinal tract, whereas endorphins are generally recognized to be opioid peptides of the pituitary gland and hypothalamus, in particular β-endorphin, a fragment of a pituitary peptide, β-lipotropin (see Chapter 22). During fetal hypoxia and acidosis both β-endorphin and β-lipotropin concentrations increase in umbilical cord blood. Release of these peptides may be a physiologic response to stress.

Though they are likely of fetal origin, the placenta may contribute a fraction of these compounds to the fetal circulation. One physiologic role for endogenous opioids might be in ventilatory control. Naloxone, an opioid antagonist, will shorten primary apnea in newborn rabbits. Because the role of endogenous opioids is not clearly understood, naloxone should not be given routinely during labor after administration of narcotics to the mother. When neonatal respiratory depression is considered to be due to maternal treatment with narcotic analgesics during labor, naloxone should prove effective to restore breathing in the newborn, but it must be remembered that its effect will disappear within 30–90 minutes and further doses usually are necessary.

A study in premature neonates (Hindmarsh et al. 1984) showed that at the same postnatal age of 3 days, babies born at a mean gestational age of 33.2 weeks had plasma β-endorphin levels more than twice as high as those in babies born after only 31.5 weeks of gestation. This appears to suggest that endorphin release increases with increasing maturation in utero. However, the gestationally older babies also had clinical evidence of acute illness. Therefore an alternative interpretation is that even premature neonates can respond to clinical stress with increased release of β-endorphin, which might affect respiratory function in these high-risk infants.

Glucocorticoids in Prophylaxis of Respiratory Distress Syndrome (RDS)

Evidence clearly shows that glucocorticoids given prenatally to mothers of premature infants will reduce the incidence of neonatal respiratory distress syndrome (RDS). Of the synthetic glucocorticoids, the most frequently used is betamethasone. Dexamethasone is also being studied. The half-life of measured biologic effects of both drugs is approximately 36–54 hours. This contrasts with their plasma half-lives of approximately 6 hours. Thus, both drugs appear to exert prolonged biologic activity and one might hypothesize that by maintaining saturation of cytosolic receptor sites in alveolar cells for sufficient time they produce continuous stimulation of surfactant production. These long-acting steroids also have a greater affinity for the type II pneumocyte receptor than does cortisol. (Type II pneumocytes are surfactant-producing alveolar cells.) Serum protein binding of cortisol (90%) is greater than that of either betamethasone or dexamethasone; free drug concentrations and activity of the latter two compounds are therefore enhanced. (Prednisolone also binds to plasma proteins to a considerable degree.)

Glucocorticoids are cleared by both hepatic and placental metabolism. Maternal metabolism contributes to elimination of the synthetic corticoids. Betamethasone was not detectable in cord blood 62–72 hours after the mother was given the drug. Infants whose mothers were treated prenatally with betamethasone have markedly reduced cord blood cortisol concentrations; however, the responses of their pituitary-adrenal axis to stress are apparently unimpaired.

Although prophylactic use of glucocorticoids may reduce the incidence of RDS, such use is not without potential danger. Thus, use in mothers with severe hypertension has resulted in an increased incidence of fetal deaths. Steroids given on the first day of life to infants with RDS were without benefit. When reviewed 5 years later, the same children were shown to have a diminished percentage of T lymphocytes, likely to be associated with an increased risk of infection. Neonates with RDS given large doses of hydrocortisone had an increased incidence of gross neurologic abnormalities. Furthermore, animal data indicate that very large doses of steroids, 12 to 300 times greater per kg of body weight than the human fetal dose, lead to fetal growth retardation and decreased brain size, possibly secondary to inhibition of cell multiplication. Hypoglycemia occurs more frequently in the newborns of mothers given betamethasone.

Theophylline in the Treatment of Apnea of Prematurity

Two methylxanthines, theophylline (a dimethylxanthine) and caffeine (a trimethylxanthine) are used in the management of neonatal apnea. They appear to exert their stimulatory effect by augmenting ventilatory responsiveness to CO_2, possibly by an interaction with, and blockade of, central adenosine receptors. It has been suggested that improved diaphragmatic contractility is an important therapeutic effect of theophylline in adults; it is possible that this mechanism is important in neonates as well.

The capacity for hepatic theophylline biotransformation is less developed in neonates than in older children and adults. The major routes of elimination of the drug in the adult include N-demethylation and C-oxidation. Very little unchanged theophylline is excreted in the urine of older patients. In the newborn, however, underdeveloped enzyme function, particularly of the N-demethylation pathway, leads to a prolonged half-life of elimination. Interestingly, one metabolic route, methylation, is quite active in the premature neonate, leading to production of caffeine as a theophylline metabolite, and hence to accumulation of caffeine in plasma to levels approaching those of theophylline. It is not until 6 months of age that clearance rates comparable to those seen in older children are reached.

Caffeine is also poorly biotransformed. Elimination of caffeine, as of theophylline, therefore depends to some degree on renal function which, as has been discussed, is limited in the newborn period. The half-life of caffeine in the newborn is approximately 100 hours. That of theophylline is 30 hours. Side effects of theophylline in the newborn include tachycardia and hyponatremia.

Anti-Prostaglandins in Neonatology

Fetal tissue (e.g., platelets, blood vessels) and placenta are capable of synthesizing prostaglandins. To date they have been reported to affect the fetus in several ways: alteration of uterine and placental blood flow; influence on organ differentiation by locally produced prostaglandins; and mediation of fetal and placental hormone production or release.

Major interest in prostaglandins in neonatology results from their action on the ductus arteriosus. Inhibitors of prostaglandin synthesis, in particular indomethacin, are used to treat persistent patent ductus arteriosus in infants of low birth weight. However, the same inhibitors may have important deleterious effects prior to birth. Maternal use of salicylates, for example, has the potential to cause constriction of the ductus arteriosus prior to birth, leading to fetal pulmonary hypertension and congestive heart failure at birth. Fortunately, this seems to be an uncommon occurrence.

The use of indomethacin for constriction of the ductus is not invariably successful, a fact that may be explained in part by the variability of drug clearance in the neonatal period. Decreased glomerular filtration rate occurs with indomethacin therapy in the neonate.

Endogenous Digoxin-like Substance in Infants and Mothers

An endogenous digoxin-like substance has been found in the serum of volume-expanded animals, neonates, women with high-risk pregnancies, and patients with hypertensive and renal disease. In all of these situations, digitalis-like activity has been measured in serum, even though the subjects have not been exposed to digoxin or to any other cardiac glycoside. Koren and others have studied this phenomenon and have shown apparent digoxin concentrations between 0.17 and 1.64 nmol/L in 30 neonates not receiving digoxin. A negative correlation has been demonstrated between gestational age and the concentration of digoxin-like substance. Neonates under 32 weeks gestational age had significantly higher levels than those over 32 weeks gestational age. Concentrations of endogenous digoxin-like substance were consistently higher in offspring than in their mothers. The substance has also been shown to have pharmacologic activity. It is capable of inhibiting the uptake of radiolabelled rubidium into red blood cells (i.e., it inhibits $(Na^+ + K^+)$-ATPase; see Chapter 34). Observations such as this cast serious doubt on the validity of previously published studies concerning digoxin pharmacokinetics and dosing in preterm infants.

CONCLUSION

It cannot be emphasized too strongly that the perinatal clinical pharmacology of drugs will be heavily influenced by the various disease states leading to drug therapy in the first instance, and by the general clinical condition including maturational status of the patient. The effects of these factors are magnified because of the limited functional reserve for biotransformation, excretion, and modulation of drug effects in the newborn infant. This is a field where knowledge is evolving rapidly, and those interested in neonatal drug therapy are well advised to consult up-to-date references.

SUGGESTED READING

Aranda JV, Turmen T, Sasyniuk BI. Pharmacokinetics of diuretics and methylxanthines in the neonate. Eur J Clin Pharmacol 1980; 18:55–63.

Ballard PL, Ballard RA. Glucocorticoids in prevention of respiratory distress syndrome. Hosp Pract 1980; 15:81–87.

Besunder JB, Reed MD, Blumer JL. Principles of drug bio-disposition in the neonate. A critical evaluation of the pharmacokinetic-pharmacodynamic interface. Clin Pharmacokinet 1988; 14:261–286.

Hindmarsh KW, Sankaran K, Watson VG. Plasma beta-endorphin concentration in neonates associated with stress. Dev Pharmacol Ther 1984; 7:198–204.

Hook JB, Bailie MD. Perinatal renal pharmacology. Ann Rev Pharmacol Toxicol 1979; 19:491–509.

Juchau MR, Chao ST, Omiecinski CJ. Drug metabolism by the human fetus. Clin Pharmacokinet 1980; 5:320–329.

Koren G, Farine D, Maresky D, et al. Significance of the endogenous digoxin-like substance in infants and mothers. Clin Pharmacol Ther 1984; 36:759–764.

Koren G, MacLeod S. Monitoring and avoiding drug and chemical teratogenicity. Can Med Ass J 1986; 135:1079–1081.

MacLeod SM, Radde IC, eds. Textbook of pediatric clinical pharmacology. Littleton, MA: PSG Publishing, 1985.

Morgan CA, Paull J. Drugs in obstetric anaesthesia. Anaesth Intens Care 1980; 8:278–288.

Morselli PL, Franco-Morselli R, Bossi L. Clinical pharmacokinetics in newborns and infants. Clin Pharmacokinet 1980; 5:485–527.

Rane A. Basic principles of drug disposition and action in infants and children. In: Yaffe SJ ed. Pediatric pharmacology: therapeutic principles in practice. New York: Grune & Stratton, 1980:7–10.

Seeds AE. Basic concepts of maternal-fetal amniotic fluid exchange. Pediatr Clin North Am 1981; 28:231–240.

Chapter 69

GERIATRIC CLINICAL PHARMACOLOGY

E.M. Sellers

Life expectancy in the Western world is becoming longer and currently stands at 69 years for men and 77 years for women. In 1980 an estimated 11% of the total population of Canada was over 65 years of age; the percentage is expected to exceed 15% by the year 2040. Compared to their young counterparts, elderly persons (namely those 65 years or older) expend on the average a higher yearly dollar amount, as well as a higher fraction of their total income, on health care. Old people have more illness and hospitalization than young individuals, and once hospitalized the elderly have a longer duration both of acute care and of total hospitalization. The need for long-term institutionalization also is greatly increased among the elderly. A recent study of patients in long-term health care facilities in Metropolitan Toronto found that average drug utilization in the elderly was 6.6 prescribed drugs per day (range 0–19). The cost of drugs was estimated to be about $105.00 per person for the 3-month study period. Therefore, the appropriate and rational use of drugs in the elderly is a problem of increasing medical and social concern.

Medical concern about drugs in the elderly is partly attributable to the development over the past 20 years of systematic epidemiologic surveillance systems for monitoring patterns of drug use and toxicity. These systems usually are hospital-based, and focus on the nature and frequency of untoward drug effects and factors predisposing to toxicity. Reports from independent monitoring systems demonstrate an overall increased frequency of adverse drug reactions associated with increasing patient age (Table 69–1).

Studies from the Boston Collaborative Drug Surveillance Program have focused specifically on the relation of age to the frequency of adverse reactions for a number of commonly used drugs. A clear relationship of age to untoward effects has been demonstrated for the benzodiazepine derivatives chlordiazepoxide, diazepam, flurazepam, and nitrazepam, and for the anticoagulant agent heparin. In the case of heparin,

TABLE 69–1 Age and Adverse Drug Reactions

Age of Patients (Years)	Incidence (%)
10–19	3.1
20–29	3.0
30–39	5.7
40–49	7.5
50–59	8.1
60–69	10.7
70–79	21.3
80–89	18.6

After Hurwitz N. Br Med J 1969; 1:536–539.

the age-related frequency of adverse effects (primarily manifested as bleeding) is greater in women than in men. For the cardiac agents lidocaine and propranolol, a relatively weak association of age to clinical toxicity occurs. For some 90 other drugs in common clinical use, age as such was not a major determinant of clinical toxicity. Administration of the same average daily dose to young adults and elderly persons would result in a higher weight-corrected dosage in the elderly due to their lower body weights, and this might increase dose-dependent adverse effects in the elderly. Conversely, a lack of association of age and clinical toxicity in epidemiologic studies does not rule out an important contribution of age as a biologic determinant of toxicity. Increased caution by clinicians when treating the elderly, such as by administration of lower doses or by more careful monitoring of drug effects, could offset an actual biologic change in drug sensitivity in the geriatric population.

Both pharmacokinetic and pharmacodynamic explanations exist for altered drug effects in the elderly.

Even if drug sensitivity in an older person were not inherently altered, changes in a drug's **pharmacokinetics** because of age-related physiologic alterations, causing higher drug concentration at the site of action, would cause an exaggerated drug response if the drug effect were proportional to receptor site concentration. Thus the ability to understand and predict clinically important age-related changes in drug disposition might be of value in designing dosage schedules for the elderly that are more likely to be therapeutically beneficial and less likely to be toxic.

The **pharmacodynamic** explanation of increased drug sensitivity in the elderly posits that at any receptor site an identical drug concentration yields a greater pharmacodynamic response in an elderly as opposed to a young individual. Rigorous testing of this hypothesis *in vivo*, particularly in humans, is difficult, and few studies convincingly demonstrate a true change of drug sensitivity in old age, but there is at least some suggestive evidence. For example, work involving the benzodiazepine derivatives, diazepam and nitrazepam, suggests greater CNS depression at any given plasma drug concentration in elderly than in young individuals. Some, but not all, studies indicate achievement of a greater anticoagulant response (evident as greater prolongation of prothrombin time) at any given dose or plasma concentration of coumarin anticoagulants in elderly than in young patients.

PHARMACOKINETIC CHANGES IN THE ELDERLY

Review of Pharmacokinetics

a. Clearance (Cl) = Dose/Area Under Curve ($AUC_{0-\infty}$).

b. Cl = Volume of Distribution (V_d) × Elimination Rate Constant (k_e).

c. Half-Life ($t\frac{1}{2}$) = $0.693/k_e$.

d. $t\frac{1}{2}$ = $(1/Cl) \times V_d \times 0.693$ (substituting (c) in (b) and rearranging). Note: If V_d increases so will $t\frac{1}{2}$.

e. Average steady state plasma drug concentration

$$\overline{C}_{pss} = \frac{Dose(D) \times Bioavailability(F)}{Dose\ Interval\ (\tau)} \times \frac{1}{Cl}$$

and

f. $$\overline{C}_{pss} = \frac{D \times F}{\tau} \times \frac{t\frac{1}{2}}{V_d} \times 1.44.$$

g. Plateau Principle: Time to reach 95% of maximum plasma concentration of a drug with a long half-life, administered in constant dose and at constant interval = $5 \times t\frac{1}{2}$.

(*See also* Chapter 5.)

Absorption

A number of changes that occur in the gastrointestinal tract with aging might be expected to alter drug absorption. They include: (1) a decrease in basal and maximal (histamine-stimulated) acid output, with consequent increase in gastric pH, thus affecting the ionization and solubility of some drugs; (2) a pronounced decrease in splanchnic blood flow, possibly reducing or delaying drug absorption; (3) a probable reduction in the number of absorbing cells; (4) a decreased rate of gastric emptying; (5) an increased incidence of duodenal diverticula that, as a result of bacterial colonization of the small intestine, appears to be the principal cause of malabsorption in this age group.

The absorption of several dietary constituents by active or specialized transport mechanisms appears to be reduced in the elderly (e.g., galactose, 3-methylglucose, calcium, and iron). Most drugs, however, are absorbed not by active transport mechanisms but by passive diffusion across the gut wall. To date, little work has been undertaken specifically to determine the rate and extent of drug absorption in the elderly and, for the most part, the information available has been obtained from the early phases of drug elimination. Definite studies on the extent of drug absorption involve comparison of the profiles of plasma drug concentration versus time following both oral and intravenous administration of the same drug dose. So far, very few age-related studies of this type have been carried out.

Despite speculation to the contrary in many reviews and secondary sources, there is essentially no evidence that drug absorption is importantly impaired in old age.

Distribution

Body Composition

Changes in body composition with age may influence drug distribution. On the average, lean body mass declines and adipose tissue mass increases relative to total body weight in the aging person. The fraction of total body weight consisting of adipose tissue may be from 18% to 36% higher in the elderly male than in the young adult male; the corresponding increase with age in the female may be 33–48% (*see* Table 69–2).

The effect of these changes on drug distribution within the body depends largely on the solubility of the particular drug in water versus lipid. Some drugs, such as acetaminophen, antipyrine, and ethanol, are relatively water-soluble and lipid-insoluble. Distribution to tissues may become less extensive in the elderly than in the young individual. Conversely, highly lipid-soluble drugs such as diazepam and other psychoactive drugs become more extensively distributed in the elderly than in the young adult. Figure 69–1 shows the

TABLE 69–2 Average Changes in Body Composition and Function (Males and Females)

	Change From Age 20 to Age 80 (%)
Body fat/total body weight	+35
Plasma volume	−8
Plasma albumin	−10
Plasma globulin	−10
Total body water	−17
Extracellular fluid (from age 20 to age 65)	−40
Conduction velocity	−20
Cardiac index	−40
Cardiac output	−30 −40
Vital capacity	−60
Glomerular filtration rate	−50
Splanchnic and renal blood flow	−40

calculated volume of distribution in subjects given diazepam or antipyrine intravenously.

Differences in body composition between male and female regardless of age may be as marked as those between young and elderly. Consequently, females show more extensive distribution of highly lipid-soluble drugs than males do and less extensive distribution of relatively water-soluble drugs.

Unless age-related changes in body composition by themselves influence the function of clearing organs, altered drug distribution in old age will not alter steady-state plasma concentrations during multiple dosage, since this depends only on dosing rate and total clearance. However, distribution has an important effect on elimination half-life (*see* Review of Pharmacokinetics and Fig. 69–2).

Protein Binding

The apparent volume of distribution of extensively protein-bound drugs may also be influenced by changes in the extent of binding to plasma proteins. Most protein-bound drugs are bound partly or entirely to plasma albumin, and a significant age-related decline in plasma albumin concentrations is consistently reported. The reduction may be large when elderly subjects are poorly nourished, have advanced illness, or are

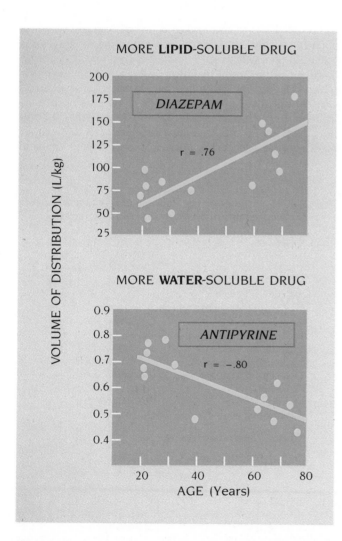

Figure 69–1 Changes in apparent volume of distribution with aging. (Modified from Greenblatt DJ, Sellers EM, Shader RI. 1982.)

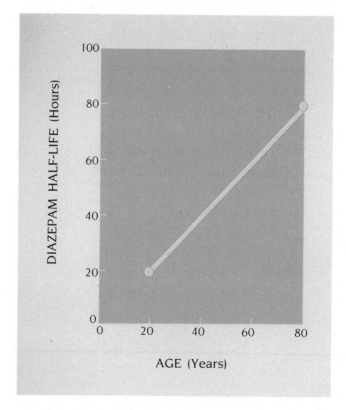

Figure 69–2 Diazepam half-life in hours happens to be approximately equal to chronologic age in years.

severely debilitated. Even in well-nourished, healthy elderly persons, however, albumin concentrations are lower than those in young individuals, even though these levels may not fall below the "usual range of normal" (Fig. 69–3). The consequence of the fall in albumin concentration for highly bound drugs is that the measured total concentration can be lower by about 10%. Free fraction is increased by 10% but free concentration is unchanged. Hence there is usually no clinical consequence of the decreased albumin. It should be emphasized, however, that neither age nor albumin concentration necessarily explains a large proportion of overall variability between individuals in protein binding of a given drug.

Drug Biotransformation and the Liver

Physiologic changes occurring in aging that might be expected to influence drug biotransformations include (1) decreased liver weight; (2) decreased number of functioning hepatic cells; (3) decreased hepatic and splanchnic blood flow; and (4) decreased liver microsomal enzyme activity (decreased in rats, but unclear in humans).

There is some evidence for lesser susceptibility to enzyme induction in the elderly, but interpretation of data is suspect because of study design. There is evidence that the apparent decrease in hepatic clearance of some drugs in older persons is really due to the

fact that the elderly smoke less, and thus diminish the level of induction of hepatic enzymes.

Hepatic Biotransformation Reactions

Mechanisms controlling hepatic biotransformation of drugs are complex, as are their alterations with old age. Hepatocytes carry out many different biotransformation reactions that contribute to the removal of drugs and other foreign chemicals. Hepatic microsomal enzymes responsible for phase 1 oxidative drug biotransformations (principally hydroxylation and N-dealkylation) may be impaired in old age, leading to reduced total drug clearance and higher steady-state plasma concentrations during multiple dosage (Table 69–3). On the other hand, studies of phase 2 biotransformations suggest that aging has a much smaller effect on glucuronide conjugating capacity.

Hepatic Blood Flow

Hepatic blood flow, rather than microsomal enzyme activity, is a major determinant of total drug clearance for a number of commonly used drugs (*i.e.*, those with high hepatic extraction ratios; see Chapter 7). Hepatic blood flow declines with age, partly because of reduced cardiac output. An estimated 40–45% reduction in total liver blood flow may occur in the elderly as compared to young adults. Likewise, liver size decreases, both in absolute terms and as a percentage of total

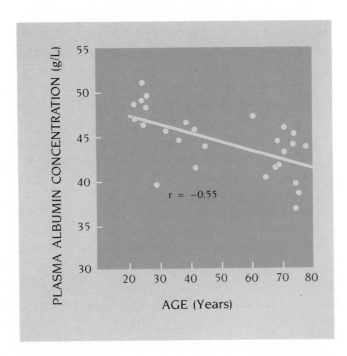

Figure 69–3 Effect of age on normal plasma albumin concentration.

TABLE 69–3 Studies on the Relation of Age and Clearance for Representative Drugs Cleared by Hepatic Biotransformation

Drug	Initial Pathway of Biotransformation*
Evidence suggestive of age-related reduction in clearance:	
Antipyrine†	Oxidation (OH, DA)
Diazepam†	Oxidation (DA)
Chlordiazepoxide	Oxidation (DA)
Desmethyldiazepam†	Oxidation (OH)
Desalkylflurazepam†	Oxidation (OH)
Clobazepam	Oxidation (DA)
Quinidine	Oxidation (OH)
Theophylline	Oxidation
Propranolol	Oxidation (OH)
Nortriptyline	Oxidation (OH)
Small or negligible age-related change in clearance:	
Oxazepam	Glucuronidation
Lorazepam	Glucuronidation
Temazepam	Glucuronidation
Isoniazid	Acetylation

* OH = hydroxylation; DA = dealkylation.
† Evidence suggestive of differential sex effect, with age-related reduction in clearance greater in men than in women.

body weight. One would expect a predictable age-related decline in total drug clearance for drugs with flow-dependent clearance, but available data are conflicting. Reduced total clearance in old age has been demonstrated for propranolol but not for lidocaine, two drugs with high and therefore flow-dependent hepatic clearance.

Hepatic Extraction

The explanation for such discrepancies may be that hepatic extraction may decrease for some drugs in the elderly. Consider the observations shown in Figure 69–4. Since the peak level and AUC of propranolol are markedly increased (about four-fold) after oral administration in the elderly, one might conclude that the hepatic extraction was decreased (*see* Chapter 7).

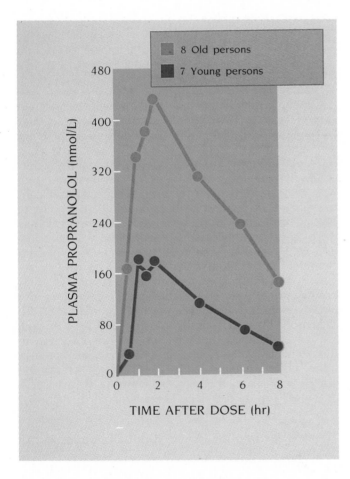

Figure 69–4 Mean plasma propranolol concentrations in two different age groups, following a single oral dose of 40 mg. Differences between age groups are statistically significant. (After Castleden CM, George CF. Br J Clin Pharmacol 1979; 7:49–54.)

Renal Elimination

Glomerular filtration rate (GFR) declines predictably in old age, with a mean 35% reduction of GFR in elderly (>65 years) compared to young (<30 years) individuals. Renal blood flow is also decreased (Table 69–2).

For drugs whose total clearance is explained partly or entirely by renal excretion of the intact drug, total clearance will predictably decline approximately in proportion to the reduced GFR. The elimination half-life is prolonged and the renal clearance and total body clearance decreased, for digoxin, lithium, penicillin G, and gentamicin, although the mechanisms of renal excretion of these drugs are not identical.

To prevent excessive accumulation of such drugs in elderly individuals, a need for downward adjustment of dosage must be anticipated. Translation of this general principle to any specific patient, however, requires knowledge of that individual's level of renal function, based upon either measurement or estimation of creatinine clearance.

Often overlooked is the decline of muscle mass and lean body mass relative to total body weight, which also declines with old age. Since serum creatinine concentration depends on creatinine turnover as well as on renal creatinine excretion, the decline in renal function in the elderly may not cause a corresponding elevation in serum creatinine concentrations. Thus, reliance on serum creatinine as the sole indicator of renal function in the elderly may be misleading. Creatinine clearance, based upon 24-hour urinary excretion as well as serum creatinine concentration, is a far more reliable indicator of renal function.

Since it is not intuitively apparent by how much the dose for a drug such as digoxin should be reduced, a specific dosage adjustment factor may be estimated. The elimination rate constant, K, is the sum of the individual rate constants from all organs involved in the elimination of the drug. As the liver and the kidney are major elimination organs, K is the sum of $k_R + k_H$, where the subscripts denote renal and hepatic, respectively.

If the fraction of drug excreted unchanged by the kidney is F (= k_R/K) and hepatic elimination is assumed to be unchanged (*i.e.*, $k_{H,1} = k_{H,2}$), the relationship between K values at two different conditions (e.g., "1" and "2") can be expressed as: $K_1/K_2 = t\frac{1}{2}(2)/t\frac{1}{2}(1)$.

The dosage-adjustment factor is the ratio between the half-life in an abnormal condition and the half-life in a normal state (e.g., in the presence of an endogenous creatinine clearance of 120 mL/min). For the present purpose $t\frac{1}{2}(2)$ is the half-life of a drug in elderly subjects and $t\frac{1}{2}(1)$ the half-life in young persons. Different values of the dosage-adjustment factor are given in Table 69–4. Practical guidelines for dosage adjustment, using this factor, are shown in Table 69–5.

TABLE 69–4   The Dosage-Adjustment Factor for Correcting for Reduced Renal Function

Percent of Drug Excreted Unchanged in the Urine	Creatinine Clearance (mL/min)						
	0	10	20	40	60†	80	120‡
10	1.1	1.1	1.1	1.1	1.1	1.0	1.0
20	1.3	1.2	1.2	1.1	1.1	1.1	1.0
30	1.5	1.3	1.3	1.2	1.2	1.1	1.0
40	1.7	1.6	1.5	1.4	1.3	1.1	1.0
50	2.0	1.8	1.7	1.5	1.3	1.2	1.0
60	2.5	2.2	2.0	1.7	1.4	1.3	1.0
70	3.3	2.8	2.3	1.9	1.5	1.3	1.0
80	5.0	3.7	3.0	2.1	1.7	1.4	1.0
90*	10.0	5.7	4.0	2.5	1.8§	1.4	1.0
100	—	12.0	6.0	3.0	2.0	1.5	1.0

* For example, digoxin.
† *i.e.*, a 70-year-old.
‡ *i.e.*, a 20-year-old.
§ Maintenance digoxin dose should be 1.8-fold *less* in a 70-year-old. Also note in this table the relative insensitivity of drugs relying upon combined renal and hepatic excretion and the critical importance of dose adjustment for drugs relying only on the kidney.

Multiple Kinetic Changes

Unfortunately the factors causing changes in kinetics in the elderly are usually multiple. The following example illustrates how changes in hepatic and renal handling of drugs and changes in protein binding can occur concurrently.

TABLE 69–5   Practical Guidelines for Adjusting the Dosage of Drugs Excreted by the Kidney in Elderly Patients

Decide the appropriate dosage regimen for the patient as if the renal function were that in a normal young patient—*i.e.*, creatinine clearance of 120 mL/min (most dosage regimens are derived from studies in younger subjects).

Ascertain the fraction of drug (and any active metabolite) that is excreted unchanged by the kidneys.

Determine the patient's renal function by measurement of endogenous creatinine clearance.

Calculate the dosage-adjustment factor as shown in Table 69–4.

Use the dosage-adjustment factor in one of the following ways (after considering which is most appropriate for the specific drug):
• Divide the dose for a patient with normal renal function by this factor and continue with the same dosage interval.
• Continue with the same dose and multiply the dosage interval determined for patients with normal renal function by this factor.
• Reduce the dose and prolong the dosage interval appropriately.

Theophylline kinetics following a single oral dose were compared in ambulatory elderly and young sex-matched control subjects (Table 69–6). Plasma levels of total drug were significantly higher in the elderly only at early sampling times (0.5 and 1 hour) and at 36 hours, while unbound theophylline levels were significantly higher at all sampling times, so that the AUC for unbound drug was 45% greater in the elderly. While no significant differences in volume of distribution (V_d) or overall plasma clearance were observed when calculations were based on total plasma theophylline, a 37% reduction in V_d and a 30% reduction in overall plasma clearance in the elderly became apparent when plasma protein binding was taken into account.

When urinary excretion patterns were compared, the elderly excreted a significantly higher fraction of the recovered dose as 1-methyluric acid and a lower fraction as unchanged theophylline. A 47% reduction in the renal clearance of unbound theophylline was also observed in the elderly (Fig. 69–5). Results were consistent with less active metabolic **and** renal excretory pathways for theophylline elimination in the elderly.

Therapeutic Implications of Kinetic Changes in the Elderly

The importance of an age-related reduction in total drug clearance depends on the therapeutic index of the particular drug. Compounds such as digoxin, quinidine, and theophylline have reasonably well defined and relatively narrow ranges of usually effective plasma concentrations, above which the likelihood of clinical toxicity increases. For such drugs, a need to reduce daily dosage in the elderly should be anticipated in order to avoid toxicity caused by excessive drug ac-

TABLE 69–6 Pharmacokinetic Parameters Derived from Plasma Concentration of Unchanged Theophylline*

	Young Controls	Elderly	Statistical Significance
Half-life (hours)	8.51 ± 1.00	9.81 ± 4.10	n.s.
V_d total (L/kg)	0.43 ± 0.06	0.32 ± 0.05	n.s.
V_d unbound (L/kg)	1.38 ± 0.23	0.86 ± 0.14	p<0.005
Total plasma clearance (mL/min)	34.9 ± 12.0	29.4 ± 9.99	n.s.
Unbound plasma clearance (mL/min)	113.5 ± 39.5	79.8 ± 29.7	p<0.02
Metabolic clearance (mL/min):			
3-Methylxanthine	14.7 ± 7.5	9.17 ± 4.25	p<0.05
Total methylurate	61.2 ± 21.1	76.0 ± 35.0	p<0.1
Renal clearance (mL/min)	17.7 ± 4.08	9.35 ± 8.19	p<0.005

* All values expressed as mean ± SD.

cumulation. Age-related changes in clearance are less likely to be important for drugs such as diazepam, for which a close relation of plasma concentration to clinical effect has not been established. Although epidemiologic studies suggest that the elderly may be more sensitive to diazepam, this is not a proven consequence of excessive drug accumulation. Also, clinicians should employ a cautious approach during the use of drugs such as lidocaine in the elderly, even though no clear age-related alteration in kinetics has been demonstrated. Definitive kinetic data unfortunately are not yet available for a number of important drugs commonly prescribed to the elderly.

PHARMACODYNAMIC CHANGES IN THE ELDERLY

In contrast to our rather detailed knowledge about pharmacokinetic changes in the elderly, very little is known about the importance or mechanism of changes in sensitivity or responsiveness to drugs in the elderly. The issue is complicated by the concurrent pharmacokinetic changes that can alter the concentration-time profile of drugs in the elderly. Clearly a basis for changes in responsiveness exists. Cardiac contractility, vital capacity, immunologic response, cellular repair, and most bodily functions decrease with age (*see* Table 69–2).

Heart and Cardiovascular System

Cardiac Glycosides and Toxicity

The elderly appear to be more sensitive to digitalis glycosides. Possible explanations for this include: (1) decreased renal function; (2) decreased extrarenal elimination; (3) frequently, concurrent administration of thiazides, which may cause an increased potassium loss compared to the young; (4) altered myocardial sensitivity and contractility (for example, the dP/dt developed after ouabain in senescent rat hearts is less than in the hearts of young animals; in this context it is of

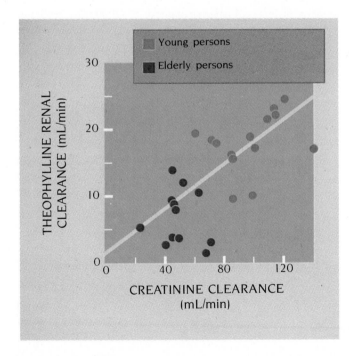

Figure 69–5 Relationship between unbound theophylline renal clearance and creatinine clearance in elderly and young volunteers. (Modified from Antal EJ, Kramer P, Mercek SA, *et al*. Br J Clin Pharmacol 1981; 12:637–645.)

interest that inhibition of $(Na^+ + K^+)$-ATPase is identical in young and old rat hearts); and (5) frequent presence of coronary artery disease.

Responsiveness to Catecholamines

Aging causes a decrease in the maximum responsiveness of the heart to catecholamines and an increase in vascular loading of the heart during exercise. This is associated with a decline in β adrenoceptor-mediated function with age; for example, heart rate responses to isoproterenol and propranolol decrease with advancing age. Lymphocytes (a model to study β receptors) from elderly people produce less cyclic AMP in the presence of isoproterenol than those from young people. However, receptor density does not differ in young and elderly people. Thus, decreases in β adrenoceptor-mediated responses in old age may be due to alterations in postreceptor events.

Central Nervous System

The elderly seem to have an inordinate number of adverse effects to CNS-active drugs, such as barbiturates, benzodiazepines, cimetidine, methyldopa, metoclopramide, opiates, propoxyphene, and tricyclic antidepressants. Perhaps such qualitative and quantitative changes in response relate to changes in the brain. Unfortunately, evidence linking these changes to altered sensitivity is circumstantial. In the elderly, brain wet weight and neuronal populations decline. In some brain areas there appears to be reduced dendritic arborization. In the aging brain, neurotransmitter metabolism is affected. Catecholamine concentrations appear to be especially reduced. More marked loss of cells and synapses is seen in senile dementia of the Alzheimer type, and there is a significant reduction in choline acetyltransferase activity and in the ability of isolated biopsy tissue to synthesize acetylcholine.

Each of these changes would be expected, in turn, to decrease the compensatory reserve of the brain when modified by drugs. As a rule of thumb, the initial dose of CNS-active drugs in the elderly should be one-half of that given to younger patients.

Analgesics and Nonsteroidal Anti-inflammatory Agents

Side effects of these drugs occur in more than 60% of patients over the age of 60, compared to 23% of patients 21–30 years old. Phenylbutazone half-life of elimination was 110 hours in a group of elderly patients (average age 81) compared to 87 hours in 24-year-old patients. [Questions for the reader: Why is the half-life longer? Does this increase in half-life explain the marked increase in toxicity? What other possibilities may exist?] A review of the side effects of phenylbuta-

zone and nonsteroidal anti-inflammatory drugs may be of help (see Chapter 33) when relating the mechanism of these adverse reactions to altered function (see Table 69–2), as well as to altered pharmacokinetics, in the elderly.

Anaesthetic Agents

Factors influencing onset and magnitude of response to anaesthetic agents or adjuncts in the elderly include: (1) longer circulation time (e.g., succinylcholine, d-tubocurarine); (2) decreased pulmonary function; (3) slower absorption from injection sites; (4) altered distribution into fat because of poorer perfusion and an increase in the proportion of body fat; (5) increased CNS sensitivity (e.g., the thiopental dose requirement falls with increased age); (6) impaired cardiovascular reflexes; and (7) decreases in renal function.

Anticoagulants (Warfarin)

Warfarin dose requirements drop by about 50% as age increases from 30 to 75 years. Also, the anticoagulant response to single doses of warfarin changes with advancing age, as shown in Figure 69–6.

Possible reasons for these differences include: (1) changed receptor sensitivity for warfarin; (2) greater vitamin K_1 clearance in the elderly in the absence of warfarin; (3) greater accumulation of vitamin K_1 oxide in the elderly in the presence of warfarin; and (4)

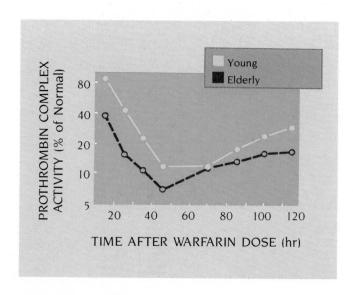

Figure 69–6 The anticoagulant response of young and elderly patients to a single dose of warfarin. Most differences are statistically significant. (Modified from Sheperd MM, Hewick DS, Moreland TA, et al. Br J Clin Pharmacol 1977; 4:315–320.)

reduced prothrombin complex activity responsiveness to vitamin K_1 in the elderly, possibly indicating reduced receptor sensitivity to vitamin K_1.

A pharmacokinetic explanation is unlikely since warfarin clearance seems not to be affected. While the elimination half-life increases 20%, the volume of distribution also increases 20%; hence total body clearance remains unchanged.

COMPLIANCE BY THE ELDERLY

In chronic diseases for which proven efficacious drug therapy exists, compliance with the treatment regimen is the major determinant of outcome. However, most studies of the influence of age on compliance (including the best ones) do not find any association of age and decreasing compliance. There is even some evidence that noncompliance protects some ambulatory geriatric patients from digoxin toxicity! The study summarized in Table 69–7 indicates that, barring dementia or physical inability to take medications, elderly patients take essential drugs and wisely exercise their free choice with respect to drugs with questionable indications or that provide insufficient symptomatic relief.

TABLE 69–7 Influence of the Type of Drug on Compliance by the Elderly

Drug	Percent Compliance
Drugs for specific indications	
Antibiotics	95
Digitalis	90
Insulin	84
Diuretics	83
Antihypertensives	75
Symptomatic drugs	
Spasmolytics	55
Psychotropics	45
Analgesics	21

n = 217; mean age = 70 years.
Data from Hemminki E, Heikkila J. Scand J Soc Med 1975; 3:87–92.

SUMMARY OF PRINCIPLES OF DRUG PRESCRIBING IN THE ELDERLY

Is Drug Therapy Required?

Many diseases from which the elderly suffer do not respond to drug treatment; use only those drugs that the patient really needs.

Drug regimens should be reviewed regularly so that unnecessary drugs are discontinued.

Be aware that drugs may cause illness.

Choice of Appropriate Drug and Preparation

Is a particular drug that is satisfactory for the younger patient suitable for the elderly? For example, is there increased likelihood of side effects?

Which preparation should be used? Consider dosage form (*e.g.*, syrup, effervescent tablet, or suppository instead of capsule or tablet); its size, shape, and color.

Dose and Dosage Regimen

In general, use smaller doses than are usually given to younger adults. For example, the initial doses of CNS-active drugs should be about 50% of the dose appropriate to younger patients. The dose can be increased thereafter on the basis of response.

Medication Instructions

Teach the patient to understand the prescribed drugs, especially their relative importance to well-being and their correct use and administration.

Drugs prescribed should be clearly labelled in large print and packaged in readily opened containers (instruction to pharmacist).

Supervision of therapy may sometimes be desirable or necessary, *e.g.*, by a responsible and interested neighbor, relative or friend, or a community nurse.

SUGGESTED READING

Crooks J. Rational therapeutics in the elderly. J Chron Dis 1983; 36:59–65.

Drug taking among the elderly. U.S. Department of Health and Human Services. DHHS Publication No. (ADM)83–1229.

Drugs and the elderly [Proceedings of symposium]. J Chron Dis 1983; 36:1–143.

Greenblatt DJ, Sellers EM, Shader RI. Drug disposition in old age. N Engl J Med 1982; 306:1081–1088.

Hershey LA. Avoiding adverse drug reactions in the elderly. Mt Sinai J Med (NY) 1988; 55:244–250.

Jenike MA. Psychoactive drugs in the elderly: antipsychotics and anxiolytics. Geriatrics 1988; 43:53–65.

Sellers EM, Bendayan R. Pharmacokinetics of psychotropic drugs in selected patient populations. In: Meltzer HY, ed. Psychopharmacology: the third generation of progress. New York: Raven Press, 1987:1397–1406.

Stewart RB, May FE, Hale WE, Marks RG. Psychotropic drug use in an ambulatory elderly population. Gerontology 1982; 18:328–335.

Thompson TL, Moran MG, Nies AL. Psychotropic drug use in the elderly. N Engl J Med 1983; 308:134–138(part I) and 194–199(part II).

Chapter 70

Sources of Variation in Drug Response

H. Kalant

In all textbooks of pharmacology, medicine, and therapeutics, recommended dosages of drugs are given in absolute amounts (*e.g.*, 10 mg three times daily) or, less frequently, in amounts relative to body weight (*e.g.*, 1 mg/kg). Such dosages are essentially statistical statements, because they are based on extensive clinical observations indicating that the recommended dosage will, in **most** patients, on **most** occasions, produce the desired therapeutic effect with an **acceptably** low risk of toxicity.

Like all statistical statements, dosage recommendations represent mean values, and imply that some individuals will require more than the mean and some will require less. This chapter deals with the following basic question: if an accepted normal dosage of a drug is prescribed, why do some patients show either too much or too little response? The answer to this question is really a composite of the answer to four subsidiary questions:

1. Was the prescribed dosage actually taken by the patient? This is dealt with below under the heading of **compliance**.

2. If it was taken as prescribed, was it properly absorbed and delivered to the systemic circulation? This is considered under **bioavailability**.

3. If absorbed and delivered to the circulation, was the drug distributed normally in the body, in such a way as to achieve the intended concentration and duration at the site(s) of action? This is examined under **pharmacokinetic** sources of variation.

4. If the drug was distributed in the expected way, did the target tissue(s) respond to it in the usual manner? This is considered under **pharmacodynamic** sources of variation.

COMPLIANCE

Most patients probably do intend to follow their physicians' instructions about prescribed medication, because most prescriptions are filled promptly. One study showed that 97% of the prescriptions written by physicians were filled within five days. If the patients did not intend to take the drugs, it is unlikely that they would go to the trouble and expense of having the prescriptions filled at a pharmacy. However, other studies have found that actual compliance with the physician's instructions is very variable: for short-term preventive medication (*i.e.*, medication intended to prevent the development of symptoms rather than to treat existing ones) the compliance rate was found to be about 80%. For long-term preventive medication (*e.g.*, for the treatment of asymptomatic hypertension), compliance was only 40%.

In efforts to examine the causes of such low compliance, investigators have assessed the possible contributions of many individual factors that might conceivably affect the patient's understanding of the physician's instructions, and the willingness or determination to follow them. A variety of **demographic factors** such as age, sex, socioeconomic level, educational level, and ethnic background do not appear to exert any statistically significant effect on the degree of compliance. There is also no significant correlation with the **specific disease** for which the medication is prescribed, except for some psychiatric illnesses, such as schizophrenia, in which the disease itself may interfere with the patient's attention to, or comprehension of, the physician's explanations, or may give rise to negative responses, apathy, or inertia. In such cases, responsibility for following the prescribed dosage schedule should probably be assigned to a family member, friend, or guardian of the patient.

The degree of **complexity** and **inconvenience** of the treatment schedule can have an important effect in decreasing compliance. The larger the number of different drugs the patient must take, the poorer is the compliance, especially if the various drugs are to be taken at different times of the day and different numbers of times each day. This may be one reason for the marketing of pharmaceutical mixtures, in which a single tablet or capsule contains fixed proportions of two or more drugs that are frequently prescribed together for patients with certain illnesses. Among the very numerous examples are mixtures of a thiazide diuretic with a hypotensive agent (for hypertension), of an atropine-like anticholinergic agent with a sedative (for peptic ulcer), and of a glucocorticoid with a β-adrenergic agonist (for bronchial asthma). It is possible that compliance is improved by such mixtures, since only a single dosage instruction has to be remembered. However, the serious disadvantage is the loss of therapeutic flexibility, since the dosages of the individual constituents of the mixture can not be separately adjusted according to the patient's needs and responses.

In contrast, several factors contribute significantly to improved compliance. One is the **continuity and ease of contact with the physician**. The longer the patient has known and trusted the physician, and the greater the convenience and promptness of scheduling of follow-up visits, the better is the physician's opportunity to remind the patient about the importance of the drugs and to strengthen the patient's motivation to use them. Closely related to this factor is the **patient's perception of the seriousness of the disease** and of the importance and efficacy of the drug therapy, both of which tend to improve compliance. In contrast, medications or treatment schedules with a high incidence of unpleasant side effects generally give rise to poor compliance.

An illustrative case. Noncompliance is a problem of particular importance for patients with arterial hypertension. On the one hand, high blood pressure *per se* does not cause symptoms in the majority of patients. On the other hand, the adverse effects of antihypertensive drugs may cause some patients to feel miserable. It is not surprising, therefore, that patients who feel quite fit frequently fail to comply with physicians' recommendations to take drugs that aim to prevent cerebral, cardiac, or renal consequences of hypertension that may occur at some unknown time in the future. Unfortunately, physicians only rarely obtain exact information on how accurately patients follow their prescriptions. In most cases, measurement of blood or urine levels of antihypertensive drugs is neither feasible nor practical to detect noncompliant patients. A study in Hamilton, Ontario [Lancet 1975;

I:1205–1207 and Lancet 1976; I:1265–1268] on improvement of compliance in hypertension brought interesting results. Of 230 hypertensive steel workers 38 were identified as noncompliant with instructions on medication. Twenty of these were placed on an experimental protocol for six months. Even when these men had more opportunity to see the doctor, for instance during working hours, or when they received instruction about the nature of hypertension, most of them remained noncompliant and their blood pressure remained elevated. However, when the patients were taught to measure their own blood pressures, asked to chart their own pressure readings and pill taking, and taught how to tailor pill taking to their daily habits, and when these manoeuvres were reinforced with supervision every two weeks, the compliance increased by 21% and the control of their blood pressures improved significantly (Fig. 70–1). This study demonstrated that compliance with medication instructions can be improved in hypertensive patients by the use of proper methods.

Important measures to assure compliance in long-term antihypertensive therapy include simplified dosage schedules, use of long-acting rather than short-acting drugs, choosing drugs with minimal side effects, and assuring continuous supervision of the patient. In addition, patients should be thoroughly familiarized with the importance of taking prescribed drugs regularly in order to prevent the serious consequences of high blood pressure. The physician can help to monitor compliance by asking patients to bring their medication bottles with them when they come for checkups. Comparison of the number of tablets or capsules prescribed and the number remaining will help to identify patients who are not taking the drugs regularly.

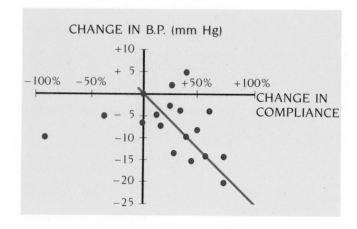

Figure 70–1   Effect of improved compliance, due to combined strategies, on improvement in blood pressure. (From Haynes RB *et al.* 1976.)

BIOAVAILABILITY

The concept of bioavailability, methods of measuring it, and the clinical significance of bioavailability are all covered in detail in Chapter 5. Therefore the topic is mentioned only briefly here, as one potentially important source of variation in drug response.

As described in Chapter 5, the term "bioavailability" refers to the fraction of an administered dose (by any route other than intravenous) that is absorbed and reaches the systemic circulation. It is most commonly measured by determining the area under the concentration-time curve after that dose and expressing it as a percentage of the corresponding area after intravenous injection of the same dose. This percentage can be reduced, for the same preparation of the same drug, by a variety of physiologic and pathologic factors in the gastrointestinal tract and liver. For example, hypermotility, diarrhea, steatorrhea, biliary obstruction, reduced gastrointestinal blood flow, or induction of hepatic drug uptake and biotransformation (*see* Chapter 4) can all reduce the fraction of an oral dose that finally reaches the systemic circulation and hence reduce the drug effect. In contrast, liver disease, especially in cases that produce intrahepatic or extrahepatic shunts (*see* Chapter 62), may result in an unusually large fraction of the dose reaching the circulation and producing an unexpectedly large effect.

Independently of the patient, however, bioavailability may vary because of differences in the formulation of the tablet, capsule, or other preparation, leading to differences in the rate and completeness of release of the active drug into solution in the gastrointestinal fluids. Dissolution is a necessary first step before the drug can be absorbed. If it does not occur rapidly enough, the undissolved part of the dose may be lost in the feces. For this reason, an overly compact tablet may show lower bioavailability than the same dose of the same drug given as a solution (Fig. 70–2). Different companies marketing the same drug may use different tablet formulations, which may differ significantly in disintegration rate and uniformity. "Brand name" drugs are often better formulated than so-called "generic" drugs, giving better and more uniform bioavailability. However, this is not always the case (Fig. 70–3), and the physician must be aware of potential differences of this type when evaluating different products in clinical practice.

PHARMACOKINETIC VARIATION

Apart from variations in drug absorption and bioavailability mentioned above, other important pharmacokinetic factors contributing to variation in drug response are differences in drug distribution, biotransformation,

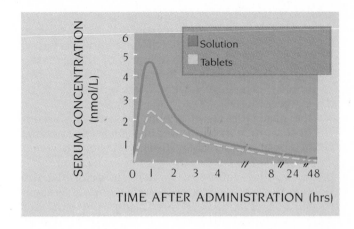

Figure 70–2 Time course of serum digoxin concentration after oral administration of 0.75 mg as an aqueous solution and as tablets.

and elimination. Some of the main sources of **variation in drug biotransformation** are reviewed in Chapter 4, in the sections on Enzyme Induction and on Sources of Variation in Drug Biotransformation. Genetically determined alterations in biotransformation are discussed in Chapter 12. The effects of liver disease on drug biotransformation and elimination are covered in some detail in Chapter 62.

The potential magnitude of these variations is illustrated by the following examples:

- in a group of geriatric inpatients, the mean plasma half-life of antipyrine was 45% greater and that of phenylbutazone was 29% greater than in young controls;

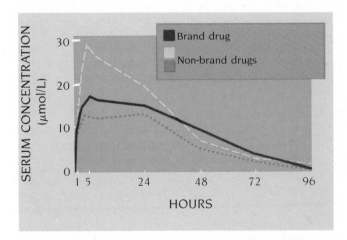

Figure 70–3 Bioavailability of different preparations of phenytoin following oral administration of 500 mg doses.

- absorption of a 400 mg oral dose of mecillinam was only slightly reduced in a group of elderly subjects (65 or more years old) compared to a group of young adults, but the elimination half-life was markedly prolonged (4 hours *vs.* 0.9 hour), and the urinary drug levels were correspondingly lower in the elderly;
- the plasma levels of phenacetin after a standard dose were markedly lower in regular smokers than in nonsmokers (Table 70-1).

The principal causes of variation in **drug distribution** are those associated with early infancy (*see* Chapter 68) and advanced age (*see* Chapter 69). However, drug distribution may also be affected by disease processes at any age. For example, normally the blood–brain barrier may prevent the passage of penicillin and various other antibiotics into the central nervous system. In the presence of inflammatory conditions (meningitis) the permeability of the blood–brain barrier is increased, and these antibiotics may pass much more readily. This improves their therapeutic value, but may also increase the risk of seizures or other toxic effects in the brain. In contrast, when an inflammatory process gives rise to a localized abscess or other walled-off infection (*e.g.*, empyema), systemic antibiotic therapy may be ineffective because the drug will not be distributed into the abscess or other cavity in which the bacteria are growing. For this reason, surgical drainage may be required, together with local application of the antibiotic directly into the affected site.

VARIATION IN REQUIRED DOSAGE IN CHILDREN

A special case of pharmacokinetic variation as a source of variation in drug response is encountered in relation to dosage in children of different ages. It is generally recognized that dosage for adults should take account of body size and body build. Obviously a large person will need more drug than a small person to achieve the same desired concentration in the blood or tissues. This is the basis for giving dosages in relative values such as mg/kg. However, the modifying factor of the percentage of body fat must be taken into account; and most differences of drug response between men and women are due to differences in body composition. An obese person can be expected to require a smaller dose of a highly water-soluble drug than a lean person of the same total body weight in order to avoid excessively high drug concentration in the body water, including the plasma water. Conversely, the obese person will probably require more of a lipid-soluble drug than the lean person to achieve the same plasma level, but the large store of drug in body fat may result in greatly prolonged drug action.

However, the required dose for a given individual is usually more strictly proportional to the metabolic rate, which in turn is more closely proportional to **body surface area** than to body weight. The discrepancy is not large for adults, but it is important for babies and small children, whose surface-to-mass ratio is considerably higher than that of adults. The relationship is described by the equation: $S \text{ (cm}^2) = W^{.425} \text{ (kg)} \times H^{.725} \text{ (cm)} \times 71.8$, but this is obviously impractical for calculating dosages in a physician's office or a patient's home. Therefore, simplified approximations have been made for calculating **children's doses** on the basis of age or surface area.

Calculation of Children's Dose by Age (Young's Rule): Age/(Age + 12) = Fraction of adult dose to be given to child.

Calculation of Children's Dose by Body Surface Area: (1.5 × Weight in kg) + 10 = Percentage of adult dose to be given to child.

Each of these calculations is based on some standard of comparison. Young's rule makes the assumption that a 12-year-old, weighing 35–40 kg, should receive one-half of an adult dose. The surface area rule is based on the assumption that the average adult has about 65 kg of metabolically active mass, and a corresponding surface area of about 1.7 m². Table 70-2 illustrates the relative doses calculated by these two methods. The younger the child, the more clearly superior is the surface area calculation.

PHARMACODYNAMIC VARIATION

Variations in drug response are probably less frequently attributable to changes in responsiveness of the target tissue than to the causes discussed in the preceding sections. Nevertheless, there are some important instances. Examples of **genetically determined abnormalities** of tissue response to drugs, such as malignant hyperthermia and warfarin insensitivity, are described in Chapter 12.

TABLE 70-1 Plasma Levels of Phenacetin in Cigarette Smokers and Nonsmokers at Various Intervals After the Oral Administration of 900 mg of Phenacetin

	Phenacetin in Plasma (µg/mL)			
Hours After Phenacetin Administration:	1	2	3.5	5
Nonsmokers	0.81	2.24	0.39	0.12
Smokers	0.33	0.48	0.09	0.02

TABLE 70–2 Some Comparisons of Age, Weight and Surface Area, and Relative Doses for Children

Age	Weight (kg)	Approximate Surface Area m²	Approximate Surface Area Percent of Adult Area	Relative Drug Dose as Percent of Adult Dose* By Young's Rule	Relative Drug Dose as Percent of Adult Dose* By Body Surface Rule
Newborn	3	0.2	12	0	15
3 months	6	0.3	18	2	19
1 year	10	0.45	26	8	25
6 years	20	0.8	47	33	40
9 years	30	1.0	59	43	55
12 years	40	1.3	76	50	70
14 years	50	1.5	88	54	85
24 years (adult)	65–70	1.7	100	100	100

* For this purpose, the "adult dose" referred to is the average dose in mg for a 65–70 kg person of normal body build.

Other changes in tissue response can be caused by **disease processes**. For example, hyperthyroidism is frequently associated with an increased number of β adrenoceptors, leading to increased sensitivity to the cardiovascular and other effects of noradrenaline and related catecholamines.

Sometimes **drug interactions** will alter pharmacodynamic sensitivity to one or more of the drugs concerned (Chapter 11). Patients with chronic left-ventricular failure, for example, are commonly given a diuretic as well as a cardiac glycoside. Improvement in cardiac output by the digitalis increases renal blood flow, and may therefore improve the urinary response to the diuretic. Conversely, if the diuretic then causes excessive loss of K+ in the urine, the hypokalemia will increase myocardial sensitivity to the digitalis glycoside and increase the risk of arrhythmia (see Chapter 34).

Previous drug history can also affect target tissue sensitivity. This is perhaps seen most clearly in relation to central nervous system depressants such as alcohol (Chapter 25), benzodiazepines and other sedatives and anxiolytics (Chapter 26), and opioid analgesics (Chapter 22). Prolonged or high-dose use of these drugs usually leads to changes in receptor number or sensitivity, or to other compensatory functional changes offsetting the drug effects, and giving rise to **tolerance** (Chapter 67). This not only decreases the response to the drug itself, but may also lead to **cross-tolerance**, i.e., decreased response to other drugs with similar effects. A well-recognized example is the decreased sensitivity to general anaesthetics that is frequently encountered in alcoholics.

CONCLUSIONS

Every aspect of drug absorption, distribution, action, and elimination is subject to greater or lesser degrees of variability, from an infinite range of causes. It is impossible to catalog all the sources of variation in this chapter. The physician prescribing drugs must be aware of their importance, and be prepared to modify the dosage in individual patients, in the light of the most probable factors operating in any given case.

SUGGESTED READING

Haynes RB, Sackett DL, Gibson ES, et al. Improvement of medication compliance in uncontrolled hypertension. Lancet 1976; 1:1265–1268.

Sackett DL, Haynes RB, Gibson ES, et al. Randomized clinical trial of strategies for improving medication compliance in primary hypertension. Lancet 1975; 1:1205–1207.

SPECIAL TOPICS

Chapter 71

PRINCIPLES OF TOXICOLOGY

M.A. McGuigan

Toxicology is the scientific discipline that is concerned with the adverse effects of (chemical) agents on biologic systems. It is a multidisciplinary field of study that draws from a number of related disciplines, including biology, chemistry, immunology, pathology, pharmacology, physiology, and public health. The vastness of the subject and the specialized approaches to its study allow only a general survey in the context of pharmacotoxicologic principles.

Various classification systems are used to designate specialized areas of interest within the field of toxicology. One such classification is based on the purpose or application to which the results of the research are to be applied (Table 71-1). Another classification is on the basis of the organ system primarily affected by the toxic reaction (e.g., cardiovascular, renal, neurotoxicology). Another classification is based on the research methods used to study the toxicity (e.g., biochemical toxicology, behavioral toxicology).

Similarly, the toxic agents themselves are classified in different ways reflecting different special interests.

One system classifies agents according to their relative potential for causing poisoning (Table 71-2). Another system, relating specifically to toxic materials of biologic origin (toxins), is based on the source of the toxin (e.g., snake venoms, spider venoms, bee-sting toxins, plant toxins, marine animal toxins). Still other classifications are by chemistry of the toxic agents (e.g., aromatic amines, halogenated hydrocarbons) or by mechanism of toxic action (e.g., sulfhydryl enzyme inhibitors, methemoglobin producers).

TABLE 71-1 Classification of Toxicology According to Areas of Application

Field of Toxicology	Area of Application
Environmental	Pollution Residues
Economic	Food additives Pesticides
Legal	Forensic Regulatory
Laboratory	Analytic
Biomedical	Human (clinical) Occupational Veterinary

TABLE 71-2 Classification of Toxicants According to Poisoning Potential

Toxicity Rating	Example	LD_{50} (mg/kg)
Slightly toxic (5–15 g/kg)	Ethanol	8,000
Moderately toxic (0.5–5 g/kg)	Sodium chloride	4,000
	Ferrous sulfate	1,500
	Malathion	1,300
	Methanol	1,000
Very toxic (50–500 mg/kg)	Acetylsalicylic acid	300
	Acetaminophen	300
	Diazinon	200
	Phenobarbital	150
	Imipramine	65
Extremely toxic (5–50 mg/kg)	Theophylline	50
	Diphenhydramine	25
Super toxic (<5 mg/kg)	Potassium cyanide	3
	Methotrexate	3
	Strychnine	2
	Nicotine	1
	Digoxin	0.2
	d-Tubocurarine	0.05
	Tetrodotoxin	0.01
	TCDD (dioxin)	0.001
	Botulinum toxin	0.00001

Despite these numerous areas of special attention, the objectives are fundamentally the same in all: to understand the mechanisms by which exogenous substances give rise to toxicity in living subjects, to define the quantitative relationships, to identify factors that increase or decrease susceptibility in individuals or populations, and to develop methods for preventing or treating the toxic reactions.

MODIFIERS OF TOXICITY

In analogy to the sources of variation in drug response (*see* Chapter 70), a number of factors can modify the manifestations of toxicity.

Age

The age of the subject is an important variable. As shown in Table 71–3 with rats of three distinct age groups, the variability in toxic response to three insecticides may depend on age-related variations in relative organ size, maturation of enzyme systems, and distribution patterns of the toxin. For example, relative toxicity of malathion in different species is inversely related to the rate of biotransformation of malathion by the hepatic cytochrome P-450 system (*see* Chapter 4). Since this system is markedly hypofunctional in the neonatal rat, this may explain the much higher toxicity of malathion in the newborn. On the other hand, β-adrenergic receptors are also hypofunctional in the newborn (*see* Chapter 68). Death by overdose of DDT in the rat is usually attributable to ventricular fibrillation, and immaturity of the catecholaminergic response system may protect the newborn against increase in myocardial irritability by DDT.

This age variability is present in human poisonings as well. Young children appear to tolerate better than adults toxic blood concentrations of acetaminophen, digoxin, and theophylline. On the other hand, children manifest more severe signs of toxicity than adults do when poisoned with antihistamines, ethanol, lead, and salicylates.

Route or Site of Administration

The route or site of administration may alter the observed toxicity of a given substance. Routes commonly used for toxicity testing and their influence on the degree of toxicity are shown in Table 71–4. Procaine toxicity depends on the rate and completeness of absorption compared to the rate of hydrolysis by plasma esterases. It is probably the variation in bioavailability that accounts for the differences in the LD_{50} found with different routes of administration. Pentobarbital toxicity is related to peak tissue concentrations. Because pentobarbital is primarily absorbed from the intestinal tract rather than from the stomach, absorption is slow and may result in relatively lower tissue levels, compared to dosing by the parenteral routes.

Duration or Frequency of Exposure

Another aspect to consider when assessing the toxicity of a substance is the duration and frequency of exposure. In toxicology, **acute** exposure is defined as exposure lasting less than 24 hours, during which time the substance may have been administered as a single, repeated, or continuous dose. **Subacute** exposure means exposure for 1 month or less. **Subchronic** exposure means a duration of 1 to 3 months, and **chronic** means more than 3 months. However, these terms are often used loosely; for example, chronic salicylate toxicity is said to develop after use of the drug for more than 2 days.

Different durations of exposure may result in different manifestations of toxicity. For example, acute exposure to benzene results in CNS depression, but chronic exposure may be associated with hematologic malignancy.

Metabolic Activation

Many toxins need to be activated through metabolic processes in order to cause toxicity. Common substances requiring activation include acetaminophen, ethylene glycol, methanol, some organophosphate in-

TABLE 71–3 Effect of Age on Acute Toxicity in Rats

Age	Malathion	DDT	Dieldrin
Newborn	+++	+	+
Preweaning	++	++	+++
Adult	+	+++	++

+, ++, +++: Increasing degrees of toxicity.

TABLE 71–4 Effect of Route of Administration on LD_{50} in Rats, Relative to Intravenous Injection

Route	Procaine	Isoniazid	Pentobarbital
Intravenous	1.0	1.0	1.0
Intraperitoneal	5.0	0.9	1.6
Intramuscular	14.0	0.9	1.5
Subcutaneous	18.0	1.0	1.6
Oral	11.0	0.9	3.5

secticides, and the herbicide paraquat. The site of activation most commonly is the liver, but other organs (*e.g.*, lung, kidney) may also produce toxic metabolites.

Nutrition

The role of nutrition in toxicology is complex but must be considered when evaluating the toxicity of a given substance. Variability in nutrition may affect the toxic response through alterations in absorption, distribution, biotransformation, and excretion of drugs and chemicals.

The presence of food in the stomach may enhance the absorption of some drugs (*e.g.*, beta-blockers, hydralazine, diazepam, lithium, carbamazepine) but may reduce the absorption of others (*e.g.*, penicillins, isoniazid, rifampin). Malnutrition appears to reduce the absorption of tetracyclines and rifampin.

The biotransformation of drugs and chemicals is affected by nutrition in various ways. Rats that were fasted for 24 hours had a decreased rate of glucuronidation of 7-hydroxycoumarin, which returned to normal after a glucose infusion. Rats fed a diet low in polyunsaturated fats and high in saturated fats have lower than normal activity of cytosolic glutathione transferase. Animals fed a low-fat high-protein diet had lower than normal elimination half-lives for antipyrine and theophylline, suggesting that substituting dietary protein for fat may accelerate some drug transformations. On the other hand, children with kwashiorkor appear to have delayed biotransformation of tetrachloroethylene, which has led to the development of toxicity from this substance when it was used as an antiparasitic agent.

DRUG-RESPONSE RELATIONSHIPS

When investigating the adverse effects of an agent on a biologic system, the toxicologist must determine the relationship between the dose and the response. The dose-response concept is defined as a correlative relationship between exposure and effect (*see* Chapter 8). Three important assumptions are implicit in this definition: (1) the observed response is, in fact, due to the chemical administered; (2) the degree of response is related to the magnitude of the dose; and (3) the response in question is precisely defined and quantifiable.

An important dose-response parameter is the **threshold dose**, *i.e.*, the lowest dose that evokes a stated all-or-none response. How the response is defined will influence the determination of the threshold dose. For example, for salicylate the threshold dose that causes gastrointestinal bleeding (1–2 tablets of ASA in an adult) is different from that which results in tinnitus (20–30 tablets), or that which is associated with systemic acidosis (40–50 tablets).

Responses develop over a period of time, so it is important to establish a fixed observation period. Some toxic effects develop quickly and are reversible (*e.g.*, inebriation and acidosis due to methanol poisoning), while others develop over several days and are irreversible (*e.g.*, blindness resulting from methanol poisoning).

Another commonly determined dose-response function, which is less susceptible to the above assumptions, is the LD_{50} (the dose causing the death of 50% of the exposed test animals; *see* Chapter 8).

A typical dose-response curve is shown in Figure 71–1 and explained in detail in Chapter 8. The dose (*e.g.*, mg/kg) is plotted on a logarithmic scale along the horizontal axis, and the response on an arithmetic scale along the vertical axis. The dose-response curves for "effective dose," "toxic dose," and "lethal dose" are generally independent of each other. Parallel dose-response curves for two substances indicate that the agents have different LD_{50} values, but that this difference is proportional over the whole scale of responses. On the other hand, intersecting dose-response curves of two substances may give one substance a lower LD_5 but a higher LD_{50}, analogous to the principle of "certain safety factor" in Chapter 8. The "potency" of a toxin is defined by the position of its dose-response curve along the "dose" axis. Thus, a substance with an LD_{50} of 8 g/kg is less potent than one with an LD_{50} of 5 g/kg.

PREDICTIVE TOXICOLOGY

Predictive toxicology assesses the risks (or evaluates the hazards) associated with a situation in which the toxic agent, the subject, and the exposure conditions are defined. The difficulties associated with risk or hazard assessment are compounded by many variables, including the interactions of several agents, the changes in subject population, and differing exposure conditions.

Two concepts are particularly important in predictive toxicology: the "**lowest observed effect level**" (LOEL) and the "**no observed effect level**" (NOEL). Increasingly sophisticated analytic techniques have steadily lowered the limits of detection and quantitation for an increasing number of chemicals. Measurable amounts of metals, aflatoxins, dioxins, pesticide residues, and chlorinated hydrocarbons are now found where none were found before, perhaps only because our ability to detect and measure them has improved. Similarly, the degree to which we can detect and observe an effect also depends on the sensitivity of the tests. For example, acceptable levels of lead in the blood of young children have dropped steadily: 40 mg/dL in 1974, 30 mg/dL in 1978, and 25 mg/dL in 1985. This reduction in acceptable blood concentrations has occurred as a result of the documentation of subtle defects by complex, sensitive neuropsychological tests.

As can be seen in the dose-response curve in Figure 71–1, the curve does not reach either axis. The difficulty at the low ends of the scales lies in extrapolating, for predictive purposes, from high-dose, high-frequency responses to low-dose, low-frequency response. Different approaches in the area of risk assessment are illustrated in Figure 71–2. Once an acceptable risk is defined, the ''virtually safe dose'' may cover a range of doses depending on the nature of the dose-response curve at the low ends of the scales. Those who believe that very low levels of chemicals in the environment pose significant risks may support the supralinearity concept. Because of the imprecision implicit in the low end of the scale, arbitrary safety factors may be used. For example, when setting a virtually safe dose of a chemical for which good human data and experience of predictive value are available, the NOEL determined in animals may be reduced by a safety factor of 10 for humans; in the absence of human data, however, the NOEL in animals might have to be reduced by a safety factor of 1000 to be virtually safe in humans.

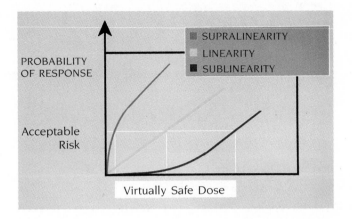

Figure 71–2 Three approaches to risk assessment.

In addition to toxicologic data, other factors may need to be considered in establishing acceptable risk levels. A chemical's beneficial effects (in terms of economics, employment, standard of living, quality of life, taxes generated) must be weighed against its known detrimental effects (health effects, loss of environmental resources, loss of work, law suits). Toxicologic risk assessment, therefore, is concerned with promoting the safety of the individual without simultaneously reducing the benefits to contemporary society.

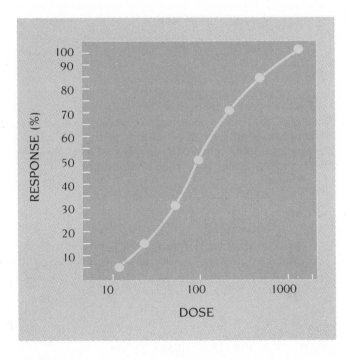

Figure 71–1 Features of the dose-response curve (*see also* Chapter 8).

SUGGESTED READING

Clayson DB, Krewski D, Munro I, eds. Toxicological risk assessment. Vols I and 2. Boca Raton: CRC Press, 1985.

Klaassen CD, Amden MO, Doull J, eds. Casarett and Doull's toxicology. The basic science of poisons. 3rd ed. New York: Macmillan, 1986.

Lu FC. Basic toxicology. New York: Hemisphere Publishing Corp, 1985.

Marquis J, ed. A guide to general toxicology. 2nd ed. Karger Cont Educ Ser. Vol 5. Basel: Karger, 1989.

SPECIAL TOPICS

Chapter 72

POISONS AND ANTIDOTES

M.A. McGuigan

Poisonings occur commonly. Over the past decade, the number of poisonings reported in Canada has increased steadily. There were 88,834 cases reported in 1985. The morbidity and mortality figures for all cases of drug and non-drug poisonings are in Table 72–1. "Drugs" include prescription (40% of all drug-related poisonings), nonprescription, and illicit drugs. Central nervous system drugs account for one-third of all drug poisonings, dermatologic drugs for 11%, antihistamines for 7%, and vitamins for 6%. The most frequently reported non-drug categories are household products (20%), plants (16%), cosmetics (12%), gases (8%), and pesticides (7.5%). Single categories associated with the highest mortality are psychotherapeutic drugs (14.5% of all deaths), gases (9.3%), cardiovascular drugs (7.8%), and sedative-hypnotic drugs (4.5%).

Poisonings affect people of all ages. In 1985, 53,392 cases of poisoning involved children under 5 years of age; 7,111 cases were in children aged 5–14 years; and the adult age group (older than 14 years) accounted for 22,301 cases.

Although most cases of poisoning are classified as inadvertent or accidental, virtually all ingestions by individuals over 10 years of age involve an intentional component.

The specific principles discussed in this chapter will aid in the treatment of a poisoning. In addition, rigorous appropriate supportive care is essential for successful treatment of a poisoned patient.

DEFINITIONS

Poison

A poison may be defined as "any substance which ... by its chemical action may cause damage to structure or disturbance of function." Based on this definition, poisons include all types of drugs as well as other synthetic and naturally occurring compounds.

Antidote

An antidote may be defined as "a remedy used for counteracting a poison." Antidotal therapy includes all varieties of therapeutic manoeuvres used to prevent, minimize, or reverse the effects of a toxin.

SOURCES OF INFORMATION

It has been recognized that optimal management of a poisoning requires personnel with experience and expertise. This awareness is resulting in the formation, in most countries, of a few large "regional" poison information centres and a consequent decrease in the number of smaller centres. These larger centres are staffed by full-time personnel who are involved with a large number and variety of poisoning cases. Available resources include data bases containing informa-

TABLE 72–1 Morbidity and Mortality Due to Poisonings in Canada—1985

	Cases	Hospitalizations	Deaths
Drugs*	42,265	21,468	333
Other agents	46,569	14,544	66
Totals	88,834	36,012	399

* Including prescription, over-the-counter, and illicit drugs.

tion on product ingredients, medically-related toxicologic information, and current information on the evaluation and treatment of poisonings. Regional poison information centres are the single best source for accurate up-to-date information on poisonings.

PRINCIPLES OF TREATMENT OF POISONINGS

In order to treat poisonings optimally, the physician must have a clear understanding of some basic principles, and therapy should be aimed at specific goals. Absorption of the toxin should be minimized. The effects of the toxin that has been absorbed should be antagonized. Metabolic processes that reduce the overall toxicity should be encouraged, while biotransformation to toxic products should be inhibited. Elimination of the toxin from the body should be enhanced. Finally, good clinical medical care of the patient must be provided.

Initial treatment should be directed towards decreasing the absorption of a poison. Once the poison is absorbed into the body and distributed to the appropriate sites, termination of its effects usually involves administration of pharmacologic agents or biotransformation and excretion from the body. This concept is depicted in Figure 72–1.

MODIFICATION OF ABSORPTION AND DISTRIBUTION

Measures for Decreasing Absorption of Toxins

The most common route by which toxins are absorbed into the body is the gastrointestinal tract, followed in decreasing frequency by the pulmonary system and the skin. Other routes include parenteral (intravenous, intramuscular, subcutaneous), rectal, and vaginal. The route of absorption dictates the initial therapy.

Oral Route

Therapeutic interventions affecting absorption of an ingested material include removing the unabsorbed toxins from the stomach and preventing absorption of remaining substances.

Emesis. Induced vomiting is the preferred means of removing most toxins from the stomach, and ipecac syrup is the drug of choice. Ipecac is a plant material containing a mixture of alkaloids, of which cephaeline and emetine are the major ones. It induces emesis through stimulation of the chemoreceptor trigger zone and through local irritation of the gastrointestinal tract. The latency period for the induction of emesis by ipecac ranges from 5 to 20 minutes, and a single dose of ipecac produces vomiting in approximately 85% of patients.

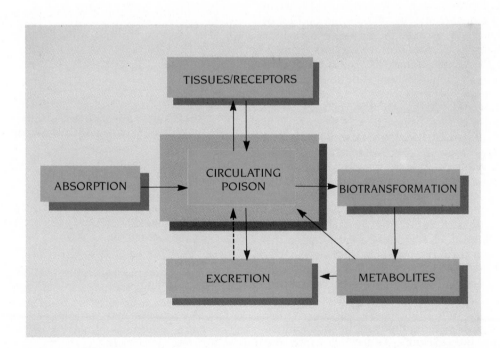

Figure 72–1 Kinetics of poisoning. Note that the various steps are qualitatively identical with those of drug kinetics.

Contraindications to the administration of ipecac include the presence of coma or convulsions, and the ingestion of a caustic (corrosive) substance. Ipecac should be used with discretion in patients who have ingested a substance that may result in the rapid onset of coma or convulsions. In patients who have ingested a petroleum hydrocarbon product (*e.g.*, kerosene) emesis may lead to a severe aspiration pneumonitis; in such patients, therefore, ipecac syrup should be used only after very careful consideration. Other relative contraindications to the use of ipecac include age less than 9 months (no clinical data available), ingestion of a nontoxic quantity of the poison, and prior administration of activated charcoal (which adsorbs ipecac and prevents its pharmacologic action).

The ingestion of antiemetic drugs (*e.g.*, phenothiazines) does not affect the efficacy with which ipecac induces vomiting. Passage of the toxin through the pylorus, or systemic absorption of toxin, reduces considerably the value of emesis, so that ipecac is not beneficial if given more than 4 hours after ingestion of the poison.

Another pharmacologic emetic is apomorphine. Subcutaneous administration of apomorphine produces forceful vomiting within five minutes, but because it also causes central nervous system and respiratory depression, the clinical usefulness of apomorphine is limited.

Gastric lavage. Intubation and lavage is currently the only other acceptable technique used to empty the stomach, but it often is less effective than ipecac-induced emesis in removing solid material. For example, in an animal study, when gastric emptying was carried out 1 hour after the ingestion of a test dose of sodium salicylate tablets, lavage removed an average of 13% while ipecac-induced emesis removed an average of 39% of the ingested salicylate. Lavage should be reserved for times when emesis is contraindicated (coma, convulsions) or when ipecac fails to induce vomiting, but care must be taken to prevent tracheal aspiration of fluids used in the lavage.

Activated charcoal. Activated charcoal (AC), when administered after emesis or lavage, will bind residual toxin within the lumen of the gastrointestinal tract and markedly reduce absorption. Activated charcoal is an inert, nonabsorbable, odorless, tasteless, fine black powder that has a high adsorptive capacity (Table 72–2). Activated charcoal should be mixed with water (25 g charcoal per 100 mL water) and administered orally or by nasogastric tube. For optimal binding, a charcoal:toxin ratio of 10:1 should be used. When the ingested dose of a toxin is a matter of speculation, the recommended dose of charcoal is 0.5–1 g/kg of body weight. The success with which activated charcoal prevents absorption of a substance depends not only on the substance itself (*see* Table 72–2), but also on the time between ingestion and administration of charcoal. As an example, the following figures illustrate the progressive decrease in efficacy against ASA with increasing delay in administration of activated charcoal:

Time of AC relative to drug ingestion	Drug adsorbed %
Simultaneous	59
+ 30 minutes	48
+ 60 minutes	21
+180 minutes	9

When the gastrointestinal absorption of a drug is delayed (ingested in large quantity or in a sustained-release formulation), the beneficial effects from the use of activated charcoal will be more significant.

Other adsorbants (cholestyramine, *etc.*) have been evaluated as binding agents, but because they effectively bind only a limited number of toxins, they are not generally useful.

"Local" antidotes. These are compounds that change the ionic form or alter the solubility of the toxin and thus reduce its toxicity. Recommended ones include sodium bicarbonate for iron ingestion (the resulting ferric carbonate is less irritating to the gastrointestinal tract and less well absorbed), and calcium (milk) for fluoride ingestion. Weak acids and alkalis should not be used to neutralize strong alkalis or acids, respectively, because temperatures of up to 100°C may occur during neutralization, which will contribute to tissue damage. (Just flushing with copious amounts of water will dilute and frequently remove acids without causing additional damage.)

Pulmonary Route

Reduction of absorption of toxic gases is accomplished simply by removing the victim from the site of exposure.

TABLE 72–2 Adsorptive Capacity of Activated Charcoal (AC) *in Vitro*

Substance	Adsorptive Capacity (g/100 g AC)
Mercuric chloride	180
Imipramine	125
Sulfanilamide	100
Strychnine nitrate	95
Nicotine	70
Barbital	70
Chlorpromazine HCl	36
Phenobarbital	30–35
Malathion (pH 1.0)	31
ASA (pH 1.0)	28
Ferrous sulfate	17
Potassium cyanide	3.5

From Hayden JW, Comstock EG. Clin Toxicol 1975; 8:515–533.

Dermal Route

Examples of toxins that are readily absorbed through the unbroken skin are given in Table 72–3.

Minimizing absorption through the skin requires removal of contaminated clothing and gentle washing of the skin with mild soap and cool water. Abrasion of the skin (*i.e.*, removing the keratin barrier) or use of hot water (*i.e.*, increasing circulation) may enhance absorption of the toxin.

Parenteral Route

Application of constricting bands or wraps proximal to the site of injection, combined with restriction of movement of the limb, may retard the systemic absorption of subcutaneously administered toxins. This is applicable primarily to snake bites.

Techniques for Altering Distribution of Toxins

The approaches to the therapy of a poisoning involve interruption of gastrointestinal recirculation of the substance and limitation of distribution of the toxin within the body.

Recirculation

Some lipid-soluble drugs (*e.g.*, phenobarbital, phencyclidine, tricyclic antidepressants) have long plasma half-lives perhaps in part because they undergo significant recirculation between the gastrointestinal tract and the portal blood. Repeated oral administration of activated charcoal will bind these drugs within the gut lumen, cause them to be excreted in the feces, and thus enhance their clearance from the body. For example, administration of repeated oral doses of activated charcoal has reduced the serum half-life of phenobarbital from 110 hours to 45 hours and has shortened the duration of phenobarbital-induced coma.

Some other drugs in which clearance from the body has been affected by repeated oral administration of activated charcoal are carbamazepine, digoxin, methotrexate, salicylates, theophylline, and thyroxine.

Limited Distribution

The distribution of some drugs is partially pH-dependent. Weak acids are less ionized as pH decreases and will cross membrane barriers more easily. The acidemia (*e.g.*, plasma pH = 7.0) that may occur in a salicylate poisoning affects the salicylate ion in this way, facilitating the entry of salicylate ($pK_a = 3.2$) into the central nervous system. Normalizing the plasma pH to 7.4 reduces the amount of nonionized salicylate, thus limiting the distribution of this particular toxin into cells.

In the same way, lowering the pH will tend to increase the proportion of the ionized forms of weak

TABLE 72–3 Toxins Absorbed Through Unbroken Skin

Nerve gas (sarin)
Carbon tetrachloride
Parathion
Phenols
Strychnine
Nicotine
Tetraethyl lead

bases, and thus hinder their diffusion. For example, the nonionized form of morphine can diffuse from the blood into the lumen of the stomach, where gastric acid ionizes it and prevents back-diffusion into the blood. Therefore gastric lavage, or activated charcoal, can help to remove morphine even after it has been administered parenterally (*see* Chapter 2).

PHARMACOLOGIC MEASURES FOR TERMINATING EFFECTS: ANTIDOTAL THERAPY

The classic antidotes for specific poisons are considered in this section. The antidotes are classified by the mechanism of action.

Competitive Antagonism

Naloxone antagonizes the sedation, respiratory depression, and miosis associated with an overdose of a morphine-like analgesic by reversibly competing with the opioid for μ and κ opioid receptors in the brain and spinal cord. A critical concentration of naloxone must be achieved and maintained at the receptor site in order for a reversal of narcotic effects to occur and persist.

Naloxone often is administered as an intravenous bolus, and the effects it produces are often of brief duration. This occurs for two reasons: (1) The relatively high central nervous system concentration of naloxone produced by the combination of bolus injection and high blood flow to the brain is rapidly reduced through redistribution of the drug. (2) The half-life of naloxone is short, approximately 30 minutes.

In the clinical setting, the brevity of action of naloxone may be countered by repeated dosing or by continuous infusion of the drug.

Noncompetitive Antagonism

Atropine therapy for carbamate insecticide poisoning is an example of noncompetitive antagonism. In other words, the antagonist (atropine) competes with the **effects** of the agonist (insecticide), not against receptor binding of the agonist itself.

Carbamate insecticides produce clinical effects by inhibiting the enzyme acetylcholinesterase. Because acetylcholine is no longer being degraded, its concentration in the nerve synapse increases, producing excessive and persistent stimulation. Clinically, this is a picture of acetylcholine excess or a "cholinergic syndrome." A sufficiently high concentration of atropine will inhibit the action of acetylcholine on the postsynaptic membrane and will reverse the clinical effects (*see* Chapter 15). Thus, atropine competes with the effect of the insecticide, but does nothing against the insecticide itself.

Chemical Neutralization

Cyanide poisoning occurs primarily in the industrial setting, but also in conjunction with therapeutic use of nitroprusside or amygdalin (a prussic acid glycoside), which can be hydrolysed to yield free cyanide. Cyanide combines strongly with ferric iron in various proteins, including cytochrome oxidase, and prevents oxidative metabolism in the mitochondria of all tissues (Equation 1; *see also* Chapter 10).

1. $CN^- + cytox\text{-}Fe^{3+} \rightleftarrows cytox\text{-}FeCN$

2. $NaNO_2 + (O) + HbFe^{2+} \rightarrow HbFe^{3+} + NaNO_3$
    $HbFe^{3+} + cytox\text{-}FeCN \rightleftarrows HbFeCN + cytox\text{-}Fe^{3+}$

3. $HbFeCN + Na_2S_2O_3 \rightleftarrows HbFe^{3+} + Na_2SO_3 + SCN^-$

In the treatment of acute cyanide poisoning, the administration of sodium nitrite creates a large circulating pool of ferric iron (methemoglobin), which attracts the cyanide ion away from the cytochrome oxidase, permitting the resumption of oxidative metabolism (Equation 2).

The next step in therapy is to supply the mitochondrial enzyme (rhodanese or sulfur transferase) that normally detoxifies cyanide, with its substrate (sodium thiosulfate), so that the enzyme can "neutralize" the cyanide ion by converting it to the nontoxic thiocyanate ion (Equation 3).

Metabolic Inhibition

Methanol itself is of relatively low toxicity, but when it is converted by the enzyme alcohol dehydrogenase to formaldehyde, which is in turn oxidized to formic acid, severe metabolic acidosis (due to the formation of formic, lactic, and α-ketobutyric acids) and blindness (formic acid causes optic nerve demyelination) may result. When ethanol is administered, it competes with methanol for alcohol dehydrogenase, markedly decreas-

ing the rate of oxidation of methanol and the subsequent development of toxicity (*see* Chapter 25). Another compound that is oxidized by alcohol dehydrogenase, with a resulting increase in toxicity, is ethylene glycol, an antifreeze. As with methanol, administration of ethanol prevents the conversion of ethylene glycol to its more toxic metabolites, glycolaldehyde and glycolic acid.

Oxidation-Reduction

Excessive amounts of certain compounds (*e.g.*, benzocaine, nitrites, or phenazopyridine) will oxidize hemoglobin (Fe^{2+}) to methemoglobin (Fe^{3+}), resulting in decreased oxygen delivery by the blood. Administered methylene blue (tetramethylthionine) acts as a cofactor to accelerate the conversion of methemoglobin to hemoglobin by methemoglobin reductase. Within one hour of administration of methylene blue, most of the methemoglobin will be reduced and tissue oxygenation restored.

Chelation

There are several examples of this type of therapy used for the treatment of intoxication with metals. In principle, a chelating agent should be able to bind tightly a specific metal and form a nontoxic chelate that can be excreted from the body. Any chelating agent should be administered as soon as possible following exposure to the toxic metal, because the agents are more efficient at preventing enzyme inhibition by the metal than they are at reactivating the enzyme. It is very difficult to evaluate the benefits of therapeutic regimens for metal poisonings.

Dimercaprol. Dimercaprol (BAL) is used to treat patients with **arsenic poisoning**. BAL (British Anti-Lewisite) is administered to form a chelate with a ratio of two molecules of BAL to one molecule of metal. The 2:1 chelate is more stable and more water-soluble than a 1:1 complex. These chelate complexes are excreted in the urine and bile. BAL increases the urinary excretion of arsenic in the first 24 hours. The magnitude of the increase depends on the "dose" of arsenic and the adequacy of renal function.

Calcium disodium EDTA. Calcium disodium edetate is used as a chelating agent because, although EDTA and Na_2EDTA would chelate many divalent and trivalent metals, they would also chelate calcium. $CaNa_2EDTA$ does not cause hypocalcemia and would chelate metals having a higher affinity for EDTA than calcium does (*e.g.*, lead, zinc). It is now used primarily to treat **lead poisoning**. Following the administration of $CaNa_2EDTA$, lead from soft tissue depots displaces the calcium ion and forms a stable $PbNa_2EDTA$ complex that is excreted in the urine. Urinary lead reaches a maximum 6 hours after administration of

CaNa$_2$EDTA, and excretion is nearly complete by 18 hours. Lead excretion decreases with subsequent doses. A "rest period" is often recommended between courses of therapy to allow for redistribution of the metal within the body.

Deferoxamine. This agent is used to treat **iron poisoning**. Following ingestion of excessive amounts of iron, plasma iron concentrations exceed the binding capacity of transferrin, and free (unbound) iron is distributed into cells where it causes disruption of the mitochondria. Deferoxamine not only binds circulating free iron and enhances its elimination in the urine, but may also remove iron from sites within hepatocytes. Although there are conflicting data on iron excretion, appropriate use of deferoxamine does reduce the mortality rate in acute iron poisoning.

Antigen-Antibody

Serum globulins with specific activity against a given substance have been used in the form of antitoxins (to treat *Clostridium botulinum* poisoning) and antivenins (to treat envenomations from poisonous snakes or spiders). Recently, the development of antigen binding fragments (Fab) derived from specific antidigoxin antibodies has improved the treatment of poisoning from the digitalis glycosides. Patients with life-threatening digoxin poisoning who receive intravenous digoxin antibody fragments demonstrate an immediate decrease in free digoxin serum concentrations; favorable changes in cardiac arrhythmias and reduction of hyperkalemia occur within 30 minutes of administration (*see* Chapter 34).

BIOTRANSFORMATION

Therapeutic interventions in metabolic processes have concentrated on preventing the development or accumulation of toxic metabolites, because there is no safe, effective way to enhance the biotransformation of a toxic substance to nontoxic metabolites rapidly enough to cause a clinically important difference in an acute intoxication. The biotransformation of chemicals occurs primarily in the liver, but it also may occur in the kidneys (acetaminophen, carbon tetrachloride), lungs (paraquat), plasma (succinylcholine), or gastrointestinal wall (oral adrenaline). The transformation products are usually intermediates of decreased toxicity and increased excretability (*see* Chapter 4), but this is not always the case. Many metabolites may be toxicologically active. Examples of compounds that are biotransformed into pharmacologically active or toxic metabolites include imipramine, parathion, methanol, and acetaminophen.

In the case of acetaminophen (N-acetyl-*p*-aminophenol), small amounts of the drug can be conjugated with glucuronic acid or sulfate, but the major route of biotransformation by the hepatic cytochrome P-450 system forms a reactive metabolite. Normally, this metabolite is "detoxified" through combination with glutathione (Fig. 72–2). When an overdose of acetaminophen is taken, glutathione reserves are depleted, the reactive metabolite accumulates, and hepatocyte damage results (*see* Chapters 4 and 62). Treatment of acute intoxication with acetaminophen currently consists of the administration of N-acetylcysteine, which helps to prevent the accumulation of toxic intermediates.

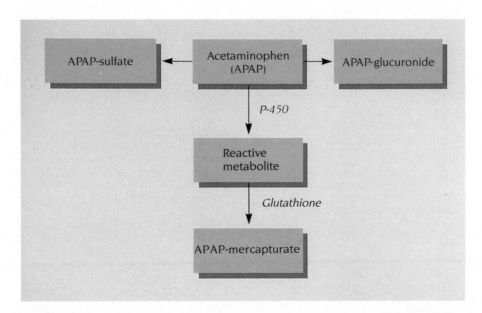

Figure72–2 Acetaminophen metabolism. (APAP = N-acetyl-*p*-aminophenol = acetaminophen.)

EXCRETION

The liver and the kidneys are the major organs responsible for drug elimination. As noted earlier, elimination of toxins can also be accomplished through the gastrointestinal tract by interrupting gastrointestinal recirculation by the use of repeated doses of activated charcoal. Most techniques used for enhancing elimination of toxic substances from the body utilize renal excretion or extracorporeal clearance.

Renal Excretion

Attempts to enhance renal excretion of a substance will be successful only if that substance is excreted in an unchanged or toxic form through the kidneys to a significant degree, *i.e.*, if a substantial portion of the total body clearance of the substance occurs through the kidneys. In order to judge this accurately, it is necessary to know the renal clearance as well as the total body clearance in the toxic or overdose state. There are relatively few substances encountered in clinical poisonings that have a significant renal excretion following an acute overdose. These compounds are listed in Table 72–4. Although the major part of a dose of amphetamines, phencyclidine, or phenobarbital undergoes biotransformation in the liver, significant portions are excreted through the kidneys. Enhanced renal excretion is usually accomplished through fluid diuresis. In other words, enough fluid is administered to produce an increased flow of urine. Often this technique is combined with systemic administration of drugs to alter the pH of the urine ("ionized diuresis"): alkalinization of the urine with sodium bicarbonate or acidification of the urine with ammonium chloride, depending on the drug to be eliminated. By the appropriate raising or lowering of the urine pH, the degree of ionization of acidic and basic drugs, respectively, is increased. Because the ionized drug is less able to cross cell membranes and be reabsorbed, it is excreted. Alkalinization of the urine may increase the excretion of salicylates and phenobarbital, whereas excretion of amphetamines and phencyclidine may be increased by acidifying the urine.

TABLE 72–4   Renally Excreted Substances

Weak Acids	Ions	Weak Bases
Phenobarbital	Bromide⁻	Phencyclidine
Salicylates	Iodide⁻	Quinidine
	Lithium⁺	Amphetamine
	Others	
	Arsenic	

Extracorporeal Clearance

Extracorporeal clearance of toxins may take two forms: dialysis or hemoperfusion.

Dialysis (Peritoneal Dialysis, Hemodialysis)

For dialysis to be effective, the toxin must have certain properties. The dialysing membrane must be permeable to the toxic molecule, and the toxin should equilibrate rapidly between the circulating plasma and the dialysis fluid. The toxin should be removed in significant quantities compared to the total body burden of toxin or to spontaneous clearance. In addition, ideally, the degree of toxicity from the poison should be related to the concentration within the body and the duration of time that this concentration is maintained. If prompt irreversible damage is produced, removal of the remaining toxin by dialysis is not likely to be of great value. From a clinical perspective, dialysis may be considered in severe intoxications (*e.g.*, deep and prolonged coma), ingestion of known lethal doses, or presence of lethal blood concentrations of the toxin. A decreased renal or hepatic clearance, or a deterioration in the clinical state due to the toxin, also constitute indications for dialysis.

Hemodialysis is usually much more effective than peritoneal dialysis.

Hemoperfusion

Hemoperfusion consists of passing blood from a blood vessel over a resin or charcoal column and then back into the circulation, so that the toxin is "bound" to the column. These techniques have essentially the same conditions and criteria for use as dialysis, with the advantage that lipophilic and highly protein-bound drugs are cleared more efficiently.

SUGGESTED READING

Bryson PD. Comprehensive review in toxicology. Rockville, MD: Aspen Publications, 1986.

Dreisbach RN, Robertson WO. Handbook of poisoning. 12th ed. Norwalk, CT: Appleton and Lange, 1987.

Ellenhorn MF, Barceloux DG. Medical toxicology. Diagnosis and treatment of human poisoning. New York: Elsevier, 1988.

Goldfrank LR, Flomenbaum NE, Lewin NA, *et al*, eds. Goldfrank's toxicologic emergencies. 3rd ed. Norwalk, CT: Appleton-Century-Crofts, 1986.

Klaassen CD, Amdur MO, Doull J, eds. Casarett and Doull's toxicology. The basic science of poisons; 3rd ed. New York: Macmillan, 1986.

Chapter 73

DRUG DEVELOPMENT AND REGULATIONS

C.A. Naranjo and E. Janecek

The first documentation of drug use occurred about 4000 years ago in the Babylonian-Assyrian culture and in Egypt. Documents from those times refer to a large number of substances, some pharmacologically active and others inert. The administration of these remedies was often accompanied by incantations indicating that magic and the supernatural played a major role in the conceptualization and treatment of diseases. The preparation of such remedies and the control of their use were usually in the hands of priests who served as exorcists, diviners and healers, and also functioned as the drug regulatory agency.

Medical papers written between 2000 and 1000 B.C. in Egypt contain information on drug formulas and instructions for preparation and use of the remedies. The emphasis on drugs and formulations in these documents suggests that in those times greater attention was paid to the pharmaceutical side of medical care than in Greek times when the emphasis was on the disease process. Hippocrates (4th century B.C., Greece) changed the concept of disease and stressed simplicity of treatment and freedom from the irrational and supernatural. Galen (2nd century A.D.) created a system of pathology and therapy that influenced Western medicine for 1500 years. Galen classified drugs according to Hippocrates' theory of four humors and described a large number of compounds used at the time.

In ancient Greece and in the Roman empire the responsibility for manufacture and use of drugs was still primarily in the hands of physicians, although drug dealers sometimes supplied ready-made medicaments to physicians. The first true pharmacopoeia "Dispensatorium" was issued in Germany in 1546. During the 15th, 16th, and 17th centuries many official and unofficial pharmacopoeias were published, most of them for local use only. The first official standard for a whole country was issued in England in 1618. Cellular pathology, medical biology, bacteriology, and experimental pharmacology originated during the 19th century and laid the basis for drug development as we know it to-

day. Now, most new drugs are developed and produced by large international corporations with headquarters primarily in Switzerland, Germany, and the United States. We have no idea how long it took the ancient Egyptians to develop the formulations for their remedies. Now it takes about 10 years and a cost of about 100 million dollars, from the time a new drug is synthesized to the time when it can be sold commercially!

METHODS OF DEVELOPING NEW DRUGS

Purification of Drugs from Natural Sources

Natural products were once the only source of drugs. Folk cures often have provided clues to plants with important pharmacologic activity. For example, cinchona alkaloids (quinine and quinidine), ephedrine, and *Rauwolfia serpentina* (the active principle of which is the antihypertensive drug reserpine) were all discovered by systematic chemical study of folk remedies, and curare was discovered by similar study of a South American arrowhead poison.

Antibiotics are particularly illustrative of the importance of natural sources. The first step in the identification and development of new antibiotics involves large-scale screening programs in which tens of thousands of samples of soil are assessed systematically for microorganisms with antibacterial or antifungal activity. Cyclosporine, an important immunosuppressant drug, was discovered by a company that required its employees to bring back a sample of soil whenever they travelled to a foreign country. Sometimes the discovery of a drug's activity comes not from a systematic program but from a chance observation, *e.g.*, Fleming's discovery of the antibiotic activity of *Penicillium notatum*. Purification of the culture media and application of modern methods of natural product chemistry are used to isolate, crystallize, and chemically characterize the active ingredients of crude fungal cultures. Antibiotics discovered in this way include streptomycin, chloramphenicol, neomycin, and erythromycin.

The isolation and identification of antileukemic alkaloids in the leaves of the periwinkle plant (*Vinca rosea*) provides another example of the serendipity involved in drug research. Crude preparations of vinca have been used in some parts of the world as antidiabetic agents. Plant extracts were assayed for hypoglycemic activity, but none was found. Some of the experimental animals, however, suffered massive leukopenia, and this effect was used as a bioassay procedure that led to the isolation of an active compound, vinblastine. Routine screening of the crude plant material in an anticancer program revealed activity against experimental leukemia in mice. This antileukemia activity was used as a bioassay procedure, and its use permitted the isolation and purification of over 30 different alkaloids in 3 years. Four, including vinblastine, were found to have antileukemic activity.

Developments in the steroid area are also of interest. Following the discovery in 1949 that cortisone was of value in the treatment of arthritis, intensive industrial competition occurred in the search for an inexpensive way to produce synthetic steroid hormones. After a couple of years of frantic searching, Mexican yams were found to contain a sterol, diosgenin, that could be converted economically to progesterone. The price of progesterone dropped from $80.00 to $1.75 per gram and now is about 15 cents a gram. A *Rhizopus* then was found that could carry out the 11-hydroxylation that was required for production of adrenal cortical hormones from progesterone, and the road was cleared for low-cost adrenal corticosteroids.

Modification of Chemical Structure

"Molecular manipulation" is widely used to obtain new drugs (*see also* Chapter 10). Often this is done to produce a patentable product to compete with one already on the market. There may, however, be more important reasons. They include:

(1) Modification to improve the desired action. For example, hundreds of modifications of the procaine molecule have been tested as local anaesthetics in attempts to produce more stable compounds with longer duration of local anaesthesia.

(2) Modification to alter absorption, distribution, or elimination. Much effort has been expended in attempts to find drug derivatives that will be absorbed effectively when given orally. Work to develop orally active progestational hormones resulted in the production of oral contraceptives.

(3) Modification to improve selectivity of action. For example, conversion of a tertiary nitrogen in atropine to a quaternary nitrogen by adding a methyl group (methatropine) reduces its ability to cross the blood–brain barrier, and thus improves selectivity for peripheral effects.

Drug distribution and hence pharmacologic activity may be markedly influenced by molecular modifications. For example, replacement of oxygen in pentobarbital by a sulfur produces thiopental, and converts the molecule from a moderately long-lasting anaesthetic to an ultra-short-acting one. The reason lies in the extreme lipid solubility of thiopental, which permits it to enter and leave the brain rapidly.

Structural modifications also can influence the length of time a drug is active. Procaine can abolish certain cardiac arrhythmias, but it is an ester and is rapidly hydrolysed by liver and plasma esterases, limiting its value. Simple substitution of the ester group by an amide group gives rise to procainamide, which has a longer duration of action because of greater resistance to hydrolysis.

Substitution to Reduce Cost

Examples include diethylstilbestrol, an inexpensive nonsteroid substitute for natural estrogens, and methadone, introduced during World War II by the Germans who needed a cheap replacement for morphine, which was unavailable to them.

De Novo Invention of New Drugs

Although there are exceptions to the rule (*e.g.*, synthesis of H_2-receptor antagonists such as cimetidine), usually new drugs are not produced as a result of highly rational programs based on complete knowledge of structure–activity relationships. Usually, serendipity and chance observations lead to identification of pharmacologic activity of a specific molecule. In recent years most pharmaceutical companies have developed systematic programs, using animal models with known predictive value, to screen chemical substances for specific pharmacologic activities. For example, several new antidepressants without the anticholinergic side effects of tricyclics have been developed in this fashion, *e.g.*, fluoxetine.

Exploitation of Side Effects of Existing Drugs

The commonest pattern in the development of new drugs is not *de novo* invention, but rather the exploitation of side effects of existing drugs. Astute exploitation of the side effects of sulfonamides (*see* Chapter 10) had led to the development of useful drugs that are not antibacterial agents, but rather, diuretics (the carbonic anhydrase inhibitors and thiazides) and antidiabetic agents (the sulfonylureas).

DRUG LEGISLATION AND REGULATIONS

There is wide cross-cultural variation in drug legislation. In general, the requirements for marketing a new drug are more strict in North America (United States, Canada) than in Europe, Asia, Africa, or Latin America. In recent years, however, there has been a trend everywhere to make the requirements for licencing a new drug more stringent. Several factors influence the drug legislation in various countries. In Canada and the United States, the following groups play a major role: multinational drug companies; nonproprietary drug companies; the federal governments; and the public. In Canada, provincial governments are also involved. Frequently these groups have conflicting goals and needs. Hence the current legislation in Canada represents an attempt, not always successful, by the federal and provincial governments to protect the interest of the public, as well as to provide incentive for drug development. Some characteristics of the drug industry in Canada may be summarized as follows.

The drug industry is dominated by multinational companies, which account for about 92% of the world sales volume at the manufacturer's level. Canada represents approximately 2% of the world market.

Like most foreign-owned industries, the drug industry carries on only limited activities in Canada. Major activities encompass the manufacturing of finished products such as tablets, capsules, liquids, ointments, powders, and injectables. Raw material synthesis, and research and development, are conducted to only a limited degree. Relatively little of the Canadian production is exported; most exportation is done by the foreign parent companies. The industry imports virtually all of its basic chemicals for the manufacture of drugs and also an increasing proportion of finished products. Drug manufacturing is not labor-intensive. In fact, the number of jobs has decreased despite the growth in the production and sales volumes.

The drug industry is relatively highly regulated *via* federal and provincial laws, compared to other industries.

With few exceptions, all "new drugs," discovered since 1960, have been discovered abroad and transferred from the parent to the subsidiary in an almost fully developed form. The innovative record of the drug industry in Canada is poor compared to that of the United States or European countries because so little basic pharmaceutical research is done in Canada. In 1982 only six of the 117 drug companies in Canada were doing basic research!

Annual profits in the drug industry average 12% after tax, based on equity.

Another characteristic is patent protection that in Canada theoretically extends for a 17-year period. However, patent protection is weakened by compulsory licencing. This means that any competitor of a major drug house, after searching the appropriate patents and by filling out an application form, can obtain a licence from the Commissioner of Patents to import the patented active ingredients. This allows a competitor to market his drug in competition with the patentee for the payment of a small royalty of 4%. Compulsory licencing became Canadian law in 1969 (Bill C-102), implementing the recommendations of the Harley Commission Report, which concluded that drug prices in Canada should be lowered and could be controlled to a degree by creating competition in the marketplace. The Commission recommended that the production of generic drugs be encouraged in order to lower drug prices for the public and the various provincial governments who pay drug costs for senior citizens, indigents, and other groups.

The Pharmaceutical Manufacturers Association of Canada claimed that Bill C-102 represents a deterrent to drug development and research. The Minister of Consumer and Corporate Affairs announced in 1983 that changes would be made to Bill C-102 to encourage pharmaceutical research in Canada. Such changes were enacted in the fall of 1987 in the form of Bill C-22. The major changes provide for 10 years of patent protection for new single-entity pharmaceuticals and the establishment of a Drug Prices Review Board. These amendments were implemented to stimulate basic and clinical pharmacologic research in Canada. They are also expected to ensure that prices of pharmaceuticals will not rise at a rate greater than those of other commodities.

In general, it has been claimed that excessive drug legislation impedes the development of new drugs. Frequently the example of the "drug lag," the lesser availability of some drugs in the United States than in the United Kingdom, is given as an example of how excessive drug legislation can impede pharmaceutical innovation. In contrast, the less stringent legislation in some European countries is cited as a way to encourage drug investigation and the earlier availability of drugs. However, these arguments are at variance with the experience of the Third World countries, which, despite minimal or nonexistent legislation, are characterized by limited innovative drug development for lack of an appropriate intellectual and/or industrial climate. The development of new drugs is a complex matter, dependent on a number of factors other than legislation. A detailed analysis of the topic is beyond the scope of this chapter.

PREMARKETING DRUG REGULATIONS

Preclinical Testing of New Drugs

Any drug that has not been sold in Canada for sufficient time and in sufficient quantity to establish satisfactorily its safety and effectiveness is defined as a "new drug" by the Regulations of the Food and Drugs Act. This same definition also applies to any new form or use for a drug that is currently on the Canadian market. (Similar legislation has been enacted in the United States, as described in Wardell WM, 1978.) Before a drug can be administered to humans, it must be tested for its pharmacologic and toxicologic activities in *in vitro* systems and in animals. The activity of pharmaceutical laboratories for developing new drugs is targeted, in the sense that chemical substances are tested systematically, depending on the type of drug, in biochemical, physiologic, behavioral, and pharmacologic screening tests designed to identify substances with the desired (expected) activity. If a substance shows such an effect, then it is possible to proceed with more detailed studies. However, an enormous amount of research is required to move from initial discovery to finished drug. Chemists may create or isolate up to 5000 different substances in order to come up with one new marketable drug. The active new drug is tested in animals and humans, in the sequence shown in Figure 73–1.

Preclinical testing determines the pharmacologic actions of the drugs as well as the mechanism of action, the specificity of effect, and the toxicity. Since all drugs have the potential to produce toxic effects, toxicity studies are conducted in animals according to well defined guidelines. Toxicologic tests are used to determine the toxicity of drugs and/or their metabolites in various biologic systems in order that predictions may be made regarding the potential risks in humans. Traditionally, toxicity testing consisted of acute, subacute, and chronic studies designed to determine the general effects of compounds on animal systems. Now there is also a requirement to assess the drug effects on reproduction as well as the potential for carcinogenic or genetic damage. Currently it is also required by the Health Protection Branch (HPB) of Health and Welfare Canada (the Food and Drug Administration [FDA] in the United States) that these tests be conducted for most drugs before clinical trials and

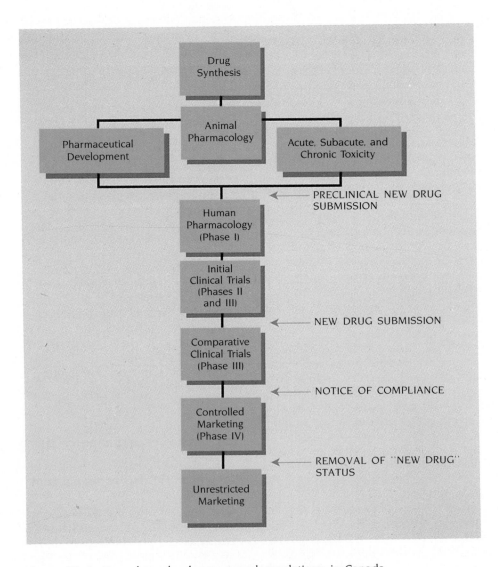

Figure 73–1 New drug development and regulations in Canada.

marketing are undertaken. The need to conduct all the toxicologic tests for a new form or for a new use of an existing drug is questionable, and is frequently a subject of debate between regulatory agencies and pharmaceutical companies.

Acute toxicity studies are those that involve the administration of a single dose, or a few equally spaced doses, within a 24-hour period. Long-term toxicity studies (subacute and chronic) are those that involve the daily administration of the drug for periods lasting from a few days to several years. In general, it is required that animal tests be carried out in at least three mammalian species (one of which must be a non-rodent). The acute (single-dose) median lethal dose (LD$_{50}$) is first determined. Then a series of tests using different dosage routes gives the lethal dose range and the nontoxic range for several species and provides some indication of an approximate dose to use in humans. At the same time the absorption, distribution, metabolism, and elimination of the drug are studied.

The long-term toxicity studies are intended to determine the toxicity (behavioral, physiologic, and histopathologic effects) when a drug is administered repeatedly, and to determine the dose-response relationship of these effects. Also important is the clear identification of the target organ of toxicity, the reversibility, and the factors influencing toxicity (sex, age, nutritional status). The first administration of a drug to humans relies heavily on animal data, and therefore depends on the belief that toxicity or the lack of it, demonstrated in animals, is relevant to humans. However, decisions on specific cases are uncertain. Therefore, it is usual to make conservative decisions, and the appearance of almost any serious toxicity in animals may be considered as sufficient evidence to reject the human administration of a drug. This decision may be faulty, because some toxicity is species-specific, and it is likely that, occasionally, potentially useful new drugs may be unnecessarily rejected. Animal toxicologic tests are usually good predictors of dose-related toxicity in humans, whereas dose-unrelated adverse drug reactions (allergic or genetically determined reactions) are not detected in traditional toxicologic tests. Thus, the first administration of a drug to a human still involves some risk, which must be carefully considered.

Evaluation of Clinical Effects (Clinical Trials)

When the new compound passes preclinical screening, clinical investigation can be conducted. The manufacturer must file a **Preclinical New Drug Submission** with the Health Protection Branch (in the United States, the FDA) and request permission to distribute the drug to qualified investigators for clinical testing in order to obtain the necessary evidence concerning the new drug's dosage, efficacy, and safety in humans. The preclinical submission must contain the following information: objectives of proposed clinical testing; name of the drug; chemical structure and source of the new drug; data on toxicity, pharmacology, and biochemistry (drug metabolism); contraindications and precautions; suggested treatment of overdose; the methods, equipment, plant, and controls used in the manufacture, processing, and packaging of the new drug; tests for potency, purity, and safety; the names and qualifications of investigators; and the institutions where the studies will be conducted. Once the application is approved, the drug is distributed with a label that states that it is an investigational drug that should be used by qualified investigators only.

Phase I Studies

This is the first administration of a drug to humans; it usually follows the completion of pharmacologic and toxicologic studies in animals. The investigational drug is given to healthy volunteers, first in single, increasing doses, and then by multiple administrations to cover the range of therapeutic use. These studies are conducted to obtain data on safety and pharmacokinetics only, since the relevant symptoms on which to test efficacy are rarely present in healthy volunteers. The selection of the initial human dose is difficult. As noted above, animal studies on drug metabolism and toxicity (e.g., LD$_{50}$) are of limited usefulness for selecting such a dose. A common rule is to begin with one-fifth or one-tenth of the maximum tolerated dose (mg/kg) in the most sensitive animal species, assuming an average human body weight of 70 kg. The drug is then given in some form of increments until the estimated therapeutically effective dose is attained or side effects develop. The protocol usually involves six to nine subjects at each dose level. Placebo and double-blind techniques are used. Multiple-dose tolerance studies are usually conducted in healthy volunteers, but it may be ethically more acceptable, as well as more efficient, to perform them in patients.

Phase I subjects are hospitalized and undergo intensive monitoring, including assessments such as daily physical examinations and determinations of blood pressure, pulse, ECG, EEG, and tests for assessing liver, kidney, and hematologic toxicity. A severe adverse event is rare in phase I. For example, in 805 studies, conducted between 1964 and 1976 in 29,000 subjects, only 55 cases of severe, definite, or probable adverse drug reactions occurred.

Phase II Studies

This is the first administration of a drug to patients. Elimination of the drug should be assessed, because patients may metabolize it differently than healthy subjects do. These trials are divided into early and late phases. The early phase II trials involve the administration of the drug to patients to observe the potential therapeutic benefits and side effects. An attempt is made to establish a dose range for more definitive therapeutic trials. Late phase II trials are intended to establish the efficacy of the drug in reducing the manifestations of the specific disease and to compare its efficacy and side effects to those of other marketed drugs used for similar purposes.

Phase III Studies

These studies include double-blind, randomized, controlled clinical trials on a sufficient number of patients to provide data permitting statistical evaluation of the drug's efficacy and safety. The procedures for assessing clinical toxicity are similar to those used in phase I. However, phase III studies provide better information because of the larger sample size.

If the human studies indicate that the compound may be an efficacious and safe therapeutic agent, the manufacturer can file a **New Drug Submission** (NDS) with the HPB (in the United States, the FDA) requesting permission to market the new drug.

The NDS must contain additional information, such as: human data to demonstrate efficacy; recommended use; safety for this use; results of further animal studies; proposed registered name, chemical name, and description; list of all ingredients; product monograph, labels, and package insert; and samples of the finished form of the new drug. An NDS often contains thousands of pages. The data are reviewed by HPB and outside consultants. NDSs are not always cleared with the first submission of data, and further information or clarifications may be required. If the documentation is acceptable to HPB, then a **Notice of Compliance** is signed by the Assistant Deputy Minister of HPB. In the United States, the corresponding official is the Director, Food and Drug Administration. This document indicates that HPB has found the content of the NDS satisfactory and in compliance with regulations. The drug can now enter the market with ''new drug'' status.

Phase IV Studies

These studies occur after the drug has obtained a marketing licence. The drug's performance is monitored in the years immediately following marketing, when widespread use may result in the discovery of relatively rare side effects, chronic toxicity developing only after many years of exposure (*e.g.*, cancer), previously unknown drug interactions, potential new therapeutic uses, or more appropriate dosage recommendations. The drug may remain in new drug status for several years until the HPB is confident that sufficient additional information has accumulated from its general use to justify release from the rigid controls applied to new drugs. While the product still has new drug status, the manufacturer is expected to report any new information concerning safety or efficacy. The HPB reserves the right to suspend the Notice of Compliance for a new drug when it is in the public interest to do so because of such findings as lack of efficacy or serious and/or frequent toxicity. Thus, the study of the performance of a new drug does not stop with its approval and marketing. Physicians must be constantly and critically assessing the clinical effects of old and new drugs.

POSTMARKETING CONTROLS

In Canada, the availability and use of drugs is controlled by both the federal and provincial governments. In the United States, all control is exercised by the federal government.

Federal Controls

Through the **Food and Drugs Act**, the federal government assumes the responsibility for protecting the public against health hazards related to the manufacture and/or sale of drugs, medical devices, cosmetics, and foods. The federal government also controls the access of new drugs to the market by requiring that the drugs meet certain standards of efficacy and safety.

This Act prohibits the sale of drugs that are manufactured or stored under unsanitary conditions, or drugs that are adulterated. The manufacturing conditions for some groups of drugs, for example insulins, vaccines, antibiotics, and radiopharmaceuticals, need to be more strictly controlled than for others, *e.g.*, ASA. Thus, the requirements for insulins, vaccines, *etc.* are spelled out in detail in the Act whereas the requirements for other drugs are described only in general.

In the Food and Drugs Act, the federal government requires that drugs provided to the public be of the highest standard. The standards for some drugs are listed in the Act itself. For other drugs the Act lists publications such as the Canadian Formulary, National Formulary, British Pharmacopoeia, United States Pharmacopeia and others, which provide an acceptable standard. Where a standard has not been provided for, in the Food and Drugs Act or in the listed publications, the manufacturer must set a standard of his own.

The government also controls advertising, labelling, packaging, and processing of drugs. For example, the Food and Drugs Act states that any advertising to the public is prohibited for prescription drugs, controlled drugs, narcotics, and any drug listed in one of the Schedules of the Act as a treatment, prevention, or cure for diseases. It also prohibits false, misleading, or deceptive claims about the efficacy, quality, or safety of the product.

With respect to labelling, the Act lists the general requirements as well as additional requirements for specific products. For example, products containing acetylsalicylic acid (ASA) must have a cautionary statement such as ''Keep Out of the Reach of Children'' on the label. An example of packaging restriction is also provided by ASA if it is intended for use in children. A container for this purpose is restricted to a maximum of 24 doses, each having no more than 81 mg of ASA per dose.

Another area covered in the Food and Drugs Act is that of drug sale or distribution and use. There are six designated groups of drugs, all of which have different levels of control concerning their distribution. The groups are: over-the-counter (OTC) products; prescription drugs; controlled drugs; narcotics; restricted drugs; and prohibited drugs.

The availability of the **OTC products** is governed by the requirements of the Food and Drugs Act with regard to packaging, labelling, conditions of manufacture, and advertising.

Drugs that may be sold only on **prescription** are listed in Schedule F of the Act. The Act specifies who may prescribe these drugs and what information must be included on the prescription. According to the federal regulations, the prescription records must be retained by the pharmacist for 2 years. In many cases, provincial legislation requires these records to be retained for a longer period of time.

Controlled drugs are listed in Schedule G of the Food and Drugs Act. They are such substances as amphetamines and barbiturates and their salts. The requirements for sale and distribution of these drugs are also included in the Act.

Restricted drugs are listed in Schedule H of the Act. These drugs are available only for investigational purposes and can be used only by the investigator according to a protocol that is approved by the appropriate bureau of the federal government. Specific handling and labelling requirements are listed in the Act.

Drugs that are classified as **narcotics** are listed in a Schedule to the Narcotic Control Act, which is separate from the Food and Drugs Act. Whereas the Food and Drugs Act is to a great extent concerned with manufacturing requirements, the Narcotic Control Act is concerned exclusively with the control of availability and use of narcotics.

To date, there is only one drug listed in the "**prohibited drugs**" category, namely, thalidomide. This drug is available only for research purposes under special permits. The only "drug combination" prohibited from sale in Canada is phenacetin and salicylates (phenacetin and salicylates can still be sold separately).

The regulations governing the distribution and use of narcotics and controlled drugs are much more stringent than those governing prescription drugs. For example, dealers require a special licence to distribute narcotics and controlled drugs. Pharmacists must keep separate records of purchases and prescriptions filled for these drugs. Both dealers and pharmacists must keep records of inventories and all transactions involving these drugs and make periodic reports to the Bureau of Dangerous Drugs (BDD; in the United States, an agency of the Food and Drug Administration). The records of dealers and pharmacies are also subject to unannounced inspections and audit by the BDD. Unautho-

rized possession of a narcotic, controlled drug, or restricted drug is a punishable offence. A physician has the onus of proving that any controlled drug or narcotic in his/her possession is for professional use, and that the drug was prescribed or administered in accordance with the regulations. The prohibition of unauthorized possession of these drugs applies not only to dealers, pharmacists, and practitioners (physicians, dentists, veterinarians), but also to patients. Patients are required to inform the prescriber if they have received a narcotic from another prescriber. Since this is not a well known fact (except among the drug-abusing population), it is advisable for the physician prescribing a narcotic to ask the patient if he was given a prescription for a narcotic in the recent past.

There are also special regulations governing the use and distribution of the narcotic, methadone. In Canada, this drug can be prescribed only by a practitioner who is authorized by the Minister of National Health and Welfare (in the United States, the Secretary of Health and Human Services). To receive this authorization, a practitioner is required to provide details of the way methadone will be prescribed in practice or provide evidence of being associated with an approved drug addiction treatment program. The practitioner or the treatment program must report the use of the drug to the BDD.

Provincial Controls

Provincial acts dealing with drug regulations are generally concerned with controls over the sale of drug products, record keeping, and licencing of pharmacists. For the most part, however, the provinces rely primarily on the federal drug regulations. The drug schedules in the provincial acts usually include more substances than the schedules in the federal act. The provincial acts also usually contain more stringent requirements regarding the distribution and use of drugs. For example, the federal regulations require prescription records to be kept for 2 years. In Ontario, pharmacists are required to retain records for 6 years. OTC substances listed in Schedule C must be sold by a pharmacist or a pharmacy student or intern under the supervision of a pharmacist (there is no such federal regulation).

While most government controls are concerned with protection of the health and well-being of the public, there are some controls in the form of public policy programs that are more related to the cost of providing drugs to the public. One such example is the PARCOST program in Ontario, which evolved into the Ontario Drug Benefit program. Its general objective is to provide medications of good quality at reasonable cost to seniors and Ontario residents who are on social welfare. The provincial government publishes the Ontario Drug Benefit Formulary which serves as a source for the selection of brands of medication of comparable efficacy and reasonable cost.

SPECIAL TOPICS

SUGGESTED READING

Bureau of Human Prescription Drugs. Pre-clinical toxicologic guidelines. Health Protection Branch, Health and Welfare Canada, 1981.

Drug Benefit Formulary and PARCOST Comparative Drug Index, No. 26, Ontario Ministry of Health. Queen's Printer for Ontario, 1989. (Periodically revised.)

Food and Drugs Act and Regulations, National Health and Welfare. Queen's Printer and Controller of Stationery, Ottawa, 1984. (Periodically amended.)

Naranjo CA. A clinical pharmacologic perspective on the detection and assessment of adverse drug reactions. Drug Info J 1986; 20:387–393.

Narcotic Control Act, Health and Welfare Canada. Printing and Publishing Supply and Services Canada, Ottawa, 1978.

Sellers EM, Sellers S. Systems for the control of therapeutic drug utilization in Canada. In: Wardell WM, ed. Controlling the use of therapeutic drugs. An international comparison. Washington, DC: American Enterprise Institute, 1978:71–95.

Wardell WM, ed. Controlling the use of therapeutic drugs. An international comparison. Washington, DC: American Enterprise Institute, 1978.

Chapter 74

PRESCRIPTION WRITING

F.A. Sunahara

A prescription is the instruction given by a physician, dentist, or veterinarian to a pharmacist. It includes directions to the pharmacist regarding the preparation and dispensing of medicinal substances, and to the patient regarding the use of the medicine. The practice of prescribing, and the form in which it is done, are subject to both legal controls and professional traditions.

LEGISLATION

In Canada, the dispensing of drugs is governed by both federal and provincial laws. At the federal level there are three areas of regulation that apply to prescriptions and prescribed drugs:
- Food and Drugs Act—Schedule F.
- Food and Drugs Act—Schedule G.
- Narcotic Control Act.

Schedule F includes drugs (except those in Schedule G and the Narcotic Control Act) that may be sold for human use only upon receipt of a prescription. Schedule G drugs are referred to as controlled drugs and include barbiturates and amphetamines alone or in combination with other drugs.

Prescriptions may be issued verbally or in writing. However, all **narcotic prescriptions must be written** except for those products containing one narcotic drug in combination with two or more non-narcotic medicinal substances and not intended for parenteral administration. These are referred to as Oral Prescription Narcotics.

In each province of Canada the practice of pharmacy is governed by the Pharmacy Act of the respective province. Provincial regulations dictating conditions under which certain drugs may be sold may vary from province to province. (For example, in Ontario, drugs listed in Schedule E to the Regulations under Part VI of The Health Disciplines Act, 1974, may only be sold by a pharmacist upon receipt of a prescription, although these drugs are not included in the relevant federal prescription schedules.)

The only restrictions governing what drugs may be prescribed by physicians or dentists are that the drug must be for a patient and that the drug must be required for a condition for which the patient is receiving treatment.

FORM OF A PRESCRIPTION

A prescription may be written on an ordinary piece of paper, but it is customary and more convenient to have prescription pads printed. The name, address, telephone number, and office hours of the practitioner are usually printed, but advertising material for, or the name of, a pharmacy should not appear on the prescription blank.

Prescriptions should be written legibly in ink, and records kept of the drugs that were prescribed for each patient. Except for certain conventional abbreviations (Table 74-1), prescriptions are best **written in modern English or French**.

SPECIAL TOPICS

TABLE 74–1 Some Commonly Encountered Abbreviations

a.c.	– before meals (*ante cibos*)
b.i.d.	– twice daily (*bis in die*)
B.P.	– British Pharmacopoeia
c̄	– with
cap.	– capsule(s)
h.s.	– at bedtime (*hora somni*)
IM *or* i.m.	– intramuscular
IV *or* i.v.	– intravenous
kg	– kilogram(s)
L	– litre(s)
mEq	– milliequivalent(s)
mg	– milligram(s)
mL	– millilitre(s)
O.D.	– right eye (*oculus dexter*)
O.S.	– left eye (*oculus sinister*)
oz.	– ounce(s)
p.c.	– after meals/food (*post cibos*)
p.o.	– orally (by mouth) (*per os*)
q.i.d.	– four times daily (*quater in die*)
q.(?)h.	– every (?) hours (*quisque (?) horae*)
SC *or* s.c.	– subcutaneous
stat.	– at once, immediately (*statim*)
supp.	– suppository(ies)
tab.	– tablet(s)
t.i.d.	– three times daily (*ter in die*)
U.S.P.	– U.S. Pharmacopeia

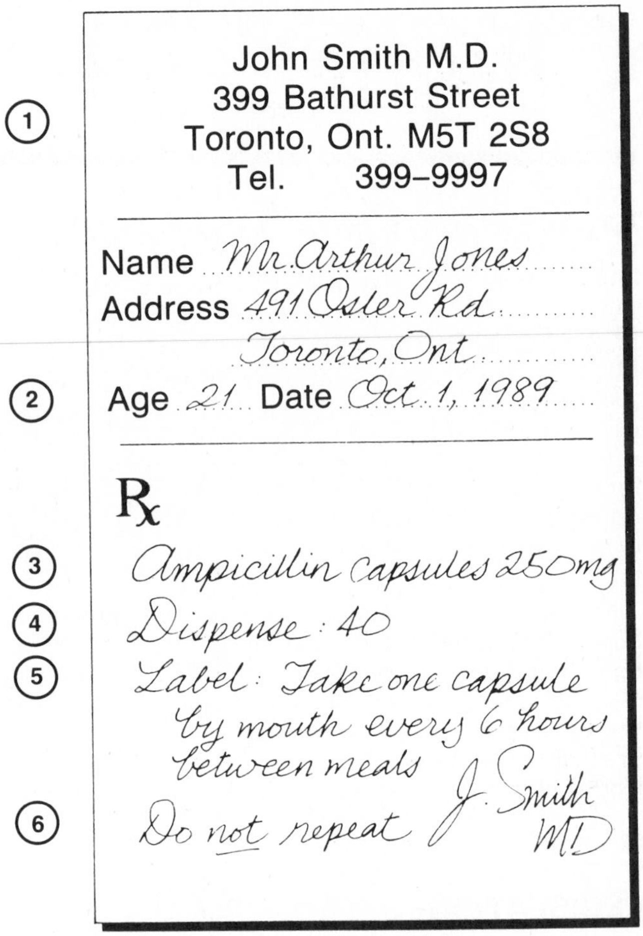

① John Smith M.D.
399 Bathurst Street
Toronto, Ont. M5T 2S8
Tel.   399–9997

Name *Mr. Arthur Jones*
Address *491 Osler Rd.*
Toronto, Ont.
② Age *21* Date *Oct. 1, 1989*

℞

③ *Ampicillin capsules 250mg*
④ *Dispense : 40*
⑤ *Label : Take one capsule*
by mouth every 6 hours
between meals
⑥ *Do not repeat*   *J. Smith*
MD

CONSTRUCTION OF THE PRESCRIPTION

Date. The date must appear on every prescription.

Patient's name and address. The full name and address of the patient must be on every prescription. In the case of a minor, the patient's **age** should also be stated.

Inscription. The sign ℞ (*recipe*, take thou) introduces the body of the prescription in which the name of the drug (or drugs) and the dosage are stated. In the case of precompounded tablets or capsules, the single dose is stated after the name of the drug. To prescribe precompounded orally administered liquids it is necessary to know the concentration of the active ingredient(s) in the preparation. Names of drugs are capitalized.

Subscription. The subscription contains directions to the pharmacist. In most cases this is limited to the number of tablets or capsules or the total volume of a liquid preparation to be dispensed.

Signature. The signature of the prescription consists of instructions to the patient, *via* the pharmacist, and is preceded by the word "Label." Latin abbreviations are often used here to save space.

Refill information. Refill instructions should be indicated on every prescription. Drugs listed in Schedule F (and E in Ontario) must not be refilled by the pharmacist unless the practitioner so directs and specifies the number of times the prescription may be refilled.

Figure 74–1 Usual form of a prescription (*see text*). Important points are: (1) Complete address and telephone number of the practitioner. (2) Although not a requirement, the age of the patient, particularly of children, may be important. (3) Nonproprietary nomenclature is preferred, unless a specific brand-name drug is specified. (4) An older notation was "Mitte." (5) An older notation was "Sig." These instructions to the patient (for which recognized abbreviations are permissible) will be typed on the label by the pharmacist. In Ontario, the nonproprietary drug name, the manufacturer, and the size of the dose are also required to be typed on the label by the pharmacist; additional recommendations regarding the use of some drugs are at the option of the pharmacist. (6) Refill instructions should always be indicated.

Controlled drugs (Schedule G) may not be repeated unless the practitioner so directs, **in writing**, the number of times and the interval between refilling, or the pharmacist contacts the prescriber directly each time a repeat is requested. An amendment made to Schedule G to the Food and Drugs Act in 1978 permits a prescriber to provide **verbal direction** to refill a prescription for a limited number of Schedule G substances, provided that the number of refills and the intervals are given verbally at the time. These substances are

- barbituric acid, its salts and derivatives **except** secobarbital and pentobarbital and their salts and derivatives;
- butorphanol;
- diethylpropion and its salts;
- methylphenidate and its salts; and
- thiobarbituric acid and its salts and derivatives.

Narcotic prescriptions are valid for one filling only. If a further quantity of an oral prescription narcotic is necessary, another verbal or written prescription must be given by the prescriber.

If the prescriber is concerned about the large quantity of a drug being dispensed at one time, the pharmacist may be authorized by the prescriber to dispense the total amount of the narcotic or controlled drug medication in portions. This direction to the pharmacist must be written into the subscription section of the prescription.

Prescriber's signature. Every prescription must be signed by the prescriber, followed by the degree (MD, DDS, DVM, *etc*.). If the prescriber's name, address, and telephone number do not appear at the top of the prescription, in the interest of clarity, the name, address, and telephone number should be printed under the signature.

(The usual form and contents of a prescription are shown in Fig. 74–1.)

WEIGHTS AND MEASURES

The metric system is used on all prescriptions. The basic units are the gram and the millilitre. Although the apothecaries' system is totally outdated, it will still be necessary to know a few simple conversions, *e.g.*, 1 fluid ounce is approximately 30 mL, 1 grain is approximately 60–65 mg, 15 grains is approximately 1 gram.

The short term for gram, "g," should not be used on prescriptions to avoid confusion with the abbreviation for grain, "gr." If no unit of measure is mentioned on a prescription, the pharmacist will assume that the basic units (grams or millilitres) are intended.

If a liquid or powder is prescribed, it is necessary to know the approximate contents of various household measures. If it is necessary to prescribe medicines for oral administration by "drops," the pharmacist should be asked to supply a calibrated dropper. One drop is approximately 0.05 mL. The size of modern spoons shows considerable variation, and critical dosages must not be prescribed in this measure. It is generally accepted that "one teaspoon" is equivalent to 5 mL, and "one tablespoon" is equivalent to 15 mL.

DRUG NAMES

Official or nonproprietary names should ordinarily be used on prescriptions. If the product of a particular manufacturer is desired, the proprietary (trade) name must be stated together with the instruction "no substitution." The nonproprietary name is sometimes incorrectly referred to as the "generic" name. ("Generic" designates a family relationship among drugs.)

ADDITIONAL GUIDELINES

- Prescribe only enough medication for the patient's particular current problem.
- Prescriptions should seldom be renewed more than two or three times without seeing the patient again.
- Minor tranquilizers and sedative-hypnotics should be prescribed in amounts not to exceed 2–4 weeks' supply.
- The instruction "Take as directed" should be avoided since verbal directions are too often misunderstood.
- Patients should get into the habit of bringing their medication with them when they come to see the physician. This allows an opportunity to review medication instructions and to check on compliance.
- Always look up information when in doubt, *e.g.*, tablet size, side effects, *etc*. Patients appreciate a careful and concerned physician.

TYPICAL PROBLEMS WITH PRESCRIPTIONS

Failure to provide a complete, legible prescription can result in patients experiencing delays in obtaining medication and pharmacists and physicians becoming involved in time-consuming telephone calls. The following are some of the more common problems.

Inappropriate or inadequate refill directions. Examples of inappropriate directions include too many refills and instructions to refill a narcotic drug. Inadequate directions can take the form of failure to indicate the time intervals as well as the number of refills for controlled drugs and the use of indefinite directions for refill, such as "refill p.r.n."

Omission of information necessary for dispensing the prescription. Although some missing information such as the age or address of the patient can be obtained from the person presenting the prescription, such necessary information as drug strength and the date on which the prescription was issued can be obtained only from the physician.

Inadequate directions for use. Such directions as "m.d.u.," "ut dict.," or "p.r.n." are often employed, presumably on the basis that the patient has received adequate instructions and no further elaboration is necessary. Unhappily, the patient often forgets how to take the drug or misunderstands the directions of the physician, and the pharmacist can neither provide much direct assistance nor properly monitor compliance when the physician's instructions are not adequately stated on the prescription. Certain drugs, such as those used for symptomatic relief of pain, diarrhea, *etc.*, may be prescribed with instructions to "use as needed." **In general, however, do not use instructions that leave it up to the patient to decide.**

Form of the prescription unclear. Unfortunately, illegible prescriptions are all too frequent. The pharmacist's experience with physicians' handwriting not-

withstanding, a clear, readable prescription is good insurance against misinterpretations.

Other problems in this area include the writing of several prescriptions on one (sometimes very small) piece of paper; the writing of refill directions or directions for use on such a "multiple prescription," making it unclear as to whether such directions refer to one or all of the prescriptions; and the writing of one prescription for several members of a family on the same form.

Difficulties are frequently experienced by pharmacists when presented with a prescription written on a hospital form. Since such forms are not imprinted with the physician's name and address, this information is often impossible to decipher. Many (but not all) hospital prescription forms have a space for printing the prescriber's name as well as signature, but this is frequently ignored, giving rise to tremendous frustrations, particularly when the patient is not aware of the name of the physician who provided treatment in the hospital.

Chapter 75

BIOMETRICS

L. Endrenyi

Physiologic characteristics of people (or of laboratory animals of a given species) are not identical: they fluctuate around some typical, average values. Similarly, different people (or different experimental animals) respond to a greater or lesser degree to a given dose of a drug (Table 75–1). It is reasonable then that, in order to describe and evaluate such scattered characteristics and responses, the medical (including in particular the pharmacologic) literature utilizes statistical methods in great abundance. Therefore, this chapter reviews some statistical terms that are used most frequently in the medical literature. This may facilitate the reading and critical assessment of the literature.

TABLE 75–1 Example of Individual Variation in Drug Response

| Patient No. | Central Venous Pressure (mm Hg) | |
	Control	Guancydine
1	8.0	3.5
2	4.0	3.0
3	2.0	1.5
4	10.5	9.0
5	4.0	3.0
6	1.7	1.7

The effect of guancydine (an investigated vasodilator and antihypertensive agent) on the central venous pressure, in mm Hg, was measured in six subjects, by comparison of the pressure before and after administration of the drug.
From Hammer J, Ulrych M, Freis ED. Clin Pharmacol Ther 1971; 12:78–80.

SELECTION AND OBSERVATION OF A SAMPLE FROM A POPULATION; EXPERIMENTAL DESIGN

In a properly executed scientific investigation the design of the study must be very carefully considered before any observations are made or experiments are performed. It is always necessary to review in advance the many factors that may affect the outcome of the study. For example, would it be possible in a given drug trial that the beneficial effect of the drug could be, in part, attributed to psychological factors, since the faith of the patients in the drug could be a major component of the cure? Could the researcher adjust for this effect by giving some patients the drug, while others would receive a dummy formulation, a placebo, similar in appearance and taste to the drug? Who should get the drug, who the placebo? One possible strategy would be to give the drug to, e.g., the first 20 patients and the placebo to the next 20. But is it not conceivable that interested young male patients would come earlier to the trials? Or that those judged particularly sick would be treated first? Surely it is more reasonable to randomize somehow the order of drug and placebo administration and, in general, the selection of subjects in the two groups.

This kind of planning is always required before the investigation is commenced: this is one of the most important research principles. Still, investigators all too often forget about it. At all times they should keep in mind the question: "Once I have my observations, what will they mean?" The same question arises in our example on the effect of guancydine, the investigated drug in Table 75–1. In five of the six subjects of that study, it appears to lower the central venous pressure. Could such an average lowering be observed even if the drug had no effect, perhaps as a result of patient-to-patient variability, or was the pressure decrease probably caused by the drug? Calculations on the data (as shown in Table 75–2) will answer this question.

Also other doubts can and should be raised about the interpretation of the results. Who were the investigated patients? What was their age? Were they elderly, in which case could the conclusions be applied only to other elderly subjects? Were the patients male or female? What was their race? What other illnesses did they have? All these questions would have to be asked, so that we could determine the range of applicability for our conclusions. In statistical terminology we would like to know: what kind of **population** does our **sample** represent (*e.g.*, Caucasian males, 40–65 years old, with hypertension but no other notable illnesses)? We would

like to answer this question because it is the (larger) population to which we would like to apply the conclusions reached on the basis of the (smaller) sample. In the published paper on guancydine, information about these questions is not provided. We do not know anything about the subjects in the sample, except that they had hypertension, and therefore we are left in uncertainty about the population, *i.e.*, about the people to whom the conclusions may be applied.

ACCURACY AND PRECISION OF THE OBSERVATIONS

We would like to evaluate a characteristic of a population; in the case of our example, this is the true mean decrease of central venous pressure attributable to

TABLE 75–2 Statistical Calculations with Direct Observations and with Paired Data

	x	$x-\bar{x}$	$(x-\bar{x})^2$	d	$d-\bar{d}$	$(d-\bar{d})^2$
	8.0	+2.97	8.82	4.5	+3.08	9.486
	4.0	−1.03	1.06	1.0	−0.42	0.176
	2.0	−3.03	9.18	0.5	−0.92	0.846
	10.5	+5.47	29.92	1.5	+0.08	0.006
	4.0	−1.03	1.06	1.0	−0.42	0.176
	1.7	−3.33	11.09	0.0	−1.42	2.016
Sum (Σ) of n values	30.2	(+0.02)*	61.13	8.5	(−0.02)*	12.706
Mean = Sum/n	5.03($\bar{x}$)			1.42($\bar{d}$)		
Sum of squares (SS) $= \Sigma(x-\bar{x})^2$						
$= \Sigma x^2 - (\Sigma x)^2/n$†	$213.14 - 30.2^2/6$	= 61.13		$24.75 - 8.5^2/6$	= 12.708	
Variance (s^2) $= SS/(n-1)$	61.13/5	= 12.23		17.708/5	= 2.542	
Standard deviation $s = \sqrt{s^2}$	$\sqrt{12.23}$	= 3.50		$\sqrt{2.542}$	= 1.59	
Standard error of mean (SEM) $s_{\bar{x}} = s/\sqrt{n}$	$3.50/\sqrt{6}$	= 1.43		$1.59/\sqrt{6}$	= 0.65	
$t_{(0.05,5)}$	From Table 75–3	= 2.57		From Table 75–3	= 2.57	
95% Probability ranges of observations $\bar{x} \pm ts$	$5.03 \pm 2.57 \times 3.50$ $\approx 5.03 \pm 8.99$	$\begin{cases} -3.96 \\ 14.02 \end{cases}$		$1.42 \pm 2.57 \times 1.59$ $\approx 1.42 \pm 4.10$	$\begin{cases} -2.68 \\ 5.52 \end{cases}$	
95% Confidence limits of mean $\bar{x} \pm ts_{\bar{x}}$	$5.03 \pm 2.57 \times 1.43$ $\approx 5.03 \pm 3.67$	$\begin{cases} 1.36 \\ 8.69 \end{cases}$		$1.42 \pm 2.57 \times 0.65$ $\approx 1.42 \pm 1.67$	$\begin{cases} -0.25 \\ 3.09 \end{cases}$	

x-Column = central venous pressure before drug administration; d-column = decrease of central venous pressure due (?) to drug administration—from Table 75–1.

* Due to rounding errors; it should be zero.

† Usual method of hand-calculation.

guancydine in subjects with hypertension. In order to **estimate** this characteristic, a sample is taken from the population, six patients in our example. A measure of the characteristic is evaluated in the sample: Most frequently we calculate the sample **average**. If this tends to be close to the true (and unknown) population mean, then we say that the experimental result is **accurate**. If, however, some systematic error distorts the result (as when the sample does not really represent the assumed population, *e.g.*, it contains five males and one female, or when a methodologic distortion, *e.g.*, a faulty instrument, is introduced), then the observed average will be inaccurate or **biased**. The experimenter must guard against these biases, which, as a rule, will not be demonstrated by the (statistical) evaluation of the experimental results.

The investigator also would like to know how uniform or how divergent his observations are among themselves. If the observed values are scattered widely around their average, then their **precision** is low and the average itself is not very reliable.

MEASURES OF PRECISION: RANGE, VARIANCE, AND STANDARD DEVIATION

A quick measure of the variability of the data, or of their precision, is provided by their **range**, the difference between the largest and the smallest observation. However, it is not easy to compare ranges of different sets of measurements since these will depend also on the number of data in each set. If we have more observations (a larger sample from a given population), their range will probably also be larger.

A more customarily used measure of precision is the **variance**, which is calculated by summing the squared deviations of the observations from their average and dividing the result by the **degrees of freedom** (df). By summing the squares of the deviations (and thus obtaining the so-called **sum of squares**, SS) we can ignore their positive or negative signs. The divisor, the degrees of freedom, is (in this simple case) one less than the number of measurements $(n-1)$ because of a restriction imposed upon the calculations: the sum of the deviations from the mean must add up to zero. [Alternatively: By definition, the mean has to be estimated (even if implicitly) before the SS is evaluated. The value of SS is, therefore, dependent on the estimation of another parameter (the mean). Thus, its df is lowered by one. In general, the mean square MS = SS/df, where the df is lowered by the number of parameters that have to be estimated for the calculation of SS.]

Statisticians prefer to evaluate the variance with its many useful theoretical characteristics. In practice, however, its square root, the **standard deviation** (s) describes the scatter of the observations more conveniently since it has the same units as the original data.

If the number of observations is fairly large and the data follow approximately the bell-shaped **normal distribution**, then the interval $\bar{x} \pm s$ (5.03 ± 3.50 mm Hg for the central venous pressure before drug administration) will contain about two-thirds of the observations, and the interval $\bar{x} \pm 2s$ about 95% of them.

For smaller samples such **probability ranges** should be calculated with the help of Student's **t-values**, which can be obtained for the desired percentages and degrees of freedom from their tabulation (Table 75–3). For a given percentage (Pc), the **significance level** (α) of the table is selected from $\alpha = (100-Pc)/100$; *e.g.*, for Pc = 95% limits, $\alpha = 0.05$ and the probability ranges are obtained from $\bar{x} \pm t_{(0.05, df)}s$, where df = $n-1$. Roughly speaking, these limits will include an average of 95% of the observations from the given population.

STANDARD ERROR OF THE MEAN (SEM)

Since the mean is calculated from several measurements, it will be known with greater precision than the individual observations. Its standard error is obtained as shown in Table 75–2. Its probability range lies between the 95% **confidence limits** of the mean. These limits (which are narrower than the probability range of the observations) will include the true mean of the population, on average, in 95% of the cases, provided

TABLE 75–3 Percentage Points of the t-Distribution

df	\multicolumn{4}{c}{Probability (α)}
	0.10	*0.05*	*0.025*	*0.01*
1	6.32	12.71	25.45	63.66
2	2.92	4.30	6.21	9.92
3	2.35	3.18	4.18	5.84
4	2.13	2.78	3.50	4.60
5	2.02	2.57	3.16	4.03
6	1.94	2.45	2.97	3.71
7	1.89	2.36	2.84	3.50
8	1.86	2.31	2.75	3.36
9	1.83	2.26	2.69	3.25
10	1.81	2.23	2.63	3.17
11	1.79	2.20	2.59	3.11
12	1.78	2.18	2.56	3.05
14	1.76	2.14	2.51	2.98
16	1.75	2.12	2.47	2.92
18	1.73	2.10	2.45	2.88
20	1.72	2.09	2.42	2.85
24	1.71	2.06	2.39	2.80
30	1.70	2.04	2.36	2.75
40	1.68	2.02	2.33	2.70
60	1.67	2.00	2.30	2.66
120	1.66	1.98	2.27	2.62
∞	1.64	1.96	2.24	2.58

the results are not influenced by some systematic error.

In our example the 95% probability range of the observations spreads from -4.0 to $+14.0$ mm Hg, implying that from this sample of observations we predict that 19 out of 20 (95 out of 100) similarly obtained probability ranges would include the true mean. But could negative central venous pressures be observed? Certainly not. This means that there is something wrong about our assumptions, in particular about our assumption of a normal distribution for these measurements. This would affect the probability ranges of the observations and of the mean, but does not change the calculated average, variance, standard deviation, or the standard error of the mean. Forgetting about the effect of the assumed distribution does not matter here because, as we shall see, we are not concerned so much with the magnitude of the venous pressure as with its change. However, similar disregard for implicit assumptions (as, for example, the normality of the distribution) is distressingly frequent in the literature: The reader must be on guard!

PAIRED DATA

The venous pressures observed in the presence and in the absence of the drug are paired: they are measured in the same patient. In this case, we are not really interested in "control" and "treated" pressures themselves but only in their differences, the pressure decreases, that could be attributed to the effects of the drug. We can evaluate this difference (d) in each patient and, from these values, assess their average, variance, *etc*. The calculations are shown in Table 75–2.

The probability range again spans a range of positive and negative values. This is reasonable now, since the evaluated quantity is the decrease of venous pressure: A negative value merely indicates an increase in the pressure. Thus (at least for this reason) we need not have doubts about the assumed distribution.

If the drug had no effect on the central venous pressure, then the true population mean of the pressure differences would be zero. Due to random fluctuations we would probably observe averages that are different from zero; still, there is a chance of $100(1 - \alpha) =$ Pc%, *i.e.*, 95%, that the confidence interval would include zero, and only 100α%, *i.e.*, 5%, that zero would be excluded. Thus, if we observe an average value that had Pc% confidence limits not including zero, then we conclude that the chance that this sample came from a population with zero mean is less than 100α%. If α is small, then this chance is also considered to be small and we could decide that the population mean is in fact probably not zero.

In our example, the 95% confidence limits of the average pressure difference do not exclude the value of zero, and therefore, we may not conclude, at the 5%

significance level or with 95% confidence, that the observed pressure decrease can not be attributed merely to random, statistical fluctuations. Note, however, that we could make such a statement at the 10% significance level. This raises the question of selecting the significance level. Since this is a matter of compromises, there is no ready answer; Pc = 95% or, equivalently, $\alpha = 0.05$ is used most frequently.

COMPARISON OF UNPAIRED DATA

Very frequently, comparison of measurements performed on two different groups (populations) is required. If paired observations (*e.g.*, samples taken from the same animal before and after treatment) are not used, then the means of the two groups can be compared by subtracting one from the other, $d = \bar{x}_2 - \bar{x}_1$, calculating the standard error of the difference (provided that the two variances are not substantially different), and evaluating the confidence limits of the differences (Expression 1). If the limits do not include the value of 0, the two means are said to be significantly different. The formulae become more simple when the number of observations in the two groups is the same, *i.e.*, when $n_1 = n_2$ and $df_1 = df_2$ (Expression 2).

Expression 1:

$$s_d = s \sqrt{\frac{1}{n_1} + \frac{1}{n_2}}, \text{ with}$$

$$s = \sqrt{(df_1 \cdot s_1{}^2 + df_2 \cdot s_2{}^2)/(df_1 + df_2)}.$$

Expression 2:

$$s_d = s \sqrt{2/n} \text{ and}$$

$$s^2 = (s_1{}^2 + s_2{}^2)/2; \text{ therefore}$$

$$s_d = \sqrt{(s_1{}^2 + s_2{}^2)/n}.$$

ENUMERATION DATA; CONTINGENCY TABLES

When the weight of an object or of an animal is measured, this may take, within a reasonable range, **any** value. Thus, if weights on a balance can be measured to 0.01 g, it is possible that the weight of an animal will be found to be between 102.35 and 102.36 g: only the low precision of the instrument prevents a more exact weighing. (It probably would not be of much use anyway.) Therefore, weight measurements are **quantitative data** that sample distributions of **continuous random variables** (*e.g.*, the normal distribution). Similar considerations apply to our central venous pressure data.

Frequently only the **number of occurrences** of certain events (the frequency of their incidence) is **counted**. For instance, 50 patients have received a drug tablet and another 50 (randomly selected) patients only placebo (Table 75–4). Of these 100 patients, after 2 weeks the condition of 10 patients deteriorated, 52 patients improved, and the remaining 38 patients had approximately unchanged disease indicators. If the condition of the patients improves or worsens **independently** of the treatment, then one would expect that the condition of $10 \times (50/100) = 5$ treated patients would deteriorate, $38 \times (50/100) = 19$ would remain unchanged, and $52 \times (50/100) = 26$ would improve. The expectations would be exactly the same in the group receiving the placebo. The test for agreement between the observed counts and those expected under the hypothesis, the **test for association** between the two factors (drug and patient condition), or the test for their independence is given by the formula appended to Table 75–4.

TABLE 75–5 Percentage Points of the χ^2-Distribution

df	Probability (α)			
	0.10	0.05	0.025	0.01
1	2.71	3.84	5.02	6.64
2	4.61	5.99	7.38	9.21
3	6.25	7.82	9.35	11.35
4	7.78	9.49	11.14	13.28
5	9.24	11.07	12.83	15.09
6	10.65	12.59	14.45	16.81
7	12.02	14.07	16.01	18.48
8	13.36	15.51	17.54	20.09
9	14.68	16.92	19.02	21.67
10	15.99	18.31	20.48	23.21
11	17.28	19.68	21.92	24.73
12	18.55	21.03	23.34	26.22
14	21.06	23.68	26.12	29.14
16	23.54	26.30	28.85	32.00
18	25.99	28.87	31.53	34.81
20	28.41	31.41	34.17	37.57
24	33.20	36.42	39.36	42.98
30	40.26	43.77	46.98	50.89
40	51.81	55.76	59.34	63.69
60	74.40	79.08	83.30	88.38

TABLE 75–4 Example of Enumeration Data and Their Analysis (*see* Text)

Condition	Observed (O)			Expected (E)			Deviation (O-E)		
	Placebo	Drug	Sum	Placebo	Drug	Sum	Placebo	Drug	Sum
Deteriorated	6	4	10	5	5	10	1	−1	0
Unchanged	24	14	38	19	19	38	5	−5	0
Improved	20	32	52	26	26	52	−6	6	0
Sum	50	50	100	50	50	100	0	0	0

$$\chi^2 = \Sigma(O\text{-}E)^2/E$$

where O = observed counts, and E = expected counts.
df = (column − 1) × (row − 1) = (2 − 1) × (3 − 1) = 2.
$\chi^2 = (1)^2/5 + (-1)^2/5 + (5)^2/19 + (-5)^2/19 + (-6)^2/26 + (6)^2/26 = 5.80$.
$\chi^2_{(2)} = 5.99$ at $\alpha = 0.05$, from the theoretical χ^2 values in Table 75–5.

Since the observed value of χ^2 is less than the tabular χ^2 at the chosen significance level, we do not reject the so-called null hypothesis for the independence of the factors. (The observed value would occur in more than 5% of the random cases by chance, by random variation alone if the factors are in fact independent.)

The χ^2-test has various other applications. Still, the basic formula for its calculation remains the same as shown in the above formula.

SUGGESTED READING

Colton T. Statistics in medicine. Boston: Little, Brown, 1974. (Introductory text, aims at the medical student, covers medical statistics in a wider sense.)

Daniel WW. Biostatistics: a foundation for analysis in the health sciences. 3rd ed. New York: Wiley, 1983. (Introductory, clear, nonmathematical, relevant presentation of statistical methods.)

Delaunois AL. Biostatistics in pharmacology. Vols 1 and 2. Oxford: Pergamon Press, 1973. (A textbook with pharmacologic orientation.)

Duncan RC, Knapp RG, Miller CM. Introductory biostatistics in the health sciences. 2nd ed. Chichester: Wiley, 1983. (Clear, nonmathematical introduction to statistical methods for medical students and those in related courses.)

Feinstein AR. Clinical biostatistics. St. Louis: CV Mosby, 1977. (Organized collection of penetrating articles printed first in Clinical Pharmacology and Therapeutics. *See* also other papers published later.)

Snedecor GW, Cochran WG. Statistical methods. 7th ed. Ames, Iowa: Iowa State University Press, 1980. (Classic, full-year first course in biostatistics.)

Appendix 1

Drug Formulary and Drug Data Summary

The drugs included in this appendix have been chosen on the basis of their relative frequency of use, or as important examples of particular classes of drugs. Entries have been organized in a format that permits the rapid survey of important drug data, familiarization with specific drug profiles, and guidelines for dosage considerations.

The pharmacokinetic data were obtained from a variety of sources in the public domain. They have been reviewed and evaluated by the editors, by members of the departmental staff, and by the authors of the respective book chapters. They are therefore considered to be accurate within the limits of accessible background information as published by a variety of investigators.

REFERENCES

Metric Commission Canada. SI manual in health care. 2nd ed. Toronto: Ontario Ministry of Health, 1982.

Moffat AC, Jackson JV, Moss MS, Widdop B, eds. Clarke's isolation and identification of drugs. 2nd ed. London: Pharmaceutical Press, 1986.

Vozeh S, Schmidlin O, Taeschner W. Pharmacokinetic drug data. Clin Pharmacokinet 1988; 15:254–282.

Windholz M, Budavari S, Blumetti RF, Otterbein ES, eds. The Merck Index, 10th ed. Rahway, NJ: Merck & Co. 1983.

This appendix contains portions of Chapter 74 in the 4th edition, compiled by P.A.J. Reilly and departmental staff. Some clinically important conversions of therapeutic plasma concentrations from traditional units to S.I. units were derived from Chapter 75 in the 4th edition, by S.G. Carruthers.

SPECIAL TOPICS

ACETAMINOPHEN (PARACETAMOL)

Brand Names: Abenol, Atasol, Campain, Exdol, Panadol, Robigesic, Rounox, Tempra, Tylenol, others.
Drug Class: Analgesic-antipyretic.
Related Drugs: Acetanilid, phenacetin.

ACTIONS: Analgesic and antipyretic effects are similar to those of ASA, but anti-inflammatory action is weak. Weak inhibitor of prostaglandin biosynthesis, possibly only of selective pathways.

PHARMACOKINETICS

pK_a: 9.5 (acidic).
Mean V_d: 1 L/kg.
Plasma Protein Binding: No binding in the therapeutic range; 15–20% at toxic levels.
Bioavailability: 60–90% (oral); may increase with large doses.
Half-Life–Normal: 2 hours. – **Disease States:** Increased in hepatic disease, neonates; fluctuates with uremia.
Absorption & Distribution: Rapid and complete absorption, peak plasma concentration in 30–60 minutes. Distributes uniformly into most body fluids; only binds to plasma proteins at toxic concentrations. Rectal absorption is poor and erratic.
Biotransformation & Elimination: 90–100% recovered in the urine as metabolites. Hepatic conjugation to glucuronide (major) and sulfate (minor) accounts for 90% of biotransformation. N-hydroxylation to hepatotoxic metabolite may occur at high doses.

ADVERSE REACTIONS AND TOXICITY

Acute: Minimal GI distress; overdose (10–15 g) can cause hepatic necrosis; 15 g or more is potentially fatal.
Chronic: Skin rash as manifestation of hypersensitivity (rare).

MAJOR DRUG INTERACTIONS: Chronic dosing may elevate prothrombin times in patients on oral anticoagulants.

THERAPEUTIC USE

Usual Effective Plasma Concentration: 10–20 µg/mL (66.2–132.4 µmol/L).
Usual Dose & Regimen: Adults, 325–1000 mg every 4–6 hours, not to exceed 4 g/day. Children, 10–15 mg/kg every 4–6 hours, not to exceed 65 mg/kg/day.
Special Considerations: Low glucuronide conjugation capacity in children may increase the risk of hepatotoxicity with overdose. Often substituted for ASA when effects on platelet function, increased bleeding times, or inhibition of uric acid excretion must be avoided.

SPECIFIC ANTIDOTE: Acetylcysteine to prevent hepatic necrosis.

ACETYLSALICYLIC ACID (ASA)

Brand Names: Ancasal, Arthrinol, Aspirin, Astrin, Coryphen, Entrophen, Novasen, Riphen-10, Sal-Adult, Sal-Infant, Supasa, Triaphen-10.
Drug Class: Nonsteroidal anti-inflammatory agent (NSAID); antithrombotic.
Related Drugs: Salicylic acid, sodium salicylate.

ACTIONS: Analgesic, antipyretic, anti-inflammatory. Inhibits the synthesis of prostaglandin endoperoxides through irreversible acetylation of cyclooxygenase; anti-inflammatory properties are due in part to formation of sodium salicylate. Inhibits platelet aggregation.

PHARMACOKINETICS

pK_a: 3.5 (acidic).
Mean V_d: 0.15 L/kg.
Plasma Protein Binding: 80% bound (as salicylate); acetylates albumin.
Bioavailability: 70% (oral); remainder absorbed as salicylate.
Half-Life–Normal: 15-20 minutes (2.5–30 hours for salicylate metabolites). – **Disease States:** Renal impairment causes accumulation of salicylate moiety.
Absorption & Distribution: Well absorbed orally from the upper part of small bowel; enteric coating of tablets delays absorption and decreases peak plasma levels. Distributes by pH-dependent passive processes.
Biotransformation & Elimination: Hydrolysed to salicylic acid by esterases in gut, blood, and other tissues. Salicylic acid is eliminated unchanged by the kidneys and by four biotransformation pathways, two of which are easily saturable; thus, high doses of ASA can lead to nonlinear kinetics and salicylate accumulation; alkaline urine (pH 8) can increase elimination over 20-fold vs. acidic urine (pH 5).

ADVERSE REACTIONS AND TOXICITY

Acute: Minor GI disturbances (nausea, vomiting, heartburn, cramps, indigestion), CNS (tinnitus, vertigo, temporary deafness), elevated prothrombin times, respiratory alkalosis, metabolic acidosis, electrolyte disturbances, hypoglycemia, hemorrhage, salicylate hypersensitivity (<0.5%).
Chronic: Major GI bleeding, benign gastric ulcer.

MAJOR DRUG INTERACTIONS: Displaces several acidic compounds which are highly bound to plasma proteins (e.g., penicillin, thyroxine, bilirubin, thiopental, phenytoin). Increased bleeding tendency if used concurrently with anticoagulants.

THERAPEUTIC USE

Usual Effective Plasma Concentration: 150–300 mg/L (1.1–2.2 mmol/L as salicylate) required for anti-inflammatory effect.
Usual Dose & Regimen: Adults, analgesic and antipyretic, 325–650 mg every 4–6 hours; anti-inflammatory, 1000 mg 4–6 times a day, maximum 10 g; stroke prevention, 325 mg every other day; inhibition of platelet aggregation, 650 mg twice a day; postmyocardial infarction, 325 mg three times a day. (Antithrombotic uses and doses are under review.)
Special Considerations: Monitoring plasma concentrations of salicylates may be useful.

SPECIFIC ANTIDOTE: None. Treatment of acid-base and electrolyte disturbances.

ADRENALINE (EPINEPHRINE)

Brand Names: Adrenalin, Bronkaid Mistometer, Dysne-Inhal, Epifrin, Glaucon, Medihaler-Epi, Sus-Phrine, Vaponefrin.
Drug Class: Sympathomimetic, catecholamine.
Related Drugs: Noradrenaline (norepinephrine), isoproterenol, dopamine, metaproterenol (orciprenaline), salbutamol (albuterol), terbutaline.

ACTIONS: Potent α - and β -adrenoceptor agonist. Strong pressor action, peripheral vasoconstriction or vasodilatation, positive chronotropic and inotropic effects. Increases blood glucose, lactic acid, and respiration.

PHARMACOKINETICS

pK$_a$: 8.7 (basic), 10.2 (acidic).
Mean V$_d$: ?
Plasma Protein Binding: About 50% bound.
Bioavailability: Nil (oral) due to biotransformation and poor absorption; 10% (aerosol).
Half-Life–Normal: A few minutes. – **Disease States:** ?
Absorption & Distribution: Poor oral absorption; hepatic catechol-O-methyl transferase (COMT) and MAO prevent significant systemic distribution. Well absorbed as aerosol in the lung; peak plasma levels in 10 minutes. Subcutaneous dose is absorbed slowly due to local vasoconstriction.
Biotransformation & Elimination: Short duration of action due to COMT and MAO activity in the liver and other tissues. Majority of a dose is excreted as metabolites in the urine.

ADVERSE REACTIONS AND TOXICITY

Acute: Anxiety, headache, fear, palpitations, tremor, dizziness, angina, arrhythmias.
Chronic: Necrotic injection sites in consequence of local vasoconstriction; tolerance.

MAJOR DRUG INTERACTIONS: Some general anaesthetics (halogenated hydrocarbons, cyclopropane) sensitize the myocardium to catecholamines. MAO inhibitors potentiate the effects, as may tricyclic antidepressants, levothyroxine, and some antihistamines.

THERAPEUTIC USE

Usual Effective Plasma Concentration: Not measured clinically.
Usual Dose & Regimen: Parenterally, 0.1–0.5 mL of 0.1% solution s.c.; or very slow, dilute i.v. injection not exceeding 0.25 mg for immediate effect. Inhalation, nebulized 1% solution as needed for symptomatic relief of bronchoconstriction. Nasal solution, 0.1% diluted for use as vasoconstrictor.
Special Considerations: Unstable in alkaline solution or when exposed to air or light. Cautious use in the elderly, cardiovascular disease, diabetes, pregnancy, psychoneurotic individuals, hyperthyroidism.

SPECIFIC ANTIDOTE: Effects controlled by rapid biotransformation (α - and β -adrenoceptor antagonists in special circumstances).

ALLOPURINOL

Brand Names: Alloprin, Apo-Allopurinol, Novopurol, Purinol, Zyloprim.
Drug Class: Xanthine oxidase inhibitor.
Related Drugs: Oxypurinol (alloxanthine).

ACTIONS: Inhibits terminal steps in uric acid biosynthesis, specifically the xanthine oxidase-catalysed reactions of xanthine and hypoxanthine; reduces the plasma concentration and excretion of uric acid, increases the excretion of its more soluble precursors.

PHARMACOKINETICS

pK$_a$: 9.4 (basic).
Mean V$_d$: 0.6 L/kg.
Plasma Protein Binding: None.
Bioavailability: 80% (oral).
Half-Life–Normal: 2–8 hours, alloxanthine metabolite 18–30 hours. – **Disease States:** Prolonged when renal function is impaired.
Absorption & Distribution: Rapid oral absorption, peaks within one hour; distributed in total body water, except the brain where concentrations of drug and metabolite are one-third of other tissues.
Biotransformation & Elimination: Rapidly converted to alloxanthine, a potent noncompetitive inhibitor of xanthine oxidase; alloxanthine accumulates in chronic treatment, causing dose-dependent elimination; 10–30% allopurinol excreted unchanged in the urine.

ADVERSE REACTIONS AND TOXICITY

Acute: Gouty attack, intestinal upset, vertigo.
Chronic: Skin reactions, hypersensitivity (3%); hematologic disorders, cataracts (rare).

MAJOR DRUG INTERACTIONS: Can decrease the hepatic inactivation of oral anticoagulants; prolongs the elimination of 6-mercaptopurine or azathioprine (their doses should be reduced by 60–75%); competes with chlorpropamide for renal excretion; probenecid (uricosuric) enhances alloxanthine excretion.

THERAPEUTIC USE

Usual Effective Plasma Concentration: Not measured clinically.
Usual Dose & Regimen: 100–800 mg/day in 1–3 doses p.o., usually with meals; maximum single dose not to exceed 300 mg.
Special Considerations: Therapy is initiated with low doses, or together with colchicine, to avoid precipitating acute gouty attack; adjust fluid intake for daily output of 2 L neutral or alkaline urine.

SPECIFIC ANTIDOTE: None. Withdraw allopurinol and maintain adequate hydration.

AMANTADINE

Brand Name: Symmetrel.
Drug Class: Antiparkinsonism agent, antiviral agent.
Related Drugs: —

ACTIONS: Releases dopamine from dopaminergic nerve terminals in the central nervous system. May counteract extrapyramidal side effects of antipsychotic drugs and supplement the action of L-dopa in Parkinson's disease.
   Antiviral activity is based on inhibition of replication of influenza A virus and possibly inhibition of viral release of nucleic acids into host cells.

PHARMACOKINETICS

pK$_a$: 10.4 (basic).
Mean V$_d$: About 1 L/kg.
Plasma Protein Binding: ?
Bioavailability: Almost 100% (oral).
Half-Life–Normal: 10–30 hours (mean 15 hours). – **Disease States:** Prolonged by renal impairment.
Absorption & Distribution: Well absorbed from GI tract and distributed in total body water. Crosses the blood–brain barrier.
Biotransformation & Elimination: No metabolites detectable in humans. Excreted unchanged in the urine (>90% of the dose).

ADVERSE REACTIONS AND TOXICITY

Acute: Insomnia, hallucinations, confusion, nightmares (generally mild, transient, reversible).
Chronic: Livido reticularis in lower extremities, orthostatic hypotensive episodes, congestive heart failure, urinary retention, depression, psychosis.

MAJOR DRUG INTERACTIONS: None observed. Adverse reactions may be more frequent in the presence of anticholinergic agents.

THERAPEUTIC USE

Usual Effective Plasma Concentration: Antiviral, 0.4 μg/mL; toxicity 1–5 μg/mL.
Usual Dose & Regimen: Parkinson's syndrome, 100 mg per day for 1–3 weeks, then 100 mg twice daily; may be combined with L-dopa. Antiviral, 200 mg per day for 3–5 days; in children, 4.4–8.8 mg/kg, not to exceed 150 mg per day.
Special Considerations: Use cautiously in patients with cerebral atherosclerosis, psychiatric disorders, or a history of epilepsy.

SPECIFIC ANTIDOTE: None. Use supportive measures.

AMPICILLIN

Brand Names: Ampicin, Ampilean, Apo-Ampi, Novo-Ampicillin, Penbritin.
Drug Class: Beta-lactam antibiotic. Semisynthetic penicillin.
Related Drugs: Amoxicillin, other penicillins.

ACTIONS: Inhibits cell wall biosynthesis in susceptible bacteria (see penicillin G). Besides Gram-positive organisms, it has bactericidal activity against several Gram-negative organisms, but resistant strains occur.

PHARMACOKINETICS

pK$_a$: 2.5 (acidic), 7.2 (basic).
Mean V$_d$: 0.3–0.4 L/kg.
Plasma Protein Binding: 20% bound.
Bioavailability: 50–75% (oral).
Half-Life–Normal: 1–1.5 hours. – **Disease States:** Increased in renal and hepatic failure and in neonates.
Absorption & Distribution: Acid stability results in good oral absorption, but can be decreased in the presence of food. Distributed to all tissues except the brain and cerebrospinal fluid. (In the presence of meningeal inflammation, CSF levels of 5% of plasma levels may be obtained.)
Biotransformation & Elimination: Primarily excreted unchanged in the urine (80–98%). A portion of ampicillin appears in the bile, undergoes enterohepatic circulation, and is excreted in the feces.

ADVERSE REACTIONS AND TOXICITY

Acute: Nausea, vomiting, diarrhea, hypersensitivity (rashes, urticaria, anaphylaxis).
Chronic: Hypersensitivity reactions (up to 10% of all patients) including serum sickness, eosinophilia, fever; superinfection.

MAJOR DRUG INTERACTIONS: Probenecid decreases renal elimination. Tetracyclines may interfere with antibacterial activity.

THERAPEUTIC USE

Usual Effective Plasma Concentration: Refer to Chapter 53.
Usual Dose & Regimen: Adults, 250–500 mg every 6–8 hours for a minimum of 7 days. Children >20 kg, 250–500 mg per day divided into 4 doses. Children 5–20 kg, 25–100 mg/kg divided into 4 doses.
Special Considerations: Dose adjustments are required in renal dysfunction. Resistant strains of many organisms abound. Contraindicated in patients allergic to penicillins or cephalosporins.

SPECIFIC ANTIDOTE: None. Anaphylaxis treated with adrenaline (epinephrine), antihistamines, glucocorticoids.

ATROPINE

Brand Names: Atropisol, Isopto Atropine, SMP Atropine.
Drug Class: Anticholinergic (antimuscarinic).
Related Drugs: Scopolamine, homatropine, propantheline, ipratropium, many others.

ACTIONS: Competitive antagonism of acetylcholine at muscarinic cholinergic receptors.

PHARMACOKINETICS

pK_a: 9.8 (basic).
Mean V_d: 2–4 L/kg.
Plasma Protein Binding: 50% bound.
Bioavailability: Estimated 80% (oral).
Half-Life–Normal: Biphasic, 2–4 hours, 13–38 hours. – **Disease States:** ?
Absorption & Distribution: Rapid absorption and distribution into all tissues. Crosses the placenta, secreted in breast milk. Antimuscarinic activity of atropine can delay gastric emptying and hence its own absorption.
Biotransformation & Elimination: Partly N-demethylated and glucuronidated. Excreted in the urine, largely as unchanged drug.

ADVERSE REACTIONS AND TOXICITY

Acute: Xerostomia (dry mouth), flushing, bradycardia, tachycardia, mydriasis, blurred vision, urinary retention, respiratory failure, delirium, convulsions.
Chronic: Same as acute.

MAJOR DRUG INTERACTIONS: Additive when used with other anticholinergic drugs or antihistamines.

THERAPEUTIC USE

Usual Effective Plasma Concentration: Not measured clinically.
Usual Dose & Regimen: Orally, 250 μg 30 minutes before meals. Parenterally, 0.4–0.6 mg. Ophthalmic solution, 1 drop of 1% solution per eye, three times daily.
Special Considerations: Contraindicated in glaucoma, paralytic ileus.

SPECIFIC ANTIDOTE: Physostigmine.

BECLOMETHASONE FOR INHALATION

Brand Names: Beclovent, Beconase, Vancenase, Vanceril.
Drug Class: Adrenocortical steroid, topical anti-inflammatory.
Related Drugs: Prednisone, betamethasone, flunisolide.

ACTIONS: Topical suppression of cell-mediated immune responses in the lungs or respiratory passages after inhalation.

PHARMACOKINETICS

pK_a: n.a. (steroid).
Mean V_d: 0.3 L/kg (estimated).
Plasma Protein Binding: 80% bound (estimated).
Bioavailability: 10–25% (inhaled). Remainder swallowed, with 75% absorption.
Half-Life–Normal: 15 hours. – **Disease States:** Prolonged in liver disease.
Absorption & Distribution: Slow oral absorption, but well absorbed from the lungs. Rapid distribution to all tissues. Only high concentrations in the lungs produce systemic effects.
Biotransformation & Elimination: Inactivation of the swallowed portion in the liver, some hydrolysis by tissue esterases. Up to 70% excreted in the bile, over 96 hours, as polar metabolites including conjugates; 10–15% excreted in the urine as metabolites.

ADVERSE REACTIONS AND TOXICITY

Acute: None.
Chronic: Candidiasis of throat and mouth, difficulty in vocalization; high doses (20 puffs/day) may induce adrenocortical suppression.

MAJOR DRUG INTERACTIONS: None known.

THERAPEUTIC USE

Usual Effective Plasma Concentration: Not measured clinically.
Usual Dose & Regimen: Adults, 2 puffs (50 μg/puff) three or four times a day, but varies from 100 to 2000 μg/day.
Special Considerations: Therapeutic effect is obtained only with continuous treatment. The aerosol does not provide immediate relief of asthma symptoms and should not be used in acute attacks.

SPECIFIC ANTIDOTE: None.

CEPHALEXIN

Brand Names: Ceporex, Keflex, Novolexin.
Drug Class: First-generation cephalosporin (beta-lactam) antibiotic.
Related Drugs: Cephalothin, cefazolin, cephradine, cefamandole, cefoxitin, cephapirin.

ACTIONS: Inhibits cell wall biosynthesis in susceptible bacteria in a manner similar to the penicillins. Same antibacterial spectrum as cephalothin, the prototype cephalosporin, but less active against penicillinase-producing staphylococci.

PHARMACOKINETICS

pK_a: 5.2 (acidic).
Mean V_d: 0.26 L/kg.
Plasma Protein Binding: Less than 15% bound.
Bioavailability: 80–100% (oral).
Half-Life–Normal: 50 minutes. – **Disease States:** Increased in renal dysfunction.
Absorption & Distribution: Acid-stable and well absorbed orally. Peak plasma levels (10–20 μg/mL after 250–500 mg) attained in 1 hour, but delayed in the presence of food. High concentrations in synovial and pericardial fluids and urine, low in the eyes, none in the brain.
Biotransformation & Elimination: More than 90% excreted unchanged in the urine within 6 hours, primarily by renal tubular secretion. Also excreted in the bile.

ADVERSE REACTIONS AND TOXICITY

Acute: Nausea, vomiting, diarrhea, abdominal cramps, headache, dizziness, drowsiness; anaphylaxis.
Chronic: Hypersensitivity reactions (rash, fever, urticaria), nephrotoxicity, superinfection.

MAJOR DRUG INTERACTIONS: Probenecid decreases renal tubular secretion.

THERAPEUTIC USE

Usual Effective Plasma Concentration: Refer to Chapter 53.
Usual Dose & Regimen: Adults, 250–500 mg every 4–6 hours, maximum 4 g per day. Children, 25–50 mg/kg/day divided into 4 doses.
Special Considerations: Cross-reactions in penicillin-hypersensitive subjects.

SPECIFIC ANTIDOTE: None.

CHLORDIAZEPOXIDE

Brand Names: Apo-Chlordiazepoxide, Librium, Medilium, Novopoxide, Solium.
Drug Class: Benzodiazepine anxiolytic, minor tranquilizer.
Related Drugs: Diazepam, oxazepam, lorazepam, triazolam.

ACTIONS: Enhances the binding of an inhibitory neurotransmitter (GABA). Depresses the brainstem reticular activating system; depresses electrical after-discharge in the limbic system; increases the seizure threshold; produces a generalized depression of the cerebral cortex.

PHARMACOKINETICS

pK_a: 4.6 (basic).
Mean V_d: 0.3 L/kg.
Plasma Protein Binding: 95% bound, decreased in cirrhosis and viral hepatitis.
Bioavailability: 100% (oral).
Half-Life–Normal: 10–14 hours. – **Disease States:** Prolonged by severe liver disease and increasing age.
Absorption & Distribution: Slowly absorbed after oral administration; poor intramuscular absorption. Long distribution phase.
Biotransformation & Elimination: Converted in the liver to an active metabolite and other oxidation products and glucuronide conjugates, which are excreted in the urine.

ADVERSE REACTIONS AND TOXICITY

Acute: Drowsiness, hypotension, dizziness, cardiopulmonary arrest (i.v.), paradoxical increase in anxiety. Impairs driving ability.
Chronic: Impairment of cognitive function.

MAJOR DRUG INTERACTIONS: Additive effects with other CNS depressants.

THERAPEUTIC USE

Usual Effective Plasma Concentration: 0.5–5.0 mg/L (2–17 μmol/L). Not measured clinically.
Usual Dose & Regimen: Orally, 15–60 mg/day in divided doses. Intravenously, 50–100 mg for acute agitation; up to 300 mg for alcohol withdrawal.
Special Considerations: Chronic use induces dependence and withdrawal symptoms such as tremor, anxiety, and (rarely) seizures.

SPECIFIC ANTIDOTE: None. (Specific receptor blockers, *e.g.*, Ro15–1788, reverse all effects of benzodiazepines, but are not yet available clinically.) General supportive care.

CHLORPROMAZINE

Brand Names: Chlorpromanyl, Largactil, Novochlorpromazine.
Drug Class: Neuroleptic, antipsychotic, major tranquilizer, phenothiazine.
Related Drugs: Promazine, triflupromazine, mesoridazine, thioridazine,* fluphenazine, trifluoperazine.†

ACTIONS: Blockade of dopamine receptors in the brain. Suppresses spontaneous movement and complex behavior; reduces the display of emotion and range of affect.

PHARMACOKINETICS

pK$_a$: 9.3 (basic).
Mean V$_d$: 20 L/kg.
Plasma Protein Binding: 95–99% bound.
Bioavailability: 15–50% (oral).
Half-Life–Normal: 15–35 hours. – **Disease States:** May be altered in hepatic cirrhosis; prolonged in the aged.
Absorption & Distribution: Well absorbed, but extensive first-pass effect causes erratic and unpredictable systemic concentrations. Highly lipophilic, binds extensively to proteins and membranes. Accumulates in brain, lungs, and other highly perfused tissues.
Biotransformation & Elimination: Oxidation and conjugation in the liver to numerous metabolites; excreted in urine and bile.

ADVERSE REACTIONS AND TOXICITY

Acute: Sedation, orthostatic hypotension, hypothermia, stuffy nose, dry mouth.
Chronic: Extrapyramidal syndromes (common), especially tardive dyskinesia; skin reactions (common), cholestatic jaundice (uncommon), blood dyscrasias (rare), elevated prolactin release.

MAJOR DRUG INTERACTIONS: Potentiation of CNS depressants, analgesics, antihistamines. Antagonizes the action of dopamine agonists (L-dopa). Hepatic enzyme inducers may decrease effects.

THERAPEUTIC USE

Usual Effective Plasma Concentration: Controversial, 30–350 ng/mL (94–1098 nmol/L).
Usual Dose & Regimen: Orally, 300–800 mg/day. Parenterally, 25–50 mg, up to 4 times/day, for acute symptomatology.
Special Considerations: Dose adjustments and addition of anticholinergic agents after chronic treatment may be necessary to minimize extrapyramidal syndromes.

SPECIFIC ANTIDOTE: Parkinsonian symptoms are treated with anticholinergic drugs. Adrenaline (epinephrine) should not be used to correct hypotension.

---

* **THIORIDAZINE** (Apo-Thioridazine, Mellaril, Novoridazine)
Similar to chlorpromazine *except*:
Less extrapyramidal effect for the same degree of antipsychotic action.

† **TRIFLUOPERAZINE** (Novoflurazine, Solazine, Stelazine, Terfluzine)
Similar to chlorpromazine *except*:
Less sedative and hypotensive effects. More extrapyramidal effect for the same degree of antipsychotic action (less cholinergic blocking action).

CHLORPROPAMIDE

Brand Names: Apo-Chlorpropamide, Diabinese, Novopropamide.
Drug Class: Oral hypoglycemic, sulfonylurea.
Related Drugs: Tolbutamide, acetohexamide, tolazamide, glibenclamide (glyburide).

ACTIONS: Stimulates pancreatic islet tissue to secrete insulin.

PHARMACOKINETICS

pK$_a$: 5.0 (acidic).
Mean V$_d$: 0.1–0.2 L/kg.
Plasma Protein Binding: 60–95% bound.
Bioavailability: Estimated 70–90% (oral).
Half-Life–Normal: 24–42 hours. – **Disease States:** Prolonged with impaired renal function.
Absorption & Distribution: Rapid absorption from GI tract.
Biotransformation & Elimination: Excreted essentially unchanged, 60% in the urine.

ADVERSE REACTIONS AND TOXICITY

Acute: Hypoglycemia.
Chronic: Hematological, cutaneous, gastrointestinal, cholestatic jaundice (0.4%, reversible), hyponatremia, enhanced renal sensitivity to ADH.

MAJOR DRUG INTERACTIONS: Alcohol intolerance. Sulfonamides, propranolol, salicylates, clofibrate, phenylbutazone and other drugs may potentiate hypoglycemia.

THERAPEUTIC USE

Usual Effective Plasma Concentration: 75–250 mg/L (270–900 µmol/L). Not measured clinically.
Usual Dose & Regimen: 125–500 mg daily as a single dose.
Special Considerations: Long half-life permits single daily dose.

SPECIFIC ANTIDOTE: Glucose for hypoglycemia.

CIMETIDINE

Brand Names: Apo-Cimetidine, Novocimetine, Peptol, Tagamet.
Drug Class: Histamine H_2-receptor antagonist, inhibitor of gastric acid secretion.
Related Drugs: Ranitidine, famotidine, nizatidine.

ACTIONS: Competitive antagonist of H_2 receptors. Suppresses gastric acid and pepsin release mediated by histamine release from mast cells in the stomach wall.

PHARMACOKINETICS

pK_a: 6.8 (basic).
Mean V_d: 1.4 L/kg.
Plasma Protein Binding: 15–25% bound.
Bioavailability: 75% (oral).
Half-Life–Normal: 1.5–3 hours. – **Disease States:** Prolonged with decreased renal, hepatic function.
Absorption & Distribution: Well absorbed orally, decreased by antacids; peak plasma concentrations in 2–3 hours. Highest concentrations in kidneys, stomach, liver. CNS penetration enhanced in liver disease. Binds extensively to hepatic cytochrome P-450.
Biotransformation & Elimination: Approximately 20–40% converted to sulfoxide. Remainder excreted unchanged, almost entirely in the urine.

ADVERSE REACTIONS AND TOXICITY

Acute: Infrequent and transient tiredness, dizziness, rash.
Chronic: Dizziness, reversible confusional states (uncommon), gynecomastia (rare), elevated serum transaminases and creatinine, increased prolactin secretion (high doses).

MAJOR DRUG INTERACTIONS: Inhibition of hepatic microsomal enzymes by cimetidine, and possibly decreased liver blood flow, increase the plasma levels of many concomitant drugs (e.g., theophylline, morphine, chlordiazepoxide, diazepam, warfarin, propranolol, phenytoin).

THERAPEUTIC USE

Usual Effective Plasma Concentration: 0.5–1 μg/mL.
Usual Dose & Regimen: Orally, 800–1200 mg/day divided into 2–4 doses for acute duodenal ulcer; 400 mg/day for ulcer prophylaxis. Parenterally, 300 mg i.v. every 6 hours.
Special Considerations: Decreased dose in hepatic, renal disease; drug interactions may require dose adjustments of other drugs.

SPECIFIC ANTIDOTE: None.

CODEINE

Brand Names: Paveral, many mixtures with caffeine and ASA or acetaminophen.
Drug Class: Opioid analgesic; antitussive.
Related Drugs: Oxycodone, morphine, many others.

ACTIONS: Binds to central endogenous opioid receptors. The affinity for these receptors is low compared to most other opioids; analgesic effects may be due partly to morphine, a metabolite of codeine.

PHARMACOKINETICS

pK_a: 8.2 (basic).
Mean V_d: 3.5 L/kg.
Plasma Protein Binding: 7–25% bound (estimated).
Bioavailability: 40–70% (oral).
Half-Life–Normal: 2–4 hours. – **Disease States:** Prolonged in hepatic disease?
Absorption & Distribution: One of the best absorbed opioid analgesics; plasma peaks are attained within 1 hour. Distribution is complete in 1.5 hours. High peripheral tissue binding.
Biotransformation & Elimination: Extensive glucuronide conjugation in the liver; 15% demethylated to morphine. Eliminated primarily in the urine as metabolites.

ADVERSE REACTIONS AND TOXICITY

Acute Overdose: Sedation, nausea, vomiting, constipation, respiratory depression, dysphoria.
Chronic: Physical dependence (low risk), constipation.

MAJOR DRUG INTERACTIONS: Additive with CNS depressants.

THERAPEUTIC USE

Usual Effective Plasma Concentration: Not measured clinically.
Usual Dose & Regimen: Analgesia, 30–60 mg in adults, 3 mg/kg/day in children in 6 doses. Antitussive, 10–15 mg, every 3–4 hours as necessary.
Special Considerations: As for all opioids.

SPECIFIC ANTIDOTE: Naloxone.

COLCHICINE

Brand Names: —
Drug Class: Plant alkaloid, anti-inflammatory, gout therapy (not a uricosuric).
Related Drugs: —

ACTIONS: Reduces inflammation and pain of gout by decreasing the mobility of granulocytes, their lactate production, phagocytosis of urate crystals, and subsequent deposition of urate crystals. Inhibits microtubule formation, arrests mitosis in metaphase; inhibits collagen formation.

PHARMACOKINETICS

pK$_a$: 1.7 (basic).
Mean V$_d$: 1–2 L/kg.
Plasma Protein Binding: 30–50% bound.
Bioavailability: Near 100% (oral).
Half-Life–Normal: About 30 minutes. – **Disease States:** 45 minutes (end-stage renal disease).
Absorption & Distribution: Rapid oral absorption; rapid distribution especially to liver, kidneys, spleen, GI tract; excluded from heart, skeletal muscle, brain. Persists in leukocytes for 8–10 days after a single dose.
Biotransformation & Elimination: Largely excreted in the feces, 10–20% in the urine.

ADVERSE REACTIONS AND TOXICITY

Acute: Abdominal pain, diarrhea, vomiting.
Chronic: Agranulocytosis, aplastic anemia, myopathy, hair loss.

MAJOR DRUG INTERACTIONS: Interferes with determinations of urinary 17-hydroxycorticosteroids.

THERAPEUTIC USE

Usual Effective Plasma Concentration: Not measured clinically.
Usual Dose & Regimen: Acute attack of gout, immediately upon first signs, 1 mg then 0.6 mg every 2 hours until pain is relieved or toxic symptoms occur (maximum 10 mg/24 hours). Prophylaxis of chronic gout, 0.5–2 mg every night or every other night.
Special Considerations: Patients with gout undergoing surgery should receive colchicine for a few days preoperatively to minimize attacks precipitated by operative procedures.

SPECIFIC ANTIDOTE: None.

CYCLOPHOSPHAMIDE

Brand Names: Cytoxan, Procytox.
Drug Class: Antineoplastic, alkylating agent.
Related Drugs: Other nitrogen mustards, ethylenimine derivatives, alkyl sulfonates, nitrosoureas.

ACTIONS: Converted to an active metabolite that causes DNA alkylation.

PHARMACOKINETICS

pK$_a$: ? (basic).
Mean V$_d$: 0.8 L/kg.
Plasma Protein Binding: 12% bound.
Bioavailability: 75–97% (oral).
Half-Life–Normal: 3–10 hours (active metabolites). – **Disease States:** ?
Absorption & Distribution: Well absorbed orally.
Biotransformation & Elimination: Extensive hepatic transformation with renal excretion of 80% of metabolites.

ADVERSE REACTIONS AND TOXICITY

Acute: Nausea, vomiting, alopecia, myelosuppression, hemorrhagic cystitis (common); water retention (uncommon).
Chronic: Leukemia.

MAJOR DRUG INTERACTIONS: n.a.

THERAPEUTIC USE

Usual Effective Plasma Concentration: Not measured clinically.
Usual Dose & Regimen: 50–100 mg/m^2 p.o. daily, or 500–1000 mg/m^2 i.v. every 7–10 days.
Special Considerations: Keep patient hydrated!

SPECIFIC ANTIDOTE: None.

DESMOPRESSIN ACETATE

Brand Name: DDAVP.
Drug Class: Antidiuretic hormone analog.
Related Drugs: Arginine vasopressin, lypressin (lysine vasopressin).

ACTIONS: Increases the water-permeability of renal distal tubular epithelium and collecting ducts, allowing increased reabsorption of free water and a decrease in urine flow. Intracellular mediator is cyclic AMP.

PHARMACOKINETICS

pK$_a$: n.a. (peptide).
Mean V$_d$: (Extracellular fluid).
Plasma Protein Binding: ?
Bioavailability: Nil (oral).
Half-Life–Normal: 1–2 hours; duration of action 8–20 hours. – **Disease States:** ?
Absorption & Distribution: Oral dose is inactivated by trypsin. Absorption from nasal mucosa (10%) is reliable. As a peptide, it is distributed only in extracellular fluid.
Biotransformation & Elimination: Cleavage of peptide bonds by peptidases in several tissues, primarily the kidneys.

ADVERSE REACTIONS AND TOXICITY

Acute: Headaches (transient), abdominal cramps, flushing, rhinitis (possibly hypertension).
Chronic: Hyponatremia, local irritation of nasal mucosa, water intoxication.

MAJOR DRUG INTERACTIONS: Chlorpropamide, acetaminophen, ASA, indomethacin enhance antidiuretic activity; demeclocycline, PGE$_1$, colchicine, and vinca alkaloids inhibit activity. Lithium causes polyuria.

THERAPEUTIC USE

Usual Effective Plasma Concentration: Not measured clinically.
Usual Dose & Regimen: Intranasal spray, 5–20 μg, 1–2 times daily. Injection (any route), 0.4–4 μg, once daily. Urine osmolality and diuresis are used to establish the dose.
Special Considerations: Use with caution in patients with coronary disease or hypertension.

SPECIFIC ANTIDOTE: None. Water restriction in overdose.

DEXTROMETHORPHAN

Brand Names: Balminil, Broncho-Grippol, Delsym, Koffex, Ornex, Robidex, Sedatuss.
Drug Class: Synthetic non-analgesic opioid, antitussive.
Related Drugs: Benzonatate, pholcodine, levopropoxyphene, noscapine.

ACTIONS: Elevates the cough threshold through central inhibition of afferent tussal impulses.

PHARMACOKINETICS

pK$_a$: 8.3 (basic).
Mean V$_d$: 3–5 L/kg.
Plasma Protein Binding: 30–50% bound.
Bioavailability: Better than 50% (oral).
Half-Life–Normal: 2–3 hours (estimated). – **Disease States:** ?
Absorption & Distribution: Well absorbed orally.
Biotransformation & Elimination: Biotransformed in the liver; excreted in the urine both as unchanged drug and demethylated morphinans.

ADVERSE REACTIONS AND TOXICITY

Acute: Slight drowsiness, dizziness or nausea (all rare). Overdose: Mental confusion, excitation, respiratory depression.
Chronic: Very occasional abuse (no physical dependence).

MAJOR DRUG INTERACTIONS: None.

THERAPEUTIC USE

Usual Effective Plasma Concentration: Not measured clinically.
Usual Dose & Regimen: Adults, 15–30 mg up to 4 times a day. Children, 1 mg/kg/day, in divided doses.
Special Considerations: Use with caution in patients with liver disease, asthma (histamine releaser).

SPECIFIC ANTIDOTE: None.

DIAZEPAM

Brand Names: Apo-Diazepam, Diazemuls, E-Pam, Meval, Novodipam, Rival, Valium, Vivol.
Drug Class: Benzodiazepine anxiolytic.
Related Drugs: Chlordiazepoxide, oxazepam, lorazepam, triazolam, temazepam, prazepam, others.

ACTIONS: Enhances binding of gamma-aminobutyric acid (GABA), an inhibitory neurotransmitter, to its receptors in the brain. Depresses the reticular activating system, electrical after-discharge in the limbic system, cerebral cortex. Increases the seizure threshold.

PHARMACOKINETICS

pK$_a$: 3.3 (basic).
Mean V$_d$: 1.1 L/kg.
Plasma Protein Binding: 98–99% bound (decreased in hypoalbuminemia).
Bioavailability: 100% (oral).
Half-Life–Normal: 40 hours (50 hours for active metabolite). – **Disease States:** Prolonged in the elderly, premature neonates, hepatic disease.
Absorption & Distribution: Rapidly absorbed, with peak plasma concentration in 30–60 minutes. Rapid distribution into the brain. Adipose tissue is depot compartment.
Biotransformation & Elimination: Hepatic oxidation to the N-demethylated form, an active metabolite which accumulates with chronic dosing. Urinary excretion of glucuronide and sulfate conjugates is the primary excretion pathway (70%). Remainder is excreted in the urine or bile as oxidized metabolites.

ADVERSE REACTIONS AND TOXICITY

Acute: Drowsiness, ataxia, hostility, irritability, nightmares, paradoxically increased anxiety, confusion.
Chronic: Same as acute; drug dependence, withdrawal seizures possible.

MAJOR DRUG INTERACTIONS: Additive with CNS depressants.

THERAPEUTIC USE

Usual Effective Plasma Concentration: 0.1–0.25 mg/L (350–900 nmol/L).
Usual Dose & Regimen: Orally, 4–40 mg per day. Intravenously, 2–20 mg per dose, *injected very slowly*.
Special Considerations: Contraindicated in myasthenia gravis.

SPECIFIC ANTIDOTE: None. (Specific receptor blockers, *e.g.,* Ro15–1788, are not yet available for clinical use.) General supportive care.

DIGOXIN

Brand Names: Lanoxin, Novodigoxin.
Drug Class: Cardiac (digitalis) glycoside.
Related Drugs: Digitoxin, ouabain, lanatoside, acetylstrophanthidin.

ACTIONS: Reversible inhibition of myocardial membrane-bound (Na$^+$+K$^+$)-ATPase. Intracellular accumulation of Na$^+$ (and decrease in intracellular K$^+$) promotes Ca^{2+} entry in exchange for Na$^+$. Subsequent release of Ca^{2+} from sarcoplasmic reticulum causes positive inotropic effect, the primary therapeutic action. Also direct and indirect effects on heart rate, cardiac excitability, conduction velocity, refractory period, automaticity.

PHARMACOKINETICS

pK$_a$: n.a. (glycoside).
Mean V$_d$: 5.3 L/kg (digitoxin 0.6 L/kg); decreased in hypothyroid, increased in hyperthyroid states.
Plasma Protein Binding: 30% bound (digitoxin 95%).
Bioavailability: 75% (oral).
Half-Life–Normal: 20–50 hours, strongly dependent on renal function. – **Disease States:** Increased in uremia, anephric patients (4.5 days), congestive heart failure.
Absorption & Distribution: Absorption varies from 40% to 90%, depending on dosage form. Peak plasma concentration in 2–3 hours; distribution to most tissues. Myocardial concentrations are 15–30 times higher than plasma concentrations (skeletal muscle is half that of cardiac muscle).
Biotransformation & Elimination: Excreted principally unchanged by the kidneys. Renal status determines clearance.

ADVERSE REACTIONS AND TOXICITY

Acute: 25% of patients may show signs of toxicity.
    Cardiac dysrhythmias: active—atrial, ventricular (*e.g.,* ventricular premature beats), atrial tachycardia; passive—block of conduction (*e.g.,* 1° block, prolonged P-R interval); combined active and passive.
    Systemic: headache, fatigue, malaise, drowsiness, nausea, anorexia, vomiting, visual disturbances, gynecomastia.
Chronic: Same as acute.

MAJOR DRUG INTERACTIONS: Concurrent administration of diuretics may cause potassium depletion, which increases digoxin toxicity. Hypomagnesemia, hypercalcemia, hypoxia also increase toxicity. Suppression of digoxin-induced dysrhythmias by lidocaine, phenytoin, atropine. Quinidine, amiodarone, spironolactone elevate plasma concentrations of digoxin.

THERAPEUTIC USE

Usual Effective Plasma Concentration: Greater than 0.8 ng/mL (1.0 nmol/L). Toxic range above 1.6 ng/mL (2.0 nmol/L), with correspondingly increasing probability of dysrhythmia.
Usual Dose & Regimen: Digitalizing dose (acute): orally, 1.5–2 mg over 24 hours; slowly i.v., 0.75–1.5 mg. Maintenance dose: 0.25–0.75 mg/day.
Special Considerations: Reduced dose requirements in older patients, in renal failure, and in patients not requiring maximal digitalization.

SPECIFIC ANTIDOTE: Specific antibody fragments are available for immediate relief of overdose effects.

DIPHENHYDRAMINE

Brand Names: Allerdryl, Benadryl, Insomnal.
Drug Class: Antihistamine (H_1-receptor blocker).
Related Drugs: Brompheniramine, chlorpheniramine, dimenhydrinate, cyclizine, promethazine, many others.

ACTIONS: Competitive, reversible blockade of histamine-H_1 receptors; also has anticholinergic (antimuscarinic) activity which may be the reason for its ability to relieve motion sickness.

PHARMACOKINETICS

pK$_a$: 9.0 (basic).
Mean V$_d$: About 8 L/kg.
Plasma Protein Binding: 80–95% bound.
Bioavailability: 60% (oral).
Half-Life–Normal: About 9 hours. – **Disease States:** ?
Absorption & Distribution: Peak plasma concentrations 2 hours after oral dose, remaining at 2-hour plateau; distributed throughout the body, including the CNS.
Biotransformation & Elimination: Biotransformed almost completely in the liver; excreted primarily in the urine, as metabolites, within 24 hours.

ADVERSE REACTIONS AND TOXICITY

Acute: Sedation (common), dizziness, dry mouth, nausea (anticholinergic). Overdose causes excitation, hallucinations, ataxia, incoordination, athetosis, convulsions.
Chronic: Allergic dermatitis, rare cases of leukopenia, agranulocytosis.

MAJOR DRUG INTERACTIONS: Sedative effects are additive with other CNS depressants. Slows gastric emptying and possibly alters absorption of other drugs.

THERAPEUTIC USE

Usual Effective Plasma Concentration: Not measured clinically.
Usual Dose & Regimen: Orally, adult, 25–30 mg, 3–4 times daily; child (under 12), half the adult dose. Parenterally, 10–50 mg i.v. or deep i.m.; up to 400 mg/day in adults.
Special Considerations: Some drugs in this class are teratogenic in animals and are contraindicated in pregnancy.

SPECIFIC ANTIDOTE: None; supportive therapy only.

ERGOTAMINE TARTRATE

Brand Names: Ergomar, Gynergen, Medihaler-Ergotamine.
Drug Class: Ergot alkaloid.
Related Drugs: Dihydroergotamine, ergonovine, bromocriptine, methysergide.

ACTIONS: Partial agonist at α-adrenergic and tryptaminergic (serotonin) receptors. Uterotonic effects; arterio- and venoconstriction.

PHARMACOKINETICS

pK$_a$: 6.3 (basic).
Mean V$_d$: 2 L/kg.
Plasma Protein Binding: Over 90% bound.
Bioavailability: About 10% (oral); erratic, enhanced by caffeine.
Half-Life–Normal: About 2 hours. – **Disease States:** Not investigated.
Absorption & Distribution: Erratically absorbed (30–60%). Extensive first-pass effect is likely to account for poor bioavailability. High concentrations in liver, lungs, kidneys. Accumulates in tissues.
Biotransformation & Elimination: Extensive conversion in the liver to unidentified metabolites. Most (90%) is eliminated in the bile, although some urinary excretion occurs.

ADVERSE REACTIONS AND TOXICITY

Acute: Nausea, vomiting, pain and weakness in extremities, transient tachycardia or bradycardia, anginal pain.
Chronic: Digital paraesthesias, vascular stasis, thrombosis, gangrene.

MAJOR DRUG INTERACTIONS: Troleandomycin or erythromycin elevate ergotamine levels.

THERAPEUTIC USE

Usual Effective Plasma Concentration: Not measured clinically.
Usual Dose & Regimen: Migraine, 2 mg at first sign of attack, 1 mg every 30 minutes, maximum 6 mg per day, limited to maximum of 10 mg in any one week.
Special Considerations: For acute migraine attacks only.

SPECIFIC ANTIDOTE: None.

FLUDROCORTISONE

Brand Name: Florinef.
Drug Class: Adrenocortical steroid, predominantly mineralocorticoid.
Related Drugs: Aldosterone, desoxycorticosterone.

ACTIONS: Binds to mineralocorticoid receptors in the kidneys. May increase the synthesis of protein controlling Na^+ uptake. Consequent loss of K^+ and H^+ in exchange for Na^+. Over 100 times more potent than cortisol (hydrocortisone) in mineralocorticoid activity, 10 times more potent in glucocorticoid activity.

PHARMACOKINETICS

pK_a: n.a. (steroid).
Mean V_d: ?
Plasma Protein Binding: 70–80% bound, to globulin and albumin.
Bioavailability: Essentially 100% (oral).
Half-Life–Normal: 6–8 hours (biologic half-life 8–12 hours). – **Disease States:** Prolonged in severe liver disease.
Absorption & Distribution: Rapid, complete absorption.
Biotransformation & Elimination: Hepatic and extrahepatic reduction, oxidation, and conjugation (sulfate or glucuronide) to several metabolites. All excreted in the urine.

ADVERSE REACTIONS AND TOXICITY

Acute: Minimal.
Chronic: Fluid retention, electrolyte disturbances, hypertension, adrenal medullary suppression, myopathy.

MAJOR DRUG INTERACTIONS: None known.

THERAPEUTIC USE

Usual Effective Plasma Concentration: Not measured clinically.
Usual Dose & Regimen: In Addison's disease, 0.1 mg/day; range 0.05–0.2 mg/day.
Special Considerations: May mask systemic infections, may suppress immune responses.

SPECIFIC ANTIDOTE: None.

FUROSEMIDE (FRUSEMIDE)

Brand Names: Apo-Furosemide, Furoside, Lasix, Novosemide, Uritol.
Drug Class: "Loop" (high-ceiling) diuretic.
Related Drugs: Ethacrynic acid, bumetanide.

ACTIONS: Inhibits Na^+ and Cl^- reabsorption in the ascending limb of the loop of Henle. Rapid onset of action, peak diuresis greater than with thiazides. May acutely decrease venous return, increase urinary potassium, decrease uric acid excretion.

PHARMACOKINETICS

pK_a: 3.8 (acidic).
Mean V_d: 0.1–0.2 L/kg.
Plasma Protein Binding: 97% bound.
Bioavailability: 65% (oral).
Half-Life–Normal: 1–3 hours. – **Disease States:** Increased in uremia (up to ten-fold), hypertension, heart failure, hepatic disease.
Absorption & Distribution: Well absorbed from GI tract, delayed by food.
Biotransformation & Elimination: Side-chain cleavage and glucuronide conjugation occur to small extent (less than 10%). Up to one-third is excreted in the feces, the remainder actively secreted into the urine. Some glomerular filtration.

ADVERSE REACTIONS AND TOXICITY

Acute: Hypotension, deafness (doses >250 mg).
Chronic: Electrolyte (K^+) and fluid disturbances; hyperuricemia.

MAJOR DRUG INTERACTIONS: Increased risk of nephrotoxicity and ototoxicity of aminoglycosides and cephalosporins. Lithium clearance is decreased. Less effective in the presence of nonsteroidal anti-inflammatory agents.

THERAPEUTIC USE

Usual Effective Plasma Concentration: Not measured clinically.
Usual Dose & Regimen: Acute, 20–40 mg i.v. in pulmonary edema. Chronic, orally, 20–80 mg/day or every other day in severe congestive heart failure.
Special Considerations: With large doses in chronic renal failure, the i.v. administration rate is restricted to 2.5–4 mg/minute.

SPECIFIC ANTIDOTE: Potassium, spironolactone are useful concomitant drugs to prevent hypokalemia.

GENTAMICIN

Brand Names: Alcomicin, Cidomycin, Garamycin, Gentamytrex.
Drug Class: Aminoglycoside antibiotic.
Related Drugs: Tobramycin, amikacin, netilmicin, kanamycin, streptomycin, neomycin.

ACTIONS: Interferes with translation of the genetic code by a direct action at the bacterial ribosome; inhibits protein synthesis. Effective primarily against aerobic Gram-negative bacilli, but resistance is common.

PHARMACOKINETICS

pK$_a$: 8.2 (basic).
Mean V$_d$: 0.25 L/kg.
Plasma Protein Binding: Less than 30% bound.
Bioavailability: Less than 1% (oral).
Half-Life–Normal: 2–3 hours. – **Disease States:** Increased in renal dysfunction.
Absorption & Distribution: Essentially nonabsorbable by the oral route. Distributes in extracellular fluid. Poor penetration into eyes, CNS, respiratory fluids.
Biotransformation & Elimination: Excreted almost entirely by glomerular filtration as unchanged drug. Tissue-bound gentamicin is excreted with a half-life in excess of 30 hours.

ADVERSE REACTIONS AND TOXICITY

Acute: Nausea, vomiting, headache.
Chronic: Superinfection, nephrotoxicity, ototoxicity. Both nephro- and ototoxicity are directly related to aminoglycoside accumulation.

MAJOR DRUG INTERACTIONS: Incompatible in solution with carbenicillin and other penicillins, cephalosporins, amphotericin B and heparin. Concomitant use with ethacrynic acid or furosemide may increase the risk of nephro- and ototoxicity. May potentiate muscle relaxants.

THERAPEUTIC USE

Usual Effective Plasma Concentration: Refer to Chapter 55. *Peak:* 4–10 μg/mL (8.6–21.6 μmol/L).
Usual Dose & Regimen: Adults, i.m., 3–5 mg/kg/day divided into 3 equal doses. Infants (and children up to two years), i.m., 2.5 mg/kg every 8 hours (7.5 mg/kg/day).
Special Considerations: Caution in patients with renal impairment.

SPECIFIC ANTIDOTE: None. Peritoneal dialysis or hemodialysis.

HALOPERIDOL

Brand Names: Apo-Haloperidol, Haldol, Novoperidol, Peridol.
Drug Class: Neuroleptic, antipsychotic, butyrophenone.
Related Drugs: Droperidol, trifluperidol.

ACTIONS: Competitive, reversible blockade of dopamine receptors in the brain. Decreases spontaneous movement and complex behavior; reduces the display of emotion and range of affect. Antiemetic effects.

PHARMACOKINETICS

pK$_a$: 8.3 (basic).
Mean V$_d$: 15–30 L/kg.
Plasma Protein Binding: 92% bound.
Bioavailability: 50–70% (oral).
Half-Life–Normal: 12–38 hours. – **Disease States:** No changes observed.
Absorption & Distribution: Good oral absorption. Rapid and extensive peripheral distribution.
Biotransformation & Elimination: Hepatic oxidative dealkylation, oxidation, and glycine conjugation are primary pathways. Metabolites are excreted in urine and bile, with 1% or less excreted as unchanged drug in the urine.

ADVERSE REACTIONS AND TOXICITY

Acute: Sedation, orthostatic hypotension (less than chlorpromazine).
Chronic: Extrapyramidal symptoms (more than chlorpromazine), hepatocellular injury, leukopenia.

MAJOR DRUG INTERACTIONS: Potentiation of sedatives, analgesics, anaesthetics.

THERAPEUTIC USE

Usual Effective Plasma Concentration: 3–10 ng/mL.
Usual Dose & Regimen: Individualized according to clinical effects. Adults, orally, 0.5–5 mg, 2–3 times daily.
Special Considerations: None.

SPECIFIC ANTIDOTE: None. Adrenaline (epinephrine) should not be used to correct hypotension.

HEPARIN

Brand Names: Calcilean, Calciparine, Hepalean.
Drug Class: Anticoagulant (direct-acting).
Related Drugs: None. Oral anticoagulants act by different mechanisms.

ACTIONS: Complex, through activation of plasma antithrombin III: inactivates clotting factors IIa, IXa, Xa, XIa, XIIa, XIIIa and complexes thrombin; neutralizes tissue thromboplastin. Activates lipoprotein lipase. Enhances endothelial electronegative charge.

PHARMACOKINETICS

pK_a: n.a. (strongly acidic).
Mean V_d: 0.06 L/kg.
Plasma Protein Binding: Extensive, at least 80% bound (to globulins, fibrinogen).
Bioavailability: Nil (oral).
Half-Life–Normal: Dose-dependent, e.g., 1 hour at 100 units/kg, 1.5 hours at 200 units/kg, 2.5 hrs at 400 units/kg. – **Disease States:** Prolonged in renal disease, cirrhosis. Shortened in pulmonary embolism, thrombophlebitis.
Absorption & Distribution: Not measurably absorbed orally, must be given parenterally. Distributed in vascular compartment.
Biotransformation & Elimination: Taken up by RES; biotransformed by heparinase; negligible urinary excretion as uroheparin.

ADVERSE REACTIONS AND TOXICITY

Acute: Bleeding (mainly from overdose).
Chronic: Hemorrhage (wound, GI tract, GU tract, etc.). Hypersensitivity, osteoporosis, alopecia (uncommon).

MAJOR DRUG INTERACTIONS: Additive effects of other agents interfering with hemostasis, e.g., oral anticoagulants, platelet inhibitors.

THERAPEUTIC USE

Usual Effective Plasma Concentration: Not measured clinically.
Usual Dose & Regimen: 5000–10,000 units i.v. injection every 6 hours; or 20,000 units/day i.v. infusion; or 5000 units s.c. (low-dose heparin) every 12 hours. Other specialized uses and dosages.
Special Considerations: Monitor blood clotting for dose adjustments.

SPECIFIC ANTIDOTE: Protamine sulfate 1:1 w/w heparin; fresh whole blood.

HYDRALAZINE

Brand Name: Apresoline.
Drug Class: Antihypertensive, smooth muscle relaxant.
Related Drugs: Minoxidil.

ACTIONS: Relaxation of vascular smooth muscle, especially arterial; decreased peripheral resistance. Diastolic pressure often drops more than systolic; minimal postural hypotension, increased cardiac output.

PHARMACOKINETICS

pK_a: 7.0 (basic).
Mean V_d: 2–7 L/kg (unreliable).
Plasma Protein Binding: ?
Bioavailability: 30–35% (oral, in slow acetylators); 10–15% (oral, in rapid acetylators).
Half-Life–Normal: 1–2 hours. – **Disease States:** Possible increase in uremia, renal failure.
Absorption & Distribution: Rapidly absorbed with plasma peak concentration occurring in 15–60 minutes. High tissue concentrations in arterial walls, kidneys, liver, blood, lungs, and adrenals.
Biotransformation & Elimination: Extensive first-pass effect, dependent on acetylator phenotype. Also hepatic oxidation and conjugation. Excreted in the urine as metabolites, less than 10% unchanged.

ADVERSE REACTIONS AND TOXICITY

Acute: Palpitation, tachycardia, anorexia, nausea, dizziness, sweating, headache.
Chronic: Rheumatoid arthritis-like syndrome, systemic lupus erythematosus (especially in slow acetylators), peripheral neuropathies (with doses of 400 mg/day).

MAJOR DRUG INTERACTIONS: Additive effects with beta-blockers (allowing reduction in hydralazine dosage).

THERAPEUTIC USE

Usual Effective Plasma Concentration: 0.5–1.5 μg/mL (3.1–9.4 μmol/L).
Usual Dose & Regimen: Orally, start with 10 mg 2–4 times a day, build up to effective dose level over several weeks; usual maintenance dose 100–200 mg/day, maximum 400 mg/day. Parenterally, 20–40 mg, i.v.
Special Considerations: Titrate slowly to minimize toxicity. Should be used with a beta-blocker to limit reflex cardiovascular responses.

SPECIFIC ANTIDOTE: None.

SPECIAL TOPICS

HYDROCHLOROTHIAZIDE

Brand Names: Apo-Hydro, Diuchlor-H, Esidrix, HydroDiuril, Natrimax, Neo-Codema, Novohydrazide, Urozide.
Drug Class: Sulfonamide (benzothiazide) diuretic.
Related Drugs: Chlorothiazide and many other thiazides, chlorthalidone, metolazone, acetazolamide. Differences are potency, cost, and degree of carbonic anhydrase inhibition.

ACTIONS: Increases renal excretion of Na^+ and Cl^-, and concurrently water, independent of acid-base status. Main site of action is the distal tubule. All drugs of this class increase urinary K^+, decrease uric acid excretion.

PHARMACOKINETICS

pK_a: 7.0, 9.2 (both acidic).
Mean V_d: About 1 L/kg.
Plasma Protein Binding: 40–60% bound.
Bioavailability: 65–75% (oral).
Half-Life–Normal: 2.5 hours. – **Disease States:** Increased in congestive heart failure, renal failure.
Absorption & Distribution: Absorption from duodenum and upper jejunum is enhanced by food and agents that delay gastric emptying. May have slow (t½ 2 hours) distribution phase. Accumulates in red blood cells.
Biotransformation & Elimination: Practically all of the drug is excreted unchanged in the urine by proximal tubular secretion.

ADVERSE REACTIONS AND TOXICITY

Acute: Hypotension.
Chronic: Hypokalemia, hyperuricemia, hyponatremia, hyperglycemia, prerenal failure, skin rashes.

MAJOR DRUG INTERACTIONS: Decreased lithium clearance.

THERAPEUTIC USE

Usual Effective Plasma Concentration: Not measured clinically.
Usual Dose & Regimen: 12.5–100 mg/day.
Special Considerations: Use with caution in borderline hepatic insufficiency. Not effective in renal insufficiency if GFR < 20 mL/minute.

SPECIFIC ANTIDOTE: None.

HYDROCORTISONE (CORTISOL)

Brand Names: Cortacet, Cortamed, Cortate, Cortef, Cortenema, Corticreme, Cortifoam, Cortiment, Cortoderm, Emo-Cort, Hycort, Hyderm, Novohydrocort, Rectocort, Solu-Cortef, Unicort, Westcort.
Drug Class: Adrenocortical steroid, glucocorticoid.
Related Drugs: Aldosterone, prednisolone, fludrocortisone, triamcinolone, dexamethasone, betamethasone.

ACTIONS: Modifies the transcription process in protein synthesis through binding of steroid-receptor complex to chromatin in the cell nucleus. Equally active in liver glycogen deposition, ACTH suppression and anti-inflammatory effects. May cause retention of sodium.

PHARMACOKINETICS

pK_a: 5.1 (as the sodium succinate).
Mean V_d: 0.5–1 L/kg.
Plasma Protein Binding: 90–95% bound.
Bioavailability: 50–60% (oral) with great individual variation.
Half-Life–Normal: 1–2 hours. – **Disease States:** Prolonged in liver disease.
Absorption & Distribution: Completely absorbed orally; transdermal absorption is variable, dependent on site, surface area, *etc.*
Biotransformation & Elimination: Transformed by several pathways, primarily (90%) to cortolones, cortols, tetrahydrocortisone, and tetrahydrocortisol. Excreted in the urine as glucuronides.

ADVERSE REACTIONS AND TOXICITY

Acute: Mental changes, euphoria.
Chronic: Cushingoid features, osteoporosis, diabetes, muscle wasting, increased susceptibility to infection, poor wound healing, adrenal suppression, salt and water retention, hypokalemic alkalosis, peptic ulceration, growth suppression in children.

MAJOR DRUG INTERACTIONS: Enzyme inducers may decrease plasma levels.

THERAPEUTIC USE

Usual Effective Plasma Concentration: 50–250 ng/mL (138–690 nmol/L).
Usual Dose & Regimen: Chronic, nonfatal diseases, start with 20–40 mg/day, up to 120 mg/day. Maintenance doses should be the minimum required for relief of symptoms. Acute, life-threatening disease, start with 100–240 mg/day, in 4 doses. Parenterally, medical emergencies, 100–500 mg i.v. over at least 30 seconds.
Special Considerations: Chronic use has all the risks. Minimize the maintenance dose. During periods of unusual stress, it may be necessary to increase the dose. After prolonged use, taper off gradually to avoid adrenal crisis. May impair patient's response to systemic infection.

SPECIFIC ANTIDOTE: None.

IBUPROFEN

Brand Names: Amersol, Apo-Ibuprofen, Motrin, Novoprofen.
Drug Class: Nonsteroidal anti-inflammatory drug (NSAID).
Related Drugs: Naproxen, ketoprofen, pirprofen, fenoprofen, many others.

ACTIONS: Anti-inflammatory, analgesic, antipyretic by virtue of reversible suppression of prostaglandin synthesis (cyclooxygenase inhibition). This effect is partially responsible for immunologic suppression in rheumatoid arthritis. Also inhibits monocyte, leukocyte migration and other functions of these cells. Potent inhibitor of platelet aggregation.

PHARMACOKINETICS

pK$_a$: 5.2 (acidic).
Mean V$_d$: 0.1 L/kg.
Plasma Protein Binding: More than 99% bound (less at high doses).
Bioavailability: 80% (oral).
Half-Life–Normal: About 2 hours. – **Disease States:** ?
Absorption & Distribution: Well absorbed, plasma peak concentration in 1–2 hours. Slow distribution to peripheral compartments due to extensive plasma protein binding. Synovial fluid concentrations equilibrate with plasma within 6 hours of dosing.
Biotransformation & Elimination: 10% excreted unchanged in the urine, remainder oxidized in the liver and rapidly cleared by the kidneys.

ADVERSE REACTIONS AND TOXICITY

Acute: Nausea, epigastric pain, heartburn (<10%); dizziness, nervousness, vomiting (infrequent).
Chronic: Visual disturbances (uncommon), headache, exacerbation of peptic ulcer, thrombocytopenia.

MAJOR DRUG INTERACTIONS: Concomitant use of ASA may decrease ibuprofen plasma levels by 50%. Increased bleeding tendency if used concurrently with anticoagulants.

THERAPEUTIC USE

Usual Effective Plasma Concentration: Not measured clinically.
Usual Dose & Regimen: Adults, for arthritis, 200–300 mg 3–4 times daily; maximum 2400 mg/day. Moderate pain or inflammation, 400 mg every 4–6 hours, as required.
Special Considerations: Antiplatelet effects can affect hemostasis in predisposed individuals.

SPECIFIC ANTIDOTE: None.

IMIPRAMINE

Brand Names: Apo-Imipramine, Impril, Novopramine, Tofranil.
Drug Class: Tricyclic antidepressant.
Related Drugs: Desipramine, amitriptyline, nortriptyline, doxepin.

ACTIONS: May potentiate the actions of noradrenaline (norepinephrine) and serotonin by blocking re-uptake of these neurotransmitters at the axon terminals. Anticholinergic actions may also be relevant.

PHARMACOKINETICS

pK$_a$: 9.5 (basic).
Mean V$_d$: 10–30 L/kg.
Plasma Protein Binding: 80–90% bound.
Bioavailability: 25–50% (oral).
Half-Life–Normal: 8–25 hours. – **Disease States:** Half-life of active metabolite prolonged in the aged.
Absorption & Distribution: Well absorbed orally, but high first-pass effect results in wide variation of plasma levels. Distributes to all tissues due to extreme lipophilicity. Extensive peripheral tissue binding.
Biotransformation & Elimination: Transformed in the liver by demethylation to desipramine, an active metabolite. Further conversion by hepatic oxidases to 2-hydroxy metabolites followed by glucuronidation. Urinary excretion is the major path of elimination.

ADVERSE REACTIONS AND TOXICITY

Acute: Drowsiness, orthostatic hypotension (adrenergic blockade); blurred vision, tachycardia, dry mouth, constipation (anticholinergic); delirium, hallucinations (central anticholinergic).
Chronic: Persistent fine tremor, occasionally mild parkinsonism, ventricular arrhythmias, conduction defects.

MAJOR DRUG INTERACTIONS: Monoamine oxidase (MAO) inhibitors together with imipramine can cause hyperpyrexia, convulsions, hypertensive crisis. Decreases uptake and effects of guanethidine, guanadrel, debrisoquine, and bethanidine. Synergistic with quinidine-like antiarrhythmics in slowing myocardial repolarization.

THERAPEUTIC USE

Usual Effective Plasma Concentration: 75–200 ng/mL (267–713 nmol/L); toxicity at >1 μg/mL (>3.56 μmol/L) (total measures of imipramine and desipramine).
Usual Dose & Regimen: Adults, 25 mg 3 times daily, up to 150 mg/day in single or divided doses.
Special Considerations: None.

SPECIFIC ANTIDOTE: None. Symptomatic and supportive treatment of overdose. Physostigmine, with great caution, for treatment of anticholinergic symptoms of overdose. Do **not** use quinidine-like antiarrhythmics to treat imipramine-induced arrhythmias.

INSULIN

Types: Crystalline zinc, Protamine zinc, Isophane, Lente, Semilente, Ultralente. Beef, Pork, Beef & Pork, Human.
Brands: Connaught Novo (Insulin, Novolin); Lilly (Iletin, Humulin); Nordisk (Velosulin, Insulatard, Mixtard, Initard).
Drug Class: Antidiabetic agent. (All preparations for treatment of insulin-dependent diabetes mellitus are formulations of insulin to impart specific pharmacokinetic characteristics or to modify antigenicity.)

ACTIONS: Stimulates transport of metabolites (glucose, amino acids) and ions (potassium, magnesium) through cell membranes, promotes biosynthesis of macromolecules (glycogen, lipids, protein) and enhances cell growth.

PHARMACOKINETICS

pK_a: n.a. (Protein with both acidic (A) and basic (B) polypeptide chains; stable at neutral or acid pH.)
Mean V_d: 0.1–0.4 L/kg.
Plasma Protein Binding: Very minor; insulin circulates as the free hormone.
Bioavailability: Nil (oral), 100% (subcutaneous).
Half-Life–Normal: Whole-body $t\frac{1}{2}=3$–4 hours; plasma $t\frac{1}{2}$ <9 minutes (no differences between normals and diabetics). – **Disease States:** Prolonged in hepatic or renal failure.
Absorption & Distribution: All insulin must be injected. Absorption depends primarily on formulation. Crystalline insulin contains zinc to promote crystal formation and gradual absorption from s.c. sites. Lente insulin is a suspension of amorphous and crystalline forms in acetate buffer, which yields a slower onset and longer duration of action. Ultralente and protamine zinc insulins are long-acting.

	CRYSTALLINE	LENTE	ULTRALENTE
ONSET (hr)	0.5–1	2–4	4–6
PEAK (hr)	3–5	7–15	10–30
DURATION (hr)	8–12	12–24	36 or more

Biotransformation & Elimination: Hepatic proteolysis and cleavage of sulfide bridges account for inactivation of 50% of secreted insulin on first pass. Renal tubules are also important sites of degradation. Constituent peptide chains and amino acids are end products. Cleared by the kidneys.

ADVERSE REACTIONS AND TOXICITY

Acute: Hypoglycemia.
Chronic: Allergic reactions (rash, urticaria, angioneurotic edema), lipoatrophy at injection sites, insulin resistance.

MAJOR DRUG INTERACTIONS: Glucagon increases blood sugar. Beta-blockers prolong hypoglycemia, mask sympathetic nervous system response to hypoglycemia (e.g., nervousness, tremor).

THERAPEUTIC USE

Usual Effective Plasma Concentration: ~ 0.4–0.8 pg/mL (~ 0.07–0.14 pmol/L). Not measured clinically, monitor blood glucose.
Usual Dose & Regimen: Entirely governed by the control of blood sugar.
Special Considerations: Labile diabetes, allergic reactions, development of resistance, and other adverse effects may require changes in dose and preparations.

SPECIFIC ANTIDOTE: Glucose, glucagon.

ISOPROTERENOL

Brand Names: Isuprel, Medihaler-Iso.
Drug Class: Sympathomimetic, catecholamine.
Related Drugs: Adrenaline (epinephrine), salbutamol (albuterol), metaproterenol (orciprenaline), many others.

ACTIONS: β-Adrenoceptor agonist. Positive cardiac chronotropic and inotropic effects; decreases peripheral resistance mainly in skeletal muscle, and renal and mesenteric vascular beds; relaxes bronchial and gastrointestinal smooth muscle and the pregnant uterus.

PHARMACOKINETICS

pK_a: 8.6 (basic), 10.1 (acidic).
Mean V_d: 0.7 L/kg.
Plasma Protein Binding: 65% bound.
Bioavailability: Nil (oral); estimated 80–100% (inhalation).
Half-Life–Normal: 2 hours. – **Disease States:** ?
Absorption & Distribution: Well absorbed when inhaled, but extensive first-pass effect orally; a large fraction of an inhaled dose is swallowed and lost. Rapid distribution to all tissues.
Biotransformation & Elimination: Sulfate conjugation in the liver, and methylation in various tissues by catechol-O-methyl transferase (COMT). Oral dose: 85% conjugated; intravenous dose: excreted in the urine as 50% free, 50% methylated; lung dose: methylated.

ADVERSE REACTIONS AND TOXICITY

Acute: Palpitations, tachycardia, headache, flushing (common). Angina, arrhythmias, tremor, sweating, nausea.
Chronic: Myocardial necrosis after chronic doses in animals, swelling of parotid glands. Increased airway resistance with chronic use.

MAJOR DRUG INTERACTIONS: Additive with other sympathomimetics. May be potentiated by tricyclic antidepressants.

THERAPEUTIC USE

Usual Effective Plasma Concentration: 0.5–2.5 ng/mL. Not measured clinically.
Usual Dose & Regimen: Subcutaneous or intramuscular dose is 200 μg. Intravenous or intracardiac dose is 20 μg. Intravenous infusion at about 5 μg/min. Inhaled dose is 1–2 inhalations (125 μg each) 4 times a day, to 1 mg maximum. (Sublingual tablets are also available.)
Special Considerations: Not to be administered together with adrenaline.

SPECIFIC ANTIDOTE: β-Adrenoceptor blockers.

LEVODOPA

Brand Name: Larodopa.
Drug Class: Catecholamine precursor. Antiparkinsonism agent.
Related Drugs: Dopamine, apomorphine, bromocriptine.

ACTIONS: Acts as metabolic precursor of dopamine, and replenishes depleted stores of this neurotransmitter in the remaining nigrostriatal neurons in brains of patients with Parkinson's disease.

PHARMACOKINETICS

pK_a: 2.3 (acidic), 8.7 (basic).
Mean V_d: About 65% of body weight.
Plasma Protein Binding: ?
Bioavailability: Estimated 10–50% (oral, erratic).
Half-Life–Normal: 1–3 hours. – **Disease States:** ?
Absorption & Distribution: Rapid absorption in the small bowel by amino acid-specific transport system. Prolonged gastric emptying time and low pH may decrease absorption because of acidic and enzymatic degradation. Distribution is extensive, but rapid peripheral decarboxylation to dopamine allows only 1% to reach the brain in unchanged form.
Biotransformation & Elimination: Decarboxylation to dopamine by peripheral (99%) and cerebral (1%) aromatic amino acid decarboxylase. Up to 30 metabolites, some active, are identified. Monoamine oxidase, followed by catechol-O-methyl transferase, is the major pathway (50% of dose). Urinary excretion of metabolites (80%) is the major route of elimination.

ADVERSE REACTIONS AND TOXICITY

Acute: Nausea, vomiting, anorexia, epigastric distress.
Chronic: Abnormal involuntary movements (up to 80% of patients), cardiac irregularities, orthostatic hypotension, psychiatric abnormalities, red or black urine.

MAJOR DRUG INTERACTIONS: Pyridoxine (in multivitamin preparations) decreases the effects. Anticholinergics, peripheral aromatic amino acid decarboxylase inhibitors potentiate the effects. Antipsychotics, reserpine, monoamine oxidase inhibitors are contraindicated.

THERAPEUTIC USE

Usual Effective Plasma Concentration: Not measured clinically.
Usual Dose & Regimen: Start with 0.5–1 g daily in 3–4 doses. Titrate to symptom improvement by weekly addition of 0.1–0.75 g/day. Maintenance dose, 3–8 g daily in at least 4 doses.
Special Considerations: Slow dose titration (1–3 months), followed by at least 3 months of maintenance dosing to determine effectiveness.

SPECIFIC ANTIDOTE: None. General supportive measures, gastric lavage for acute overdose.

LEVOTHYROXINE SODIUM

Brand Names: Eltroxin, Synthroid.
Drug Class: Thyroid hormone.
Related Drugs: Thyroid U.S.P., Thyroglobulin U.S.P., L-triiodothyronine, thyronine.

ACTIONS: Acts as a substrate for deiodination to T_3 (active form), which binds with high affinity to receptors in cell nuclei. Acts to promote growth and development and increases the basal metabolic rate.

PHARMACOKINETICS

pK_a: 2.2, 6.7, 10.1.
Mean V_d: 0.15 L/kg.
Plasma Protein Binding: More than 99.9% bound.
Bioavailability: 40–75% (oral).
Half-Life–Normal: 6–7 days. – **Disease States:** Increased in myxedema, pregnancy. Decreased in hyperthyroidism, nephrosis, hepatic cirrhosis.
Absorption & Distribution: Oral absorption is good but somewhat erratic, dependent on intestinal contents. Systemic distribution is limited to the extracellular space, except for the free fraction of 0.05%. Remainder is bound to specific globulin and prealbumin proteins.
Biotransformation & Elimination: Approximately 35% is converted to T_3, and approximately 45% is converted to rT_3 (inactive) in peripheral tissues. Hepatic conjugation to glucuronic acid, enterohepatic recirculation, deiodination, and other hepatic transformations occur. 20–40% excreted in the feces.

ADVERSE REACTIONS AND TOXICITY

Acute: Induced hyperthyroidism due to overdose.
Chronic: Same as acute.

MAJOR DRUG INTERACTIONS: Salicylate, dicumarol decrease protein binding and shorten half-life.

THERAPEUTIC USE

Usual Effective Plasma Concentration: Representative normal values in adult serum: T_4, 4–11 μg/dL (51–142 nmol/L); T_3, 60–180 ng/dL (0.92–2.76 nmol/L); TSH, <6 μU/mL (<6 mU/L) (may differ in different laboratories).
Usual Dose & Regimen: Adults, 100–200 μg daily, occasionally up to 400 μg. Children, often up to 300–400 μg daily. Intravenously, 200–500 μg single dose.
Special Considerations: Severe myxedema may require slow, careful titration of the dose. Caution in the presence of heart disease.

SPECIFIC ANTIDOTE: None. Propranolol is useful in suppressing sympathomimetic symptoms.

SPECIAL TOPICS

LIDOCAINE (LIGNOCAINE)

Brand Names: Xylocaine, Xylocard.
Drug Class: Antiarrhythmic. Local anaesthetic.
Related Drugs: Bupivacaine, mepivacaine.

ACTIONS: *In the heart:* Decreases the slope of phase 4 depolarization in Purkinje fibres. Also increases the diastolic electrical current threshold in Purkinje fibres and the threshold for fibrillation. No effect on conduction velocity in normal tissues, but it may be decreased in ischemic tissues. Decreases action potential duration only in Purkinje fibres and ventricular muscle. Abolishes ventricular reentry. Little effect on atria or atrial arrhythmias.

In neurons: Lidocaine inhibits the conduction of action potentials by blocking sodium channels when applied directly to the nerve.

PHARMACOKINETICS

pK_a: 7.9 (basic).
Mean V_d: 1.3 L/kg, reduced in heart failure.
Plasma Protein Binding: 65–75% bound (concentration dependent); decreased in neonates.
Bioavailability: 25–50% (oral).
Half-Life–Normal: 1–2 hours. – **Disease States:** Elevated in cirrhosis, myocardial infarction with congestive failure, neonates.
Absorption & Distribution: Oral absorption is too unreliable for antiarrhythmic effect. Therefore used only intravenously or intramuscularly. Rapid distribution except in congestive heart failure. Rapid onset of action and redistribution make it useful in acute situations.
Biotransformation & Elimination: Dealkylated by hepatic cytochrome P–450; one metabolite is active. None is excreted unchanged in the urine.

ADVERSE REACTIONS AND TOXICITY

Acute: Drowsiness, hypotension, coma, paraesthesias, convulsions, respiratory arrest.
Chronic: Same as acute.

MAJOR DRUG INTERACTIONS: Propranolol may prolong half-life in cardiac patients.

THERAPEUTIC USE (as antiarrhythmic)

Usual Effective Plasma Concentration: 1–5 μg/mL (4.3–21.3 μmol/L), toxic at >6 μg/mL (>25.8 μmol/L).
Usual Dose & Regimen: Intravenous loading dose, 1–1.5 mg/kg; intravenous infusion, 20–50 μg/kg/min. Intramuscular single dose, 4–5 mg/kg (onset in 15 min).
Special Considerations: Drug of choice for ventricular arrhythmias, early postmyocardial infarction.

SPECIFIC ANTIDOTE: None.

LITHIUM CARBONATE

Brand Names: Carbolith, Duralith, Lithane, Lithizine.
Drug Class: Alkali metal. Mood stabilizer.
Related Drugs: —

ACTIONS: The mechanisms are unknown. It is suggested that lithium acts on the phosphoinositol system involved in neurotransmission; that it inhibits cAMP synthesis in several tissues; that it is an inhibitor of membrane $(Na^+ + K^+)$-ATPase activity; that it facilitates central catecholamine re-uptake.

PHARMACOKINETICS

pK_a: 6.8.
Mean V_d: 0.4–1.4 L/kg.
Plasma Protein Binding: None.
Bioavailability: Approximately 100% (oral).
Half-Life–Normal: 20–40 hours. – **Disease States:** Half-life correlates with creatinine clearance; sodium depletion causes retention (= cumulation) of lithium.
Absorption & Distribution: Slow absorption, but complete by 8 hours; plasma peak concentration at 2–4 hours. Distribution in extracellular space followed by redistribution into intracellular fluid. Cerebrospinal fluid concentrations 40% of plasma levels at steady state.
Biotransformation & Elimination: Urinary excretion of unchanged lithium ion is the major pathway, dependent upon renal glomerular filtration. This appears to be biphasic. Elimination continues for 10–14 days after termination of therapy. Secreted in sweat, saliva, breast milk.

ADVERSE REACTIONS AND TOXICITY

Acute: Edema, sodium retention, nausea, GI discomfort, vertigo.
Chronic: Hand tremor, fatigue, thirst, polyuria, thyroid enlargement, ECG changes, leukocytosis, allergic reactions, renal function changes.

MAJOR DRUG INTERACTIONS: Diuretics producing hyponatremia increase the half-life of lithium. Nonsteroidal anti-inflammatory drugs decrease renal elimination of lithium, and can cause accumulation.

THERAPEUTIC USE

Usual Effective Plasma Concentration: Outpatients, 0.8–1 mmol/L, 8–12 hours after last daily dose. Inpatients, 1–1.5 mmol/L. Toxicity above 2 mmol/L.
Usual Dose & Regimen: Outpatients, 900–1500 mg daily. Hospitalized patients, 1200–2700 mg daily depending on desired plasma concentration.
Special Considerations: Plasma concentrations must be monitored due to low therapeutic index.

SPECIFIC ANTIDOTE: None, but sodium loading hastens urinary elimination of lithium, and lithium is readily removed by hemodialysis.

MEPERIDINE (PETHIDINE)

Brand Name: Demerol.
Drug Class: Opioid analgesic (synthetic).
Related Drugs: Alphaprodine, anileridine, diphenoxylate, loperamide, fentanyl, morphine.

ACTIONS: Agonist at opioid μ receptors in CNS and spinal cord. Depresses adenylate cyclase activity and inhibits neurotransmitter release in CNS and myenteric plexus. Produces analgesia, gastrointestinal stasis. Depresses respiratory and cough centres, stimulates the chemoreceptor trigger zone. Various effects on mood and neuroendocrine function.

PHARMACOKINETICS

pK$_a$: 8.7 (basic).
Mean V$_d$: 3–5 L/kg.
Plasma Protein Binding: 50–60% bound.
Bioavailability: 50–60% (oral); up to 90% in cirrhosis.
Half-Life–Normal: 3–4 hours. – **Disease States:** Increased by 25% postoperatively, by up to 100% in cirrhosis.
Absorption & Distribution: Absorbed orally, but extensive (50%) first-pass effect. Erratic absorption from intramuscular sites. Highly bound in plasma to α_1-acid glycoproteins.
Biotransformation & Elimination: Less than 5% of a dose excreted unchanged in the urine; primarily converted in the liver to several metabolites (hydrolysis, N-demethylation, conjugation) and largely excreted in the bile. Renal excretion is pH-dependent, normally about 20%.

ADVERSE REACTIONS AND TOXICITY

Acute: Drowsiness, euphoria, dry mouth, urinary retention, nausea, vomiting, sweating, syncope. Overdose: respiratory depression, coma, shock, cardiac arrest.
Chronic: Physical dependence, hypogonadism (male and female).

MAJOR DRUG INTERACTIONS: CNS depressants may enhance the central toxicity of meperidine.

THERAPEUTIC USE

Usual Effective Plasma Concentration: 2–6 μg/mL.
Usual Dose & Regimen: 50–100 mg, i.m., s.c. or p.o. Dose repeated at 3–4 hour intervals, as necessary.
Special Considerations: High abuse potential. Does not produce pinpoint pupils observed with natural opioids.

SPECIFIC ANTIDOTES: Naloxone, levallorphan tartrate. Their use in physically dependent patients can precipitate acute withdrawal syndrome.

METHOTREXATE (AMETHOPTERIN)

Brand Names: Folex, Mexate, Abitrexate, and others.
Drug Class: Antineoplastic, antimetabolite, antifol, purine synthesis inhibitor.
Related Drugs: Other antimetabolites (pyrimidine analogs, purine analogs).

ACTIONS: Inhibits dihydrofolic acid reductase; inhibits DNA synthesis.

PHARMACOKINETICS

pK$_a$: 4.8 (acidic).
Mean V$_d$: About 1 L/kg.
Plasma Protein Binding: 50–60% bound.
Bioavailability: 60–100% (variable with oral administration).
Half-Life–Normal: 5–10 hours. – **Disease States:** Increases with renal insufficiency.
Absorption & Distribution: Absorbed from all routes. Enterohepatic circulation occurs. Crosses blood–brain barrier readily.
Biotransformation & Elimination: Renal excretion; about 10% biotransformed in the liver.

ADVERSE REACTIONS AND TOXICITY

Acute: Nausea, vomiting, alopecia, myelosuppression, mucositis (common); skin rash, renal failure (uncommon).
Chronic: Cirrhosis (uncommon).

MAJOR DRUG INTERACTIONS: ASA reduces renal excretion, displaces the drug from albumin binding sites. Probenecid decreases renal clearance.

THERAPEUTIC USE

Usual Effective Plasma Concentration: Not usually measured clinically. However, levels often measured during high-dose cancer chemotherapy for prevention or treatment of toxicity: toxic level varies with dosage and schedule.
Usual Dose & Regimen: 25 mg/m^2 p.o. 2 times per week.
Special Considerations: Avoid severe leukopenia, thrombocytopenia, bone marrow aplasia.

SPECIFIC ANTIDOTE: Folinic acid (Leucovorin).

METHYLDOPA

Brand Names: Aldomet, Apo-Methyldopa, Dopamet, Novomedopa.
Drug Class: Sympathoplegic. Central α_2-adrenoceptor agonist.
Related Drugs: Clonidine, guanfacine, guanabenz.

ACTIONS: Central stimulation of α_2-adrenoceptors in the nucleus tractus solitarius by its metabolite α-methylnoradrenaline (α-methylnorepinephrine) decreases sympathetic outflow from the CNS. The peripheral release of noradrenaline (norepinephrine) is inhibited. Because the action depends on a metabolite, two or three days are required to reach maximum therapeutic effects.

PHARMACOKINETICS

pK$_a$: 2.2(COOH), 9.2(OH), 10.6(NH$_2$), 12.0(OH).
Mean V$_d$: 0.4–0.7 L/kg.
Plasma Protein Binding: 10–15% bound.
Bioavailability: 10–60%, mean 25% (oral).
Half-Life–Normal: 1.5–2 hours. – **Disease States:** Increased with impaired renal function.
Absorption & Distribution: Large variation in oral bioavailability, partly due to first-pass effect. Peak plasma concentration at 2 hours. Absorption decreased by food. Rapid distribution to all tissues, especially kidneys, heart, brain.
Biotransformation & Elimination: An orally administered dose is excreted in the urine 50% unchanged and 50% as sulfate conjugates and several other metabolites. Liver enzyme induction increases elimination. α-Methylnoradrenaline is the primary active metabolite, which may be slowly eliminated.

ADVERSE REACTIONS AND TOXICITY

Acute: Sedation, headache, weakness, dizziness, fever, dry mouth, bradycardia.
Chronic: Edema, positive Coombs test (10–20%), hemolytic anemia (rare), abnormal liver function, jaundice, hepatic necrosis (rare), leukopenia, thrombocytopenia (rare).

MAJOR DRUG INTERACTIONS: Potentiated by other antihypertensive drugs.

THERAPEUTIC USE

Usual Effective Plasma Concentration: No correlation with therapeutic effect.
Usual Dose & Regimen: Initially, 250 mg, 2–3 times daily; dosage then adjusted gradually, according to response, to maintenance dose of 500–2000 mg/day; maximum 3000 mg/day.
Special Considerations: Interferes with urinary catecholamine analysis.

SPECIFIC ANTIDOTE: None. General supportive treatment. Sympathomimetics may be indicated.

METOCLOPRAMIDE

Brand Names: Emex, Maxeran, Reglan.
Drug Class: Antiemetic and modifier of gastrointestinal motility.
Related Drugs: Sulpiride, procainamide (structural similarities).

ACTIONS: Central dopamine receptor blockade, possibly D$_2$ (not linked to adenylate cyclase), may account for many effects, but increased peripheral release of acetylcholine and increased muscarinic receptor sensitivity also contribute. Behavioral, motor, and neuroendocrine effects relate to antidopaminergic activity. Increases the amplitude of peristaltic waves, enhances esophageal clearance, shortens gastric emptying and GI transit times.

PHARMACOKINETICS

pK$_a$: 9.0 (basic).
Mean V$_d$: 2–3 L/kg.
Plasma Protein Binding: 60–70% bound.
Bioavailability: 32–98% (oral). Variation due to first-pass effect.
Half-Life–Normal: 3–6 hours. – **Disease States:** Increased (to 14 hours) in renal failure, possibly also in the elderly.
Absorption & Distribution: Rapid absorption on empty stomach, peak plasma concentration by 1 hour. Distribution half-life 5–20 minutes, into all tissues. Elimination half-life 35 hours.
Biotransformation & Elimination: Extensive sulfate conjugation in the gut wall or liver determines the bioavailability and the wide range (ten-fold) of plasma concentrations. Hepatic conjugation (glucuronide) and oxidation also occur. About 65–85% of an oral dose is excreted in the urine, up to 20% as unchanged drug.

ADVERSE REACTIONS AND TOXICITY

Acute: Sedation, drowsiness, lassitude, insomnia, headache, dizziness, GI disturbances, skin rash, galactorrhea, menstrual disorders, methemoglobinemia.
Chronic: Parkinsonian and/or extrapyramidal reactions, acute dystonias, tardive dyskinesia.

MAJOR DRUG INTERACTIONS: May potentiate extrapyramidal side effects of neuroleptics; additive sedative effects with sedatives, hypnotics, opioids.

THERAPEUTIC USE

Usual Effective Plasma Concentration: Peak plasma levels above 120 ng/mL cause akathisia.
Usual Dose & Regimen: Adults, 5–10 mg orally 3–4 times a day before meals. Children, 2.5–5 mg orally 3 times a day before meals. Maximum dose not to exceed 0.5 mg/kg/day.
Special Considerations: Increased frequency of seizures in epileptics; higher incidence of extrapyramidal reactions in children.

SPECIFIC ANTIDOTES: Anticholinergics for specific symptoms.

MORPHINE

Brand Names: Epimorph, Morphine HP, Morphitec, M.O.S., MS Contin, Roxanol, Statex.
Drug Class: Opioid analgesic.
Related Drugs: Heroin, codeine, hydromorphone, oxycodone, meperidine, many others.

ACTIONS: Agonist at endorphin and enkephalin receptors, localized primarily in synaptic areas of the limbic system, thalamus, striatum, hypothalamus, midbrain, and spinal cord. Stereospecific binding causes decreased adenylate cyclase activity and inhibits the release of some neurotransmitters in CNS and myenteric plexus. Produces analgesia, gastrointestinal stasis. Depresses respiratory and cough centres, stimulates the chemoreceptor trigger zone.

PHARMACOKINETICS

pK_a: 7.9 (basic), 9.9 (acidic).
Mean V_d: 3 L/kg.
Plasma Protein Binding: 35% bound.
Bioavailability: 20–33% (oral).
Half-Life–Normal: 2–3 hours. – **Disease States:** Decreased protein binding in hepatic failure.
Absorption & Distribution: Well absorbed orally, but significant first-pass effect. Also absorbed from the nasal mucosa and lungs. Route of administration determines the plasma time course-effect curve. Rapid distribution from blood into lungs, liver, kidneys, spleen. Slow passage across the blood–brain barrier.
Biotransformation & Elimination: Primary metabolite is glucuronic acid conjugate. 90% of a dose is excreted in the urine within 24 hours, largely conjugated; less than 10% in bile. Renal clearance of unchanged morphine is pH-dependent.

ADVERSE REACTIONS AND TOXICITY

Acute: Drowsiness, respiratory depression, coma, hypothermia, hypotension, pupillary constriction, constipation, nausea, dysphoria, allergic rash (uncommon).
Chronic: Physical and psychological dependence, hypogonadism (male and female).

MAJOR DRUG INTERACTIONS: Sedative agents enhance CNS-depressant effects.

THERAPEUTIC USE

Usual Effective Plasma Concentration: 30–130 ng/mL. Not measured clinically.
Usual Dose & Regimen: Analgesic for severe pain, 5–15 mg i.m. every 3–4 hours. Intravenous use only in emergencies, slowly, in dilute solution.
Special Considerations: High abuse potential.

SPECIFIC ANTIDOTES: Naloxone, naltrexone. Use in physically dependent patients can precipitate acute withdrawal syndrome.

NALOXONE

Brand Name: Narcan.
Drug Class: Opioid antagonist.
Related Drugs: Nalorphine, pentazocine, buprenorphine, nalbuphine, naltrexone.

ACTIONS: Relatively pure competitive antagonist of morphine and its endogenous and exogenous analogs at all subtypes (especially μ) of opiate receptors. The profile of pharmacologic effects depends on affinities at each site, the presence of an opiate, and whether or not physical dependence has developed.

PHARMACOKINETICS

pK_a: 7.9 (basic).
Mean V_d: 2–3 L/kg.
Plasma Protein Binding: About 40% bound.
Bioavailability: Less than 5% (oral).
Half-Life–Normal: Adults, 1–1.5 hour; infants 2.5–3.5 hours. – **Disease States:** ?
Absorption & Distribution: Well absorbed, but poor bioavailability due to extensive hepatic first-pass effect. Rapid CNS distribution after i.v. dose (0.5–2 minutes), or by s.c. or i.m. routes (2–3 minutes).
Biotransformation & Elimination: Extensive and rapid hepatic glucuronidation; other oxidative metabolites occur to a minor extent. Glomerular filtration of glucuronide is the major excretory pathway; some biliary excretion occurs (profile like morphine).

ADVERSE REACTIONS AND TOXICITY

Acute: In normal subjects, no marked effects, but may cause dysphoria; withdrawal reaction in the presence of narcotic dependence; in narcotic overdose, abrupt reversal of opioid effects may cause nausea, vomiting, sweating, tachycardia, hypertension, tremor, pulmonary edema (rarely).
Chronic: None recorded in normal subjects after chronic doses of 90 mg/day, s.c.

MAJOR DRUG INTERACTIONS: Morphine and congeners.

THERAPEUTIC USE

Usual Effective Plasma Concentration: Not measured clinically.
Usual Dose & Regimen: Narcotic overdose, adult, 400 μg i.v., i.m. or s.c.; children 5–10 μg/kg. Postoperative narcotic depression, 100–200 μg i.v., i.m., or s.c.
Special Considerations: Can produce narcotic withdrawal reaction in narcotic abusers.

SPECIFIC ANTIDOTE: None (no recorded overdose).

SPECIAL TOPICS

NEOSTIGMINE

Brand Name: Prostigmin.
Drug Class: Parasympathomimetic, anticholinesterase.
Related Drugs: Physostigmine, pyridostigmine, edrophonium, demecarium, carbaryl.

ACTIONS: Reversible inhibition of acetylcholinesterase. Direct effect on nicotinic receptors in skeletal muscle.

PHARMACOKINETICS

pK$_a$: 12.0 (basic).
Mean V$_d$: 0.5–1 L/kg.
Plasma Protein Binding: None.
Bioavailability: Unclear, probably less than 5%.
Half-Life–Normal: 50–90 minutes. – **Disease States:** Increased in uremia, renal disease.
Absorption & Distribution: Poor oral absorption because of quaternary nitrogen. Crosses membrane barriers poorly and slowly. Does not cross the blood–brain barrier sufficiently to have significant CNS effects.

Biotransformation & Elimination: Slow hydrolysis by acetylcholinesterase (t½ 15–30 minutes) and also by plasma esterases. Unchanged drug (up to 70%) and alcoholic metabolite (30%) are excreted in the urine.

ADVERSE REACTIONS AND TOXICITY

Acute: *Muscarinic*—nausea, vomiting, diarrhea, abdominal cramps, salivation, bronchial secretion, miosis, sweating.
Nicotinic—muscle cramps, fasciculation, weakness. Hypotension and bradycardia in the presence of curare.
Chronic: Same as acute.

MAJOR DRUG INTERACTIONS: Additive with other parasympathomimetics.

THERAPEUTIC USE

Usual Effective Plasma Concentration: Not measured clinically.
Usual Dose & Regimen: Intestinal atony or urinary retention, 0.5 mg s.c. or i.m. every 4–6 hours. Myasthenia gravis, 75–300 mg orally over 24 hours, spaced as required; up to 1 mg i.m. every hour in myasthenic crisis. To antagonize curare, 0.5–2 mg i.v.
Special Considerations: Contraindicated in bronchial asthma.

SPECIFIC ANTIDOTE: Atropine.

NIFEDIPINE

Brand Names: Adalat, Procardia.
Drug Class: Calcium entry (channel) blocker.
Related Drugs: Diltiazem, verapamil; many others (e.g., nicardipine, felodipine) not available in North America.

ACTIONS: Specifically inhibits transmembrane influx of Ca^{2+} into cardiac muscle and vascular smooth muscle. Blocks the "slow-channel" calcium influx without blocking "fast-channel" sodium influx. Reduces afterload.

PHARMACOKINETICS

pK$_a$: ?
Mean V$_d$: 1.2 L/kg.
Plasma Protein Binding: 95% bound.
Bioavailability: About 50% (oral).
Half-Life–Normal: Distribution half-life 2.5–3 hours, elimination half-life 5 hours. – **Disease States:** Possibly prolonged in cirrhosis.
Absorption & Distribution: Well absorbed orally with onset of action in less than 20 minutes, plasma peaks in 1–2 hours.

Biotransformation & Elimination: Almost completely transformed by hepatic enzymes and excreted *via* renal (75%) and biliary (15%) pathways.

ADVERSE REACTIONS AND TOXICITY

Acute: Headache, dizziness, flushing, nausea, vomiting or GI distress, hypotension.
Chronic: Peripheral edema, skin rash, hypersensitivity.

MAJOR DRUG INTERACTIONS: Augments beta-blocker effects on blood pressure.

THERAPEUTIC USE

Usual Effective Plasma Concentration: Not measured clinically.
Usual Dose & Regimen: Start with 10 mg 3 times a day. Increase until symptoms are relieved or side effects occur. Maximum 120 mg/day.
Special Considerations: Use with care in hypotension.

SPECIFIC ANTIDOTES: Calcium salts infused i.v. Catecholamines.

NITROGLYCERIN (GLYCERYL TRINITRATE)

Brand Names: Nitro-Bid, Nitrogard-SR, Nitrol, Nitrolingual, Nitrong-SR, Nitrostat, Tridil. Nitrol (ointment).
Drug Class: Organic nitrate vasodilator.
Related Drugs: Isosorbide dinitrate, pentaerythritol nitrate, amyl nitrite (inhalation), erythrityl tetranitrate.

ACTIONS: Relaxation of vascular smooth muscle, thereby reducing myocardial oxygen demand (*not* increasing oxygen supply). Venous effects appear to predominate.

PHARMACOKINETICS

pK$_a$: ?
Mean V$_d$: 3 L/kg.
Plasma Protein Binding: At plasma levels of 50–500 ng/mL, about 60% bound.
Bioavailability: 10% (oral).
Half-Life–Normal: 2–5 minutes (1.5–2 hours for active metabolite). – **Disease States:** ?
Absorption & Distribution: Highly lipid-soluble, well absorbed sublingually and transdermally (also orally, but subject to first-pass effect). Rapid distribution to all tissues.
Biotransformation & Elimination: Reductive hydrolysis in the liver to nitrite and dinitrates (partially active), which requires hepatic glutathione. Glucuronidation of a large fraction of metabolites precedes elimination in the urine. Duration of action is determined by the rate of biotransformation.

ADVERSE REACTIONS AND TOXICITY

Acute: Headaches, hypotension (weakness, dizziness), flushing, nausea, methemoglobinemia.
Chronic: Tolerance to therapeutic effects develops with constant dosing; dermatitis.

MAJOR DRUG INTERACTIONS: Cross-tolerance to other nitrates.

THERAPEUTIC USE

Usual Effective Plasma Concentration: Not measured clinically.
Usual Dose & Regimen: Sublingually, 0.2–0.3 mg for relief of angina pectoris. Oral slow-release preparations, 1.3–6.5 mg every 8–12 hours. Ointment, 1–10 cm of 2% preparation on the skin, as required.
Special Considerations: Contraindicated in severe anemia, increased intraocular or intracranial pressure, hypotension.

SPECIFIC ANTIDOTE: None.

PENICILLIN G

Brand Names: Ayercillin, Bicillin, Crystapen, Megacillin, Novopen G, Penioral-500, P.G.A., P-50, Wycillin.
Drug Class: Beta-lactam antibiotic. Native penicillin.
Related Drugs: Penicillin V, phenethicillin, others.

ACTIONS: Kills susceptible microorganisms by inhibiting bacterial cell wall synthesis through reaction with transpeptidase, thereby preventing cross-linking of peptidoglycan strands and causing osmotic lysis of bacteria.

PHARMACOKINETICS

pK$_a$: 2.8 (acidic).
Mean V$_d$: 0.5 L/kg.
Plasma Protein Binding: 45–65% bound.
Bioavailability: About 30% (oral).
Half-Life–Normal: 0.5–1 hour. – **Disease States:** Prolonged in renal dysfunction, neonates.
Absorption & Distribution: Acid-labile (pH 2 or less) properties cause variation in absorption dependent on gastric acidity. Oral doses producing plasma levels equivalent to those after i.m. dosing must be at least four-fold higher. Food decreases oral bioavailability. (Penicillin V is more acid-resistant.) Distributes poorly to brain, except in the presence of meningitis.
Biotransformation & Elimination: Excreted unchanged in the urine, largely by tubular secretion. Biliary secretion also occurs, but renal secretory mechanisms predominate.

ADVERSE REACTIONS AND TOXICITY

Acute: Hypersensitivity reactions (rash, urticaria, fever, anaphylaxis); nausea, vomiting, epigastric distress, diarrhea, black hairy tongue.
Chronic: Same as acute; superinfection; nephropathy.

MAJOR DRUG INTERACTIONS: Probenecid decreases renal secretion; used clinically to prolong the half-life of penicillin. Tetracyclines may interfere with antibacterial activity.

THERAPEUTIC USE

Usual Effective Plasma Concentration: Refer to Chapter 53.
Usual Dose & Regimen: Orally, 0.6–3 million units daily, maximum 20 million units. Parenterally, 0.3–1.2 million units daily, maximum 20 million units (i.v. infusion).
Special Considerations: Oral doses should be taken on empty stomach.

SPECIFIC ANTIDOTE: None. Anaphylaxis treated with adrenaline (epinephrine), antihistamines, glucocorticoids.

SPECIAL TOPICS

PHENOBARBITAL

Brand Names: Gardenal, Luminal.
Drug Class: Barbiturate, antiseizure drug.
Related Drugs: Mephobarbital, methabarbital, amobarbital, pentobarbital, secobarbital, others.

ACTIONS: Limits the spread of seizure activity and elevates the seizure threshold, possibly by potentiation of inhibitory pathways involved in seizures. Sedative effects may relate to generalized stimulation of receptors for gamma-aminobutyric acid (GABA).

PHARMACOKINETICS

pK_a: 7.4 (acidic).
Mean V_d: 0.6 L/kg.
Plasma Protein Binding: About 50% bound.
Bioavailability: Better than 80% (oral, estimated).
Half-Life–Normal: 72–120 hours (mean 96 hours). – **Disease States:** Shortened in children, prolonged in the elderly and in cirrhosis.
Absorption & Distribution: Nearly complete but slow absorption; peak plasma concentrations several hours after an oral dose. Moderate protein binding and tissue binding (including brain).
Biotransformation & Elimination: Hepatic oxidation to the para-hydroxyphenyl metabolite, then glucuronide and sulfate conjugation. Eliminated unchanged in the urine (25%) by a pH-dependent process; metabolites excreted in urine and bile.

ADVERSE REACTIONS AND TOXICITY

Acute: Sedation, nystagmus, ataxia, confusion; irritability and hyperactivity in children.
Chronic: Megaloblastic anemia, osteomalacia, rash (1–2%). Tolerance to sedative effects, withdrawal reaction.

MAJOR DRUG INTERACTIONS: Valproic acid elevates plasma levels by up to 40%. Hepatic enzyme induction by phenobarbital may decrease levels of other drugs. Ethanol may result in severe CNS depression.

THERAPEUTIC USE

Usual Effective Plasma Concentration: 10–25 µg/mL (43.1–107.7 µmol/L). Toxicity above 40 µg/mL (>172.2 µmol/L).
Usual Dose & Regimen: Orally, sedative, 15–30 mg 2–3 times a day (2 mg/kg 3 times a day in children). Orally, anticonvulsant, 50–100 mg 2–3 times a day (15–50 mg, 2–3 times a day in children). Intravenously, anticonvulsant, 200–300 mg every 6 hours as necessary.
Special Considerations: Contraindicated in porphyria.

SPECIFIC ANTIDOTE: Picrotoxin (?). Forced diuresis and alkalinization of the urine increase excretion.

PHENYLBUTAZONE

Brand Names: Apo-Phenylbutazone, Butazolidin, Intrabutazone, Novobutazone, Phenbuff.
Drug Class: Pyrazolone, nonsteroidal anti-inflammatory drug (NSAID).
Related Drugs: Oxyphenbutazone, antipyrine, aminopyrine, azapropazone, acetylsalicylic acid.

ACTIONS: Inhibits prostaglandin synthesis through inhibition of cyclooxygenase and other enzymes involved in prostaglandin pathways. Anti-inflammatory effects are prominent, analgesic and antipyretic effects are weaker than those of acetylsalicylic acid.

PHARMACOKINETICS

pK_a: 4.5 (acidic).
Mean V_d: 0.1 L/kg.
Plasma Protein Binding: 97–99% bound.
Bioavailability: 100% (oral).
Half-Life–Normal: 50–100 hours (dose dependent). – **Disease States:** Prolonged in the elderly, and in hepatic, cardiac, renal diseases (contraindicated).
Absorption & Distribution: Rapid, complete absorption, with good distribution into synovial spaces (50% of plasma concentrations), despite high plasma protein binding.
Biotransformation & Elimination: Hydroxylation and glucuronidation in the liver. The hydroxy metabolite, oxyphenbutazone, is active with a long plasma half-life. Conjugates are eliminated slowly in the urine due to high protein binding and extensive tubular reabsorption.

ADVERSE REACTIONS AND TOXICITY

Acute: Nausea, vomiting, diarrhea, vertigo, insomnia.
Chronic: Agranulocytosis, aplastic anemia, skin rashes, hematuria, water and electrolyte retention, edema, peptic ulceration, hypersensitivity. (Not recommended for long-term use in the U.S.)

MAJOR DRUG INTERACTIONS: Displaces anticoagulants, sulfonylurea hypoglycemic agents, methotrexate, other anti-inflammatory drugs from protein binding sites; displaces thyroid hormones; additive with anticoagulants because of platelet effects. Inhibits hydroxylation of warfarin initially, but induces hepatic microsomal enzymes when used chronically.

THERAPEUTIC USE

Usual Effective Plasma Concentration: Not measured clinically.
Usual Dose & Regimen: Orally, 300–800 mg daily for short periods, 100–400 mg when longer-term use necessary. In acute gout, 800 mg daily for 2 days, then 300–400 mg per day.
Special Considerations: Contraindicated in hypertension, cardiac, renal, hepatic dysfunction, or with a history of peptic ulcer. Monitor patient's blood and weight for signs of toxicity (agranulocytosis, edema).

SPECIFIC ANTIDOTE: None.

PHENYTOIN

Brand Name: Dilantin.
Drug Class: Anticonvulsant, antiarrhythmic.
Related Drugs: Mephenytoin, ethotoin.

ACTIONS: A large number of mechanisms have been proposed, most of them stressing effects on basic membrane properties (sodium pump, ion flux, *etc.*). Recently, the discovery of a phenytoin binding site has suggested the possibility of a specific receptor mechanism, but its pharmacologic relevance remains to be established.

PHARMACOKINETICS

pK_a: 8.3 (acidic).
Mean V_d: About 0.7 L/kg.
Plasma Protein Binding: 70–95% bound (decreased in uremia, hypoalbuminemia, neonates).
Bioavailability: Variable, up to 98% (oral).
Half-Life–Normal: 24 hours, but concentration-dependent, varies four-fold. – **Disease States:** Reduced in hypoalbuminemia.
Absorption & Distribution: Slow and variable absorption, differing among brands. Peak plasma levels 2–6 hours after an oral dose. Distributes to all tissues.
Biotransformation & Elimination: Hepatic microsomal biotransformation, primarily to the *p*-hydroxyphenyl metabolite. Excreted in bile and urine, also glucuronide-conjugated. Less than 2% excreted unchanged. Below 10 μg/mL, elimination is first-order process.

ADVERSE REACTIONS AND TOXICITY

Acute: Nystagmus, incoordination, ataxia, drowsiness and lethargy (concentration-dependent).
Chronic: Same as acute, plus rash, gum hyperplasia, hirsutism, hypocalcemia with or without rickets or osteomalacia, megaloblastic anemia, lymphadenopathy, hepatic toxicity, cerebellar damage, risk of congenital abnormalities.

MAJOR DRUG INTERACTIONS: Disulfiram, isoniazid (in slow acetylators) both increase the risk of phenytoin intoxication.

THERAPEUTIC USE

Usual Effective Plasma Concentration: 10–20 μg/mL (39.6–79.2 μmol/L); toxic at >20 μg/mL (>79.2 μmol/L).
Usual Dose & Regimen: Loading dose, if necessary, 10–15 mg/kg p.o. or slowly i.v. Maintenance dose, 300 mg (range 200–600 mg) daily in single or divided doses. Adjustments by clinical effect; measuring plasma concentrations is useful.
Special Considerations: Caution in pregnancy.

SPECIFIC ANTIDOTE: None.

PRAZOSIN

Brand Name: Minipress.
Drug Class: Vasodilator.
Related Drugs: Terazosin (not available in Canada). Nitroprusside, hydralazine relax vascular smooth muscle.

ACTIONS: Blocks noradrenaline-mediated vasoconstriction of resistance vessels, most likely by direct α_1-adrenoceptor blockade. Also decreases venous tone.

PHARMACOKINETICS

pK_a: 6.5 (basic).
Mean V_d: 0.6 L/kg.
Plasma Protein Binding: 95% bound.
Bioavailability: 45–70% (oral).
Half-Life–Normal: 3 hours. – **Disease States:** Prolonged in congestive heart failure.
Absorption & Distribution: Adequate oral absorption; may be subject to first-pass effect.
Biotransformation & Elimination: All but 10% or less undergoes hepatic demethylation and conjugation. Pathways of elimination are primarily the bile and feces.

ADVERSE REACTIONS AND TOXICITY

Acute: Postural hypotension and/or syncope (first-dose effect), drowsiness, dry mouth, dizziness, fatigue, headache, palpitations.
Chronic: Same as acute (excluding hypotension, syncope), plus sexual dysfunction (uncommon), fluid retention, positive test for antinuclear factor.

MAJOR DRUG INTERACTIONS: Increased effectiveness when added to diuretic or beta-blocker.

THERAPEUTIC USE

Usual Effective Plasma Concentration: Not measured clinically.
Usual Dose & Regimen: Start with 0.5 mg, with meals, 2–3 times daily for 3 days. Increase to 1 mg, 2–3 times daily for another 3 days. Then add increments to obtain blood pressure control, to a maximum of 20 mg/day.
Special Considerations: First-dose effect of hypotension and syncope avoided by slow titration with small doses.

SPECIFIC ANTIDOTE: None. Cardiovascular support.

PREDNISONE

Brand Names: Apo-Prednisone, Deltasone, Novoprednisone, Winpred.
Drug Class: Adrenocortical steroid, glucocorticoid.
Related Drugs: Prednisolone, dexamethasone, hydrocortisone (cortisol), beclomethasone.

ACTIONS: *See* hydrocortisone (cortisol). Anti-inflammatory and antiallergic action through suppression of immune-mediated cell response and other agents of inflammation and hypersensitivity reactions.

PHARMACOKINETICS

pK$_a$: n.a. (steroid).
Mean V$_d$: 0.97 L/kg.
Plasma Protein Binding: 75%, decreased with liver disease.
Bioavailability: 80% (oral).
Half-Life–Normal: 3–4 hours. – **Disease States:** Prolonged in liver disease.
Absorption & Distribution: Absorbed orally and converted in the liver to prednisolone.
Biotransformation & Elimination: Converted to prednisolone (active form). Reduction of 4,5 double bond occurs in several tissues; oxidation at 3-position, sulfate and glucuronide conjugation in the liver. Elimination almost entirely in the urine as conjugates.

ADVERSE REACTIONS AND TOXICITY

Acute: Mental changes.
Chronic: Cushingoid features, osteoporosis, diabetes, muscle wasting, increased susceptibility to infection, poor wound healing, adrenal suppression, salt and water retention with large doses.

MAJOR DRUG INTERACTIONS: Drugs which induce hepatic enzymes may enhance the rates of biotransformation and clearance; this may increase dosage requirements.

THERAPEUTIC USE

Usual Effective Plasma Concentration: Not measured clinically.
Usual Dose & Regimen: In chronic, nonfatal diseases, 5–30 mg/day divided into 3–4 doses, but can be higher. Acute, nonfatal diseases or episodes of exacerbation, 20–30 mg/day up to 250 mg/day.
Special Considerations: Chronic use in children can suppress growth. May decrease patient's host-response to systemic infections or immunization. Has less mineralocorticoid activity than hydrocortisone. Discontinuation of chronic therapy should be tapered to avoid secondary adrenocortical insufficiency. For some groups of diseases, an alternate-day dosage regimen can be effective while minimizing Cushingoid side effects and adrenal suppression.

SPECIFIC ANTIDOTE: None.

PROCAINAMIDE

Brand Names: Procan, Pronestyl.
Drug Class: Antiarrhythmic.
Related Drugs: Quinidine, disopyramide, procaine.

ACTIONS: Decreases the slope of phase 4 depolarization, reduces conduction velocity in atria, bundle of His, and ventricles; vagolytic. Excitability of cardiac muscle by stimulation is decreased; refractory period, especially atrial, is prolonged. No effect on contractility.

PHARMACOKINETICS

pK$_a$: 9.2 (basic).
Mean V$_d$: 1.7–2.2 L/kg.
Plasma Protein Binding: 15–20% bound.
Bioavailability: 75–95% (oral), good intramuscular absorption.
Half-Life–Normal: 2–4 hours. – **Disease States:** Prolonged in heart failure, renal insufficiency, and myocardial infarction.
Absorption & Distribution: Well absorbed, with capsules producing more rapid peak plasma levels than tablets. Sustained-release formulations increase the duration of action to 6–8 hours. Rapid distribution, but not into brain. Decreased distribution in cardiac failure, shock. Poor absorption for 24 hours following myocardial infarction.
Biotransformation & Elimination: Up to two-thirds of a dose can be excreted unchanged in the urine by glomerular filtration and tubular secretion. Decreased in renal incompetence. Up to 40% of a dose is acetylated and renally excreted. The metabolite is active and also accumulates in renal failure.

ADVERSE REACTIONS AND TOXICITY

Acute: Anorexia, diarrhea, nausea, vomiting, A-V block, hypotension, oliguria, confusion.
Chronic: High incidence of cardiotoxicity, lupus erythematosus-like syndrome (uncommon), agranulocytosis (rare).

MAJOR DRUG INTERACTIONS: Possible potentiation of neuromuscular blockers, and of the myocardial depressant effects of beta-blockers. Unpredictable effects in digitalis-intoxicated patients. May interact with kanamycin, neomycin, streptomycin to produce apnea, muscle weakness (neuromuscular blockade). Renal elimination impaired by cimetidine and ranitidine.

THERAPEUTIC USE

Usual Effective Plasma Concentration: 4–8 µg/mL (17–34 µmol/L); major toxicity at 14 µg/mL (60 µmol/L).
Usual Dose & Regimen: Orally, loading dose of 500–1000 mg, followed by maintenance doses of 250–500 mg every 4 hours. Intravenously, 25–50 mg/min maximum rate. Intramuscularly, 500–1000 mg every 3 hours until oral therapy possible.
Special Considerations: Precipitous fall in blood pressure may occur with i.v. dose in cardiac failure.

SPECIFIC ANTIDOTE: None.

PROPRANOLOL

Brand Names: Apo-Propranolol, Detensol, Inderal, Inderal-LA, Novopranol.
Drug Class: Nonselective β-adrenoceptor blocker.
Related Drugs: Metoprolol, timolol, acebutolol, pindolol, atenolol, nadolol.

ACTIONS: Competitive, reversible antagonist of β_1 and β_2 adrenoceptors. Also has membrane-stabilizing properties (equivalent to lidocaine in local anaesthetic potency).

PHARMACOKINETICS

pK$_a$: 9.45 (basic).
Mean V$_d$: 3 L/kg.
Plasma Protein Binding: 93% bound.
Bioavailability: 25–50% (oral), large first-pass effect with great individual variation; bioavailability greatly increased in cirrhosis.
Half-Life–Normal: 3–5 hours. – **Disease States:** Prolonged by hepatitis and cirrhosis.
Absorption & Distribution: Almost complete oral absorption, with peak plasma concentrations 30–90 minutes after oral dose. Highly bound to α_1-acid glycoproteins in plasma. Twenty-fold variations in peak plasma concentrations are possible. Widely distributed in body tissues, CNS, placenta, milk.
Biotransformation & Elimination: Completely biotransformed in the liver before excretion in the urine. Oxidation and glucuronidation are primary processes. 4-Hydroxypropranolol is active but has a short half-life. Possibly saturable extraction site in the liver.

ADVERSE REACTIONS AND TOXICITY

Acute: Nausea, vomiting, diarrhea, fatigue, bradycardia, cardiac failure, heart block, bronchoconstriction.
Chronic: Hallucinations, sleep disorders, depression, cold extremities, Raynaud's phenomenon. Increased likelihood of ischemic cardiac events after sudden withdrawal from prolonged propranolol use.

MAJOR DRUG INTERACTIONS: Possibly prolonged insulin hypoglycemia.

THERAPEUTIC USE

Usual Effective Plasma Concentration: 20 ng/mL (77 nmol/L); maximal β-adrenoceptor blockade at 50 ng/mL (193 nmol/L).
Usual Dose & Regimen: Hypertension, start with 40 mg twice daily, raise gradually to 160–480 mg/day as single or divided doses. Angina pectoris, arrhythmias, 10 mg 4 times a day, raise gradually to 320 mg/day. Doses up to 2 g/day have been used. For secondary prevention after acute myocardial infarction, 40 mg 3–4 times a day.
Special Considerations: Numerous absolute or relative contraindications, all related to the pharmacologic actions of the drug.

SPECIFIC ANTIDOTES: β-Adrenoceptor agonists, atropine for bradycardia; digitalis and diuretics for cardiac failure; vasopressors for hypotension.

PROPYLTHIOURACIL

Brand Name: Propyl-Thyracil.
Drug Class: Antithyroid, thionamide.
Related Drugs: Methimazole, carbimazole.

ACTIONS: Decreases the formation of thyroid hormones by interfering with incorporation of iodine into tyrosyl residues of thyroglobulin, and by inhibiting coupling of iodotyrosyl residues to form iodothyronines. Blocks T_3 formation from T_4.

PHARMACOKINETICS

pK$_a$: 8.3 (acidic).
Mean V$_d$: 0.4 L/kg.
Plasma Protein Binding: 85% bound.
Bioavailability: 60–90% (oral).
Half-Life–Normal: 1–2 hours. – **Disease States:** Increased in renal failure.
Absorption & Distribution: Well absorbed orally. Effective plasma concentrations attained in 20–30 minutes; rapidly distributed.
Biotransformation & Elimination: Hepatic transformation with renal excretion of unchanged drug and metabolites; effects wane within 8 hours.

ADVERSE REACTIONS AND TOXICITY

Acute: Headaches, nausea.
Chronic: Total incidence about 3%. Hypothyroidism, agranulocytosis (0.5%), usually reversible; purpuric and papular rash, arthralgia, paraesthesias, alopecia, hair depigmentation.

MAJOR DRUG INTERACTIONS: The induced hypothyroidism may cause decreased response to warfarin, increased response to digitalis.

THERAPEUTIC USE

Usual Effective Plasma Concentration: Not measured clinically.
Usual Dose & Regimen: Controlling dose, 200–600 mg/day. Maintenance dose, 50–200 mg/day.
Special Considerations: Cautious use in pregnancy, no breast-feeding (crosses the placenta and is secreted into milk during lactation).

SPECIFIC ANTIDOTES: T_4, T_3.

SPECIAL TOPICS

QUINIDINE

Brand Names: Apo-Quinidine (sulfate), Biquin Durules (bisulfate), Cardioquin (polygalacturonate), Novoquinidin (sulfate), Quinate and Quinaglute (gluconates), Quinidex Extentabs (sulfate).
Drug Class: Antiarrhythmic agent.
Related Drugs: Procainamide, disopyramide.

ACTIONS: Decreases the slope of phase 4 depolarization and the amplitude of phase 0 of the action potential. Depresses excitability, conduction velocity and contractility of the myocardium through a direct myo-cardial depressant effect. Indirect anticholinergic effects also occur. Antimalarial, antipyretic, and oxytocic effects of quinine (the levorotatory isomer) can be observed with quinidine.

PHARMACOKINETICS

pK_a: 4.2, 8.8 (both basic).
Mean V_d: 2–3 L/kg.
Plasma Protein Binding: 75–90% bound.
Bioavailability: 70–80% (oral). Gluconate slightly less than sulfate.
Half-Life–Normal: 4–8 hours; shortened by microsomal enzyme inducers (e.g., phenobarbital, phenytoin). – **Disease States:** Increased in cirrhosis, elderly patients, possibly in renal disease.
Absorption & Distribution: Absorption occurs very rapidly, primarily from the duodenum. Distribution is mainly extravascular (although hemoglobin binds it) and accumulation occurs in most tissues except the brain. In the heart, the drug is localized in sarcolemma and mitochondria.
Biotransformation & Elimination: Hydroxylation in the liver to several metabolites, some active. About 20% cleared unchanged in the kidneys by glomerular filtration and tubular secretion. Metabolites excreted in the urine; less than 5% in bile.

ADVERSE REACTIONS AND TOXICITY

Acute: Nausea, vomiting, diarrhea, cinchonism (tinnitus, visual blurring, GI distress), hypotension. (One-third of patients may not be able to tolerate GI reactions.)
Chronic: Cardiotoxicity (prolonged QRS duration, S-A or A-V block, arrhythmias, ventricular tachycardia), GI disturbances, arterial embolism, hypersensitivity, cinchonism.

MAJOR DRUG INTERACTIONS: Renal excretion is decreased, and plasma levels elevated, by alkalinization of the urine. Elevates plasma digoxin concentrations. Potentiates neuromuscular blockade by skeletal muscle relaxants. Antagonizes neostigmine, physostigmine. Potentiates anticoagulants.

THERAPEUTIC USE

Usual Effective Plasma Concentration: 2–6 μg/mL (7.3–21.9 μmol/L).
Usual Dose & Regimen: Orally, 300–500 mg, 4 times a day. Large interindividual variation requires dose adjustments, monitoring of plasma concentration.
Special Considerations: Gastrointestinal disturbances may be modified by using different formulations.

SPECIFIC ANTIDOTE: None. Gastric lavage; prevention of tubular precipitation and acidifying the urine may help in overdose.

RESERPINE

Brand Names: Novoreserpine, Reserfia, Serpasil.
Drug Class: Rauwolfia alkaloid. Adrenergic neuron blocker.
Related Drugs: —

ACTIONS: Depletes neuronal storage sites of catecholamines and serotonin. Also depresses myocardial function and releases gastrin.

PHARMACOKINETICS

pK_a: 6.6 (basic).
Mean V_d: ?
Plasma Protein Binding: About 95% bound.
Bioavailability: Probably greater than 80%.
Half-Life–Normal: 46–168 hours. – **Disease States:** ?
Absorption & Distribution: Kinetics are poorly defined, but the structure suggests high lipophilicity. High peripheral tissue binding, especially in adipose tissue and in adrenergic and serotonergic neurons in CNS and periphery. Crosses the blood–brain barrier, appears in milk.
Biotransformation & Elimination: Not evaluated. Probably extensive hepatic demethylation occurs. Undergoes considerable first-pass effect in the liver.

ADVERSE REACTIONS AND TOXICITY

Acute: Sedation, gastrointestinal cramps, diarrhea, flushing, hypotension, nasal congestion (frequent).
Chronic: Nightmares, psychic depression, extrapyramidal symptoms (rare), arrhythmias, hypersensitivity, weight gain, supersensitivity to catecholamines.

MAJOR DRUG INTERACTIONS: MAO inhibitors prevent catecholamine depletion. Digitalis or quinidine may induce arrhythmias. Potentiates the effects of guanethidine.

THERAPEUTIC USE

Usual Effective Plasma Concentration: Not measured clinically.
Usual Dose & Regimen: Hypertension, 0.5 mg daily for 2 weeks, then reduced to 0.1–0.25 mg daily p.o. Tachycardia, 0.1–0.5 mg daily p.o. Special dosage regimens for psychiatric use.
Special Considerations: Contraindicated in depressed patients, active peptic ulcer, ulcerative colitis, digitalis intoxication, and electroconvulsive therapy.

SPECIFIC ANTIDOTES: Directly acting vasopressors (levarterenol, phenylephrine, dopamine).

SALBUTAMOL (ALBUTEROL)

Brand Names: Novosalmol, Ventolin.
Drug Class: Sympathomimetic, relatively selective β_2-adrenoceptor agonist.
Related Drugs: Fenoterol, terbutaline, isoproterenol, adrenaline (epinephrine), isoetharine.

ACTIONS: Dilates large and small airways through β_2 adrenoceptor-mediated relaxation of bronchial and bronchiolar smooth muscle; also suppresses the release of mast-cell mediators of bronchoconstriction; may also modulate mucus output.

PHARMACOKINETICS

pK$_a$: 9.3 (basic).
Mean V$_d$: 1 L/kg.
Plasma Protein Binding: Not significantly bound.
Bioavailability: 30% (oral), 10% (inhaled).
Half-Life–Normal: Terminal half-life is 3–8 hours. – **Disease States:** Duration of effect 4–6 hours in asthma.
Absorption & Distribution: Relatively slowly absorbed after oral administration (peak plasma concentration at 3 hours); absorption from the lungs is poor; distribution half-life is long (1–2 hours).
Biotransformation & Elimination: Extensively transformed in the gut wall and liver (less than 20% may reach the systemic circulation unchanged). Urinary excretion.

ADVERSE REACTIONS AND TOXICITY

Acute: Increased cardiac output, heart rate and pulse pressure; hypoxemia, peripheral vasodilatation, arrhythmia (rare), skeletal muscle tremor, metabolic alterations.
Chronic: Tolerance to bronchodilatation may occur; paradoxical increase in airway resistance (rare).

MAJOR DRUG INTERACTIONS: In acute asthma attacks, the responsiveness to salbutamol may be enhanced when given in conjunction with a corticosteroid.

THERAPEUTIC USE

Usual Effective Plasma Concentration: Not measured clinically.
Usual Dose & Regimen: Orally, 2–4 mg 3–4 times a day in adults. Inhalation, 1–2 puffs (100 μg per puff) every 4 hours or as needed for relief of symptoms.
Special Considerations: Excessive use (> 20–30 puffs) during status asthmaticus may provoke arrhythmias or cardiovascular toxicity.

SPECIFIC ANTIDOTE: A β-adrenoceptor blocker, *e.g.*, propranolol.

SODIUM CROMOGLYCATE (CROMOLYN SODIUM)

Brand Names: Fivent, Intal, Nalcrom, Opticrom, Rynacrom, Vistacrom.
Drug Class: Mast cell stabilizer.
Related Drugs: —

ACTIONS: Antiallergic. Inhibits secretion of mast cell contents in response to antigen-antibody (Type I) reaction.

PHARMACOKINETICS

pK$_a$: 2.5 (acidic).
Mean V$_d$: 0.13 L/kg.
Plasma Protein Binding: 60–75% bound.
Bioavailability: 10% (inhaled), less than 1% (oral).
Half-Life–Normal: About 1 hour. – **Disease States:** ?
Absorption & Distribution: 10% of an inhaled dose is absorbed in the lung. (Mucus and bronchoconstriction may decrease the absorption of an inhaled dose.) Peak plasma levels are obtained in 10 minutes. Rapid distribution to tissues, especially liver and kidneys.
Biotransformation & Elimination: No detectable metabolites. The absorbed portion of a dose is eliminated equally in bile and urine, with elimination half-life of 80 minutes.

ADVERSE REACTIONS AND TOXICITY

Acute: Transient throat irritation or bronchospasm; rash, nausea (uncommon).
Chronic: Possible rebound of allergic symptoms upon withdrawal.

MAJOR DRUG INTERACTIONS: None observed.

THERAPEUTIC USE

Usual Effective Plasma Concentration: Not measured clinically.
Usual Dose & Regimen: Powder inhaler, 20 mg 4 times daily, maximum 160 mg/day. Aerosol inhaler, 2 mg 4 times daily, maximum 32 mg/day. Ophthalmic solution, 1–2 drops of 2% solution per eye, 4 times daily, maximum 12.8 mg/day. Nasal, 1–2 squeezes per nostril 6 times daily (0.8 mg/squeeze).
Special Considerations: Must be used prophylactically on a regular basis regardless of symptoms.

SPECIFIC ANTIDOTE: None (no recorded overdose).

SODIUM NITROPRUSSIDE

Brand Name: Nipride.
Drug Class: Antihypertensive agent. Direct-acting smooth muscle relaxant.
Related Drugs: —

ACTIONS: Direct relaxation of vascular smooth muscle, both arteriolar and venous. Minimal effects on gastrointestinal or uterine muscle. Decreased preload and afterload, decreased or unchanged cardiac output. Blood pressure effect is modulated by the rate of infusion.

PHARMACOKINETICS

pK_a: ?
Mean V_d: ?
Plasma Protein Binding: ?
Bioavailability: n.a.
Half-Life–Normal: Few minutes. – **Disease States:** Decreased thiocyanate excretion in renal impairment.
Absorption & Distribution: Given only as intravenous infusion. Rapid equilibration into vascular smooth muscle.
Biotransformation & Elimination: Sodium nitroprusside degrades nonenzymatically to cyanogen (CN), which is metabolized by rhodanese to thiocyanate, excreted in the urine.

ADVERSE REACTIONS AND TOXICITY

Acute: Hypotension, anorexia, nausea, vomiting, metabolic acidosis.
Chronic: Cyanide toxicity. Thiocyanate accumulates in chronic therapy; hypothyroidism.

MAJOR DRUG INTERACTIONS: Blockers of α and β adrenoceptors augment the hypotensive effect.

THERAPEUTIC USE

Usual Effective Plasma Concentration: Thiocyanate toxicity at >100 $\mu g/mL$.
Usual Dose & Regimen: Only by intravenous infusion, 3 $\mu g/kg/min$, but broad dose range, maximum 800 $\mu g/min$. Continuous monitoring of blood pressure is required.
Special Considerations: Solution is light-sensitive; discard diluted solutions that are more than 4 hours old. Avoid extravasation.

SPECIFIC ANTIDOTE: Hydroxycobalamin to decrease cyanide effects.

SPIRONOLACTONE

Brand Names: Aldactone, Novospiroton, Sincomen.
Drug Class: Aldosterone antagonist, diuretic.
Related Drugs: Triamterene, amiloride.

ACTIONS: Promotes the excretion of water and sodium, and retention of potassium, by competitive binding to receptors at the aldosterone-dependent sodium/potassium exchange sites in distal tubules.

PHARMACOKINETICS

pK_a: ?
Mean V_d: ?
Plasma Protein Binding: 98% bound (as canrenone).
Bioavailability: Better than 90% (oral).
Half-Life–Normal: Rapid (within minutes) conversion to active metabolites with half-lives of 13–24 hours. – **Disease States:** Prolonged in liver disease, congestive heart failure.
Absorption & Distribution: Well absorbed from oral administration.
Biotransformation & Elimination: Hepatic transformation to the active metabolites canrenone (aldadiene) and canrenoate. Metabolites are excreted primarily in the urine, but also in bile. Long half-life of active metabolites results in peak diuretic effects 2–3 days after onset of dosing, and 2–3 days decline after stopping the drug.

ADVERSE REACTIONS AND TOXICITY

Acute: GI symptoms (nausea, cramping, diarrhea).
Chronic: Hyperkalemia, gynecomastia.

MAJOR DRUG INTERACTIONS: Potassium supplements can cause hyperkalemia. Additive or supra-additive effect with other diuretic or hypotensive agents.

THERAPEUTIC USE

Usual Effective Plasma Concentration: Not measured clinically.
Usual Dose & Regimen: 50–400 mg/day. Initial doses 50–100 mg/day. Three days are required for peak diuretic effect.
Special Considerations: Contraindicated in acute renal insufficiency or renal impairment. Spironolactone should not be administered together with potassium supplements (including dietary).

SPECIFIC ANTIDOTE: None.

SUCCINYLCHOLINE (SUXAMETHONIUM)

Brand Names: Anectine, Quelicin Chloride.
Drug Class: Depolarizing (desensitizing) neuromuscular blocking agent.
Related Drugs: Decamethonium, benzoquinonium.

ACTIONS: Combines with cholinergic receptors on muscle endplates to produce depolarization resulting in initial muscle contraction (fasciculations), followed by prolonged neuromuscular blockade and flaccid paralysis (desensitization).

PHARMACOKINETICS

pK$_a$: n.a. (strongly basic).
Mean V$_d$: ? (Highly bound to peripheral sites.)
Plasma Protein Binding: ?
Bioavailability: Nil (oral); 100% (i.m. or i.v.).
Half-Life–Normal: Approximately 2–3 minutes. – **Disease States:** Variably prolonged in patients with atypical, or reduced levels of, plasma cholinesterase.
Absorption & Distribution: Not active orally because of quaternary ammonium groups. Intramuscular injection delays the onset of action for about three minutes. Equilibrium between receptor-bound molecules and plasma succinylcholine determines the duration of action, normally 8–10 minutes.
Biotransformation & Elimination: Hydrolysed by plasma cholinesterases to monosuccinylcholine, which has competitive neuromuscular blocking activity. Succinic acid and choline are ultimate metabolic products. About 10% is excreted in the urine as unchanged drug.

ADVERSE REACTIONS AND TOXICITY

Acute: Extension of pharmacologic effects, such as profound muscle relaxation, respiratory paralysis, apnea; hyperthermia (genetic variant), increased intraocular pressure, salivation, bradycardia, tachycardia, hypertension, hypotension, arrhythmias.
Chronic: Same as acute.

MAJOR DRUG INTERACTIONS: Cyclophosphamide, neostigmine, procaine inhibit or compete for plasma cholinesterase. Neomycin, streptomycin, kanamycin, and similar aminoglycoside antibiotics may act as weak depolarizing agents. Hypokalemia, hypocalcemia potentiate the effects.

THERAPEUTIC USE

Usual Effective Plasma Concentration: Not measured clinically.
Usual Dose & Regimen: Single i.v. injection, 20 mg given over 10–30 seconds. Infusion, 0.2% solution in 5% dextrose or isotonic sodium chloride at 2–4 mg/min. Adjust flow for desired degree of muscle relaxation.
Special Considerations: Stable only in acidic solution. Specialized uses only.

SPECIFIC ANTIDOTE: None. Artificial ventilation during periods of prolonged apnea.

SULFISOXAZOLE (SULFAFURAZOLE)

Brand Names: Apo-Sulfisoxazole, Gantrisin, Novosoxazole.
Drug Class: Antibacterial sulfonamide.
Related Drugs: Sulfanilamide, sulfadiazine, sulfamethoxazole; sulfacetamide.

ACTIONS: Sulfonamides are structural analogs of p-aminobenzoic acid and are competitive antagonists at bacterial sites synthesizing folic acid from PABA. This has a bacteriostatic effect; host defences and immune systems are essential for eradication of the infection.

PHARMACOKINETICS

pK$_a$: 4.9 (acidic).
Mean V$_d$: 0.15 L/kg.
Plasma Protein Binding: 85–95% bound.
Bioavailability: 100% (oral).
Half-Life–Normal: 5–7 hours. – **Disease States:** Increased in uremia.
Absorption & Distribution: Excellent absorption of oral dose, with plasma peak at 2–4 hours. Distributed in extracellular fluid. High solubility permits high urinary concentrations without correspondingly high renal toxicity. Cerebrospinal fluid levels are one-third of plasma levels.
Biotransformation & Elimination: N-Acetylation in the liver (major) and glucuronidation (minor) are the biotransformation pathways. Excreted primarily by the kidneys in both unchanged (70%) and acetylated (5–20%) forms, mainly by glomerular filtration.

ADVERSE REACTIONS AND TOXICITY

Acute: Nausea, vomiting, abdominal pain, headache.
Chronic: Hematuria and crystalluria (0.2–0.3%), anuria, blood dyscrasias, allergic reactions. Superinfections.

MAJOR DRUG INTERACTIONS: Trimethoprim, acting on another step of the bacterial folate pathway, produces synergistic effects. The effects of oral hypoglycemics and diuretics of the sulfonamide class may be potentiated.

THERAPEUTIC USE

Usual Effective Plasma Concentration: Refer to Chapter 56.
Usual Dose & Regimen: Adults, 2–4 g initially, then 4–8 g/day, divided into 4–6 doses. Children over 2 months, start with half the maintenance dose, then 150 mg/kg/day or 4 g/m^2/day, maximum 6 g/day.
Special Considerations: Patients should ingest the drug with adequate quantities of water to minimize potential renal damage. Contraindicated in renal, hepatic, hematologic disease; prematures, newborns, uremia, porphyria, G-6-PD deficiency.

SPECIFIC ANTIDOTE: None. Gastric lavage, symptomatic treatment.

TETRACYCLINE

Brand Names: Achromycin, Apo-Tetra, Neo-Tetrine, Novotetra, Tetracyn.
Drug Class: Tetracycline antibiotic.
Related Drugs: Chlortetracycline, oxytetracycline, demeclocycline, methacycline, doxycycline, minocycline.

ACTIONS: Crosses bacterial cell membranes through active transport processes, reversibly binds to ribosomes and inhibits protein synthesis. Bacteriostatic activity at normal *in vivo* concentration range.

PHARMACOKINETICS

pK$_a$: 3.3, 7.7 (both acidic), 9.7 (basic).
Mean V$_d$: 1.5 L/kg.
Plasma Protein Binding: 25–65% bound.
Bioavailability: 77% (oral).
Half-Life–Normal: 8–12 hours. – **Disease States:** Increased in uremia.
Absorption & Distribution: Gastrointestinal absorption is inhibited in the presence of milk products; aluminum hydroxide gels; sodium bicarbonate; calcium, magnesium, and iron preparations; elevated gastric pH. Peripheral tissue binding and plasma protein binding both occur. Bile concentration is elevated five-fold over plasma; other fluids including CSF have some free drug.
Biotransformation & Elimination: Tetracycline is eliminated by renal glomerular filtration of active drug (20–50% of dose), and by hepatic concentration and excretion into the bile (50–75%). Enterohepatic recirculation occurs.

ADVERSE REACTIONS AND TOXICITY

Acute: Nausea, vomiting, epigastric distress, and diarrhea are dose-related.
Chronic: Superinfections, candidiasis, photosensitivity (less than 2%), hepatotoxicity (jaundice, azotemia, acidosis), renal toxicity, brownish discoloration of teeth in children less than 10 years old, deposition in bone, hypersensitivity, leukocytosis, elevated BUN.

MAJOR DRUG INTERACTIONS: Tetracyclines chelate calcium, iron, magnesium, *etc.* Antacids, bicarbonate interfere with absorption; the effects of anticoagulants are potentiated; with methoxyflurane, tetracycline causes impairment of renal function; the antibacterial activity of penicillins is inhibited.

THERAPEUTIC USE

Usual Effective Plasma Concentration: Refer to Chapter 55.
Usual Dose & Regimen: Orally, adults, 250–500 mg 4 times a day; children, 25–50 mg/kg/day in divided doses. Intravenously, adults, 250–500 mg every 12 hours, maximum 1 g/day.
Special Considerations: Do not use in pregnancy, children under 10, renal insufficiency. Expiry dating on drug labels should be closely followed.

SPECIFIC ANTIDOTE: None. Calcium for inactivation by chelate formation in oral overdose.

THEOPHYLLINE

Brand Names: Elixophyllin, Pulmophylline, Quibron-T, Slo-Bid, Somophyllin, Theochron, Theo-Dur, Theolair, Theo-SR, Uniphyl.
Drug Class: Methylated xanthine. Bronchodilator.
Related Drugs: Aminophylline, caffeine, theobromine, oxtriphylline, dyphylline.

ACTIONS: Relaxation of bronchial smooth muscle, possibly through intracellular phosphodiesterase inhibition. Also stimulates the CNS respiratory centre and reduces fatigue of diaphragmatic muscles.

PHARMACOKINETICS

pK$_a$: 8.8 (acidic), 0.7 (basic).
Mean V$_d$: About 0.5 L/kg.
Plasma Protein Binding: 40–60% bound.
Bioavailability: 90–100% (oral).
Half-Life–Normal: 6–12 hours (mean 9 hours, decreased in smokers). – **Disease States:** Prolonged in neonates, the elderly, cirrhosis (7–60 hours), and acute heart failure (up to 80 hours).
Absorption & Distribution: Uncoated tablets are rapidly and well absorbed. Slow-release products delay absorption because of slowly dissolving coatings. Distributes in total body water.
Biotransformation & Elimination: Hepatic mixed-function oxidases transform 80–90% of a dose. Metabolites are actively secreted into the urine, but 10% of a dose is excreted unchanged, dependent on urine flow rates. Elimination rates are affected by many factors (age, metabolic status, *etc.*).

ADVERSE REACTIONS AND TOXICITY

Acute: Anorexia, nausea, vomiting, irritability, headache, arrhythmias, tachycardia. Overdose: epigastric pain, vomiting, diarrhea, convulsions, hypotension.
Chronic: Same as acute.

MAJOR DRUG INTERACTIONS: Cimetidine, erythromycin, large doses of allopurinol decrease clearance. Potentiates diuretics, digitalis, ephedrine; increases lithium, phenytoin clearance.

THERAPEUTIC USE

Usual Effective Plasma Concentration: 10–20 μg/mL (55.5–111 μmol/L).
Usual Dose & Regimen: Must be individualized. Intravenously, as aminophylline (= 80% theophylline) 5.6 mg/kg load over 20 minutes, 0.9 mg/kg/hour infusion. Orally, adults, 250 mg 3–4 times daily; children, 12–20 mg/kg/day.
Special Considerations: Large variations in metabolic rate and narrow therapeutic window require monitoring of plasma concentrations for effective therapy.

SPECIFIC ANTIDOTE: None.

THIOPENTAL SODIUM

Brand Name: Pentothal Sodium.
Drug Class: Ultra-short-acting barbiturate; anaesthetic.
Related Drugs: Methohexital.

ACTIONS: Generalized CNS depression.

PHARMACOKINETICS

pK$_a$: 7.6 (acidic).
Mean V$_d$: 2.5 L/kg.
Plasma Protein Binding: 75–85% bound (dose-dependent).
Bioavailability: n.a.
Half-Life–Normal: 3–5 minutes (redistribution); 7–15 hours (elimination). – **Disease States:** ?
Absorption & Distribution: Only used by intravenous injection. Distributed into all tissues with initial distribution into brain, heart, kidneys, then redistributed into muscle and fat.
Biotransformation & Elimination: Slow transformation in the liver; renal excretion.

ADVERSE REACTIONS AND TOXICITY

Acute: Pain and tissue destruction from improper injection. Depression of respiratory and cardiovascular systems (overdose).
Chronic: n.a.

MAJOR DRUG INTERACTIONS: Other CNS depressants.

THERAPEUTIC USE

Usual Effective Plasma Concentration: Not measured clinically.

Usual Dose & Regimen: 3–5 mg/kg as a 2.5% solution i.v. to induce general anaesthesia.
Special Considerations: Avoid repeated use at short intervals—cumulation. Avoid drug in shock and cardiovascular disease. Contraindicated in porphyria, status asthmaticus.

SPECIFIC ANTIDOTE: None. Life support in overdose.

TOLBUTAMIDE

Brand Names: Apo-Tolbutamide, Mobenol, Novobutamide, Orinase.
Drug Class: Oral hypoglycemic, sulfonylurea.
Related Drugs: Acetohexamide, tolazamide, chlorpropamide, glibenclamide (glyburide).

ACTIONS: Stimulates pancreatic islet tissue to secrete insulin, enhances the antilipolytic action of insulin.

PHARMACOKINETICS

pK$_a$: 5.3 (acidic).
Mean V$_d$: 0.15 L/kg.
Plasma Protein Binding: 95–97% bound.
Bioavailability: 93% (oral).
Half-Life–Normal: 6 hours. – **Disease States:** Decreased in acute viral hepatitis, chronic respiratory insufficiency.
Absorption & Distribution: Rapidly and nearly completely absorbed.
Biotransformation & Elimination: Hepatic oxidation to carboxylated metabolite, which is excreted in the urine.

ADVERSE REACTIONS AND TOXICITY

Acute: Hypoglycemia.
Chronic: Total incidence is approximately 3%. Cutaneous (rash, photosensitivity) and gastrointestinal (GI upset, cholestatic jaundice) are most common. Leukopenia, thrombocytopenia (about 1 in 500). Possible increased risk of cardiovascular complications.

MAJOR DRUG INTERACTIONS: Potentiated by dicumarol, oxyphenbutazone, phenylbutazone, sulfonamides, salicylates, propranolol. Disulfiram-like reaction with alcohol.

THERAPEUTIC USE

Usual Effective Plasma Concentration: 80–240 µg/mL lowers blood glucose by 25% or more.
Usual Dose & Regimen: 250–2000 mg per day, as determined by blood glucose response.
Special Considerations: None.

SPECIFIC ANTIDOTE: Glucose for hypoglycemia.

TUBOCURARINE

Brand Name: Tubarine.
Drug Class: Competitive (nondepolarizing) neuromuscular blocker.
Related Drugs: Alcuronium, gallamine, pancuronium, fazadinium.

ACTIONS: Competitive antagonist of acetylcholine at postjunctional nicotinic cholinergic receptor sites in skeletal muscle. Weak effects also at autonomic ganglionic transmission sites.

PHARMACOKINETICS

pK$_a$: 8.0, 9.2 (basic).
Mean V$_d$: 0.2–0.4 L/kg.
Plasma Protein Binding: 40–60% bound.
Bioavailability: Nil (oral); complete absorption from i.m. sites.
Half-Life–Normal: 2–4 hours. – **Disease States:** Increased in uremia, renal insufficiency.
Absorption & Distribution: Quaternary nitrogens prevent oral absorption almost completely. Rapid redistribution after i.v. injection is responsible for the initially short duration of action. Saturation of tissue receptor sites occurs after repeated doses.
Biotransformation & Elimination: About 35–50% of a dose is excreted unchanged in the urine. Some biliary excretion and variable degrees of hepatic biotransformation occur.

ADVERSE REACTIONS AND TOXICITY

Acute: Extension of pharmacologic effects, such as respiratory paralysis and prolonged apnea. Release of histamine and heparin can cause bronchospasm, hypotension, bronchial and salivary secretion, blood hypocoagulability, cardiovascular collapse.
Chronic: Same as acute.

MAJOR DRUG INTERACTIONS: Potassium depletion by thiazide diuretics increases the effects. Neomycin, streptomycin, kanamycin, and similar aminoglycoside antibiotics may act as weak depolarizing agents. Succinylcholine (additive). Anticholinesterases (inhibitory).

THERAPEUTIC USE

Usual Effective Plasma Concentration: 0.4–0.8 μg/mL.
Usual Dose & Regimen: Anaesthesia beyond Stage 2, 6–9 mg i.v. followed by 3–4.5 mg 5 minutes later, repeated when necessary. Other specialized uses.
Special Considerations: Do not mix with thiopental in the same syringe in a ratio greater than 1 mg per 25 mg thiopental.

SPECIFIC ANTIDOTES: Neostigmine, physostigmine.

WARFARIN

Brand Names: Athrombin-K, Coumadin, Warfilone.
Drug Class: Anticoagulant (indirect-acting).
Related Drugs: Dicumarol (bishydroxycoumarin), acenocoumarol, phenprocoumon.

ACTIONS: Interferes with hepatic vitamin K-dependent synthesis of clotting factors II, VII, IX, X.

PHARMACOKINETICS

pK$_a$: 5.05 (acidic).
Mean V$_d$: 0.1 L/kg.
Plasma Protein Binding: More than 99% bound.
Bioavailability: 100% (oral).
Half-Life–Normal: 20–70 hours. – **Disease States:** Prolonged in liver disease.
Absorption & Distribution: Rapidly and completely absorbed; crosses placenta, secreted in milk.
Biotransformation & Elimination: Racemic warfarin is converted in the liver to (a) secondary alcohol and (b) 7-hydroxywarfarin. Inactive metabolites are excreted in urine and stool.

ADVERSE REACTIONS AND TOXICITY

Acute: None.
Chronic: Hemorrhage.

MAJOR DRUG INTERACTIONS: All other agents interfering with hemostasis:
  Potentiation: Platelet inhibitors, clofibrate, co-trimoxazole, D-thyroxine, cimetidine, phenylbutazone.
  Inhibition: Barbiturates, glutethimide, cholestyramine, rifampin, vitamin K.

THERAPEUTIC USE

Usual Effective Plasma Concentration: 1–3 mg/L (3.3–9.8 μmol/L). Not measured clinically.
Usual Dose & Regimen: 10–15 mg/day for 3 days, then adjusted on the basis of prothrombin time response (target is 1½–2 times normal).
Special Considerations: Monitor prothrombin times; adjust the dose whenever interacting drugs are used.

SPECIFIC ANTIDOTE: Vitamin K$_1$ (phytonadione; AquaMephyton, Konakion).

Appendix 2

SELECTED LIST OF EQUIVALENT DRUG NAMES IN AMERICAN, BRITISH, AND CANADIAN USAGE
(Prepared by Dr. D. Kadar)

U.S.A.	Canada	U.K.
acetaminophen	acetaminophen	paracetamol
albuterol	salbutamol	salbutamol
amobarbital	amobarbital	amylobarbitone
antipyrine	antipyrine	phenazone
apazone	apazone	azapropazone
arginine vasopressin	arginine vasopressin	argipressin
articane	articane	carticane
aspirin	acetylsalicylic acid	aspirin
bendroflumethiazide	bendroflumethiazide	bendrofluazide
benzothiazides	benzothiazides	benzthiazides
corticosterone	corticosterone	deoxycortone
cromolyn sodium	sodium cromoglycate	sodium cromoglycate
dibucaine	dibucaine	cinchocaine
diethylstilbestrol	diethylstilbestrol	stilboestrol
epinephrine	adrenaline	adrenaline
estradiol	estradiol	oestradiol
estriol	estriol	oestriol
estrogen	estrogen	oestrogen
estrone	estrone	oestrone
fluoroprednisolone	fluoroprednisolone	fluprednisolone
furosemide	furosemide	frusemide
heroin	heroin	diamorphine
hexobarbital	hexobarbital	hexobarbitone
isoproterenol	isoproterenol	isoprenaline
lidocaine	lidocaine	lignocaine
meperidine	meperidine	pethidine
mesalamine	5-aminosalicylic acid	mesalazine
metaproterenol	metaproterenol, orciprenaline	orciprenaline
methohexital	methohexital	methohexitone
methotrexate	amethopterin, methotrexate	methotrexate
moxalactam	moxalactam	latamoxef
norepinephrine	noradrenaline	noradrenaline
pentobarbital	pentobarbital	pentobarbitone
pentylenetetrazole	pentylenetetrazole	leptazole
phenobarbital	phenobarbital	phenobarbitone
pipotiazine	pipotiazine	pipothiazine
pizotyline	pizotyline	pizotifen
quinacrine	quinacrine, mepacrine	mepacrine
ribavirin	ribavirin	tribavirin
riboflavin	riboflavin	riboflavine
rifampin	rifampin	rifampicin
secobarbital	secobarbital	quinalbarbitone
sodium carboxymethylcellulose	sodium carboxymethylcellulose	carmellose sodium
sulfisoxazole *	sulfisoxazole	sulphafurazole
sulfonamide	sulfonamide	sulphonamide
tetracaine	tetracaine	amethocaine
thiamin	thiamin	thiamine
thiopental	thiopental	thiopentone

* Names beginning with sulf- in Canada and the United States are generally written with sulph- in the U.K.

Index